Liver Diseases

Florentina Radu-Ionita • Nikolaos T. Pyrsopoulos
Mariana Jinga • Ion C. Tintoiu
Zhonghua Sun • Ecaterina Bontas
Editors

Liver Diseases

A Multidisciplinary Textbook

Springer

Editors
Florentina Radu-Ionita
Faculty of Medicine, "Titu Maiorescu" University
Central Military Emergency University Hospital
"Dr. Carol Davila"
Bucharest
Romania

Mariana Jinga
Carol Davila University of Medicine and Pharmacy
Central Military Emergency University Hospital
"Dr. Carol Davila"
Bucharest
Romania

Zhonghua Sun
Medical Radiation Sciences
Curtin University
Perth, WA
Australia

Nikolaos T. Pyrsopoulos
New Jersey Medical School
Rutgers University New Jersey Medical School
Newark, NJ
USA

Ion C. Tintoiu
Faculty of Medicine, "Titu Maiorescu" University
Central Military Emergency University Hospital
"Dr. Carol Davila"
Bucharest
Romania

Ecaterina Bontas
"Prof. C.C. Iliescu" Emergency Institute for Cardiovascular Diseases
Bucharest
Romania

ISBN 978-3-030-24431-6   ISBN 978-3-030-24432-3 (eBook)
https://doi.org/10.1007/978-3-030-24432-3

This Springer imprint is published by the registered company Springer Nature Switzerland AG
The registered company address is: Gewerbestrasse 11, 6330 Cham, Switzerland

Preface

Let me teach you something
—Hans Popper

The complexity of managing patients with liver disease, liver failure, and advanced fibrosis requires a multidisciplinary approach. Physicians and scientists today are specialized in a variety of fields, including gastroenterology, internal medicine, radiology, pathology, surgery, and nutrition, and along with leaders in other fields they together constitute the multidisciplinary team.

The importance and input of the multidisciplinary team is clear during the time of pre-transplant evaluation as well as post-transplant management. In large liver centers, the members of the "Liver Team" are creating the strategy regarding patient management at multiple levels.

Ideally, this concept can be instituted at an earlier stage with a focus on prevention and appropriate screening in order to avoid and prevent the detrimental complications of advanced liver diseases.

Liver Diseases: A Multidisciplinary Textbook has been written by an international assembly of outstanding experts in their field. These scientists have shared their knowledge on key elements such as an overview of basic liver concepts, functions and mechanisms of liver injury/regeneration, epidemiologic data, clinical manifestations of the various stages of liver diseases, and diagnostic tools and algorithms along with current and future treatment strategies.

The chapters are structured in a unique fashion incorporating key concepts and didactic elements, along with practical examples and exercises. A significant number of tables, figures, and illustrations have been included in each chapter.

We believe that this book, supported by the current international literature, written by distinguished leaders of hepatology and other research fields, will provide a platform for readers to better understand liver diseases and the opportunity to find the answers they are looking for and enhance their knowledge in the field of liver disease.

Bucharest, Romania — Florentina Radu-Ionita
Newark, NJ, USA — Nikolaos T. Pyrsopoulos
Bucharest, Romania — Mariana Jinga
Bucharest, Romania — Ion C. Tintoiu
Perth, WA, Australia — Zhonghua Sun
Bucharest, Romania — Ecaterina Bontas

Contents

Part I

Overview

Anatomy and Embryology of the Liver

1

Sergio Morini, Guido Carpino, Simone Carotti, and Eugenio Gaudio

Key Concepts

- The liver is a gland that exerts both an exocrine and endocrine function, as well as a regulation of almost all the metabolic homeostasis.
- To support all these functions, it has a particular circulatory system with blood supply from many abdominal organs via the portal vein.
- The division of the parenchyma into functionally independent segments, based on the vascular internal subdivision, is of importance in clinical practice.
- An amount of genes and transcription factors, activated by interaction with mesenchymal signals, regulate the embryonic development of the liver, until it progressively assumes its final configuration and function.

1.1 Introduction

The liver is the largest organ in the human body and represents 2–5% of body weight in adults.

It can perform both exocrine and endocrine-metabolic functions. A unique feature of the liver is that its cells, the hepatocytes, are able to exercise both exocrine and endocrine functions on their own, unlike the pancreas where the two functions are performed by different cells. The liver exercises the exocrine function like a gland attached to the duodenum, from which it has its embryological origin, and in which it secretes the bile. Instead, endocrine functions include the secretion of some hormones such as Insulin-like growth factors, angiotensinogen and thrombopoietin.

The endocrine-metabolic function is made possible by the particular position of the liver in relation to the circulatory system: it is in fact interposed between the portal circle and the inferior vena cava. It therefore receives venous blood from the abdominal organs of the digestive system and from the spleen, containing the metabolites absorbed in the intestine and the products of the splenic metabolism.

The liver can therefore play a key role in the metabolic homeostasis of the whole organism. It is in fact essential for the control of several metabolic functions, including glucose homeostasis, gluconeogenesis and glycogenolysis, fatty acid and cholesterol synthesis and processing of dietary fats to lipoproteins, drug detoxification, urea metabolism. Beside glycogen, it can storage iron, copper and some vitamins like vitamin A, D, K and B12. Finally, it secrets an extensive array of plasma proteins, among which albumin, binding proteins, apolipoproteins, fibrinogens and other coagulation factors.

1.2 Clinical Anatomy of the Liver

The liver is positioned in the right upper abdomen, corresponding to the right hypochondrium, part of the epigastrium and of the left hypochondrium. It is therefore below the diaphragm, which separates it from the pleurae, the lungs and the heart, and above the stomach and the transverse colon; posteriorly it is in relationship with the last thoracic vertebrae and with the retroperitoneal organs, such as the kidney, the right adrenal gland and the inferior vena cava.

Despite the advent of the modern diagnostic imaging techniques, the surface and clinical anatomy of the abdominal organs continues to be quite relevant in the clinical semeiotics. Due to variable shape and extension of the liver through different subjects, also the surface margins of the organ are variable. The projection of the liver on the anterior

S. Morini (✉) · S. Carotti
Department of Medicine and Surgery, University Campus Bio-Medico of Rome, Rome, Italy
e-mail: s.morini@unicampus.it

G. Carpino
Department of Motor, Human and Health Sciences, University of Rome "Foro Italico", Rome, Italy

E. Gaudio
Department of Anatomical, Histological, Locomotor and Legal Medicine Sciences, Sapienza University, Rome, Italy

F. Radu-Ionita et al. (eds.), *Liver Diseases*, https://doi.org/10.1007/978-3-030-24432-3_1

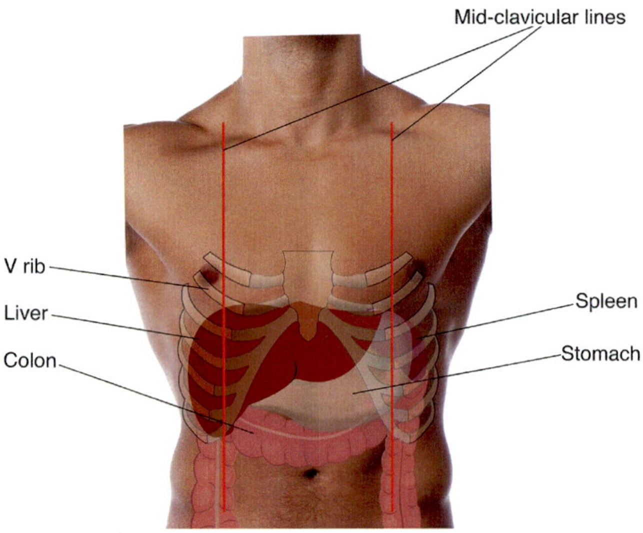

Fig. 1.1 Projection of the liver on the anterior surface of the abdomen

abdominal wall assumes a roughly triangular shape (Fig. 1.1). The upper margin corresponds to the contour of the diaphragm and, after a normal expiration, is represented by a line passes between the right fifth rib at the right mid-clavicular line, and the fifth intercostal space at the left mid-clavicular line. This line is slightly concave upward at the central tendon of the diaphragm on which the heart rests, and crosses the midline behind the xiphisternal joint. The lower margin correspond to a line passes between the intersection of the tenth costal cartilage at the right mid-clavicular line, and the intersection of the fifth intercostal space and the left mid-clavicular line. This margin crosses the right costal arch at the level of the tenth coast and the left one at the level of the seventh coast. In healthy subjects, this margin is appreciable during a deep inspiration, lowering about 1–2 cm. The right border of the liver correspond to a slightly concave curve that joins the two right ends of the other margins.

The fundus of the gallbladder normally corresponds to a point between the tenth right costal cartilage and the lateral margin of the rectus abdominis (linea semilunaris).

1.3 Gross Anatomy and Surfaces of the Liver

The liver occupies a proper space of the peritoneal cavity (Fig. 1.2a). It has the shape of a horizontally arranged ovoid, cut from an oblique plane with the removal of the posterior-inferior portion. It measures about 25–28 cm in width, 8 in height and 16–17 in the anterior-posterior diameter; it weighs about 2000 g in living (slightly lower in females), and about 1500 g, when eliminating the contained blood.

Its surface is smooth, surrounded by the Glisson connective capsule and largely coated by the peritoneum. It presents a diaphragmatic face, with anterior-superior extension, and a

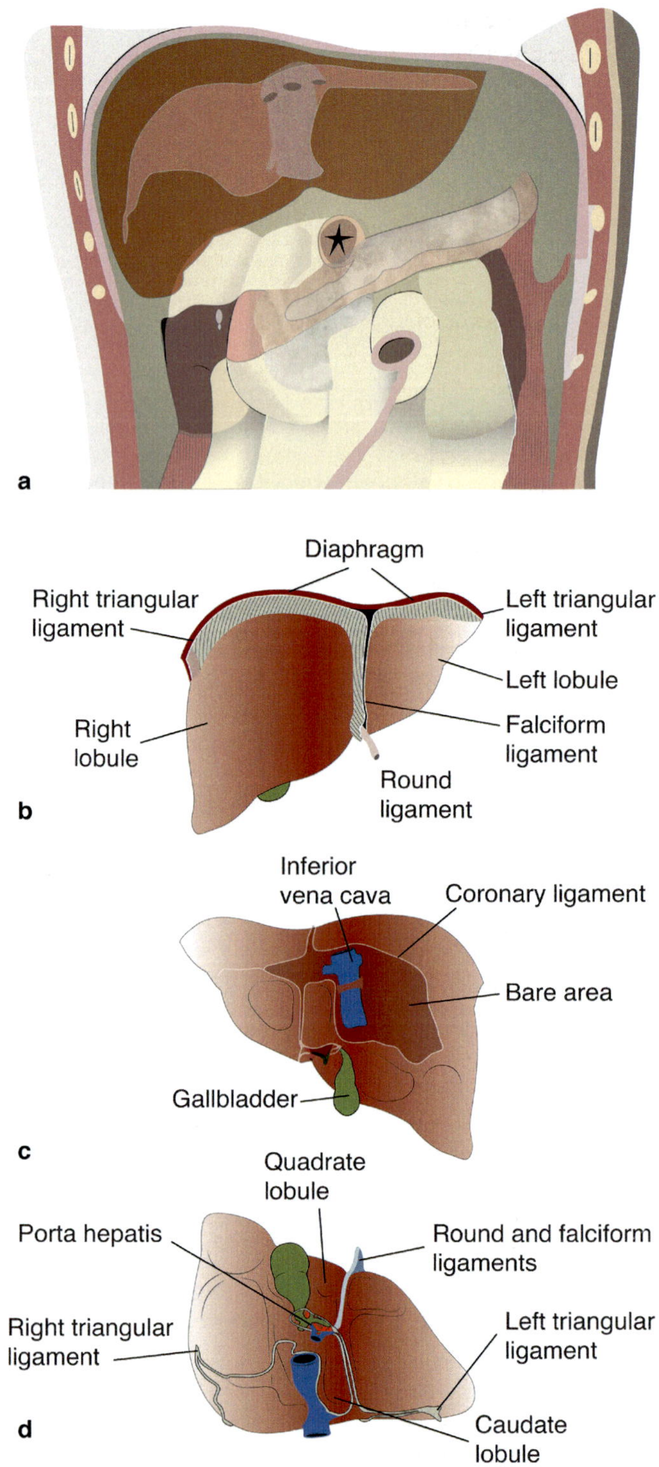

Fig. 1.2 Position of the liver in the abdomen (**a**) and its relationship with the retroperitoneal organs. The inferior vena cava and the line of reflection of the peritoneum, forming the coronary ligament and delimiting the bare face (clearer area), are visible in transparency behind the liver; the stomach and the spleen have been removed. The anterior (**b**), posterior (**c**) and inferior (**d**) surfaces of the liver with the peritoneal ligaments

lower visceral face. The two sides meet in the thin anterior margin, corresponding to the lower projection line of the liver, and in the posterior margin. The latter is thin in the left portion, but becomes thicker to the right, where it can be also considered as a back face of the liver.

The anterior-superior face, or diaphragmatic face, is limited by the anterior margin and at the top by the reflection of the peritoneum that forms the upper part of the coronary ligament. The face is subdivided in a right lobe and a left lobe by a sagittal furrow. Along this furrow the peritoneum rises to form the falciform ligament. The inferior face, or visceral face, is turned backwards and downwards. It appears irregular due to the presence of three grooves and some imprints. The right sagittal groove, that corresponds to the main portal fissure or Cantlie's line, is broad and contains the gallbladder anteriorly and the inferior vena cava in the posterior portion. The left sagittal groove is deep and thin: in its anterior portion, the umbilical fissure, it contains the round ligament, while in the posterior portion it assume the name of venous fissure containing the venous ligament. The deep transverse fissure included between the two sagittal ones constitutes the porta hepatis and contains all the structures of the hepatic peduncle that reach the liver. The three grooves delimit four lobes on the visceral face of the liver: right lobe, left lobe, square lobe, in front of the porta hepatis, and caudate lobe placed behind it. On the visceral face are also present the imprints of the abdominal organs: on the right the flexure of the ascendant colon, the duodenum, the right kidney and the adrenal gland; on the left the stomach and the esophagus; on the square lobe the impression of the pylorus. The posterior face of the liver is in relationship with the diaphragm, the last thoracic vertebrae, the large abdominal vessels and the esophagus. It is bounded by the lines of reflection of the peritoneum that form the two parts of the coronary ligament of the liver: on the right the two sheets move away leaving a large surface of the liver free from the peritoneum and in contact with the diaphragm, the bare area.

1.4 Peritoneum and Ligaments of the Liver

The liver is closely linked to the diaphragm and the inferior vena cava. The adhesion to the diaphragm through the coronary ligament and the bare face, where the Glisson capsule merges with the fascia of the muscle, allows the liver to remain as hanging to the diaphragm and to follow its movements. The inferior vena cava, which at the top is fixed to the orifice of the diaphragm, constitutes as a support pylon for the liver, which surrounds the vena and adheres to it in particular through the outlet of the hepatic veins. These two systems can be considered the true structures for the liver fixity, while the ligaments are formed by thin sheets of peritoneum and have the meaning of connection with the neighboring organs (Fig. 1.2b–d). In addition, the support provided by the right kidney and the duodenum-pancreatic complex, as well as the abdominal pressure, contributes to maintain the position of the liver.

The *coronary ligament* is considered to be a suspensory ligament of the liver. It is formed by the reflection of the two upper and lower peritoneal sheets which, separated from each other, delimit the bare area of the liver. At both extremities, the upper and lower peritoneal sheets come closer together and become thicker, forming the two right and left *triangular ligaments*. The upper sheet of the coronary ligament divides into two parts that rise up to form the two peritoneal sheets of the falciform ligament.

The *falciform ligament* originates at the upper sagittal groove of the liver where the peritoneum rises in two sheets that form the base of the scythe. The anterior margin of the ligament continues with the parietal peritoneum along a line extending between the diaphragm and the anterior abdominal wall, up to the navel; the free margin, facing towards the internal abdominal cavity and extending from the navel up to the anterior-inferior margin of the liver contains in its thickness the *round ligament of the liver*. This ligament, residual of the umbilical vein, has the appearance of a fibrous cord that reaches the liver from the navel, and runs along the left sagittal sulcus up to the hilum of the organ; its continuation is the venous ligament, the residue of the venous duct (Aranzian duct) that connects to the inferior vena cava.

Finally, the *lesser omentum* is the remnant of the original ventral mesogastrium. It extends from the transverse sulcus at the porta hepatis to the small curvature of the stomach and to the upper margin of the first portion of the duodenum. It consists of two portions: the *gastrohepatic ligament* (*pars flaccida*), that is very thin and anteriorly delimits the *superior recess of the lesser sac*, and the *hepatoduodenal ligament* (*pars tensa*). The latter is much thicker and contains all the structures that reach the liver: the portal vein, the hepatic artery, the extrahepatic biliary tract, as well as lymphatic and nervous trunks. Inside the ligament, the portal vein occupies the rearmost position, while normally the artery is located on the left anterior position and the *common bile duct* on the right anterior one.

1.5 Vessels and Nerves

The blood reaches the liver through two vessels, the portal vein and the hepatic artery, which penetrate the organ at the level of the hilum; a single venous system comes out of the organ, consisting of the hepatic veins that flow into the inferior vena cava.

The *portal vein* is a large vessel, with a lumen of about 1 cm, which forms behind the head or isthmus of the pancreas due to the confluence of the superior mesenteric vein, the inferior mesenteric vein and the splenic vein (Fig. 1.3). The last two usually converge to form a common trunk, although different variants of vein union exist with very different percentages in the literature. In particular, in the most frequent case the inferior mesenteric vein enters the splenic

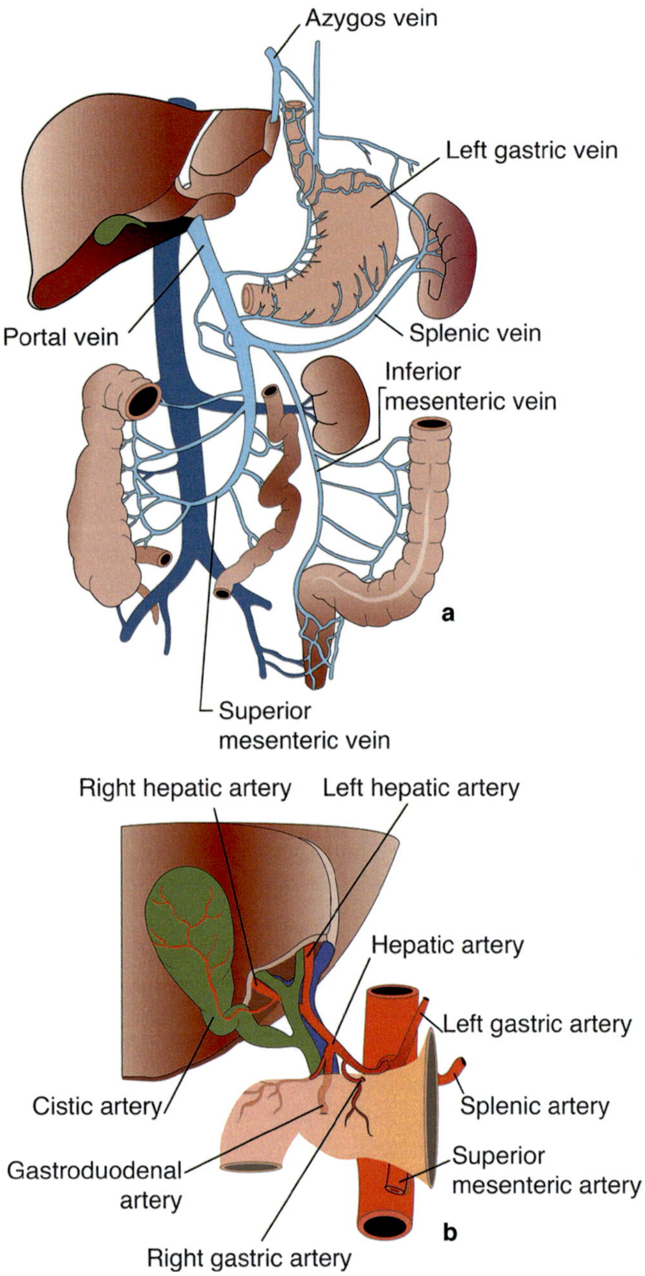

Fig. 1.3 Representation of the portal vein with tributaries (**a**) and the hepatic artery with its divisions (**b**), according to the most frequent mode of organization

vein; in the variations it can converge at the angle of confluence of the splenic vein and the superior mesenteric vein, or enter into the superior mesenteric vein; other variants are very rare [1, 2]. After covering the entire hepatoduodenal ligament, the portal vein reaches the liver where it first subdivides into a right and a left branch; from these branches, an arborization originates with successive branches of progressively smaller calibre, at the end of which the network of hepatic sinusoids originates.

Accessory portal veins are defined as veins that carry venous blood to the hepatic parenchyma without reaching the portal vein. These are the cystic veins, the veins accompanying the falciform ligament and the round ligament, and the veins of the lesser omentum.

The veins tributaries of the portal vein present some anastomoses with veins that directly are headed to the district of the inferior vena cava, thus constituting collateral circles that bypass the liver. It deals of anastomoses with the esophageal, hemorrhoidal, paraumbilical veins, with the parietal veins of the Retzius' circle, and with the accessory portal veins. All these anastomosis can constitute porto-systemic shunts that have no relevance under normal conditions, but acquire much relief in chronic hepatic diseases and in portal hypertension.

The *hepatic artery* (Fig. 1.3) originates from the celiac trunk, first as a common hepatic artery, which divides into the gastroduodenal artery and the proper hepatic artery. The latter joins the portal vein and reaches the liver. Within the organ, the artery subdivides following the way of branching of the portal vein. Before arriving at the liver, the hepatic artery gives rise to the cystic artery and to other branches for the extrahepatic biliary tract. Inside the liver, in addition to the branches destined to the capsule and the connective tissue of the periportal spaces, the artery supplies the peribiliary plexus, a capillary network to nourish the intrahepatic bile ducts. The blood drained from the peribiliary plexus eventually flows into the network of the hepatic sinusoids. In about one third of subjects, variant of the left or the right hepatic arteries are present, and only few patients show a variant anatomy involving both arteries. The origin of the common hepatic artery from the superior mesenteric artery or from the aorta is rare. These anatomical variants of the hepatic artery have relevance for surgical and interventional radiological procedure [3, 4].

The portal vein is responsible for about 70–80% of the blood supply to the liver, while the remaining is due to the hepatic artery. The portal blood has a saturation of about 80% and can give oxygen to the hepatocytes.

The *hepatic veins* constitute a system of veins that carries blood from the liver. They originate from the progressive confluence of the central veins of the lobules in ever larger trunks that form the roots of the hepatic veins. At the end three main venous trunks are formed. In vivo studies showed that the prevailing pattern of the three hepatic veins is a right hepatic vein and a common trunk for the middle and left hepatic veins (61%), while in the remaining patients the three veins drain independently into the inferior vena cava [5].

The right hepatic vein is the largest, but also the most variable in size, sometimes accompanied by a right inferior hepatic vein (21.0%), or an accessory vein (8%); it drains the whole segments VI and VII, and partially the segments V and VIII. The middle hepatic vein drains the central part of the liver with variable blood supply from the segments IV, V and VIII, while the left hepatic vein collects blood from the segments II, III and IV, although intrahepatic venous anastomoses are frequently reported [6]. Some minor hepatic veins drain blood from segment I, or caudate lobe. All the veins of the liver flow into the inferior vena cava. The knowledge of the venous hepatic anatomy of the right lobe is particularly important in living hepatic donors.

The lymphatic vessels are present in the liver only in correspondence with the connective of the portal spaces [7]. The lymphatic ways of the liver may have different destinies. Most of thc intrahepatic deep lymphatic vessels converge towards the hilum where the hepatic lymph nodes are present. Other lymphatic vessels can follow the hepatic veins and the inferior vena cava, joining the diaphragmatic groups of lymph nodes. Finally, the superficial lymphatic vessels that run under the peritoneum, can reach different stations of lymph nodes at the esophageal hiatus and cardias, around the vena cava and the coeliac nodes or drain directly into the thoracic duct, according to their position.

The liver is innervated by sympathetic fibers from the celiac plexus and parasympathetic fibers of the vagus nerve; despite having different origins, they unite in the hepatic plexus that surrounds the hepatic artery, distinguishing itself in an anterior and posterior plexus. Partly, nerve fibers reach the wall of the vessels, where regulate blood flow through the hepatic sinusoids, and the bile ducts; they also extend into the lobule in close relationship to stellate cells and hepatic parenchymal cells, exerting a direct stimulation and regulation of the metabolic function on both hepatocytes and cholangiocytes. Aminergic, cholinergic, peptidergic and also nitrergic fibers are present in the liver [8], but their role does not seem to be essential, as it is shown in the transplanted and denervated livers.

1.6 Segmental Anatomy of the Liver

The division and distribution of the branches of the portal vein within the liver, accompanied by ramifications of the hepatic artery and the bile ducts, follows a quite constant organization, although variants [9, 10] should be taken into account by radiologists and surgeons.

It is therefore possible to describe within the liver some hepatic territories or sectors, classically described by Couinaud [11]; these sectors possess blood supply and biliary drainage independent of neighboring territories, allowing a partial surgical resection of the organ. The portal vein, the main afferent vessel, divides into two branches that supply the right side and the left side of the liver. On the visceral surface of the organ, a line identifies the left and right territories, going from the cystic fossa to the left margin of the inferior vena cava (Cantlie's line). The two main portal branches in turn divide into secondary branches: schematically, the left branch gives rise to a lateral and a paramedian branch, and a branch for the caudate lobe; the right branch, of larger caliber, divides into the lateral and the paramedian branches, each giving front and rear branches. Four sectors are thus distinguished: two right sectors, lateral and medial, and two left lateral and medial sectors. Among these sectors the three hepatic veins run following vertical planes called portal fissures: right portal fissure, main (middle) portal fissure, left portal fissure. The further subdivision of the portal branches gives rise to two segments for each sector; veins distribute to more restricted parts of the parenchyma, without exchanging anastomoses. Thus, we describe eight functionally independent segments of the liver [12] (Fig. 1.4).

- Segment I. It corresponds to the caudate lobe. It is in a dorsal position compared to segment IV, and adjacent to segment II, while on the right it enfolds the inferior vena cava. According to different classifications, two or three territories can be recognize within the segment, receiving vessels mainly from the left branch of the portal vein, and partly also from the right one. The efferent veins drain directly into the inferior vena cava. The bile ducts usually flow into the left hepatic duct very close to the point of confluence with the right one.
- Segment II. It is located laterally to the left portal fissure in a superior-lateral position in the left lobe of the liver.
- Segment III. It is on the left of the umbilical fissure, in an inferior-lateral position of the left lobe of the liver. It receives blood from one to two left portal branches, but it can also receive from a small right branch. It drains into the left hepatic vein.
- Segment IV. Located in front of the caudate lobe, at the right of the umbilical fissure and medially to the main or middle portal fissure. It is supplied with blood from the right branch of the portal vein and only occasionally also from a small left branch, and drains into the mean hepatic vein. An upper and a lower part are distinguished, respectively IVa and IVb.
- Segment V. It is in anterior-inferior position, between the middle and right hepatic veins, where the blood drains from the parenchyma. It is vascularized by the right portal branches.
- Segment VI. It correspond to the lower part of the lateral or posterior right sector. It receives blood from the right lateral branch of the portal vein and drains into the right hepatic vein.
- Segment VII. Located above segment VI, it is supplied by lateral upper right branches of the portal vein and drains into the right hepatic vein.
- Segment VIII. It is in anterior position above segment V, supplied by upper branches of the vein of the medial sector, while it follows the drainage modalities of the segment V.

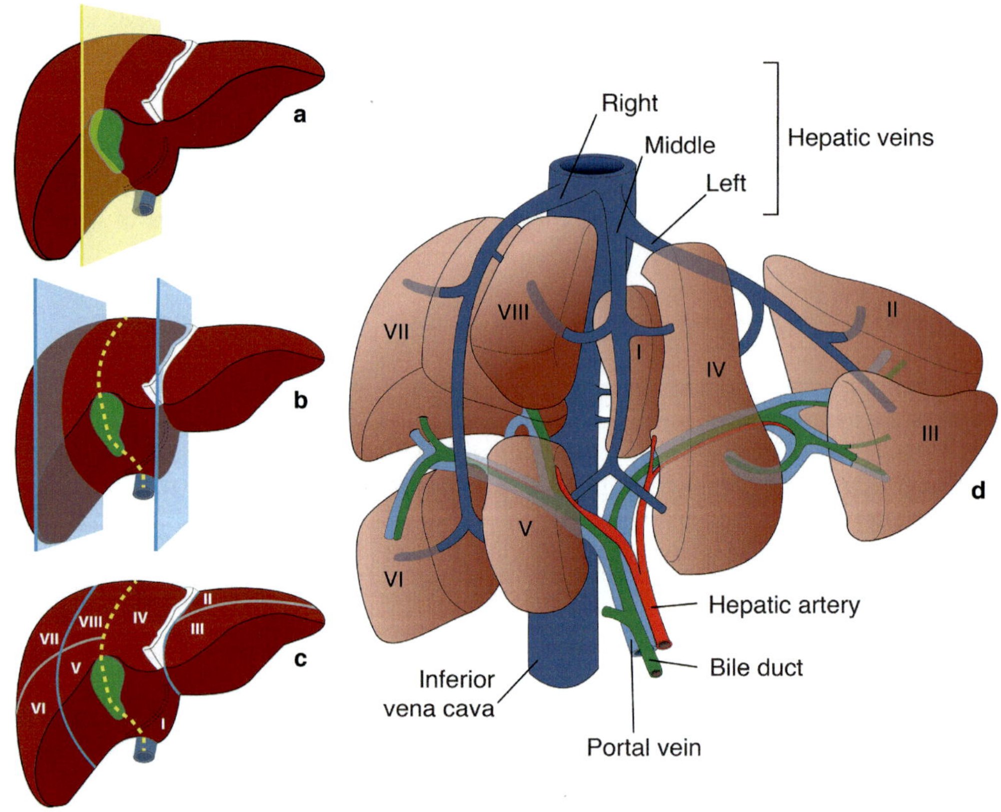

Fig. 1.4 Segmental Anatomy of the Liver. (**a**) A midplane divides the liver in left and right hemi-livers. (**b**) Two intersectional planes divide the liver in four sections. (**c**) Eight segments of the liver. (**d**) The branches of the portal vein, supplying each segments of the liver, with the corresponding subdivisions of the hepatic artery and the bile ducts; the hepatic veins drain the liver determining the sectors

1.7 Extrahepatic Biliary Tract

The biliary ways constitute the system of excretory ducts of the liver that convey the bile towards the duodenum. About the biliary ways, we can distinguish an intrahepatic course, which originates in the hepatic lobules and ends in the porta hepatis, and an extrahepatic course.

The extrahepatic biliary tract originates from the two right and left hepatic ducts, which receive bile from the respective portions of the liver. Inside the liver, the ducts generally follow the ways of dividing of the portal vein, but frequent variations are possible, especially for the right duct. The two most common variations are the right anterior and posterior hepatic ducts converging to form the right hepatic duct, or a trifurcation where they join directly to the confluence with the left hepatic duct to form the common hepatic duct. For the left hepatic duct, the two most common variations are segment IV drainage to the left or right hepatic ducts [13].

The gallbladder is a container attached to the main bile duct with the function of accumulation and concentration of bile. It is located in the anterior part of the right sagittal groove of the visceral surface of the liver. Three portions are recognized in the gallbladder: the fundus, which protrudes beyond the anterior margin of the liver at the level of the tenth coast; the body that adheres to the liver and elongates backwards where it is thinned forming the neck of the gallbladder from which the cystic duct originates.

At the porta hepatis the right and left bile ducts are located in front of the corresponding portal branches and shortly after the exit from the liver they converge to form the common hepatic duct. In the adults the duct has a length of about 3 centimeters, and a luminary diameter of less than 5 mm; it is included in the hepatoduodenal ligament and ends where it receives the confluence of the cystic duct.

The cystic duct comes from the gallbladder and joins the common hepatic duct giving rise to the common bile duct. It has a length and behavior that varies widely in different subjects often showing a tortuous course [14].

The common bile duct has a length of about 6–8 cm. It runs downwards initially into the hepatoduodenal ligament where it is in relation to the portal vein and the hepatic artery. Then it passes behind the first portion of the duodenum and the head of the pancreas, and finally it crosses the pancreas to penetrate the second portion of the duodenum and to finish into the major duodenal papilla. In the distal portion the duct is provided with a proper sphincter. Together with the pancreatic duct, the common bile duct converge in the hepatopancreatic ampulla, where the two ducts are provided with a common sphincter that measures approximately 15–20 mm in length. This region deserves clinical importance because it can be affected by both congenital and acquired disorders like gallstone obstruction, periampullary tumors and recurrent pancreatitis.

The arteries supplying the gallbladder are branches of the cystic artery, which in turn originates from the right hepatic artery, or from the proper hepatic artery; however variations are frequent. The biliary duct system is supplied by several arteries: the major arteries are the cystic artery, the posterior superior pancreaticoduodenal artery, the right hepatic artery, and the retroportal artery. All these arteries form different types of anastomotic patterns on the walls of the ducts [15].

1.8 Liver Development

The fundamental processes that govern the development of the liver was widely studied in the last decades: liver diseases are one of the leading cause of death in the middle-aged population, and the knowledge of their mechanism might open potential perspectives on future therapies. Many genes that contribute to hepatogenesis are now known, but signaling pathways and transcription factors that regulate their expression show different functions at different times of development [16], and their precise temporal sequence and interaction is object of studies [17–20]. Here we propose a brief overview of the liver development.

The liver begins to develop early in the embryo, in the middle of the third week of gestation. At the tenth week of gestation its weight is about 10% of body weight and it rapidly grows to become one of the most voluminous organs in the fetus, due to its essential functions as metabolic organ and as site for hematopoiesis during fetal life. At birth its weight is about 5% of body weight.

The liver and the gastrointestinal tract derive from the definitive endoderm. During the formation of the primitive gut tube, the endoderm is patterned along the anterior-posterior axis into foregut, midgut and hindgut by a concentration gradient of retinoic acid (RA) and secreted factors from the mesoderm. As a result, in each of these portions several transcription factors specify different tissues along both the anterior-posterior and the dorsal-ventral axes of the embryo (Fig. 1.5).

The dorsal endoderm does not activate liver genes, since FGF4 and Wnt ligands from mesoderm and ectoderm of the embryonic dorsal domain inhibit the liver development [21, 22]. The only tract of the primitive intestine that exhibit the capacity to develop into liver is the anterior-ventral domain of endoderm [23].

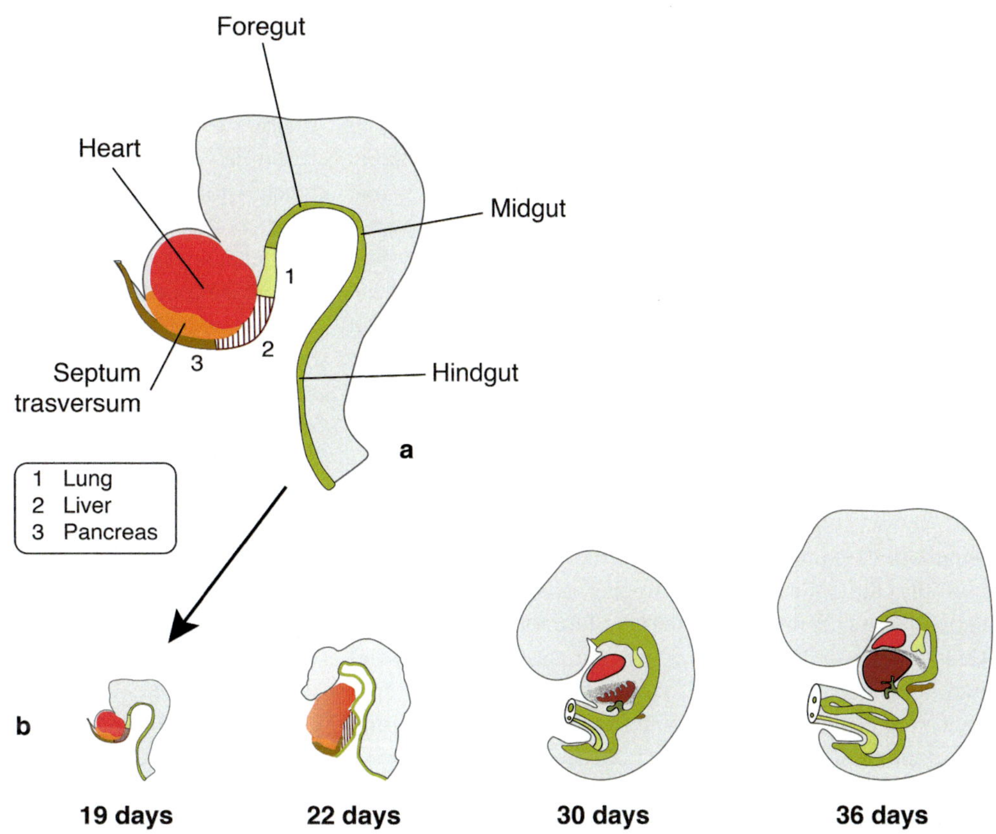

Fig. 1.5 Schematic representation of the stages of liver formation: (**a**) the anterior-ventral endoderm (green) forms the foregut from which the lung, liver and pancreas give origin; (**b**) subsequent stages of development of the liver

1.8.1 Hepatic Competence

Before cell type differentiation, a network of transcription factors activates the transcription of the genes involved in the acquisition of hepatic developmental competence: at least HNFs (Foxa2), GATA4-6 and Hhex are implicated. Moreover, other factors, such as SOX transcription factors and Foxa family, play important roles in several phases of liver development and physiology [20, 24]. GATA4 in the septum transversum parenchyma regulates BMP4 [25], a secreted bone morphogenetic protein member of the transforming growth factor (TGF) family; both GATA and BMP regulate hepatic development [26]. The homeobox transcription factor Hhex, an essential transcriptional regulator of hepatic development, is involved at multiple time points [16, 27], being expressed in both the endoderm and the liver. Wnt signaling acts in the posterior ectoderm to repress the expression of Hhex in early stage, but following specification in the ventral foregut, when cells are not yet determined to a specific fate and can be reversed to another fate, it promotes hepatogenesis [28, 29].

1.8.2 Hepatic Induction

The induction of hepatic fate in the ventral foregut occurs as result of signaling from the cardiac mesoderm and the septum transversum mesenchyma [22]. The developing hearth is in close proximity to the ventral foregut endoderm, so that different concentrations of several fibroblast growth factors (FGFs) signaling promote the development of lung, liver and ventral pancreas in the foregut [30]. The cardiac mesoderm expression of FGF-1, FGF-2 and FGF-8 is necessary and sufficient to induce hepatic gene activity within the endoderm. At the same time, the ventral foregut endoderm expresses FGF receptors (FGFR).

1.8.3 Liver Bud Formation and Growth

Few hours after liver genes activation the newly specified hepatic cells express liver genes. As the hepatic cells begin to multiply, the endoderm layer thicken and the proliferating cells emerge from the epithelium, forming the liver bud. Cells initiate to migrate and concentrate into the septum transversum mesenchyme. The cell migration is accompanied by interruption and loss of the basement membrane, and by remodeling of the surrounding extracellular matrix. Prox1 and Onecut factors (OC-1 and 2) downregulate E-cadherin in hepatoblasts and regulate the expression of enzymes (MMPs) for the remodeling of extracellular matrix and the control of hepatoblast migration [31]. Cells localized in the caudal part of the liver bud, maintaining the initial connection with the original epithelium, will give rise to the bile ducts, and those in the ventral portion to the gallbladder.

The growing liver progressively invades the septum transversum mesenchyme, while cells are going to organize like cords of hepatoblasts. Once again, mesenchymal signals are essential: the extracellular matrix of the septum transversum mesenchyme further promotes hepatic cells proliferation, differentiation and migration through a large number of signals. Among these, FGF, BMP, Hepatocytes Growth Factor (HGF), Wnt, TGFβ, retinoic acid, stress-activated kinases SEK1/MKK4 and some other factors coordinate the hepatic growth through an extensive cross talk that activate a number of genes encoding regulators of proliferation and cell survival [16, 32, 33].

Endothelial cells also contribute to the liver formation [34]. The migrating hepatoblasts progressively settle around the capillary network and veins. The hepatoblast cords form the liver plates interspersed with capillaries, and will give rise to the sinusoidal architecture of the liver. This particular structure is critical for supporting both mature liver function, and fetal hematopoiesis. Sinusoids and hepatocytes growth supporting each other [35]: VEGF secret by hepatocytes promotes both angiogenesis of endothelial cells and their maturation up to reach the structural, molecular and functional characteristics of mature sinusoids; in response to their activation, endothelial cells secret some mitogen factors, such as HGF and IL6.

Starting from the fifth week, hematopoietic cells initiate to migrate to the liver from the yolk sack, and subsequently from the aorta-gonad-mesonephros region. Their activity reaches the maximum in the third month and progressively decreases until it ends in the seventh month. Hepatoblasts, but not hepatocytes, support hematopoiesis [36], so that hematopoietic stem cells move from the fetal liver to the adult bone marrow while hepatocytes differentiate. Endothelial cells and hematopoietic cells provide signals for hepatocytes growth and differentiation: oncostatin M [37] is the most effective, but some others have been described, like HNF-4α and metal-responsive transcription factor-1 (MTF-1) [38].

1.8.4 Hepatoblasts Fate and Function

At the fourth to fifth week the endodermal cells of the ventral foregut specified as hepatic cells express only a few liver genes, including albumin, α-fetoprotein (Afp), transthyretin (Ttr), retinol binding protein (Rbp) and the transcription factor Hnf4α. Later, the activity of the hepatoblasts increases, other specific liver genes are expressed, and several transcription factors allow the expression of all the proteins that characterize the hepatic function: HNF1α and β, C/EBPα, HNF4α, and some others transcription factors act in combination for controlling hepatocytes differentiation and liver function [39]. During embryogenesis HNF-4α plays a central role in transforming the fetal liver into an epithelial parenchyma [40]; later it maintains a differentiated hepatocyte phenotype [41] and coordinates a transcription factor network regulating hepatic fatty acid metabolism essential for the maintenance of lipid homeostasis [42]. Hepatoblasts are quite immature cells as morphology and function, characterized by the expression of cytokeratin-8, 18 and 19, and able to differentiate into hepatocytes and cholangiocytes.

The establishment of the hepatic architecture and the maturation of the parenchyma is a complex phenomenon [27]. It requires an expansion of the hepatocyte compartment until it reaches the definitive volume, together with a concomitant extensive differentiation of parenchymal and non-parenchymal cell types, and with organization of the extracellular matrix. Concurrently we observe the maturation of the sinusoidal network and of the hepatic vasculature, the formation of the biliary tract and the re-organization of the hepatocytes in epithelial polarized cells. Extensive interaction among the hepatoblasts and several types of mesenchymal cell are necessary.

1.8.5 Differentiation of Hepatocytes and Biliary Epithelial Cells

The hepatoblasts are bipotential cells [43]: initially they express genes associated with fetal liver, adult hepatocytes and biliary epithelial cells. Hepatocyte Growth Factor (HGF) inhibit biliary cells and promotes hepatocytes [44]. SOX4 and SOX9 [45], TGFβ, Notch signaling pattern and Wnt promote the differentiation into biliary epithelial cells: these signals downregulate pro-hepatic factors (HNF4α, Tbx3 and C/EBPα), and increase the expression of OC1-2 and HNF1β. Moreover, OC1 (HNF6) seems to control both the timing of differentiation for biliary cells, and their position close to the portal mesenchyme [46, 47], but also other transcription factors act to control cholangiocytes differentiation [35]. Recently, microRNAs have been identified as fine modulators of both hepatocytes and cholangiocytes differentiation and of liver development and function [48].

The intrahepatic biliary tree develops in association to the portal vein starting from the hilum and extending towards the periphery of the liver. It gives rise to the definitive intrahepatic ducts, which remains in continuity with the extrahepatic tree; its complete maturation occurs after birth.

The periportal extracellular matrix, that is reach in laminin, collagen and fibronectin, can influence the cell fate. The hepatoblasts close to the portal vein mesenchyme initially form a monolayer of cuboidal cells around the vessels. While the single layer duplicates the cells acquire a biliary phenotype by increasing cytokeratin-19 (CK-19) expression. In the bi-layer, focal dilations appear crowning a lumen of tubular structures that identify the primitive ducts surrounded by portal mesenchyme, while the remaining bi-layer cells regress. The process of ductal plate remodeling, involving tubulogenesis, apoptosis and outgrowth of the mesenchyme that separate biliary cells from the limiting plate of hepatocytes, continues until near birth (Fig. 1.6) [49]. At about 20 weeks of gestation the expression of cytokeratin-7 (CK-7), another marker of biliary cells, begins in large bile ducts and reaches the entire biliary tree after birth.

The hepatoblasts that are not in close contact with portal veins differentiate into mature hepatocytes under oncostatin M, glucocorticoid hormones, HGF and Wnt signaling. Moreover, a role for HNF4α, C/EBPα and HNF1α in hepatocyte differentiation has been described [16]. Oncostatin M and HGF induce metabolic maturation and promote morphological maturation into polarized epithelial cells. The inhibition of this activity by TNFα maintains the proliferative capability of the cells, allowing liver growth up to the appropriate size [50].

While the entire parenchyma express hepatic genes, different expression of some genes characterizes zonal regions in relation to the proximity to the portal triad or the central vein [51]. The compartmentalized zonal expression may be due to the action of transcriptional repressors, among which a contribution of HNF4α and the WNT/β-catenin signaling pathway in controlling the positional identity of hepatocytes within the hepatic lobule has been described [52–54].

Hepatocytes express cytokeratin-8 and 18, but not cytokeratin-19 and gradually acquire the characteristic morphology arranged in epithelial chords. Starting from the 7–8 week of gestation bile canaliculi appear on the apical surfaces of the cells. The bile canaliculi network inside the hepatocytes plates links the intrahepatic bile ducts of the portal spaces, allowing the continuity of the biliary tree up to the smallest canaliculi.

Hepatocytes progressively assume their metabolic functions: albumin and α-fetoprotein synthesis is precocious, the latter rapidly decreasing after birth; bile acid synthesis begins at 12 weeks, followed by bile secretion a few time later. Glycogen granules and glycogenesis are present within 12–14 weeks. Glycerol and lipid synthesis occurs in parallel to glycogenesis. Cytochrome P-450, the most common drug metabolizing enzymes, are also expressed in liver fetus, although at low rate. The heterogeneity of most enzyme in relation to the zonal position of the cells will develop gradually during early post-natal life.

A quote of undifferentiated stem cells, the hepatic progenitor cells, will remain in the adult liver. They reside in the small terminal bile ducts, and they can proliferate and differentiate both in hepatocytes and in biliary cells under appropriate stimulation, such as in severe diseases.

In the growing liver, the hepatocytes initially form thick epithelial plates that persists during the fetal life and the first

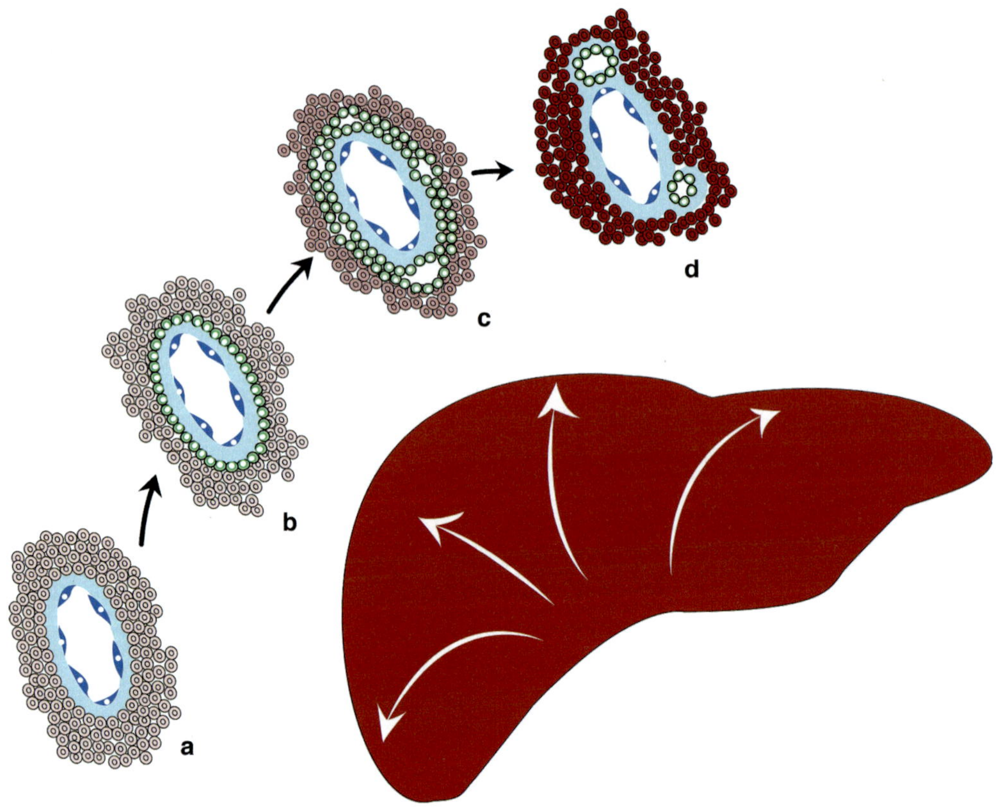

Fig. 1.6 Development of the intrahepatic biliary system. The process begins at the hilum and progressively advances towards the periphery along the portal branches. The hepatoblasts at the limiting plate (**a**) acquire a biliary phenotype (**b**), then form a second layer with some lumens of tubular aspect (**c**), the ductal plate; remodeling of the ductal plate give rise to the definitive bile ducts (**d**) surrounded by mature hepatocytes

years postpartum: some months after bird the sheets are two cells thick, to reach the single cell thickness around about 5 years. Continuous growth of the sinusoids and remodeling of the parenchyma accompanies the changes in the structure of the liver.

The hepatic stellate cells reside in the perisinusoidal space. They are essential for sinusoids formation and maintenance, and for extracellular matrix deposition. They appear at 6–8 weeks of gestation, and their origin is still debated: an endodermal, neural crest, or mesenchymal origin have been reported, but more recent evidences have suggested that they are of mesenchymal origin [55]. During embryogenesis they contribute to the liver development. In adults they are able to store vitamin A, to modulate hepatic microcirculation and, when activated, to adopt a myofibroblast phenotype and to secrete collagen.

Kupffer cells are resident macrophages of the liver. They do not seem to be directly involved in liver development, but they contribute to the maturation of erythrocytes during fetal liver hematopoiesis.

1.8.6 Hepatic Vascular Development

When the hepatoblasts invade the transverse septum mesenchyme, they are arranged around a network of vessels that arises from the two vitelline veins. After forming the vascular plexus inside the liver, the vitelline veins flow into the venous sinus of the heart together with the adjacent umbilical veins. These latter come from the placenta, carrying oxygenated blood, and initially they constitute the major afferent vessels to the liver (Fig. 1.7). Subsequently the vitelline veins form various anastomoses inside and outside the liver, and the umbilical veins participate to the anastomosis with the sinusoids. Part of the vitelline veins and their anastomoses obliterate over time; only a venous trunk will remain, which will become the portal vein, and progressively it begins responsible for most of the supply of the liver [56]. The proximal portion of the vitelline veins, between the plexus of the liver and the venous sinus, will form the hepatic veins. The right umbilical vein and part of the left vein collapse and atrophy. For some time the blood from the placenta passes through the liver into the right vitelline vein. Then the venous duct develops from the left umbilical vein as an independent venous trunk that runs diagonally to the inferior edge of the liver and enters the heart, and in a later period into the inferior vena cava: only a part of its blood passes through the liver. At birth, the venous duct is obliterated forming the venous ligament, and the residue of the by now occluded umbilical vein forms the round ligament.

The arterial supply of the liver competes to the hepatic artery, which arise from the celiac axis. The artery accompanies the growth of the liver bud. It is directed from the hilum to the periphery, closely parallel to the growing bile ducts, a

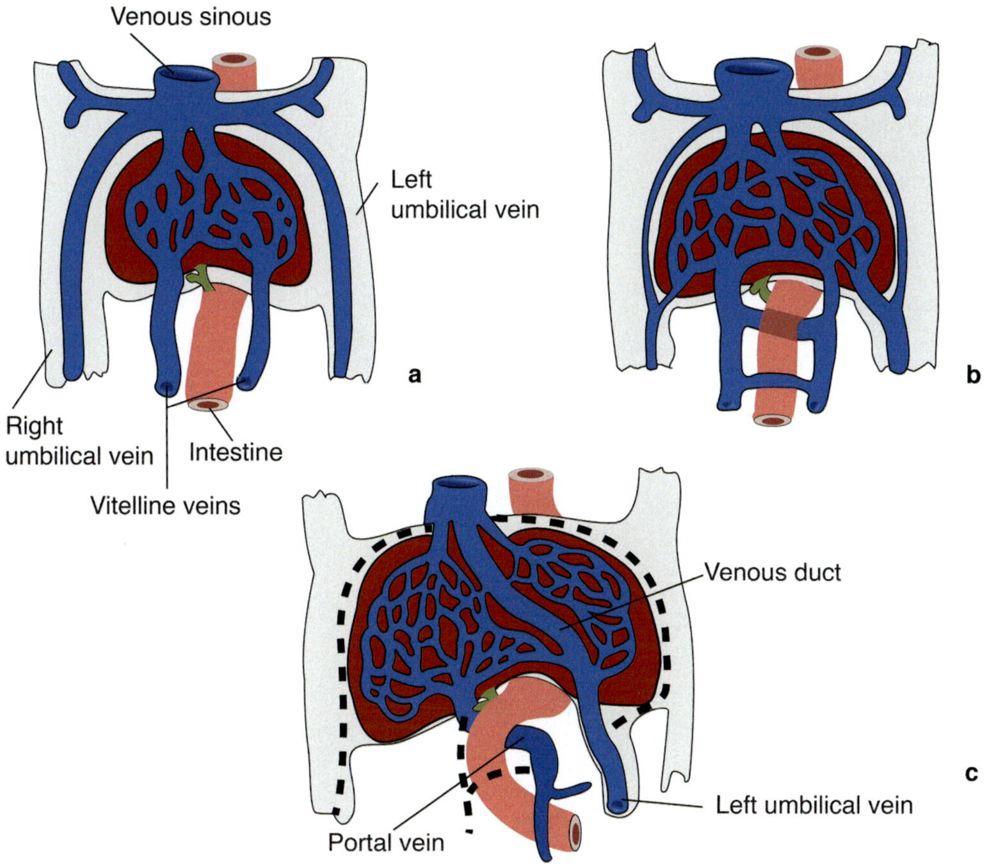

Fig. 1.7 Vascular development in the liver: schematic events are sequentially presented in figures **a–c**. The dotted lines correspond to the umbilical and vitelline veins after their obliteration

source of VEGF. The artery divisions mimics and follows the pattern of development of the biliary tract, providing a loose capillary plexus around the single ducts. The peribiliary plexus will differentiate into a double layer where the wall of the ducts is thicker, like in the extrahepatic tract.

1.8.7 Morphogenetic Events Accompanying the Liver Growth

The liver growths rapidly and gradually protrudes ventrally into the abdominal cavity. The ventral mesogastrium, together with the residue of the septum transversum mesenchyme placed between the liver and the anterior intestine, will form the lesser omentum (Fig. 1.8). The portion placed between the liver and the anterior abdominal wall, will form the falciform ligament, whose free margin extends to the entrance of the yolk sac and contains the umbilical vein. The mesoderm that delimits the septum transversum in the ventral portion and envelops the liver will differ in the visceral peritoneum. The septum transversum will become the diaphragm and the portion of the liver adhering to it remains without peritoneal lining forming the bare area of the liver.

In the meantime, the rotation of the stomach and the lengthening of the duodenum cause the latter to assume a handle conformation with rotation towards the right. The head of the pancreas develops inside the duodenal loop. Following the duodenal rotation, the end of the biliary tract from anterior becomes posterior; the caudal portion of the common bile duct runs into the free margin of the lesser omentum (hepatoduodenal ligament), the ventral portion lying behind the duodenum and the head of the pancreas.

The morphogenetic events of liver and biliary tract formation could be considered completed at the end of the seventh week.

1.9 Conclusions

The anatomy of the liver has acquired an increasingly important meaning for the modern physicians with both diagnostic and therapeutic implications. Especially the advancement in surgical techniques and the advent of the modern diagnostic techniques of imaging, has induced renewal of studies for deepening several aspects of the liver and bile tract anatomy. In particular, the knowledge of the modalities of vascularization, has allowed to develop the modern surgical techniques of partial resection and selective catheterization, that are widely used in the treatment of primary and secondary lesions of the liver. On the other hand, the knowledge of the

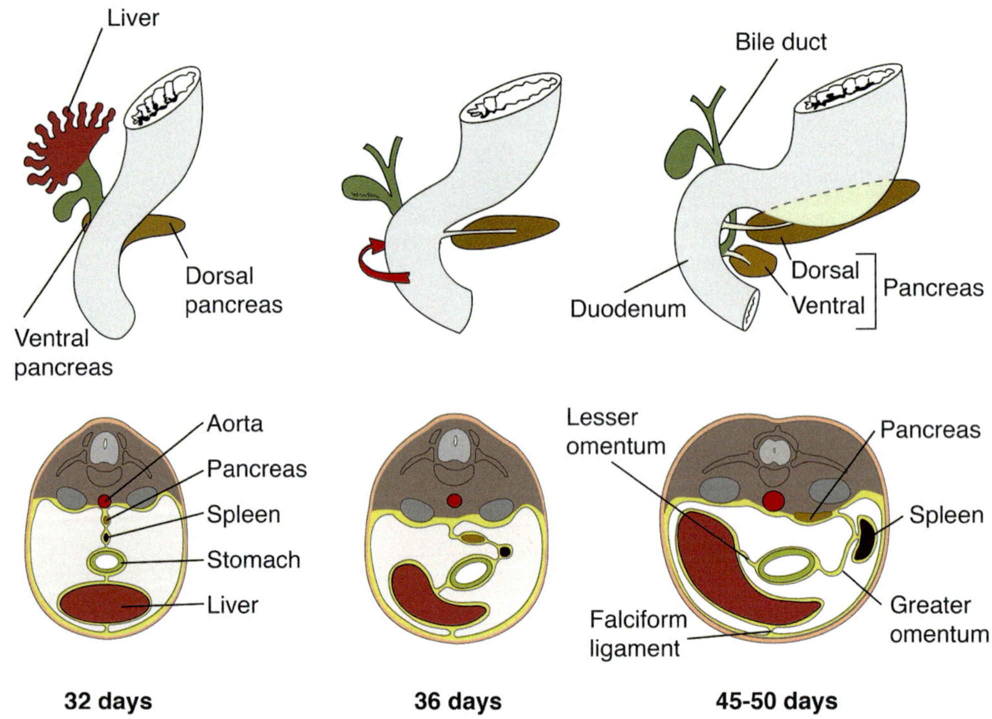

Fig. 1.8 Development and final position of the liver and the organs of the upper abdomen following the rotation of the stomach and the lengthening of the duodenum

molecular mechanisms that regulate the embryonic development of the liver opens new perspectives also to the possibility of molecular and gene therapies for liver diseases.

Acknowledgments Thanks are due to Mr. Francesco Mastrostefano for his help in the artwork generation.

Self Study

Questions

1. Which statement(s) is/are true?
   (a) The liver occupies the entire upper abdomen (right and left hypochondrium).
   (b) Liver fixation structures are the coronary ligament, the falciform ligament, the gastrocolic ligament, the adhesion to the diaphragm and the inferior vena cava.
   (c) In physiologic conditions the portal vein is responsible for more than 70% of the blood supply to the liver.
   (d) A focal lesion of the VIII segment of the liver is located in the lower part of the lateral or posterior left sector.
   (e) The extrahepatic biliary tract connects the liver with the gallbladder, pancreas and duodenum.
2. Which statement(s) is/are true?
   (a) The liver begins to develop during the third week of gestation and completes its morphological formation after birth.
   (b) The liver develops from the primitive endoderm without the contribution of cells from other embryonic tissues.
   (c) Undifferentiated stem cells completely disappear in the adult liver.
   (d) Different gene expression characterizes compartmentalized zonal regions in relation to the proximity to the portal triad or the central vein.
   (e) Hepatoblasts are bi-potential cells able to differentiate into hepatocytes and biliary epithelial cells.

Answers

1. Which statement(s) is/are true?
   (a) The liver occupies the entire right hypochondrium, and only part of the epigastrium and of the left hypochondrium.
   (b) The main fixation structures of the liver are the adhesion to the diaphragm through the coronary ligament and the bare area, and the vena cava. Other ligaments have little significance as fixation structures, and connect the liver to other organs allowing the passage of blood vessels. The gastrocolic ligament is not properly a ligament of the liver and connects the stomach and the transverse colon.
   (c) The portal vein is responsible for 70–80% of the blood supply to the liver in physiologic conditions (**CORRECT**), while the hepatic artery provides the remaining supply.

(d) The VIII segment of the liver is located in the anterior superior position of the right sector.
(e) The extrahepatic biliary tract include the gallbladder, and connects the liver with duodenum.

2. Which statement(s) is/are true?
   (a) The liver begins to develop in the middle of the third week of gestation and completes its formation at the end of the seventh week. However, it continues to acquire and increase its functions even after birth.
   (b) In the liver there are different populations of cells that come from various embryonic tissues (certainly at least from the endoderm and mesoderm): their interactions are essential for the correct development of the organ.
   (c) A little quote of undifferentiated stem cells, the hepatic progenitor cells, still remain in the adult liver.
   (d) (**CORRECT**) The heterogeneity of most enzyme in relation to the zonal position of the cells will develop gradually during early post-natal life. This phenomenon is the basis for the metabolic zonation of the adult liver.
   (e) Hepatoblasts are bi-potential cells that can differentiate into hepatocytes and biliary epithelial cells in relation to their position near or far to the branches of the portal vein and the extracellular matrix (**CORRECT**).

References

1. Krumm P, Schraml C, Bretschneider C, Seeger A, Klumpp B, Kramer U, Claussen CD, Miller S. Depiction of variants of the portal confluence venous system using multidetector row CT: analysis of 916 cases. Rofo. 2011;183:1123–9. https://doi.org/10.1055/s-0031-1281745.
2. Sakaguchi T, Suzuki S, Morita Y, Oishi K, Suzuki A, Fukumoto K, Inaba K, Kamiya K, Ota M, Setoguchi T, Takehara Y, Nasu H, Nakamura S, Konno H. Analysis of anatomic variants of mesenteric veins by 3-dimensional portography using multidetector-row computed tomography. Am J Surg. 2010;200:15–22. https://doi.org/10.1016/j.amjsurg.2009.05.017.
3. Covey AM, Brody LA, Maluccio MA, Getrajdman GI, Brown KT. Variant hepatic arterial anatomy revisited: digital subtraction angiography performed in 600 patients. Radiology. 2002;224:542–7. https://doi.org/10.1148/radiol.2242011283.
4. Saba L, Mallarini G. Anatomic variations of arterial liver vascularization: an analysis by using MDCTA. Surg Radiol Anat. 2011;33:559–68. https://doi.org/10.1007/s00276-011-0778-x.
5. Fang CH, You JH, Lau WY, Lai EC, Fan YF, Zhong SZ, Li KX, Chen ZX, Su ZH, Bao SS. Anatomical variations of hepatic veins: three-dimensional computed tomography scans of 200 subjects. World J Surg. 2012;36:120–4. https://doi.org/10.1007/s00268-011-1297-y.
6. Hribernik M, Trotovšek B. Intrahepatic venous anastomoses with a focus on the middle hepatic vein anastomoses in normal human livers: anatomical study on liver corrosion casts. Surg Radiol Anat. 2014;36:231–7. https://doi.org/10.1007/s00276-013-1198-x.
7. Ohtani O, Ohtani Y. Lymph circulation in the liver. Anat Rec (Hoboken). 2008;291:643–52. https://doi.org/10.1002/ar.20681.
8. McCuskey RS. Anatomy of efferent hepatic nerves. Anat Rec A Discov Mol Cell Evol Biol. 2004;280:821–6. https://doi.org/10.1002/ar.a.20087.
9. Covey AM, Brody LA, Getrajdman GI, Sofocleous CT, Brown KT. Incidence, patterns, and clinical relevance of variant portal vein anatomy. AJR Am J Roentgenol. 2004;183:1055–64. https://doi.org/10.2214/ajr.183.4.1831055.
10. Onishi H, Kawarada Y, Das BC, Nakano K, Gadzijev EM, Ravnik D, Isaji S. Surgical anatomy of the medial segment (S4) of the liver with special reference to bile ducts and vessels. Hepato-Gastroenterology. 2000;47:143–50.
11. Couinaud C. Le foie; études anatomiques et chirurgicales. Paris: Masson; 1957.
12. Delattre JF, Avisse C, Flament JB. Anatomic basis of hepatic surgery. Surg Clin North Am. 2000;80:345–62. https://doi.org/10.1016/S0039-6109(05)70409-6.
13. Chaib E, Kanas AF, Galvão FH, D'Albuquerque LA. Bile duct confluence: anatomic variations and its classification. Surg Radiol Anat. 2014;36:105–9. https://doi.org/10.1007/s00276-013-1157-6.
14. Lamah M, Karanjia ND, Dickson GH. Anatomical variations of the extrahepatic biliary tree: review of the world literature. Clin Anat. 2001;14:167–72. https://doi.org/10.1002/ca.1028.
15. Chen WJ, Ying DJ, Liu ZJ, He ZP. Analysis of the arterial supply of the extrahepatic bile ducts and its clinical significance. Clin Anat. 1999;12:245–9. https://doi.org/10.1002/(SICI)1098-2353(1999)12:4<245::AID-CA2>3.0.CO;2-W.
16. Zorn AM. Liver development. In: StemBook, editor. The stem cell research community. Cambridge: StemBook; 2008. https://doi.org/10.3824/stembook.1.25.1. http://www.stembook.org.
17. Gordillo M, Evans T, Gouon-Evans V. Orchestrating liver development. Development. 2015;142:2094–108. https://doi.org/10.1242/dev.114215.
18. Gruppuso PA, Sanders JA. Regulation of liver development: implications for liver biology across the lifespan. J Mol Endocrinol. 2016;56:R115–25. https://doi.org/10.1530/JME-15-0313.
19. Ober EA, Lemaigre FP. Development of the liver: Insights into organ and tissue morphogenesis. J Hepatol. 2018;68:1049–62. https://doi.org/10.1016/j.jhep.2018.01.005.
20. Yin C. Molecular mechanisms of Sox transcription factors during the development of liver, bile duct, and pancreas. Semin Cell Dev Biol. 2017;63:68–78. https://doi.org/10.1016/j.semcdb.2016.08.015.
21. Bossard P, Zaret KS. GATA transcription factors as potentiators of gut endoderm differentiation. Development. 1998;125:4909–17.
22. Gualdi R, Bossard P, Zheng M, Hamada Y, Coleman JR, Zaret KS. Hepatic specification of the gut endoderm in vitro: cell signaling and transcriptional control. Genes Dev. 1996;10:1670–82.
23. Tremblay KD, Zaret KS. Distinct populations of endoderm cells converge to generate the embryonic liver bud and ventral foregut tissues. Dev Biol. 2005;280:87–99. https://doi.org/10.1016/j.ydbio.2005.01.003.
24. Wilkins BJ, Pack M. Zebrafish Models of Human Liver Development and Disease. Compr Physiol. 2013;3:1213–30. https://doi.org/10.1002/cphy.c120021.
25. Nemer G, Nemer M. Transcriptional activation of BMP-4 and regulation of mammalian organogenesis by GATA-4 and -6. Dev Biol. 2003;254:131–48. https://doi.org/10.1016/S0012-1606(02)00026-X.
26. Shin D, Shin CH, Tucker J, Ober EA, Rentzsch F, Poss KD, Hammerschmidt M, Mullins MC, Stainier DY. Bmp and Fgf signaling are essential for liver specification in zebrafish. Development. 2007;134:2041–50. https://doi.org/10.1242/dev.000281.
27. Zhao R, Duncan SA. Embryonic development of the liver. Hepatology. 2005;41:956–67. https://doi.org/10.1002/hep.20691.
28. McLin VA, Rankin SA, Zorn AM. Repression of Wnt/beta-catenin signaling in the anterior endoderm is essential for liver and pancreas development. Development. 2007;134:2207–17. https://doi.org/10.1242/dev.001230.

29. Ober EA, Verkade H, Field HA, Stainier DY. Mesodermal Wnt2b signalling positively regulates liver specification. Nature. 2006;442:688–91. https://doi.org/10.1038/nature04888.
30. Serls AE, Doherty S, Parvatiyar P, Wells JM, Deutsch GH. Different thresholds of fibroblast growth factors pattern the ventral foregut into liver and lung. Development. 2005;132:35–47. https://doi.org/10.1242/dev.01570.
31. Margagliotti S, Clotman F, Pierreux CE, Beaudry JB, Jacquemin P, Rousseau GG, Lemaigre FP. The Onecut transcription factors HNF-6/OC-1 and OC-2 regulate early liver expansion by controlling hepatoblast migration. Dev Biol. 2007;311:579–89. https://doi.org/10.1016/j.ydbio.2007.09.013.
32. Ganiatsas S, Kwee L, Fujiwara Y, Perkins A, Ikeda T, Labow MA, Zon LI. SEK1 deficiency reveals mitogen-activated protein kinase cascade crossregulation and leads to abnormal hepatogenesis. Proc Natl Acad Sci U S A. 1998;95:6881–6.
33. Kyrmizi I, Hatzis P, Katrakili N, Tronche F, Gonzalez FJ, Talianidis I. Plasticity and expanding complexity of the hepatic transcription factor network during liver development. Genes Dev. 2006;20:2293–305. https://doi.org/10.1101/gad.390906.
34. Matsumoto K, Yoshitomi H, Rossant J, Zaret KS. Liver organogenesis promoted by endothelial cells prior to vascular function. Science. 2001;294:559–63. https://doi.org/10.1126/science.1063889.
35. Si-Tayeb K, Lemaigre FP, Duncan SA. Organogenesis and development of the liver. Dev Cell. 2010;18:175–89. https://doi.org/10.1016/j.devcel.2010.01.011.
36. Hata M, Nanno M, Doi H, Satomi S, Sakata T, Suzuki R, Itoh T. Establishment of a hepatocytic epithelial cell line from the murine fetal liver capable of promoting hemopoietic cell proliferation. J Cell Physiol. 1993;154:381–92. https://doi.org/10.1002/jcp.1041540222.
37. Miyajima A, Kinoshita T, Tanaka M, Kamiya A, Mukouyama Y, Hara T. Role of Oncostatin M in hematopoiesis and liver development. Cytokine Growth Factor Rev. 2000;11:177–83.
38. Wang Y, Wimmer U, Lichtlen P, Inderbitzin D, Stieger B, Meier PJ, Hunziker L, Stallmach T, Forrer R, Rülicke T, Georgiev O, Schaffner W. Metal-responsive transcription factor-1 (MTF-1) is essential for embryonic liver development and heavy metal detoxification in the adult liver. FASEB J. 2004;18:1071–9. https://doi.org/10.1096/fj.03-1282com.
39. Zaret KS. Regulatory phases of early liver development: paradigms of organogenesis. Nat Rev Genet. 2002;3:499–512. https://doi.org/10.1038/nrg837.
40. Parviz F, Matullo C, Garrison WD, Savatski L, Adamson JW, Ning G, Kaestner KH, Rossi JM, Zaret KS, Duncan SA. Hepatocyte nuclear factor 4alpha controls the development of a hepatic epithelium and liver morphogenesis. Nat Genet. 2003;34:292–6. https://doi.org/10.1038/ng1175.
41. Hayhurst GP, Lee YH, Lambert G, Ward JM, Gonzalez FJ. Hepatocyte nuclear factor 4alpha (nuclear receptor 2A1) is essential for maintenance of hepatic gene expression and lipid homeostasis. Mol Cell Biol. 2001;21:1393–403. https://doi.org/10.1128/MCB.21.4.1393-1403.2001.
42. Martinez-Jimenez CP, Kyrmizi I, Cardot P, Gonzalez FJ, Talianidis I. Hepatocyte nuclear factor 4alpha coordinates a transcription factor network regulating hepatic fatty acid metabolism. Mol Cell Biol. 2010;30:565–77. https://doi.org/10.1128/MCB.00927-09.
43. Lemaigre F, Zaret KS. Liver development update: new embryo models, cell lineage control, and morphogenesis. Curr Opin Genet Dev. 2004;14:582–90. https://doi.org/10.1016/j.gde.2004.08.004.
44. Tchorz JS, Kinter J, Müller M, Tornillo L, Heim MH, Bettler B. Notch2 signaling promotes biliary epithelial cell fate specification and tubulogenesis during bile duct development in mice. Hepatology. 2009;50:871–9. https://doi.org/10.1002/hep.23048.
45. Poncy A, Antoniou A, Cordi S, Pierreux CE, Jacquemin P, Lemaigre FP. Transcription factors SOX4 and SOX9 cooperatively control development of bile ducts. Dev Biol. 2015;404:136–48. https://doi.org/10.1016/j.ydbio.2015.05.012.
46. Clotman F, Lannoy VJ, Reber M, Cereghini S, Cassiman D, Jacquemin P, et al. The onecut transcription factor HNF6 is required for normal development of the biliary tract. Development. 2002;129:1819–28.
47. Coffinier C, Gresh L, Fiette L, Tronche F, Schutz G, Babinet C, et al. Bile system morphogenesis defects and liver dysfunction upon targeted deletion of HNF1beta. Development. 2002;129:1829–38.
48. Chen Y, Verfaillie CM. MicroRNAs: the fine modulators of liver development and function. Liver Int. 2014;34:976–90. https://doi.org/10.1111/liv.12496.
49. Lemaigre FP. Development of the biliary tract. Mech Dev. 2003;120:81–7. https://doi.org/10.1016/S0925-4773(02)00334-9.
50. Kamiya A, Gonzalez FJ. TNF-alpha regulates mouse fetal hepatic maturation induced by oncostatin M and extracellular matrices. Hepatology. 2004;40:527–36. https://doi.org/10.1002/hep.20362.
51. Jungermann K, Katz N. Functional specialization of different hepatocyte populations. Physiol Rev. 1989;69:708–64. https://doi.org/10.1152/physrev.1989.69.3.708.
52. Birchmeier W. Orchestrating Wnt signalling for metabolic liver zonation. Nat Cell Biol. 2016;18:463–5. https://doi.org/10.1038/ncb3349.
53. Kaestner KH. In the zone: how a hepatocyte knows where it is. Gastroenterology. 2009;137:425–7. https://doi.org/10.1053/j.gastro.2009.06.020.
54. Stanulović VS, Kyrmizi I, Kruithof-de Julio M, Hoogenkamp M, Vermeulen JL, Ruijter JM, Talianidis I, Hakvoort TB, Lamers WH. Hepatic HNF4alpha deficiency induces periportal expression of glutamine synthetase and other pericentral enzymes. Hepatology. 2007;45:433–44. https://doi.org/10.1002/hep.21456.
55. Loo CK, Wu XJ. Origin of stellate cells from submesothelial cells in a developing human liver. Liver Int. 2008;28:1437–45. https://doi.org/10.1111/j.1478-3231.2008.01788.x.
56. Collardeau-Frachon S, Scoazec JY. Vascular development and differentiation during human liver organogenesis. Anat Rec (Hoboken). 2008;291:614–27. https://doi.org/10.1002/ar.20679.

Liver Histology

2

Simone Carotti, Sergio Morini, Guido Carpino, and Eugenio Gaudio

Key Concepts

- Different hepatic morpho-functional units are postulated, including the hepatic lobule and acinus, through which microcirculatory and metabolic features of liver parenchyma are described in terms of functional heterogeneity and liver zonation.
- Different cell types contribute to hepatic lobule organization: hepatocytes, forming epithelial laminae; sinusoidal cells lining the fenestrated sinusoids; Kupffer cells belonging to monocyte/macrophage system responsible for immune tolerance and surveillance together with lymphocytic cells; finally, the hepatic stellate cells, vitamin A storing cells, able to activate in a pro-fibrogenic and contractile phenotype.
- The biliary system is composed by ducts and ductules lined by cholangiocyte heterogeneous in size and function with different sensibility to hormones, growth factors and hepatic damage.
- The peribiliary plexus is furnished by terminal branches of hepatic artery and supplies the bile ducts; it constitutes a microcirculatory system through which bile components could be reabsorbed and regulate their own production.

S. Carotti · S. Morini (✉)
Department of Medicine and Surgery, University Campus Bio-Medico of Rome, Rome, Italy
e-mail: s.morini@unicampus.it

G. Carpino
Department of Motor, Human and Health Sciences, University of Rome "Foro Italico", Rome, Italy

E. Gaudio
Department of Anatomical, Histological, Locomotor and Legal Medicine Sciences, Sapienza University, Rome, Italy

2.1 Introduction: The Microstructure of the Liver

The liver is a parenchymal organ, covered for the greater part of its extension by a peritoneal lining consisting of a single-layer mesothelium disposed on a thin layer of sub-mesothelial connective tissue. Below the peritoneum, the organ surface consists of a thin but dense layer of connective tissue with rare elastic fibers, the fibrous capsule of Glisson. The Glisson's capsule is adherent to the underlying parenchymal tissue, in which it sends short connective septa; at the level of the hepatic hilum, the connective tissue thickens and penetrates inside the organ following the ramification of the blood vessels, the bile ducts and the nerves, without however separating autonomous areas of parenchyma inside the organ. The basic histological structure of the liver consists of closely intertwined epithelial cell cords that make it a cordonal gland.

2.2 Hepatic Morpho-functional Units: Hepatic Lobule, Portal Lobule, Hepatic Acinus

The lack of connective septa in humans cannot clearly identify structural units such as lobes and lobules. This has meant that the definition of the morpho-functional unit of the liver parenchyma has been the subject of countless studies over the centuries.

In 1833 Kiernan [1] came to the definition of classic hepatic lobule with the portal spaces in the periphery and the centrilobular vein in the center. The hepatic lobule, with a diameter of about 1 mm and a height of about 1.5–2 mm, in cross-section appears as an area of polygonal shape to identify which, in humans, it is necessary to join with virtual lines the portal spaces surrounding a centrilobular vein (Fig. 2.1a). Each lobule is made up of laminae of epithelial cells, the hepatocytes, which are anastomosed to each other, forming a labyrinthine system of regular spaces in which the vascular network consists of capillaries with a tortuous course, the

F. Radu-Ionita et al. (eds.), *Liver Diseases*, https://doi.org/10.1007/978-3-030-24432-3_2

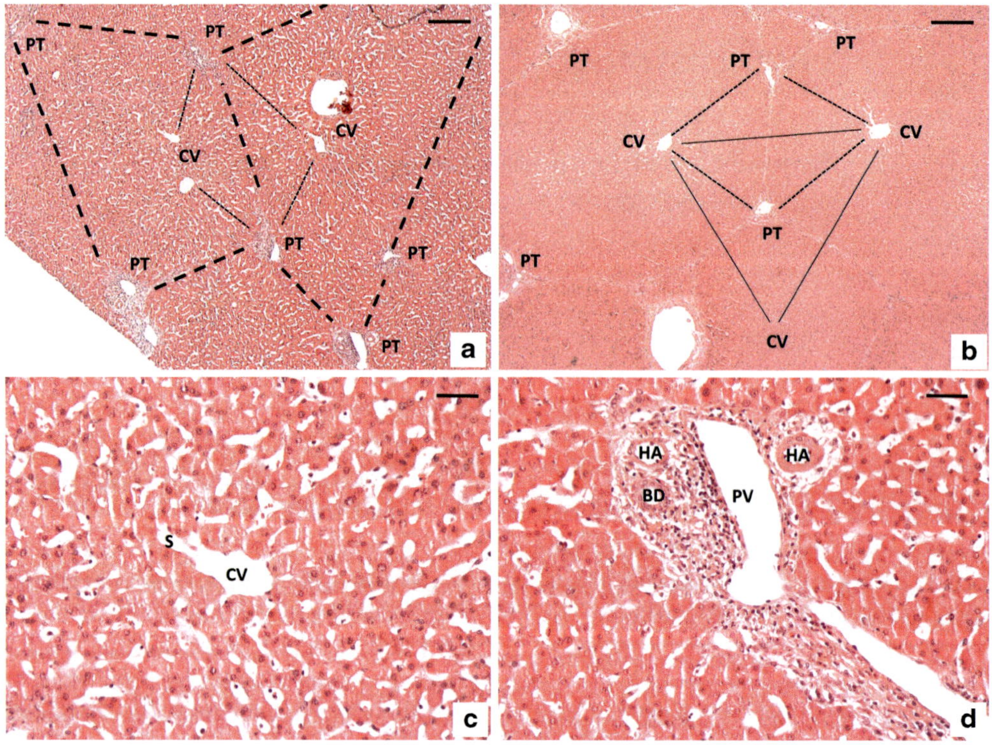

Fig. 2.1 Normal histology of the liver and hepatic morpho-functional units. (**a**) The classic lobule (thick dashed line) obtained by joining some portal tracts (PT) around a centilobular vein (CV); the acinus (thin dashed line) joining two portal tracts to two adjacent centrilobular veins. (**b**) In the porcine liver, the delimitation of the classic hepatic lobule is facilitated by the presence of interlobular connective septa. An acinus (thin dashed line) and a portal lobule (thin continuous line). (**c**) A centrilobular vein (CV) with the wall characteristically pitted by the openings of the sinusoids (S). (**d**) Portal space: branches of the portal vein (PV), branches of the hepatic artery (HA), bile interlobular ducts (BD). Original magnification: ×40 (**a**, **b**), ×200 (**c**, **d**). Scale bar: 250 μm (**a**, **b**), 50 μm (**c**, **d**)

hepatic sinusoids. The laminae of hepatocytes and the sinusoids from the periphery of the lobule converge towards the center, where the central (centrilobular) vein is located, whose wall is pitted by the opening of the sinusoids that converge there (Fig. 2.1c). The perilobular connective thickens to form an envelope at the terminal branches of the portal vein and of the hepatic artery and to collect the initial formations of the bile ducts and lymphatic vessels, forming the portal or porto-biliary spaces located at the periphery of the hepatic lobule (Fig. 2.1d). The blood coming from the portal space is introduced into the sinusoidal capillaries, conveys towards the centrilobular vein and subsequently flows into the sub-lobular veins; the latter form the roots of the hepatic veins through which the blood reaches the inferior vena cava.

In 1906 Mall [2] proposed the portal lobule as a structural unit, considering the portal space at the center and the centrilobular veins in the periphery (Fig. 2.1b). The exocrine function of the organ was thus placed at the center of the hepatic organization, constituted by the elaboration of the bile by the hepatocytes.

The observed histopathological outcomes of microcirculatory hepatic pathologies led in the 50's Rappaport [3] to propose a new morphofunctional unit, identified as the hepatic acinus. The hepatic acinus is an area of roughly quadrangular shape in a cross-section, supplied by a terminal branch of the portal vein and of the hepatic artery and drained by the centrilobular vein. The hepatic acinus is obtained by joining with imaginary lines two portal spaces to the two centrilobular veins immediately adjacent (Fig. 2.1a, b).

Many aspects of liver physiology and metabolism show a heterogeneous distribution along the porto-central axis of the lobule. This functional heterogeneity is the basis of the metabolic zonation. Three zones can be individuated in the hepatic lobule or acinus: the periportal zone (zone 1) at the periphery of the lobule, the centrilobular zone (zone 3) near the central vein, and a midzonal area (zone 2) between the previous ones. Hepatocytes located in the periportal area are more involved in lipid metabolism whereas those located in the pericentral one are the most able to detoxify. Also, glucose metabolism at the hepatocytes level shows heterogeneous localization, with gluconeogenesis occurring mainly in the periportal while glycolysis in the pericentral region. There are several mechanisms responsible for metabolic zonation, ranging from the different blood solutes availability in the different regions of the lobule, to the presence of oxygen and hormones gradients across the lobular parenchyma. At the molecular level, the Wnt/beta-catenin pathway seems to play a major role in the determination of hepatic zonation [4]. Apc is able to control the precise zonal localization of several genes regulated by beta-catenin such as GS, transporter-1 of glutamate (Glt1) and ornithine aminotransferase (Oat) [5]. If the inhibition performed by Apc is interrupted selectively or the constitutive activation of the Wnt/beta-catenin signaling pathway is promoted, the panlobular expression of genes involved in ammonium metabolism is determined.

Based on the microcirculatory and metabolic features of the liver, alternative functional unit has been proposed. Matsumoto and Kawakami [6] proposed a functional structural unit, the primary lobule: the classic lobule, or secondary lobule, consisted of the union of six to eight primary cone-shaped lobules. The metabolic lobule substantially coincides with it. Hofmann [7] identified a further morphofunctional unit that defined a choleon, consisting of a group of hepatocytes whose bile canaliculi drain into a single biliary duct. The hepatic microcirculatory subunit (HMS) [8] occupies a volume of tissue that coincides with the choleon. It consists of a group of sinusoids and related hepatocytes arranged in a cone with the apex towards the centrilobular vein, perfused by a terminal portal vein. The fusion of the choleon with HMS generates the most modern morphofunctional subunit that can be drawn inside the classic hepatic lobule, the choleohepaton.

2.3 Hepatic Cytotypes

The main cytotypes within the liver are hepatocytes, sinusoidal cells, Kupffer cells, stellate cells, lymphocytic cells.

2.3.1 Hepatocytes

The hepatocyte is a polygonal epithelial cell with a diameter between 30 and 40 µm. Like other epithelial cells, it has a high polarization with a transport directed from the sinusoidal surface to the one facing the biliary canaliculi (Fig. 2.2a). Three different specialized regions or domains of the plasma membrane can be described in the hepatocyte: the sinusoidal, facing the sinusoid and the perisinusoidal space, the lateral, facing the intercellular space between two hepatocytes and the canalicular, which surrounds that specific portion of

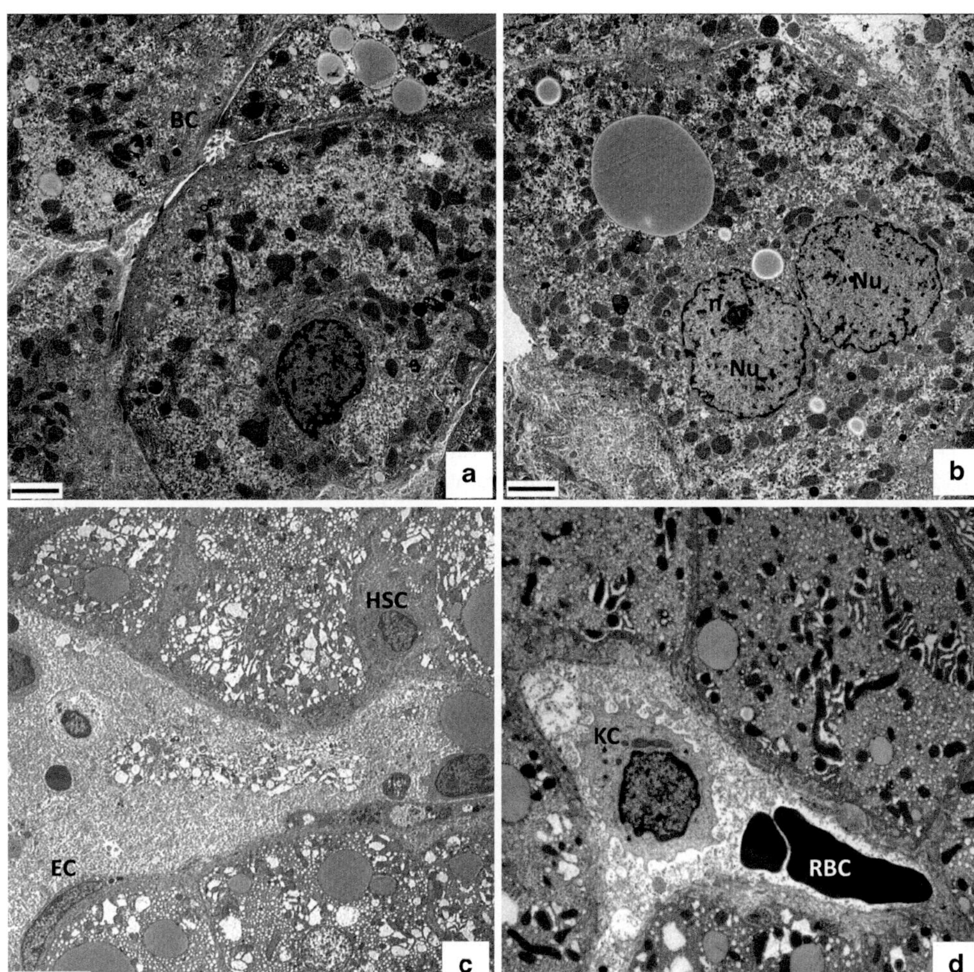

Fig. 2.2 (**a**) Two adjacent hepatocytes face each other, delimiting a biliary canaliculus (BC). (**b**) Bi-nucleated (Nu) hepatocyte with a nucleolus (n). (**c**) Hepatic sinusoid lined by an endothelial cell (EC) with elongated nucleus. Outside the sinusoid, a hepatic stellate cell (HSC) is embedded between two hepatocytes in the perisinusoidal space of Disse. (**d**) Within a sinusoid, a Kupffer cell (KC) with its typical dendroid shape near a red blood cell (RBC). Original magnification: ×3000 (**a**, **b**, **d**), ×1100 (**c**). Scale bar: 2 µm (**a**, **b**, **d**), 5 µm (**c**). (Transmission electron microscopy images, courtesy of Dr. Maria Zingariello, Laboratory of microscopic and ultrastructural anatomy, University Campus Bio-Medico of Rome)

the intercellular space that constitutes the biliary canaliculus. The demarcation of the different cellular domains is guaranteed by tight junction which delimit the sinusoidal and lateral domains from the canalicular one. In addition to tight junctions, the lateral domain also houses other junctional devices such as desmosomes and gap junctions, the latter responsible for intercellular communication.

The sinusoidal domain of the hepatocyte is directed towards the perisinusoidal space of Disse between the hepatocytes and the endothelial cells that line the sinusoids. At this level, the plasma membrane of the hepatocyte presents abundant microvilli of about 0.5 μm in length, which can be pushed through the fenestrations of the endothelial cells inside the sinusoidal lumen. The sinusoidal domain through microvilli and secretory vacuoles that open at their base, allows both absorption and secretion functions. Also at the base of microvilli there are clathrin-coated dimples involved in selective endocytosis mediated by receptors and caveolae, membrane microdomains rich in cholesterol, sphingolipids and caveolin that are responsible for selective trafficking from the membrane inside the cell [9, 10].

The lateral surface of the hepatocyte extends from the edge of the sinusoidal surface to the biliary canaliculus and presents intercellular junctions. Its surface is irregular for the presence of occasional folds and openings of pinocytosis vesicle and hosts gap junctions. Between the surfaces of two hepatocytes a depressed area forms a half-channel which, joining an adjacent analogous structure, constitutes the lumen of the biliary canaliculus: it is delimited by tight junctions and isolated from the rest of the intercellular surface also by junctional complexes such as desmosomes, intermediate junctions and gap junctions. The diameter of the bile canaliculi varies between 0.5 and 1 μm at pericentral and between 1 and 2.5 at periportal level. The lumen is abundantly characterized by the extroversion of microvilli (Fig. 2.2a).

The nucleus of hepatocytes is actively involved in protein synthesis. It occupies 5–10% of the cell volume; it is spherical in shape with one or more prominent nucleoli and dispersed chromatin. At birth, almost all hepatocytes are mononuclear with uniform size, while at least about 25% of adult hepatocytes are binucleated (Fig. 2.2b). Moreover, the DNA content is variable, since at birth almost all hepatocytes are diploid, but from 8 years of age the number of tetraploid nuclei increases to reach 15% at the age of 15 years [11]. The mitotic divisions of the hepatocytes determine a significant increase in the size of the organ in intrauterine and neonatal life, continue during childhood and then decrease in adulthood, when the liver has a very low mitotic index.

The endoplasmic reticulum constitutes 15% of the cell volume with a 35 times greater surface than that of the plasma membrane. The rough endoplasmic reticulum usually dominates the smooth reticulum; the relationship between the two types varies according to the physiological state and the position of the hepatocytes in the acinus. The surface of the smooth reticulum is double in zone 3 compared to zone 1 of the acinus. A precise topographic relationship was observed between glycogen deposits and smooth endoplasmic reticulum membranes; such membranes with their enzymatic kit (glucose-6-phosphatase) can contribute to the glycogenolysis process, followed by the release of glucose into the blood. In addition, the lipids, absorbed from the blood, are conveyed into the smooth endoplasmic reticulum whose membranes are linked to part of the enzymes responsible for the synthesis of cholesterol and the degradation of many liposoluble drugs. The rough endoplasmic reticulum and free ribosomes are responsible for the synthesis of albumin, fibrinogen and plasma proteins released into the circulation. The endoplasmic reticulum of hepatocytes also performs the function of assembling lipoprotein molecules such as VLDL (very low-density lipoprotein), protein complexes consisting of a nucleus of triglycerides and an envelope formed by proteins and a mixture of cholesterol and phospholipids. Cytochrome P-450 is located on the membrane of the smooth endoplasmic reticulum and represents an inducible way by which liver cells metabolize and detoxify xenobiotics. The preponderance of smooth endoplasmic reticulum in the centrilobular region and the presence of heme in cytochrome P-450 enzymes explain the darker color that this region of the lobule presents in a macroscopic inspection of fresh liver slices.

The Golgi apparatus has about 50 complexes that can be connected to each other. It locates more frequently near the nucleus or near the biliary canaliculus. From its concave edge originate secretory vesicles containing secretory proteins, such as lipoproteins, for release in the sinusoidal surface or, less commonly, in the canalicular domain. Also, the membrane proteins, before their final destination, are transported to the Golgi complex which possesses a considerable quantity of glycosylation enzymes.

Lysosomes are vesicles coated with a single membrane and contain about 60 types of acidic hydrolases such as acid phosphatase, aryl-sulfatase, esterase and beta-glucuronidase. The hepatocyte plays a pivotal role in the metabolism of cholesterol and lipids in general and has a subpopulation of lysosomes accompanied by hydrolases that are especially concerned with that function. In the inner side of lysosomal membrane is located the glycocalyx, a thick layer of polysaccharides protecting the lysosomal membrane from the degradation of acidic hydrolases. Lysosomes are metabolic regulator of the cell, entertaining different networks with nucleus, cell membrane and other organelles such as lipid droplets and mitochondria and is involved in the phenomena of cell autophagy/lipophagy [12, 13].

The peroxisomes occupy 1.5–2% of the cell volume; they contain oxidases that use molecular oxygen to oxidize different compounds with the production of hydrogen peroxide then hydrolyzed by peroxisomal catalase. Through this mechanism, peroxisomes are capable of metabolizing an overload of alcohol via their catalase.

The mitochondria, which can reach a diameter of 1.5 μm and a length of 4 μm form about 20% of the cytoplasmic volume of hepatocytes. They are provided with an external membrane that is separated by an additional internal membrane from which the mitochondrial crests are projected towards the inner lumen of the organ which contains the so-called matrix. A peculiar aspect of the hepatocyte mitochondria is that their ridges make up about a third of the total cell membranes. The inner membrane and lamellar crests host the respiratory chain enzymes responsible for the oxidative phosphorylation necessary for the production of ATP. Within the matrix there are instead most of the components of the citric acid cycle, the enzymes involved in the beta-oxidation of fatty acids and in the urea cycle. In the matrix, circular DNA is depositary of genetic information for the synthesis of a portion of mitochondrial proteins, the rest of which is encoded by nuclear DNA. The distribution of mitochondria is subject to a certain variability on the basis of hepatic zonation: at the centrilobular level the mitochondria are smaller and less numerous than the periportal area.

2.3.2 Endothelial Cells

The cells forming the sinusoidal wall are flattened endothelial cells, which protrude into the lumen only with their dilated portion that contains the nucleus (Fig. 2.2c). The sinusoidal wall is discontinuous due to the presence of numerous pores and fenestrations of variable size and position. The pores, with a diameter less than 0.1–0.2 μm, may be isolated or grouped together, while the larger fenestrations may reach a diameter of more than 1 micrometer and are more abundant at the distal end of the sinusoid. The discontinuities are so abundant that most of the cell is pitted like a net and forms the slender wall of the sinusoid, reinforced sometime by the overlap of adjacent endothelial cells that apparently do not seem to form junctions between them. The porosity of the endothelial cell is greater in the perivenular area than in the periportal area. The fenestrations appear to be structures of variable diameter in response to both endogenous and exogenous mediators such as serotonin or alcohol. The extracellular matrix present in the space of Disse is itself capable of modulating the fenestrae. Since the fenestrations are not provided with diaphragms and the basal membrane is lacking on the deep surface of the endothelial cell, the solutes pass freely through the fenestrations within the space of Disse and arrive in contact with the basal-lateral membrane of hepatocytes. Furthermore, the sinusoidal cells of the liver show a series of peculiar phenotypic characteristics. In physiological conditions, they do not express, for example, the von Willebrand factor, which they acquire only in conditions of chronic liver disease. Moreover, they express at very low levels other characteristic molecules of the endothelium such as E-selectin, CD 31 and CD 34 [14]. They instead express ICAM-1 whose ligand, LFA-1, is present on cells of inflammatory processes such as Kupffer cells and lymphocytes and this involves sinusoidal cells in the dynamics of inflammatory processes affecting the liver [15]. The sinusoidal endothelial cells are heterogeneous within the lobule as regard the cell size, the ability to bind lectin, the expression of different receptors and the endocytotic capacity. The endocytosis is largely aimed at capturing and degrading compounds circulating within the blood, molecules that are removed from the circulation as proteoglycans of the hyaluronic acid or chondroitin sulfate type or soluble immune complexes. Another part of the molecules that are taken by endocytosis are instead modified and reach the hepatocytes by transcitosis, thus achieving a more selective mode of transport of macromolecular solutes compared to transport through fenestrations. Endothelial cells also have an active synthesis function and produce nitric oxide (NO), endothelin, prostaglandins and cytokines such as interleukin-1 and interleukin-6, all mediators that have potent effects on vascular tone and the functions of surrounding cells. Sinusoidal endothelial by paracrine activity also regulates hepatic regeneration and fibrosis through the production of growth factors and mediators such as Wnt2 and hepatocyte growth factor (HGF) that promote hepatocyte proliferation [16]. Moreover, sinusoidal endothelial cells are able to modify the surrounding extracellular matrix in response to tissue damage, for example through the production of the fibronectin cell isoform, a potent activator of hepatic stellate cells at the level of which stimulates endothelin-1 synthesis (ET-1) which in turn has a paracrine effect on stellate cells themselves. Soluble factors, including growth factors such as VEGF and others mediators such as angiopoietins, ephrines and fibroblast growth factors, are responsible for the regulation of the sinusoidal endothelial cell phenotype. The phenotype of sinusoidal endothelial cells is also regulated by biomechanical forces such as shear stress, the most significant effect of which is to modulate the activity of nitric oxide synthase of the endothelium (eNOS) thereby regulating the flow and vascular tone in the sinusoids.

2.3.3 Hepatic Stellate Cells

The hepatic stellate cells are also known as perisinusoidal cells, Ito cells, fat-storing cells or lipocytes. They are localized close to the sinusoidal endothelial cells, within the perisinusoidal space of Disse and are probably of mesenchymal origin with a pericyte-like function (Fig. 2.2c). They share features with fibroblasts and myofibroblasts

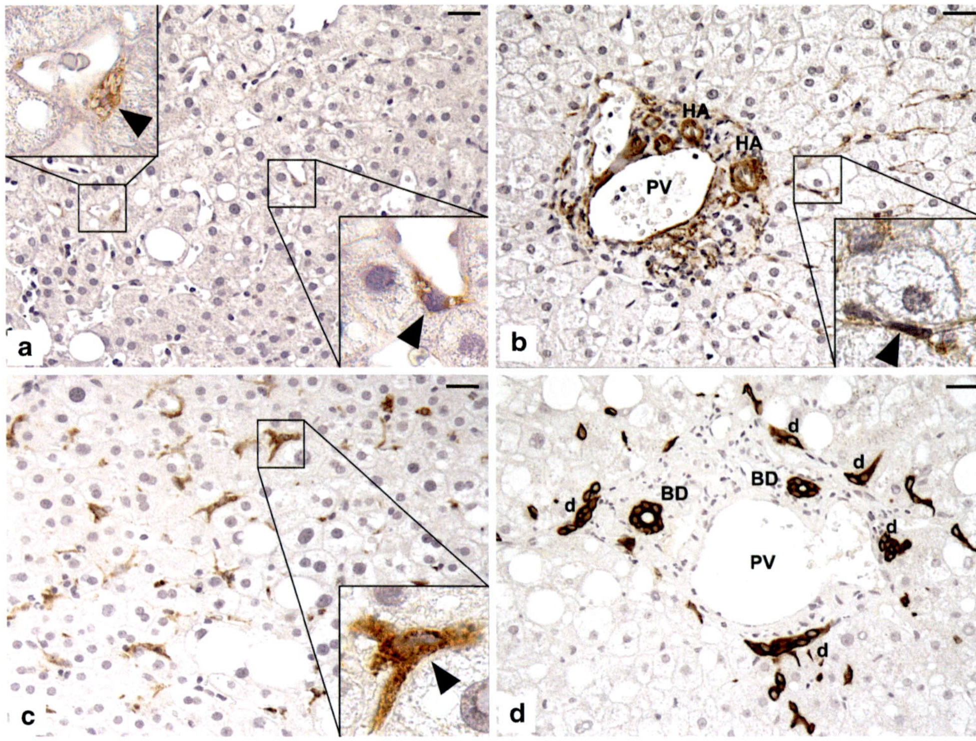

Fig. 2.3 Hepatic cell types. (**a**) Quiescent hepatic stellate cells characterized by little droplets in their cytoplasm (high power fields, arrowheads) in which vitamin A is stored (immunohistochemistry for reelin). (**b**) Hepatic stellate cells near to a portal tract exhibit the typical features of activated phenotype (high power field, arrowhead), with immunohistochemical positivity for alpha-smooth muscle actin. Portal vein (PV); hepatic arteries (HA); the smooth muscle cells in the arteries wall are also positive for alpha-smooth muscle actin. (**c**) CD68-positive hepatic macrophages with the typical dendroid shape (high power field, arrowhead). (**d**) Bile ducts (BD) and ductules (d) are identified by cytokeratin 7-positivity in a portal tract in a steatosic liver, in larger number than normal, due to a mild ductular reaction. Original magnification: ×300, high power filed ×1000. Scale bar: 25 μm

and, due to the expression of some neural markers such as glial fibrillary acidic protein and reelin (Fig. 2.3a), with cells of neural origin [17, 18]. In addition, fibers of the autonomic nervous system seem to terminate on them. Finally, like most pericytes, they store vitamin A esters, containing about 90% of the total body retinoids. In the normal liver, the stellate cells are quiescent, showing by electron microscopy paucity of rough endoplasmic reticulum and a small Golgi apparatus. They only produce moderate levels of collagen proteins and matrix glycoproteins (mainly laminin, entactin and fibronectin). The liver damage induces rapid and pleiotropic changes in the function of stellate cells that affect aspects such as proliferation, migration, contractility and increased matrix production, resulting in alterations generally referred to activation [19]. A salient aspect of stellate cell activation is the de novo expression of the muscle-smooth isoform of α-actin (α-SMA) (Fig. 2.3b) that has been extensively used as an activation marker [20]. Retinoid reserves decrease rapidly during activation and surface receptors for growth factors and cytokines, such as PDGF receptors that appear during activation to allow proliferation, mediated by PDGF, are also regulated. The major subunits of the TGF beta receptor despite being present also in the quiescent and transition cells, change their expression in fully activated cells. Similarly, the endothelin receptors change during the activation of stellate cells being their contraction mediated by endothelial cells derived endothelin. Modifications also occur at the level of cell adhesion molecules, such as ICAM-1, VCAM-1 and NCAM-1, which increasing levels help interaction with leukocyte integrins and mediate firm adhesion and transendothelial migration. Finally, the activation of stellate cells is characterized by the synthesis and secretion of matrix proteins, among which the type I and III collagen increase prevalently. Parallel to the secretion of a fibrillar matrix, the stellate cells produce metalloproteinases (MMPs) that degrade the basal membrane-like extracellular matrix with the result of a gradual substitution within the Disse's space of the normal extracellular matrix with repair tissue. Among the cytokines produced by stellate cells are endothelin, PDGF, CTGF, TGFbeta, PAF and several peptide chemokines some of the which perform an autocrine action, other paracrine. Evidence has also shown that activated stellate cells are able to express the vascular factor of endothelial origin (VEGF) and its receptors [19].

2.3.4 Kupffer Cells

Hepatic macrophages are represented by Kupffer cells (Fig. 2.2d): they originate from the fetal yolk sac, forming the permanently resident macrophage population, and from medullary-derived monocytes/macrophages, which subsequently infiltrate the organ and settle there when needed [21, 22]. While it was believed for a long time that tissue macrophages originated from circulating blood monocytes, it is now fairly established that tissue macrophages are established at the organ level during embryonic development and remain independent of the contribution of circulating monocytes under homeostasis conditions. This results in a situation of high concentration of macrophage cells in the organ, since the liver accommodates about 80% of all macrophages present in the organism and is also guarded by populations of monocytes circulating in the blood. Circulating monocytes in case of damage infiltrate the organ and give rise to new macrophages. In homeostatic conditions, the macrophages residing in the liver self-renew their population thanks to resident stem cells originating from the fetal yolk sac. CD 68 is traditionally used in the liver as a marker, although not exclusive, of Kupffer cells (Fig. 2.3c), while more recently CD163L has been proposed as a marker of tissue macrophages resident differently from CLC5A which would identify monocyte-derived macrophages with pro-inflammatory function [23]. Under hepatic injury subpopulations of circulating monocytes are massively recruited into the liver and become the predominant fraction of organ macrophages. Although these monocyte-derived macrophages initially exert pro-inflammatory and pro-fibrogenic actions, they may differentiate into another sub-population likely to promote tissue repair and damage resolution.

Kupffer cells represent the first line of defense against hepatic damage and constitute a highly dynamic cellular complex able to counteract microorganisms and identify alterations in tissue integrity. Since the liver is constantly exposed to antigens of intestinal origin, as well as to low levels of bacterial endotoxins, mechanisms have been developed that can regulate the activation of the immune system; Kupffer cells play a significant role in the maintenance of immune tolerance in the liver exerting an anti-inflammatory action under conditions of homeostasis [24]. In fact, Kupffer cells secrete anti-inflammatory cytokines such as interleukin 10 and express MHC II molecules through which they are able to regulate T cells in particular by promoting the development of regulatory T cells stimulating immune tolerance. The Kupffer cells recruit monocyte populations in the liver during damage, thus preparing the tissue conditions for hepatic regeneration. In addition, Kupffer cells interact with stellate cells regulating the phenomena that may eventually lead to hepatic fibrosis in case of persistent damage.

2.3.5 Lymphocytes or Pit Cells

As an organ with a lymphoid attitude, the liver contains several lymphocyte populations dedicated to innate immunity such as NK cells, natural killer T (NKT) cells, gamma-delta T cells, which in humans can represent up to 65% of all liver lymphocytes. Only a minor part consists of lymphocyte populations of adaptive immunity such as alpha-beta T cells and B cells. Overall lymphocyte cells represent a percentage of 5% on the total liver cells. NK cells of rat liver, the "pit cells", have a diameter between that of lymphocytes and granulocytes, similar to Kupffer cells with which they share an irregular and dynamic shape. The pit cells adhere to the endothelial lining; small microvillary structures can pass through endothelial discontinuities and contact similar microvilli of the parenchymal cells in order to anchor themselves to them. The most peculiar ultrastructural characteristic are the numerous granules, 0.3 μm in diameter, which tend to be grouped in discrete areas of cytoplasm. These granules are rounded and provided with an electron-dense content surrounded by a light halo and a single membrane. The rest of the cytoplasm contains scant organelles, free ribosomes and few and small mitochondria. Unlike Kupffer cells, pit cells do not exhibit phagocytic or endocytic functions and do not react to most experimental conditions except for partial hepatectomy, a condition in which such cells undergo mitosis in the remaining liver portion [25].

2.4 Cholangiocytes and the Intrahepatic Bile Ducts

The intrahepatic bile ducts have their roots in the bile canaliculi that run between adjacent hepatocytes forming a complex network within the lobule. The diameter of the canaliculi gradually increases from the pericentral to the periportal region and physiologically enlarge under conditions of increased bile flow. At the boundary of the portal space the canaliculi continue in the channels of Hering or bile ductules, whose wall initially consists partly of hepatocytes and partly of cholangiocytes, where the ductule-canalicular junction is formed. In the channels of Hering a resident progenitor cell compartment is present. Hepatic stem/progenitor cells are bipotential stem cells, able to differentiate under appropriate stimuli towards mature hepatocytes and cholangiocytes. The topic is extensively treated in Chap. 62.

The ductules present an intralobular portion of variable length, and a more peripheral extremity within the portal space, where they are coated by a basal membrane and have their own complete wall consisting of three to six cholangiocytes. Their terminal portions join the interlobular bile ducts, whose minor branches have a diameter of 15–20 μm (Fig. 2.3d).

The interlobular bile ducts are coated with a single layer of cubic epithelium, possess a basal membrane and are further coated by the connective tissue of the portal space. As they merge with each other, their size increases and constitute septal ducts with a diameter of more than 100 μm covered by a simple columnar epithelium with basal nuclei. The major ducts are further anastomosed to form intrahepatic bile ducts of a diameter ranging from 1 to 1.5 mm which give rise to the main hepatic ducts. The presence of glandular elements around the larger intrahepatic bile ducts has recently been described and confirmed. These glandular elements consist of a population of intramural mucous glands in direct continuity with the lumen of the bile duct and a component of extramural mixed serum glands formed by branched tubulo-alveolar lobules and secretory ducts that drain into the lumen of the bile duct.

The cholangiocytes represent 35% of the cells in the liver and line the intrahepatic and extrahepatic bile ducts. Cholangiocytes are responsible for the modification of the bile composition during its course along the biliary tree, being able to secrete and absorb water, electrolytes and other organic solutes. At an ultrastructural level, cholangiocytes consist of a prominent Golgi complex, numerous cytoplasmic vesicles and short luminal microvilli. It is likely that between 20 and 40% of the basal biliary flow is produced by the epithelium of the ducts in humans. The secretion is regulated by secretin and somatostatin; in particular, secretin is released from the duodenum following vagal stimulation and the presence of acid, and stimulates the secretion of a bile rich in bicarbonate. The reabsorption concerns water, glucose, glutamate and urate. Bile acids reabsorbed through the biliary epithelium recirculate thanks to the hepatic-biliary shunt via the peribiliary plexus. Cholangiocytes have a sodium dependent apical biliary transporter (ASBT) and are able to collect bile salts from within the lumen of the duct and direct them to the peribiliary circulatory plexus, which via a hepatic-biliary shunt puts them available again for the hepatocytes to stimulate a further secretion of bile [26].

The intrahepatic bile ducts can be classified in humans according to their diameter in large ducts (>800 μm), and then segmental, zonal, sepal, interlobular ducts (15–100 μm) and finally in ductules (<15 μm) [26, 27].

Cholangiocytes are heterogeneous in size and a direct correlation between diameter of the ducts and size of cholangiocytes has been demonstrated. Large cholangiocytes, located in the bile ducts up to the portal spaces, have a reduced nucleus/cytoplasm ratio, while the nucleus/cytoplasm ratio is greater in small cholangiocytes. Large cholangiocytes, about 15 μm in diameter, and small cholangiocytes, about 8 μm in diameter, both express cytokeratin CK19. However, they show differences in the expression of important genes and proteins in the regulation of biliary function. The expression of molecules involved in secretion stimulated by secretin differs in fact along the different segments of the biliary tree [28]. Secretin receptor (SR), cystic fibrosis transmembrane conductance regulator (CFTR) and anion exchanger 2 (AE2) are expressed only by large cholangiocytes and are responsible for most of the biliary fluid secretion that occurs through the activation of a cyclic dependent AMP pathway. On the other hand, in small cholangiocytes the Ca^{2+} activated signaling pathways seem predominant [29]. From a functional point of view, large cyclic AMP cholangiocytes are more susceptible to hepatic injury while small cholangiocytes are more resistant to it [30]. The proliferative response to hepatic injury is different as cholangiocytes of the large ducts proliferate as a result of cholestatic stimuli, such as obstruction or ligation of the main bile duct, or hormonal, such as stimulation by estrogen, and are damaged by administration of toxic substances such as carbon tetrachloride. Following the functional loss of the large ducts, the cholangiocytes of the ductules undergo proliferation and become sensitive to the stimulation of secretin replacing the larger cholangiocytes [31].

2.5 Hepatic Microcirculation

The blood supplying the hepatic lobule and its morphofunctional units is distributed to the hepatic parenchyma by the branches of the portal vein and the hepatic artery. Inside the liver, the portal vein is divided into successive generations of portal branches that form interlobar, segmental and interlobular branches in succession. The further branching of this last generation of portal vessels provide preterminal and terminal branches that distribute the blood inside the sinusoids through venules that leave the portal space and penetrate into the parenchyma to open in the sinusoids. The portal system comprehends about 17–20 branching orders to supply the entire mass of the liver. However, the subdivisions are not strictly dichotomous and therefore the different branches do not have the same number of ramifications, giving a certain degree of irregularity to the general lobular organization.

The geometry of the hepatic sinusoidal network is highly complex (Fig. 2.4a). Its normal morphological organization supports the efficiency of exchanges between blood and hepatocytes, while the rearrangements of the microvascular organization in chronic pathological conditions are related with reduction or loss of liver function [32].

The ramifications of the hepatic artery follow substantially those of the portal system penetrating the organ through it. The termination of the hepatic artery is a peribiliary vascular plexus (Fig. 2.4b) with trophic functions at the level of all intrahepatic bile ducts [33]. Around the larger ducts the peribiliary plexus is disposed in two layers, one of which is more internal located at the sub-epithelial level made up of thin capillaries and another more external, periductular, con-

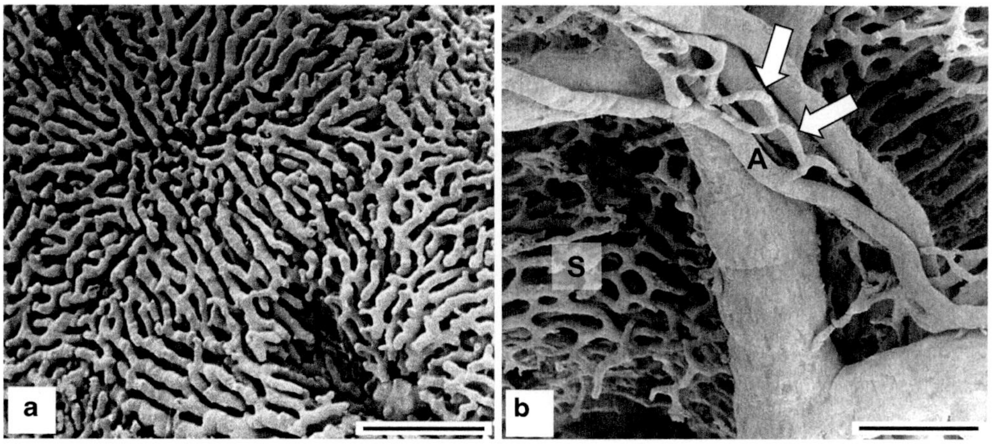

Fig. 2.4 Scanning electronic microscopy vascular corrosion casts of normal liver. (**a**) Lobular microvascular pattern is featured by a network of tortuous sinusoids. (**b**) Separated from the sinusoidal network (S), a peribiliary plexus (arrows) run at the periphery of the lobule along with portal vein branches and furnished by terminal branches of hepatic artery (A). Original magnification: ×30 (**a**), ×60 (**b**). Scale bar: 300 μm (**a**), 150 μm (**b**). ((**a**) From Journal of Anatomy, 2005, vol. 207, p. 107–115; From Gaudio E, Chaberek S, Montella A, Pannarale L, Morini S, Novelli G, Borghese F, Conte D, Ostrowski K. Fractal and Fourier analysis of the hepatic sinusoidal network in normal and cirrhotic rat liver. J Anat. 2005 Aug; 207 (26):107–15. DOI: https://doi.org/10.1111/j.1469-7580.2005.00436.x. **With permission**. (**b**) The Italian Journal of Anatomy and Embryology, 2007, vol. 112, p. 1–12)

sisting of a venous plexus receiving blood from the innermost layer. All smaller terminal bile ducts have only one capillary plexus. The peribiliary plexus drains mainly in the hepatic sinusoids and its embryological development takes place parallel to that of the intrahepatic bile ducts. The peribiliary plexus originates from the hepatic hilum and moves towards the peripheral portions of the liver, reaching full development with complete maturation of the biliary system. In addition to providing trophic support for the bile ducts, the peribiliary plexus is involved in the reabsorption of bile components, including bile acids; these are captured by cholangiocytes and secreted in the interstitium of the portal tract, where are reabsorbed into the capillaries plexus, providing the bases for bilio-hepatic re-circulation. In this way, in case of downstream biliary tract obstruction, the reabsorption of bile solutes can direct them into the systemic circulation to be eliminated by the kidneys.

After having perfused the lobule, the blood penetrates into the central veins placed at the center of the classic hepatic lobule, whose wall presents the sinusoid openings. The centrilobular veins flow together forming, first, the sublobular hepatic veins and then the tributaries of the hepatic veins. The arrangement of the hepatic vein system does not correspond to that of the portal system following alternative routes that intersect the portal system.

Total hepatic blood flow in the adult under resting conditions is between 1500 and 1900 ml/minute, i.e. approximately 25% of the cardiac output. About two-thirds of this is provided by the portal vein while the remaining third by the hepatic artery. The venous flow coming from the portal vein is subject to changes that are determined by the splanchnic blood flow, increasing after meals and decreasing during exercise and sleep. For this reason, a direct external regulation of hepatic blood flow can be mainly obtained through the hepatic artery [34, 35]. On the other hand, the intrinsic regulation of blood flow within the liver is rather complex and the precise mechanism that regulates liver microcirculation remains controversial. Although the portal and hepatic veins and the hepatic arterioles have an endowment of smooth muscle cells in their wall that can provide a certain degree of regulation of the diameter through their contractile capacity, the main site of the regulation of hepatic microcirculation seems to be the sinusoids themselves. The sinusoidal endothelial cells are able to respond to a series of vasoactive substances which, by determining their partial contraction or their relative relaxation, modify the sinusoidal diameter. Even the stellate cells with their long processes that embrace the sinusoidal wall, are able to respond to mediators with a vasoconstricting action. Moreover, it has been observed that reductions in the portal blood flow decrease the blood flow inside the sinusoids with a significant reduction of their diameter [36].

2.6 Microstructure of the Extrahepatic Biliary Tract

Extra hepatic biliary tracts are primarily composed by the right and left hepatic ducts. These, at the level of the liver, get together to form the common hepatic duct; the latter, in turn, joins the cystic duct coming from the gallbladder. From this confluence, the common bile duct originates and, after a long course, ends in the second (descending) duodenal portion. The main biliary tract, therefore, consists of the

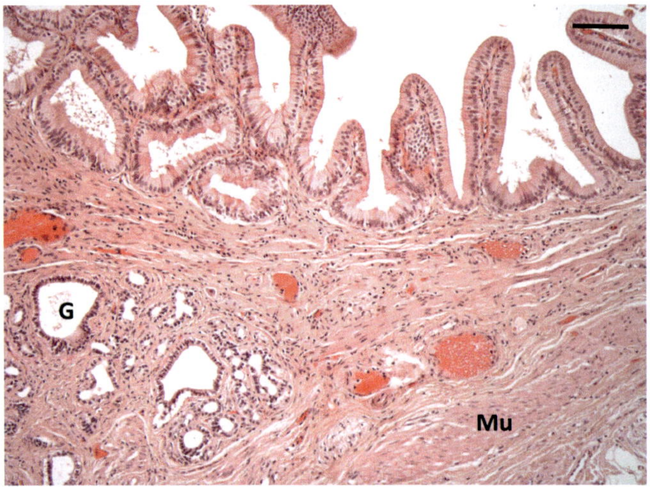

Fig. 2.5 Normal histology of the gallbladder wall with the mucosa raised in folds and the muscle bundles (Mu) close to the lamina propria. Glandular structures (G) are more frequent in the gallbladder neck. Original magnification: ×100. Scale bar: 50 μm

axis formed by the right and left hepatic ducts, the common hepatic duct and the common bile duct. The accessory biliary pathway, which can be considered a diverticulum of the main way, is represented by the gallbladder and the cystic duct. The structure of the right and left hepatic ducts, of the common hepatic duct and of the common bile duct is constituted externally by a fibromuscular layer and internally by a mucosal one. The fibromuscular layer has numerous connective, collagen and elastic fibers, mixed with poor smooth muscle fibers with a plexiform pattern. The mucosa is constituted internally by a simple cylindrical epithelium with two types of cells: cells with microvilli and mucous secretion cells. In the lamina propria of the mucosa, especially in the common bile duct, there are the biliary glands, simple or branched tubule-acinar with mucous secretion, going deep into the fibromuscular layer. The fibromuscular layer progressively increases consistency towards the duodenal opening, where the circular component thickens, helping to form the Oddi's sphincter apparatus and in particular the proper sphincter of the common bile duct. The mucosa of gallbladder is raised in ridges who are anastomosed to each other delimiting irregular recesses and diverticula that give to its internal surface a labyrinthine aspect (Fig. 2.5). The lining epithelium is constituted by a single layer of high cylindrical cells with microvilli and glycocalyx. The cells are tightly joined to each other at the apical level by means of junction complexes that create a barrier impermeable to bile. At the basal level, these cells by means of deep interdigitations delimit an intercellular canalicular space that accounts for the remarkable absorbing activity of these cells. The reabsorption of water and solutes fluids for the concentration of bile, begins at the apical level through pinocytosis and terminate in the blood and lymphatic circulation. The mucosa presents numerous glands with mucous secretion only at the neck of the gallbladder, while in the other portions the mucosa adheres directly to the underlying muscular layer. The smooth muscle cells that compose the muscular layer alternate with elastic fibers and their course is predominantly arranged in a spiral pattern. The serosal layer rests on a thin layer of loose connective tissue more or less richly infiltrated by fat cells. The cystic duct, with a general structure similar to that of the other parts of the biliary tract, presents a characteristic lifting of the mucous membrane internally reinforced by smooth muscle fibers coming from the fibromuscular layer, which forms the Heister's spiral valve involved in the regulation of biliary flow.

2.7 Conclusions

The knowledge of the morphological and ultrastructural bases of the liver complex functions opens perspectives on the further understanding of the mechanisms driving the development and the progression of the liver diseases. Significant developments are expected in the treatment of serious conditions such as fibrosis and liver tumors from going insight into the comprehension of the molecular bases of hepatic zonation and heterogeneity of liver cells and systems.

Self Study

Questions

1. Which statement(s) is/are true?
   (a) The portal lobule is a morpho-functional liver unit obtained by joining different portal tracts each other and placing in the center the centri-lobular vein.
   (b) Glucose metabolism at the hepatocytes level shows heterogeneous localization, with gluconeogenesis occurring mainly in the periportal while glycolysis in the pericentral region.
   (c) The sinusoidal domain of hepatocyte through microvilli has only functions of absorption.
   (d) The fenestrations of sinusoidal endothelial cells are provided with diaphragms; hence the solutes don't pass freely within the space of Disse and selective transcitosis is always required.
   (e) In the normal liver hepatic stellate cells are α-SMA-expressing cells that produce large amount of collagen and matrix proteins.
2. Which statement(s) is/are true?
   (a) The intrahepatic bile ducts have their roots in the bile canaliculi with cholangiocytes lining their wall.
   (b) Secretin receptor (SR), cystic fibrosis transmembrane conductance regulator (CFTR) and anion exchanger

2 (AE2) are expressed both by large and small cholangiocytes and are responsible for most of the biliary fluid secretion that occurs through the Ca^{2+} activated signaling pathways.

(c) The ramifications of the hepatic artery follow substantially those of the portal system penetrating the organ through it and directly terminating into sinusoidal bed.

(d) The main site of the regulation of hepatic microcirculation seems to be represented by sinusoids themselves.

(e) The function of the gallbladder is only to contain the bile waiting for the bile to be pushed into the common bile duct and fed into the duodenum after a meal.

Answer

1. Which statement(s) is/are true?

(a) The portal lobule is a structural unit in which the portal space is at the center and the centrilobular veins in the periphery. The morpho-functional unit with the portal spaces in the periphery and the centrilobular vein in the center is the classic hepatic lobule.

(b) (**CORRECT**) Many aspects of liver physiology and metabolism show a heterogeneous distribution along the porto-central axis of the lobule determining the *so-called* liver zonation. Hepatocytes located in the periportal area are more involved in gluconeogenesis and lipid metabolism whereas those located in the pericentral are the most able to detoxify and are involved in glycolysis.

(c) At the level of the sinusoidal domain of the hepatocyte, the plasma membrane has abundant microvilli and secretion vacuoles that open at their base, responsible for the processes of exocytosis; hence both functions of absorption and secretion are exerted.

(d) The fenestrations of sinusoidal cells are not provided with diaphragms and the basal membrane is lacking on the deep surface of the endothelial cell; hence, the solutes pass freely through the fenestrations within the space of Disse and arrive in contact with the plasma membrane of hepatocytes. However, sinusoidal endothelial cells exhibit also endocytotic capacity and part of the molecules that are taken by endocytosis are modified and reach the hepatocytes by transcytosis.

(e) In the normal liver, the stellate cells are quiescent; they only produce moderate levels of collagen proteins and matrix glycoproteins. The liver damage induces activation of stellate cells affecting aspects such as proliferation, migration, contractility and increased matrix production; a feature of stellate cell activation is the de novo expression of the muscle-smooth isoform of α-actin (α-SMA).

2. Which statement(s) is/are true?

(a) The bile canaliculi run between adjacent hepatocytes that form the canaliculi's wall with their canalicular domain; at the boundary of the portal space the canaliculi continue in the bile ductules, whose wall initially consists partly of hepatocytes and partly of cholangiocytes; then interlobular bile ducts in the portal tract are lined by cholangiocytes.

(b) Secretin receptor (SR), cystic fibrosis transmembrane conductance regulator (CFTR) and anion exchanger 2 (AE2) are expressed only by large cholangiocytes and are responsible for most of the biliary fluid secretion that occurs through the activation of a cyclic dependent AMP pathway; on the other hand, in small cholangiocytes, the Ca^{2+} activated signaling pathways is predominant.

(c) The ramifications of the hepatic artery follow substantially those of the portal system; however, the termination of the hepatic artery is a peribiliary vascular plexus at the level of the intrahepatic bile ducts; then the peribiliary plexus drains mainly in the hepatic sinusoids.

(d) (**CORRECT**) The sinusoidal endothelial cells are able to respond to a series of vasoactive substances which modify the sinusoidal diameter, by determining their partial contraction or their relative relaxation. Even the stellate cells with their long processes that embrace the sinusoidal wall, are able to respond to mediators with a vasoconstricting action.

(e) The reabsorption of water and solutes fluids for the concentration of bile is a fundamental role of the gallbladder; thus, it is not designed only to storing bile.

References

1. Kiernan F. The anatomy and physiology of the liver. Philos Trans R Soc Lond. 1833;123:711–70.
2. Mall FP. A study of the structural unit of the liver. Am J Anat. 1906;5:227–308.
3. Rappaport AM. The structural and functional unit in the human liver (liver acinus). Anat Rec. 1958;130:673–89.
4. Monga SP. β-Catenin signaling and roles in liver homeostasis, injury, and tumorigenesis. Gastroenterology. 2015;148:1294–310. https://doi.org/10.1053/j.gastro.2015.02.056.
5. Benhamouche S, Decaens T, Godard C, Chambrey R, Rickman DS, Moinard C, Vasseur-Cognet M, Kuo CJ, Kahn A, Perret C, Colnot S. Apc tumor suppressor gene is the "zonation-keeper" of mouse liver. Dev Cell. 2006;10:759–70.
6. Matsumoto T, Kawakami M. The unit-concept of hepatic parenchyma—a re-examination based on angioarchitectural studies. Acta Pathol Jpn. 1982;32(Suppl 2):285–314.
7. Hofmann AF. The choleohepatic circulation of unconjugated bile acids: an update. In: Paumgartner G, Stiehl A, Gerok W, editors. Bile acids and the hepatobiliary system: from basic science to

clinical practice. Dordrecht: Kluwer Academic Publishers; 1993. p. 143–60.
8. Ekataksin W, Zou ZZ, Wake K, et al. HMS, hepatic microcirculatory subunits in mammalian species. Intralobular grouping of liver tissue with definition enhanced by drop out sinusoids. In: Wisse E, Knook DL, Wake K, editors. Cells of the hepatic sinusoid. Leiden: Kupffer Cell Foundation; 1995. p. 247–51.
9. Cao H, Krueger EW, McNiven MA. Hepatocytes internalize trophic receptors at large endocytic “Hot Spots”. Hepatology. 2011;54:1819–29. https://doi.org/10.1002/hep.24572.
10. Mazzone A, Tietz P, Jefferson J, Pagano R, LaRusso NF. Isolation and characterization of lipid microdomains from apical and basolateral plasma membranes of rat hepatocytes. Hepatology. 2006;43:287–96.
11. Wang MJ, Chen F, Lau JTY, Hu YP. Hepatocyte polyploidization and its association with pathophysiological processes. Cell Death Dis. 2017;8:e2805. https://doi.org/10.1038/cddis.2017.167.
12. Czaja MJ. Functions of autophagy in hepatic and pancreatic physiology and disease. Gastroenterology. 2011;140:1895–908. https://doi.org/10.1053/j.gastro.2011.04.038.
13. Liu K, Czaja MJ. Regulation of lipid stores and metabolism by lipophagy. Cell Death Differ. 2013;20:3–11. https://doi.org/10.1038/cdd.2012.63.
14. Couvelard A, Scoazec JY, Dauge MC, Bringuier AF, Potet F, Feldmann G. Structural and functional differentiation of sinusoidal endothelial cells during liver organogenesis in humans. Blood. 1996;87:4568–80.
15. Poisson J, Lemoinne S, Boulanger C, Durand F, Moreau R, Valla D, Rautou PE. Liver sinusoidal endothelial cells: physiology and role in liver diseases. J Hepatol. 2017;66:212–27. https://doi.org/10.1016/j.jhep.2016.07.009.
16. Ding BS, Nolan DJ, Butler JM, James D, Babazadeh AO, Rosenwaks Z, Mittal V, Kobayashi H, Shido K, Lyden D, Sato TN, Rabbany SY, Rafii S. Inductive angiocrine signals from sinusoidal endothelium are required for liver regeneration. Nature. 2010;468(7321):310–5. https://doi.org/10.1038/nature09493.
17. Carotti S, Morini S, Corradini SG, Burza MA, Molinaro A, Carpino G, Merli M, De Santis A, Muda AO, Rossi M, Attili AF, Gaudio E. Glial fibrillary acidic protein as an early marker of hepatic stellate cell activation in chronic and posttransplant recurrent hepatitis C. Liver Transpl. 2008;14:806–14. https://doi.org/10.1002/lt.21436.
18. Carotti S, Perrone G, Amato M, Vespasiani Gentilucci U, Righi D, Francesconi M, Pellegrini C, Zalfa F, Zingariello M, Picardi A, Onetti Muda A, Morini S. Reelin expression in human liver of patients with chronic hepatitis C infection. Eur J Histochem. 2017;61:2745. https://doi.org/10.4081/ejh.2017.2745.
19. Friedman SL. Hepatic stellate cells: protean, multifunctional, and enigmatic cells of the liver. Physiol Rev. 2008;88:125–72. https://doi.org/10.1152/physrev.00013.2007.
20. Carpino G, Franchitto A, Morini S, Corradini SG, Merli M, Gaudio E. Activated hepatic stellate cells in liver cirrhosis. A morphologic and morphometrical study. Ital J Anat Embryol. 2004;109(4):225–38.
21. Gomez Perdiguero E, Klapproth K, Schulz C, Busch K, Azzoni E, Crozet L, Garner H, Trouillet C, de Bruijn MF, Geissmann F, Rodewald HR. Tissue-resident macrophages originate from yolk-sac-derived erythro-myeloid progenitors. Nature. 2015;518(7540):547–51. https://doi.org/10.1038/nature13989.
22. Karlmark KR, Weiskirchen R, Zimmermann HW, Gassler N, Ginhoux F, Weber C, Merad M, Luedde T, Trautwein C, Tacke F. Hepatic recruitment of the inflammatory Gr1+ monocyte subset upon liver injury promotes hepatic fibrosis. Hepatology. 2009;50:261–74. https://doi.org/10.1002/hep.22950.
23. González-Domínguez É, Samaniego R, Flores-Sevilla JL, Campos-Campos SF, Gómez-Campos G, Salas A, Campos-Peña V, Corbí ÁL, Sánchez-Mateos P, Sánchez-Torres C. CD163L1 and CLEC5A discriminate subsets of human resident and inflammatory macrophages in vivo. J Leukoc Biol. 2015;98:453–66. https://doi.org/10.1189/jlb.3HI1114-531R.
24. Jenne CN, Kubes P. Immune surveillance by the liver. Nat Immunol. 2013;14:996–1006.
25. Peng H, Wisse E, Tian Z. Liver natural killer cells: subsets and roles in liver immunity. Cell Mol Immunol. 2016;13:328–36. https://doi.org/10.1038/cmi.2015.96.
26. Alvaro D, Mancino MG, Glaser S, Gaudio E, Marzioni M, Francis H, Alpini G. Proliferating cholangiocytes: a neuroendocrine compartment in the diseased liver. Gastroenterology. 2007;132:415–31.
27. Roskams TA, Theise ND, Balabaud C, Bhagat G, Bhathal PS, Bioulac-Sage P, Brunt EM, Crawford JM, Crosby HA, Desmet V, Finegold MJ, Geller SA, Gouw AS, Hytiroglou P, Knisely AS, Kojiro M, Lefkowitch JH, Nakanuma Y, Olynyk JK, Park YN, Portmann B, Saxena R, Scheuer PJ, Strain AJ, Thung SN, Wanless IR, West AB. Nomenclature of the finer branches of the biliary tree: canals, ductules, and ductular reactions in human livers. Hepatology. 2004;39:1739–45.
28. Alpini G, Roberts S, Kuntz SM, Ueno Y, Gubba S, Podila PV, LeSage G, LaRusso NF. Morphological, molecular, and functional heterogeneity of cholangiocytes from normal rat liver. Gastroenterology. 1996;110:1636–43.
29. Maroni L, Haibo B, Ray D, Zhou T, Wan Y, Meng F, Marzioni M, Alpini G. Functional and structural features of cholangiocytes in health and disease. Cell Mol Gastroenterol Hepatol. 2015;1:368–80.
30. Glaser SS, Gaudio E, Rao A, Pierce LM, Onori P, Franchitto A, Francis HL, Dostal DE, Venter JK, DeMorrow S, Mancinelli R, Carpino G, Alvaro D, Kopriva SE, Savage JM, Alpini GD. Morphological and functional heterogeneity of the mouse intrahepatic biliary epithelium. Lab Investig. 2009;89:456–69. https://doi.org/10.1038/labinvest.2009.6.
31. Mancinelli R, Franchitto A, Gaudio E, Onori P, Glaser S, Francis H, Venter J, Demorrow S, Carpino G, Kopriva S, White M, Fava G, Alvaro D, Alpini G. After damage of large bile ducts by gamma-aminobutyric acid, small ducts replenish the biliary tree by amplification of calcium-dependent signaling and de novo acquisition of large cholangiocyte phenotypes. Am J Pathol. 2010;176:1790–800. https://doi.org/10.2353/ajpath.2010.090677.
32. Gaudio E, Chaberek S, Montella A, Pannarale L, Morini S, Novelli G, Borghese F, Conte D, Ostrowski K. Fractal and Fourier analysis of the hepatic sinusoidal network in normal and cirrhotic rat liver. J Anat. 2005;207:107–15.
33. Gaudio E, Onori P, Pannarale L, Alvaro D. Hepatic microcirculation and peribiliary plexus in experimental biliary cirrhosis: a morphological study. Gastroenterology. 1996;111:1118–24.
34. Eipel C, Abshagen K, Vollmar B. Regulation of hepatic blood flow: the hepatic arterial buffer response revisited. World J Gastroenterol. 2010;16:6046–57.
35. Lautt WW. Relationship between hepatic blood flow and overall metabolism: the hepatic arterial buffer response. Fed Proc. 1983;42:1662–6.
36. Reynaert H, Thompson MG, Thomas T, Geerts A. Hepatic stellate cells: role in microcirculation and pathophysiology of portal hypertension. Gut. 2002;50:571–81.

Hepatic Progenitor Cells and Biliary Tree Stem Cells

3

Guido Carpino, Sergio Morini, Simone Carotti, and Eugenio Gaudio

Key Concepts
- Hepatic Progenitor Cells are facultative bipotential stem cells within the human liver.
- Hepatic Progenitor Cells are quiescent in normal conditions and activated in disease states.
- Hepatic Progenitor Cells are activated in human chronic liver diseases, including NAFLD, alcoholic hepatitis, viral hepatitis and cholangiopathies.
- Biliary tree stem/progenitor cells reside within peribiliary glands along the biliary tree and are activated in human primary sclerosing cholangitis, participating in the progression of biliary strictures.
- Hepatic Progenitor Cells and Biliary tree stem/progenitor cells could be a source for clinical programs in regenerative medicine of the liver and pancreas.

3.1 Hepatic Progenitor Cells: Embryology Derivation and Anatomical Location

In the adult human liver, a resident progenitor cell compartment is present in Canals of Hering (Fig. 3.1), which represent the smaller branches of intrahepatic biliary tree [1]. Hepatic stem/progenitor cells (HPCs or HpSCs) are facultative bipotential stem cells, which are capable to differentiate towards mature hepatocytes and cholangiocytes [2]. HPCs have unique phenotype (Figs. 3.1b and 3.2) since they can express stem cell (e.g. Sox9, CD44, CD133, EpCAM, NCAM), mature cholangiocyte (e.g. CK7, CK19), and hepatocyte (Albumin, CK18) markers [3]. The differentiation toward a more mature phenotype is characterized by the progressive acquisition of mature traits and the appearance of cells with an intermediate phenotype, such as intermediate hepatocyte and immature bile ducts: intermediate hepatocytes are cells with a size between progenitor cells and mature hepatocytes, they express biliary cytokeratins (i.e. CK7 with a membranous pattern) and are positive for EpCAM; on the other side, immature bile ducts are characterized by maintenance of stem cell markers and lack of specific mature markers (i.e. CFTR, SRCTR) [4].

The HpSC compartment embryologically derives from the ductal plate; at earlier stages of development, a common precursor for the liver and the bile duct system exists in the forming foregut [3]. In the human embryo, the primitive hepatoblasts around the mesenchyme of portal tracts become immunoreactive for Sox9 and biliary cytokeratins; this layer of cells is termed the ductal plate. The ductal plate undergoes a process of remodeling leading to the formation of intrahepatic bile duct system. At the end of this process, the canals of Hering is the remnant of the ductal plate in pediatric and adult liver and represents the Sox9+ HPC niche [3].

3.2 Role of Hepatic Progenitor Cells and Regeneration Pathways in Human Liver Pathologies

In adult organ, mature parenchymal cells (i.e. hepatocytes and cholangiocytes) have high proliferative capabilities and their proliferation supports the physiological turnover of liver parenchyma. Thus, a significant contribution from stem/progenitor cell niche in liver physiological renewal has

G. Carpino
Department of Motor, Human and Health Sciences, University of Rome "Foro Italico", Rome, Italy

S. Morini (✉) · S. Carotti
Department of Medicine and Surgery, University Campus Bio-Medico of Rome, Rome, Italy
e-mail: s.morini@unicampus.it

E. Gaudio
Department of Anatomical, Histological, Locomotor and Legal Medicine Sciences, Sapienza University, Rome, Italy

F. Radu-Ionita et al. (eds.), *Liver Diseases*, https://doi.org/10.1007/978-3-030-24432-3_3

A

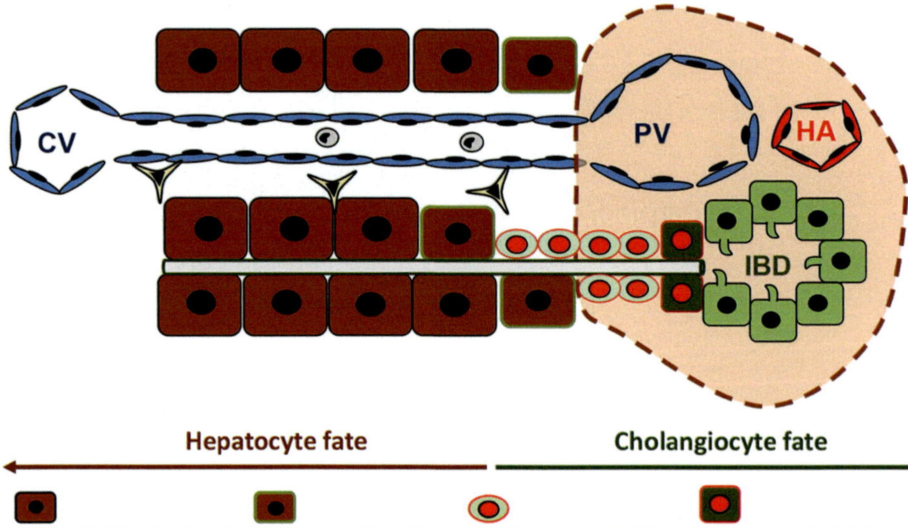

B

	Hepatocytes	Intermediate Hepatocytes	HPC	Immature Cholangiocytes	Cholangiocyte
K7	-	+	+	+	+
K19	-	-	+	+	+
Sox9	-	-	+	+	-
EpCAM	-	+	+	+	-
CD133	-	-	+	-	-
ALB	+	+	+/-	-	-
HNF4α	+	+	-	-	-
PC	-	-	-	-	+
CFTR	-	-	-	-	+
SCTR	-	-	-	-	+

Fig. 3.1 Hepatic Progenitor Cells: anatomical position and progeny. (**a**) The cartoon shows the position of Hepatic Progenitor Cells (HPCs) within bile ductules and Canal of Hering. The HPC progeny comprises intermediate hepatocytes and immature cholangiocytes. *CV* central vein, *PV* portal vein, *HA* hepatic artery, *IBD* interlobular bile ducts. (**b**) The table summarizes key markers which distinguish HPCs from their progeny and mature parenchymal cells. *K* cytokeratin, *EpCAM* epithelial cell adhesion molecule, *ALB* albumin, *HNF* hepatocyte nuclear factor, *PC* primary cilium, *CFTR* cystic fibrosis transmembrane regulator, *SCTR* secretin receptor

been excluded and the normal turnover is ensured by the proliferation of mature cells. However, the activation of a stem/progenitor cell compartment in human livers has been described in disease conditions [3]. Human liver diseases are characterized by a severe and progressive impairment of hepatocyte or cholangiocyte proliferation capabilities [5]. This is due to chronic long-term damage and prolonged cell death or cell cycle arrest induced by specific insults (e.g. oxidative stress in NAFLD) [2, 5]. Thus, end-stage chronic liver pathologies are characterized by an increase of proliferative senescence in hepatocytes and, in parallel, chronic cholangiopathies are characterized by increasing apoptosis and senescence of cholangiocytes [6]. Consequently, HPC compartment can be activated in a variety of human diseases on the basis of specific insults and pathogenesis [2, 5].

The hallmark of HPC activation is represented by the appearance of the so-called ductular reaction (DR) [7]; DR consists of strings of cells with irregular lumina (*reactive ductules*) and composed of cells with a highly variable phenotype [4]. Virtually, the emergence of DRs characterizes all chronic liver diseases and acute (or acute-on-chronic) liver failure [5]. Interestingly, the etiology of the disease strictly influences the variable phenotypes of DR. In chronic biliary diseases (Fig. 3.3), DR is mostly composed of cells expressing biliary, neuroendocrine, and stem cell markers (such as Sox9, CD133) [4, 5]. On the other hand, in liver diseases of non-biliary origin, the cells within reactive ductules show hepatocyte-like features [4, 5].

DR in humans is strongly correlated with the severity of liver damage and is associated with fibrogenesis. In adult and

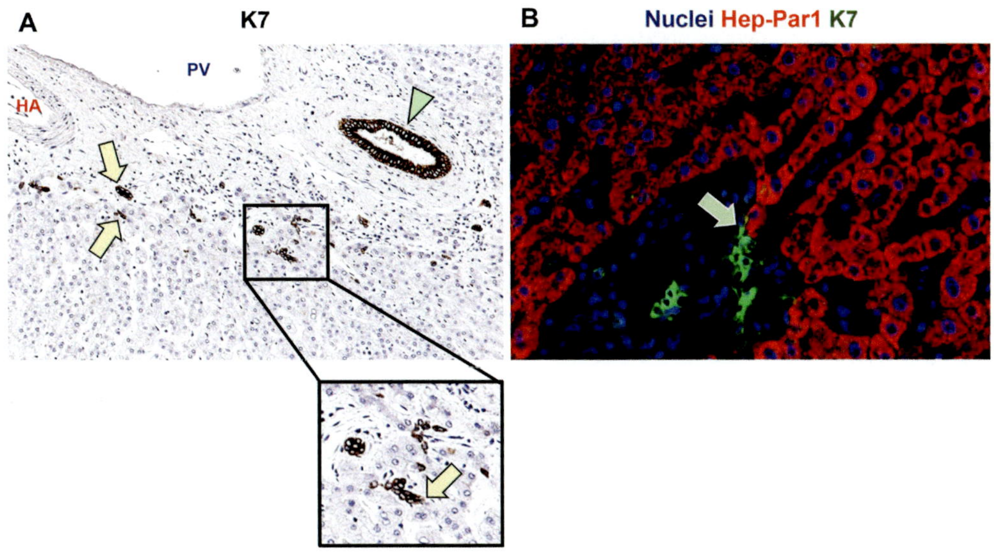

Fig. 3.2 Hepatic progenitor cells in normal human liver. (**a**) Immunohistochemistry for cytokeratin 7 (K7). Single Hepatic Progenitor cells (HPCs) and bile ductules are located at the interface between liver parenchyma and portal tracts (arrow). Area in the box is magnified to show the anatomical continuity between bile ductule and hepatocyte plate (arrow) at the level of Canal of Hering where HPC are located. The green arrowhead individuates an interlobular bile duct within portal tract. *PV* portal vein, *HA* hepatic artery. Original Magnification: ×10. (**b**) Immunofluorescence for K7 and Hep-Par1 (hepatocyte marker). The anatomical continuity between bile ductule and hepatocyte plate at the level of Canal of Hering was indicated by the arrow. Nuclei are displayed in blue color. Original Magnification: ×20

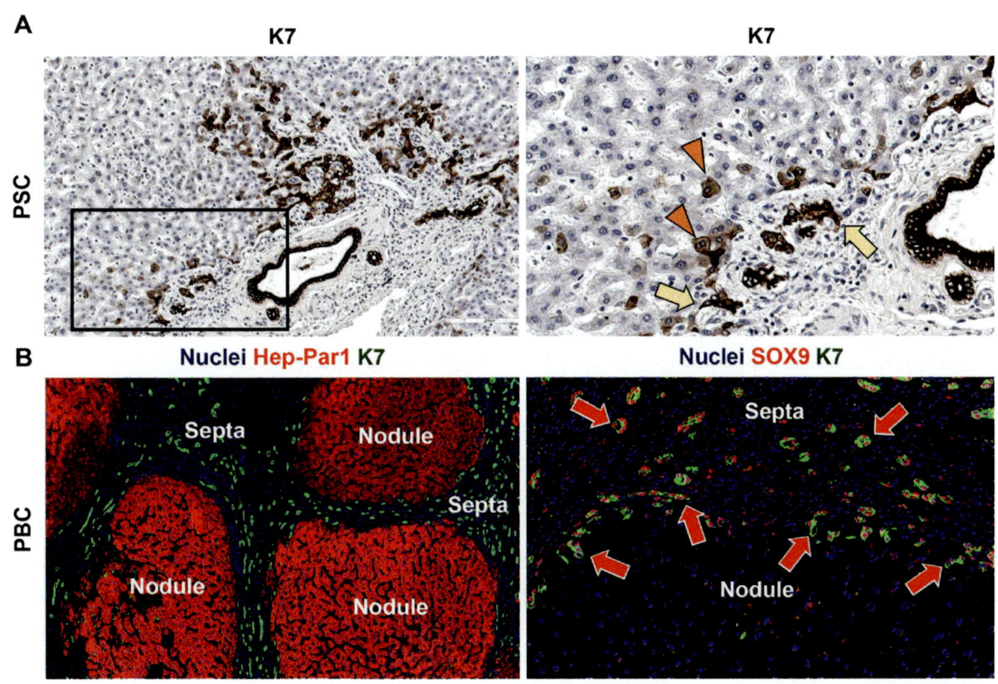

Fig. 3.3 Hepatic progenitor cell and ductular reaction in human cholangiopathies. (**a**) Immunohistochemistry for cytokeratin 7 (K7). In Primary Sclerosing Cholangitis (PSC), a human cholangiopathy, Hepatic Progenitor Cells (HPCs) are activated and reactive ductules appear (Ductular Reaction: DR; arrows in the right image). Area in the box is magnified on the right. In magnified image, intermediate hepatocytes (arrowheads) are recognized for their shape and the K7 patter expression (low expression in cytoplasm with membranous reinforcement). (**b**) Immunofluorescence for K7 and Hep-Par1 (left) or SOX9 (right). In Primary Biliary Cholangitis (PBC), DR is prominent in cirrhotic stage and located in fibrous septa between cirrhotic nodules (green cellular strings) and at the interface with nodules (arrows in right). In PBC, DR is mostly composed by SOX9+ cells (arrows)

pediatric [8] patients with Non Alcoholic Fatty Liver Disease (NAFLD), DR is prominent in steatohepatitis but not in simple steatosis; in this disease, DR appearance and signs of differentiation are associated with hepatocyte cell cycle arrest and apoptosis, and DR extension is correlated with portal fibrosis [8] and portal inflammation [9]; from a clinical point of view, DR extension is predictive of clinical manifestations [10]. Alcoholic hepatitis (AH) represents a disease condition exemplificative for activation of HPC niche in human pathologies [11]. AH is a severe complication of alcoholic liver disease occurring in heavy drinkers and is associated with high morbidity and mortality [11]. Biopsies obtained from AH patients at the diagnosis are characterized by HPC expansion, and the expression of HPC marker individuates a more severe liver damaging and can predict short-term mortality [11].

The inefficient maturation of HPC is a common feature in human liver disease where the inflammatory milieu alters signals within the niche. This is also the case of acute massive hepatocellular necrosis (fulminant hepatitis); in this condition, signs of differentiation toward hepatocytes are minimal in acute liver failure patients [12] and, when present, are a negative prognostic factor; moreover, in acute hepatitis, HPCs predominantly proliferate rather than differentiate [4], and their differentiation starts not earlier than 1 week after the initial liver injury [12]. Interestingly, in acute-on-chronic liver failure, HPC activation and differentiation are more prominent in comparison with acute liver failure and in decompensated cirrhosis [12].

Finally, in chronic cholangiopathies such as Primary Biliary Cholangitis (PBC) and Primary Sclerosing Cholangitis (PSC), HPC activation (Fig. 3.3) is massive and is strongly correlated with fibrosis [13]. Moreover, in PBC, HPC ductular reaction was strongly correlated with clinical prognostic scores [13]. Interestingly, progenitor cell activation differs between PSC and PBC and is characterized by a divergent fate commitment, suggesting a different pathogenetic pathway in the two diseases [3, 13].

Taken together, evidence obtained from human liver disease indicates that the activation of the secondary pathway of HPC takes place in almost all human disease. HPCs are implicated in the formation of cirrhotic nodules and their potential to generate mature cells could be engaged by the inflammatory milieu or un-orchestrated signals within the niche. These alterations can be at the basis of pro-fibrogenic loop leading to the progression of liver fibrosis.

3.3 HPCs Activation Is Driven by a Specialized Niche and Signaling Pathways

Hepatic stem/progenitor cell response is surrounded by a specialized niche [14]. This niche furnishes several key signals driving HPC activity. The cellular components of the niche are represented by portal myofibroblasts (MFs), hepatic stellate cells (HSC), and resident macrophages (i.e. Kupffer cells) [14]. In pathological conditions, HSCs/MFs and macrophages can produce a variety of signals able to drive HPC response. Interestingly, macrophages are a main source of cytokines; among them, TNF-like weak inducer of apoptosis (TWEAK) has a key role in the prominent expansion of undifferentiated HPCs [2]. Beside cytokine production, macrophages can activate canonical Wnt pathway in HPCs triggering their differentiation towards hepatocyte [14]. On the other side, in biliary diseases, fibrogenetic cells secrete Notch ligands (e.g. Jagged1), thus inducing the activation of Notch signaling in HPC niche. Notch signaling pathway has been associated with promotion of biliary differentiation [4]. In sum, Notch and Wnt signaling pathways have a key role in HPC proliferation and response [13, 14]. Furthermore, a key member of HPC niche is represented by the extra-cellular matrix (ECM) composition [15]; both macrophages and myofibroblasts contribute to the precise composition of ECM around HPC through the secretion of ECM elements and by the production of several matrix metalloproteinases and their tissue inhibitors [14]. In this context, the formation of a laminin-rich niche is essential in inducing HPC proliferation and maintaining an undifferentiated phenotype [16]. By contrast, the differentiation into hepatocytes is determined by the leave of the laminin-rich niche [15, 16]. Interestingly, in alcoholic hepatitis, livers predominantly express laminin and, consequently, HPC expansion is inefficient at yielding mature hepatocytes [17].

In addition to signals from the niche, HPC may furnish signals to influence niche composition [14]; thus, HPCs could activate the myofibroblast pools via activation of the Hedgehog (Hh) pathway or by the secretion of Osteopontin and Transforming growth factor-β1 (TGF-β1). In chronic pathological conditions, this cellular cross-talk could be responsible of inducing collagen-I deposition and establishing a pro-fibrogenic loop [1]; the myofibroblast activation follows the expansion of HPC compartment and this process is mediated by the Hedgehog pathway [18].

In general, the expansion of the HPC niche represents an attempt to participate in the regeneration of damaged liver; unfortunately, the persistent injury and the chronic inflammatory milieu activate pro-fibrogenetic pathways and lead to matrix deposition and fibrosis.

3.4 Biliary Tree Stem Cells and Peribiliary Glands

Beside HPCs in bile ductules and Canals of Hering, large intrahepatic bile ducts and extrahepatic biliary tree contain a large population of progenitor/stem cells named biliary tree stem/progenitor cells (BTSCs) [19]. Anatomically, BTSCs reside within peribiliary glands, glandular elements located along the biliary tree [19]; embryologically, BTSCs are considered the remnant in the adult organs of the common biliopancreatic progenitors of the ventral endoderm in the primitive duodenum [3]. BTSCs can be easily isolated from adult or fetal organs, showed clonal expansion capability and are multipotent since they can differentiate toward hepatocytes, cholangiocytes and pancreatic endocrine cells [19]. BTSCs and peribiliary glands are involved in the pathogenesis of human biliary disease; in liver transplantation procedures, ischemia-reperfusion injury of the PBGs has been associated with the loss of epithelial cells and the development of non-anastomotic biliary strictures [1, 3]. Furthermore, BTSCs are activated to proliferate in primary sclerosing cholangitis and have a key role in progression of biliary strictures. Finally, they have been suggested as a cell of origin for cholangiocarcinoma [1, 14].

3.5 Stem Cells in Regenerative Medicine for Liver Diseases

In the field of liver diseases, orthotopic liver transplantation (OLT) represents the only curative treatment for acute liver failure and end-stage chronic liver disease [20]. Unfortunately, a major point is represented by the severe shortage of organ donors for OLT [21]. This has opened the need of innovative therapeutic strategies based on cell therapy as a possible option to support liver function. Cell therapies with mature hepatocytes have demonstrated that hepatocyte transplantation achieve only transient effects and hepatocyte cell function declines few months after cell transplantation. Moreover, a main obstacle to the clinical application of hepatocyte transplantation resides in sourcing of cells; given the competition with OLT procedures, current sources of tissue for hepatocyte isolation are limited and of poor quality, such as marginal organs unsuitable for OLT, livers that have undergone aggressive therapies, or surrounding parenchyma from tumor resection [21].

Thus, the identification of sustainable and readily available cell sources is required [20]. In keeping, the possibility of reprogramming adult somatic cells attracted attention for the possibility to generate mature hepatocyte readily available for transplantation. Recently, induced hepatocytes (iHeps) have been directly reprogrammed from fibroblasts by forcing the expression of specific hepatic transcription factors [22]. Unfortunately, the application of reprogrammed cells in clinics have major concern regarding the possible uncontrolled tumorigenic expansion within the recipient [20]. This aspect is crucial in pediatric patients for the long-life expectancy of recipient and in chronic liver diseases characterized by an "adverse" inflammatory niche which can favor mutations and tumorigenesis [20].

Besides cell reprogramming, the use of hepatic stem/progenitor cells isolated from adult or fetal human organs has been proposed for the regenerative medicine of the liver and pancreas [21]. HPCs and BTSCs have the key advantage to require minimal manipulation with respect to reprogrammed cells and they can be easily isolate from human organs by immune-selection for specific surface antigens such as Epithelial Cell Adhesion Molecule (EpCAM) and single Leucine-rich repeat-containing G-protein coupled receptor 5 (Lgr5). Isolated cells can be expanded in vitro and are able to differentiate into functional hepatocytes and β-pancreatic cells in vitro and in vivo [3, 23]. Long-term expansion of adult bile duct-derived bipotent progenitor cells has been achieved and indicated a high stability at the chromosome and structural level and the single base changes occur at very low rates and have null tumorigenic potential [23]. However, few clinical trials were started with the use of human HPCs and, to date, the only completed was conducted at the Liver Institute in Hyderabad (India) [24]. Furthermore, a preliminary clinical report indicated the feasibility and safety of BTSC transplantation into the liver of patients with end-stage chronic liver disease [25]. In general, the use of determined stem cells has the advantage of lower manipulation in comparison with reprogrammed cells and no need of immunosuppression in comparison with mature cells.

3.6 Conclusions

The liver and the extrahepatic biliary tree contain distinct niches of stem/progenitor cells. HPCs and BTSCs are quiescent and are activated in human liver and biliary pathologies, participating in tissue regeneration after massive acute and chronic injuries. These cells can be easily isolated from adult or fetal human livers and could represent a possible source for cell therapy program for liver and pancreatic diseases.

Self Study

Questions

1. Which statement is true?
   (a) Hepatic Progenitor Cells are located in Bile Canaliculi.
   (b) Hepatic Progenitor Cells are pluripotent stem cells.
   (c) Hepatic Progenitor Cells are facultative stem cells.
   (d) Hepatic Progenitor Cells do not express biliary markers.
2. Which statement/statements is/are true?
   (a) Hepatic Progenitor Cells participate in hepatocyte physiological turnover.

(b) Hepatic Progenitor Cells are activated in human cholangiopathies.
(c) Hepatic Progenitor Cells are quiescent in Non-alcoholic Fatty Liver Diseases.
(d) Ductular Reaction represents the histological hallmark of hepatocyte apoptosis

Answers

1. Which statement is true?
   (a) False. Hepatic Progenitor Cells are located in bile ductules and Canal of Hering. Bile Canaliculi are comprised between adjacent hepatocytes
   (b) False. Hepatic Progenitor Cells are bipotential.
   (c) **True**. Hepatic Progenitor Cells are quiescent in normal conditions and activated in pathological conditions.
   (d) False. Hepatic Progenitor Cells express biliary cytokeratins (7 and 19).
2. Which statement is true?
   (a) False. Hepatocytes have high proliferative potentialities and their proliferation supports parenchymal physiological turnover.
   (b) **True**. Both in primary biliary and primary sclerosing cholangitis Hepatic Progenitor Cells are activated to support biliary and hepatocyte regeneration in late stages.
   (c) False. Hepatic Progenitor Cell activation has been described in Non-alcoholic Fatty liver Disease both in adult and in pediatric patients. This activation was associated with portal fibrogenesis and with steatohepatitis.
   (d) False. Ductular Reaction represents the histological hallmark of Hepatic Progenitor Cell activation.

References

1. Alvaro D, Gaudio E. Liver capsule: biliary tree stem cell subpopulations. Hepatology. 2016;64:644.
2. Carpino G, Renzi A, Franchitto A, Cardinale V, Onori P, Reid L, Alvaro D, Gaudio E. Stem/progenitor cell niches involved in hepatic and biliary regeneration. Stem Cells Int. 2016;2016:3658013.
3. Lanzoni G, Cardinale V, Carpino G. The hepatic, biliary, and pancreatic network of stem/progenitor cell niches in humans: a new reference frame for disease and regeneration. Hepatology. 2016;64:277–86.
4. Spee B, Carpino G, Schotanus BA, Katoonizadeh A, Vander Borght S, Gaudio E, Roskams T. Characterisation of the liver progenitor cell niche in liver diseases: potential involvement of Wnt and Notch signalling. Gut. 2010;59:247–57.
5. Gouw AS, Clouston AD, Theise ND. Ductular reactions in human liver: diversity at the interface. Hepatology. 2011;54:1853–63.
6. Nakanuma Y, Sasaki M, Harada K. Autophagy and senescence in fibrosing cholangiopathies. J Hepatol. 2015;62:934–45.
7. Williams MJ, Clouston AD, Forbes SJ. Links between hepatic fibrosis, ductular reaction, and progenitor cell expansion. Gastroenterology. 2014;146:349–56.
8. Nobili V, Carpino G, Alisi A, Franchitto A, Alpini G, De Vito R, Onori P, Alvaro D, Gaudio E. Hepatic progenitor cells activation, fibrosis and adipokines production in pediatric nonalcoholic fatty liver disease. Hepatology. 2012;56:2142–53.
9. Gadd VL, Skoien R, Powell EE, Fagan KJ, Winterford C, Horsfall L, Irvine K, Clouston AD. The portal inflammatory infiltrate and ductular reaction in human nonalcoholic fatty liver disease. Hepatology. 2014;59:1393–405.
10. Nobili V, Alisi A, Cutrera R, Carpino G, De Stefanis C, D'Oria V, De Vito R, Cucchiara S, Gaudio E, Musso G. Altered gut-liver axis and hepatic adiponectin expression in OSAS: novel mediators of liver injury in paediatric non-alcoholic fatty liver. Thorax. 2015;70:769–81.
11. Sancho-Bru P, Altamirano J, Rodrigo-Torres D, Coll M, Millan C, Jose Lozano J, Miquel R, Arroyo V, Caballeria J, Gines P, et al. Liver progenitor cell markers correlate with liver damage and predict short-term mortality in patients with alcoholic hepatitis. Hepatology. 2012;55:1931–41.
12. Rastogi A, Maiwall R, Bihari C, Trehanpati N, Pamecha V, Sarin SK. Two-tier regenerative response in liver failure in humans. Virchows Arch. 2014;464:565–73.
13. Carpino G, Cardinale V, Folseraas T, Overi D, Floreani A, Franchitto A, Onori P, Cazzagon N, Berloco PB, Karlsen TH, et al. Hepatic stem/progenitor cell activation differs between primary sclerosing and primary biliary cholangitis. Am J Pathol. 2018;188:627–39.
14. Boulter L, Lu WY, Forbes SJ. Differentiation of progenitors in the liver: a matter of local choice. J Clin Invest. 2013;123:1867–73.
15. Lorenzini S, Bird TG, Boulter L, Bellamy C, Samuel K, Aucott R, Clayton E, Andreone P, Bernardi M, Golding M, et al. Characterisation of a stereotypical cellular and extracellular adult liver progenitor cell niche in rodents and diseased human liver. Gut. 2010;59:645–54.
16. Kallis YN, Robson AJ, Fallowfield JA, Thomas HC, Alison MR, Wright NA, Goldin RD, Iredale JP, Forbes SJ. Remodelling of extracellular matrix is a requirement for the hepatic progenitor cell response. Gut. 2011;60:525–33.
17. Dubuquoy L, Louvet A, Lassailly G, Truant S, Boleslawski E, Artru F, Maggiotto F, Gantier E, Buob D, Leteurtre E, et al. Progenitor cell expansion and impaired hepatocyte regeneration in explanted livers from alcoholic hepatitis. Gut. 2015;64(12):1949–60.
18. Grzelak CA, Martelotto LG, Sigglekow ND, Patkunanathan B, Ajami K, Calabro SR, Dwyer BJ, Tirnitz-Parker JE, Watkins DN, Warner FJ, et al. The intrahepatic signalling niche of hedgehog is defined by primary cilia positive cells during chronic liver injury. J Hepatol. 2014;60:143–51.
19. Cardinale V, Wang Y, Carpino G, Cui CB, Gatto M, Rossi M, Bartolomeo Berloco P, Cantafora A, Wauthier E, Furth ME, et al. Multipotent stem/progenitor cells in human biliary tree give rise to hepatocytes, cholangiocytes, and pancreatic islets. Hepatology. 2011;54:2159–72.
20. Forbes SJ, Gupta S, Dhawan A. Cell therapy for liver disease: from liver transplantation to cell factory. J Hepatol. 2015;62:S157–69.
21. Lanzoni G, Oikawa T, Wang Y, Cui CB, Carpino G, Cardinale V, Gerber D, Gabriel M, Dominguez-Bendala J, Furth ME, et al. Concise review: clinical programs of stem cell therapies for liver and pancreas. Stem Cells. 2013;31:2047–60.
22. Rezvani M, Grimm AA, Willenbring H. Assessing the therapeutic potential of lab-made hepatocytes. Hepatology. 2016;64:287–94.
23. Huch M, Gehart H, van Boxtel R, Hamer K, Blokzijl F, Verstegen MM, Ellis E, van Wenum M, Fuchs SA, de Ligt J, et al. Long-term culture of genome-stable bipotent stem cells from adult human liver. Cell. 2015;160:299–312.

24. Khan AA, Shaik MV, Parveen N, Rajendraprasad A, Aleem MA, Habeeb MA, Srinivas G, Raj TA, Tiwari SK, Kumaresan K, et al. Human fetal liver-derived stem cell transplantation as supportive modality in the management of end-stage decompensated liver cirrhosis. Cell Transplant. 2010;19:409–18.

25. Cardinale V, Carpino G, Gentile R, Napoletano C, Rahimi H, Franchitto A, Semeraro R, Nuti M, Onori P, Berloco PB, et al. Transplantation of human fetal biliary tree stem/progenitor cells into two patients with advanced liver cirrhosis. BMC Gastroenterol. 2014;14:204.

Hepatocellular Death: Apoptosis, Autophagy, Necrosis and Necroptosis

4

Florentina Radu-Ionita, Ecaterina Bontas, and Ion C. Tintoiu

Abbreviations

AIF	Apoptosis-inducing factor
ALD	Alcoholic liver disease
AP-1	Activator protein-1
AP-1	The activation protein-1
APAF-1	Apoptosis protease-activating factor-1
Atg	Autophagy-related proteins
ATP	Adenosine triphosphate
ATP	Deoxyadenosine triphosphate
Bcl-2	(B-cell lymphoma-2)
c-FLIP	Cellular FLICE-like inhibitory protein
DAMPs	Damage-associated molecular patterns
DISC	The death-inducing signaling complex
FADD	Fas-associated protein with a death domain
FasL	Fas Ligand
HMGB1	Protein (high-mobility group box-1) or HMG-1 (high—mobility group)1
Hsc70	The chaperone heat shock cognate 70
IAP	Inhibitors of apoptotic proteins
IKK complex	I-kappa B kinase complex
JNK	c-Jun N-terminal kinase
LAMP2A	Lysosome-associated membrane protein 2A
LUBAC	Linear ubiquitin chain assembly complex
MAPK	Mitogen-activated protein kinase
MAPK	Mitogen-activated protein kinases
MLKL	Mixed-lineage kinase domain-like
MOMP	Mitochondrial outer membrane permeabilization
MOMP	Mitochondrial outer membrane permeabilization
mTOR kinase	The mammalian target of rapamycin kinase
NAFLD	Nonalcoholic fatty liver disease
NASH	Non-alcoholic steatohepatitis
NF-KB	Transcription factor nuclear factor
PCD	Programmed cell death
PI3K	Class III phosphatidyl inositol-3 kinase
PRRs	The pathogen recognition receptors
PS	Phosphatidylserine
RIPK	Receptor interacting protein kinase or receptor interacting serine-threonine kinase
RIPs	Receptor interacting proteins
ROS	Reactive oxygen species
Smac	Second activator of mitochondrial apoptosis
TFEB	Transcription factor EB
TGF-β1	Transforming growth factor
TNF	Tumor necrosis factor
TNFR1	TNF receptor type 1
TNFR2	TNF receptor type
TNF-α	Tumor necrosis factor
TRADD	TNF receptor associated death domain protein
TRAF2	TNF receptor-associated factor 2
TRAIL	TNF related apoptosis-inducing ligand
TRAIL	TNF-released apoptosis-inducing ligand
TRAIL-R	TNF-related apoptosis-inducing ligand receptor
UTP	Uridine triphosphate

F. Radu-Ionita
Department of Gastroenterology, Central Military Emergency University Hospital "Dr. Carol Davila", Bucharest, Romania

Internal Medicine Department, Faculty of Medicine, "Titu Maiorescu" University, Bucharest, Romania

E. Bontas (✉)
"Prof. C.C. Iliescu" Emergency Institute for Cardiovascular Diseases, Bucharest, Romania

I. C. Tintoiu
Internal Medicine Department, Faculty of Medicine, "Titu Maiorescu" University, Bucharest, Romania

Cardiology Department, "Carol Davila" Central Military Emergency University Hospital, Bucharest, Romania

F. Radu-Ionita et al. (eds.), *Liver Diseases*, https://doi.org/10.1007/978-3-030-24432-3_4

Key Concepts

- Cell death is classified into three morphotypes apoptosis, autophagy and necrosis.
- Apoptosis and necrosis represent the two major modes of hepatocyte death, and apoptosis assures tissue homeostasis by the physiologic removal of damaged hepatocytes.
- Hepatocyte autophagy is a protective pathway as survival mechanism in starvation.
- Cytoprotective autophagy inhibits apoptosis, whereas cytotoxic autophagy promotes apoptosis.
- Signaling death pathways of liver might carry significant information for a correct treatment of hepatic disorders.

4.1 Introduction

Hepatic tissue homeostasis is a based on the equilibrium between cell growth and cell death [1]. According to the known evidence, a number of hepatocellular death mechanisms have been observed including apoptosis, autophagy, necrosis and necroptosis. Without a doubt, hepatocellular death exists in all types of human liver disease such as viral, metabolic, autoimmune and toxic conditions [2]. Consistent with this, hepatocyte death is the hallmark of liver disease development such as inflammation, fibrosis, cirrhosis, and hepatocellular carcinoma.

Presently, the recommendations of the Nomenclature Committee on Cell Death 2018 are grading cell death into three morphotypes (Fig. 4.1, Table 4.1) [3]:

1. Type I cell death (***apoptosis***) is characterized by plasma membrane blebbing, reduction of cytoplasma, pyknosis or karyopyknosis (irreversible chromatin condensation) followed by karyorrhexis (nuclear fragmentation), and formation of "apoptotic bodies" (small vesicles) that are broke down inside of lysosomes;
2. Type II cell death (***autophagy***) shows broad "cytoplasmic vacuolization" removed in same way inside of lysosomes; and
3. Type III cell death (***necrosis***) without characteristics of type I or II cell death.

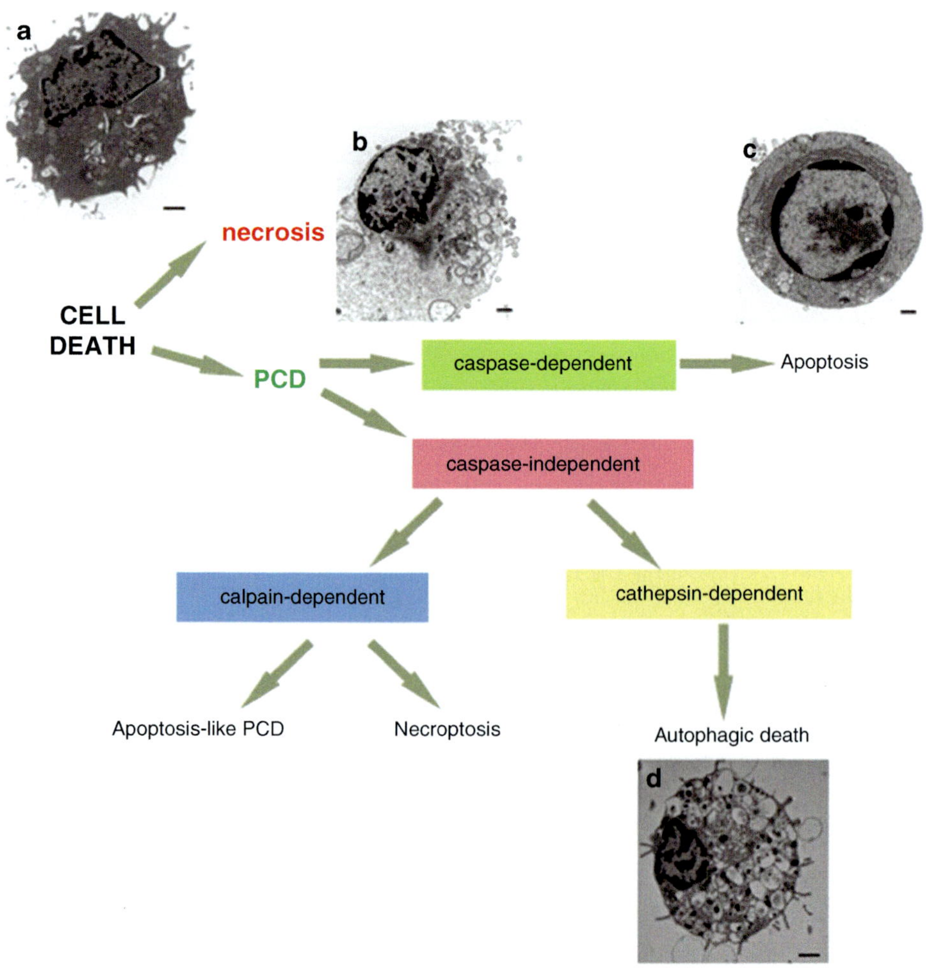

Fig. 4.1 Types of cell death and their morphological hallmarks. Diagrammatic classification of different types of cell death. PCD: programmed cell death. Morphological features of (**a**) a healthy cell, (**b**) a necrotic cell, (**c**) an apoptotic cell and (**d**) an autophagic cell. [(Electron micrograph pictures adapted from ref. [4]. Scale bar: 1 mm.) [5]. With permission]

Table 4.1 Cell death mechanisms. (Adapted from [3, 6, 7])

Cell death	Characteristics of process
Apoptosis	Cellular shrinkage, caspase-3 activation, cytochrome c release, nuclear/nucleus condensation, DNA fragmentation, blebbing of cytoplasm/membrane, secretion of cellular components; main pathway caspase -3,-6, -7
Autophagy	Nucleus condensation in late stage, Atgs recruit, autophagic vesicles, phagolysosome fusion, autophagosomes, chromatin condensation, autolysosomes, main pathway mTOR, Atg
Necrosis/ oncosis	Mild DNA damage, cell swelling, membrane blebbing, release of cellular components, main pathway ROS
Necroptosis	Normal nucleus, cell swelling, membrane rupture with cellular components release, main pathway is RIP/RIP3
Pyroptosis	Nucleus condensation, DNA fragmentation, cell swelling, membrane pores, release of cellular components, inflammasome, caspase-1 activation, pore formation, cell swelling and lysis; main pathway caspase -1
Apoptosis/ autophagy interrelation	Energy metabolism change, membrane asymmetry, PS exposure, membrane blebbing, small sealed membrane vesicles

DNA deoxyribonucleic acid, *RIP1/RIP3* receptor interacting proteins, *Atgs* autophagy-related proteins, *mTOR kinase* the mammalian target of rapamycin kinase, *PS* phospholipid phosphatidylserine, *ROS* reactive oxygen production

Generally, apoptosis, necroptosis, and necrosis are a feature of acute and chronic liver diseases. Obviously, there is no separation between apoptosis, necrosis, and necroptosis in vivo. Moreover, all together may evolve in same time in acute and chronic liver disease [2]. However, all above mentioned death mechanisms can support inflammation with activation of liver stellate cells (HSC) and further proliferation of hepatocytes. Cell death is a constructive mechanism in acute liver disease. Subsequently, blocking of cell death pathways may be associated with no development of chronic liver disease. The process by which phagocytic cells engulf the apoptotic bodies with the removal of cellular debris is termed efferocytosis [8]. In this regard, *efferocytosis* by Kupffer cells (liver macrophages) can lead to their activation with death ligands exhibition and liver injury. Efferocytes assure removal of apoptotic cells and necrotic cells [8]. The absence of apoptotic bodies engulfing is termed "defective efferocytosis" and causes further necrosis. Ferroptosis is an intracellular iron-dependent cell death [9]. As a side note, the extremely difficult molecular biology and genetic taxonomy differentiates a gene from a protein by a general agreement [10, 11]. A human gene is described in italic uppercase letters (e.g., *GATA4*), while the protein obtained from this gene is described in nonitalic uppercase letters (e.g., GATA4) [10, 11].

4.2 Apoptosis

Apoptosis is the physiologically exclusion of unnecessary cells (impaired cells, senescent cells) through liver development or mature liver [12]. It is a vital process that runs liver growth and regeneration, along with the hepatic tissue homeostasis through normal cell turnover. Nonetheless, apoptosis supports liver regeneration by producing of growth signals that increase the development of progenitor cells. Lastly, apoptosis is a final step during genetically programmed cell death (PCD) supporting adult tissue homeostasis, morphogenesis and removal of senescent cells [6].

As expected, there is an increased apoptosis in cholestasis, alcoholic hepatitis, non-alcoholic steatohepatitis, autoimmune hepatitis, viral hepatitis, fulminate hepatic failure, ischemia-reperfusion injury, fibrosis and cirrhosis [1, 13]. In case of hepatitis, apoptosis is the major cell death [14], being a cytoprotective mechanism in clearance from infections. Importantly, it occurs mainly in perivenous acinar area of hepatocytes [1].

So, apoptotic cells are smaller than normal hepatocytes [8]. **Morphologically**, hepatocyte apoptosis is defined by a smaller spheric cell, reduction of cell or "cell shrinkage", plasma membrane blebbing, chromatin condensation (pyknosis or small pyknotic nucleus), nuclear fragmentation (karyorrhexis), DNA splitting, mitochondrial permeabilization, cytoplasmic condensation (hypereosinophilic cytoplasm), followed by cell fragmentation into apoptotic bodies that are removed within lysosomes [12, 15]. Specifically, the apoptotic bodies present "nuclear fragments" or "micronuclei" [16]. Typically, these apoptotic bodies exhibit on the external/outer cell membrane phospholipid phosphatidylserine (PS) [8]. By definition, apoptotic bodies are fragments of apoptotic cells resulting from caspase 3 activation which have a pyknotic nuclear fragment with/without cytoplasm [15].

In fact, the elimination of apoptotic bodies is quickly being induced by PS that covers apoptotic bodies. Liver macrophages (i.e. Kupffer cells, liver stellate cells) engulf apoptotic bodies with no discharge of cellular components and therefore with **reduced inflammation** [2, 16]. Also, the engulfment of apoptotic bodies leads to exhibition of death ligands: (1) TNF-α; (2) TRAIL (TNF-released apoptosis-inducing ligand); (3) FasL (Fas Ligand) which further trigger "death receptor-mediated apoptosis" [16]. In chronic liver injury, hepatic stellate cells become activated with apoptotic bodies engulfment that leads to secretion of profibrogenic cytokines (TGF-β1 or Transforming growth factor, collagen type 1). Initially, liver stellate cells transform into myofibroblasts when phagocytose apoptotic bodies. These myofibroblasts secrete TGF-β1 and collagen type 1 with fibrosis and cirrhosis.

It should be stressed that in apoptosis, apoptotic bodies discharge decreased proinflammatory mediators (i.e. ATP—adenosine triphosphate, UTP or uridine triphosphate, adenosine, fractalkaline, and lysophosphatidyl choline, chemokines, sphingosine-1-phosphate) to be detected by phagocytes. Specifically, the discharge of nucleotides (UTP, ATP) modulate the P2Y2 purinergic receptors from myofibroblasts with increased collagen secretion [16]. The process by which phagocytic cells engulf the apoptotic bodies with the removal of the cellular debris by the process termed efferocytosis. In this regard, efferocytosis by Kupffer cells (liver macrophages) can lead to their activation with death ligands exhibition and liver injury.

Biochemically, liver apoptosis is characterized by exposing of PS on outer leaflet of the plasma membrane bilayer, increased permeability of mitochondrial membrane permeability, and caspases activation [12]. Caspases are intracellular enzymes (cysteine-dependent aspartate or cysteinyl aspartate-specific proteases) that undergo proteolytic cleavage [1]. *Initiator caspases* are caspases 2, 8, 9, and 10. Caspases 8 and 10 modulate death receptor-mediated apoptosis whereas mitochondrial dysfunction is followed by caspase 9-induced apoptosis. *Effector or executioner caspases* are represented by caspases 3, 7, and 6.

Caspase-independent apoptosis comprises (see Fig. 4.1) (1) mitochondrial malfunction caused by ROS; (2) mitochondrial release of AIF (apoptosis-inducing factor) into cytoplasm where activates DNA splitting with chromatin condensation; and (3) TNFα (tumor necrosis factor) inhibits caspases [13].

Apoptosis has three pathways (1) extrinsic apoptosis or death receptors pathway, (2) intrinsic apoptosis or mitochondrial pathway; and (3) perforin/granzyme pathway (Fig. 4.2) [15].

All forms of apoptosis present integrity of plasma membrane until late in the process [15] with no cellular components release into cytoplasm therefore **no inflammation**. The **reduced inflammatory response** of apoptosis is caused by *decreased* discharge of DAMPs (Damage-associated molecular patterns) and rapid exclusion of apoptotic bodies [2]. DAMPs induces the **apoptotic** inflammation from chronic liver diseases (i.e. ALD, NAFLD, viral hepatitis). However, the mainly discharge of DAMPs appears in necrosis and necroptosis.

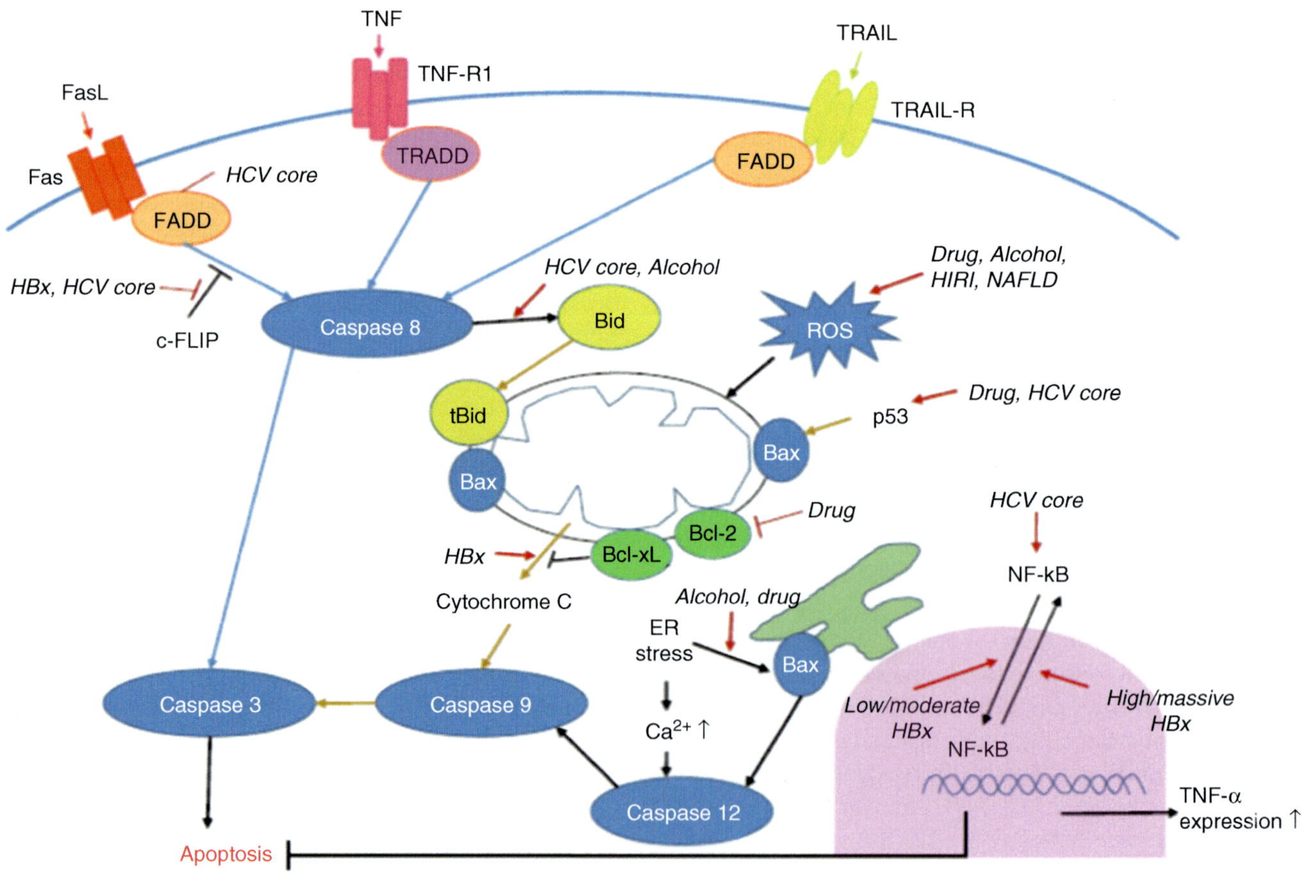

Fig. 4.2 The schematic diagram of apoptotic pathways in hepatocytes. Blue lines indicate extrinsic pathways, whereas light brown lines indicate intrinsic pathways. The influence of virus infection, alcohol, fat, ischemia reperfusion, and drug on hepatocyte apoptosis is also indicated by italics and red arrows [13].

1. **Extrinsic apoptosis or death receptors pathway**. Presently, the Nomenclature Committee on Cell Death 2018 defines **extrinsic apoptosis** as a form of regulated cell death induced or triggered by " *perturbations of the extracellular microenvironment that are detected by plasma membrane receptors, propagated by **caspase-8** (with the optional involvement of MOMP), and precipitated by executioner caspases, mainly caspase-3*" [3]. Briefly, **extrinsic apoptosis** comprises death receptors, pro-apoptotic ligands, transduction of intracellular signals, adaptor proteins, DISC (the death-inducing signaling complex) formation, and initiation of caspases through **caspase 8** [15].

Extrinsic apoptosis is based on the triggering of death transmembrane receptors (TNF receptor gene superfamily) [15]. The **death receptors** are universally distributed in all liver and belongs to a family of cytokines receptors named the TNF/nerve growth factor (NGF) receptor family mainly type I transmembrane proteins [16]. Specifically, death receptors are "cysteine-rich extracellular domain and intracellular cytosol death domain" [17].

Collectively, *death receptors* and their corresponding *ligands* are represented by (1) *Fas* (CD95/APO1/DR2) with its cognate ligand FasL (CD95L); (2) *TNFR1* (or TNF receptor type 1, p55/CD120a/DR1) with its cognate ligand TNF; (3) *TNFR2* (TNF receptor type 2, p75/80, CD120b); (4) *TRAIL-R1* (death receptor 4, DR4); (5) *TRAIL-R2* (death receptor 5-DR5/APO-2/KILLER/TRAILCK2) and its cognate ligand TRAIL or Apo2L; and (6) *DR6* with its cognate ligand TRADD (TNF receptor associated death domain protein) [3, 16, 17]. The death receptors TRAIL-R (TNF-related apoptosis-inducing ligand receptor), TRAIL-R1 and TRAIL-R2 are highly expressed in cirrhosis, acute HBV hepatitis, and chronic HCV hepatitis. Subsequently, death receptors attach special ligands or cognate ligands TNF family that are mainly type II transmembrane proteins. The ligands of these death receptors are Fas ligand or FasL/CD95L, TNF (tumor necrosis factor) family or TNF-α, and TRAIL (TNF related apoptosis-inducing ligand), and are mostly displayed by immune system cells that further remove impaired hepatocytes [12]. These ligands initiate the **extrinsic pathways** of liver apoptosis "that overlap a part of intrinsic/mitochondrial pathway by the cleavage and activation of Bid" [16].

As well, the membrane associated **Fas receptors** have a soluble form (sFas) produced by alternative mRNA splicing. Both sFas and sFasL are non-invasive serum biomarkers of cell death. For the instance, studies proven that sFasL are boosted in hepatitis, acute liver failure, sepsis. sFas levels are increased in NASH and steatosis [7]. Hence, **Fas/FasL signaling pathway** is linked with several disorders such as acute fulminant hepatitis, alcoholic liver disease (ALD), Wilson's disease, chronic viral hepatitis, fatty liver/steatosis caused by obesity [7].

Characteristically, **Fas signaling** triggers apoptosis via caspase-8 complexed with FADD. Both Fas ligand and TNF elicit cell death by using a common signal transduction with final activation of caspase-8 and effector caspases. RIP1 (receptor interacting proteins) characterizes the TNF pathway and it is a signaling molecule in cytotoxic/cytoprotective pathways. Activation of TNF receptor is a feature of many cellular reactions such as survival, inflammation, proliferation, and cell death.

A keynote factor, **TNF-α** is a pleiotropic monocyte-derived cytokine. In normal hepatocytes, TNFα is not able to produce liver injury. It is related with the outcomes of liver injury. Respectively, TNF-α attaches two types of receptors TNFR1 and TNFR2. All tissue expresses TNFR1, whereas inflammatory cells exhibit TNFR2. Additionally, the association of TNF-α to TNFR1 induces the binding of TRADD to the death domain of TNFR1 (TNF receptor type 1) [7].

As a matter of fact, within **TNF signaling pathway**, TRADD triggers at least three different signaling pathways (1) I-kappa B kinase (IKK) complex that triggers further pro-inflammatory and anti-apoptotic target genes; (2) DISC; and (3) c-Jun N-terminal kinase (JNK) [7]. DISC and JNK trigger apoptosis. MAPK (mitogen-activated protein kinases) through TNF signaling pathway activates apoptosis [3]. In fact, JNK is a member MAPK (mitogen-activated protein kinases). Triggered JNK phosphorylates including the activation protein-1 (AP-1) transcription factor subunit c-JUN, that leads to the raised transcriptional activity of AP1 (the activation protein-1) [3].

Hence, the association of *death receptor-cognate ligand* at the cellular plasma membrane leads to conformational changes with trimerization of death receptor, with further recruitment of cytosol adaptor proteins (i.e. FADD, Fas-associated protein with a death domain; also known as MORT-1 or mediator of receptor-induced toxicity) and activation of signaling pathways (i.e. caspase-8) [3]. Association of FADD with TRAIL-R1 (TNF-related apoptosis-inducing ligand receptor) and TRAIL-R2 activate **caspase-8**. As described above, the attachment of TNF to TNFR1 induces trimerization and recruits the adaptor molecule TRADD that further enables the FADD binding with activation of *caspase-8*. Therefore, *caspase-8* binds to the adaptor protein FADD at the DISC with its conformational changes and its activation by proteolytic cleavage [3]. In fact, caspases 8 and 10 activate further a proteolytic cascade that finally generates caspases 3, 6 and 7 with cellular proteins alteration and cell death.

Hepatocytes (type II cells) can activate procaspase 8 only in minimal amounts [1]. Its deubiquination diminishes the activity of caspase-8 and stops extrinsic apoptosis [3]. Correspondingly, caspase-8 is inhibited by c-FLIP [17]. Besides, NF-KB (transcription factor nuclear factor) causes the exhibition of c-FLIP. What is more, the forms of c-FLIP (c-FLIP$_S$-short form; c-FLIP$_L$-long form) regulate the conformational changes of caspase-8 with its activation or inhibition. In summary, caspase-8 and c-FLIP isoforms are enrolled to DISC [3].

In **the death pathway** autoproteolytic activation of procaspases-8 results in the **DISC** (Fig. 4.2) [18]. Activation of initiator caspases (caspase 8) splits pro-apoptotic protein Bid producing truncated Bid (t-Bid) that gets inside mitochondria by translocation via N-myristoylation. Herein, tBid functions as a BH3-only protein activator and merges with the proapoptotic Bcl-2 proteins Bax and Bak [1]. The activation of proapoptotic Bcl-2 family members Bax and Bak by caspase-8 leads to their oligomerization and incorporation into the mitochondrial membrane [18]. It has to be underlined that the complex formed by t-Bid and activated proapoptotic Bax and Bak leads to **mitochondrial outer membrane permeabilization (MOMP)** with cytochrome c release [16]. In same time, triggering of caspase-8 causes the discharge of the lysosomal enzyme cathepsin B known as an activator of intrinsic apoptosis [18]. Furthermore, the Bax/Bak-dependent MOMP with further activation of caspase-9 happens [3]. Mitochondrial cytochrome c activates **apoptosome** formation that is a complex containing cytochrome c, APAF-1 (apoptosis protease-activating factor-1), ATP and procaspases-9. Caspase 9 activates further caspase 3 [1]. In same time with apoptosome formation, proteins Smac/DIABLO with low PI attach the XIAP (X chromosome linked inhibitor of apoptosis protein) with its deactivation [3]. This results in activation of apoptotic cascade.

As mentioned, the association of death receptors, adaptor proteins and apoptotic signaling pathways represents **DISC** [3] with the initiation of effector caspases (-3, -6, and -7). It is also important to acknowledge that DISC activates type I or type II signaling cascade [7]. In case of **extrinsic apoptosis**, DISC is triggering **type I death receptor** signaling (i.e., lymphocytes) where there is the activation of effector caspases by direct cleavage from the initiator caspases. So that, **type I signaling pathway** is characterized by the development of initiator caspase-8 that leads to the activation of apoptotic executioner/effector caspases (caspase-3,-6, and -7) [7].

2. **Intrinsic apoptosis or *mitochondrial pathway*** which can be activated by p53 upon DNA damage, is triggered by DISC that activates **type II death receptor signaling** (i.e., hepatocytes, cholangiocytes) [12]. Importantly, Bcl-2 proteins family regulates mitochondrial-mediated intrinsic apoptosis pathway. Briefly, the activation of DISC leads to MOMP with discharge of cytochrome c (mitochondrial proapoptogenic factor). This process is mediated by Bcl-2 proteins which can act either pro-apoptotic (e.g. Bid and Bax) or anti-apoptotic (e.g. Bcl-xL and Bcl-2). Characteristically, **Bcl-2 family proteins** are triggered by MOMP with the discharge of cytosol proapoptotic factors such as cytochrome c, Smac/DIABLO, endonuclease G, HrtA2 (high temperature requirement A2) and AIF (Apoptosis inducing factor) [16]. Cytochrome c induces APAF1 (apoptosis protease-activating factor-1) to undergo conformational changes (oligomerization) into apoptosome. As described above, released cytochrome c forms an apoptosome with APAF-1, dATP and procaspase 9. The subsequent activation of caspase 9 can be counteracted by the proteins IAPs (inhibitors of apoptotic proteins) family, which itself can be blocked by the Smac/DIABLO protein [1]. It is documented that mitochondria releases IAPs represented by cIAP1, cIAP2, NIAP, SURVIVIN, BRUCE [17]. The Smac/DIABLO proteins released from mitochondria isolate IAPs with activation of caspases [17]. Further, caspase 9 triggers then **caspase 3**, which is a major executor of apoptosis by cleavage of a broad spectrum of cellular proteins [1]. Therefore, **type II signaling pathway** is based on mitochondrial dysfunction and apoptosome complex formation. To sum up, **intrinsic apoptosis** has an enhanced mitochondrial permeability, cytochrome c is released, apoptosome formation, and activation of caspases through caspases 9 [15].

It is well documented that intrinsic pathway is initiated by various *intracellular stress inducers* (i.e. DNA damage, oxidative stress, UV and γ-irradiation, toxins, absence of growth factors, p53 and endoplasmic reticulum (ER) stress) [8, 12]. It should be stressed that ER stress is a possible another pathway of apoptosis. *Misfolded proteins* are a feature of ER stress. Furthermore, ER stress is induced by misfolded protein or damaged calcium homeostasis. Mild ER stress assures protection for cells, whereas important ER stress stimulate cell death through CHOP (the transcription factor C/EBP homologous protein) and JNK [2]. Importantly, ER stress causes Bax activation with apoptosis.

It is important to remember that **p53** named the "guardian of genome" is another intracellular regulator that decides if damaged DNA from an ongoing apoptosis may be removed or repaired [2]. In fact, altered DNA and senescence trigger oncogenes with further activation of p53. As such, p53 is triggered by damaged DNA, ischemia, oxidative stress, hypoxia and heat shock [5, 12]. Respectively, the apoptosis -related genes (i.e. Bcl-2,

Apaf1) are controlled by p53 [19]. Furthermore, p53 regulates MOMP dependent Bcl-2 family proteins with apoptosis [5]. A pivotal determinant, mTOR kinase (the mammalian target of rapamycin kinase) triggers apoptosis through p53, BAD, Bcl-2 proteins, PRAS40 (the proline-rich AKT substrate) and protein FLJ14213 [5].

As mentioned above, ***Bcl-2* protein family** modulates the *mitochondrial pathway of apoptosis*. Activated **intrinsic pathway** results in activation of Bcl-2 family within mitochondria. Hepatocytes do not express Bcl-2 family proteins. There are **three types of Bcl-2 proteins**: (1) *antiapoptotic proteins* (Bcl-2, Bcl-XL, Bcl-W, Mcl-1 and A1); (2) *Pro-apoptotic proteins* (Bax, Bak, Bok); and (3) *BH3-only proteins* (Bid, Bim, Bad, Bik, Bmf, Hrk, Noxa, and Puma) [16].

Anti-apoptotic Bcl-2 family (Bcl-2, Bcl-XL) inhibit the activation of Bid and Bax and further inhibits apoptosis in hepatocytes [3]. Bcl-2 and Bcl-XL are anti-apoptotic by inhibition of cytochrome c release [17]. Anti-apoptotic Bcl-2 family (i.e. Bcl-XL, Bcl-2, Bcl-W, Mcl-1) inhibits the release of pro-apoptotic factors from mitochondria [5]. It should be reiterated that antiapoptotic Bcl-2 family proteins attach to the outer mitochondrial membrane with its decreasing permeability that leads to the absence of cytochrome c in cytosol.

Pro-apoptotic proteins (Bax, Bak) induce the pore development in the outer mitochondrial membrane [5]. The pro-apoptotic proteins are vital for MOMP. NF-KB mediates with upregulation the antiapoptotic genes (i.e. Bcl-xl, c-FLIP), intervenes to stop sustained JNK activation that it is coregulated by antioxidant proteins (i.e. ferritin, SOD2) [2]. Blocking of NF-KB is associated with TNF pathway activation that further results in triggered JNK, cFLIP alteration, stimulation of proapoptotic Bcl2 family with antiapoptotic Bcl2 family inhibition. TNF apoptotic death pathway is blocked by the NF-kB-regulated gene products. Moreover, TNF is regulating the cellular proliferation via the TNF-R1 (Fig. 4.2) [18]. In fact, activated IKKs leads to IkB phosphorylation with its proteasome-dependent degradation with further discharging of NF-kB heterodimers. By translocation, NF-kB heterodimers get into the cellular nucleus with genes activation required for TNF-induced hepatocyte proliferation [18]. Moreover, the JNK/c-Jun/AP-1 pathway activation can support hepatocyte proliferation through AP-1-dependent gene expression. On the other hand, the prolonged and sustained activation of AP-1 can trigger apoptosis via death pathway [18].

BH3-only proteins interrelate with pro-apoptotic and anti-apoptotic Bcl2-proteins and cause programmed cell death [5]. As described above, the BH3-only proteins represent the triggers of the mitochondrial cell death pathway.

3. **Perforin or granzyme apoptosis pathway**. Perforin/granzyme apoptosis pathway is a cytotoxic pathway regulated by T-cells [15].

In fact, Elmore et al. defined the **perforin or granzyme apoptosis pathway** as the process that "it is characterized by secretion of the transmembrane pore-forming molecule perforin, exophytic release of cytoplasmic granules containing serine proteases (granzymes) through the pore and into the target cell" [15]. This type of apoptosis is followed by either (1) dependent caspases pathway, or (2) caspases independent DNA splitting through a SET complex formed from nucleosome, protein SET, Ape1, pp32, and HMBG2 (HMG2) (high- mobility group box-1) proteins [15].

Apoptosis biomarkers. Hepatocyte apoptosis is characterized by the elevation of serum AST, ALT, cytokeratin 18 (CK18) fragments (Fig. 4.3). Nonetheless, the acute hepatocyte apoptosis has an elevation of inflammatory markers. Importantly, in apoptosis the serum release of CK18 can occur [7]. CK18 (cytokeratin-18) is the mainly filament protein in the liver [7]. For instance, Mallory bodies from hepatocytes of alcoholic hepatitis or cirrhosis have cytokeratin 18. As such, CK-18 is degraded via caspase 6/7/8 pathway and discharged into blood vessels. Increased CK18 and CK18 fragments occur in acute and chronic liver injury [7]. It remains to be firmly demonstrated that the determination of ALFSG index (with CK18 fragments) predicts outcomes in patients with acute liver failure much better than both the King's College criteria (KCC) and MELD score [7]. Importantly, future studies on cell death biomarkers may establish more precisely information regarding the treatment and prognosis from acute and chronic liver diseases [2].

4.3 Autophagy

In fact, it is Greek for "self-digestion", "eating of self" or "self eating". Hepatocyte autophagy is a protective pathway as survival mechanism in starvation [16]. It maintains cellular homeostasis being a catabolic cellular process in starvation [16]. Overall, autophagy is triggered by starvation (nutrient deprivation), hypoxia, energy metabolism deficiency and growth factor deficiency [5] with further triggering of LKB1-AMPK pathway. As a result, it is a vital process for normal development, metabolic balance and prevention of degenerative disease [6]. Hence, it is related with immunity (innate, adaptive), developmental defects, tumorigenesis and cell death [6]. ER stress induces autophagy as an adaptive response [5]. Autophagy keeps ER function by removal of misfolded/unfolded proteins complexes [6]. However, autophagy characterizes many liver diseases such as ischemia-reperfusion injury, drugs (acetaminophen), alcoholic liver disease, TNF-mediated liver injury, fatty diet.

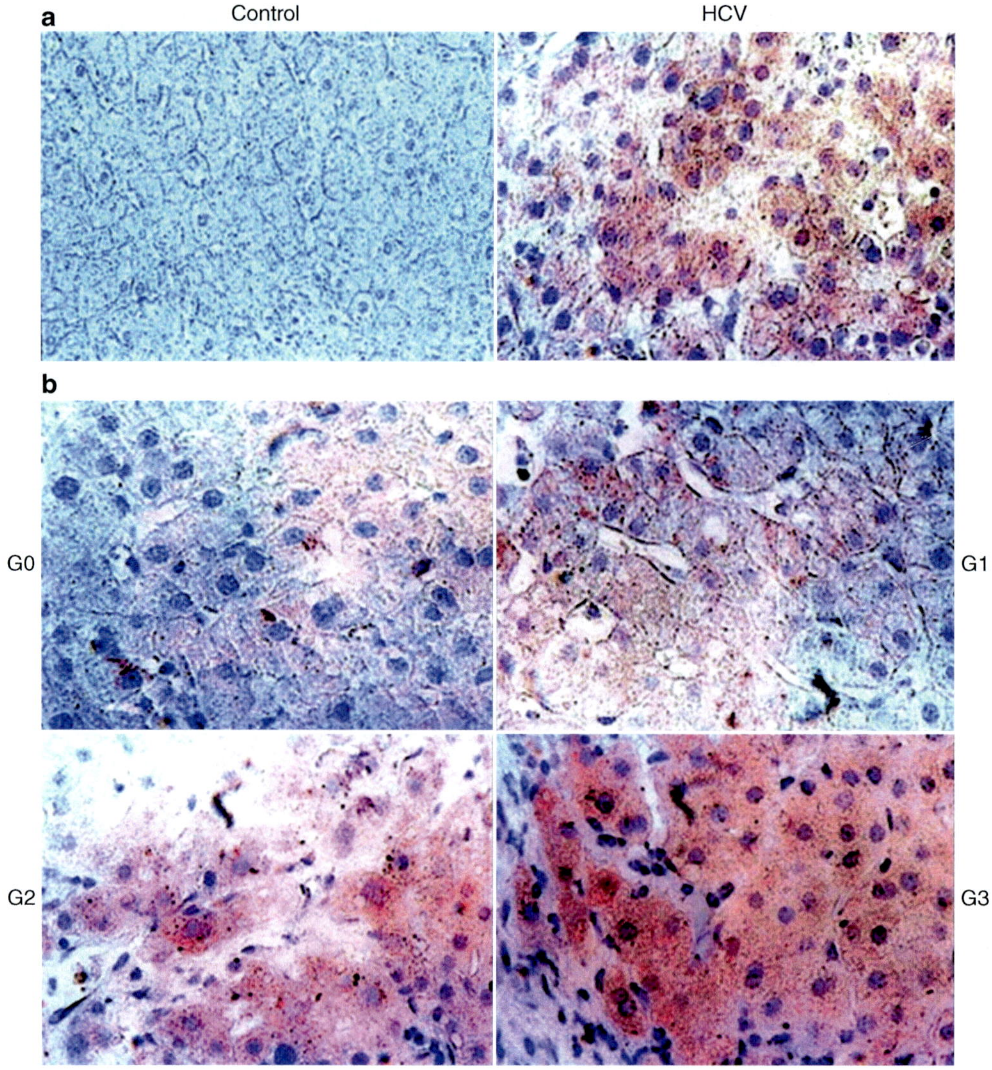

Fig. 4.3 Detection of caspase-mediated CK-18 cleavage in HCV-infected liver biopsies. (**a**) Pattern of CK-18 cleavage in liver from a healthy control and HCV patient as assessed via immunostaining (red color) with a monoclonal antibody recognizing a specific caspase-generated neoepitope of CK-18 (original magnification ×400). (**b**) Paraffin-fixed liver tissue sections with grades 0, 1, 2, and 3 of disease activity according to Batts and Ludwig [20] were analyzed. Immunoreactivity is elevated in tissue sections with higher grades of inflammatory liver injury. Note that many hepatocytes, though positive for caspase activation, do not exhibit an overt apoptotic morphology, indicating that CK-18 cleavage marks a very early event in the apoptotic process. *HCV* hepatitis C virus, *G* grade of disease activity [21]. (**With permission**)

By definition, it represents a cytoprotective mechanism by which damaged intracellular components are eliminated through proteolytic digestion inside lysosomes [22]. Also, it is the only one removal mechanism of protein complexes and bulky intracellular organelle; eliminates large intracellular organelle and regulates hepatic apoptosis via mitochondrial pathway with recycle of mitochondria [6]. It should be reiterated that lysosome is an important system of degradation from the eukaryotic cells including hepatocytes. Extracellular components get inside lysosomes by endocytosis. Further, their final degradation is accomplished by autophagy. As a side note, mitophagy is defined as a special or selective autophagy implied in mitochondrial regulation [23]. ER-phagy is degradation of ER by autophagy. One major function of liver is to assure drug metabolism. For instance, drugs which cause P-450 system activation cause increased catabolism in ER with is important proliferation. As a result, autophagy clears extra ER membranes.

The development of ***autophagosomes*** characterizes autophagy. In fact, autophagosomes present a similar morphology with apoptotic bodies (Fig. 4.4). Morphologically, autophagic cell death has significant increase of autophagosomes in cellular cytoplasm in the absence of chromatin condensation (**Note**: chromatin condensation is a hallmark of apoptosis). On the other hand, the presence of autophagosomes in dying cells is not correlated with the fact that cell death is mediated by autophagy [16].

Generally, cellular **autophagic signaling pathways** comprise: (1) stress signaling kinases (JNK-1) that supports Bcl-2 phosphorylation with further interrelation of Beclin1-VPS34; (2) inhibition by mTOR kinase of the Atg1/Ulk-1/Ulk-2 complexes during the onset of phagophore development; (3) diminished cellular ATP levels and hypoxia trigger autophagia inhibition via mTOR kinase activity by decreased Rheb GTPase activity. Increased Rheb GTPase activity such as boosted growth factor signaling inhibits autophagy [22].

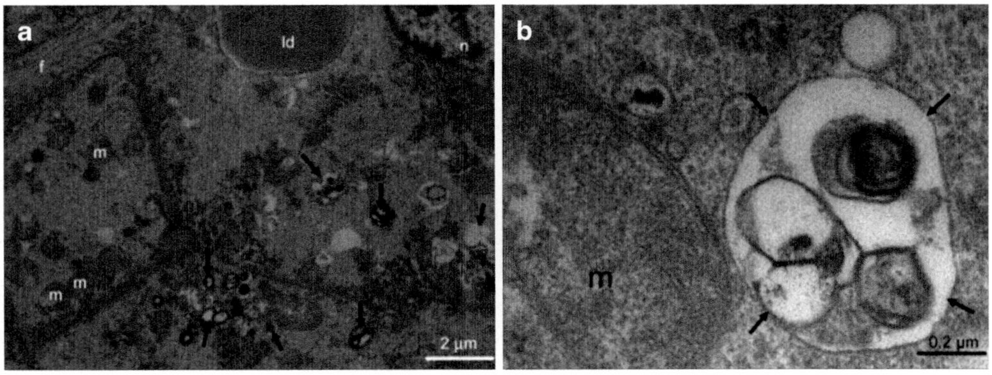

Fig. 4.4 Electron micrographs showing ultrastructure of hepatocytes from a chronic hepatitis C patient. Black arrows point to **autophagic vacuoles**. (**a**) Low-magnification image showing hepatocytes containing several autophagic vacuoles (original magnification, ×8000). (**b**) Partial view of a hepatocyte containing an autophagic vacuole (original magnification, ×100,000). *F* fibrosis, *ld* lipid droplet, *m* mitochondria, *n* nucleus [24]. (**With permission**)

There are three types of autophagy: macroautophagy, microautophagy, and chaperone-mediated autophagy (Fig. 4.5).

Macroautophagy (Fig. 4.5). In general, macroautophagy is activated in physiological and pathological processes such as embryogenesis (removal of apoptotic cells), stress (starvation) or removal of infections, altered organelles and misfolded proteins. Starvation activates autophagy. In fact, amino acids deprivation stimulate autophagy in liver with intense proteolysis. Glucagon activates autophagy. On the other hand, autophagy is inhibited by amino acids, and insulin. In starvation, macroautophagy triggers cellular catabolism. As already mentioned, this form of autophagy is based on formation of **autophagosomes** which are structures with double membrane inside of cellular cytoplasm that contain intracellular organelle and cytoplasm. Autophagic digestion by lysosomal hydrolases delivers into cytosol amino acids, glucose and other small molecules used for energy production or recycling in hepatocytes [24]. Typically it has the smallest cell death phagocytosis [22].

It is well documented that **autophagosome** development comprises (1) ***ULK1 complex*** generation from ULK1Ser/Thr protein kinase, Atg13 (autophagy-related proteins), and FIP200 (where ULK1, uncoordinated 51-like kinase 1; FIP200, 200-kDa focal adhesion kinase family-interacting protein); (2) ***Beclin 1****-class III phosphatidylinositol 3-kinase (PI3K)* complex; and (3) **phagophore** formation [3]. **Beclin 1** has a vital role in autophagosome development and it is a component of multiprotein PI3K complex [5]. In fact, multiprotein class PI3K complex is formed from VPS34, Beclin 1, and VPS15 multiprotein class III phosphatidyl inositol -3 kinase (PI3K) complex [3].

To begin with, stress autophagic signaling pathways trigger **phagophore** formation by Beclin-1/VPS34 at the ER and other membranes [22]. Atgs (autophagy-related protein) genes mediate the phagophore formation. In line with this, TFEB (transcription factor EB) is an important transcriptional factor that mediates autophagy, and one of its role is to regulate **Atgs gene** expression [23]. **Phagophores** are lipidic bilayer structures that develops from lipids and proteins originated from cell organelles (i.e. mitochondria, Golgi, ER, plasma membrane and endocytic system or endosomes) [23]. LC3B-II are receptors of the phagophore. ***Phagophore*** engulf intracellular components (ribosomes, organelles, protein aggregates) and become double-membrane **autophagosomes**. Further, autophagosomes merge with lysosomes, constitute **autophagolysosome** or *autolysosome (unilayer structures)* so that its outer membrane fit in the structure of lysosome but the inner membrane is degraded by acidic lysosomal hydrolases inside the lysosome [16, 22]. As a result, the autophagosomes components are degraded by lysosomal acid proteases into amino acids and other products which get back into cytosol as energy source.

Importantly, signaling pathways (i.e. Sonic Hedgehog pathway) located in the primary cilia detect starvation. In fact, activation of these signaling pathways is made by **Atgs** (autophagy-related proteins) genes. Moreover, **Atgs** mediate every step of autophagy [23]. Beclin 1 (Atg6) joins to VPS34, VPS15 and Atg14. Bcl-2 inhibits Beclin 1/VPS34 complex formation. Essentially, Atgs proteins are necessary for the phagophore and the autophagosome formation [24].

Presently, the Nomenclature Committee on Cell Death 2018 sustains that the development of autophagosome involves the joining of Atg5 and Atg12 in the presence of Atg7 and Atg10 [3]. The Atg5-Atg12 is a multimer complex. Further, the adding of Atg16L leads to the complex Atg5-Atg12-Atg16. In same time, LC3 interrelates with PE (phosphatidylethanolamine) at phagophore membrane. Once the complex Atg5-Atg-12-Atg16 is formed, the conjugated form of Atg8 (ubiquitin-like protein)/LC3-II (microtubule-associated protein 1 light chain 3) select the autophagosomal membrane. It results "autophagic vesicle-associated form (LC3-II)" with the autophagic vacuole development [3].

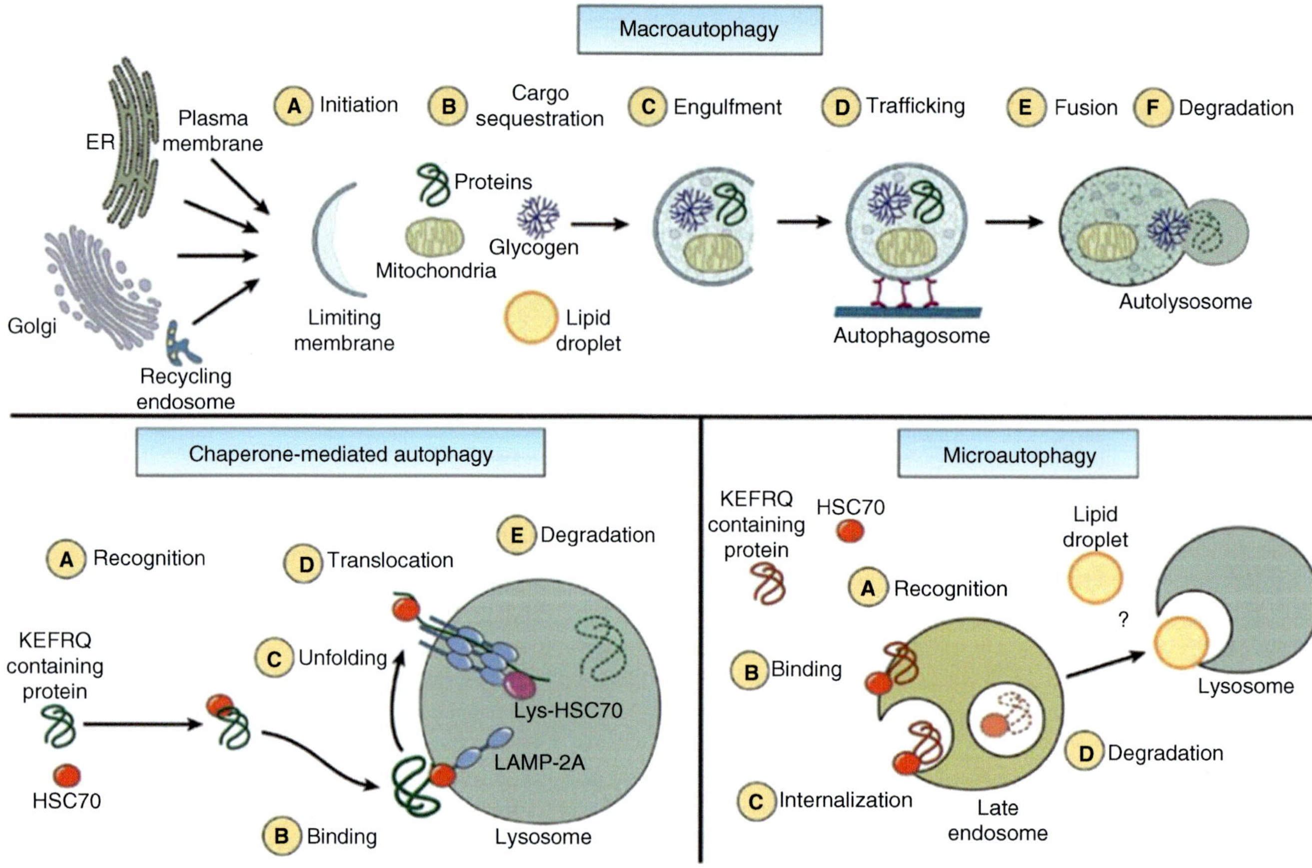

Fig. 4.5 Scheme of autophagy pathways in the liver. Schematic depiction of the 3 types of autophagy that co-exist in liver. (Upper panel) **Macroautophagy** is (A) initiated with the formation of the limiting membrane using lipids and proteins from different organelles. Cargo sequestration (B) can occur in bulk or in a selective manner mediated by soluble protein receptors. After engulfment (C), the sealed vesicle (autophagosome) traffics (D) via microtubules and delivers cargo to lysosomes through membrane fusion (E) to form an autolysosome where cargo is degraded by lysosomal hydrolases (F). (Lower left panel) In CMA, all substrates carry a pentapeptide (KFERQ-like) recognized (A) by the cytosolic chaperone HSC70. The substrate-chaperone complex binds (B) to the CMA receptor LAMP-2A at the lysosomal membrane. The substrate must be unfolded (C) before translocation (D) through the multimeric complex formed by LAMP-2A at the lysosomal membrane. A luminal HSC70 assists in substrate translocation into a lysosome, where the substrate finally is degraded (E). (Lower right panel) **Microautophagy** in liver has been observed in late endosomes where proteins also carrying KFERQ-like motifs are internalized in small microvesicles that form through invagination of the endosomal membrane. As in **CMA**, the consensus motif allows HSC70 recognition (A), but in this case the substrate/chaperone complex binds directly to lipids at the endosomal membrane (B). Microvesicles trapping this cargo that form in an endosomal sorting complex required for transport (ESCRT)-dependent manner are internalized (C) into the endosome lumen where degradation takes place (D). Some degradation also may be completed upon endosome/lysosomal fusion. In the case of yeast, direct trapping of lipid droplets by the vacuole (yeast lysosome equivalent) through a microautophagy-like process has been described, but whether or not this process also takes place in mammalian lysosomes requires future investigation [23]. (**With permission**)

Likewise, mTOR kinase mediates growth for early development or ageing. Upregulation of autophagy results from *mTOR inhibition* (i.e. starvation, increased ATP levels, decreased growth factors). Inhibition of mTOR causes diminishing of mRNA translation with autophagy activation [5]. As well, starvation inhibits TOR with autophagy activation. Starvation is also associated with decreased growth factory receptor activity that inhibits TOR kinase via Tsc1 and Tsc2. Also, sustained starvation re-triggers mTOR signaling with rebuilding of normal lysosome homeostasis [24]. Moreover, hypoxia generates unfolded protein response with ER stress and reduced oxidative phosphorylation with autophagic process. Low **ATP levels** trigger the activation of adenosine 5-monophosphate (AMP), activated protein kinase (AMPK) that further activates Tsc1/Tsc2 tumour suppressor proteins with inhibition of a GTase (Rheb) necessary for mTOR activity [22].

Microautophagy describes unilayer invaginations of lysosomal membrane while engulfing cytosolic components (Fig. 4.5) [23]. Shortly, the cytoplasmic components (cytosol, organelles, nuclear fragments) get inside lysosome by invaginations. As a result, cytoplasmic components are absorbed by lysosomes via the lysosomal membrane invaginations [22]. Herein, lysosomal hydrolases degrade these invaginations. This endosomal microautophagy characterizes hepatocytes. Hsc70 (the chaperone heat shock cognate 70) binds selectively the proteins cargo. It should be pointed that the development of invaginating vesicles in the late endosomes is based on ESCRTI and ESCRTIII (the endosomal sorting complexes required for transport) pathway [23].

Chaperone-mediated autophagy (CMA). Madrigal-Matute et al. defines CMA as the "direct transport of soluble proteins with the consensus pentapeptide sequence KFERQ via Hsc70 (the cytoplasmic chaperone heat shock cognate 70) to the lysosomal docking protein LAMP2A (lysosomal membrane receptor lysosomal-associated membrane protein 2A) followed by translocation into the lysosomal for degradation" (Fig. 4.5) [16, 23]. In fact, complexes formed from proteins with KFERQ motif firstly associate Hsc70 and co-chaperones (Hsp40, Hsp90, Hip so on) and binds to lysosomal membrane via LAMP-2A with their transportation across the lysosomal membrane. Within lysosomes, these proteins complexes are unfolded with digestion [22]. Shortly, CMA is a (1) cytoprotective mechanism in case of hepatocytes injury with the scope of proteins removal; and (2) is a hepatocyte mechanism in starvation [23].

CMA is regulated by unknown signaling mechanisms. Despite this, it turns out that CMA is triggered by NFAT-calcineurin axis (during T-cell activation), free fatty acids (FFA) and ketone bodies [23]. Moreover, CMA is inhibited by increased FFA and by the nuclear retinoic acid receptor alpha [23].

4.4 Necrosis

The term necrosis comes from the Greek "necros" for cadaver. It is also named "oncotic necrosis" or "oncosis" [7]. It is an irreversible incidental form or **unprogrammed cell death** due to physiochemical stress [2, 15]. Necrosis is a vital feature of APAP-induced liver injury (Acetaminophen-Induced Liver Necrosis) [12], of ischemia or hypoxic cell injury (ischemia-reperfusion injury) with diminished levels of ATP and increased ROS; other toxins (xenobiotics) and acute fulminant liver failure.

As briefly described, plasma membrane alteration and energy reduction are the major etiologies of necrosis [8]. It is also caused by acute cellular injury with metabolic failure [15] and ROS formation with mitochondrial damage and failure of ATP levels [7]. Basically, in necrosis there is an alteration of ion homeostasis with cell enlargement, the cellular free calcium upsurges, initiation of multiple proteases and phospholipases with mitochondrial damage. This further leads to decreased **ATP** and malfunction of ATP-dependent ion pumps. Also, the oncosis process (swelling of cell organelles and cells) is followed by cellular membrane blebbing with its rupture.

Morphologically, necrosis presents cell swelling (oncosis), plasma membrane blebbing *without cellular organelles*, intact and swollen nucleus with nuclear fragmentation unstained by hematoxylin, organelles swelling (mitochondria, ER), rupture of organelle and plasma membrane rupture, with cellular components discharge (Fig. 4.6, Table 4.2) [5, 7, 8]. (**Note**: in apoptosis—plasma membrane blebs contain organelle). This leads to inflammatory process through release of HMGB1 and HDGF (Hepatoma Derived Growth Factor). NLRP3 is the main protein of inflammasome and activates **inflammasome** with further discharge of IL1β that is an pro-inflammatory cytokine. The activation of NLRP3 inflammasome is caused by released mitochondrial ATP from altered cells [5]. The **morphologic hallmark** of necrosis is the damage of plasma membrane and release of intracellular components including *increased* discharge of inflammatory **DAMPs** into extracellular environment [2]. Subsequently, important inflammatory reaction is triggered. Importantly, the inflammatory reaction from necrosis is *higher than* of apoptosis [12].

It should be stressed that the **biochemical** feature of necrosis is the lack of mitochondrial oxidative phosphorylation. In fact, the absence of mitochondrial oxidative phosphorylation involves rapid drop of cellular ATP, and further the alteration of ion pumps, intracellular calcium homeostasis, and other cellular processes. Additionally, alteration of the ion gradients through the inner mitochondrial membrane produces loss of the mitochondrial membrane potential with the **mitochondrial permeability transition (MPT)**. MPT (mitochondrial permeability transition) comprises the permeabilization of both mitochondrial membranes (outer, inner) with mitochondrial dysfunction or uncoupling of oxidative phosphorylation [2, 16]. When inner mitochondrial membrane is losing its permeability, it follows the failure of ion gradients, the intracellular cytosol is getting alkaline, the fall of mitochondrial membrane potential and failure of oxidative phosphorylation, failure of cellular ATP and final blebbing and swelling of cell with membrane rupture. (**Note**: mitochondrial dysfunction is a significant feature for both apoptosis and necrosis but with different molecular mechanisms). Mitochondrial ROS induces signaling pathways (JNK, cyclophilin D) with MPT pore and necrosis [14]. By definition, **MPT-driven necrosis** is usually a regulated cell death triggered often by increased cytoplasmic calcium overload or severe oxidative stress that leads to necrosis [3]. Protein cyclophilin D (CYPD, PPIF, peptidylprolyl isomerase F) has to be present for MPT forming [3].

All nuclear cells (eukaryotic cells) exhibit HMGB1. On the whole, **necrosis** comprises (1) cellular membrane integrity failure with cellular swelling and organelle swelling; (2) organelle membrane damage; lysosomes release proteolytic enzymes in cellular cytoplasm with cellular degradation; cell swelling can cause plasma membrane rupture with release of pro-inflammatory cell components into cytoplasm and interstitial space. Obviously, this leads to the recruitment of inflammatory cells (macrophages, natural killer cells, neutrophils, mature dendritic cells) which release *HMGB1* protein in necrosis. HMGB1 protein is also known as amphoterin

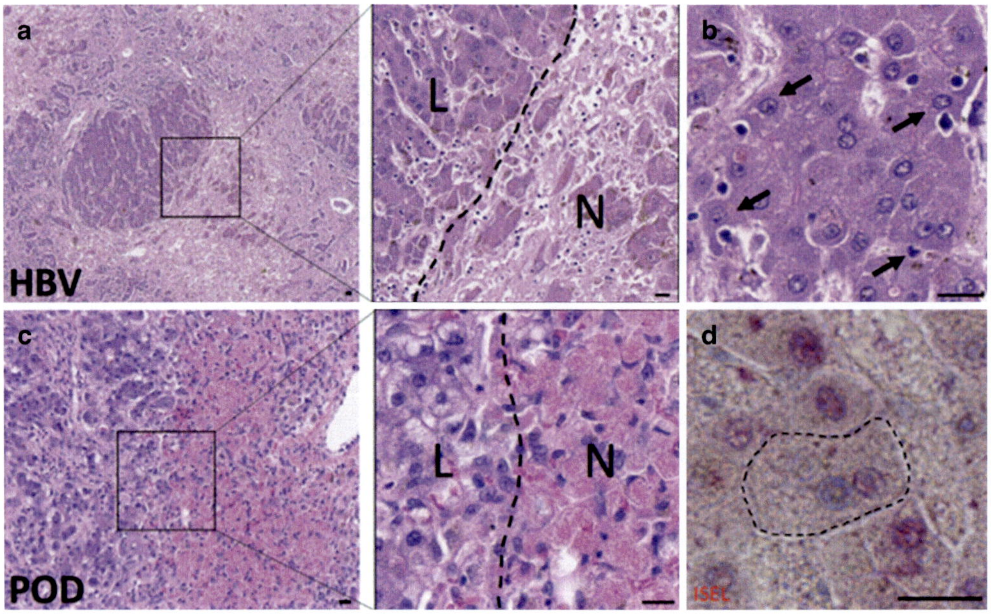

Fig. 4.6 Hepatocytes engulf necrotic and apoptotic cells in **acute-on-chronic liver injury** caused by hepatitis B infection (HBV) and in paracetamol injury (POD). (**a**) Hematoxylin–eosin staining of acute-on-chronic liver injury in a patient with HBV infection. Large areas of hepatocyte **necrosis** are evident. Inset image shows dark stained hepatocyte nuclei in live hepatocytes (L) and pyknotic or karyolytic nuclei in necrotic hepatocytes (N). (**b**) Healthy hepatocytes with clearly marked nuclei are seen phagocytosing small **apoptotic** cells (arrows). Note hepatocyte invaginations which have formed to enable capture of apoptotic cells. (**c**) Hematoxylin-eosin staining of liver with paracetamol-induced injury, which causes centrilobular **necrosis**. Inset shows pink cytoplasm in necrotic hepatocytes (N) compared to surviving non-discolored hepatocytes with clearly defined nuclei (L). (**d**) In situ end labeling (ISEL) of **apoptotic cell nuclei** is seen here in pink, in a liver with ischemia-reperfusion injury. The marked hepatocyte has a non-apoptotic nucleus seen in blue, and has engulfed an apoptotic cell with a pink nucleus. Neighboring **apoptotic hepatocytes** can be seen with pink nuclei, and non-apoptotic cells with blue nuclei. The bars show 20 μm [7].

(non-histone nuclear protein). HMGB1 activate RAGE (receptor for advanced glycan end products) and TLR4 (toll-like receptor 4) [7]. Further, RAGE and TLR4 trigger NF-KB. HMGB1 attaches TLR4 for advanced glycation end products with further involvement of (1) MyD88 with NF-KB activation via TRAF6, IRAK1 (interleukin-1 receptor-associated kinase 1), and IRAK4; (2) attaches RAGE with NF-KB activation via CDC42/Rac1 or Ras/p38 activation [7]. Specifically, inflammation with further injury in case of acute liver diseases (i.e. acetaminophen, ischemia-reperfusion injury) evolves when HMGB1 acts (1) by TLR4; (2) formyl peptides via FPR1; and via (3) ATP [2].

Within nucleus, HMGB1 protein suffers acetylation via NF-KB, MAPKM, and NFA; and regulates nucleosomes and favour genes transcription. Acetylated HMGB1 is discharged into blood vessel being interrelated with the activation of inflammasome via PKR activation [7].

4.5 Necroptosis

When necrosis happens in vitro as programmed cell death is named ***necroptosis*** or aponecrosis [15, 26]. On the whole, necroptosis is a protective mechanism implied in stress, nor-

Table 4.2 Patterns of necrosis in liver disease [25]. (**With permission**)

Pattern of necrosis	Description	Underlying cause
Apoptosis (apoptotic body, acidophil body, or Councilman body)	Necrosis of single cells	Hepatitis (viral, autoimmune, drug)
Focal/spotty	Necrosis involving small clusters of hepatocytes	Hepatitis (viral, autoimmune, drug)
Zonal necrosis		
Centrilobular	Necrosis around central vein (acinar zone 3)	Ischemia, drugs, VOI, P/R injury
Periportal (IH/piecemeal necrosis)	Necrosis of periportal zone (acinar zone 1)	Hepatitis (viral, autoimmune, drug)
Confluent necrosis		
Localized (multilobular) necrosis	Necrosis of a part of the liver	Localized ischemia, transarterial embolization treatment
Submassive/massive necrosis	Subtotal/total hepatocellular necrosis (often with prominent ductular reaction)	Hepatitis (viral, autoimmune, drug), acute allograft failure, fulminant Wilson's disease

Abbreviations: *P/R* preservation/reperfusion, *VOI* venous outflow impairment mal development (before parturition) and adult T-cell homeostasis [3].

Presently, the *Nomenclature Committee on Cell Death 2018* defines **necroptosis** as a "form of regulated cell death initiated by perturbations of the extracellular or intracellular microenvironment detected by specific death receptors, including Fas and TNFR1, or pathogen recognition receptors (PRRs), including TLR3, TLR4, and ZBP1 (Z-DNA binding protein1, DAI)" [3]. Likewise, it is a cell death mechanism same to necrosis triggered by blocked apoptosis [9]. Overall, necroptosis has same signaling pathways of apoptosis.

It is defined as the cytotoxic death cell due to the inhibition of caspase 8. As mentioned, necroptosis can be induced via PRR family from immunity system. It is mediated by PARP1 activation, Ca^{2+} dependent calpain Cys-proteases, and pro-apoptotic Bax [5]. Furthermore, necroptosis is activated by TNF family factors with caspase -8 inhibition and development of **necrosome** (RIPK1-RIPK3 complex IIb) [15]. Necroptosis has the death receptors (TNFR1, Fas, TNFR2, TRAILR1, TRAILR2). The spontaneous trimerization of TNFR1 subunits leads to the recruitment of TRADD, RIP1, cIAP1, cIAP2, TRAF2 and TRAF5 with the complex I formation and NF-KB signaling pathway activation [5]. Essentially, liver necroptosis is a kinase-dependent cell death. Likewise, it is a process determined by the activity of kinases such as MLKL and RIPK3 [3].

Kinases family have proteins RIPs. RIP1 phosphorylates and activates RIP3 that together form with MLKL (mixed lineage kinase domain-like) a complex [3, 9]. RIP1 and RIP3 interrelate each other. As a result, the complex **necrosome** is formed from RIPK1/RIPK3 and MLKL; it induces the MLKL phosphorylation mediated by RIPK3 with its oligomerization that ultimately causes the lipid bilayer permeabilization [14]. Finally, Bid mediates Bax activation and **necroptosis** [5]. Presently, the Nomenclature Committee on Cell Death 2018 states that signaling pathway of necroptosis happens ***without*** *the involvement* of mitochondria. As a consequence, there are no involvements in necroptosis of mitochondrial phosphoglycerate mutase (PGAM) family member 5, serine/threonine protein phosphatase, PGAM5 and dynamin-related protein (DRP1)-driven mitochondrial fragmentation [3].

TNFα triggers PARP1 with diminishing ATP and necrosis [5]. The nuclear enzyme PARP1 regulates DNA being triggered by altered DNA [5]. **TNF pathway** is used in **necroptosis** and it is a feature of ischemia-reperfusion injury.

Necroptosis induced by **TNF pathway** (Fig. 4.7). The association of TNF with TNFR leads to an complex formed

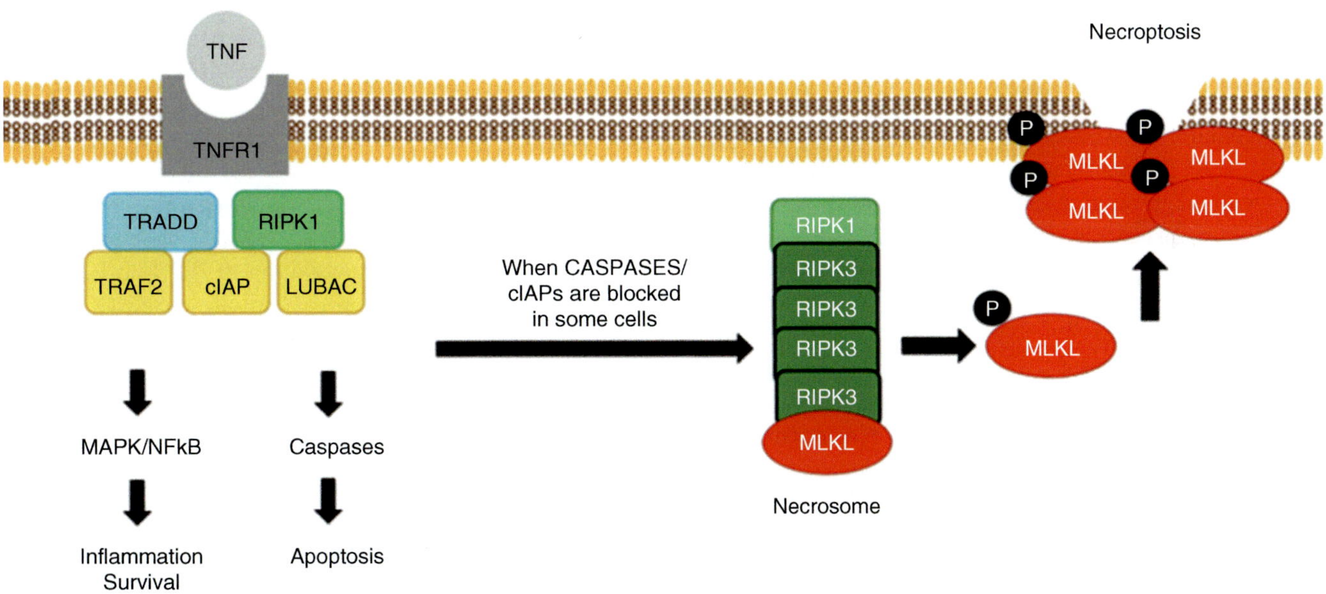

Fig. 4.7 A simplified depiction of **necroptosis** induction by TNF. When TNF binds to its receptor (TNFR), complex 1 forms, which consists of the adaptor protein TRADD and ubiquitin ligases TRAF2 (also an adaptor), cIAPs, and LUBAC as well as the kinase, RIPK1. Ubiquitination of RIPK1 forms a platform to approximate key proteins leading to NFκB and MAPK activation and transcription of pro-survival and pro-inflammatory genes. Complex I internalization leads to the formation of the cytosolic complex II (not shown), which ultimately results in Caspase-8 activation culminating in apoptosis. When caspases +/− cIAPs are inhibited in certain cells, RIPK1 then forms a complex with RIPK3, which oligomerizes and recruits the pseudokinase, MLKL. RIPK3 phosphorylates MLKL that activates the protein leading to its translocation to cell membrane where it forms tetramers to permeate the lipid bilayer. TNF, tumor necrosis factor; TRADD, tumor necrosis factor receptor type 1-associated death domain; TRAF2, TNF receptor-associated factor 2, cIAP, cellular inhibitors of apoptosis; LUBAC, linear ubiquitin chain assembly complex; RIPK1, receptor interacting protein kinase 1; NFκB, nuclear factor κB; MAPK, mitogen-activated protein kinase; RIPK3, receptor Interacting protein kinase 3; MLKL, mixed-lineage kinase domain-like [27]. **Attribution 4.0 International (CC BY 4.0)**

from (1) the adaptor protein TRADD; (2) the adaptor ubiquitin ligases TRAF2 (TRAF2, TNF receptor-associated factor 2), (3) cellular IAPs, (4) LUBAC, linear ubiquitin chain assembly complex, (5) RIPK1 [14]. Necroptosis usually is regulated by TNFR1 [14]. Intracellular segment of TNFR1 binds TRADD, and RIPK1 [9]. As already described, the association of TNFα with TNFR1 causes complex II DISC formation [5]. It seems that FADD-RIP1/3-NEMO complex leads to Bax/Bak-dependent mitochondrial damages with ***TNF α-dependent necroptosis*** [5]. The inactivation of caspase 8 induces necroptosis [5]. In fact, caspase-8 is inhibited with RIP1/RIP3 association and induces the development of **necrosome** with necroptosis. As a result, RIPK3 triggers the production of ROS with membrane permeability by activation and production of MLKL oligomers. The complex **necrosome** is formed from RIPK1/RIPK3 and MLKL [9]. The generated MLKL bind at plasma membrane the phosphatidylinositol phosphate with further activation of plasma membrane permeabilization [3]. Also, RIPK3 can be activated by innate immunity proteins (i.e. TRIF, ZBP1) [3].

Importantly, a key mediator of necroptosis is **MLKL** that can support the production of mitochondrial ROS. p-MLKL is an activated tetramer form of MLKL that can induce necroptosis [14]. Currently, the Nomenclature Committee on Cell Death 2018 states that the mechanism by which *MLKL induces necroptosis is not well-defined*. However, oligomerization and translocation of MLKL is promoted by HSP90 (the heat shock protein 90 kDa alpha family class A member 1) [3]. Oligomerization of MLKL is followed by calcium influx, exhibition of PS on plasma membrane bubbles. Also, MLKL from plasma membrane triggers ADAM family proteins with magnesium channels generation [3].

Lastly, **necroptosis** may be inhibited by (1) caspase-8, FADD, and c-FLIP, and (2) c-IAPs (they ubiquitinate RIPK1) [3].

4.6 The Crosstalk Between Apoptosis, Autophagy, Necrosis and Necroptosis

Even if autophagy and apoptosis are independent processes, they overlap and crosstalk at many levels. Both **apoptosis** and **autophagy** may cause cell death. Importantly, these mechanisms may interrelate when autophagy stimulate via cytotoxic pathway or inhibit **apoptosis** (cytoprotective pathway). Cytoprotective autophagy inhibits **apoptosis**, whereas cytotoxic autophagy promotes apoptosis [6].

As already mentioned, apoptosis is *triggered* by (1) activation of caspase-8 and caspase-3, or (2) pro-apoptotic proteins activation (Bid, Bax). It leads to formation of the apoptosome complex (cytochrome C, Apaf-1, caspase-9) with further caspase-3 activation [7]. Regulatory genes p53, Atg5, Bcl-2 represent the interconnection **between apoptosis and autophagy**. As well, the subcellular localization of Bcl-2 can have two outcomes: (1) Bcl-2 reduces the discharge of cytochrome c with pro-survival mitochondrial function and **inhibited apoptosis**; (2) Bcl-2 inhibits ER **autophagy** via Beclin1 [22]. As well, cleavage of Atg5 calpain-mediated is followed by its translocation into mitochondria with Bcl-XL interaction and discharge of cytochrome c, activation of caspase and **apoptosis** [22]. Additionally, Mcl1 known as anti-apoptotic Bcl-2 family regulates apoptosis and autophagy [5]. Moreover, the interrelation between **Beclin 1** and the anti-apoptotic proteins Bcl-2 and Bcl-XL mediates the **crosstalk between apoptosis and autophagy** [5, 6].

Bcl-2 proteins (Bcl-2, BclXL, BcljB) attach Beclin-1 with PI3KC3 complex and **blocking of autophagy**. Bcl-2 proteins "downregulate" **apoptosis** and act together with Beclin-1 to **block autophagy** [6]. The ongoing interaction between Bcl-2 and Beclin-2 is interrupted by BNIP3 that increases **apoptosis** via Bax/Bad although isolates Bcl-2 proteins [6]. Lastly, p53 regulates both **autophagy** signaling pathways (i.e. AMPK/mTOR, Bmf/Beclin-1) [19].

Apoptosis and **necroptosis** have same initiators of cell death: TNF-α, FasL, and TRAIL. Moreover, apoptosis may develop secondary necrosis [2]. Notably, RIP1/RIP3 kinase cascade activates JNK with mitochondrial oxidative stress modulation. On the other hand, RIP1 and RIP3 can induce the switch from **apoptosis** to **necroptosis**. Both kinases named RIP1 and RIP3 switch death receptors activation toward **apoptosis** or **necroptosis**. RIP1 activation can further lead to NF-KB, MAPK, **apoptosis** or **necrosis** [9].

If caspase-8 is triggered with the cleavage of RIP1/RIP3, cell death is switched on **apoptosis**. RIP1/RIP3 forms together with TRADD, FADD and caspase-8. Within complex II, the inactivation of RIP1 and RIP3 by caspase 8 is followed by pro-apoptotic caspases triggering. Cellular IAPs inhibition leads to inhibition of RIP ubiquitylation with complex II development and further caspase 8 activation [5]. What is more, serine-threonine kinase Akt **inhibits apoptosis. This kinase** triggers the transcription factor CREB and IKK complex with further inhibition of pro-apoptotic proteins Bad and caspase-9 with **necroptosis** [5].

Increased intracellular ATP favours **apoptosis**, while diminished intracellular ATP facilitates **necrosis** [5]. It is important to underline that **secondary necrosis** defines switching of apoptotic cells into necrotic cells in case of ATP depletion [8].

Pyroptosis. It is a caspase-1 dependent cell death with morphologic features of **apoptosis** and/or **necrosis**. It is supported by activation of caspase-1, formation of inflammasome dependent caspase-1 activation, followed by pyroptotic cell death. Therefore, **inflammasome** triggers the caspase-1 activation with further discharge of proinflammatory cytokines IL-1β, and IL-18 [3].

4.7 Conclusions

Without a doubt, cell death is a major determinant factor regarding the tissue injury severity and consequent organ and systems functions [14]. Regardless, hepatocyte death is the hallmark of liver disease development such as inflammation, fibrosis, cirrhosis, and hepatocellular carcinoma. Apoptosis and necrosis represent the two major modes of hepatocyte death, and apoptosis assures tissue homeostasis by the physiologic removal of damaged hepatocytes. It is now clear that apoptosis is a significant finding of numerous liver disorders. Upcoming studies should reveal knowledge regarding the liver regulation of hepatic signaling death pathways. For instance, signaling death pathways with activation of hepatocyte proliferation may bring benefits in acute liver disease, while inhibition of chronic liver disease development may be obtained by interruption of profibrogenic, proliferative, and proinflammatory cell death pathways [2]. Correspondingly, signaling death pathways of liver might carry significant findings for a correct treatment of hepatic disorders [2]. For this reason, therapeutic modulation of liver cell death "holds promise" [12].

Self Study

Questions

1. **Which statement is true?**
   (a) Cell death is grading into four morphotypes apoptosis, autophagy, necrosis and necroptosis.
   (b) Apoptosis is morphologically defined by a smaller spheric cell with plasma membrane blebbing.
   (c) Extrinsic apoptosis as a form of incidental cell death.
   (d) p53 is blocked by damaged DNA.
2. **Which statement/statements is/are true?**
   (a) Mitochondrial dysfunction is a feature for both apoptosis and necrosis.
   (b) Apoptosis is a feature of cholestasis, alcoholic hepatitis, non-alcoholic steatohepatitis, autoimmune hepatitis, viral hepatitis, fulminate hepatic failure, ischemia-reperfusion injury, fibrosis and cirrhosis.
   (c) DAMPs have low release in apoptosis, necrosis and necroptosis.
   (d) Extracellular cytochrome c activates apoptosome formation.

Answers

1. **Which statement is true?**
   (a) Cell death is grading into three morphotypes apoptosis, autophagy and necrosis.
   (b) Hepatocyte apoptosis is morphologically defined by a smaller spheric cell, reduction of cell or ''cell shrinkage", plasma membrane blebbing, chromatin condensation (pyknosis or small pyknotic nucleus), nuclear fragmentation (karyorrhexis), DNA splitting, mitochondrial permeabilization, cytoplasmic condensation (hypereosinophilic cytoplasm), followed by cell fragmentation into apoptotic bodies that are removed within lysosomes. **Note**: chromatin condensation is a hallmark of apoptosis **CORRECT**.
   (c) Extrinsic apoptosis as a form of regulated cell death induced or triggered by perturbations of the extracellular microenvironment that are detected by plasma membrane receptors, propagated by caspase-8 (with the optional involvement of MOMP), and precipitated by executioner caspases, mainly caspase-3.
   (d) p53 named the ''guardian of genome" is another intracellular regulator that decides if damaged DNA from undergoing apoptosis may be removed or repaired. As such, p53 is triggered by damaged DNA, ischemia, oxidative stress, hypoxia and heat shock.
2. **Which statement/statements is/are true?**
   (a) Mitochondrial dysfunction is a significant feature for both apoptosis and necrosis but with different molecular mechanisms. **CORRECT.**
   (b) There is an increased apoptosis in cholestasis, alcoholic hepatitis, non-alcoholic steatohepatitis, autoimmune hepatitis, viral hepatitis, fulminate hepatic failure, ischemia-reperfusion injury, fibrosis and cirrhosis. In case of hepatitis, apoptosis is the major cell death, being a cytoprotective mechanism in the liver clearance from infections. **CORRECT.**
   (c) The reduced inflammatory response of apoptosis is caused by decreased discharge of DAMPs (Damage-associated molecular patterns) and rapid exclusion of apoptotic bodies. However, the mainly discharge of DAMPs appears in necrosis and necroptosis.
   (d) Mitochondrial cytochrome c activates apoptosome formation that is a complex containing cytochrome c, APAF-1 (apoptosis protease-activating factor-1), ATP and procaspases-9. Caspase 9 activates further caspase 3.

References

1. Vinken M, Maes M, Oliveira AG, Cogliati B, Marques PE, Menezes GB, Dagli ML, Vanhaecke T, Rogiers V. Primary hepatocytes and their cultures in liver apoptosis research. Arch Toxicol. 2014;88(2):199–212. https://doi.org/10.1007/s00204-013-1123-4.
2. Luedde T, Kaplowitz N, Schwabe RF. Cell death and cell death responses in liver disease: mechanisms and clinical relevance. Gastroenterology. 2014;147(4):765–783.e4. https://doi.org/10.1053/j.gastro.2014.07.018.
3. Galluzzi L, Vitale I, Aaronson SA. Molecular mechanisms of cell death: recommendations of the Nomenclature Committee on Cell Death 2018. Cell Death Differ. 2018;25(3):486–541. https://doi.org/10.1038/s41418-017-0012-4.

4. Edinger AL, Thompson CB. Death by design: apoptosis, necrosis and autophagy. Curr Opin Cell Biol. 2004;16:663–9.
5. Nikoletopoulou V, Markaki M, Palikaras K, Tavernarakis N. Crosstalk between apoptosis, necrosis and autophagy. Biochim Biophys Acta. 2013;1833(12):3448–59. https://doi.org/10.1016/j.bbamcr.2013.06.001.
6. Wang K. Autophagy and apoptosis in liver injury. Cell Cycle. 2015;14(11):1631–42. https://doi.org/10.1080/15384101.2015.1038685.
7. Eguchi A, Wree A, Feldstein AE. Biomarkers of liver cell death. J Hepatol. 2014;60(5):1063–74. https://doi.org/10.1016/j.jhep.2013.12.026.
8. Davies SP, Reynolds GM, Stamataki Z. Clearance of apoptotic cells by tissue epithelia: a putative role for hepatocytes in liver efferocytosis. Front Immunol. 2018;9:44. https://doi.org/10.3389/fimmu.2018.00044.
9. Saeed WK, Jun DW. Necroptosis: an emerging type of cell death in liver diseases. World J Gastroenterol. 2014;20(35):12526–32. https://doi.org/10.3748/wjg.v20.i35.12526.
10. Radu-Ionita F, Bontas E, Goleanu V, Circiumaru B, Bartos D, Parepa I, Tintoiu IC, Popa A. Heart embryology—overview. In: Dumitrescu S, Tintoiu IC, Underwood MJ, editors. Right heart pathology from mechanism to management. New York: Springer; 2018. p. 3–24. isbn:978-3-319-73763-8.
11. Kloesel B, DiNardo JA, Body SC. Cardiac embryology and molecular mechanisms of congenital heart disease: a primer for anesthesiologists. Anesth Analg. 2016;123:551–69. https://doi.org/10.1213/ANE.00000000000014.
12. Guicciardi ME, Malhi H, Mott JL, Gores GJ. Apoptosis and necrosis in the liver. Compr Physiol. 2013 Apr;3(2):977–1010. https://doi.org/10.1002/cphy.c120020.
13. Cao L, et al. Mechanism of hepatocyte apoptosis. J Cell Death. 2016;9:19–29. https://doi.org/10.4137/JCD.S39824.
14. Dara L, Liu ZX, Kaplowitz N. A murder mystery in the liver: who done it and how? J Clin Invest. 2016;126(11):4068–71. https://doi.org/10.1172/JCI90830.
15. Elmore SA, Dixon D, Hailey JR, Harada T, Herbert RA, Maronpot RR, Nolte T, Rehg JE, Rittinghausen S, Rosol TJ, Satoh H, Vidal JD, Willard-Mack CL, Creasy DM. Recommendations from the INHAND apoptosis/necrosis working group. Toxicol Pathol. 2016;44(2):173–88. https://doi.org/10.1177/0192623315625859.
16. Malhi H, Guicciardi ME, Gores GJ. Hepatocyte death: a clear and present danger. Physiol Rev. 2010;90(3):1165–94. https://doi.org/10.1152/physrev.00061.2009.
17. Ku NO, Strnad P, Bantel H, Omary MB. Keratins: biomarkers and modulators of apoptotic and necrotic cell death in the liver. Hepatology. 2016;64(3):966–76. https://doi.org/10.1002/hep.28493.
18. Schattenberg JM, Galle PR, Schuchmann M. Apoptosis in liver disease. Liver Int. 2006;26(8):904–11.
19. Guo W, Yan L, Yang L, Liu X, E Q, Gao P, Ye X, Liu W, Zuo J. Targeting GRP75 improves HSP90 inhibitor efficacy by enhancing p53-mediated apoptosis in hepatocellular carcinoma. PLoS One. 2014;9(1): e85766. https://doi.org/10.1371/journal.pone.0085766.
20. Batts KP, Ludwig J. Chronic hepatitis. An update on terminology and reporting. Am Surg Pathol. 1995;19:1409–17.
21. Bantel H, Lügering A, Heidemann J, Volkmann X, Poremba C, Strassburg CP, Manns MP, Schulze-Osthoff K. Detection of apoptotic caspase activation in sera from patients with chronic HCV infection is associated with fibrotic liver injury. Hepatology. 2004;40(5):1078–87.
22. Glick D, Barth S, Macleod KF. Autophagy: cellular and molecular mechanisms. J Pathol. 2010;221(1):3–12. https://doi.org/10.1002/path.2697.
23. Madrigal-Matute J, Cuervo AM. Regulation of liver metabolism by autophagy. Gastroenterology. 2016;150(2):328–39. https://doi.org/10.1053/j.gastro.2015.09.042.
24. Rautou PE, Mansouri A, Lebrec D, Durand F, Valla D, Moreau R. Autophagy in liver diseases. J Hepatol. 2010;53(6):1123–34. https://doi.org/10.1016/j.jhep.2010.07.006.
25. Krishna M. Patterns of necrosis in liver disease. Clin Liver Dis. 2017;10:53–6. https://doi.org/10.1002/cld.653.
26. Linkermann A, Green DR. Necroptosis. N Engl J Med. 2014;370:455–65.
27. Dara L, Liu Z-X, Kaplowitz N. Questions and controversies: the role of necroptosis in liver disease. Cell Death Discov. 2016;2:16089. https://doi.org/10.1038/cddiscovery.2016.89.

5 Liver Inflammation: Short Uptodate

Mariana Mihaila, Ecaterina Bontas, and Cecilia Patru

Abbreviations

ALD	Alcoholic liver disease
DCs	Dendritic cells
HMGB1	Protein (high-mobility group box-1) or HMG-1 (high—mobility group)1
IL	Interleukin
NAFLD	Nonalcoholic fatty liver disease
NASH	Non-alcoholic steatohepatitis
PAMPs	Pathogen Associated Molecular Patterns
PRRs	The pathogen recognition receptors
TNF	Tumor necrosis factor

Key Concepts

- Human liver is a tolerogenical immune organ with increased number of myeloid and lymphoid immune cells.
- Liver has specific immune mechanisms of tolerance because it is primarily exposed to gut microbiome, dietary products and environmental antigens.
- Liver fibrosis is considered a pathological feature, and it is an essential feature for liver wound repair or liver regeneration.
- Hepatic tolerogenic mechanisms are lost in the presence of severe inflammation.

M. Mihaila
Fundeni Clinical Institute, București, Romania

E. Bontas (✉)
"Prof. C.C. Iliescu" Emergency Institute for Cardiovascular Diseases, Bucharest, Romania

C. Patru
"Carol Davila" Central Military Emergency University Hospital, Bucharest, Romania

5.1 Introduction

According to current evidence the ***inflammation*** represents a complex immune reaction subsequent to an aggression. It is now well accepted that the innate immune cells are monocytes, macrophages, mast cells, neutrophils and natural killer (NK) cells, which identify PAMPs (Pathogen Associated Molecular Patterns) and endogenous ligands [1]. Briefly, PAMPs are represented by glycolipids, flagellin, lipopolysaccharide (LPS), lipoproteins, bacterial DNA, and viral RNA. Endogenous ligands (heat shock proteins) are identified by innate immune cells via PRRs (Pattern-Recognition receptors) [1].

Human liver has specific immune mechanisms of tolerance because it is primarily exposed to gut microbiome, dietary products and environmental antigens. Moreover, the liver is usually subject to a permanent aggression from bacteria or viruses that have an inflammatory potential. Antimicrobial factors are represented by complement system, acute phase proteins, inflammatory cytokines and chemokines as well [1]. Under this perspective, the liver is considered a tolerogenical organ. In a simplified manner, liver innate cells are resident macrophages (Kupffer cells), dendritic cells, NK cells, and NKT cells [1]. Therefore, in case of liver, the local immune system detects hepatotropic pathogens. These molecules are tolerated by the immune system of the liver, which, at the same time, must respond to danger. It means that this aggression leads to a persistent inflammation of the liver. Furthermore, the inflammation itself triggers the capillary permeability, leukocytes migration into tissue and the secretion of inflammatory mediators. To date, a healthy liver is characterized by (1) pro-inflammatory cytokines (IFNγ, IL-2, IL-7, IL-15), and (2) anti-inflammatory cytokines such as TGFβ, IL-10 and IL-13 [2].

F. Radu-Ionita et al. (eds.), *Liver Diseases*, https://doi.org/10.1007/978-3-030-24432-3_5

5.2 Liver Inflammation

If it is of note, the inflammation of the liver is due to a diversity of causes, where the viral infection (hepatitis A, hepatitis B, hepatitis C, hepatitis D and E viruses) is the most important of them. At the same time, there are other causes of liver damage such as autoimmune hepatitis, alcohol liver disease, nonalcoholic steatohepatitis or drug-toxicity. Liver inflammation is also metabolically regulated, being evident in non-alcoholic fatty liver disease (NAFLD), hepatitis B virus and hepatitis C virus infections [2]. Moreover, as described above, the human liver has a constant exposure to gut microbiota and dietary components [1].

By definition liver inflammation requires the presence of inflammatory cells [1]. Liver has ***resident immune cells*** represented mainly by (1) antigen presenting cells (APC); (2) Kupffer cells or liver resident macrophages; (3) lymphocytes; (4) MDSC (myeloid-derived suppressor cells); and (5) dendritic cells (Fig. 5.1) [2]. Initially, hepatic inflammation recruits the innate immune cells (monocytes, neutrophils and NK cells). Liver resident dendritic cells evaluate and transport the foreign antigens into "local draining lymph nodes" presenting antigens to adaptative naïve T cells [1]. Accordingly, ***acute liver inflammation*** determines the leukocytes recruitment, with the activation and induction of fibrotic responses [3]. As a side note, the fibrosis present in the acute phase of liver inflammation protects the liver cells by cutting down the pro-apoptotic signaling [4]. While ***chronic inflammation*** can progress to fibrosis, cirrhosis and even liver cancer [2].

Another useful classification of liver immunological cells are myeloid and lymphoid cells [5]. Myeloid cells of liver are represented by Kupffer cells and DCs (dendritic cells) known also as hepatic non-lymphoid cells [5]. The main antigen-presenting cells in liver are dendritic cells. Overall, the antigen-presenting cells of liver are hepatic parenchymal cells represented by cholangiocytes and dendritic cells [5]. Liver Kupffer cells represent the biggest population of mononuclear phagocytes from human body [5]. Diseases and liver damage trigger the differentiation of resident monocytes into mature Kupffer cells [5]. If is of note Kupffer cells have their location at the luminal side of the liver sinusoidal endothelium [5].

Hepatic lymphoid cells are liver resident lymphocytes and are represented by B cells, CD4+ T cells, CD8+ T cells, natural Killer (NK) cells and non-conventional lymphoid cells such as NK T cells, gamma delta TCR+ T cells, CD4-CD8- T cells [5].

5.2.1 Macrophages

They are defined also as myeloid cells. Briefly, as stated above, myeloid cells comprise Kupffer cells, MDSC (myeloid-derived suppressor cells), and dendritic cells [2]. Resident myeloid cells are implied in the preservation of hepatic tolerance [2]. Importantly, the Kupffer cells are the liver resident macrophages. They have the capacity of auto-renewing and may also come from local progenitor liver cells [6]. Also, they express PRRs, Fc receptors and complement receptors [2]. Their role in "immune regulation, tissue repair, and liver regeneration" is well demonstrated [2].

When liver injury is initiated, the Kupffer cells get activated and may secrete powerful pro-inflammatory cytokines. In fact, Kupffer cells receive signals for recognizing and discarding the pathogen agent through PRRs (pattern recognition receptors) that are TLRs (Toll like Receptors) and NLR (NOD like receptors). During the acute liver damage, the activated Kupffer cells produce pro-inflammatory cytokines (IL-1, IL-6, GM-CSF and TNF-α), and chemokines: MIP-1α (macrophage inflammatory protein-1α) and RANTES (*Regulated upon activation normal T cell expressed and secreted*) [7]. Also, Kupffer cells have a key role in liver regeneration through IL-6 and TNF-α with hepatocyte proliferation [2].

As well as the other macrophages, the Kupffer cells secret Il-1α and IL-1β and initiate the passage from phase G0 to G1 of the cellular cycle. All this leads to hepatocytes proliferation. IL-1 has an essential role both in initiating some hepatic pathologic processes including inflammatory response and in hepatic regeneration [8].

In case of macrophages, that are derived from monocytes, both are essential cells in the acute and chronic liver inflammation. Their classification comprises M1 macrophages responsible for inflammation initiation, also called pro-inflammatory; and M2 macrophages known as cellular healing and immunosuppressive macrophages. M1 macrophages are implied in the chronic inflammation initiation through the pro-inflammatory cytokines: IL1, IL6 and TNF. On the other side, M2 macrophages have anti-inflammatory effects and initiate cellular healing process [9].

5.2.2 Dendritic Cells (DCs)

They are characterizing the healthy liver and they can trigger powerful stimulation of T-cells [2]. Published data support the fact that the dendritic cells are the main antigen presenting cells. They are involved in both the innate and acquired immune responses. There are three types of dendritic cells: type 1, type 2 and the plasmacytoid dendritic cells, each having a different function: type 1 dendritic cells present the antigen to T lymphocyte, type 2 dendritic cells have tolerogenic functions, and the plasmacytoid dendritic cells produce INF in viral infections [10]. Published data support the role of dendritic cells in viral infections, autoimmune diseases, hepatocellular carcinoma, and liver transplantation [1].

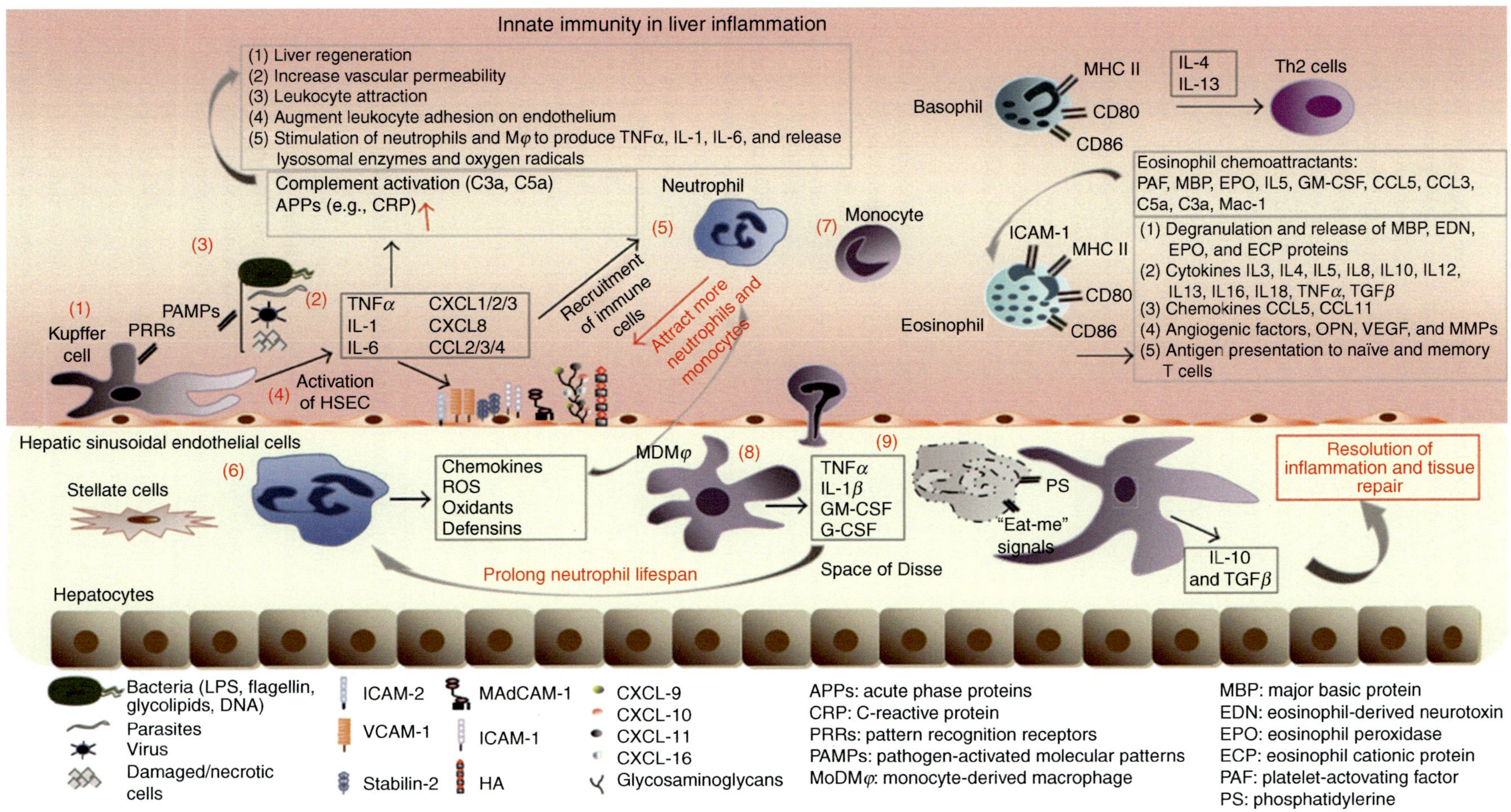

Fig. 5.1 Innate immune cells in liver inflammation. During an infectious insult in the liver (1) resident macrophages, Kupffer cells, are the first immune cells to detect the presence of invading pathogens (bacteria, parasites, viruses, damaged, and/or necrotic cells) via PRRs/PAMPs. (2) Upon activation Kupffer cells release cytokines TNFα, IL-1, and IL-6 as well as chemokines CXCL1–3, CXCL-8, CCL-2–4 that initiate (3) the acute-phase response and inflammation. Acute inflammation is characterized by the rise in plasma proteins, collectively named acute phase proteins (APPs) that include C-reactive protein (CRP) and complement components. (4) Proinflammatory cytokines released from activated Kupffer cells can activate hepatic sinusoidal endothelial cells to upregulate adhesion molecules (ICAM 1 and 2, VCAM-1, MAdCAM etc.) and in combination with the chemokines secreted from Kupffer cells can stimulate the recruitment of neutrophils and monocytes to the liver. (5) Neutrophils are the initial phagocytes to arrive at the site of microbial invasion, where (6) they change their phenotype, they become activated and release powerful and cytotoxic antimicrobial molecules such as reactive oxygen species (ROS), oxidants, defensins, as well as chemokines to attract more neutrophils and monocytes. (7) Following their recruitment to the tissue, monocytes undergo differentiation into (8) tissue macrophages (MDMϕ), which release TNFα, IL-1β, G-CSF, and GM-CSF factors that can extend the lifespan of neutrophils thus sustaining their presence at the site of inflammation. (9) In order for inflammation to be resolved, the dangerous neutrophils at the inflammatory loci undergo apoptosis and terminate the inflammatory process quickly. Apoptotic neutrophils represent an important antiinflammatory stimulus to other cells involved in there solution of inflammation by producing "eat-me" signals recognized by the surrounding phagocytes. Phosphatidylserine (PS) residues on the apoptotic neutrophil membrane allow recognition by its receptor on macrophages, which not only initiates phagocytosis but also modifies the transcriptional profile of the Macrophages, increasing the production of IL-10 and TGF-b, cytokines associated with resolution of inflammatory response and tissue repair. Basophils are short-lived cells that express MHC II and CD80/CD86 costimulatory molecules, thus are able to present antigens to CD4+ T cells promoting their differentiation into Th2 cells via release of IL-4 and IL-13. Eosinophils recruited to the liver release proinflammatory mediators including granule-stored cationic proteins, cytokines, and chemokines. They also express MHC II, CD80/CD86, CD40, and ICAM-1; thus they are able to present antigens to T cells initiating or amplifying antigenic-specific immune responses. (From [1]. **It is open access**)

5.2.3 Lymphocytes

Among lymphocytes, those belonging to innate immune response are involved in the hepatic inflammation. Innate liver lymphocytes comprise natural killer (NK) cells, NKT cells, and MAIT (mucosal associated invariant T cells) [2]. Basically, all these lymphocytes produce powerful cytokines which activate liver immunity (innate or adaptive) [2]. On the other side, healthy liver has adaptive lymphocytes such as MHC-restricted $CD4^+$ *and CD8+ T cells, and lesser B cells* [2]. Majority of the hepatic T cells are (1) apoptosing peripheral T cells; (2) moderate expression of the TCR; and (3) coexpress NK cell markers [5]. *Particularly T-cells accumulate in liver with the onset of apoptosis process* [2].

Of note, NK cells and NKT cells stand for the first line against infections and tumor growth and contribute to the development of the hepatic chronic inflammation [11]. Moreover, both NK cells and NKT cells contribute to the liver aggression either by producing pro-inflammatory cytokines or by making the hepatocytes to die [12].

NK cells or "pit cells" have an important role being involved in viral infections, liver regeneration, liver fibrosis, antitumour activity and hepatic tolerance [1]. Importantly, half of hepatic NK cells from human adult liver is formed from $CD56^{bright}$ NK cells [2]. Also, in the presence of NK cells, dendritic cells trigger tolerogenic regulatory T cells [1].

It is well demonstrated that NKT cells take part in the alcohol produced liver injury [13, 14]. By contrast, NKT cells may protect against the acute liver inflammation and damage induced by CCl_4 [15]. Nonetheless, Treg (Regulatory T cells) populations sustain the balance between activation and immuno-tolerance [5]. In fact, modulation of Treg in therapeutic methodologies is ongoing [5].

5.2.4 Mucosal-Associated Invariant T (MAIT)

MAIT cells are innate-like T cell populations; and they represent 20–50% of intrahepatic T cells [16]. These MAIT cells represent a greatly specialized T cell population with specific immunological activity in the liver vessels [5].

MAIT are involving in inflammatory and autoimmune disease. For example, they appear in a reduced number in HCV chronic infection, but they remain reduced after the virus clearance with DAA (Direct Acting Antiviral) therapy [17, 18]. In obese NASH patients, MAIT cells appear in great numbers in the adipose tissue as compared to peripheral blood. Moreover, they secret IL-17. As a fact, after the bariatric surgery, the number of circulating MAIT cell is restored in 3 months [19], while their normal function comes back in 6 months [20].

5.2.5 Leukocytes

They accumulate in liver only in the presence of inflammation and infection [2]. They release the inflammatory cytokines and growth factors that regulate the fibrotic process. These cytokines are: TNFα, IL-6, platelet derived growth factor and TGFβ. As a result, the hepatic stellate cells are activated by these cytokines and produce extracellular matrix components (α smooth muscle actin and type I collagen) [21].

The presence of neutrophils has been described in acute liver injury such as alcohol hepatitis, ischemia reperfusion injury, and sepsis [1]. As stated above, leukocytes accumulate in liver in the presence of chemotactic factors which produce their migration into liver. Only that, too much accumulation of neutrophils in liver may cause pathological pro-inflammation [1].

5.2.6 HMGB1 (High Mobility Group Box 1) Protein

It is defined as a nuclear and cytoplasmatic protein, and it is a compulsory mediator of the inflammation. It is released by necrotic liver cells [22]. Its presence as both actively and passively forms in the extracellular environment, it is observed after the hepatocyte necrosis. HMGB1 acts like cytokines, and chemokines which play an important part in the inflammation [23]. At present, HMGB1 is considered to be an essential protein both in acute and chronic liver injury. It is released from the injured hepatocytes and mediate the leucocytes attraction by connecting extracellular HMGB1 with RAGE—a high specificity receptor [24].

As to the acute inflammation, HMGB1 is involved in ischemic/reperfusion lesions, sepsis and drug-toxicity. In chronic inflammation HMGB1 is observed in alcoholic and nonalcoholic liver disease. HMGB1 is also implied in the fibrosis process and liver cancer.

5.3 Pathological Liver Inflammation

Pathological liver inflammation enhances the development of liver fibrosis into cirrhosis. Even if liver fibrosis is considered a pathological feature, it is an essential feature for liver wound repair or liver regeneration [2]. Conversely, fibrosis becomes pathological as a result of a persistent inflammation with liver damage.

By definition, pathological inflammation is the constant triggering or activation of innate immune system pathways [2]. Further, alcohol, fat, chronic infection or tissue injury cause pathological liver inflammation. But then continual inflammation in liver leads to the permanent activation of hepatic myofibroblasts produced by hepatic stellate cells [2]. Tolerogenical liver is supported by resident myeloid cells such as Kupffer cells, hepatic myeloid dendritic cells, liver sinusoidal endothelial cells (LSECs) and MDSCs (myeloid-derived suppressor cells) [2]. The anti-inflammatory cytokine IL-10 is released by Kupffer cells, dendritic cells, and MDSCs. On the other hand, hepatic tolerogenic mechanisms are lost in the presence of severe inflammation [2].

5.3.1 Cholangiocyte Immune Response

The first barrier against components translocated from the gut to liver is represented by biliary epithelial cells [25]. In healthy liver, cholangiocytes protect against gut-derived molecules or gut microbiota. Cholangiocytes present secretory, apoptotic and proliferative functions [5].

In general, they have the ability to release sIgA (secretory immunoglobulin A) that protects against microbial attachment. Importantly, these biliary cells express PRRs which are activated by PAMPs. They also attach DAMPs (damage-associated molecular patterns) discharged by damaged cells [25]. A major component of PRRs is TLRs (Toll-like receptors). When cholangiocytes are exposed to PAMPs, it happens the activation of TLR4, that finally activate genes of pro-inflammatory cytokines such as AP-1 (activator protein-1) and Nf-kB (nuclear factor-kappa B) [25]. As a result, cholangiocytes secrete cytokines and chemokines with the activation of resident liver cells and immune cells (Fig. 5.2) [25].

Initial injury activates cholangiocytes into "reactive cholangiocytes" or "biliary epithelitis" to release IL-6 with proliferation of cholangiocytes [25]. These reactive cholangiocytes secrete pro-inflammatory and fibrogenic mediators. On the other hand, chronic biliary injury is associated with fibrogenesis (periportal fibrosis) and ductopenia [25]. Particularly, cytokine TGFβ inhibits the proliferation of cholangiocytes with loss of biliary ducts or ductopenia [25]. To sum up, "biliary epithelitis" is a finding of PBC (primary biliary cirrhosis) and PSC (primary sclerosing cholangites) [5].

5.3.2 Steatosis and Steatohepatitis

Nowadays, the commonest liver disorder is NAFLD (non-alcoholic fatty liver disease) [26]. Briefly, its evolution is characterized by liver ***inflammation***, ***steatosis*** to non-alcoholic ***steatohepatitis*** (NASH), cirrhosis and hepatocellular carcinoma [26, 27]. It is already established that liver steatosis is a marker of insulin resistance and metabolic syndrome [7].

Importantly, liver ***inflammation*** triggers the stress response in hepatocytes with further lipid addition [28]. According to this logic, hepatic steatosis may be "bystander phenomenon" secondary to inflammation [28]. However, **liver steatosis** may be a benign process or may further develop along with the stimulation of inflammation. As a result, liver inflammation is set up by resident Kupffer cells and innate immune cells such as infiltrating macrophages, T lymphocytes, neutrophils, and dendritic cells [7]. Moreover, steatosis continues with inflammation [29].

Hepatosteatosis or **steatosis** is the main histological feature in NAFLD (nonalcoholic fatty liver disease) and describes the excessive storage of triglycerides within hepatocytes [26]. The minimum criterion for the histological diagnosis of NAFLD is the existence of >5% hepatocytes with steatosis or "steatotic hepatocytes" (Fig. 5.3) [26, 30].

Usually, NAFLD has a ***macrovesicular steatosis*** that describes the hepatocyte uploaded with one/many intracytoplasmatic fat droplets with its nucleus located to the cell periphery [26]. Furthermore, this macrovesicular steatosis has a panacinar or zone 3 distribution [31].

Macrovesicular steatosis is a histological finding in excessive alcohol consumption, parenteral nutrition, starvation, hepatitis C (genotype 3), Wilson's disease, lipodystrophy, abetalipoproteinemia, and medication (amiodarone, methotrexate, tamoxifen, corticosteroids) [26]. On the other hand, ***microvesicular steatosis*** is a histological finding in Reye's syndrome, of medications (valproate, and anti-retroviral medicines), acute fatty liver of pregnancy and for inborn errors of metabolism (LCAT deficiency, cholesterol ester storage disease, Wolman disease) [26].

Importantly, nonalcoholic fatty liver disease usually presents the commonest form of histological steatohepatitis at liver biopsy, that it is a zone 3 borderline steatohepatitis [26]. It comprises inflammation, steatosis, ballooned hepatocytes frequently with Mallory-Denk bodies, with or without fibrosis [26]. If is of note, children have zone 1-borderline pattern that defines a steatohepatitis with portal inflammation, zone 1 steatosis, sometimes zone 1-ballooned hepatocytes, and portal fibrosis [26].

In general, ***steatohepatitis*** is a marker of liver injury. And portal inflammation, liver distribution of steatosis, Mallory bodies (Mallory-Denk Bodies), and megamitochondria are correlated with steatohepatitis [26].

Non-alcoholic **steatohepatitis** (NASH) is described by *inflammation with macrovesicular steatosis and apoptosis, with or without fibrosis* [28]. On the other side, hepatocyte ballooning or **ballooning injury** is a key marker for non-alcoholic steatohepatitis (Fig. 5.4) [32–34].

Hepatocellular ballooning or "ballooned hepatocytes" are a marker of lipotoxic liver damage [35]. It is a key marker used in the diagnosis of NAFLD and NASH by liver biopsy [35].

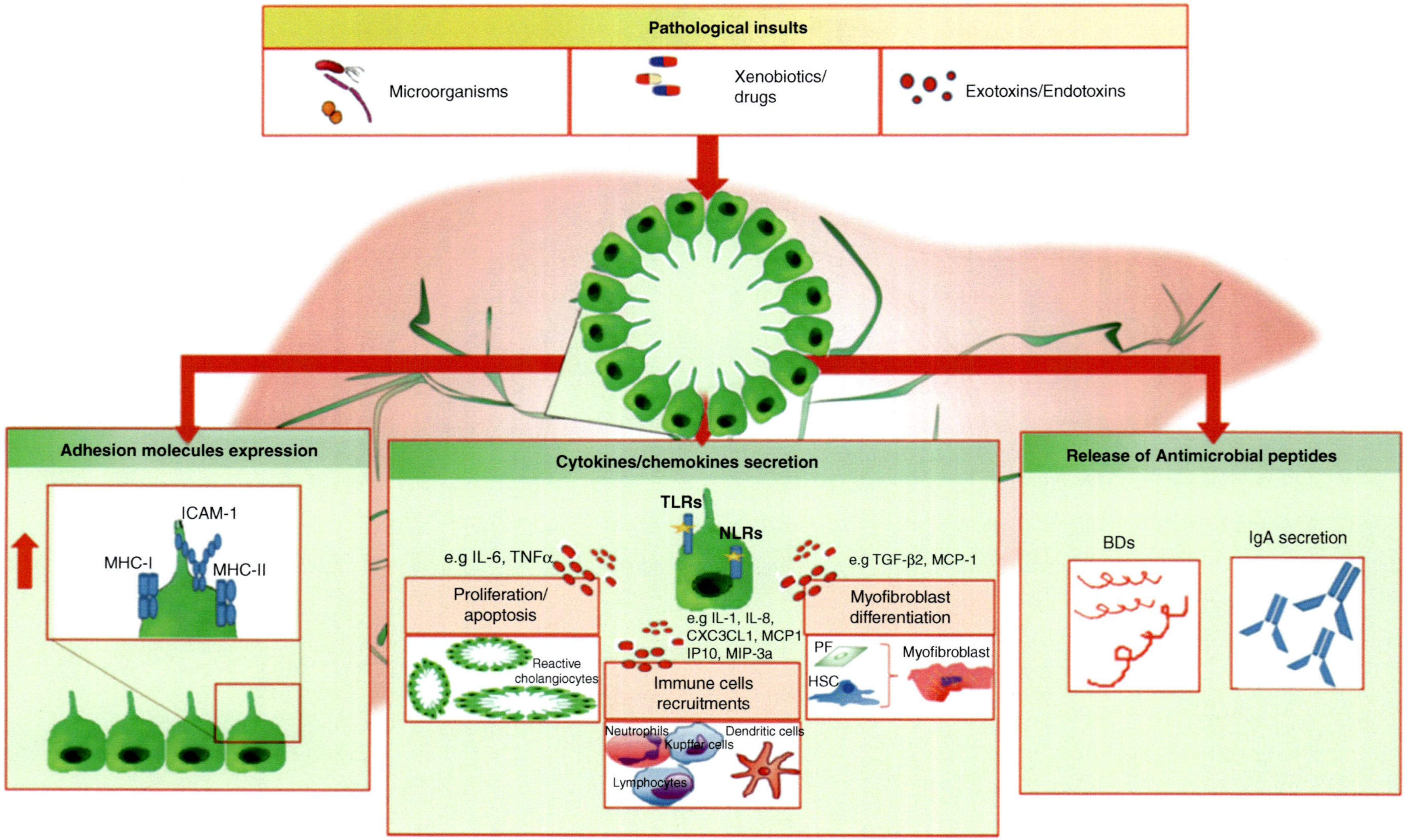

Fig. 5.2 Cholangiocyte immune response. Biliary epithelial cells are exposed to different dangerous stimuli such as microorganisms, drugs or toxins, and others exotoxins/endotoxins which trigger tissue damage. In this setting, cholangiocytes may modify their biology and phenotype by increasing the release of proinflammatory mediators (e.g., IL-6, IL-8, IL-1), which act in autocrine/paracrine fashion on both resident and non-resident cells, by upregulating the expression of surface proteins (i.e., MHC-I, MHC-II and ICAM-1) and by releasing antimicrobial molecules such as beta-defensins (BDs) or IgA following epithelial transcytosis. These events lead to ductules' proliferation, immune cells chemotaxis and myofibroblast differentiation. In case of persistent biliary damage, these processes could lead to chronic inflammation and fibrosis establishment. *PF* portal fibroblast, *HSC* hepatic stellate cell. (From [25]. **It is open access**. This is an **open access article** distributed under the Creative Commons Attribution License which permits unrestricted use, distribution, and reproduction in any medium, provided the original work is properly cited (CC BY 4.0))

Ballooned hepatocyte is the undead degenerated hepatocyte with hepatocyte swelling, reticulated cytoplasm, central nucleus, hepatocyte polarity is dysregulated, and ubiquitination of proteins with further decreasing of keratin 8 and keratin 18 (Fig. 5.5) [33, 35].

Hepatocyte ballooning is a process linked with the activation of "hedgehog signaling pathway" [35]. This Hedgehog pathway is crucial for hepatic repair and regeneration but its chronic activation causes liver fibrosis [35]. Mallory-Denk bodies are another histological feature of NASH, and represent ubiquitinated proteins [35]. In fact, apoptosis is triggered in liver by Mallory bodies and hepatocyte ballooning [26]. Mallory bodies have a prognostic role in ***steatohepatitis***, and are importantly correlated with liver mortality [26, 36, 37].

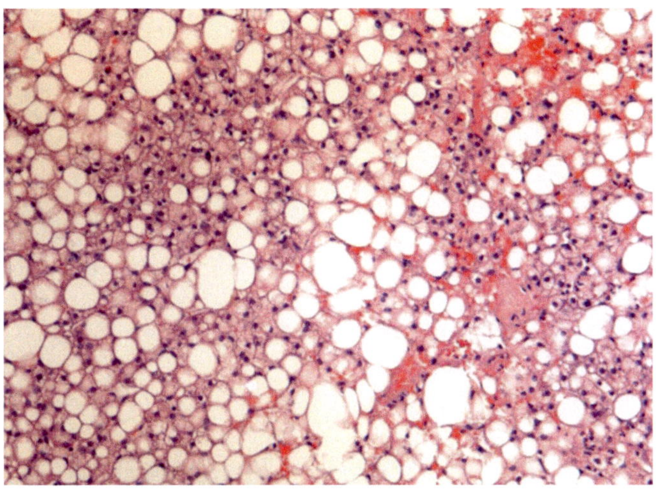

Fig. 5.3 Steatosis. Hematoxylin-eosin stain [30]. (**It is open access**)

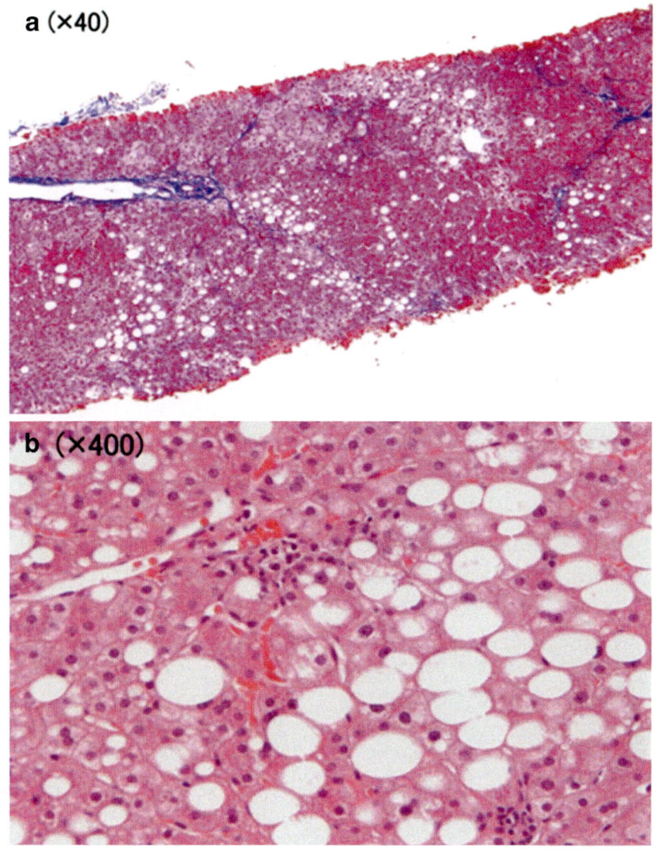

Fig. 5.5 Liver biopsy. (**a**) Moderate fibrosis was observed in the low-power field (Azan-Mallory stain, ×40). (**b**) Higher magnification showed hepatic steatosis, hepatocyte ballooning, and polymorphonuclear cell inflammation (HE staining, ×400). (From [33]. **It is open access**. This is an open access article under the terms of the http://creativecommons.org/licenses/by/4.0/ License, which permits use, distribution and reproduction in any medium, provided the original work is properly cited)

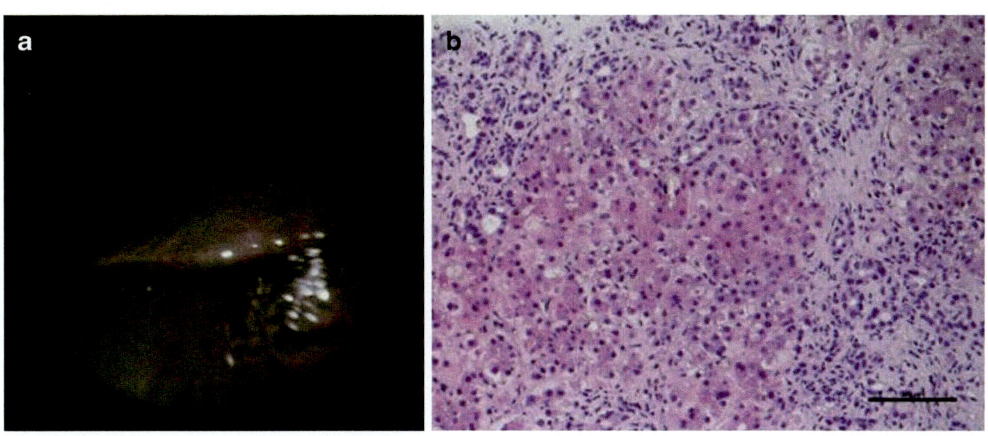

Fig. 5.4 (**a**) Mini-laparoscopy showing the right liver lobe with cholestatic changes of the parenchyma, regenerative nodules, and capsular fibrosis. (**b**) Liver biopsy (HE, ×200) showing cholestasis, **hepatocyte ballooning**, ductular proliferation, and increasing fibrosis [34]. [**Open Access** . This article is distributed under the terms of the Creative Commons Attribution 4.0 International License (http://creativecommons.org/licenses/by/4.0/), which permits unrestricted use, distribution, and reproduction in any medium, provided you give appropriate credit to the original author(s) and the source, provide a link to the Creative Commons license, and indicate if changes were made. The Creative Commons Public Domain Dedication waiver (http://creativecommons.org/publicdomain/zero/1.0/) applies to the data made available in this article, unless otherwise stated]

5.3.3 Inflammation in NASH

It is characterized by powerful recruitment of neutrophils, monocytes and monocyte-derived macrophages and NK cells (Fig. 5.6) [35]. Furthermore, Fig. 5.7 shows "satelitosis" defined as the liver infiltration with neutrophils (polymorphs) in the vicinity of ballooned hepatocytes [26].

In fact, any type of steatohepatitis has hepatic neutrophil infiltration being higher in alcoholic steatohepatitis [35]. Characteristically, the chemokine receptors of monocytes such as C-C chemokine receptor (CCR)2 and CXCR3 are triggering monocytes with their activation and liver infiltration [35]. Also, in case of NASH, resident Kupffer cells eliminate by phagocytosis the dead cells, eliminate pathogens and their products; release proinflammatory cytokines (TNF, chemokines such as CXCL10 and IL-8) and trigger further liver inflammation and fibrosis by the continual ongoing and recruitment of immune cells in liver [35].

5.3.4 Metaflammation

It is defined as the low-grade inflammation caused by gradually expression of cytokines and the infiltration with immune cells [27]. This metaflammation is described for white adipose tissue, liver, pancreas and gut cells. Basically, adipocytes release TNFα, MCP1 (Macrophage Chemoattractant Protein 1) also known as CCL2 (CC-motif Chemokine Ligand 2), IL6 and IL18. Correspondingly adipocytes secrete adipokines such as adiponectin, leptin and resistin. Leptin is a pro-inflammatory adipokine that regulates food intake through the central nervous system [27].

In ***overnutrition***, adipocytes release pro-inflammatory cytokines such as IL15, CCL2, CCL3, CCL4, CXL10, with the activation of innate and adaptive immune cells. Monocytes turn into M1 macrophages with final release of TNFα, IL6, iNOS, IFNγ, and IgGs (Fig. 5.8b). Recruitment of NK cells by adipocytes it is followed by increased secre-

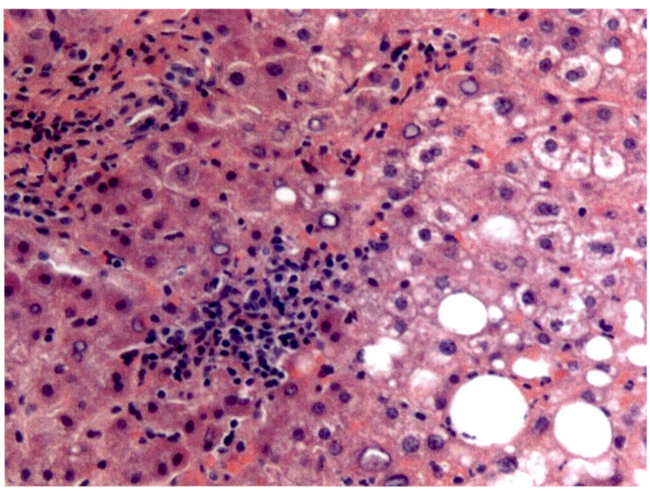

Fig. 5.6 Mononuclear inflammatory infiltration. Hematoxylin-eosin stain. (From [26]. **It is open access**)

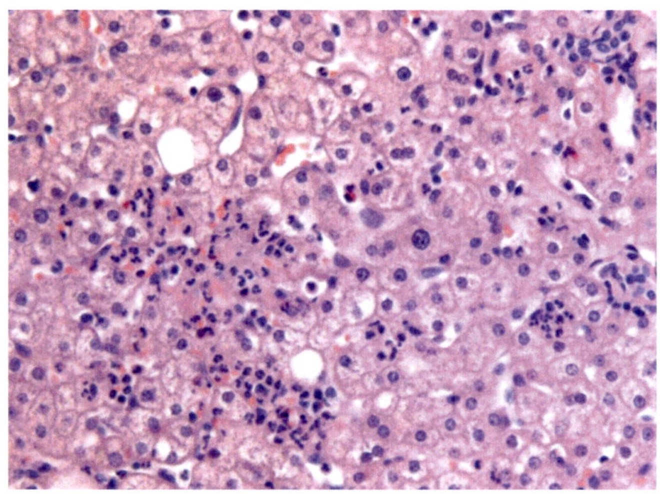

Fig. 5.7 Polymorph around ballooned hepatocytes, "satelitosis". (From [26]. **It is open access**)

Fig. 5.8 Liver-adipose tissue cross-talk in lean and overnutrition state. (**a**) Lean state. Insulin signaling in the liver induces phosphorylation of the protein kinase AKT. AKT-dependent downregulation of forkhead box (Foxo) transcription factor reduces the transcription of gluconeogenic genes, such as PhosphoEnolPyruvate CarboxyKinase (PEPCK), and hepatic glucose production (HGP). AKT-dependent upregulation of the mammalian target of rapamycin complex (mTORC) upregulates Sterol Regulatory Element-Binding Protein 1c (SREBP1c) thus inducing de novo lipogenesis (DNL) and triglyceride (TG) synthesis. DNL inhibits both the transport of fatty acids in the mitochondria via carnitine palmitoyl transferase carrier (CPT) and the β-oxidation (β-ox), which is controlled by peroxisome proliferator-activated receptors α (PPARα). Hepatic TGs are secreted in the circulation in form of very low-density lipoproteins (VLDLs) to reach muscle and adipose tissue where they are taken up, through the action of CD36 and lipoprotein lipase (LPL). In adipose tissue, insulin inhibits the release of nonesterified fatty acids (NEFAs). (**b**) Overnutrition. In obesity, hepatic DNL and HGP are both active. PPARγ is upregulated in hepatosteatosis, further inducing DNL and hepatic TG content. Amino acids (AA) derived from the diet influence mTORC/S6 kinase (S6K) pathway that, through an intertissue connection, affects LPL activity in the adipose tissue and thus increases circulating TGs. Hepatic VLDL secretion increases, but their uptake by adipose tissue is reduced because of the low expression of CD36 and LPL. Conversely, CD36 and LPL are more expressed in muscles and liver that therefore internalize more VLDLs. HGP upregulation is due to different processes: (a) lower utilization of glucose due to reduced glucokinase (GCK) activity, (b) increased adipose tissue lipolysis due to insulin resistance and consequent increase in the releasing of NEFAs in the circulation. Hepatic acetyl-CoA content and pyruvate carboxylase (PC) activity increase, with consequent higher transformation of pyruvate into glucose. In obesity, both liver and adipose tissue undergo an inflammatory response with production of proinflammatory cytokines: interleukin 6 (IL6), tumor necrosis factor alpha (TNF-α), C-reactive protein (CRP), plasminogen activator inhibitor 1 (PAI-1). (From [27] with **permission**)

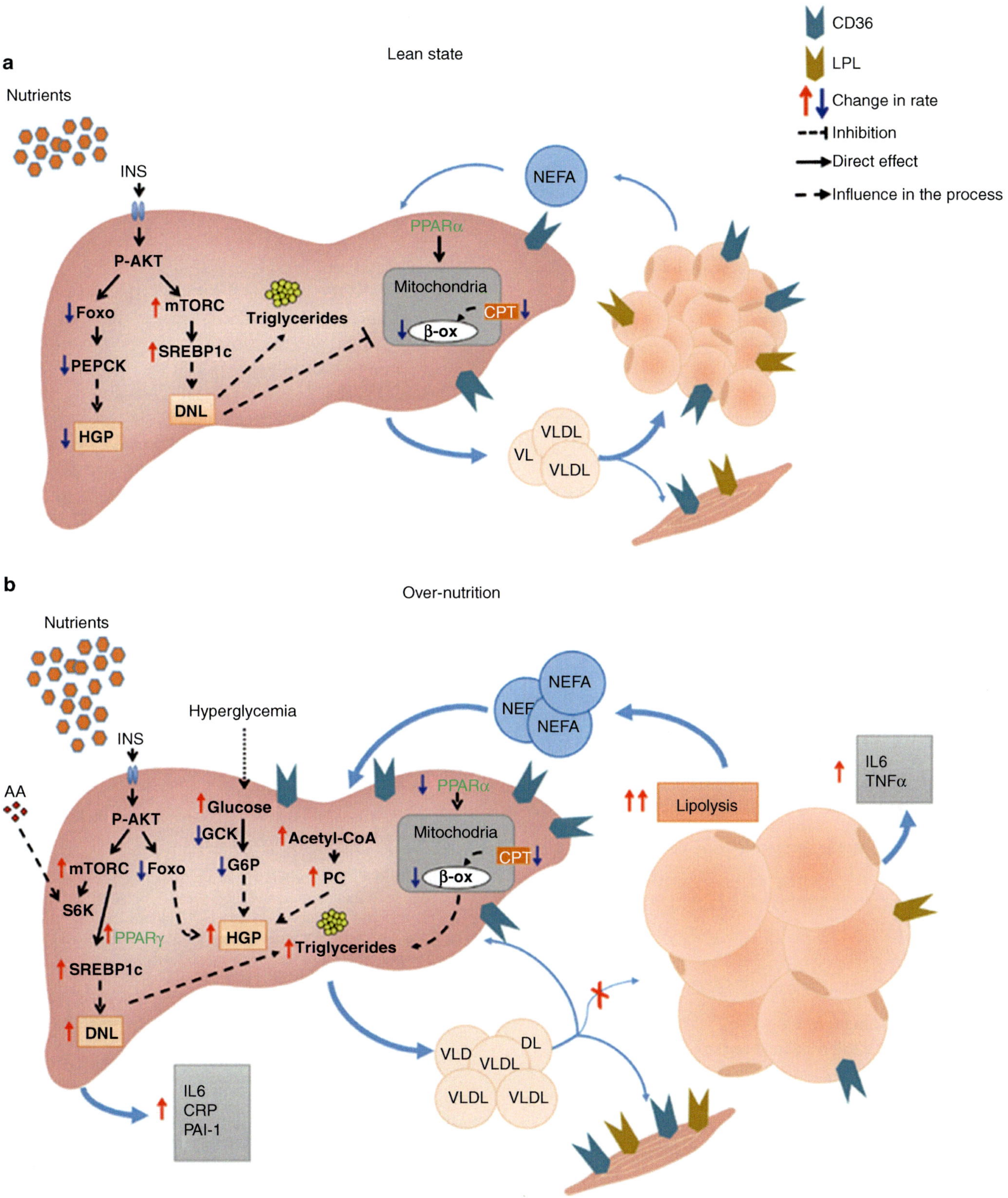
CD36
LPL
Change in rate
Inhibition
Direct effect
Influence in the process
a
Lean state
Nutrients
INS
P-AKT
Foxo
mTORC
PEPCK
SREBP1c
HGP
DNL
Triglycerides
PPARα
Mitochondria
CPT
β-ox
NEFA
VLDL
VL
VLDL
b
Over-nutrition
Nutrients
INS
AA
Hyperglycemia
P-AKT
mTORC
Foxo
S6K
PPARγ
SREBP1c
DNL
Glucose
GCK
G6P
HGP
Acetyl-CoA
PC
Triglycerides
PPARα
Mitochondria
CPT
β-ox
NEFA
NEF
NEFA
Lipolysis
IL6
TNFα
IL6
CRP
PAI-1
VLD
DL
VLDL
VLDL
VLDL

tion of leptin. The final outcome is worsening of inflammation because leptin activate CD4+ cells [27].

Conversely, ***fasting*** is defined by glycogenolysis, gluconeogenesis, and increased release of FFAs by lipolysis of adipose tissue (Fig. 5.8a). If it is of note, the key factor in fasting is PPARα (peroxisome proliferator—activated receptors) that is a "lipid sensor". The nuclear receptor PPARα regulates liver for the duration of fasting, including mitochondrial β-oxidation and peroxisomal β-oxidation. As a result, fasting is correlated with raised afflux of FFAs to the liver by lipolysis, along with inhibited activity of LPL [27].

5.4 Conclusions

It is now well accepted that liver is a lymphoid organ with complex immunological mechanisms which assure a vital balance between immune tolerance and overreaction [5].

In healthy liver, inflammatory mechanisms have a broad spectrum of functions being vital to maintain a balanced tissue and organ homeostasis [2]. The molecular mechanisms of the hepatic inflammation are involved in the maintenance of the liver homeostasis, by protecting the liver against pathogen agents (viral infections, tumors, alcohol and drug toxicity). Even if liver fibrosis is considered a pathological feature, it is an essential feature for liver wound repair or liver regeneration. Conversely, fibrosis becomes pathological as a result of a persistent inflammation with liver damage. On the other hand, hepatic tolerogenic mechanisms are lost in the presence of severe inflammation [2].

Conflicts of Interest The authors declare no conflict of interest.

Self Study

Questions

1. **Which statement is true?**
   (a) Liver is a tolerogenical organ
   (b) Liver resident immune cells are represented only by Kupffer cells.
   (c) Macrophages are myeloid cells.
   (d) M2 macrophages have anti-inflammatory effects and initiate cellular healing process.
2. **Which statement/statements is/are true?**
   (a) Pathological liver inflammation enhances the development of liver fibrosis into cirrhosis.
   (b) Cholangiocytes present secretory, apoptotic and proliferative functions.
   (c) The spectrum of NAFLD (nonalcoholic fatty liver disease) is characterized by liver inflammation, steatosis to non-alcoholic steatohepatitis (NASH), cirrhosis and hepatocellular carcinoma.
   (d) Hepatosteatosis or steatosis is the main histological feature in NAFLD (nonalcoholic fatty liver disease).

Answers

1. **Which statement is true?**
   (a) **CORRECT**. Human liver has specific immune mechanisms of tolerance because it is primarily exposed to gut microbiome, dietary products and environmental antigens.
   (b) **INCORRECT**. Liver resident immune cells are represented by Kupffer cells, dendritic cells, and resident lymphocytes and are represented by B cells, CD4+ T cells, CD8+ T cells, natural Killer (NK) cells and non-conventional lymphoid cells such as NK T cells, gamma delta TCR+ T cells, CD4-CD8- T cells.
   (c) **Correct**.
   (d) **Correct**.
2. **Which statement/statements is/are true?**
   (a) **CORRECT**.
   (b) **CORRECT**.
   (c) **CORRECT**.
   (d) **CORRECT**.

References

1. Liaskou E, Wilson DV, Oo YH. Innate immune cells in liver inflammation. Mediat Inflamm. 2012;2012:949157,. 21 pages. https://doi.org/10.1155/2012/949157.
2. Robinson MW, Harmon C, O'Farrelly C. Liver immunology and its role in inflammation and homeostasis. Cell Mol Immunol. 2016;13(3):267–76. https://doi.org/10.1038/cmi.2016.3.
3. Pellicoro A, Ramachandran P, Iredale JP, Fallowfield JA. Liver fibrosis and repair: immune regulation of wound healing in a solid organ. Nat Rev Immunol. 2014;14:181–94.
4. Bourbonnais E, Raymond V-A, Ethier C, Nguyen BN, El-Leil MS, Meloche S, et al. Liver fibrosis protects mice from acute hepatocellular injury. Gastroenterology. 2012;142:130–9.
5. Invernizzi P. Liver auto-immunology: the paradox of autoimmunity in a tolerogenic organ. J Autoimmun. 2013 Oct;46:1–6. https://doi.org/10.1016/j.jaut.2013.08.006.
6. Gomez Perdiguero E, et al. Tissue-resident macrophages originate from yolk-sac-derived erythro-myeloid progenitors. Nature. 2015;518(7540):547–51.
7. Koyama Y, Brenner D. Liver inflammation and fibrosis. J Clin Invest. 2017;127(1):55–64.
8. Tau Q, Hu J, Yu X, Lu H, Yu Y, Yu Y, Zang G, Tang Z. The role of IL-1 family members and Kupffer cells in liver regeneration. Biomed Res Int. 2016;2016(1):1–6.
9. Zhang F, Wang H, Wang X, Jiang G, Liu H, Zhang G, Wang H, Fang R, Bu X, Cai S, Du J. TGF-β induces M2-like macrophage polariza-

tion via SNAIL-mediated suppression of a pro-inflammatory phenotype. Oncotarget. 2016;7(32):52294–306.
10. Kayama Y, Brenner D. Liver inflammation and fibrosis. J ClinInvest. 2017;127(1):55–64.
11. Gao B, Radaeva S, Park O. Liver natural killer and natural killer T cells: immunobiology and emerging roles in liver disease. J Leukoc Biol. 2009;86(3):513–28.
12. Wang H, Yin S. Natural killer T cells in liver injury, inflammation and cancer. Expert Rev Gastroenterol Hepatol. 2015;9(8):1077–85.
13. Minagawa M, Deng Q, Liu ZX, Tsukamoto H, Dennert G. Activated natural killer T cells induce liver injury by Fas and tumor necrosis factor-alpha during alcohol consumption. Gastroenterology. 2004;126(5):1387–99.
14. Jaruga B, Hong F, Kim WH, Sun R, Fan S, Gao B. Chronic alcohol consumption accelerates liver injury in T cell-mediated hepatitis: alcohol disregulation of NF-kappaB and STAT3 signaling pathways. Am J Physiol Gastrointest Liver Physiol. 2004;287(2):G471–9.
15. Park O, Wang L, Jeong W, Wang H, Lian Z, Gershwin M, Gao B. Diverse roles of invariant natural killer T cells in liver injury and fibrosis induced by carbon tetrachloride. Hepatology. 2009;49:1683–94.
16. Dusseaux M, Martin E, Serriari N, Péguillet I, Premel V, Louis D, Milder M, Le Bourhis L, Soudais C, Treiner E, Lantz O. Human MAIT cells are xenobiotic-resistant, tissue-targeted, CD161hi IL-17-secreting T cells. Blood. 2011;117(4):1250–9.
17. van Wilgenburg B, Scherwitzl I, Hutchinson EC, Leng T, Kurioka A, Kulicke C, et al. MAIT cells are activated during human viral infections. Nat Commun. 2016;7(11653):20.
18. Hengst J, Strunz B, Deterding K, Ljunggren H-G, Leeansyah E, Manns MP, et al. Nonreversible MAIT cell-dysfunction in chronic hepatitis C virus infection despite successful interferon-free therapy. Eur J Immunol. 2016;46(9):2204–1.
19. Magalhaes I, Pingris K, Poitou C, Bessoles S, Venteclef N, Kiaf B, Beaudoin L. Mucosal-associated invariant T cell alterations in obese and type 2 diabetic patients. J Clin Invest. 2015;125:1752–62.
20. Kurioka A, Walker LJ, Klenerman P, Willberg CB. MAIT cells: new guardians of the liver. Clin Transl Immunol. 2016;5(8):e98.
21. Hellerbrand C, Stefanovic B, Giordano F, Burchardt ER, Brenner DA. The role of TGFbeta1 in initiating hepatic stellate cell activation in vivo. J Hepatol. 1999;30:77–87.
22. Jaeschke H. Mechanisms of liver injury. II. Mechanisms of neutrophil-induced liver cell injury during hepatic ischemia-reperfusion and other acute inflammatory conditions. Am J Physiol Gastrointest Liver Physiol. 2006;290(6):G1083–8. https://doi.org/10.1152/ajpgi.00568.2005.
23. Yang H, Wang H, Chavan SS, Andersson V. High Mobility Group Box Protein1 (HMGB1): the prototypical endogenous danger molecule. Mol Med. 2015;21(Suppl 1):S6–S12.
24. Huebener P, et al. The HMGB1/RAGE axis triggers neutrophil-mediated injury amplification following necrosis. J Clin Invest. 2015;125(2):539–50.
25. Giordano DM, Pinto C, Maroni L, Benedetti A, Marzioni M. Inflammation and the gut-liver axis in the pathophysiology of cholangiopathies. Int J Mol Sci. 2018;19(10):3003. https://doi.org/10.3390/ijms1910300.
26. Cabezas J, Mayorga M, Crespo J (2012). Nonalcoholic fatty liver disease: a pathological view, liver biopsy, Nobumi Tagaya, IntechOpen. https://doi.org/10.5772/52622. Available from: https://www.intechopen.com/books/liver-biopsy-indications-procedures-results/nonalcoholic-fatty-liver-disease-a-pathological-view.
27. Caputo T, Gilardi F, Desvergne B. From chronic overnutrition to metaflammation and insulin resistance: adipose tissue and liver contributions. FEBS Lett. 2017;591(19):3061–88. https://doi.org/10.1002/1873-3468.12742.
28. Parkash O, Saeed S (2018). Molecular basis for pathogenesis of steatohepatitis: contemporary understanding and new insights, nonalcoholic fatty liver disease, Rodrigo Valenzuela, IntechOpen. https://doi.org/10.5772/intechopen.71405. Available from: https://www.intechopen.com/books/non-alcoholic-fatty-liver-disease-molecular-bases-prevention-and-treatment/molecular-basis-for-pathogenesis-of-steatohepatitis-contemporary-understanding-and-new-insights.
29. Tilg H, Moschen AR. Evolution of inflammation in nonalcoholic fatty liver disease: the multiple parallel hits hypothesis. Hepatology. 2010;52(5):1836–46.
30. Kleiner DE, Brunt EM, Van Natta M, Behling C, Contos MJ, Cummings OW, et al. Design and validation of a histological scoring system for nonalcoholic fatty liver disease. Hepatology. 2005;41(6):1313–21.
31. Chalasani N, Wilson L, Kleiner DE, Cummings OW, Brunt EM, Unalp A. Relationship of steatosis grade and zonal location to histological features of steatohepatitis in adult patients with non-alcoholic fatty liver disease. J Hepatol. 2008;48(5):829–34.
32. Malhi H, Gores GJ, Lemasters JJ. Apoptosis and necrosis in the liver: a tale of two deaths? Hepatology. 2006;43(2 Suppl 1): S31–44.
33. Minohara S, Bae SK, Sugiyama S, Shibata N, Gushima T, Motoshita J, Shimoda S, Takagi A, Ikeda Y, Takahashi K. A case of non-alcoholic steatohepatitis complicated with severe acute pancreatitis induced by decreased lipoprotein lipase and hepatic triglyceride lipase activity levels in a young Japanese woman. Clin Case Rep. 2018;6(9):1769–73. https://doi.org/10.1002/ccr3.1706.
34. Buechter M, Gerken G, Hoyer DP, Bertram S, Theysohn JM, Thodou V, Kahraman A. Liver maximum capacity (LiMAx) test as a helpful prognostic tool in acute liver failure with sepsis: a case report. BMC Anesthesiol. 2018;18(1):71. https://doi.org/10.1186/s12871-018-0538-0.
35. Ibrahim SH, Hirsova P, Gores GJ. Non-alcoholic steatohepatitis pathogenesis: sublethal hepatocyte injury as a driver of liver inflammation. Gut. 2018;67(5):963–72. https://doi.org/10.1136/gutjnl-2017-315691.
36. Matteoni CA, Younossi ZM, Gramlich T, Boparai N, Liu YC, McCullough AJ. Nonalcoholic fatty liver disease: a spectrum of clinical and pathological severity. Gastroenterology. 1999;116(6):1413–9.
37. Younossi ZM, Stepanova M, Rafiq N, Makhlouf H, Younoszai Z, Agrawal R, et al. Pathologic criteria for nonalcoholic steatohepatitis: interprotocol agreement and ability to predict liver-related mortality. Hepatology. 2011;53(6):1874–82.

Molecular Basis of Fibrogenesis and Angiogenesis During Chronic Liver Disease: Impact of TGF-β and VEGF on Pathogenic Pathways

6

Shinya Mizuno and Eriko Osaki

Key Concepts

- TGF-β plays multiple roles in establishing liver cirrhosis through inducing hepatocyte apoptosis and differentiation of liver cells to myofibroblasts for the efficient collagenous deposition.
- Recent studies delineated that VEGF-induced pathogenic angiogenesis is associated with TGF-β-conducted cirrhotic lesions.
- With regard to this, TGF-β-induced endothelin-1 is responsible for hypoxia and VEGF induction, whereas VEGF activates latent form of TGF-β, hence indicating a crosstalk between TGF-β-induced fibrogenesis and VEGF-induced angiogenesis.
- Not only TGF-β-antagonism but also anti-angiogenic treatments can be a reasonable strategy to delay or arrest the progression of liver cirrhosis, a common final feature of chronic liver disease.

6.1 Introduction

Chronic liver disease (CLD) is a comprehensive terminology that includes persistent hepatitis, induced by hepatitis viruses such as HBV and HCV, alcoholic and non-alcoholic steatohepatitis, biliary atresia and so on. Regardless of the initial causes, liver cirrhosis (LC) is a common hallmark of CLD and is characterized by the progressive loss of functional hepatocytes [1]. The defection of parenchymal area is replaced with the interstitial deposition of extracellular matrix (ECM) proteins, such as type-I and type-III collagens. In other words, impairment of hepatocyte repair system allows for unfavorable response of collagen deposition, and it takes longer than 10 years for injured livers to acquire the LC-like phenotypes, and LC is believed to be a precancerous lesion leading to the progression of hepatocellular carcinoma. The cancer-associated fibroblasts are associated with LC lesions [2], such as hepatocyte loss, epithelial-to-mesenchymal transition (EMT) and ECM overproduction. Thus, it is important to elucidate the molecular mechanism of LC during CLD progression.

Transforming growth factor-β (TGF-β) is one of the most important cytokines for the onset and progression of LC [3]. TGF-β secreted from Kupffer cells (KCs) converts sinusoidal cells, such as hepatic stellate cells (HSCs) and endothelial cells (ECs), to smooth muscle cell (SMC)-like myofibroblasts (MyoFBs). TGF-β is also important to induce ECM production in interstitial MyoFBs [3]. Several lines of clinical studies indicate an increase in blood and hepatic TGF-β levels of LC patients [4]. Of note, liver-specific activation of TGF-β transgene induces the LC-like lesions in mice [5]. Indeed, TGF-β is involved in multiple pathological steps, such as hepatocyte apoptosis, EMT, MyoFB conversion and ECM overproduction [3]. The studies of twentieth century identified TGF-β as a pivotal player for LC during CLD.

Recent emerging evidence indicates the important role of pathogenic angiogenesis during CLD [6]. Portal hypertension is, in part, a result of persistent fibrosis, and is responsible for intrahepatic and extrahepatic angiogenesis that cause LC-associated complications, such as esophageal varices [7]. TGF-β (and its inducer, angiotensin-II) may induce hepatic hypoxia via recruiting vasoconstrictors, such as

S. Mizuno (✉)
Department of Zoology, Faculty of Science, Okayama University of Science, Okayama, Japan

Department of Microbiology and Immunology, Osaka University Graduate School of Medicine, Suita, Japan

E. Osaki
Department of Microbiology and Immunology, Osaka University Graduate School of Medicine, Suita, Japan

F. Radu-Ionita et al. (eds.), *Liver Diseases*, https://doi.org/10.1007/978-3-030-24432-3_6

endothelins. Under such a pathological circuit, vascular endothelial growth factor (VEGF) is upregulated, possibly as an adaptation to hypoxia, but VEGF-induced angiogenesis results in permeability and subsequent inflammation. With regard to this, Sakata et al. delineated a novel role of VEGF in facilitating TGF-β activation [8], hence suggesting a feedback loop between angiogenesis and fibrogenesis.

In this chapter, we will discuss the potential linkage of angiogenesis to fibrogenesis, with a special focus on TGF-β and VEGF as fibrogenic and angiogenic cytokine, respectively. Indeed, TGF-β and VEGF cooperatively contribute to progression of LC, a common final outcome of CLDs. Antagonism of this cooperative pathway may open up a new avenue for arresting the progression of LC (and carcinoma) during CLDs.

6.2 Biology of TGF-β Signaling Pathway

TGF-β is a unique cytokine that elicits a multiple function required for controlling cellular growth and ECM homeostasis (see, Sects. 6.3 and 6.4). In the injured livers, TGF-β is secreted from hepatocytes and interstitial cells (including HSCs, KCs and macrophages) [9]. The transcriptional regulators, such as AP1 and Sp1, play a critical role in activating the TGF-β gene promoter region, as described in Sect. 6.4. The epigenetic histone methylation regulates TGF-β gene expression, and the increased levels of active chromatin marks (such as H3K4me1, H3K4me2 and H3K4me3) and decreased levels of repressive marks (including H3K9me2 and H3K9me3) participate in TGF-β mRNA expression during LC [10], possibly via the concerted activation of a transcriptional modulator, MKL [11].

The latent form of TGF-β is bound for inhibitory anchors, such as LAP and LTBP1, and is enzymatically activated by thrombospondin-1 or plasma kallikrein [12]. In this process, $\alpha_v\beta_1$, $\alpha_v\beta_3$, $\alpha_v\beta_5$ and $\alpha_v\beta_6$-integrins are involved in the cleavage of LAP-TGF-β at cell surfaces. Interestingly, $\alpha_v\beta_6$ antagonist inhibited the TGF-β activation in a mouse model of LC, induced by bile duct ligation (BDL) [13], suggesting a pivotal role of this integrin in TGF-β activation during CLD. Thrombospondin-1 binds to PAR-1 receptor for intracellular Rho→ROCK activation, and such a small-G protein-derived cascade is necessary for α_v-type integrins to activate the latent form TGF-β [14]. Plasma kallikrein is known to activate pro-urokinase and enhance urokinase type plasminogen activator production [15]. This effect is also contributable for TGF-β activation, especially after VEGF induction [8] (see, Sect. 6.7).

After cleavage of the LAP-bound latent form, TGF-β induces biological functions via two types of receptors. The type-II receptor, TβR-II is a ligand-trapping receptor, while type-I receptor, TβR-I (also known as ALK5) acts as a signaling transduction receptor. Once TGF-β binds to TβR-II, ALK5/serine- and threonine-type receptor is recruited to ligand-TβR-II complex. Immediately after the ALK5 phosphorylation, ALK5-targeted downstream effectors, such as Smad2 and Smad3, are also phosphorylated and moved into nucleus (i.e., canonical pathway) [3]. As a result, phosphorylated Smad3 acts like a transcriptional switch for initiating mRNA synthesis of TGF-β-targeted genes, such as NOX4. Noncanonical pathway is also important for TGF-β-mediated fibrotic events. Actually, JAK1-STAT3 and ERK activation are necessary for the induction of connective tissue growth factor (CTGF) [16] and Sp1-mediated activation of HSCs, including MyoFB conversion and ECM production [17]. Both canonical and noncanonical cascades additively contribute to the acceleration of LC [3].

The sequential crosstalk among liver cells is important for LC during chronic hepatitis. For instance, hepatocyte-derived Activin-A elicits TGF-β production in KCs via a paracrine loop, and then HSCs are differentiated to MyoFBs for the efficient production of ECMs [18]. Oncostatin-M promotes TGF-β production in hepatic macrophages and induces tissue inhibitor of metalloproteinase-1 (TIMP1) in HSCs, and both activities are necessary for LC progression through accelerating ECM synthesis and inhibiting its degradation [19]. HSCs highly express toll-like receptor-4 (TLR4), and bacterial components, such as LPS, stimulate TLR4, resulting in the secretion of several chemokines. Under infection, TLR4-primed event is critical for the activation of KCs, a key source of TGF-β. In addition, LPS-TLR4 axis on HSCs causes the downregulation of BAMBI, a pseudoreceptor of TGF-β. As a result, TGF-β-primed signaling transduction was enhanced in HSCs after bacterial challenge [20]. Hypoxia and oxidative stress are key events to link fibrogenesis to angiogenesis during CLD [21], and TGF-β production is also enhanced by hypoxia, especially in hepatocytes and hepatic macrophages.

Herein, we described the biological information on transcription, activation and signaling pathway of TGF-β, related to LC progression. In addition, we emphasized the importance of intracellular network for understanding of molecular basis during LC process. In other words, there are some targeted points in each step for delaying LC progression, as discussed later.

6.3 Apoptotic and Fibrotic Effects of TGF-β on Hepatocytes

Tissue fibrosis progresses as a result of a decrease in functional parenchymal cells, and defected epithelial cells must be replaced with pathogenic ECMs, such as collagens. Thus, chronic activation of epithelial death system is responsible for tissue fibrosis with dysfunction. Actually, apoptotic removal of hepatocytes induces liver fibrosis. For instance, Bcl-xL is a key anti-apoptotic molecule to stabilize mitochondrial membrane, and hepatocyte-specific deletion of Bcl-xL elicits liver fibrosis in mice [22]. TGF-β induces apoptotic death in hepatocytes, possibly via Bcl-xL downregulation in vivo. This section describes recent information on cytotoxic mechanisms of TGF-β in hepatic parenchymal cells.

Oberhammer et al. found that active form TGF-β induced apoptotic changes in the primary culture of rat hepatocyte [23]. This effect was also reproduced in vivo: administration of adenovirus vector containing TGF-β1 plasmid induced apoptosis in hepatocytes (TGF-β1 group: 14.1% versus control group: 0.25%) after 70%-partial hepatectomy in rats [24]. In a chronic model of CCl_4-induced liver fibrosis, hepatocyte apoptosis becomes evident, and this result was associated with the upregulation of TGF-β1. Importantly, neutralization of TGF-β1 by vaccination led to a decrease in apoptotic hepatocytes in the CCl_4-treated mice [25], hence suggesting that TGF-β can be a target for inhibiting hepatocyte apoptosis during CLD. CCl_4 is a hepatocyte-selective toxin. Thus, inflammation-induced TGF-β enhances this toxin-induced cell death (and in part, directly induces apoptosis).

TGF-β is now a key regulator for enhancing hepatocyte death under injurious conditions. Thus, it is important to elucidate the mechanism that underlies the TGF-β-induced apoptosis. Hepatocyte apoptosis depends on mitochondrial stresses, including cytochrome-c-conducted caspase activation for DNA fragmentation. TGF-β induces reactive oxygen species (ROS) through recruiting NOX4, a typical NADPH oxidase for cytoplasmic generation of hydrogen peroxide [26]. Such an oxidant stress leads to decreased Bcl-xL levels, loss of mitochondrial transmembrane potential, cytochrome-c release and caspase-3 activation (Fig. 6.1). Indeed, TGF-β-induced hepatocyte apoptosis was diminished by Z-VAD, a pan-caspase inhibitor. The possible involvement of p53 stabilization, E2F transcriptional activation and PKA-STAT3 phosphorylation is a critical event for TGF-β to induce apoptosis [27, 28].

In addition to apoptotic action, TGF-β can induce EMT in hepatocytes to acquire MyoFB-like phenotypes for interstitial ECM production. TGF-β induces G_1/S phase-dependent EMT (and G_2/M phase-related apoptosis) [29]. With regard to this, Snail or Slung are a typical transcriptional switch to induce EMT in numerous organs. Overproduction of Snail

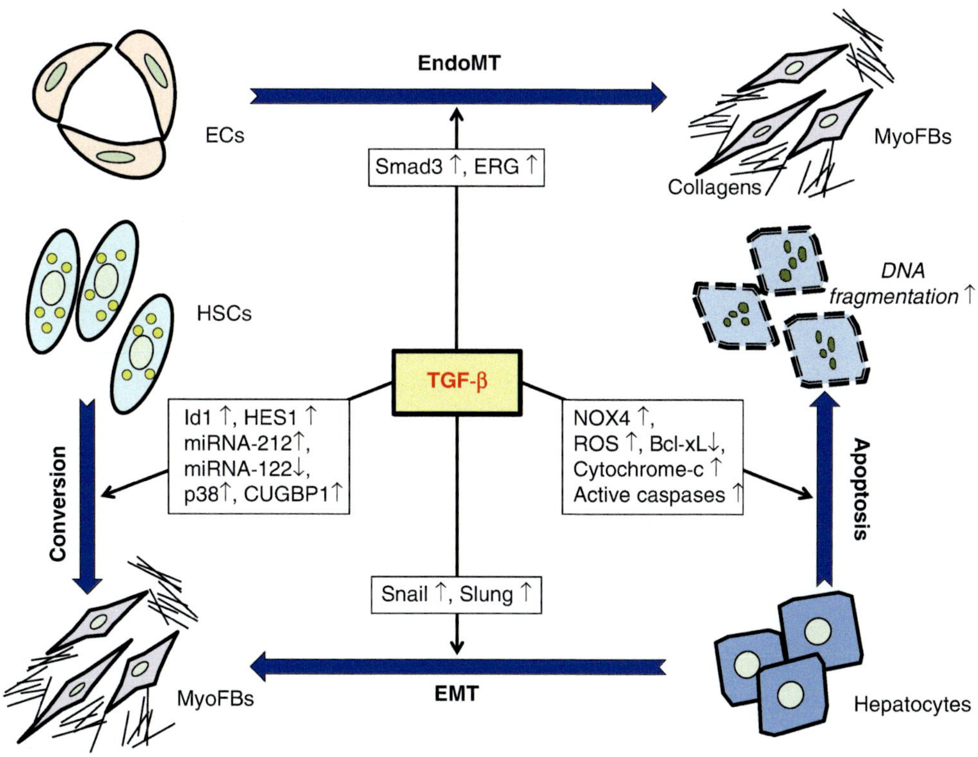

Fig. 6.1 Multiple effects of TGF-β on hepatic cells. TGF-β is highly produced by KCs, HCSs and hepatocytes during CLD progression. TGF-β plays a key role in differentiation of ECs to MyoFBs (i.e., EndoMT) via Smad3- or ERG-dependent mechanisms. Furthermore, TGF-β induces MyoFB-like phenotypes in HSCs, whereas Id1 and Notch-induced HES1 are critically involved in the HSC → MyoFB conversion as transcriptional regulators. MicroRNAs, such as miRNA-212 and miRNA-122 participate in this process as positive and negative regulator, respectively. MAPK-p38-induced production of CUGBP1 enhances HSC → MyoFB conversion via downregulation of IFN-γ, a counterpart of TGF-β. TGF-β has a dual effect on hepatocytes: one is induction of apoptotic cell death via an oxidative stress-dependent pathway (i.e., NOX4 → ROS → Bcl-xL loss → caspase-3 activation → DNA fragmentation). Another effect is EMT that depends on Snail or Slung-primed mechanisms. TGF-β-mediated hepatocyte death and MyoFB deposition lead to parenchymal reduction and interstitial expansion, a common histological finding of LC

confers resistance to TGF-β-induced apoptosis and is sufficient to induce EMT in the primary culture of hepatocytes [30]. Thus, TGF-β contributes to LC progression via a dual function of apoptosis and EMT (Fig. 6.1), eventually leading to reduced epithelium and expanded interstitium.

6.4 Molecular Basis for Phenotypic Changes of HSCs to MyoFBs

Liver regeneration means a replacement of defected hepatocytes with newly generated hepatocytes, but such a repair system is impaired by TGF-β-mediated apoptosis and cell cycle arrest [3], resulting in collagenous deposition, rather than hepatocyte replication. In this process, interstitial MyoFBs play a central role in accumulation of ECM, and canonical signaling of TGF-β is critical for resident interstitial cells (such as HSCs and portal fibroblasts) to acquire SMC-like phenotypes (i.e., MyoFBs). In this section, we will focus on HSCs to discuss the molecular mechanism of MyoFB transition.

Epigenetic regulation is important for differentiation, including conversion of HSCs to MyoFBs. Activation of TGF-β1 promoter region by AP1 and Sp1 is necessary for HSC → MyoFB transition [31]. Smad7 is a dominant suppressor of TGF-β pathway [3]. In contrast, Id1 is identified as a negative regulator of Smad7 and is an essential mediator for TGF-β-induced conversion of HSCs to MyoFBs [32]. Smad7 inhibits MyoFB differentiation via suppressing Id1 production. Conversely, TGF-β upregulates Id1 via an ALK1-Smad1 pathway, and this noncanonical pathway has a critical part in the release of Smad7-mediated inhibition, leading to the efficient conversion to MyoFBs. Several lines of evidence indicate a role of Notch signaling for HSC → MyoFB transition. Noch1 and its ligand, Jagged1 expression were increased during LC progression in rodents, while an inhibitor of Notch signaling cascade diminished HSC → MyoFB conversion [33]. Notably, TGF-β induces HES1, a downstream effector of Notch signaling that activates DNA promoter regions of α-SMA and type-I collagen [34]. Overall, signaling cascade of TGF-β → Jagged1-Notch→HES1 between HSC-HSC was shown to be necessary for the HSC → MyoFB differentiation (i.e., juxtacrine pathway) (Fig. 6.1).

MicroRNA (miRNA) is a small Noncording RNA and is important for RNA silencing and post-transcriptional regulation. A recent report identified miRNA-212 as a Smad7-inhibiting regulator [35]. Actually, forced induction of miRNA-212 in HSCs enhanced the MyoFB differentiation. Of importance, TGF-β induces miRNA-212 expression. Thus, induction of miRNA-212 is necessary for TGF-β to induce MyoFB-like phenotypes in HSCs. In contrast to this miRNA, miRNA-122 is shown to reduce the transcription of α-SMA, a marker of MyoFBs, by inhibiting the expression of serum response factor that is a key transcription factor for tissue fibrogenesis. Of interest, TGF-β decreases miRNA-122 levels in HSCs [36], and such an inhibitory cascade participates in MyoFB conversion (Fig. 6.1). RNA-binding proteins are also involved in the fibrotic events. SphK1 kinase is a downstream effector for TGF-β-induced HSC activation, while RNA-binding protein, HuR stabilizes SphK1 mRNA, resulting in the enhanced activity of this kinase [37]. Further studies on the roles of miRNAs or RNA-binding proteins will provide a molecular basis of MyoFB differentiation.

We next discuss the TGF-β-transduced downstream pathway, with a focus on intracellular signaling kinases. MAPK-p38 kinase is necessary for TGF-β-induced MyoFB conversion. Upregulation of NOX4 by TGF-β results in ROS synthesis [26]. Under such an oxidative stress, p38 is activated via a noncanonical pathway, while Smad3 phosphorylation is also enhanced. The synchronized activation of noncanonical and canonical pathways leads to induction of differentiation-inducible master switches, such as Snail and Slung, for MyoFB transition [38]. IFN-γ is a counterpart of TGF-β to block MyoFB conversion. Recently, TGF-β-mediated p38 activation was shown to be critical for induction of CUG-binding protein 1 (CUGBP1) that suppress IFN-γ transcription via a direct binding to 3′-UTR region of IFN-γ mRNA. Overall, TGF-β → p38 axis was demonstrated to be necessary for MyoFB conversion, at least in part, via a CUGBP1-dependent decrease of IFN-γ levels [39] (Fig. 6.1). JNK kinase is also critical for MyoFB conversion through the enhancement of TGF-β-mediated NOX4 induction [40].

Finally, it is important to discuss the extracellular substances that trigger TGF-β production in HSCs. The local renin-angiotensin system is involved in TGF-β upregulation as an upstream effector beyond organs [41]. Pharmacological inhibitors of angiotensin-II conversion enzyme or angiotensin-II receptor antagonist delays the progression of LC in rodent models, associated with the lowered levels of TGF-β and suppressed accumulation of interstitial MyoFBs [42]. Regardless of initial etiology, angiotensin-II may be a common trigger of TGF-β production in injured livers (Fig. 6.2). Tryptophan metabolism is also involved in TGF-β production. Serotonin is a tryptophan intermediate metabolite and stimulates de novo synthesis of TGF-β1 in HSCs. 5-hydroxytryptamine 2B receptor (5-HT_{2B}-Rc) is the first gate for uptake of serotonin into HSCs [43]. Notably, 5-HT_{2B}-Rc antagonist was shown to delay the progression of LC in rodents. Pharmacological targeting of 5-HT_{2B}-Rc may be therapeutic in human CLD.

In summary, biochemical analysis revealed the potential mechanisms of TGF-β-mediated MyoFB conversion. CTGF is a downstream target of TGF-β/STAT3 axis [16]. Once HSCs are converted to MyoFBs, TGF-β-induced CTGF elicits production of ECMs, such as type-I collagen, in MyoFBs [44], and these sequential events are critical for LC progression.

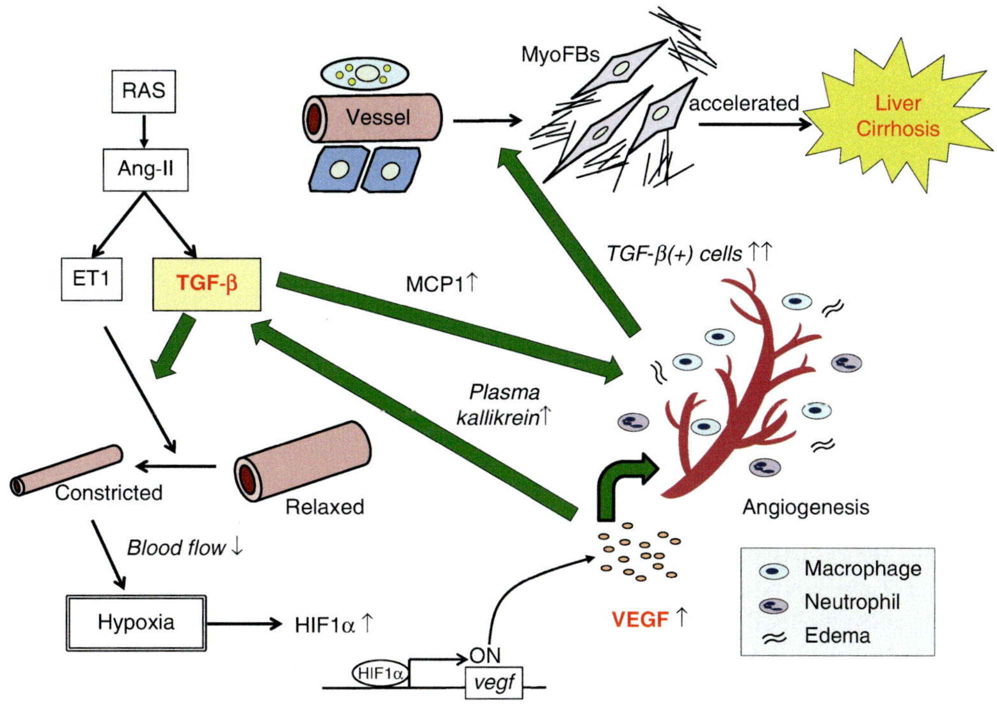

Fig. 6.2 Potential linkage of angiogenesis with fibrogenesis during LC progression. Renin angiotensin system (RAS) is locally activated in liver tissues, in response to persistent injuries, and then ET1 and TGF-β are upregulated via angiotensin II (Ang-II)-mediated pathway. ET1 induces hepatic hypoxia by inducing constriction of vascular SMCs. HIF1α is upregulated under hypoxia, and then VEGF promoter regions are activated, followed by VEGF upregulation. During CLD progression, there are sequential circuits between TGF-β and VEGF: (1) Hypoxia-primed VEGF induces pathogenic angiogenesis with edema formation; (2) VEGF is able to activate latent form TGF-β via recruiting plasma kallikrein; and (3) TGF-β-induced MCP1 can induce perivascular infiltration of macrophages (i.e., a major source of TGF-β), resulting in an increase in hepatic TGF-β levels. Under such a hypoxic condition, differentiation of liver cells to MyoFBs (i.e., EndoMT, EMT and HSC-MyoFB conversion) becomes evident, in response to TGF-β upregulation. Overall, LC progression is accelerated via a crosstalk between VEGF-induced angiogenesis and TGF-β-conducted fibrogenesis during CLDs

6.5 Linkage of VEGF-Induced Angiogenesis with TGF-β-Induced Fibrogenesis

TGF-β is one of the most important cytokine for the pathogenesis of LC. Local hypoxia is closely associated with the progression of LC during chronic hepatitis [45]. Under hypoxia, VEGF mRNA is upregulated via a hypoxia-inducible factor-1 (HIF1)-dependent pathway [45]. Indeed, VEGF is a potent mitogenic factor for ECs, but not pericytes. Thus, loss of pericyte recruitment leads to an increase in vascular permeability and leucocyte extravasation (i.e., pathological angiogenesis due to edema and inflammation). Recent reports identify the pathological angiogenesis as a risk factor for accelerating LC, as described below.

Hypoxia is a result of persistent LC, but inversely, it can be a causative factor to enhance the fibrogenic events in injured livers [45]. Thus, it is important to discuss how TGF-β induces local hypoxia in response to persistent injuries. Endothelin-1 (ET1) is a typical vasoconstrictor via selective contraction of SMCs. Clinical and experimental evidence have revealed that ET1 levels increase in the injured liver of humans [46]. Indeed, administration of recombinant ET1 induced local hypoxia in the liver of piglets [47]. Conversely, ET1-blocking agent attenuated the hepatic hypoxia in a rat model of LC [48]. These studies identified ET1 as a critical hypoxia-inducing factor. Of note, TGF-β enhances the production and secretion of ET1 in vascular cells [49]. Together, TGF-β likely contributes to vasoconstriction-based hepatic hypoxia, partly via recruiting ET1 in hepatic sinusoidal vessels (Fig. 6.2).

As repeated, local VEGF expression depends on HIF1-conducted transcriptional cascade. Under hypoxic condition, cytoplasmic HIF1 becomes active for nuclear translocation, while VEGF gene promoter region contains HIF1-responsive element. As a result, RNA polymerase is recruited near the HIF1-binding site, followed by an initiation of VEGF transcription. Given that VEGF induces perivascular edema, it is important to discuss how VEGF elicits vascular permeability. Cytoskeletal structural components, such as focal adhesion kinase and its adaptor, paxillin are required for sustaining endothelial barrier function. In this process, VEGF disrupts the barrier stability via Rho activation and paxillin dysfunction [50]. Cell surface VE-cadherin is also critical for maintaining endothelial integrity. Of interest, VEGF enhances internalization of VE-cadherin via VEGFR2/KDR-Src-PAK-mediated signaling cascades [51]. Interaction of angiopoietin-2 with VEGF leads to enhanced edema formation [52]. Such a hypoxia-induced molecular crosstalk participates in VEGF-triggered edematous lesions.

Local inflammation is characterized by infiltrated macrophages and is an important step for accelerating LC, especially after the onset of vascular permeability. Monocyte chemoattractant protein-1 (MCP1/CCL2) is a key cytokine to link local inflammation with hepatic fibrosis [53]. In an advanced stage, MCP1 is upregulated in injured livers, especially in bile duct epithelium near portal zones. Importantly, MCP1 antagonism produces anti-fibrotic outcomes in animal models of LC [54], thus establishing a major role of macrophages during LC progression. TGF-β → Smad3 canonical pathway phosphorylates MAPK-p42/p44, resulting in MCP1 mRNA production. Inversely, recruitment of macrophages (i.e., TGF-β-producing cells) by MCP1 leads to an increase in hepatic TGF-β levels. Such a loop between MCP1-producing bile ducts and TGF-β-secreting macrophages contributes to fibrogenesis post-angiogenic stage (Fig. 6.2).

How infiltrated leucocytes contribute to LC progression? After the successful extravasation from pathogenic vessels, macrophages play a central role in oxidant stress-based damage in inflamed organs. In this process, ROS is involved in induction of fibrogenic events, including MyoFB differentiation and collagen production. ROS is generated in cytosol by NADPH oxidases, such as NOX4 [55]. Notably, TGF-β signaling transduction initiates NOX4 mRNA synthesis. Indeed, NOX4 promoter region contains Smad2/3-responsive element, and after recruitment of Smad2/3 onto the element [56], NOX4 mRNA synthesis is initiated. Thus, TGF-β-induced NOX4 elicits generation and release of ROS from the infiltrated macrophages, and then ROS activates biological functions of TGF-β. Such a positive feedback between TGF-β and ROS is also responsible for LC formation.

Another possibility of angiogenesis- or hypoxia-enhanced LC is that VEGF activates latent form of TGF-β on HSCs (i.e., direct action). Sakata et al. reported that recombinant VEGF induced liver fibrosis in normal mice, associated with an increase in the number of ECs [8]. Using the primary culture, they found that VEGF enhances kallikrein production in sinusoidal ECs. The EC-derived condition medium enhanced TGF-β activation and MyoFB conversion in the culture of HSCs, and this effect was abolished by a kallikrein inhibitor. Overall, VEGF was shown to be critical not only for vessel formation but also for fibrosis via TGF-β activation on HSCs (Fig. 6.2). Local hypoxia upregulates VEGF and thrombospondin-1 through HIF1-based cascades, while thrombospondin-1 is also important for activation of TGF-β [12, 57].

VEGF induces TGF-β activation on HSCs [8], whereas TGF-β enhances VEGF production in several organs. P300/CREB-binding protein (CBP) is known to potentiate histone acetylation at nucleosomes and act as a coactivator to facilitate HIF1-primed transcription of VEGF mRNA. Of interest, TGF-β-phosphorylated smad2/3 directly binds to and activates CBP, resulting in the efficient production of VEGF mRNA [58]. A recent report described that hepatic MyoFBs promote vascular remodeling during CLDs in rodents through the release of VEGF-containing microparticles [59]. TGF-β-mediated induction of Jagged1 (i.e., a Notch ligand) onto MyoFBs leads to vascularization of ECs through VEGF-A production [60], and such a cell contact-based system between "Jagged1 on MyoFBs" and "Notch on ECs" may be a critical event to explain the possible linkage of fibrogenesis with angiogenesis.

In summary, TGF-β promotes VEGF production via TGF-β-ET1-induced hypoxia (i.e., indirect effect) and enhances VEGF mRNA transcription via the CBP function (i.e., direct effect), contributing to the onset of pathogenic angiogenesis during LC. VEGF has a direct effect on pathogenic angiogenesis and contributes to fibrogenesis through the following indirect events: (1) MCP1-based infiltration of macrophages; (2) production of NOX4 and ROS by infiltrated leukocytes; and (3) kallikrein-mediated enhancement of latent TGF-β activation. Such direct or indirect actions of TGF-β and VEGF provide a complicated crosstalk between ECs and MyoFBs for the potential linkage of angiogenesis with fibrogenesis (Fig. 6.2).

6.6 Endothelial to Mesenchymal Transition (EndoMT) for LC

The major origins of collagen-producing MyoFBs during LC development are divided into three groups: (1) in situ activated HSCs; (2) resident fibroblasts around portal zones (i.e., portal MyoFBs); and (3) functional hepatocytes prior to EMT. In addition to these origins, ECs can be differentiated to MyoFB, associated with the loss of cell-cell contact and the acquisition of a contractile phenotype, like SMCs. This pathological change is defined as EndoMT. In addition to EMT, TGF-β plays a key role in EndoMT during CLD in rodents and humans [61]. TGF-β-mediated induction of fibrogenic master switches, such as Snail and Slung, leads to EndoMT in vitro [62], and possibly in vivo. EndoMT is detected in a mouse model of diabetic nephropathy. Of importance, Smad3 inhibitor delayed the renal damages, at least in part, via a decrease in the number of EndoMT-positive cells [63], hence suggesting the contribution of TGF-β-Smad3 axis to the appearance of EndoMT in vivo.

EndoMT is, more or less, involved in fibrogenesis in injured organs, such as the kidney, skin and lungs. Until the mid 2000s, little information was available about EndoMT in the liver. Kitao et al. for the first time reported in 2009 that

EndoMT is also detectable in the livers of patients suffering from idiopathic portal hypertension (IPH) [64]. This group found the $CD34^+/S100A4^+$ cells (i.e., histological markers of EndoMT) in the portal vein endothelium of IPH-affected livers and emphasized that EndoMT is one of the key mechanisms of IPH-related portal venous stenosis. It is, indeed, possible that pathogenic angiogenesis causes IPH [65], and VEGF is critical for the angiogenic response to persistent IPH. VEGF enhances bioactivity of TGF-β [8]. Thus, angiogenetic induction by VEGF may lead to an increase in opportunity for ECs to undergo EndoMT, in particular, under the condition of IPH.

The possible contribution of EndoMT to liver fibrosis is now reproduced not only in IPH but also in other types of hepatitis in human and animals [66]. Ets-related gene (ERG) is known to control canonical signaling of TGF-β-Smad by repressing access of Smad3 to DNA. Using the EC-specific ERG-knockout mice, Dufton et al. demonstrated that ERG is necessary for protecting ECs from EndoMT [66]. Strikingly, genetic ablation of ERG expression in ECs led to the spontaneous occurrence of EndoMT, along with accelerated liver fibrosis in mice. This result was associated with the marked increase in Smad3 activity. Indeed, decreased ERG expression also correlated with the EndoMT score in the hepatic samples obtained from patients with CLDs. Overall, ERG was demonstrated to be a physiological regulator that is required for sustaining vascular homeostasis and avoiding overactivation of TGF-β-Smad3 axis.

TGF-β-induced EndoMT is a newly recognized source of activated MyoFBs, while HSCs are a major source of ECM-producing MyoFBs. Recently, Ribera et al. reported the small population of EndoMT-positive cells (less than 4%) in a mouse model of CCl_4-induced liver fibrosis [67]. The contribution of EndoMT to human CLDs has not yet been accepted, except for IPH. Thus, it is still controversial whether inhibition of EndoMT can be a primary choice for delaying LC, and future studies would shed more light on this notion.

6.7 Summary and Perspective

TGF-β is now an essential conductor for promoting tissue fibrosis beyond types of organs. In the liver, TGF-β induces apoptotic and fibrogenic phenotypes in hepatocytes. Under chronic inflammation, resident KC-derived or infiltrated macrophage-produced TGF-β differentiates sinusoidal HSCs or ECs to MyoFBs that produce pathogenic ECM proteins, such as type-I collagen. Thus, TGF-β neutralization is a reasonable strategy for delaying the LC progression. For example, anti-TGF-β antibody (1D11/CG1008) blocked the fibrotic lesions in a rat model of LC [68], and safety of this antibody was carefully evaluated in a phase-I clinical trial for patients bearing melanoma [69]. The chemical blocker of the TGF-β type-I receptor/ALK5 (i.e., EW-7197) is also promising for retarding LC progression, at least in rodents [70].

Emerging evidence delineated the major role of pathogenic angiogenesis in LC progression. For the potential explanation, we focused on VEGF to link the hypoxia to fibrogenesis. Actually, TGF-β can promote VEGF production via ET1-induced local hypoxia (i.e., indirect effect) and enhances VEGF mRNA transcription via Smad3-based activation of CBP function (i.e., direct effect), leading to the onset of pathogenic angiogenesis. Another terminology of VEGF is vascular permeability factor (VPF). As its name indicated, VPF/VEGF has a direct intractable effect on angiogenesis, leading to the perivascular edema formation.

There is now emerging evidence to show that anti-angiogenic treatment is reasonable for retarding the LC progression in animal models [6]. Not only anti-VEGF receptor antibodies but also chemical inhibitors to block the signaling transduction of VEGF reduced LC-like changes in rodents [6, 71]. Antagonism of angiotensin-II-TGF-β axis by candesartan may be practical as a FDA-approved drug-repositioning therapy for delaying LC [72]. In addition, ET1-blocker may be a primary choice for attenuating IPH that causes extrahepatic angiogenesis, a common cause of esophageal varices and ascetic fluid accumulation in advanced stage of CLD [7, 65]. The potential target molecules for delaying LC progression are summarized in Table 6.1.

Self Study

Questions

1. Which statement is true?
   (a) MicroRNA (miRNA) is a small non-coding RNA and is important for RNA silencing and post-transcriptional regulation.
   (b) miRNA-122 decreases the transcription of α-SMA. **CORRECT**.
   (c) TGF-β increases miRNA-122 levels in HSCs.
   (d) TGF-β inhibits EMT in hepatocytes to acquire MyoFB-like phenotypes for interstitial ECM production.
2. Which statement is true?
   (a) Transforming growth factor-β (TGF-β) is one of the most important cytokines for the onset and progression of liver cirrhosis.
   (b) TGF-β secreted from Kupffer cells (KCs) converts sinusoidal cells, such as hepatic stellate cells (HSCs) and endothelial cells (ECs), to smooth muscle cell (SMC)-like myofibroblasts (MyoFBs).
   (c) In the injured livers, TGF-β is protective toward hepatocytes.
   (d) Oncostatin-M induces tissue inhibitor of metalloproteinase-1 (TIMP1) in HSCs, and further stimulates liver cirrhosis regression.

Table 6.1 Pathogenic molecule-targeting strategies for suppressing liver fibrogenesis and angiogenesis in animal models

Targets	Agents	Animal models	Outcomes	Investigators (Year)	Ref no.
TGF-β1	Poly-peptide vaccine	CCl_4 (i.p.) → Mice	Suppressed fibrosis,	Fan X et al. (2015)	[25]
	TGF-β1-[41-65]		Suppressed apoptosis,		
	TGF-β1-[83-112]		Enhanced regeneration		
TGF-β1,2,3	Anti-panTGF-β mAB	TAA (i.p.) → Mice	Reversed fibrosis post-onset,	Ling H et al. (2013)	[68]
	(1D11)		Decreased TGF-β1 and PAI-1 levels		
$\alpha_v\beta_6$ integrin antagonist	EMD527040	BDL → Rats	Suppressed fibrosis,	Patsenker E et al. (2008)	[13]
			Improved hepatic failure,		
			Suppressed cholangiopathy		
Notch inhibitor	Avagacestat	CCl_4 (i.p.) → Mice	Suppressed MyoFB conversion,	Bansal R et al. (2015)	[33]
			Decreased M1-type macrophages		
Angiotensin II receptor	Candesartan	BDL → Mice	Suppressed fibrosis,	Ueki M et al. (2006)	[42]
			Decreased TGF-β1 and CTGF levels		
5-HT_{2B} receptor	SB-204741	CCl_4 (i.p.) → Mice	Suppressed MyoFB conversion,	Ebrahimkhani MR et al. (2011)	[43]
			Decreased TGF-β1 and TIMP levels		
CTGF	FG-3019	TGF-β2 and CTGF (i.p.)	Decreased fibrosis scores,	Wang Q et al. (2011)	[44]
	(Anti-CTGF mAB)	→ Neonatal mice	Decreased hydroxyproline levels		
ET1 blocker	Bosentan	BDL → Rats	Decreased VEGF levels,	Hsu SJ et al. (2016)	[48]
	Ambrisentan		Suppressed shunting and angiogenesis		
MCP1	NOX-E36	CCl_4 (i.p.) → Mice	Suppressed macrophage infiltration,	Baeck C et al. (2014)	[54]
(CCL2)	(CCL2 receptor-binder)		Decreased TNF-α levels		
TGF-β type-I receptor	EW-7197	CCl_4 (i.p.) → Mice	Suppressed fibrosis,	Park SA et al. (2015)	[70]
(ALK5)		BDL → Rats	Suppressed ROS accumulation		
VEGF receptor	Anti-VEGFR1 mAB,	CCl_4 (i.p.) → Mice	Suppressed fibrosis,	Yoshiji H et al. (2003)	[71]
(VEGFR1, VEGFR2)	Anti-VEGFR2 mAB		Suppressed angiogenesis		

Abbreviations are listed as followed: *CCl_4* carbon tetrachloride, *i.p.* intraperitoneal injection, *mAB* monoclonal antibody, *TAA* thioacetamide, *PAI-1* plasminogen activator inhibitor-1, *VEGFR1* VEGF type-I receptor, *VEGFR2* VEGF type-II receptor. See text for other abbreviations

Answers

1. Which statement is true?
   (a) MicroRNA (miRNA) is a small non-coding RNA and is important for RNA silencing and post-transcriptional regulation. **CORRECT.**
   (b) miRNA-122 decreases the transcription of α-SMA. **CORRECT.**
   (c) TGF-β decreases miRNA-122 levels in HSCs.
   (d) TGF-β can induce EMT in hepatocytes to acquire MyoFB-like phenotypes for interstitial ECM production.

2. Which statement is true?
   (a) Transforming growth factor-β (TGF-β) is one of the most important cytokines for the onset and progression of liver cirrhosis. **CORRECT.**
   (b) TGF-β secreted from Kupffer cells (KCs) converts sinusoidal cells, such as hepatic stellate cells (HSCs) and endothelial cells (ECs), to smooth muscle cell (SMC)-like myofibroblasts (MyoFBs). **CORRECT.**
   (c) In the injured livers, TGF-β is apoptotic toward hepatocytes.

(d) Oncostatin-M induces tissue inhibitor of metalloproteinase-1 (TIMP1) in HSCs, and further stimulates liver cirrhosis progression.

References

1. Ramachandran P, Henderson NC. Antifibrotics in chronic liver disease: tractable targets and translational challenges. Lancet Gastroenterol Hepatol. 2016;1:328–40.
2. Kubo N, Araki K, Kuwano H, et al. Cancer-associated fibroblasts in hepatocellular carcinoma. World J Gastroenterol. 2016;22:6841–50.
3. Dooley S, ten Dijke P. TGF-β in progression of liver disease. Cell Tissue Res. 2012;347:245–56.
4. Annoni G, Weiner FR, Zern MA. Increased transforming growth factor-β1 gene expression in human liver disease. J Hepatol. 1992;14:259–64.
5. Kanzler S, Lohse AW, Keil A, et al. TGF-β1 in liver fibrosis: an inducible transgenic mouse model to study liver fibrogenesis. Am J Phys. 1999;276:G1059–68.
6. Bocca C, Novo E, Miglietta A, et al. Angiogenesis and fibrogenesis in chronic liver diseases. Cell Mol Gastroenterol Hepatol. 2015;1:477–88.
7. Gana JC, Serrano CA, Ling SC. Angiogenesis and portal-systemic collaterals in portal hypertension. Ann Hepatol. 2016;15:303–13.
8. Sakata K, Eda S, Lee ES, et al. Neovessel formation promotes liver fibrosis via providing latent transforming growth factor-β. Biochem Biophys Res Commun. 2014;443:950–6.
9. De Bleser PJ, Niki T, Rogiers V, et al. Transforming growth factor-β gene expression in normal and fibrotic rat liver. J Hepatol. 1997;26:886–93.
10. Sheen-Chen SM, Lin CR, Chen KH, et al. Epigenetic histone methylation regulates transforming growth factor-β1 expression following bile duct ligation in rats. J Gastroenterol. 2014;49:1285–97.
11. Fan Z, Hao C, Li M, et al. MKL1 is an epigenetic modulator of TGF-β induced fibrogenesis. Biochim Biophys Acta. 2015;1849:1219–28.
12. Murphy-Ullrich JE, Suto MJ. Thrombospondin-1 regulation of latent TGF-β activation: a therapeutic target for fibrotic disease. Matrix Biol. 2018;68-9:28–43.
13. Patsenker E, Popov Y, Stickel F, et al. Inhibition of integrin alphavbeta6 on cholangiocytes blocks transforming growth factor-β activation and retards biliary fibrosis progression. Gastroenterology. 2008;135:660–70.
14. Cattaneo F, Guerra G, Parisi M, et al. Cell-surface receptors transactivation mediated by G protein-coupled receptors. Int J Mol Sci. 2014;29:19700–28.
15. Emami N, Diamandis EP. New insights into the functional mechanisms and clinical applications of the kallikrein-related peptidase family. Mol Oncol. 2007;1:269–87.
16. Liu Y, Liu H, Meyer C, et al. Transforming growth factor-β (TGF-β)-mediated connective tissue growth factor (CTGF) expression in hepatic stellate cells requires Stat3 signaling activation. J Biol Chem. 2013;288:30708–19.
17. Li HY, Ju D, Zhang DW, et al. Activation of TGF-β1-CD147 positive feedback loop in hepatic stellate cells promotes liver fibrosis. Sci Rep. 2015;5:16552.
18. Kiagiadaki F, Kampa M, Voumvouraki A, et al. Activin-A causes hepatic stellate cell activation via the induction of TNFα and TGF-β in Kupffer cells. Biochim Biophys Acta. 2018;1864:891–9.
19. Matsuda M, Tsurusaki S, Miyata N, et al. Oncostatin-M causes liver fibrosis by regulating cooperation between hepatic stellate cells and macrophages in mice. Hepatology. 2018;67:296–312.
20. Seki E, De Minicis S, Osterreicher CH, et al. TLR4 enhances TGF-β signaling and hepatic fibrosis. Nat Med. 2007;13:1324–32.
21. Copple BL. Hypoxia stimulates hepatocyte epithelial to mesenchymal transition by hypoxia-inducible factor and transforming growth factor-β-dependent mechanisms. Liver Int. 2010;30:669–82.
22. Takehara T, Tatsumi T, Suzuki T, et al. Hepatocyte-specific disruption of Bcl-xL leads to continuous hepatocyte apoptosis and liver fibrotic responses. Gastroenterology. 2004;127:1189–97.
23. Oberhammer FA, Pavelka M, Sharma S, et al. Induction of apoptosis in cultured hepatocytes and in regressing liver by transforming growth factor-β1. Proc Natl Acad Sci U S A. 1992;89:5408–12.
24. Schrum LW, Bird MA, Salcher O, et al. Autocrine expression of activated transforming growth factor-β1 induces apoptosis in normal rat liver. Am J Physiol Gastrointest Liver Physiol. 2001;280:G139–48.
25. Fan X, Zhang Q, Li S, et al. Attenuation of CCl_4-induced hepatic fibrosis in mice by vaccinating against TGF-β1. PLoS One. 2013;8:e82190.
26. Herrera B, Fernández M, Alvarez AM, et al. Activation of caspases occurs downstream from radical oxygen species production, Bcl-xL down-regulation, and early cytochrome C release in apoptosis induced by transforming growth factor-β in rat fetal hepatocytes. Hepatology. 2001;34:548–56.
27. Sola S, Ma X, Castro RE, et al. Ursodeoxycholic acid modulates E2F-1 and p53 expression through a caspase-independent mechanism in transforming growth factor-β1-induced apoptosis of rat hepatocytes. J Biol Chem. 2003;278:48831–8.
28. Yang Y, Pan X, Lei W, et al. Regulation of transforming growth factor-β1-induced apoptosis and epithelial-to-mesenchymal transition by protein kinase A and signal transducers and activators of transcription 3. Cancer Res. 2006;66:8617–24.
29. Tian HY, Zhang KH, Gao X, et al. Comparative proteomic analysis of cell cycle-dependent apoptosis induced by transforming growth factor-β. Biochim Biophys Acta. 2009;1794:1387–97.
30. Franco DL, Mainez J, Vega S, et al. Snail1 suppresses TGF-β-induced apoptosis and is sufficient to trigger EMT in hepatocytes. J Cell Sci. 2010;123:3467–77.
31. Presser LD, McRae S, Waris G. Activation of TGF-β1 promoter by hepatitis C virus-induced AP-1 and Sp1: role of TGF-β1 in hepatic stellate cell activation and invasion. PLoS One. 2013;8:e56367.
32. Wiercinska E, Wickert L, Denecke B, et al. Id1 is a critical mediator in TGF-β-induced transdifferentiation of rat hepatic stellate cells. Hepatology. 2006;43:1032–41.
33. Bansal R, van Baarlen J, Storm G, et al. The interplay of the Notch signaling in hepatic stellate cells and macrophages determines the fate of liver fibrogenesis. Sci Rep. 2015;5:18272.
34. Zhang K, Zhang YQ, Ai WB, et al. Hes1, an important gene for activation of hepatic stellate cells, is regulated by Notch1 and TGF-β/BMP signaling. World J Gastroenterol. 2015;21:878–87.
35. Zhu J, Zhang Z, Zhang Y, et al. MicroRNA-212 activates hepatic stellate cells and promotes liver fibrosis via targeting SMAD7. Biochem Biophys Res Commun. 2018;496:176–83.
36. Zeng C, Wang YL, Xie C, et al. Identification of a novel TGF-β-miR-122-fibronectin 1/serum response factor signaling cascade and its implication in hepatic fibrogenesis. Oncotarget. 2015;6:12224–33.
37. Ge J, Chang N, Zhao Z, et al. Essential roles of RNA-binding protein HuR in activation of hepatic stellate cells induced by transforming growth factor-β1. Sci Rep. 2016;6:22141.
38. Colak S, ten Dijke P. Targeting TGF-β signaling in cancer. Trends Cancer. 2017;3:56–71.
39. Wu X, Wu X, Ma Y, et al. CUG-binding protein 1 regulates HSC activation and liver fibrogenesis. Nat Commun. 2016;7:13498.
40. Tobar N, Toyos M, Urra C, et al. c-Jun N terminal kinase modulates NOX-4 derived ROS production and myofibroblasts differentiation in human breast stromal cells. BMC Cancer. 2014;14:640.
41. Kim G, Kim J, Lim YL, et al. Renin-angiotensin system inhibitors and fibrosis in chronic liver disease: a systematic review. Hepatol Int. 2016;10:819–28.

42. Ueki M, Koda M, Yamamoto S, et al. Preventive and therapeutic effects of angiotensin II type 1 receptor blocker on hepatic fibrosis induced by bile duct ligation in rats. J Gastroenterol. 2006;41:996–1004.
43. Ebrahimkhani MR, Oakley F, Murphy LB, et al. Stimulating healthy tissue regeneration by targeting the 5-HT_2B receptor in chronic liver disease. Nat Med. 2011;17:1668–73.
44. Wang Q, Usinger W, Nichols B, et al. Cooperative interaction of CTGF and TGF-β in animal models of fibrotic disease. Fibrogenesis Tissue Repair. 2011;4:4.
45. Rosmorduc O, Housset C. Hypoxia: a link between fibrogenesis, angiogenesis, and carcinogenesis in liver disease. Semin Liver Dis. 2010;30:258–70.
46. Wereszczynka-Siemiatkowska U, Swidnicka-Siergiejko A, Siemiatkowski A, et al. Endothelin-1 and transforming growth factor-β1 correlate with liver function and portal pressure in cirrhotic patients. Cytokine. 2015;76:144–51.
47. Unneberg K, Mjaaland M, Helseth E, et al. Effects of endothelin-1 on hepatic blood flow. HPB Surg. 1996;9:153–9.
48. Hsu SJ, Lin TY, Wang SS, et al. Endothelin receptor blockers reduce shunting and angiogenesis in cirrhotic rats. Eur J Clin Investig. 2016;46:572–80.
49. Shimada H, Staten NR, Rajagopalan LE. TGF-β1 mediated activation of Rho kinase induces TGF-β2 and endothelin-1 expression in human hepatic stellate cells. J Hepatol. 2011;54:521–8.
50. Birukova AA, Cokic I, Moldobaeva N, et al. Paxillin is involved in the differential regulation of endothelial barrier by HGF and VEGF. Am J Respir Cell Mol Biol. 2009;40:99–107.
51. Azzi S, Hebda JK, Gavard J. Vascular permeability and drug delivery in cancers. Front Oncol. 2013;3:211.
52. Melgar-Lesmes P, Tugues S, Ros J, et al. Vascular endothelial growth factor and angiopoietin-2 play a major role in the pathogenesis of vascular leakage in cirrhotic rats. Gut. 2009;58:285–92.
53. Affò S, Sancho-Bru P. CCL2: a link between hepatic inflammation, fibrosis and angiogenesis? Gut. 2014;63:1834–5.
54. Baeck C, Wei X, Bartneck M, et al. Pharmacological inhibition of the chemokine C-C motif chemokine ligand 2 (monocyte chemoattractant protein 1) accelerates liver fibrosis regression by suppressing Ly-6C(+) macrophage infiltration in mice. Hepatology. 2014;59:1060–72.
55. Morry J, Ngamcherdtrakul W, Yantasee W. Oxidative stress in cancer and fibrosis: opportunity for therapeutic intervention with antioxidant compounds, enzymes, and nanoparticles. Redox Biol. 2017;11:240–53.
56. Jiang F, Liu GS, Dusting GJ, et al. NADPH oxidase-dependent redox signaling in TGF-β-mediated fibrotic responses. Redox Biol. 2014;2:267–72.
57. Gressner OA, Weiskirchen R, Gressner AM. Evolving concepts of liver fibrogenesis provide new diagnostic and therapeutic options. Comp Hepatol. 2007;6:7.
58. Ji H, Li Y, Jiang F, et al. Inhibition of transforming growth factor-β/SMAD signal by MiR-155 is involved in arsenic trioxide-induced anti-angiogenesis in prostate cancer. Cancer Sci. 2014;105:1541–9.
59. Lemoinne S, Cadoret A, Rautou PE, et al. Portal myofibroblasts promote vascular remodeling underlying cirrhosis formation through the release of microparticles. Hepatology. 2015;61:1041–55.
60. Jin X, Aimaiti Y, Chen Z, et al. Hepatic stellate cells promote angiogenesis via the TGF-β1-Jagged1/VEGFA axis. Exp Cell Res. 2018;373:34–43.
61. Piera-Velazquez S, Mendoza FA, Jimenez SA. Endothelial to mesenchymal transition (EndoMT) in the pathogenesis of human fibrotic diseases. J Clin Med. 2016;5:45.
62. Doerr M, Morrison J, Bergeron L, et al. Differential effect of hypoxia on early endothelial mesenchymal transition response to transforming growth-β isoforms 1 and 2. Microvasc Res. 2016;108:48–63.
63. Li J, Qu X, Yao J, et al. Blockade of endothelial-mesenchymal transition by a Smad3 inhibitor delays the early development of streptozotocin-induced diabetic nephropathy. Diabetes. 2010;59:2612–24.
64. Kitao A, Sato Y, Sawada-Kitamura S, et al. Endothelial to mesenchymal transition via transforming growth factor-β1/Smad activation is associated with portal venous stenosis in idiopathic portal hypertension. Am J Pathol. 2009;175:616–26.
65. Thabut D, Shah V. Intrahepatic angiogenesis and sinusoidal remodeling in chronic liver disease: new targets for the treatment of portal hypertension? J Hepatol. 2010;53:976–80.
66. Dufton NP, Peghaire CR, Osuna-Almagro L, et al. Dynamic regulation of canonical TGFβ signalling by endothelial transcription factor ERG protects from liver fibrogenesis. Nat Commun. 2017;8:895.
67. Ribera J, Pauta M, Melgar-Lesmes P, et al. A small population of liver endothelial cells undergoes endothelial-to-mesenchymal transition in response to chronic liver injury. Am J Physiol Gastrointest Liver Physiol. 2017;313:G492–504.
68. Ling H, Roux E, Hempel D, et al. Transforming growth factor-β neutralization ameliorates pre-existing hepatic fibrosis and reduces cholangiocarcinoma in thioacetamide-treated rats. PLoS One. 2013;8:e54499.
69. Morris JC, Tan AR, Olencki TE, et al. Phase I study of GC1008 (fresolimumab): a human anti-transforming growth factor-β (TGF-β) monoclonal antibody in patients with advanced malignant melanoma or renal cell carcinoma. PLoS One. 2014;9:e90353.
70. Park SA, Kim MJ, Park SY, et al. EW-7197 inhibits hepatic, renal, and pulmonary fibrosis by blocking TGF-β/Smad and ROS signaling. Cell Mol Life Sci. 2015;72:2023–39.
71. Yoshiji H, Kuriyama S, Yoshii J, et al. Vascular endothelial growth factor and receptor interaction is a prerequisite for murine hepatic fibrogenesis. Gut. 2003;52:1347–54.
72. Kim MY, Cho MY, Baik SK, et al. Beneficial effects of candesartan, an angiotensin blocking agent, on compensated alcoholic liver fibrosis—a randomized open-label controlled study. Liver Int. 2012;32:977–87.

7 Hepatotoxicity: Mechanisms of Liver Injury

Manuela G. Neuman

Abbreviations

ALP	Alkaline phosphatase
ALT	Alanine aminotransferase (glutamic-pyruvic transaminase, SGPT)
AST	Aspartate aminotransferase (glutamic-oxaloacetic aminotransferases, SGOT)
CB	Conjugated (direct) bilirubin
GGT	γ-Glutamyltransferase (γ-glutamyltranspeptidase, GGTP)
ICH	International Conference on Harmonisation
INR	International Normalized Ratio
TB	Total bilirubin (sum of conjugated and non-conjugated serum bilirubin)
ULN	Upper limit of the normal reference range (or N)

7.1 Introduction

Chemical injury to the liver presents diverse aspects including the nature of the toxic agents, the character of the injury, the mechanism for the toxic effects, the conditions of exposure, and the medical and social importance [1–5]. Some hepatotoxins are found in nature as products of plants or animals, fungal or bacterial metabolism [6–10]. Many hepatotoxicants are products of the chemical, food or pharmaceutical industry [11, 12]. Other hepatotoxins are industrial byproducts or waste materials that, by polluting the environment, access humans [13–15]. Several agents have been shown to be synthesized in humans [16].

Morbidity and mortality caused by medications or inappropriate administration created a concern to health policy makers, and even patients [17, 18]. Hepatotoxicity caused by exposure to an agent produces injury to the liver that may be associated with impaired liver function [19].

The exposure to a drug that leads to histological or functional damage to the liver and is associated with impaired liver role is defined as hepatocytotoxicity [20–23]. Drug-induced hepatic reactions may produce liver injury to engage liver cells' function such as detoxification and transport. Moreover, DILI is the source of impaired bilirubin transport. The hepatotoxicity of this severity is likely to result in liver failure, especially if the offending drug is not stopped [3]. Other drugs lead to cholestatic injury by mechanistically impairing bile flow, which may lead to jaundice. However, the parenchymal injury is small [24]. Some therapeutic agents may produce degeneration of liver cells or vascular lesions of the liver [25, 26].

Other agents direct to a mixed type with simultaneous features of cytotoxic and cholestatic injury. Therefore, there may be considerable variability in causation and frequency of injury because of differences in the intrinsic and extrinsic factors, and the availability and prescribing patterns of the health products. Genetic polymorphisms affecting metabolic and transport pathways may affect the local concentration of the product or reactive metabolite at the cellular level, which in some instances may either form a covalent complex or trigger damage directly [27, 28]. Susceptibility may also be increased by the presence of another condition that impairs function in one or more metabolic or regulatory pathways. Product-induced hepatotoxicity may occur as an expected dose-dependent hepatic toxicity or as an unexpected idiosyncratic reaction. Consequently, there is a connection between the stimulus, the individual response and risk of hepatotoxicity. Diagnosis of chemically-induced hepatotoxicity relies on the exclusion of multiple elements, such as the medical history (risk factors, exclusion of other diseases), and presentation (time to onset of symptoms, jaundice or laboratory findings, and clinical features [29].

Detection of drug-induced liver injury depends on valid causality assessment and a sufficient number of subjects.

M. G. Neuman (✉)
In Vitro Drug Safety and Biotechnology, Department of Pharmacology and Toxicology, Banting Institute, University of Toronto, Toronto, ON, Canada
e-mail: manuela.neuman@utoronto.ca

F. Radu-Ionita et al. (eds.), *Liver Diseases*, https://doi.org/10.1007/978-3-030-24432-3_7

Absence of hepatotoxicity in clinical trials may only make available a limited predictive value on whether a product is hepatotoxic [3].

7.2 Hepatic Injury

Hepatic injury may result from direct damage to the hepatocytes, or from damage to bile canalicular cells, sinusoidal epithelial, stellate or Kupffer cells which alter function or indirectly damage the hepatocytes [21–26].

The liver has regenerative properties as an adaptive response to many agents. As a result, a range of clinical and pathological manifestations exist. Biochemical functions, metabolism and transport should be considered in assessing a drug's potential for causing hepatotoxicity [27–31].

Table 7.1 defines terminology utilised in this chapter while Table 7.2 describes the names of enzymes and proteins important for healthy liver function.

Table 7.1 Definitions

Definition	Explanation
Abnormal liver test	Any AST, ALT, Bilirubin test value greater than the population-defined upper limit of the normal reference range (ULN).
Adverse event	Any problematic medical occurrence in a patient administered a health product and which does not necessarily have a causal relationship with this treatment. An adverse event can therefore be any unfavourable and unintended sign (for example, an abnormal laboratory finding), symptom, or disease temporally associated with the use of a medicinal product, whether or not considered related to this medicinal product.
Adverse reaction	A noxious and unintended response to a drug used for prophylactic, therapeutic or withdraw and includes an unwanted effect
Enzymes	Alanine aminotransferase (ALT), aspartate aminotransferase (AST), alkaline phosphatase (ALP), and gamma-glutamyl transpeptidase (GGT)
Idiosyncratic	Host response where the individual is unable to tolerate usually prescribed doses of a product that may be safe in others. The reaction is not predicted by the pharmacokinetic or pharmacodynamic properties of the stimulus, it is not dose dependent, and is independent of the frequency of the drug administration.
Liver failure	Clinical manifestation of severe liver injury. The phenomenon encompasses both fulminant (within 8 weeks of symptoms) and sub-fulminant (late-onset) hepatic failure in a previously healthy liver.
Serious adverse reaction	A noxious and unintended response to a health product that occurs at any dose and that requires in-patient hospitalization or a prolongation of existing hospitalization; that results in significant disability or incapacity that is life-threatening, or that results in death.
Xenobiotic	A chemical that produces environmental contaminants.

The mechanisms of hepatotoxicity may cause presentations ranging from asymptomatic elevations of enzymes to severe dysfunction. Adverse drug reaction (ADR) can be consider any noxious, unintended and undesired effect of a drug, which occurs at doses used in humans for prophylaxis, diagnosis or therapy. This definition excludes therapeutic failures, intentional and accidental poisoning and drug abuse. Adverse drug reactions are classified as Type A and Type B. Type A reactions represent an extension of the drug's therapeutic effect. Type A, ADR occur frequently and are dose-related [5]. By contrast, type B reactions are unpredictable, occurring only in susceptible individuals. Type B 'idiosyncratic' reactions are dose-independent. Pirmohamed and Park's review ADR and make a classification of enzymes, transporters and immune response genes with associations to genetic individual susceptibility [32]. Table 7.3 presents a link between gene susceptibility and sensitivity specific medication.

ADRs are considered serious adverse drug reactions (SADRs) if they require hospitalization, prolonged hospitalization, and/or result in permanent disability or are fatal [33]. SADRs can arise via Type A or B mechanisms. The overall incidence of SADRs in hospitalized patients in the United States has been estimated at 6.2–6.7% and the incidence of fatal ADRs is estimated to be 0.15–0.3% [32]. This results in over two million estimated SADRs among hospitalized patients annually, with more than 100,000 deaths, in USA. Studies in Europe and Australia have yielded similar estimates [34]. The resulting cost has an impact on both the healthcare and the pharmaceutical industry internationally [35].

Pharmacokinetics relates to the absorption, distribution, metabolism and excretion of a drug and its metabolites in the body. Pharmacodynamics involves mechanism of action of a drug, including receptor binding and signal transduction [36].

Regarding morphology, the hepatic injury is classed as hepatocellular, cholestatic, mixed (cholestatic and hepatocellular), immunologic and mitochondrial. The mechanisms of hepatic injury may include: disruption of intracellular calcium homeostasis (membrane); disruption of actin filaments (canaliculus); covalent binding of a substance to cellular proteins resulting in immune injury, inhibition of cell metabolic pathways, blockage of cellular transport pumps, induction of apoptosis, and interference with mitochondrial function [37, 38].

Liver injury may develop within days or after several weeks after exposure to the incriminated agent. The injury pattern may be consistent for a class of products, but not all products have a characteristic time to onset, pattern of biochemical values, clinical course, or degree of severity [3].

Hepatocellular injury leading to hepatic necrosis is detected by increases in activity of serum aminotransferases, alanine aminotransferase (ALT) and aspartate aminotransferase (AST).

Table 7.2 Liver enzymes and proteins as laboratory tools in DILI

Enzyme/protein	Origin, importance and role in toxic reaction
Alanine aminotransferase (ALT)	ALT is present in hepatocytes, and in smaller amounts in skeletal muscle and intestinal epithelium. ALT is more sensitive and specific than AST for liver inflammation and hepatocyte necrosis. It rises rapidly in patients with acute damage to the hepatocytes. The absolute value of ALT increase is not directly proportional to the degree of liver damage, the value of 3×ULN can always be considered to be abnormal if the value persists. The value usually correlates well with the development of disease. If the hepatic injury is caused by biliary obstruction, then the increase in ALT is slower and is accompanied by increased ALP and GGT.
Aspartate aminotransferase (AST)	AST is found in many tissues (liver, skeletal muscle, heart, kidney, brain, erythrocytes, lung and pancreas) and may increase even if there is no hepatic injury. The increase in AST is usually less than the increase in ALT. AST higher than ALT may suggest, but not prove, alcohol-induced injury.
Alkaline Phosphatase (ALP)	ALP is a nonspecific screening test and may be increased by causes unrelated to liver (e.g. bone, kidney, breast, etc.). High ALP usually means that either the liver has bile duct damage or blockage or a condition causing increased bone cell activity is present. If other liver tests such as bilirubin, AST, or ALT are also high, usually the ALP is coming from the liver. If GGT or 5′-nucleotidase is also increased, then the high ALP is likely due to liver disease. If either of these two tests is normal, then the high ALP is likely due to a bone condition.
γ-Glutamyl-transferase (GGT)	Although present in many different organs, GGT is found in particularly high concentrations in the epithelial cells lining biliary ductules. It is a very sensitive indicator of hepatobiliary disease, but is not specific. Levels are elevated in other conditions including renal failure, myocardial infarction, pancreatic disease, alcohol use, and diabetes mellitus. Its major clinical use is to exclude a skeletal source of an elevated serum alkaline phosphatase level.
Bilirubin	Hepatocytotoxicity leads to increase of conjugated bilirubin (CB). Increased total or unconjugated bilirubin may be a result of hemolytic, sickle cell or pernicious anemias or a transfusion reaction. If conjugated bilirubin is elevated, there is an obstruction of the vascular path or bile ducts, hepatitis, trauma to the liver, cirrhosis, a drug reaction, or long-term alcohol abuse. Drug-induced hyperbilirubinemia may occur as a side effect due to inhibition of bilirubin UDP-glucuronyl-transferase 1A1 (UGT1A1) activity by certain drugs. Predominantly unconjugated bilirubin and is not associated with liver injury or indicators of hepatobiliary damage. If total bilirubin (TB) is elevated due to CB in order to differentiate cholestasis from hepatocellular injury. ALP should be determined for the same reason. An increase in INR may precede an increase in serum TB level. TB increase due to liver toxicity it is accompanied by a rapid increase in ALT. Increased bilirubin due to biliary obstruction, is accompanied by increased ALP and GGT,
Prothrombin time and International Normalized Ratio (INR)	Coagulation factor I (fibrinogen), II (prothrombin), V, VII, IX, and X. The prothrombin time is useful in assessing severity and prognosis of acute live disease. Deficiency of one or more of the liver-produced factors results in a prolonged prothrombin time. Prolongation of the prothrombin time in cholestatic liver disease may result from vitamin K deficiency. Other explanations for a prolonged prothrombin time apart from hepatocellular disease or vitamin K deficiency include consumptive coagulopathies, inherited deficiencies of a coagulation factor, medications that antagonize the prothrombin complex. Vitamin K deficiency diagnosis can be excluded if an administration of vitamin K 10 mg corrects or improves the prothrombin time within 24 h. This implies that hepatic synthetic function is intact. Prolongation of the prothrombin time that is unresponsive to vitamin K infusions suggests a fulminant liver disease.
Bile acids	Bile acids are synthesized from cholesterol in the liver, conjugated to glycine or taurine, and excreted in the bile. Bile acids facilitate fat digestion and absorption within the small intestine. They recycle through the enterohepatic circulation; secondary bile acids form by the action of intestinal bacteria. Elevated level of serum bile acids indicates biliary dysfunction. Normal bile acid levels in the presence of hyper-bilirubinemia suggests haemolysis or Gilbert's syndrome. High bile acid indicates chemical/drug/herbal-induced hepatotoxicity. This test provides diagnosis of hepatocellular dysfunction, but will not provide a definitive diagnosis of the nature of the hepatotoxicity. Additional test to establish or rule out liver failure are decreased albumin and clotting factors.

Cholestatic injury is due to disease or bile duct blockage or stricture among other reasons. The intrahepatic cholestasis causes include drugs, toxins, viral hepatitis, alcoholic liver disease, hemochromatosis, primary biliary cirrhosis, primary sclerosing cholangitis, steatohepatitis, and Wilson's disease. From the biochemical perspective, cholestatic injury shows increases in alkaline phosphatase (ALP) and gamma-glutamyl transpeptidase (GGT) activity, and bilirubin level. Cholestasis is due to specific agents like terbinafine is chronic. In order to diagnose a hepatic damage, it is necessary to look at all the enzymes (ALT, AST, ALP, GGT) and bilirubin [5].

The immunologic mechanism of hepatotoxicity involves formation of a covalent complex between the product or its reactive metabolite and cellular protein. Human leukocyte antigen (HLA) polymorphism leads to an inappropriate local T-cell response. In addition, mitochondrial injury develops due to oxidative phosphorylation, mitochondrial adenosine triphosphate (ATP) depletion, interference of lipid metabolism. This may be identified by the presence of lactic acidosis and microvesicular steatosis; and enzymatic activities of respiratory chain complexes II–IV, manganese superoxide dismutase

Table 7.3 Gene susceptibility to drug-induced liver injury

Drug	Gene	Drug class	Toxicity
Ximelagatran	*DRB1*07*	Thrombin	Elevation in transaminase
	*DQA1*02*	Inhibitor	
Tolcapone	*UGT1A16*	Catechol-O-methyl-transferase inhibitor	Transaminases
			Elevation
Amoxicillin/clavulanic acid	*DRB1*1501DRB5**	Antibiotic/amino-penicillin β-lactamase inhibitor	Jaundice
	*0101DQA1*0102D*		Serum bilirubin
	*QB1*0602*		
Diclofenac	*UGT2B7*	NSAID	High transaminase to acute liver failure
	CYP2C8		
Tranilast	*UGT1A1*	TGF-β-antagonist	Unconjugated hyper-bilirubinaemia
Rifampin	*DRB1*03*	Antibiotic	*High transaminase*
			Bilirubin > 3.0 mg/dL
Isoniazid	*CYP2E1*	Anti-tuberculosis antibiotic	*High transaminase*
	NAT2		Bilirubin > 3.0 mg/dL

(SOD2) and glutathione peroxidase (GPX1), which are involved in mitochondrial oxidative stress management [39–45].

7.3 Hepatic Function

The hepatic functions can be determined by measurement of total bilirubin (TB), conjugated (direct) bilirubin (CB), serum albumin and prolonged blood prothrombin time [5]. Clinically, acute liver failure is divided into: fulminant hepatic failure, with hepatic encephalopathy developing within 8 weeks of the onset of illness and subfulminant hepatic failure, with hepatic encephalopathy developing 8 weeks to 6 months after the onset of illness. Subfulminant hepatic failure is more often caused by product-induced hepatotoxicity or unknown factors [5].

In chronic liver failure, there is progression of the hepatic injury leading to end-stage signs and symptoms like cirrhosis, ascites, malnutrition, encephalopathy, coagulopathy, malaise and fatigue, with bilirubin, decreased albumin, and increased International normalized ratio (INR).

7.4 Hy's Law

Hy's Law or rule can be used to estimate severity and the likelihood that a therapeutic will cause an incidence of severe hepatotoxicity. Hy's Law is based on the combined evidence of hepatic injury, decreased hepatic function, and the absence of disease-induced damage [5, 46].

Criteria are: 1-injury: elevation of >3 × ULN ALT or AST activity; 2-function: >2 × ULN TB (another clinical marker for function, such as >1.5 × ULN INR may be acceptable if the change is clinically significant in the absence of obstruction) without >2 × ULN ALP; and 3-clinical verification to ensure that the liver injury is or is not induced by other diseases or another cause.

However, there are limitations since ALT is sensitive but not specific for liver injury, and TB is specific but insensitive for determining liver function [17]. A combination of both predicts the development of severe hepatotoxicity. The degree of ALT elevation determines serious liver injury. ALP >2 × ULN can be associated with subsequent liver failure. Sometimes a combination of the ratio: ALT [× ULN]/ALP [× ULN]) ≥5 with total bilirubin ≥2 × ULN at time of peak ALT may be considered a better and more predictive definition of Hy's Law [47]. However, a single case of drug-induced hepatotoxicity meeting Hy's Law should be considered as a signal of hepatotoxicity for the product.

7.5 Detecting and Assessing Hepatotoxicity

Clinical signs, clinical chemistry and microscopic changes should be made at multiple time intervals to determine the effect of exposure. When clinical chemistry or histologic evaluations indicate hepatic changes, studies on the mechanism of action should be conducted with serial specimens of blood, urine or tissues, including samples from matched asymptomatic treated individuals.

The identification of mechanisms and characterization of sub-population differences that result in hepatotoxicity, in vitro studies may help to identify the mechanism and the specific drugs, chemicals or natural product that induced liver injury. Factors such as timing, concomitant and/or preexisting liver disease, concomitant medications, the exclusion of alternative causes of liver damage, the response to dechallenge, and where appropriate, rechallenge of the treatment should be considered [47–49]. The risk profile may also be equally broad, and vary with factors including age, gender, ethnicity and concomitant diseases [50].

Assessment of hepatotoxicity requires a thorough clinical review of the patient and a systematic exclusion of other potential causes for the hepatic abnormalities as outlined in the chapter on DILI. Methods have been proposed for the assessment of hepatotoxicity in individual subjects, including but not limited to: Clinical Diagnostic Scale, Council for International Organizations of Medical Sciences (CIOMS)/RUCAM scale, Maria and Victorino Scales, the Naranjo Adverse Drug Reactions Probability Scale, and World Health Organization (WHO) causality algorithm [50–56]. European Medicines Agency and FDA present additional guidance for pharmaceutical industry [57–60].

Other factors and diseases may mimic or increase sensitivity towards drugs, or natural product-induced liver disease. These include: non-alcoholic steatotic hepatitis (NASH); Gilbert's syndrome; co-morbidity; paraneoplastic phenomena; metastases; viral hepatitis (A, B, C or E); alcohol and drugs of misuse; biliary abnormalities; autoimmune disease or immunosuppression; haemodynamic, genetic and metabolic disorders; concurrent and previous therapy, environmental and occupational exposures to xenobiotics including plant and animal toxins [5].

7.6 Morphologic Pathology

Nonspecific histologic lesions typically include: hepatitis, hepatocellular necrosis, granulomas, inflammatory cell infiltrates, zonal distribution of lesions, hepatocellular degenerative effects, apoptosis, cholestasis, steatosis, vascular lesions and neoplasia. Liver biopsy is required to assess structural changes. Additional assessments may include ultra-structural pathology, morphometrics, special histological stains, or antibody detection. The pattern of cellular injury, the presence of cellular infiltrates, and the presence of necrotic and/or apoptotic cells should all be assessed. The exclusion of other causes of liver injury requires a complete case report description, clinical laboratory radiology, and medical history to allow the evaluation of alternative causes [22, 23].

Hepatotoxins are found in nature as products of plants, fungal or bacterial metabolism, or as minerals [61–65]. Some toxins are products of the chemical or pharmaceutical industry [66, 67]. Still others are industrial byproducts or waste materials that, by polluting the environment, may gain access to humans [68, 69]. The injury also includes necrosis or apoptosis. Others lead only to interference with bile secretion and to jaundice with little injury to the hepatocytes [70].

A general scheme of toxin-induced liver injury is shown in Fig. 7.1.

Acetaminophen, may be safe in ordinarily therapeutic doses but hepatotoxic for a number of species in overdose or in

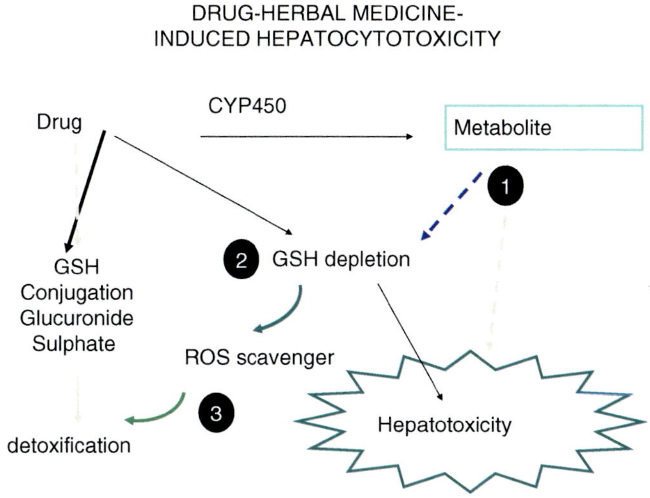

Fig. 7.1 Drug-herbal medicine induced hepatotoxicity. The drug at the therapeutical plasma concentration arriving to the liver is 1—glucuronate or sulphated to the non-toxic metabolite that is detoxify immediately or 2—undergo metabolization via Cyp 450 to the toxic metabolite. 3—Glutathione depletion does not permit detoxification leading to hepatotoxicity or a reactive oxygen scavenger can help to detoxification

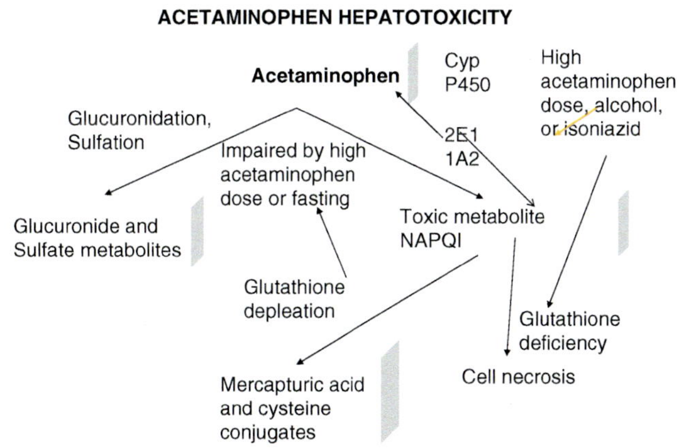

Fig. 7.2 Acetaminophen-induced liver injury. A small fraction of a dose is metabolized by a cytochrome P450 oxidase to a reactive intermediate. The metabolite is detoxified by conjugation with glutathione. If the dose given depletes glutathione reserves, metabolites may then covalently bind to cell macromolecules with resultant hepatotoxicity. High doses of acetaminophen or a combination of acetaminophen with alcohol deplete further the glutathione leading to hepatotoxicity

individuals with increased susceptibility [71]. Acetaminophen mechanism of toxicity has been extensively studied [72]. A fraction of a dose is metabolized by a cytochrome P450 oxidase to a reactive intermediate. The metabolite is detoxified by conjugation with glutathione. If the dose given depletes glutathione reserves, metabolites may then covalently bind to cell macromolecules with resultant hepatotoxicity [73].

Schematically acetaminophen-induced toxicity is presented in Fig. 7.2.

Increased toxicity could result from cytochrome P450 enzyme induction or deficits in glutathione detoxification from dietary deficiency or inborn errors of metabolism such as glutathione synthetase deficiency or regular alcohol consumption [74–76].

There is a wide range of hepatotoxic potency among intrinsic toxins. Moreover, within the group of "true" toxins and the group that depends on idiosyncrasy, several different mechanisms may be responsible for the production of hepatic injury [5].

Some phytotoxins, like the amanitin from *Amanita phalloides* and the pyrrolizidine alkaloids from *Caleolepis laureola*, are environmental hazards [77]. The phytotoxins are taken as "natural" medicines [78–81].

Important contributors to liver damage are environmental and occupational hazards. Ingestion of toxic agents (e.g. CCl_4) [82–86], were reported. Bromobenzene, phosphorus, ethionine and dimethyl-nitrosamine may play a role in the production of hepatic injury [87–90].

Microbiome attention focused on the demonstration the nitrosamines may be formed by intestinal bacteria in animals that ingest food preserved with nitrites. These observations have led to the concern that ingestion of nitrites and secondary amines by humans might provide exposure to the powerful hepatotoxic and hepatocarcinogenic effects of dimethylnitrosamine. Some strains of *Escherichia coli* can produce ethionine. This implies a microbiome-induced hepatotoxic effect. The production of lithocholate by microbiome should also be included [91].

The role of drug-induced hepatic injury becomes ever more important among elderly patients because of frequency of drug use and perhaps susceptibility.

The advances in the understanding of hepatotoxicity are due to revealing the enzyme mechanisms. The critical role of the cytochrome P-450 and its isoforms in drug metabolism as well as the development of molecular biology and the identification of cytokines have shed important light on the mechanisms of toxic hepatic injury.

7.7 Direct Hepatotoxins

Hepatotoxins that damage the liver by a directly destructive effect on the membranes of the hepatocyte are *direct* hepatotoxins. An example is carbon tetrachloride [82–86]. The halogenated aliphatic compounds are used in industry and the home and are found in the environment. Chloroform ($CHCl_3$) and carbon tetrachloride (CCl_4) are hepatotoxins. CCl_4 is a potent hepatotoxin leading to hepatic zonal necrosis [5].

Alcohol and drugs of use and misuse induced hepatotoxicity.

The pathological consequences of acute and chronic alcohol abuse are multi-factorial and multi-systemic. The dynamic interaction between chronic and acute alcohol abuse appears to play differential roles in the patterns of tissue injury and fibrogenesis between young individuals and elderly individuals [92–95].

Table 7.4 Elements to determine chemical or drug induce-toxicity

Pathology	Histopathology	Critical for identification of certain hepatic changes
	Gross pathology	Critical for determination of pathogenesis/mechanism of change
	Biochemistry	
Clinical	Clinical observations	In itself does not identify selected hepatic change, but does provide complementary data and clinical consequence to hepatic changes, includes accumulation of parent substrate and metabolite(s)
	Body weight, Diet Alcohol consumption,	
	Other drugs of use and misuse or complementary and alternative medicine	
Expression	Metabolism and transport: inhibition/induction	Provides complementary data for morphologic pathology findings
		Critical for determining certain potential interactions

CYP2E1 induction leads to increased metabolism of acetaminophen, valproic acid and methotrexate. Their toxic intermediates result in hepatocytes injury [96].

The interaction between alcohol and the anti-TB drug, isoniazid, also presents clinical importance since the metabolism of this drug involves acetylation. Since acyl transferase, the enzyme responsible for this step, is polymorphic, individuals who possess an acyl transferase with low activity may accumulate an intermediate which is then activated by CYP2E1 [97].

The interplay between alcohol and cytokine-mediated cellular effects is also important in the mechanism of liver injury. Chronic alcohol consumption may damage the liver by inhibiting the hepatoprotective actions of some cytokines, while adding to the pro-inflammatory effect of other cytokines. The co-morbidity of ALD and hepatitis C virus (HCV) infection, hepatitis B virus (HBV) infection or human immunodeficiency virus (HIV) infection leads to enhanced liver damage. Moreover, medications used to treat viral infections or other co-morbidities can interact with alcohol [98, 99].

Table 7.4 presents some elements that may help to determine chemical or drug induce-toxicity.

Phenotypic both chemical-drug and herbal induce injury present as immuno-hepatitis autoimmune hepatitis, hepatic necrosis/apoptosis, Acute liver failure, Cholestatic hepatitis, Steatosis/Steatohepatitis Sinusoidal obstruction syndrome, Vanishing bile duct syndrome.

The micrographs (Figs. 7.3, 7.4, 7.5, and 7.6) present the biopsies of individuals diagnosed with hepatotoxicity due to interactions between alcohol consumption and drugs of use or misuse.

Acknowledgements All the micrographs presented are cases that consulted Dr. Neuman and belong to In Vitro Drug Safety and Biotechnology.

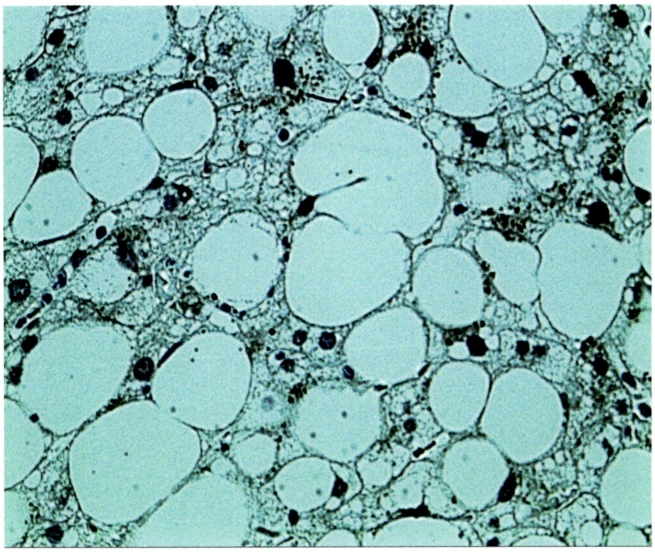

Fig. 7.3 Micrograph of a liver biopsy from a patient that consume alcohol and took risperidone. The diagnostic is non-alcoholic steatohepatitis. Large lipid droplets cover almost the entire hepatocyte and necrotic cells can be seen (magnification ×60)

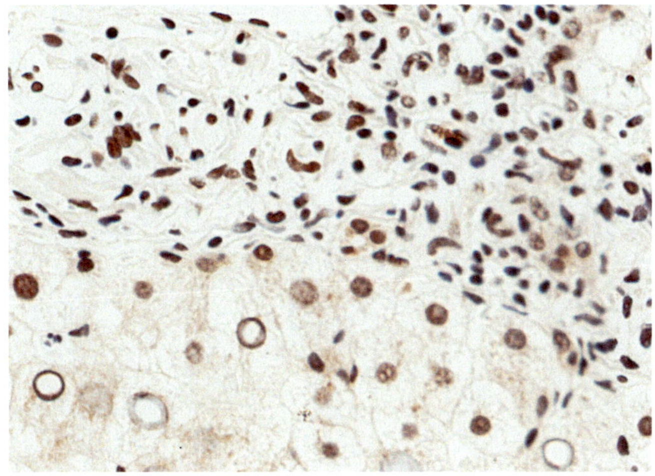

Fig. 7.4 Micrograph of a liver biopsy from a patient that consume alcohol and took phenytoin. The patient is ethnic Han-Chinese. He has a alcohol dehydrogenase polymorphism and a human leucocyte antigen polymorphism. Diagnosis is liver failure

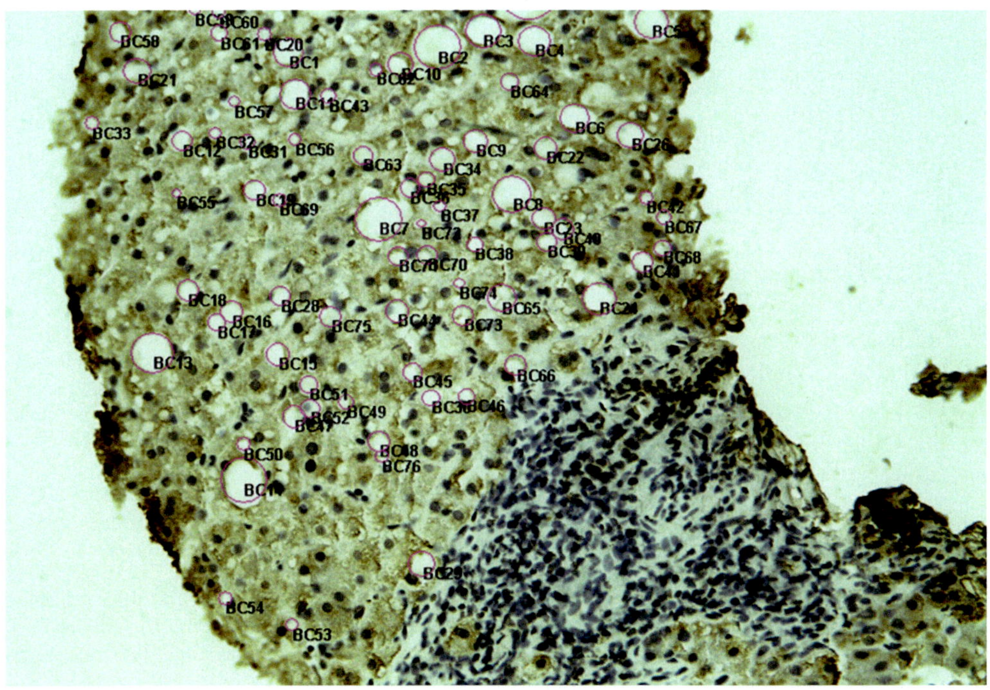

Fig. 7.5 Micrograph of a liver biopsy of a patient that combine consumption of alcohol and *Cannabis* sp. Diagnosis is massive necrosis (Magnification ×20)

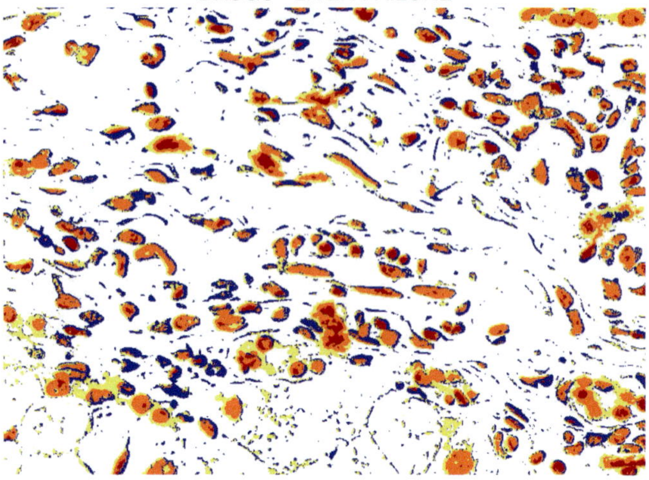

Fig. 7.6 Micrograph of a liver biopsy from a patient that consume alcohol and recreational drugs. Diagnosis is liver failure

Self Study

Questions and Answers

Which statement is true

1. Acetaminophen at therapeutic concentration taken concomitantly with alcohol in normal doses is
   (a) not harmful
   (b) a deadly combination
   Response correct (b)
2. In drug-induced hepatitis, which of the following is correct?
   (a) ALT is higher than AST
   (b) AST is higher than ALT
   Response correct (a)
3. Herbal and complementary medicine may produce:
   (a) Liver damage
   (b) Enhancement of liver function
   (c) Liver failure
   (d) All of the above
   Response correct (a)

References

1. Ch R. Experimental toxic injury of the liver. In: Ch R, editor. The liver. New York: Academic; 1964. p. 335–476.
2. Benhamou JP. Drug-induced hepatitis: clinical aspects. In: Fillastre JP, editor. Hepatotoxicity of drugs. Rouen: Universite de Rouen; 1986. p. 26–30.
3. Zimmerman HJ. The spectrum of hepatotoxicity. Perspect Biol Med. 1968;12:135–61.
4. Zimmerman HJ, Maddrey WC. Toxic and drug-induced hepatitis. In: Schiff L, Schiff ER, editors. Diseases of the liver. Philadelphia: JB Lippincott Company; 1993. p. 707–69.
5. Zimmerman HJ. Hepatotoxicity: the adverse effects of drug and other chemicals on the liver. 2nd ed. Philadelphia: Lippincott Williams and Wilkins; 1999. Chapters 4, 5 and 16
6. McCuskey RS, Earnest DL. Hepatic and gastrointestinal toxicology, vol 9. In: Sipes IG, CA MQ, Gandolfi AJ, editors. Comprehensive toxicology. Cambridge: Pergamen Press; 1997.
7. Wieland T. Poisonous principles of mushrooms of the genus Amanita. Science. 1968;159:946.
8. Goldblatt LA. Aflatoxins—scientific background control and implications. New York: Academic; 1969.
9. Neuman MG, Eshchar J, Cotariu D, Ishay J, Barr-Nea L. Hepatotoxicity of Hornet's venom sac extract, after repeated *in vivo* and *in vitro* envenomation. Acta Pharmacol Toxicol Scand. 1983;53:314–9.
10. Neuman MG, Ishay J, Zimmerman HJ, Eshchar J. Hepatotoxicity of the oriental hornet venom. Harefuah. 1990;118(2):78–80.
11. Teschke R, Danan G. Review: drug induced liver injury with analysis of alternative causes as confounding variables. Br J Clin Pharmacol. 2018;84:1467–77.
12. Chuttani HK, Gupta PS, Gulati S, Gupta DN. Acute copper sulfate poisoning. Am J Med. 1965;39:849.
13. Goldstein BD, Witz G. Benzene. In: Lippman M, editor. Environmental toxicants: human exposures and their health effects. 2nd ed. New York: Wiley Interscience; 2000. p. 121–51.
14. Kenna JG. Immunological allergic drug-induced hepatitis. Lessons from halothane. J Hepatol. 1997;26(Suppl):5.
15. Ludwig J, Kim CH, Wiesner RH, Krom RI. Floxuridine-induced sclerosing cholangitis. An ischemic cholangiopathy? Hepatology. 1989;9:215–8.
16. Neuman MG, French SW, Zakhari S, Malnick S, Seitz HK, Cohen LB, Salaspuro M, Voinea-Griffin A, Barasch A, Kirpich IA, Thomes PS, Schrum LW, Donohue TM Jr, Kharbanda K, Cruz M, Opris M. Alcohol, microbiome, life style influence alcohol and non-alcoholic organ damage. Exp Mol Pathol. 2017;102(1):162–80. https://doi.org/10.1016/j.yexmp.2017.01.003.
17. Navarro VJ, Senior JR. Drug-related hepatotoxicity. N Engl J Med. 2006;354(7):731–9.
18. Hoofnagle JH, Carithers RL, Shapiro C, Ascher N. Fulminant hepatic failure. Summary of a workshop. Hepatology. 1995;21:240–52.
19. Zafrani E, Pinaudeau Y, Dhumeaux D. Drug-induced vascular lesions of the liver. Arch Intern Med. 1983;143:195–200.
20. Daly A. Drug-induced liver injury: past, present and future. Pharmacogenomics. 2010;11:607–11.
21. Lee WM, Senior JR. Recognizing drug-induced liver injury: current problems, possible solutions. Toxicol Pathol. 2005;33(1):155–64.
22. Rappaport AM. Acinar units and pathophysiology of the liver. In: Rouiller C, editor. The liver, vol. I. New York: Academic; 1963. p. 265–328.
23. Zimmerman HJ, Ishak KG. Hepatic injury due to drugs and toxins. In: MacSween RNM, Anthony PP, Scheuer PJ, Burt AD, Portman BC, editors. Pathology of the liver. 3rd ed. Edinburgh: Churchill-Livingstone; 1994. p. 563–634.
24. Ishak KG, Mullick FG. Drug-induced and toxic injury. In: Peters RL, Craig JR, editors. Liver pathology. New York: Churchill-Livingstone; 1986. p. 221–54.
25. Neuman MG, Winkler R. Veno-occlusive disease of the liver induced by traditional herbal medicine Roumanian. J Rev Hepatol. 2008;4(2):3, 7-9.
26. Loyke HF. Experimental hypertension treated with CCl4: measurement of adrenal function, vascular responsiveness, and angiotensinase converting enzyme. Proc Soc Exp Biol Med. 1964;115:1035.
27. Andrade RJ, Robles M, Lucena MI. Rechallenge in drug-induced liver injury: the attractive hazard. Expert Opin Drug Saf. 2009;8(6):709–14.

28. Watkins PB. Role of cytochrome P450 in drug metabolism and hepatotoxicity. Semin Liver Dis. 1990;10:235–50.
29. Plaa GL, Hewitt WR. Quantitative evaluation of indices of hepatotoxicity. In: Plaa GL, Hewitt WR, editors. Toxicology of the liver. New York: Raven Press; 1982. p. 103–20.
30. Ishak KG, Zimmerman HJ. Morphologic spectrum of drug-induced hepatic disease. Gastroenterol Clin No Am. 1995;24:759–78.
31. Wilke RA, Reif DM, Moore JH. Combinatorial pharmacogenetics. Nature Rev Drug Discov. 2005;4:911–8.
32. Pirmohamed M, Park BK. Genetic susceptibility to adverse drug reactions. Trends Pharmacol Sci. 2001;22:298–305.
33. Severino G, Del Zompo M. Adverse drug reactions: role of pharmacogenomics. Pharmacol Res. 2004;49:363–73.
34. Lazarou J, Pomeranz BH, Corey PN. Incidence of adverse drug reactions in hospitalized patients: a meta-analysis of prospective studies. JAMA. 1998;279:1200–5.
35. Pasanen MK, Neuvonen M, Neuvonen PJ, Niemi M. *SLCO1B1* polymorphism markedly affects the pharmacokinetics of simvastatin acid. Pharmacogenet Gen. 2006;16:873–9.
36. Bissell DM, Gores GJ, Laskin DL, Hoofnagle JH. Drug-induced liver injury: mechanisms and test systems. Hepatology. 2001;33:1009–13.
37. Neuman MG. Apoptosis in liver disease. Rom J Gastroenterol. 2002;11(1):3–7.
38. Phillips MJ, Latham PS, Poucell-Halton S. Electron microscopy of human liver disease. In: Schiff L, Schiff ER, editors. Diseases of the liver. 7th ed. Philadelphia: J.B. Lippincott; 1993. p. 189–216.
39. Apostolova N, Lj G-S, Moran A, Alvarez A, Blas-Garcia A, Esplugues J. Enhanced oxidative stress and increased mitochondrial mass during Efavirenz-induced apoptosis in human hepatic cells. Br J Pharmacol. 2010;160(8):2069–84.
40. Assis DN, Navarro VJ. Human drug hepatotoxicity: a contemporary clinical perspective. Expert Opin Drug Metab Toxicol. 2009;5(5):463–73.
41. De Bus L, Depuydt P, Libbrecht L, Vandekerckhove L, Nollet J, Benoit D, Vogelaers D, Van Vlierberghe H. Severe drug-induced liver injury associated with prolonged use of linezolid. J Med Toxicol. 2010;6(3):322–6.
42. Jones DP, Lemasters JJ, Han D, Boelsterli UA, Kaplowitz N. Mechanisms of pathogenesis in drug hepatotoxicity putting the stress on mitochondria. Mol Interv. 2010;10(2):98–111.
43. Kaplowitz N, LD DL. Drug-induced hepatic disease. New York: Marcel Decker Inc; 2003.
44. Lucena MI, Garca-Martín E, Andrade RJ, Martínez C, Stephens C, Ruiz JD, Ulzurrun E, Fernandez MC, Romero-Gomez M, Castiella A, Planas R, Durán JA, De Dios AM, Guarner C, Soriano G, Borraz Y, Agundez JA. Mitochondrial superoxide dismutase and glutathione peroxidase in idiosyncratic drug-induced liver injury. Hepatology. 2010;52(1):303–12.
45. Neuman MG. Cytokines and Inflamed Liver. Clin Biochem. 1999;33:601–5.
46. Lewis J. 'Hy's law', the 'Rezulin Rule' and other predictors of severe drug-induced hepatotoxicity; putting risk-benefit into perspective. Pharmacoepiol Drug Safety. 2006;15:221–9.
47. Neuman MG, Malkiewicz IM, Shear NH. A novel lymphocyte toxicity assay to assess drug hypersensitivity syndromes. Clin Biochem. 2000;33(7):517–24.
48. Neuman MG, Shear NH, Jacobson-Brown PM, Katz GG, Neilson HK, Malkiewicz IM, Cameron RG, Abbott F. CYP2E1-mediated modulation of valproic acid-induced hepatocytotoxicity. Clin Biochem. 2001;34(3):211–8.
49. Krivoy N, Taeri M, Neuman MG. Antiepileptic drug-induced hypersensitivity syndrome reactions mechanisms. Curr Drug Safety. 2006;1(3):289–99.
50. Aithal GP, Rawlins MD, Day CP. Clinical diagnostic scale: a useful tool in the evaluation of suspected hepatotoxic adverse drug reactions. J Hepatol. 2000;33(6):949–52.
51. Danan G, Benichou C. Causality assessment of adverse reactions to drugs—I. A novel method based on the conclusions of international consensus meetings: application to drug-induced liver injuries. J Clin Epidemiol. 1993;46(11):1323–30.
52. Fontana RJ, Seeff LB, Andrade RJ, Björnsson E, Day CP, Serrano J, Hoofnagle JH. Standardization of nomenclature and causality assessment in drug-induced liver injury: summary of a clinical research workshop. Hepatology. 2010;52(2):730–42.
53. Food and Drug Administration Warning Working Group. Nonclinical assessment of potential hepatotoxicity in man. p. 1–12, appendix, November 2000. Food and Drug Administration Warning Working Group. Clinical white paper. November 2000.
54. Lee WM. Drug-induced hepatotoxicity. N Engl J Med. 2003;349:474–85.
55. Maria VA, Victorino RM. Development and validation of a clinical scale for the diagnosis of drug-induced hepatitis. Hepatology. 1997;26(3):664–9.
56. Naranjo CA, Busto U, Sellers EM, Sandor P, Ruiz I, Roberts EA, Janecek E, Domecq C, Greenblatt DJ. A method for estimating the probability of adverse drug reactions. Clin Pharmacol Ther. 1981;30(2):239–45.
57. European Medicines Agency, Committee for Medicinal Products for Human Use, Draft Guideline on Detection of Early Signals of Drug-induced Hepatotoxicity in Non-clinical Studies. Doc. Ref. EMEA/CHMP/SWP/150115/2006. 2006.
58. Food and Drug Administration Warning. 2004. www.fda.gov/medwatch/SAFETY/2004/Viramune_PI.pdf
59. Food and Drug Administration. Warning concept paper. Premarketing evaluation of drug-induced liver injury. 2007.
60. Food and Drug Administration. Guidance for industry, drug-induced liver injury: premarketing clinical evaluation. 2009.
61. McLean EK. The toxic actions of pyrrolizidine (Senecio) alkaloids. Pharmacol Rev. 1970;22:429–83.
62. Neuman MG, Cameron RG, Shear NH, Feuer G. Drug-induced apoptosis of skin cells and liver. In: Cameron RG, Fauer G, editors. Handbook of experimental pharmacology: apoptosis modulation by drugs. Vol. 142, Chapter 13. Heidelberg: Springer Verlag Publishers; 1999. p. 344–55.
63. Neuman MG, Cohen L, Opris M, Nanau RM, Jeong H. Hepatotoxicity of pyrrolizidine alkaloids. J Pharm Pharm Sci. 2015;18(4):825–43.
64. Neuman MG, Ishay J, Zimmerman HJ, Eshchar J. Hepatotoxicity of *Vespa orientalis* venom sac extract. Pharmacol Toxicol. 1991;69(1):1–36.
65. Schoepfer AM, Engel A, Fattinger K, Marbet UA, Criblez D, Reichen J, Zimmermann A, Oneta CM. Herbal does not mean innocuous: ten cases of severe hepatotoxicity associated with dietary supplements from Herbalife products. J Hepatol. 2007;47(4):521–6.
66. Fischl J. Aminoaciduria in thallium poisoning. Am J Med Sci. 1966;251:40.
67. Luongo MA, Bjornson SS. The liver in ferrous sulfate poisoning. A report of three fatal cases in children and an experimental study. N Engl J Med. 1954;251:995.
68. Bagberi SA, Boyer JL. Peliosis hepatis associated with androgen-anabolic steroid therapy. A severe form of hepatic injury. Ann Intern Med. 1974;81:6100618.
69. Benjamin SB, Ishak KG, Zimmerman H, Agron M. Phenylbutazone liver injury: a clinical pathologic survey of 23 cases and review of the of the literature. Hepatology. 1981;1:255–63.
70. McLean AEM, McLean ER, Judah JD. Cellular necrosis in the liver induced and modified by drugs. Internat Rev Exp Pathol. 1965;4:127.
71. Schiodt FV, Rochling FA, Casey DL, Lee WM. Acetaminophen toxicity in a urban county hospital. N Engl J Med. 1997;337:112–7.
72. Vale JA, Proudfoot AT. Paracetamol (acetaminophen) poisoning. Lancet. 1995;346:547–52.

73. Wendel A, Feuerstein S, Konz KH. Acute paracetamol intoxication of starved mice leads to lipid peroxidation in vivo. Biochem Pharmacol. 1979;28:2051.
74. Artwohl JE, Henne-Bruns O, Carter E, Cara LM. Acetaminophen toxicosis: a potential model for liver failure in swine. Vet Hum Toxicol. 1988;30:324.
75. Zimmerman HJ. Effects of aspirin and acetaminophen on the liver. Arch Intern Med. 1981;141:333–8.
76. Zimmmerman HJ, Maddrey WC. Acetaminophen (paracetamol) hepatotoxicity with regular intake of alcohol. Analysis of instances of a therapeutic misadventure. Hepatology. 1995;22:767–2.
77. Schiano TD. Liver injury from herbs and other botanicals. Clin Liver Dis. 1998;2:607–36.
78. Javaid A, Bonkovsky HL. Hepatotoxicity due to extracts of Chinese green tea (*Camellia sinensis*): a growing concern. J Hepatol. 2006;45(2):334–5.
79. Jimenez-Saenz M, Martinez-Sanchez MC. Acute hepatitis associated with the use of green tea infusions. J Hepatol. 2006;44(3):616–7.
80. Molinari M, Watt KD, Kruszyna T, Nelson R, Walsh M, Huang WY, Nashan B, Peltekian K. Acute liver failure induced by green tea extracts: case report and review of the literature. Liver Transpl. 2006;12(12):1892–5.
81. Teschke R, Andrade RJ. Special Issue "Drug, Herb, and Dietary Supplement Hepatotoxicity". Int J Mol Sci. 2016;17(9):1488. https://doi.org/10.3390/ijms17091488.
82. Cornish HM, Block WD. A study of carbon tetrachloride. II. The effect of carbon tetrachloride on serum and tissue enzymes. Arch Environ Hlth. 1960;1:96.
83. Kosrud GO, Price HG, McLaughlin JM. Sensitivity of several serum enzymes in detecting carbon tetrachloride-induced liver damage in rats. Toxicol Appl Pharmacol. 1972;22:474.
84. Fox CF, Dinman BD, Frajola WJ. CCl4 poisoning. II. Serum enzymes, free fatty acids and liver pathology: effects of phenoxybenzamine and phenergan. Proc Soc Exp Biol Med. 1962;111:731.
85. Recknagel RO. Carbon tetrachloride hepatotoxicity. Pharmacol Rev. 1967;19:145.
86. Recknagel RO, Glende EA Jr. Carbon tetrachloride hepatotoxicity: an example of lethal cleavage. CRC Crit Rev Toxicol. 1973;2:263.
87. Lai KK, Gang DL, Zawacki JK, Cooley TP. Fulminant hepatic failure associated with 2′3′dideoxyinosine (ddI). Ann Intern Med. 1991;165:382–284.
88. Davis DC, Hashimoto M, Gillette JR. Effects of bromobenzene and carbon tetrachloride on the synthesis and release of proteins by the perfused rat liver. Biochem Pharmacol. 1973;22:1989.
89. Althausen TL, Thoenes E. Influence on carbohydrate metabolism of experimentally induced hepatic changes in phosphorus poisoning. Arch Intern Med. 1932;50:58.
90. Suzuki S, Ogawa W, Shibata KL, Tsuzuki H. Changes in Zn and Fe metabolism and carbonic anhydrase and catalase activity in animals with liver damage by carbon tetrachloride or ethionine. Jpn J Pharmacol. 1967;17:393.
91. Gumucio JJ, Katz ME, Miller DL, et al. Bile salt transport after selective damage to acinar zone 3 hepatocytes by bromobenzene in the rat. Toxicol Appl Pharmacol. 1979;50:77.
92. Haddad P, Gascon-Barr M, Dumont A. Comparative hepatic response to bromobenzene and allyl alcohol in the vitamin D-replete and vitamin D depleted rat. J Pharmacol Exp Ther. 1985;233:499.
93. Mallory FB. Phosphorous poisoning and alcoholic cirrhosis. Am J Pathol. 1933;9:557.
94. Rojkind A. Collagen metabolism in the liver. In: Hall P, editor. Alcoholic liver disease pathobiology, epidemiology and clinical aspects. London: Edward Arnold; 1985. p. 90–112.
95. Maker JJ, Friedman SL. Pathogenesis of hepatic fibrosis. In: Hall P, editor. Alcoholic liver disease. 2nd ed. London: Edward Arnold; 1995. p. 71–8.
96. Seeff LB, Cuccherini BA, Zimmerman HJ, Adler E, Benjamin SB. Acetaminophen hepatotoxicity in alcoholics: a therapeutic misadventure. Ann Intern Med. 1986;104:399–404.
97. Neuman MG, Cohen LB, Steenkamp V. Pyrrolizidine alkaloids enhance alcohol-induced hepatocytotoxicity *in vitro* in normal human hepatocytes. Eur Rev Med Pharmacol Sci. 2017;21(1 Suppl):53–68.
98. Katz GG, Shear NH, Malkiewicz IM, Valentino K, Neuman MG. Signaling for ethanol-induced apoptosis and repair *in vitro*. Clin Biochem. 2001;34:219–27.
99. Malnick S, Maor Y, Melzer E, Ziv-Sokolowskaia N, Neuman MG. Severe hepatotoxicity link to denosumab. Eur Rev Med Pharmacol Sci. 2017;21(1):78–85.

Crosstalk of Molecular Signaling in Hepatocellular Carcinoma

8

Huarong Chen and Jun Yu

Key Concepts

- Hepatocellular carcinoma is one of the most common cancers with high mortality worldwide.
- The development of sorafenib represents a breakthrough in molecular targeted therapy for HCC. However, high rate of sorafenib resistance greatly limits its beneficial effects.
- HCC is a highly heterogeneous malignancy, characterized by alteration of a multitude of different signaling pathways.
- Crosstalk among signaling pathways may play a pivotal role in affecting efficacy of molecular targeted therapy for HCC.

8.1 Introduction

Hepatocellular carcinoma (HCC) is the most common primary liver malignancy, which accounts for around 782,000 new cancer cases and 745,000 deaths worldwide in 2012 [1]. The major known risk factors for the development of HCC are chronic hepatitis B virus or hepatitis C virus infections, alcohol abuse, obesity and nonalcoholic fatty liver disease [2]. Surgical resection or percutaneous ablation is considered first-line treatment option for HCC patients in early stage, whereas the recurrence rate is nearly 50% at 5 years [3–6]. In addition, more than 50% of patients with HCC present an advanced or unresectable disease at diagnosis, whose prognosis is very poor and the therapeutic options are limited [7]. For the past decade, sorafenib is the only molecular target drug approved for first-line treatment of advanced primary liver cancer, which extends median overall survival from 7.9 months to 10.7 months [8]. However, most patients are highly refractory to sorafenib treatment, inferring the existence of resistance factors in primary HCC tissues [9]. In this case, regorafenib and nivolumab were approved last year as second-line treatment for HCC patients who have previously received sorafenib. Even so, the objective response rate was only 10.6% in patients treated with regorafenib and 15–20% with nivolumab [10, 11], underlining the importance of systematical investigations of therapeutic strategies for HCC.

The development of HCC is a complex multistep process, characterized by alteration of multiple genetic and epigenetic events. Over the last few decades, a series of studies has unraveled several oncogenic signaling pathways implicated in HCC that regulate cell survival, proliferation, invasion, angiogenesis, and metastasis. These include mitogen activated protein kinase/extracellular-signal-regulated kinase (MAPK/ERK) pathway, phosphatidylinositol 3-kinase/protein kinase B/mammalian target of rapamycin (PI3K/Akt/mTOR) pathway, Wnt/β-catenin signaling pathway, Transforming growth factor beta (TGF-β) pathway, Janus kinase/signal transducers and activators of transcription (JAK/STAT) pathway, and Mouse double minute 2 homolog (MDM2)-p53 pathway. Moreover, the advent of next-generation sequencing techniques vastly accelerate the acquisition of genomic data to decipher the mutational landscape of HCC and lead to the identification of main potential drivers with associated dysregulated pathways that trigger hepatocarcinogenesis. All these emerge as potential therapeutic targets. Importantly, signaling pathways within cells can crosstalk with each other. Alteration of one pathway may signal to either enhance or suppress another pathway. The crosstalk between pathways and feedback inhibition constitutes a complex network of signal transduction that drives dynamic and adaptive cellular responses [12]. In cancer, aberrant regulation of crosstalk has been demonstrated, in

H. Chen · J. Yu (✉)
Institute of Digestive Disease and Department of Medicine and Therapeutics, State Key laboratory of Digestive Disease, Li Ka Shing Institute of Health Sciences, CUHK Shenzhen Research Institute, The Chinese University of Hong Kong, Sha Tin, Hong Kong, China
e-mail: hchen2@cuhk.edu.hk; junyu@cuhk.edu.hk

F. Radu-Ionita et al. (eds.), *Liver Diseases*, https://doi.org/10.1007/978-3-030-24432-3_8

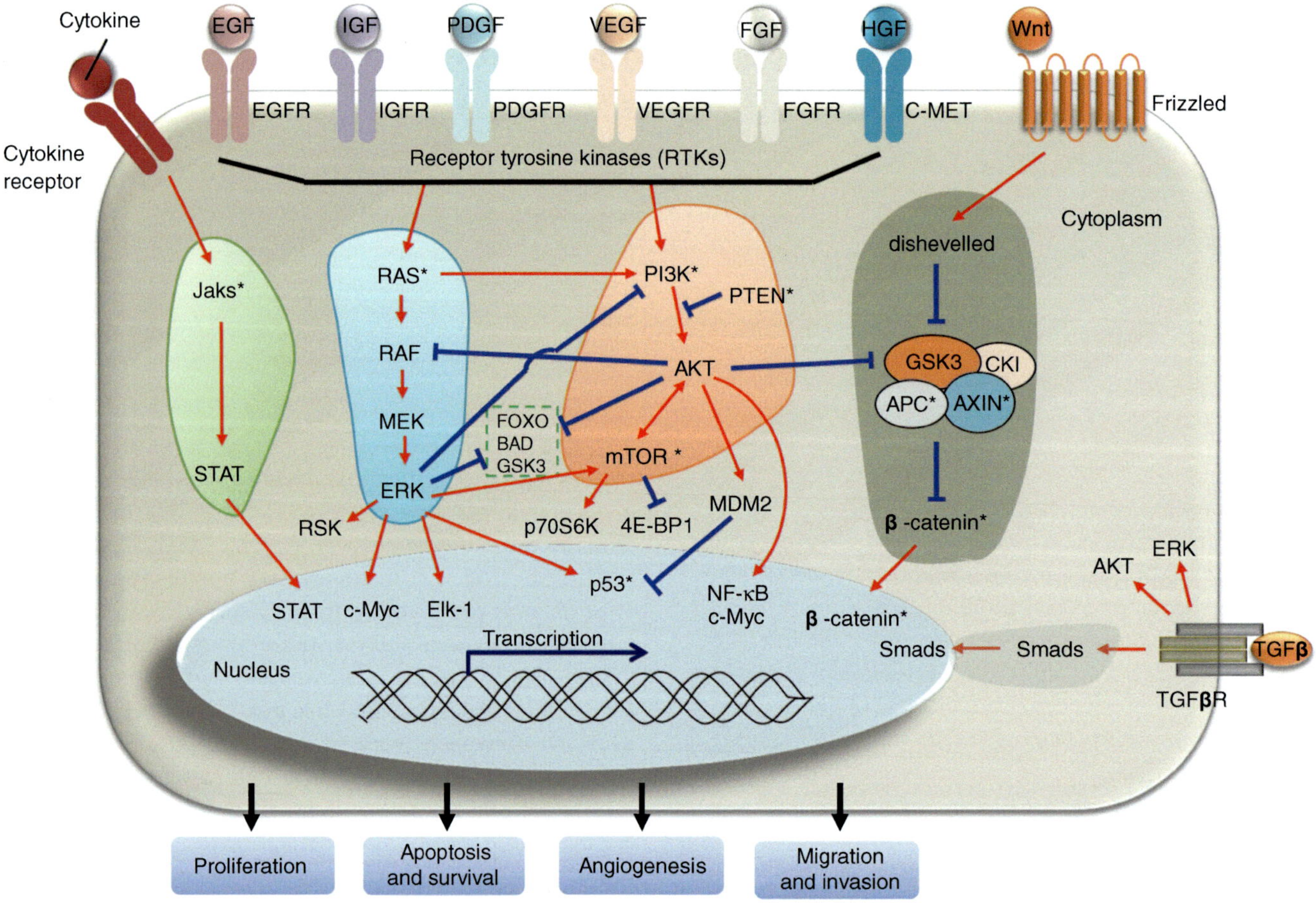

Fig. 8.1. Cellular signaling pathways implicated in the pathogenesis of hepatocellular carcinoma (HCC). Asterisks indicate mutated genes in HCC. Positive and negative regulation of the substrate protein is shown as red arrow and green blunt-ended line, respectively

which oncogenic factors can cause rewiring of signaling networks [13]. This turns out to favor the adaptation of cancer cells to drug treatment, emphasizing the need and importance to illustrate crosstalk between major signaling pathways inside cancer. The purpose of this paper is to discuss the major dysregulated pathways, relevant somatic driver mutations, and the signaling crosstalk implicated in the pathogenesis of HCC (Fig. 8.1).

8.2 Receptor Tyrosine Kinases Signaling

Receptor tyrosine kinases (RTKs) are the high-affinity and single-pass transmembrane receptors, which bind various polypeptide growth factors, cytokines, and hormones [14]. In human genome, 58 of the 90 unique tyrosine kinase genes are identified to encode receptor tyrosine kinase proteins, e.g., epidermal growth factor receptor (EGFR), vascular endothelial growth factor receptor (VEGFR), platelet-derived growth factor receptors (PDGFR), fibroblast growth factor receptor (FGFR), hepatocyte growth factor receptor (HGFR or c-MET) and insulin growth factor receptor (IGFR) [15]. All RTKs have a similar molecular architecture comprising a ligand-binding domain of the extracellular region, a transmembrane helix, and a cytoplasmic region recognized as catalytic domains and protein-protein interaction sites [16]. Upon binding growth factor ligands, the "inactive" RTKs undergo a substantial conformational change that allows it to be stabilized in an "active" dimer or oligomer, which in turn activate the intracellular signaling pathways [17]. A large body of evidence suggests that RTKs function as key regulatory nodes of critical cellular processes, such as proliferation, survival, differentiation, metabolism, motility and cell-cycle control [18]. Mutations and aberrant activation of RTKs signaling pathways have been demonstrated in HCC, including MAPK/ERK and PI3K/Akt/mTOR pathway [19–21].

8.3 MAPK/ERK Pathway

The MAPK/ERK pathway, also known as Ras-Raf-MAP/ERK kinase (MEK)-ERK pathway, is one of the most important signaling cascades for liver tumorigenesis. The MAPK/ERK pathway is activated in 50% of HCC patients in early stage and almost all HCC patients in advanced-stage [22–24]. MAPK/ERK pathway transduces extracellular signals from "active" RTKs to the cell nucleus through a series of phosphorylation events regulated by specific kinases and GTP/GDP exchange proteins. Upon epidermal growth factor (EGF) binding, EGFR can form active homo or hetero dimmers to stimulate its intrinsic intracellular protein-tyrosine kinase activity, resulting in autophosphorylation of tyrosine residues in its C-terminal domain [25]. Several adaptor proteins that contain Src-homology 2 domains (SH2), e.g., growth factor receptor-bound protein 2 (Grb2) and Src homology 2 domain-containing transforming protein (SHC), can bind to the phosphorylated tyrosine residues of EGFR [26, 27]. Meanwhile, Grb2 also binds to the guanine nucleotide exchange factor Son of Sevenless (SOS) to form a complex. Once the Grb2-SOS complex is recruited to activated receptors, SOS becomes active and subsequently promotes the switch of Ras from an inactive GDP-bound state to an active GTP-bound state [28]. Activation of Ras then stimulates a series of phosphorylation events downstream the MAPK cascade. Although mutations of RAS are frequent in human cancers, it is rare in HCC patients with a reported frequency of less than 3% [9, 29, 30]. Active Ras recruits Raf from the cytoplasm to the plasma membrane for activation. Raf is the best characterized Ras effector that functions as essential connector between Ras and the downstream MEK-ERK signaling [31]. Active Raf induces the phosphorylation of MEK1 and MEK2 which successively phosphorylate and activate ERK1 and ERK2 [32]. Upon activation, ERK can phosphorylate target proteins in cytoplasm, e.g., ribosomal protein S6 kinases (RSKs), which in turn phosphorylate several cytoplasmic targets and transcriptional regulators [33]. Furthermore, phosphorylated ERK can translocate to nucleus and directly phosphorylates transcription factor substrates that promote cellular growth and inhibit apoptosis [34]. Proto-oncogene c-myc is one of direct target of ERK which is involved in multiple aspects of growth control. ERK-induced phosphorylation of c-Myc at serine (Ser) 62 promotes c-Myc protein stabilization, thus enhancing its expression and activity [35].

8.4 PI3K/Akt/mTOR Pathway

PI3K/Akt/mTOR pathway is another key mechanism for controlling cell proliferation, survival, and metabolism in HCC. Binding of growth factors, e.g., IGF and EGF, to their receptors can activate class I PI3Ks through either direct recruitment of PI3K or indirect recruitment involving the insulin receptor substrate (IRS) or GRB2-associated binder (GAB) docking proteins [20]. Activating mutations of PIK3CA, which encodes p110α catalytic subunit of PI3K, are also found to activate PI3K/Akt/mTOR signaling. Somatic mutations of PIK3CA are common in many cancer types [36], whilst a low frequency of 3% is observed in HCC [9, 29, 30]. The class I PI3Ks can phosphorylate phosphatidylinositol (4,5)-bisphosphate (PIP2) to produce phosphatidylinositol-3,4,5-trisphosphate (PIP3), a phospholipid that resides on the plasma membrane [37]. PIP3 recruits the protein kinase Akt and 3-phosphoinositide-dependent kinase 1 (PDK1) to the cell membrane, where Akt is phosphorylated on threonine (Thr) 308 and Ser473 by PDK1 and mTOR Complex 2 (mTORC2), respectively [38]. Once activated, Akt phosphorylates and inactivates several substrates, such as forkhead box O (FOXO), BCL2-associated agonist of cell death (BAD) and Glycogen synthase kinase 3 beta (GSK3β), to enhance cell growth and survival [38]. Loss of phosphatase and tensin homolog (PTEN) function also leads to overactivation of Akt in cancer cells. PTEN is a lipid phosphatase that negatively regulates PI3K/Akt signaling by dephosphorylating the PIP3 [39]. Frequent loss of PTEN through gene deletion, mutation, or epigenetic silencing has been demonstrated in human HCC [40]. Targeted deletion of PTEN in mouse hepatocytes leads to the development of steatohepatitis and liver tumors [41]. In addition, we recently explore the role of squalene epoxidase, a rate-limiting enzyme in cholesterol biosynthesis, in promoting the development of non-alcoholic fatty liver disease-HCC through suppressing the expression of PTEN followed by activation of PI3K/Akt/mTOR pathway [42]. The critical downstream effector of Akt, mTOR, is a serine/threonine kinase that exerts profound effects on gene expression by translational control and plays a pivotal role in HCC [43]. mTOR protein serves as a core component of protein kinase complex mTOR complex 1 (mTORC1) by linking other proteins including regulatory-associated protein of mTOR (Raptor), mammalian lethal with SEC13 protein 8 (MLST8), proline-rich Akt substrate of 40 kDa (PRAS40) and DEP domain-containing mTOR-interacting protein (DEPTOR) [44–46]. Akt activates mTORC1 through the phosphorylation and inactivation of tuberous sclerosis complex 2 (TSC2), thus relieving the inhibitory effects of the TSC1-TSC2 complex on mTORC1 [47]. Inactivating mutations in TSC1 and TSC2, as well as activating mutations in MTOR have been identified in HCC with the estimated frequency of 3%, 5% and 2%, respectively [29, 30]. Activated mTORC1 phosphorylates two major downstream effectors, eukaryotic initiation factor 4E-binding protein 1 (4E-BP1) and 40S ribosomal protein S6 kinase (p70s6k), which are critical for translational regulation.

8.5 Crosstalk of ERK/MAPK and PI3K/Akt/mTOR Pathway

Recent findings have uncovered modes of crosstalk between ERK/MAPK and PI3K/Akt/mTOR pathway, including cross-activation, cross-inhibition and pathway convergence. Extensive negative- and positive-feedback loops exist between these two pathways, leading to sensitive pathway responses and multi-stability. In case of cross-activation, Ras-GTP can directly bind and activate PI3K [48]. The interaction of RAS with PI3K p110 subunit is required for RAS-driven tumorigenesis, as shown in KRAS-induced lung tumorigenesis mouse model and HRAS-induced skin carcinogenesis mouse model [49, 50]. Co-expression of activated forms of Ras and Akt in the mouse liver promotes rapid hepatocarcinogenesis in mice, mainly through induction of mTORC1 [51]. Under these circumstances, activation of ERK/MAPK pathway can stimulate mTOR signaling. The phosphorylation and inactivation of TSC2 by active Erk and RSK disrupt the association of TSC1-TSC2, thus relieving the inhibition of mTORC1 [52, 53]. Besides, Erk and RSK can induce RAPTOR phosphorylation, which subsequently elevates mTORC1 activity [54, 55]. In addition to cross-activation, ERK/MAPK and PI3K/Akt/mTOR pathways can negatively act on each other. In response to a selective small molecule inhibitor of MEK, feedback upregulation of the PI3K/Akt pathway is observed in basal-like breast cancer cells [56]. In keeping with this, blocking EGF-stimulated ERK activation by MEK inhibitor can enhance the association between Gab1 and PI3K p85 subunit, resulting in increased phosphorylation of Akt and PI3K activity [57]. On the contrary, endogenous activation of ERK reduces insulin-stimulated Akt activation via inducing Gab1 phosphorylation [58]. Another analogous cross-inhibition occurs between Akt and Raf. Strong IGF1 stimulation quickly activates Akt but induces phosphorylation of Raf at Ser259 to suppress its kinase activity [59]. Akt binds and antagonizes Raf activity by direct phosphorylation on Ser259 in the regulatory domain of Raf, thus causing inhibition of the ERK/MAPK pathway [60]. Protein phosphatases 1 (PP1) and 2A (PP2A) may remove these inhibitory phosphorylations to promote Raf-1 activation [61]. In addition to the negative- and positive-feedback loops, activation of ERK/MAPK and PI3K/Akt/mTOR signaling often converge on the same substrate, e.g., c-Myc, FoxO, BAD and GSK3 [51, 62, 63]. In response to arginine deprivation, ERK/MAPK and PI3K/Akt signaling cascades are activated to promote phosphorylation and stabilization of c-Myc [64]. There are two phosphorylation sites in the N-terminal of Myc, Thr58 and Ser62 that are critical for stability of Myc protein. As mentioned earlier, phosphorylation of Ser62 is required for Ras-induced stabilization of Myc. Conversely, GSK-3-mediated phosphorylation of c-Myc at Thr58, a process that is dependent on Ser62 phosphorylation, primes c-Myc for degradation [65]. Activation of PI3K/Akt phosphorylates GSK-3 and held its activity in check [38]. In HCC, HBV-X protein can activate Erk to interact with GSK-3β, priming GSK-3β for subsequent phosphorylation and inactivation [63]. Another mechanism by which ERK/MAPK and PI3K/Akt signaling promotes the transcriptional activity of Myc is through accelerating the ubiquitination and degradation of Mad1, an important cellular antagonist of Myc [66]. FoxO transcription factors are other common substrates of ERK/MAPK and PI3K/Akt/mTOR pathway. Phosphorylation of FoxOs by Akt inhibits their transcriptional activity and contributes to cell proliferation and survival [67]. Activated ERK directly interacts with FOXO3a to induce FOXO3a phosphorylation at Ser 294, Ser 344 and Ser 425, leading to inactivation of FOXO3a which consequently promotes tumorigenesis [68].

8.6 Wnt/β-Catenin Signaling

HCC is characterized by the aberrant up-regulation of WNT/β-catenin pathway. Wnt proteins are a large family of secreted glycoproteins that bind to the Frizzled (Fz) receptor family [69]. The Fz receptor is a seven trans-membrane span protein similar to G-protein coupled receptors [70]. In addition to the interaction between Wnt and Fz, single transmembrane proteins low-density-lipoprotein-related protein 5 (LRP5) and LRP6 act as co-receptors for activating canonical Wnt pathway. In the absence of Wnt ligands, LRP5/6 and Frizzled remain inactive. The cytoplasmic pool of β-catenin is restrained by a multiprotein destruction complex consisting of Axin, adenomatosis polyposis coli (APC), GSK3 and casein kinase 1 (CK1) [71]. Axin1 is considered as the rate-limiting factor of the destruction complex which functions as central scaffold and direct interacts with all other core components of the destruction complex [72]. CK1 phosphorylates β-catenin at Ser45, which in turn primes GSK3-dependent phosphorylation of β-catenin on the N-terminal Thr41, Ser37, and Ser33 residues [73]. Phosphorylated β-catenin is then targeted by β-TrCP ubiquitin E3 ligase for proteasome-mediated protein degradation [74]. To activate the canonical Wnt signaling pathway, Wnt ligands bind to the Frizzled and LRP5/6 coreceptor complex. The activated receptors dissociate the destruction complex involved by dishevelled (Dvl), which in turn prevent the β-catenin degradation. As a consequence, active β-catenin accumulates and translocates to nucleus where it binds to T-cell factor/lymphoid enhancer factor (TCF/LEF) and acts as a co-activator to drive the transcription of downstream genes involved in cell differentiation, proliferation and migration [75]. In addition to ligand-induced activation, mutations of major components for Wnt/β-catenin signaling are demonstrated in HCC. Activating mutations in β-catenin (20–40%), as well as inactivating mutations of AXIN1 (11%), AXIN2 (1%) and APC (1%) are described in human HCC samples, leading to stabilization and intracellular accumulation of β-catenin [76–80].

8.7 Crosstalk of Wnt/β-Catenin Pathway with Other Pathways

Crosstalk between Wnt/β-catenin pathway and the other pathways might contribute to HCC progression. Activation of the canonical Wnt signaling not only induces β-catenin accumulation and transcription activation, but also stimulates the mTOR pathway. Wnt-induced mTOR activation is through inhibiting the sequential phosphorylation of TSC2 by AMPK and GSK3, which is independent of β-catenin-dependent transcription [81, 82]. It is worth noting that TSC2 is also phosphorylated by Akt, ERK and RSK as mentioned above. Thus stimulation of phosphorylation events on TSC1-TSC2 complex by distinct signaling pathways could either inhibit or activate the complex to modulate mTORC1 activity [83]. In HCC, activation of Erk by HBV-X can upregulate β-catenin in a manner dependent on phosphorylation and inactivation of GSK-3β [63]. Similarly, in response to insulin stimulation, active Akt phosphorylates and inactivates GSK-3β, leading to increased β-catenin-TCF/LEF-1 transactivation [84]. Meanwhile, Akt may directly induce phosphorylation of β-catenin, thus stimulate Wnt/β-catenin signaling [85]. Crosstalk between Wnt/β-catenin and TGF-β pathways may also occur in HCC. Treatment of TGF-β in HCC cell lines augments Wnt/β-catenin activity via altering subcellular localization of β-catenin [86, 87]. Consistently, phosphorylation of Smad3 by TGF-β1 induces rapid nuclear translocation of β-catenin in adult mesenchymal stem cells [88].

8.8 TGF-β Signaling

TGFβ is a growth factor and cytokine that belongs to the transforming growth factor superfamily. Three types of TGF-β ligands have been demonstrated: TGF-β1, TGF-β2 and TGF-β3 [89]. All three ligands can bind to a transmembrane serine-threonine kinase receptor TGFβ type II receptor that recruits the type I receptor to form heterodimers [90]. Activated receptors then propagate the signal intracellularly through phosphorylation of the Smad proteins. There are eight distinct Smad proteins that are divided into three functional classes: receptor-regulated Smads (R-Smads), common partner Smads (Co-Smads), and inhibitory Smads (I-Smads). Activated type I receptor kinases directly phosphorylate and activate R-Smads (Smad1, 2, 3, 5, and 8) which now undergo homotrimerization and form heteromeric complexes with the Co-Smad (Smad4) [90]. The activated Smad complexes then translocate into the nucleus and act as transcription factors to regulate the expression of target genes. I-Smads (Smad6 and Smad7) act as antagonists of TGF-β signaling by preventing association of R-Smads with receptor complex or Co-Smad and by targeting the receptors for degradation [91, 92]. Activation of TGF-β signaling is closely linked with liver fibrosis, cirrhosis and subsequent development of HCC. Although TGF-β functions as a tumor suppressor to inhibit cell growth and induce apoptosis in the healthy liver and during tumor initiation, it promotes cell migration and invasion once cancer cells evade the growth inhibitory effects of TGF-β. TGF-β1 promotes the epithelial-to-mesenchymal transformation (EMT) in HCC cells through down-regulation of E-cadherin and inducing nuclear translocation of β-catenin [93]. EMT is known to mediate the drug resistance of tumor cells. In HCC, different studies have demonstrated that sorafenib resistance mechanisms may involve EMT [94, 95], although the exact mechanism remains unknown.

8.9 Crosstalk of TGF-β Signaling with Other Pathways

Besides Smad-mediated transcription, TGF-β also stimulates other oncogenic signals, e.g., PI3K/Akt and ERK/MAPK pathway [96]. TGF-β can induce PI3K-dependent Akt activation by a mechanism that may involve RhoA [97]. In addition, activation of PI3K/Akt signaling may also result from TGF-β-induced TGF-α expression and consequent phosphorylation and activation of EGFR [98]. Akt activation has been demonstrated to protect HCC cell line from TGF-β1-induced apoptosis [99]. Inactivation of PI3K signaling reduces TGF-β-induced Smad2 phosphorylation and transcription [98]. TGF-β can also activate the ERK/MAPK pathways. Rapid activation of Ras by TGF-β in epithelial cells recruits Raf to the plasma membrane, leading to activation of Erk [100]. TGF-β-induced ERK/MAPK signaling is found to promote invasion and metastasis of cancer cells [101]. Conversely, treatment of TGF-β inhibitor in HCC cells has been shown to dephosphorylate Akt, mTOR, MEK and ERK, but activate PTEN [102].

8.10 JAK/STAT Pathway

Jak/Stat pathway is universally activated in human HCC and play a pivotal role for HCC development [23]. JAKs, STATs, and receptors are three key components of JAK-STAT pathway to transmit intercellular signals. The binding of cytokines to cell-surface receptors results in the formation of receptor dimers, which brings the receptor-associated JAKs into close proximity for transphosphorylation and activation [103]. JAK proteins are intracellular, nonreceptor tyrosine kinases, comprising JAK1, JAK2, JAK3 and TYK2 [104]. The cytokine-activated JAKs phosphorylate the cytokine receptors, creating a docking site for the SH2 domain which is present among STATs family members (STAT1, STAT2, STAT3, STAT4, STAT5A, STAT5B and STAT6). After phosphorylation by the JAKs, these STAT transcription factors form hetero- or homodimers and translocate to nucleus to induce transcription of target genes involved in cell differentiation, proliferation and apoptosis. Among the downstream targets, positive and negative regulators of JAK/STAT pathway have been identified which can modulate the magnitude and/or duration of signaling [105, 106]. Suppressors of cytokine signaling (SOCS) proteins are reported to be a part of a negative feedback loop in the JAK/STAT pathway. In HCC, SOCS-1 is silenced by methylation, which may contribute to the constitutive activation of JAK/STAT pathway [107]. Next-generation sequencing of HCC leads to identification of a low-frequency somatic mutation of JAK1 (around 1%) [9, 29, 30], which may also cause the activation of JAK1/STAT signaling.

8.11 Crosstalk of JAK/STAT Pathway with Other Pathways

JAK-STAT pathway may interconnect with other pathways such as ERK/MAPK and PI3K/Akt/mTOR [108]. Overexpression of EGFR in primary esophageal keratinocytes activates STAT in a manner dependent on JAK [109]. Activated JAKs can phosphorylate tyrosine residues on receptors which can serve as docking sites for SH2-containing adapter proteins. Both Grb2 and PI3K protein contain an SH2 domain, implying the possibility that activated JAK-STAT pathway may also regulate ERK/MAPK and PI3K/Akt/mTOR signaling. However, the crosstalk of JAK/STAT pathway with other pathways in HCC remains largely unknown.

8.12 MDM2-p53 Pathway

The MDM2-p53 pathway is frequently altered in HCC [9, 29, 30]. The p53 transcription factor serves as an important tumor suppressor regulating DNA repair, cell cycle, apoptosis and senescence to maintain the integrity of the genome. The E3 ubiquitin ligase Mdm2 is the major and essential negative regulator to hold the activity of p53 in check. On the one hand, Mdm2 can bind p53 at its transactivation domain to inhibit the activity of p53 [110]. On the other hand, Mdm2 can promote the polyubiquitination of p53 for subsequent proteasome-dependent protein degradation [111]. It is worth noting that p53 also enhances Mdm2 transcription through binding and activating the internal P2 promoter of Mdm2, thus leading to the formation of autoregulatory feedback loop between p53 and Mdm2 to maintain their balance [112]. Somatic mutations of p53 occur in approximately 30% of HCC, causing the loss of p53 suppressor function as exemplified by a lower affinity to bind its target genes at the sequence-specific response elements [113]. In addition, mutant p53 proteins often accumulate in the nucleus of in situ and metastatic cancer cells, exerting oncogenic gain-of-function properties to promote proliferation, survival, and metastasis of cancer cells or conferring a dominant-negative activity over remaining wild-type p53 [114].

8.13 Crosstalk of MDM2-p53 Pathway with Other Pathways

ERK activation may cooperate with p53 protein to regulate cell cycle arrest and apoptosis. ERK protein is capable to bind p53 and induce phosphorylation of p53 at Ser15 in vitro [115, 116]. Phosphorylation of p53 on Ser15 inhibits the p53-Mdm2 interaction to stabilize p53 protein and promotes its accumulation [116]. Thr55 is another important site of p53, the phosphorylation of which by activated ERK2 promotes DNA-binding activity of p53 [117]. Moreover, sustained ERK activation also induces phosphorylation of Mdm2 at Ser166, thus inhibiting its ubiquitin ligase activity toward p53 [118]. Cooperation of ERK activation with enhanced p53 activity induces cellular senescence in murine fibroblasts [119]. A negative-feedback loop exists between the p53 and Akt signaling to balance the pro-apoptotic and anti-apoptotic signals [120]. On the one hand, p53-dependent destruction of Akt promotes apoptotic cell death. On the other hand, the survival signals are effective for recruiting Akt to activate Mdm2, leading to inhibition of p53 and consequent p53-dependent apoptosis. Akt-mediated phosphorylation of Mdm2 at Ser186 enhances the ubiquitination-promoting function of Mdm2, resulting in a reduction of p53 protein [121].

8.14 Other Signaling Pathways

There are several other molecular events that are involved in hepatocarcinogenesis such as telomere stability, NF-κB signaling and Hedgehog (Hh) pathway. High frequency (over 50%) of telomerase reverse transcriptase (TERT) promoter mutations, which are associated with an increase expression of TERT, are considered cancer drivers for HCC development [9, 29, 122]. TERT is a catalytic subunit of telomerase that is responsible for maintaining telomere length. Telomere shortening plays a dual role in hepatocarcinogenesis, leading to chromosomal instability and tumor initiation, but providing a barrier for tumor progression [123]. Reactivation of telomerase and maintenance of telomere are important for liver carcinogenesis. Activation of NF-κB signaling is a frequent and early event in HCC, which might be contributed by different factors, e.g., HBV-X protein, HCV core protein, LPS, and fatty acids [124]. However, to date no oncogenic mutations have been reported to be responsible for NF-κB activation in carcinomas [125]. We recently identified OGT, a unique glycosyltransferase enzyme, plays an oncogenic role in non-alcoholic fatty liver disease-HCC through activating oncogenic JNK/c-jun/AP-1 and NF-κB cascades [126]. Activation of NF-κB signaling might facilitate HCC progression through promoting the survival and expansion of tumor cells. Aberrant activations of Hh signaling are also demonstrated in HCC, which may be contributed by the overexpression of the 7-transmembrane protein Smoothened (SMO) or induction of Sonic hedgehog (SHH) ligand [127, 128]. Reactivation of Hh pathway in HCC is reported to sustain cancer cell growth and progression [129]. Hh signaling may promote the invasion and metastasis of HCC by a mechanism mediated by ERK-driven MMP-9 expression [130]. For the above-mentioned pathways, further attention should be paid to assess their significance and potential therapeutic value for HCC.

8.15 Conclusions and Perspectives

HCC is a highly heterogeneous malignancy, both clinically and biologically. With the advances of next-generation sequencing, genomic landscape of HCC has been identified to favor the understanding of genetic and epigenetic changes involved in the development of HCC. Among these changes, RTKs have emerged as attractive targets in molecular targeted therapy for HCC. Sorafenib, an oral multikinase inhibitor of VEGFR, PDGFR and Raf, is the first effective systemic treatment in HCC, representing a landmark advancement in therapy of HCC. However, the overall treatment outcomes are far from satisfactory since most of patients are highly refractory to sorafenib treatment because of primary or adaptive resistance. The fact that a multitude of different signaling pathways emerge in liver cancer cells makes it difficult for effective treatment of HCC. The tumor easily develops resistance against the blockade of a specific target via rewiring cell signaling. EGFR activation may interfere with the response of HCC to sorafenib [131–133]. As a consequence, some patients do not respond to the sorafenib treatment at all. In addition, several mechanisms have been proposed to explain the acquired resistance of HCC to sorafenib, of which the cross-talk between effector pathways and feedback inhibition has been attracting attention. Activation of PI3K/Akt pathway may be associated with sorafenib resistance, considering the existing crosstalk between the PI3K/Akt and ERK/MAPK pathways. Treatment of sorafenib in HCC cell lines has been demonstrated to activate PI3K/Akt/mTOR pathway, as evidenced by increased phosphorylation of 4E-BP1 and p70s6k [134, 135]. In keeping with this, sorafenib-resistant HCC cells show increased phosphorylation of Akt and PI3K p85 subunit [136]. Other mechanisms such as JAK-STAT pathway may also contribute to the acquired resistance to sorafenib [137]. Therefore, exploring biomarkers to identify responders and non-responders to therapy for HCC is a priority for future study. Meanwhile, combinational therapy using other anticancer agents with sorafenib may improve the therapeutic efficacy for HCC.

In summary, multiple signaling pathways are frequently dysregulated in HCC. The aberrant regulation of crosstalk between pathways may confer the resistance of HCC to molecular targeted therapy.

Self Study

Questions

(a) The process by which molecular signals are transmitted from a cell's exterior to its interior as a series of molecular events is called ________.

(b) Instances in which one or more components of one signal transduction pathway affects another are called ________.

Answers

(a) Signal transduction

(b) Crosstalk

References

1. Ferlay J, Soerjomataram I, Dikshit R, Eser S, Mathers C, Rebelo M, et al. Cancer incidence and mortality worldwide: sources, methods and major patterns in GLOBOCAN 2012. Int J Cancer. 2015;136(5):E359–86.
2. Gomaa AI, Khan SA, Toledano MB, Waked I, Taylor-Robinson SD. Hepatocellular carcinoma: epidemiology, risk factors and pathogenesis. World J Gastroenterol. 2008;14(27):4300–8.
3. Liu PH, Hsu CY, Hsia CY, Lee YH, Huang YH, Chiou YY, et al. Surgical resection versus radiofrequency ablation for single hepatocellular carcinoma </= 2 cm in a propensity score model. Ann Surg. 2016;263(3):538–45.
4. Kao WY, Chao Y, Chang CC, Li CP, Su CW, Huo TI, et al. Prognosis of early-stage hepatocellular carcinoma: the clinical implications of substages of Barcelona clinic liver cancer system based on a cohort of 1265 patients. Medicine. 2015;94(43):e1929.
5. Wang Y, Luo Q, Li Y, Deng S, Wei S, Li X. Radiofrequency ablation versus hepatic resection for small hepatocellular carcinomas: a meta-analysis of randomized and nonrandomized controlled trials. PLoS One. 2014;9(1):e84484.
6. Peng ZW, Lin XJ, Zhang YJ, Liang HH, Guo RP, Shi M, et al. Radiofrequency ablation versus hepatic resection for the treatment of hepatocellular carcinomas 2 cm or smaller: a retrospective comparative study. Radiology. 2012;262(3):1022–33.
7. Colagrande S, Inghilesi AL, Aburas S, Taliani GG, Nardi C, Marra F. Challenges of advanced hepatocellular carcinoma. World J Gastroenterol. 2016;22(34):7645–59.
8. Llovet JM, Ricci S, Mazzaferro V, Hilgard P, Gane E, Blanc JF, et al. Sorafenib in advanced hepatocellular carcinoma. N Engl J Med. 2008;359(4):378–90.
9. Llovet JM, Villanueva A, Lachenmayer A, Finn RS. Advances in targeted therapies for hepatocellular carcinoma in the genomic era. Nat Rev Clin Oncol. 2015;12(8):436.
10. Bruix J, Qin S, Merle P, Granito A, Huang YH, Bodoky G, et al. Regorafenib for patients with hepatocellular carcinoma who progressed on sorafenib treatment (RESORCE): a randomised, double-blind, placebo-controlled, phase 3 trial. Lancet. 2017;389(10064):56–66.
11. El-Khoueiry AB, Sangro B, Yau T, Crocenzi TS, Kudo M, Hsu C, et al. Nivolumab in patients with advanced hepatocellular carcinoma (CheckMate 040): an open-label, non-comparative, phase 1/2 dose escalation and expansion trial. Lancet. 2017;389(10088):2492–502.

12. Mendoza MC, Er EE, Blenis J. The Ras-ERK and PI3K-mTOR pathways: cross-talk and compensation. Trends Biochem Sci. 2011;36(6):320–8.
13. Logue JS, Morrison DK. Complexity in the signaling network: insights from the use of targeted inhibitors in cancer therapy. Genes Dev. 2012;26(7):641–50.
14. Hubbard SR, Miller WT. Receptor tyrosine kinases: mechanisms of activation and signaling. Curr Opin Cell Biol. 2007;19(2):117–23.
15. Robinson DR, Wu YM, Lin SF. The protein tyrosine kinase family of the human genome. Oncogene. 2000;19(49):5548–57.
16. Hubbard SR. Structural analysis of receptor tyrosine kinases. Prog Biophys Mol Biol. 1999;71(3–4):343–58.
17. Ullrich A, Schlessinger J. Signal transduction by receptors with tyrosine kinase activity. Cell. 1990;61(2):203–12.
18. Lemmon MA, Schlessinger J. Cell signaling by receptor tyrosine kinases. Cell. 2010;141(7):1117–34.
19. Muntane J, De la Rosa AJ, Docobo F, Garcia-Carbonero R, Padillo FJ. Targeting tyrosine kinase receptors in hepatocellular carcinoma. Curr Cancer Drug Targets. 2013;13(3):300–12.
20. Avila MA, Berasain C, Sangro B, Prieto J. New therapies for hepatocellular carcinoma. Oncogene. 2006;25(27):3866–84.
21. Villanueva A, Newell P, Chiang DY, Friedman SL, Llovet JM. Genomics and signaling pathways in hepatocellular carcinoma. Semin Liver Dis. 2007;27(1):55–76.
22. Huynh H, Nguyen TT, Chow KH, Tan PH, Soo KC, Tran E. Over-expression of the mitogen-activated protein kinase (MAPK) kinase (MEK)-MAPK in hepatocellular carcinoma: its role in tumor progression and apoptosis. BMC Gastroenterol. 2003;3:19.
23. Calvisi DF, Ladu S, Gorden A, Farina M, Conner EA, Lee JS, et al. Ubiquitous activation of Ras and Jak/Stat pathways in human HCC. Gastroenterology. 2006;130(4):1117–28.
24. Newell P, Toffanin S, Villanueva A, Chiang DY, Minguez B, Cabellos L, et al. Ras pathway activation in hepatocellular carcinoma and anti-tumoral effect of combined sorafenib and rapamycin in vivo. J Hepatol. 2009;51(4):725–33.
25. Schlessinger J. Ligand-induced, receptor-mediated dimerization and activation of EGF receptor. Cell. 2002;110(6):669–72.
26. Lowenstein EJ, Daly RJ, Batzer AG, Li W, Margolis B, Lammers R, et al. The SH2 and SH3 domain-containing protein GRB2 links receptor tyrosine kinases to ras signaling. Cell. 1992;70(3):431–42.
27. Zheng Y, Zhang C, Croucher DR, Soliman MA, St-Denis N, Pasculescu A, et al. Temporal regulation of EGF signalling networks by the scaffold protein Shc1. Nature. 2013;499(7457):166–71.
28. Zarich N, Oliva JL, Martinez N, Jorge R, Ballester A, Gutierrez-Eisman S, et al. Grb2 is a negative modulator of the intrinsic Ras-GEF activity of hSos1. Mol Biol Cell. 2006;17(8):3591–7.
29. Schulze K, Nault JC, Villanueva A. Genetic profiling of hepatocellular carcinoma using next-generation sequencing. J Hepatol. 2016;65(5):1031–42.
30. Li X, Xu W, Kang W, Wong SH, Wang M, Zhou Y, et al. Genomic analysis of liver cancer unveils novel driver genes and distinct prognostic features. Theranostics. 2018;8(6):1740–51.
31. Matallanas D, Birtwistle M, Romano D, Zebisch A, Rauch J, von Kriegsheim A, et al. Raf family kinases: old dogs have learned new tricks. Genes Cancer. 2011;2(3):232–60.
32. Pearson G, Robinson F, Beers Gibson T, Xu BE, Karandikar M, Berman K, et al. Mitogen-activated protein (MAP) kinase pathways: regulation and physiological functions. Endocr Rev. 2001;22(2):153–83.
33. Chen RH, Sarnecki C, Blenis J. Nuclear localization and regulation of erk- and rsk-encoded protein kinases. Mol Cell Biol. 1992;12(3):915–27.
34. Xing J, Ginty DD, Greenberg ME. Coupling of the RAS-MAPK pathway to gene activation by RSK2, a growth factor-regulated CREB kinase. Science. 1996;273(5277):959–63.
35. Sears R, Nuckolls F, Haura E, Taya Y, Tamai K, Nevins JR. Multiple Ras-dependent phosphorylation pathways regulate Myc protein stability. Genes Dev. 2000;14(19):2501–14.
36. Zhang Y, Kwok-Shing Ng P, Kucherlapati M, Chen F, Liu Y, Tsang YH, et al. A pan-cancer proteogenomic atlas of PI3K/AKT/mTOR pathway alterations. Cancer Cell. 2017;31(6):820–32. e3
37. Czech MP. PIP2 and PIP3: complex roles at the cell surface. Cell. 2000;100(6):603–6.
38. Manning BD, Cantley LC. AKT/PKB signaling: navigating downstream. Cell. 2007;129(7):1261–74.
39. Cantley LC, Neel BG. New insights into tumor suppression: PTEN suppresses tumor formation by restraining the phosphoinositide 3-kinase/AKT pathway. Proc Natl Acad Sci U S A. 1999;96(8):4240–5.
40. Peyrou M, Bourgoin L, Foti M. PTEN in liver diseases and cancer. World J Gastroenterol. 2010;16(37):4627–33.
41. Horie Y, Suzuki A, Kataoka E, Sasaki T, Hamada K, Sasaki J, et al. Hepatocyte-specific Pten deficiency results in steatohepatitis and hepatocellular carcinomas. J Clin Invest. 2004; 113(12):1774–83.
42. Liu D, Wong CC, Fu L, Chen H, Zhao L, Li C, et al. Squalene epoxidase drives NAFLD-induced hepatocellular carcinoma and is a pharmaceutical target. Sci Transl Med. 2018;10(437):pii: eaap9840.
43. Villanueva A, Chiang DY, Newell P, Peix J, Thung S, Alsinet C, et al. Pivotal role of mTOR signaling in hepatocellular carcinoma. Gastroenterology. 2008;135(6):1972–83. 83.e1–11
44. Wullschleger S, Loewith R, Hall MN. TOR signaling in growth and metabolism. Cell. 2006;124(3):471–84.
45. Sancak Y, Thoreen CC, Peterson TR, Lindquist RA, Kang SA, Spooner E, et al. PRAS40 is an insulin-regulated inhibitor of the mTORC1 protein kinase. Mol Cell. 2007;25(6):903–15.
46. Peterson TR, Laplante M, Thoreen CC, Sancak Y, Kang SA, Kuehl WM, et al. DEPTOR is an mTOR inhibitor frequently overexpressed in multiple myeloma cells and required for their survival. Cell. 2009;137(5):873–86.
47. Inoki K, Li Y, Zhu T, Wu J, Guan KL. TSC2 is phosphorylated and inhibited by Akt and suppresses mTOR signalling. Nat Cell Biol. 2002;4(9):648–57.
48. Kodaki T, Woscholski R, Hallberg B, Rodriguez-Viciana P, Downward J, Parker PJ. The activation of phosphatidylinositol 3-kinase by Ras. Curr Biol. 1994;4(9):798–806.
49. Gupta S, Ramjaun AR, Haiko P, Wang Y, Warne PH, Nicke B, et al. Binding of ras to phosphoinositide 3-kinase p110alpha is required for ras-driven tumorigenesis in mice. Cell. 2007;129(5):957–68.
50. Johnson L, Mercer K, Greenbaum D, Bronson RT, Crowley D, Tuveson DA, et al. Somatic activation of the K-ras oncogene causes early onset lung cancer in mice. Nature. 2001;410(6832):1111–6.
51. Wang C, Cigliano A, Delogu S, Armbruster J, Dombrowski F, Evert M, et al. Functional crosstalk between AKT/mTOR and Ras/MAPK pathways in hepatocarcinogenesis: implications for the treatment of human liver cancer. Cell Cycle. 2013;12(13):1999–2010.
52. Ma L, Chen Z, Erdjument-Bromage H, Tempst P, Pandolfi PP. Phosphorylation and functional inactivation of TSC2 by Erk implications for tuberous sclerosis and cancer pathogenesis. Cell. 2005;121(2):179–93.
53. Roux PP, Ballif BA, Anjum R, Gygi SP, Blenis J. Tumor-promoting phorbol esters and activated Ras inactivate the tuberous sclerosis tumor suppressor complex via p90 ribosomal S6 kinase. Proc Natl Acad Sci U S A. 2004;101(37):13489–94.
54. Carriere A, Cargnello M, Julien LA, Gao H, Bonneil E, Thibault P, et al. Oncogenic MAPK signaling stimulates mTORC1 activity by promoting RSK-mediated raptor phosphorylation. Curr Biol. 2008;18(17):1269–77.
55. Carriere A, Romeo Y, Acosta-Jaquez HA, Moreau J, Bonneil E, Thibault P, et al. ERK1/2 phosphorylate Raptor to promote Ras-dependent activation of mTOR complex 1 (mTORC1). J Biol Chem. 2011;286(1):567–77.

56. Hoeflich KP, O'Brien C, Boyd Z, Cavet G, Guerrero S, Jung K, et al. In vivo antitumor activity of MEK and phosphatidylinositol 3-kinase inhibitors in basal-like breast cancer models. Clin Cancer Res. 2009;15(14):4649–64.
57. Yu CF, Liu ZX, Cantley LG. ERK negatively regulates the epidermal growth factor-mediated interaction of Gab1 and the phosphatidylinositol 3-kinase. J Biol Chem. 2002;277(22):19382–8.
58. Lehr S, Kotzka J, Avci H, Sickmann A, Meyer HE, Herkner A, et al. Identification of major ERK-related phosphorylation sites in Gab1. Biochemistry. 2004;43(38):12133–40.
59. Moelling K, Schad K, Bosse M, Zimmermann S, Schweneker M. Regulation of Raf-Akt Cross-talk. J Biol Chem. 2002;277(34):31099–106.
60. Zimmermann S, Moelling K. Phosphorylation and regulation of Raf by Akt (protein kinase B). Science. 1999;286(5445):1741–4.
61. Jaumot M, Hancock JF. Protein phosphatases 1 and 2A promote Raf-1 activation by regulating 14-3-3 interactions. Oncogene. 2001;20(30):3949–58.
62. Xin B, Yamamoto M, Fujii K, Ooshio T, Chen X, Okada Y, et al. Critical role of Myc activation in mouse hepatocarcinogenesis induced by the activation of AKT and RAS pathways. Oncogene. 2017;36(36):5087–97.
63. Ding Q, Xia W, Liu JC, Yang JY, Lee DF, Xia J, et al. Erk associates with and primes GSK-3beta for its inactivation resulting in upregulation of beta-catenin. Mol Cell. 2005;19(2):159–70.
64. Tsai WB, Aiba I, Long Y, Lin HK, Feun L, Savaraj N, et al. Activation of Ras/PI3K/ERK pathway induces c-Myc stabilization to upregulate argininosuccinate synthetase, leading to arginine deiminase resistance in melanoma cells. Cancer Res. 2012;72(10):2622–33.
65. Gregory MA, Qi Y, Hann SR. Phosphorylation by glycogen synthase kinase-3 controls c-myc proteolysis and subnuclear localization. J Biol Chem. 2003;278(51):51606–12.
66. Zhu J, Blenis J, Yuan J. Activation of PI3K/Akt and MAPK pathways regulates Myc-mediated transcription by phosphorylating and promoting the degradation of Mad1. Proc Natl Acad Sci U S A. 2008;105(18):6584–9.
67. Zhang X, Tang N, Hadden TJ, Rishi AK. Akt, FoxO and regulation of apoptosis. Biochim Biophys Acta. 2011;1813(11):1978–86.
68. Yang JY, Zong CS, Xia W, Yamaguchi H, Ding Q, Xie X, et al. ERK promotes tumorigenesis by inhibiting FOXO3a via MDM2-mediated degradation. Nat Cell Biol. 2008;10(2):138–48.
69. Komiya Y, Habas R. Wnt signal transduction pathways. Organogenesis. 2008;4(2):68–75.
70. Huang HC, Klein PS. The Frizzled family: receptors for multiple signal transduction pathways. Genome Biol. 2004;5(7):234.
71. Li VS, Ng SS, Boersema PJ, Low TY, Karthaus WR, Gerlach JP, et al. Wnt signaling through inhibition of beta-catenin degradation in an intact Axin1 complex. Cell. 2012;149(6):1245–56.
72. Kishida S, Yamamoto H, Ikeda S, Kishida M, Sakamoto I, Koyama S, et al. Axin, a negative regulator of the wnt signaling pathway, directly interacts with adenomatous polyposis coli and regulates the stabilization of beta-catenin. J Biol Chem. 1998;273(18):10823–6.
73. Liu C, Li Y, Semenov M, Han C, Baeg GH, Tan Y, et al. Control of beta-catenin phosphorylation/degradation by a dual-kinase mechanism. Cell. 2002;108(6):837–47.
74. Aberle H, Bauer A, Stappert J, Kispert A, Kemler R. beta-catenin is a target for the ubiquitin-proteasome pathway. EMBO J. 1997;16(13):3797–804.
75. MacDonald BT, Tamai K, He X. Wnt/beta-catenin signaling: components, mechanisms, and diseases. Dev Cell. 2009;17(1):9–26.
76. Laurent-Puig P, Zucman-Rossi J. Genetics of hepatocellular tumors. Oncogene. 2006;25(27):3778–86.
77. Breuhahn K, Longerich T, Schirmacher P. Dysregulation of growth factor signaling in human hepatocellular carcinoma. Oncogene. 2006;25(27):3787–800.
78. Anastas JN, Moon RT. WNT signalling pathways as therapeutic targets in cancer. Nat Rev Cancer. 2013;13(1):11–26.
79. Schulze K, Imbeaud S, Letouze E, Alexandrov LB, Calderaro J, Rebouissou S, et al. Exome sequencing of hepatocellular carcinomas identifies new mutational signatures and potential therapeutic targets. Nat Genet. 2015;47(5):505–11.
80. Totoki Y, Tatsuno K, Covington KR, Ueda H, Creighton CJ, Kato M, et al. Trans-ancestry mutational landscape of hepatocellular carcinoma genomes. Nat Genet. 2014;46(12):1267–73.
81. Inoki K, Ouyang H, Zhu T, Lindvall C, Wang Y, Zhang X, et al. TSC2 integrates Wnt and energy signals via a coordinated phosphorylation by AMPK and GSK3 to regulate cell growth. Cell. 2006;126(5):955–68.
82. Castilho RM, Squarize CH, Chodosh LA, Williams BO, Gutkind JS. mTOR mediates Wnt-induced epidermal stem cell exhaustion and aging. Cell Stem Cell. 2009;5(3):279–89.
83. Huang J, Manning BD. The TSC1-TSC2 complex: a molecular switchboard controlling cell growth. Biochem J. 2008;412(2):179–90.
84. Cross DA, Alessi DR, Cohen P, Andjelkovich M, Hemmings BA. Inhibition of glycogen synthase kinase-3 by insulin mediated by protein kinase B. Nature. 1995;378(6559):785–9.
85. Fang D, Hawke D, Zheng Y, Xia Y, Meisenhelder J, Nika H, et al. Phosphorylation of beta-catenin by AKT promotes beta-catenin transcriptional activity. J Biol Chem. 2007;282(15):11221–9.
86. Hoshida Y, Nijman SM, Kobayashi M, Chan JA, Brunet JP, Chiang DY, et al. Integrative transcriptome analysis reveals common molecular subclasses of human hepatocellular carcinoma. Cancer Res. 2009;69(18):7385–92.
87. Steinway SN, Zanudo JG, Ding W, Rountree CB, Feith DJ, Loughran TP Jr, et al. Network modeling of TGFbeta signaling in hepatocellular carcinoma epithelial-to-mesenchymal transition reveals joint sonic hedgehog and Wnt pathway activation. Cancer Res. 2014;74(21):5963–77.
88. Jian H, Shen X, Liu I, Semenov M, He X, Wang XF. Smad3-dependent nuclear translocation of beta-catenin is required for TGF-beta1-induced proliferation of bone marrow-derived adult human mesenchymal stem cells. Genes Dev. 2006;20(6):666–74.
89. Goumans MJ, Mummery C. Functional analysis of the TGFbeta receptor/Smad pathway through gene ablation in mice. Int J Dev Biol. 2000;44(3):253–65.
90. Shi Y, Massague J. Mechanisms of TGF-beta signaling from cell membrane to the nucleus. Cell. 2003;113(6):685–700.
91. Imamura T, Takase M, Nishihara A, Oeda E, Hanai J, Kawabata M, et al. Smad6 inhibits signalling by the TGF-beta superfamily. Nature. 1997;389(6651):622–6.
92. Nakao A, Afrakhte M, Moren A, Nakayama T, Christian JL, Heuchel R, et al. Identification of Smad7, a TGFbeta-inducible antagonist of TGF-beta signalling. Nature. 1997;389(6651):631–5.
93. Xu Z, Shen MX, Ma DZ, Wang LY, Zha XL. TGF-beta1-promoted epithelial-to-mesenchymal transformation and cell adhesion contribute to TGF-beta1-enhanced cell migration in SMMC-7721 cells. Cell Res. 2003;13(5):343–50.
94. van Malenstein H, Dekervel J, Verslype C, Van Cutsem E, Windmolders P, Nevens F, et al. Long-term exposure to sorafenib of liver cancer cells induces resistance with epithelial-to-mesenchymal transition, increased invasion and risk of rebound growth. Cancer Lett. 2013;329(1):74–83.
95. Dazert E, Colombi M, Boldanova T, Moes S, Adametz D, Quagliata L, et al. Quantitative proteomics and phosphoproteomics on serial tumor biopsies from a sorafenib-treated HCC patient. Proc Natl Acad Sci U S A. 2016;113(5):1381–6.
96. Derynck R, Zhang YE. Smad-dependent and Smad-independent pathways in TGF-beta family signalling. Nature. 2003;425(6958):577–84.
97. Bakin AV, Tomlinson AK, Bhowmick NA, Moses HL, Arteaga CL. Phosphatidylinositol 3-kinase function is required for transforming

growth factor beta-mediated epithelial to mesenchymal transition and cell migration. J Biol Chem. 2000;275(47):36803–10.
98. Vinals F, Pouyssegur J. Transforming growth factor beta1 (TGF-beta1) promotes endothelial cell survival during in vitro angiogenesis via an autocrine mechanism implicating TGF-alpha signaling. Mol Cell Biol. 2001;21(21):7218–30.
99. Chen RH, Su YH, Chuang RL, Chang TY. Suppression of transforming growth factor-beta-induced apoptosis through a phosphatidylinositol 3-kinase/Akt-dependent pathway. Oncogene. 1998;17(15):1959–68.
100. Yue J, Mulder KM. Activation of the mitogen-activated protein kinase pathway by transforming growth factor-beta. Methods Mol Biol. 2000;142:125–31.
101. Mulder KM, Morris SL. Activation of p21ras by transforming growth factor beta in epithelial cells. J Biol Chem. 1992;267(8):5029–31.
102. Fransvea E, Mazzocca A, Santamato A, Azzariti A, Antonaci S, Giannelli G. Kinase activation profile associated with TGF-beta-dependent migration of HCC cells: a preclinical study. Cancer Chemother Pharmacol. 2011;68(1):79–86.
103. Jatiani SS, Baker SJ, Silverman LR, Reddy EP. Jak/STAT pathways in cytokine signaling and myeloproliferative disorders: approaches for targeted therapies. Genes Cancer. 2010;1(10):979–93.
104. Aaronson DS, Horvath CM. A road map for those who don't know JAK-STAT. Science. 2002;296(5573):1653–5.
105. Shuai K, Liu B. Regulation of JAK-STAT signalling in the immune system. Nat Rev Immunol. 2003;3(11):900–11.
106. Levy DE, Darnell JE Jr. Stats: transcriptional control and biological impact. Nat Rev Mol Cell Biol. 2002;3(9):651–62.
107. Yoshikawa H, Matsubara K, Qian GS, Jackson P, Groopman JD, Manning JE, et al. SOCS-1, a negative regulator of the JAK/STAT pathway, is silenced by methylation in human hepatocellular carcinoma and shows growth-suppression activity. Nat Genet. 2001;28(1):29–35.
108. Rawlings JS, Rosler KM, Harrison DA. The JAK/STAT signaling pathway. J Cell Sci. 2004;117(Pt 8):1281–3.
109. Andl CD, Mizushima T, Oyama K, Bowser M, Nakagawa H, Rustgi AK. EGFR-induced cell migration is mediated predominantly by the JAK-STAT pathway in primary esophageal keratinocytes. Am J Physiol Gastrointest Liver Physiol. 2004;287(6):G1227–37.
110. Kussie PH, Gorina S, Marechal V, Elenbaas B, Moreau J, Levine AJ, et al. Structure of the MDM2 oncoprotein bound to the p53 tumor suppressor transactivation domain. Science. 1996;274(5289):948–53.
111. Toledo F, Wahl GM. Regulating the p53 pathway: in vitro hypotheses, in vivo veritas. Nat Rev Cancer. 2006;6(12):909–23.
112. Barak Y, Gottlieb E, Juven-Gershon T, Oren M. Regulation of mdm2 expression by p53: alternative promoters produce transcripts with nonidentical translation potential. Genes Dev. 1994;8(15):1739–49.
113. Muller PA, Vousden KH. Mutant p53 in cancer: new functions and therapeutic opportunities. Cancer Cell. 2014;25(3):304–17.
114. Willis A, Jung EJ, Wakefield T, Chen X. Mutant p53 exerts a dominant negative effect by preventing wild-type p53 from binding to the promoter of its target genes. Oncogene. 2004;23(13):2330–8.
115. Persons DL, Yazlovitskaya EM, Pelling JC. Effect of extracellular signal-regulated kinase on p53 accumulation in response to cisplatin. J Biol Chem. 2000;275(46):35778–85.
116. She QB, Chen N, Dong Z. ERKs and p38 kinase phosphorylate p53 protein at serine 15 in response to UV radiation. J Biol Chem. 2000;275(27):20444–9.
117. Yeh PY, Chuang SE, Yeh KH, Song YC, Chang LL, Cheng AL. Phosphorylation of p53 on Thr55 by ERK2 is necessary for doxorubicin-induced p53 activation and cell death. Oncogene. 2004;23(20):3580–8.
118. Courtois-Cox S, Genther Williams SM, Reczek EE, Johnson BW, McGillicuddy LT, Johannessen CM, et al. A negative feedback signaling network underlies oncogene-induced senescence. Cancer Cell. 2006;10(6):459–72.
119. Ferbeyre G, de Stanchina E, Lin AW, Querido E, McCurrach ME, Hannon GJ, et al. Oncogenic ras and p53 cooperate to induce cellular senescence. Mol Cell Biol. 2002;22(10):3497–508.
120. Gottlieb TM, Leal JF, Seger R, Taya Y, Oren M. Cross-talk between Akt, p53 and Mdm2: possible implications for the regulation of apoptosis. Oncogene. 2002;21(8):1299–303.
121. Ogawara Y, Kishishita S, Obata T, Isazawa Y, Suzuki T, Tanaka K, et al. Akt enhances Mdm2-mediated ubiquitination and degradation of p53. J Biol Chem. 2002;277(24):21843–50.
122. Nault JC, Zucman-Rossi J. TERT promoter mutations in primary liver tumors. Clin Res Hepatol Gastroenterol. 2016;40(1):9–14.
123. Satyanarayana A, Manns MP, Rudolph KL. Telomeres and telomerase: a dual role in hepatocarcinogenesis. Hepatology. 2004;40(2):276–83.
124. Luedde T, Schwabe RF. NF-kappaB in the liver—linking injury, fibrosis and hepatocellular carcinoma. Nat Rev Gastroenterol Hepatol. 2011;8(2):108–18.
125. Karin M. NF-kappaB as a critical link between inflammation and cancer. Cold Spring Harb Perspect Biol. 2009;1(5):a000141.
126. Xu W, Zhang X, Wu JL, Fu L, Liu K, Liu D, et al. O-GlcNAc transferase promotes fatty liver-associated liver cancer through inducing palmitic acid and activating endoplasmic reticulum stress. J Hepatol. 2017;67(2):310–20.
127. Sicklick JK, Li YX, Jayaraman A, Kannangai R, Qi Y, Vivekanandan P, et al. Dysregulation of the Hedgehog pathway in human hepatocarcinogenesis. Carcinogenesis. 2006;27(4):748–57.
128. Huang S, He J, Zhang X, Bian Y, Yang L, Xie G, et al. Activation of the hedgehog pathway in human hepatocellular carcinomas. Carcinogenesis. 2006;27(7):1334–40.
129. Della Corte CM, Viscardi G, Papaccio F, Esposito G, Martini G, Ciardiello D, et al. Implication of the Hedgehog pathway in hepatocellular carcinoma. World J Gastroenterol. 2017;23(24):4330–40.
130. Lu JT, Zhao WD, He W, Wei W. Hedgehog signaling pathway mediates invasion and metastasis of hepatocellular carcinoma via ERK pathway. Acta Pharmacol Sin. 2012;33(5):691–700.
131. Blivet-Van Eggelpoel MJ, Chettouh H, Fartoux L, Aoudjehane L, Barbu V, Rey C, et al. Epidermal growth factor receptor and HER-3 restrict cell response to sorafenib in hepatocellular carcinoma cells. J Hepatol. 2012;57(1):108–15.
132. Ito Y, Takeda T, Sakon M, Tsujimoto M, Higashiyama S, Noda K, et al. Expression and clinical significance of erb-B receptor family in hepatocellular carcinoma. Br J Cancer. 2001;84(10):1377–83.
133. Ezzoukhry Z, Louandre C, Trecherel E, Godin C, Chauffert B, Dupont S, et al. EGFR activation is a potential determinant of primary resistance of hepatocellular carcinoma cells to sorafenib. Int J Cancer. 2012;131(12):2961–9.
134. Gedaly R, Angulo P, Hundley J, Daily MF, Chen C, Koch A, et al. PI-103 and sorafenib inhibit hepatocellular carcinoma cell proliferation by blocking Ras/Raf/MAPK and PI3K/AKT/mTOR pathways. Anticancer Res. 2010;30(12):4951–8.
135. Huynh H, Ngo VC, Koong HN, Poon D, Choo SP, Thng CH, et al. Sorafenib and rapamycin induce growth suppression in mouse models of hepatocellular carcinoma. J Cell Mol Med. 2009;13(8B):2673–83.
136. Chen KF, Chen HL, Tai WT, Feng WC, Hsu CH, Chen PJ, et al. Activation of phosphatidylinositol 3-kinase/Akt signaling pathway mediates acquired resistance to sorafenib in hepatocellular carcinoma cells. J Pharmacol Exp Ther. 2011;337(1):155–61.
137. Chen KF, Tai WT, Hsu CY, Huang JW, Liu CY, Chen PJ, et al. Blockade of STAT3 activation by sorafenib derivatives through enhancing SHP-1 phosphatase activity. Eur J Med Chem. 2012;55:220–7.

Drug Induced Liver Injury: Mechanisms, Diagnosis, and Clinical Management

9

Rolf Teschke and Gaby Danan

Key Concepts

- Drug-induced liver injury (DILI) is the first cause of stopping drug development and withdrawal of marketed products.
- At therapeutic doses, many drugs can lead to idiosyncratic DILI in susceptible individuals, whereas intrinsic DILI is caused by overdosed drugs such as acetaminophen.
- The diagnosis of DILI requires chronological criteria and the exclusion of alternative causes, both best achieved by using a transparent, specific, quantitative, and validated causality assessment method (CAM) such as RUCAM (Roussel Uclaf Causality Assessment Method).
- The diagnosis of DILI should lead to quick discontinuation of the suspected drug and most commonly to a favorable clinical outcome.
- Drug-induced acute liver failure (ALF) develops rarely, especially when the diagnosis is missed and drug discontinuation is delayed. It accounts for almost half of the ALF cases mostly attributed to overdosed acetaminophen, and remains the first cause of liver transplantation.

9.1 Introduction

Diagnostic challenges in clinical medicine are patients with liver injury by chemicals such as alcohol [1], organic solvents [2], and drugs [3–8]. It is the first cause of stopping drug development and drug withdrawal from the market. As compared to other causes of liver diseases, liver injury by drugs is a rare event in the general population and occurs with an annual estimated incidence of around 14 cases per 100,000 inhabitants [7]. Consequently, physicians caring for patients with suspected drug induced liver injury (DILI) are confronted with a wide range of alternative diagnoses [7–9] that require a liver specific, validated, quantitative and scoring diagnostic algorithm such as the Roussel Uclaf Causality Assessment Method (RUCAM) [3–8]. This is a tool to verify or revoke the diagnosis of DILI, an approach that should also followed by authors of DILI case reports or case series [3, 8]. Only DILI cases with a probable or highly probable causality level qualify for a correct characterization of clinical features and DILI risk factors [9]. In the past, many DILI cases were indeed not DILI but the liver injuries were likely due to another cause [4, 7], representing a problem for authors, editors, clinicians, pharmaceutical companies, and most importantly, for patients [7].

This chapter provides a critical insight in essential key elements of DILI including causality assessment.

9.2 Definitions

9.2.1 Idiosyncratic Versus Intrinsic Toxicity

Drugs are rare causes of liver injury, whether the toxicity is due to the interaction between the drug and patient factors (idiosyncrasy) or the drug only (intrinsic toxicity) [3, 9–12]. DILI commonly stands for idiosyncratic DILI, which is caused by drugs at therapeutic dosages in a few exposed patients and triggered by unpredictable, mostly immunologic and less frequently metabolic drug reactions [3, 8, 9, 12]. This

R. Teschke (✉)
Department of Internal Medicine II, Division of Gastroenterology and Hepatology, Klinikum Hanau, Hanau, Academic Teaching Hospital of the Medical Faculty, Goethe University Frankfurt/Main, Frankfurt/Main, Germany

G. Danan
Pharmacovigilance Consultancy, Paris, France

F. Radu-Ionita et al. (eds.), *Liver Diseases*, https://doi.org/10.1007/978-3-030-24432-3_9

is in contrast to intrinsic DILI characterized by a dose dependent and therefore predictable reaction related to overdosed drugs such as acetaminophen [3, 9, 10]. Idiosyncratic and intrinsic DILI share the risk of acute liver failure (ALF) with high mortality rate or need for liver transplantation. However, the identification of offending drug(s) often remains uncertain essentially because the principles of diagnosis including causality assessment are not based on a quantitative and transparent scoring system such as RUCAM [3].

9.3 DILI Mechanisms and Hypothetical Cascade of Events

Hepatic drug metabolism proceeds along two phases, these reactions lead to conjugated products ready for biliary or renal excretion, unless there is a drug overdose. Conversely, conditions are different in acetaminophen (syn. paracetamol) overdose [10], because toxic metabolites are produced in excess that initiate liver injury following covalent binding with macromolecules. Liver injury is prevented if paracetamol sulfation and glucuronidation is sufficient or hepatic glutathione levels are high enough to bind toxic metabolites.

In analogy to human and experimental liver injury by alcohol [1] and other hepatotoxins such as aliphatic halogenated hydrocarbons [2], non-parenchymal cells of the liver like Kupffer cells, stellate cells, and sinusoidal cells likely play a contributory pathogenetic role for DILI whereas the focus is clearly on the hepatocyte [11, 12], with its endoplasmic reticulum and mitochondria that are considered as the major cell organelle targets of liver injury [11, 12]. Most drugs are metabolized in the hepatocyte, mainly in the endoplasmic reticulum, which corresponds to the microsomal fraction of the biochemists obtained by ultracentrifugation of liver homogenates. Within the endoplasmic reticulum, drugs compete metabolically with other chemicals at the site of cytochrome P450 (CYP 450) [1]. This cytochrome is present in various isoenzymes such as CYP1A1, CYP1A2, CYP2B6, CYP2C9, CYP2C19, CYP2D6, CYP2E1, CYP3A4, CYP3A5 and CYP3A7. Drugs enter as substrates in the microsomal CYP 450 circle and usually leave it as oxidized drugs. However, the introduction of electrons and O_2 is risky if the reactions proceed incompletely and generate reactive oxygen species (ROS), in line with similar toxic intermediates observed in liver injury by alcohol [1] or aliphatic halogenated hydrocarbons [2].

Elucidating pathogenetic details of idiosyncratic DILI is hampered by the lack of experimental animal models, whereas those of intrinsic DILI are better investigated [12]. A body of evidence suggests that both, idiosyncratic and intrinsic DILI, are caused by drug metabolites rather than by the parent drug [5, 10–12] and may follow a three-step working model including a cascade of events [11, 12]. In the first step of this model, common to idiosyncratic and intrinsic toxicity, drugs or their toxic intermediates generated through microsomal metabolism cause injury of the endoplasmic reticulum and mitochondria of the hepatocyte (Fig. 9.1). The second hit is different in the two DILI types: in the idiosyncratic toxicity, the innate and adaptive immunity system triggers immune

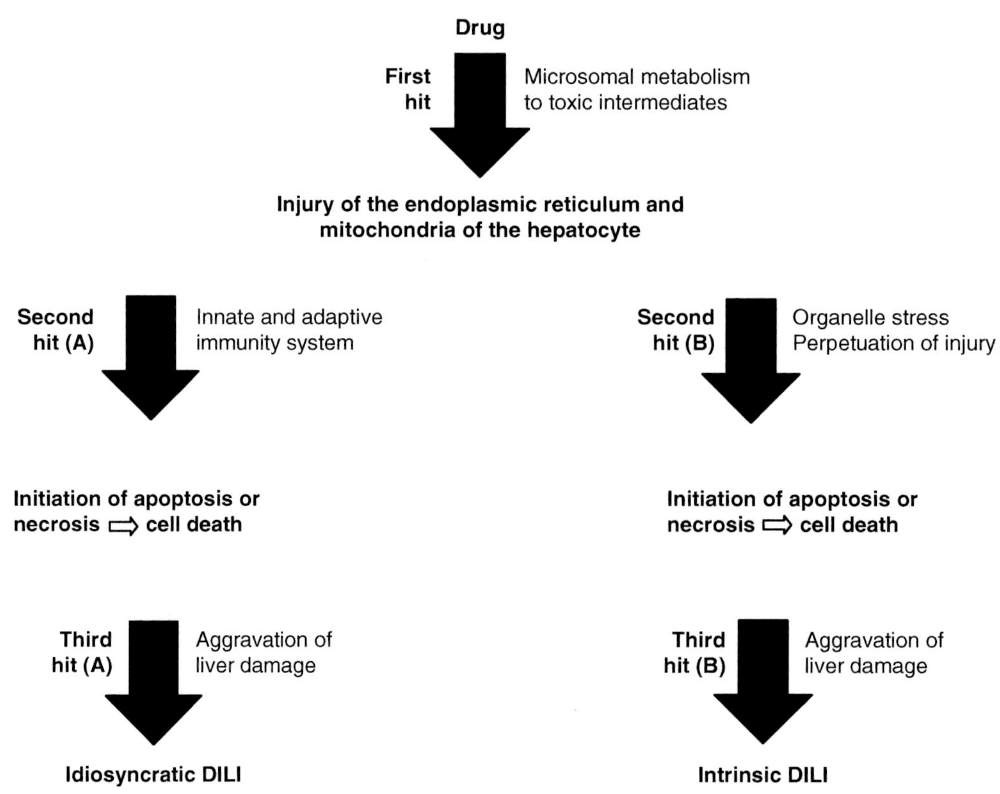

Fig. 9.1 Hypothetical cascade of events involving three hits and leading to cell death and DILI

reactions whereas in the intrinsic toxicity, organelle stress of the endoplasmic reticulum and mitochondria is caused by reactive oxygen species (ROS) (Fig. 9.1). The second hit initiates apoptosis, necrosis, and cell death, though not uniformly but at various degrees. For both types of toxicity the third hit is characterized by aggravation of the liver damage.

9.4 Clinical Aspects

9.4.1 Most Implicated Drugs

Considering published DILI cases with high causality levels assessed by RUCAM, consensus exists that most drugs are potential cause of liver injury in susceptible users [16–18]. However, the number of reported DILI cases in a given country or region is highly dependent on the use of the drugs in the same geographic area. This is the reason why the ranking of the most implicated drugs should be interpreted with the use of those drugs. For example, in Germany the drugs most commonly implicated were in descending order flupirtine, clarithromycin, fluoroquinolones, oestrogen + diogenoest, irbesartan, terbinafine, and metamizole [16], while in India, these drugs are antituberculosis drugs (49%), antiepileptic drugs (12%), complementary and alternative medicine (10%), antiretroviral drugs (9%), and non-steroidal anti-inflammatory drugs (6%) [17]. In China, DILI is most frequently reported with antibiotics, antituberculosis drugs, antithyroid drugs, antineoplastic drugs, hypolipidemic drugs, antipyretic analgesics, antiepileptics, hypoglycemic drugs, antivirals, glucocorticoids, antithrombotics, and antihypertensive drugs [18]. It is therefore important for the clinician in a specific region to be aware of the likely cases of liver injury induced by the drugs, herbs or complementary medicines used in the same region. This information is usually provided by the regulatory agencies and by specialized DILI databases such as U.S. NIH LiverTox database. Nevertheless, despite the great attention given to the published cases, the site did assess the causality with a method mainly based on a mere opinion. For some cases it is hard to rely on cases poorly documented and assessed. It would be suitable to reassess the cases with a more transparent and quantitative method such as RUCAM [4].

9.4.2 Genetic and Non-genetic Risk Factors

Several risk factors of idiosyncratic DILI have been proposed, but some are still under discussion because the data derived from questionable DILI cases were not assessed with a robust CAM such as RUCAM [8, 9, 12–14]. In short, among the proposed but not necessarily validated risk factors are drug lipophilicity, high daily dosage (>50 mg or 100 mg), high hepatic metabolism, comedications, and HLA alleles due to genetic variability. Although based on high profile studies, risk factors such as age > 55 years [3, 8], alcohol use [3, 8, 9], and some preexisting liver disease including nonalcoholic or alcoholic liver disease [15] are still subject to discussion. Because genetic factors, ethnicity, race, gender, and age are likely major contributors to idiosyncratic DILI, our knowledge should be expanded by enlarging population analysis with prospective and scoring causality assessment such as RUCAM [6].

9.4.3 DILI Signatures for Specific Drugs

For some drugs, clinical and laboratory characteristics have been identified. They are called "signatures" such as the time to onset of the liver injury, the type of the liver injury and associated signs or symptoms. Although not necessarily validated by a CAM, this profile may be obtained from the NIH LiverTox website and could help determine the offending drug; however, one drug can induce various types of liver injury that limits the interpretation of website-based signatures [16–18]. The general rule is that DILI signatures for specific drugs must be validated by several cases of DILI cases with confirmed high causality levels using RUCAM.

9.4.4 Demographics and DILI Characteristics

Based on DILI cases with causality assessment by RUCAM, features of idiosyncratic DILI have been published [16–18]. These reports originating from Germany [16], India [17], and China [18], enable deep analysis through comparisons across populations. According to the DILI results of the hospital-based Berlin Case-Control Surveillance Study from Germany, mean age was 55 years, and there was preponderance of females with 58% and the hepatocellular type of injury with 46–69% [16]. Comedication with another hepatotoxic drug and compatible time course was described with 49–66% [16]. In half of the patients of the study from Germany, time from beginning of the drug administration was within a period ranging from 5 days up to 90 days [16]. Somewhat different results have been reported in the DILI study from India, with a mean age of 40 years, an equal distribution of females and males, a mean duration of drug exposure of 34 days, a mean interval between symptom onset and DILI recognition of 14 days [17]. There was a predominance of hepatocellular injury (50%) as compared to cholestatic injury (15%) and mixed injury (35%) [17]. Analyses of DILI cases in China provided a mean age of 43 years and a predominance of the female gender (51%) and hepatocellular injury (62%) [18].

9.4.5 Clinical Spectrum

A typical clinical example for idiosyncratic DILI is triggered by the anesthetic halothane. Risk factors for halothane liver injury and ALF included age, obesity, female gender, and especially reexposure with halothane within a short period, a known risk often not considered by professionals. Liver histology usually shows confluent liver cell necrosis without intact hepatocytes. Today, other fluorinated anesthetics have replaced halothane, but the risks of liver injury remained though at a lower level.

Early clinical recognition of DILI is essential in order to discontinue the therapy with the suspect drug and to facilitate a complete resolution. Physicians should inform patients about possible symptoms that may emerge under a drug therapy especially when the drug is known to induce acute liver injury. Patients with DILI may experience a variety of signs and symptoms, which are not specific and require further diagnostic evaluation. In detail, in Germany, fatigue was described in 50–66%, jaundice in 25–44%, and pale stool/dark urine in 16–34% of the series [16]. Most common symptoms in India were nausea (91%), vomiting (85%), abdominal pain (73%), and anorexia (69%), with lower frequencies of dark urine (58%) and jaundice (55%) [17]. Non-survivors commonly experienced jaundice, vomiting, dark urine, and abdominal pain, whereas these signs and symptoms were less frequently observed in survivors [17], in China the frequency of signs and symptoms was not specified [18].

The mortality rate of DILI was 5% in Germany [16], 16% in India [17], and 2.8% in China [18]. Liver transplantation rate was variable: Germany (0.5%) [16], India (0%) [17], and China (0.8%) [18]. For ALF by idiosyncratic DILI, no proven antidotes or other therapy options are available [5, 19, 20], whereas N-acetylcysteine is an established treatment to prevent aggravation of the acute liver injury to ALF due to acetaminophen overdose [10]. This treatment should be initiated immediately after admission, even if the overdose is only suspected. Despite options of specific and effective therapy, ALF remains a clinical issue, as evidenced by the fact that the most common cause of liver transplantation is DILI caused by acetaminophen overdose.

Otherwise, the clinical outcome of DILI is usually a complete resolution after cessation of the suspected drug. In rare instances, DILI may evolve to chronic liver disease [18]. However, once the offending drug is discontinued, the lesion becomes inactive but the sequelae are irreversible such as a vanishing bile duct syndrome or extensive liver fibrosis with the serious complications of these conditions. Overall prognosis of DILI can certainly be improved if the offending drug is early discontinued, but this requires quick diagnosis of DILI after alternative causes have been ruled out that are considered as confounding factors [7].

9.4.6 Alternative Causes

DILI is, by essence, a diagnosis of exclusion, requiring consideration of other liver diseases mimicked by DILI. In practice, they are compiled in a check list (Table 9.1), which is not a comprehensive list and should be adapted to the clinical context [3, 8]. Alternative causes were identified as so called DILI cases in 22 published DILI series, ranging from 4% to 47%. Among 13,336 cases of initially suspected DILI, alternative causes were found more likely in 4556 patients (34.2%) [7]. Biliary diseases such as biliary obstruction, cholangitis, choledocholithiasis, primary biliary cholangitis, and primary sclerosing cholangitis were among the most missed diagnoses. Alternative liver diseases included hepatitis B, C, and E, CMV, EBV, ischemic hepatitis, cardiac hepatopathy, autoimmune hepatitis, non-alcoholic fatty liver disease, non-alcoholic steatohepatitis, and alcoholic liver disease [7]. For reasons of transparency, in publications on DILI case series the presentation of a flow chart signifying alternative causes is recommended [7].

9.5 Biomarkers

Biomarkers cannot solve the problems of alternative diagnoses confounding DILI. No valid diagnostic or prognostic biomarker currently exists for idiosyncratic DILI, and several studies failed to show good performance indicators of candidates [12]. The main reasons would be that idiosyncratic DILI is (1) typically a human disease hardly reproducible in animals, and (2) DILI cases used for testing the new biomarkers are not correctly assessed for causality that would decrease substantially the power of the tested biomarker [8]. Here also RUCAM-based assessment will ensure homogeneity of cases tested with the new biomarker. However, diagnostic biomarkers as blood (or urine) tests would be of great help for clinicians and regulators, and pharmaceutical industry would be more comfortable if, in addition to RUCAM, causality of DILI can be objectively confirmed [12].

Among the potential biomarkers under discussion [12] are CK-18 (Cytokeratin-18), microRNA-122 (microarray RNA-122), total HMGB-1 (High Mobility Group Box protein-1), GLDH (Glutamate dehydrogenase), SDH (Sorbitol dehydrogenase) proposed as marker for hepatocyte necrosis, ccCK-18 (caspase-cleaved CytoKeratin-18) proposed as marker for apoptosis, hyperacetylated HMGB-1, and MCSFR-1 (Macrophage colony-stimulating factor receptor-1) proposed as marker for immune activation [8, 12]. Other proposals included M-30 (apoptosis), M-65 (apoptosis/necrosis), and microRNA-192 (unspecified liver damage). Some of the proposed biomarkers are not liver or not drug specific, others are difficult to be assessed due to the requirement of mass spectroscopy [8, 12]. Microarray RNAs (microRNAs) including microRNA-122 have been evaluated in experimental liver injury and in human intrinsic DILI caused by acetaminophen or paracetamol, but uncertainty exists on their diagnostic value in human idiosyncratic DILI [12].

Table 9.1 Checklist of differential diagnoses of DILI

Differential diagnosis	Diagnostic parameters	Done		
		Yes	No	Partially
Group I				
Hepatitis A virus (HAV)	Anti-HAV-IgM	□	□	□
Hepatitis B virus (HBV) (Hepatitis D virus, HDV)	Anti-HBc-IgM and HBV-DNA (specific marker of HDV)	□	□	□
Hepatitis C virus (HCV)	Anti-HCV and HCV-RNA	□	□	□
Hepatitis E virus (HEV)	Anti-HEV-IgM and HEV-RNA	□	□	□
Ischemic liver necrosis	Episode of severe hypotension, shock, hypoxia or heart failure within 3 days before the onset of liver injury	□	□	□
Biliary obstruction	Liver imaging (e.g., ultrasound, CT, ERCP, MRC)	□	□	□
Alcoholic liver disease (ALD)	History, clinical and laboratory assessment (AST/ALT>2), other alcoholic disease(s)	□	□	□
Group II				
• Cytomegalovirus (CMV)	CMV-PCR, titer change for anti-CMV-IgM/anti-CMV-IgG	□	□	□
• Epstein Barr virus (EBV)	EBV-PCR, titer change for anti-EBV-IgM/anti-EBV-IgG	□	□	□
• Herpes simplex virus (HSV)	HSV-PCR, titer change for anti-HSV-IgM/anti-HSV-IgG	□	□	□
• Varicella zoster virus (VZV)	VZV-PCR, titer change for anti-VZV-IgM/anti-VZV-IgG	□	□	□
• Other viral infections	Specific serology of HIV, Adenovirus, Coxsackie-B-Virus, Echovirus, Measles virus, Rubella virus, Flavivirus, Arenavirus, Filovirus, Parvovirus	□	□	□
• Other infectious diseases	Specific assessment of bacteria, fungi, parasites, worms, and others	□	□	□
• Autoimmune hepatitis (AIH) type I	Gamma globulins, ANA, SMA, AAA, SLA/LP, Anti-LSP, Anti-ASGPR	□	□	□
• Autoimmune hepatitis (AIH) type II	Gamma globulins, Anti-LKM-1 (CYP 2D6), Anti-LKM-2 (CYP 2C9), Anti-LKM-3	□	□	□
• Primary biliary cirrhosis (PBC)	AMA, Anti PDH-E2	□	□	□
• Primary sclerosing cholangitis (PSC)	p-ANCA, MRC	□	□	□
• Autoimmune cholangitis (AIC)	ANA, SMA	□	□	□
• Overlap syndromes	See AIH, PBC, PSC, and AIC	□	□	□
• Non alcoholic steatohepatitis (NASH)	BMI, insulin resistance, hepatomegaly, echogenicity of the liver	□	□	□
• Cocaine, ecstasy and other amphetamines	Toxin screening	□	□	□
• Rare intoxications	Toxin screening for household and occupational toxins	□	□	□
• Hereditary hemochromatosis	Serum ferritin, total iron-binding capacity, genotyping for C2824 and H63D mutation, hepatic iron content	□	□	□
• Wilson's disease	Copper excretion (24 h urine), Ceruloplasmin in serum, Free copper in serum, Coombs-negative hemolytic anemia, hepatic copper Content, Kayser-Fleischer-ring, neurologic-psychiatric Work-up, genotyping	□	□	□
• Porphyria	Porphobilinogen in urine, total porphyrins in urine	□	□	□
• α_1-Antitrypsin deficiency	α_1-Antitrypsin in serum	□	□	□
• Pancreatic diseases	Clinical and laboratory assessment, sonography, CT, MRT	□	□	□
• Celiac disease	TTG antibodies, endomysium antibodies, duodenal biopsy	□	□	□
• Anorexia nervosa	Clinical context	□	□	□
• Parenteral nutrition	Clinical context	□	□	□
• Cardiopulmonary diseases	E.g., Assessment of congestive heart disease, myocardial infarction, cardiomyopathy, cardiac valvular dysfunction, pulmonary embolism, pericardial diseases, arrhythmia, hemorrhagic shock	□	□	□
• Addison's disease	Plasma cortisol	□	□	□
• Thyroid diseases	TSH basal, T4, T3	□	□	□

(continued)

Table 9.1 (continued)

Differential diagnosis	Diagnostic parameters	Done Yes	No	Partially
• Grand mal seizures	Clinical context of epileptic seizure	□	□	□
• Heat stroke	Shock, hyperthermia	□	□	□
• Polytrauma	Shock, liver injury	□	□	□
• Systemic diseases	Liver cancer, sarcoidosis, amyloidosis, liver metastases, sepsis	□	□	□

This tabular listing, although not comprehensive, is to be used as a guide and in connection with the updated RUCAM (Tables 9.2 and 9.3), derived from a previous publication [3]. Abbreviations: *AAA* anti-actin antibodies, *AMA* antimitochondrial antibodies, *ANA* antinuclear antibodies, *ASGPR* asialo-glycoprotein-receptor, *BMI* body mass index, *CT* computed tomography, *CYP* cytochrome P450, *DPH* pyruvate dehydrogenase, *HAV* hepatitis A virus, *HBc* hepatitis B core, *HBV* hepatitis B virus, *HCV* hepatitis C virus, *HEV* hepatitis E virus, *HILI* herb induced liver injury, *HIV* human immunodeficiency virus, *LKM* liver kidney microsomes, *LP* liver-pancreas antigen, *LSP* liver specific protein, *MRC* magnetic resonance cholangiography, *MRT* magnetic resonance tomography, *p-ANCA* perinuclear antineutrophil cytoplasmatic antibodies, *PCR* polymerase chain reaction, *RUCAM* Roussel Uclaf Causality Assessment Method, *SLA* soluble liver antigen, *SMA* smooth muscle antibodies, *TSH* thyroid stimulating hormone, *TTG* tissue transglutaminase

9.6 RUCAM-Based Causality Assessment

9.6.1 Principles

RUCAM is characterized by seven well-defined and scored key elements, the sum of which provides a final score with causality grading [3]. In addition to the tables providing the key elements and the score (Tables 9.2 and 9.3), working instructions are available in order to consider the vast majority of situations and therefore reduce inter rater variability [8].

Before assessing causality, the first step is to define a liver injury. Current definitions are based on serum activity of alanine aminotransferase (ALT) of at least 5 x ULN (upper limit of normal) and/or hepatic alkaline phosphatase (ALP) of at least 2 x ULN [3].

The second step is to determine the type of the liver injury according to the R ratio. The numerator is the ALT value expressed as a multiple of ULN (ALT/ALT ULN) and the denominator the ALP value expressed also as a multiple of the ULN (ALP/ALP ULN). The ratio R should be calculated at the beginning of the liver injury as the initial type could evolve over time towards another type that would change the criteria for causality assessment. In practice, two types of liver injury are considered for evaluation: hepatocellular injury ($R > 5$) and cholestatic/mixed liver injury ($R \leq 5$) [3] as they have different risk factors and time courses of ALT and ALP.

Key elements of RUCAM and their respective scores are provided for the hepatocellular injury (Table 9.2) and the cholestatic/mixed liver injury (Table 9.3).

The discussion on each key elements has been detailed elsewhere [8]. In brief, the key elements are: the timing of events, dechallenge, risk factors, comedications, search for alternative causes, known hepatotoxicity of the suspect drug and the results of rechallenge. In any case of suspected DILI it is possible to give a score to each element even when there is no information on this element (score null). The final score for each suspect drug indicates causality degrees: ≤0 point, excluded causality; 1–2, unlikely; 3–5, possible; 6–8, probable; ≥9, highly probable. In case of suspected drug-drug interaction, RUCAM should be applied to the suspected combination as a single product.

9.6.2 Alternative Approaches of Causality Assessment

CAMs such as Naranjo scale or WHO-UMC causality assessment method are not liver specific, and they should be seen as guide for any adverse event [3, 8]. A suspected DILI needs a more specific approach with precise elements as described in RUCAM. Other CAMs proposed only some RUCAM elements and their scores [3, 8, 9] but due to shortcomings none was recommended for use [3, 8]. The global introspection method used by DILIN considers some RUCAM items but without formal algorithm [3, 8]. This approach results in a subjective causality grading expressed as arbitrary percentage ranges and leaves questions open as to how key elements and missing data were taken into consideration. Finally due to the absence of items definition and scores it is not easy or even possible to re-assess independently the cases [3, 8, 9]. Instead, RUCAM was designed to be a user-friendly method with a simple form to go through and associated recommendations to users [3, 8].

9.6.3 Global Usage

There is much international support using RUCAM to assess causality for drugs and herbs in suspected DILI and HILI cases [3, 8, 9] as evidenced by the large number of RUCAM-

Table 9.2 Drug or herb induced liver injury. RUCAM scale for hepatocellular injury

Suspected product:	Date:	
Items for hepatocellular injury	Score	Result
1. Time to onset from the beginning of the drug/herb		
• 5–90 days (rechallenge: 1–15 days)	+2	□
• <5 or >90 days (rechallenge: > 15 days)	+1	□
Alternative: Time to onset from cessation of the drug/herb		
• ≤ 15 days (except for slowly metabolized chemicals: > 15 days)	+1	□
2. Course of ALT after cessation of the drug/herb		
Percentage difference between ALT peak and ULN		
• Decrease ≥50% within 8 days	+3	□
• Decrease ≥50% within 30 days	+2	□
• No information or continued drug use	0	□
• Decrease ≥50% after the 30th day	0	□
• Decrease <50% after the 30th day or recurrent increase	−2	□
3. Risk factors		
• Alcohol use (current drinks/day: > for women, > 3 for men)	+1	□
• Alcohol use (current drinks/day: ≤ 2 for women, ≤ 3 for men)	0	□
• Age ≥ 55 years	+1	□
• Age < 55 years	0	□
4. Concomitant drug(s)/herb(s)		
• None or no information	0	□
• Concomitant drug/herb with incompatible time to onset	0	□
• Concomitant drug/herb with time to onset 5–90 days	−1	□
• Concomitant drug/herb known as hepatotoxin and with time to onset 5–90 days	−2	□
• Concomitant drug/herb with evidence for its role in this case (positive rechallenge or validated test)	−3	□
5. Search for alternative causes	Tick if negative	Tick if not done
Group I (7 causes)		
• HAV: Anti-HAV-IgM	□	□
• HBV: HBsAg, anti-HBc-IgM, HBV-DNA	□	□
• HCV: Anti-HCV, HCV-RNA	□	□
• HEV: Anti-HEV-IgM, anti-HEV-IgG, HEV-RNA	□	□
• Hepatobiliary sonography/Doppler/CT/MRC	□	□
• Alcoholism (AST/ALT ≥2)	□	□
• Acute recent hypotension history (particularly if underlying heart disease)	□	□
Group II (5 causes)		
• Complications of underlying disease(s) such as sepsis, metastatic malignancy, autoimmune hepatitis, chronic hepatitis B or C, primary biliary cholangitis or sclerosing cholangitis, genetic liver diseases	□	□
• Infection suggested by PCR and titer change for	□	□
• CMV (anti-CMV-IgM, anti-CMV-IgG)	□	□
• EBV (anti-EBV-IgM, anti-EBV-IgG)	□	□
• HSV (anti-HSV-IgM, anti-HSV-IgG)	□	□
• VZV (anti-VZV-IgM, anti-VZV-IgG)	□	□
Evaluation of groups I and II		
• All causes-groups I and II—reasonably ruled out	+2	□
• The 7 causes of group I ruled out	+1	□
• 6 or 5 causes of group I ruled out	0	□
• Less than 5 causes of group I ruled out	−2	□
• Alternative cause highly probable	−3	□
6. Previous hepatotoxicity of the drug/herb		
• Reaction labelled in the product characteristics	+2	□
• Reaction published but unlabelled		

(continued)

Table 9.2 (continued)

Suspected product:	Date:	
Items for hepatocellular injury	Score	Result
• Reaction unknown	0	□
7. Response to unintentional reexposure		
• Doubling of ALT with the drug/herb alone, provided ALT below 5ULN before reexposure	+3	□
• Doubling of ALT with the drug(s)/herb(s) already given at the time of first reaction	+1	□
• Increase of ALT but less than ULN in the same conditions as for the first administration	−2	□
• Other situations	0	□
Total score		

The above items specifically refer to the hepatocellular injury rather than to the cholestatic or mixed liver injury, adapted from a previous detailed report on the updated RUCAM [3]. Abbreviations: *ALT* alanine aminotransferase, *AST* aspartate aminotransferase, *CMV* cytomegalovirus, *CT* computer tomography, *DILI* drug induced liver injury, *EBV* Epstein Barr virus, *HAV* hepatitis A virus, *HBc* hepatitis B core, *HBsAg* hepatitis B surface antigen, *HBV* hepatitis B virus, *HCV* hepatitis C virus, *HEV* hepatitis E virus, *HSV* herpes simplex virus, *MRC* magnetic resonance cholangiography, *RUCAM* Roussel Uclaf Causality Assessment Method, *ULN* upper limit of the normal range, *VZV* Varicella zoster virus. Total score and resulting causality grading: ≤0, excluded; 1–2, unlikely; 3–5, possible; 6–8, probable; ≥9, highly probable

Table 9.3 Drug or herb induced liver injury. RUCAM scale for cholestatic/mixed liver injury

Suspected product:	Date:	
Items for cholestatic or mixed liver injury	Score	Result
1. Time to onset from the beginning of the drug/herb		
• 5–90 days (rechallenge: 1–90 days)	+2	□
• <5 or >90 days (rechallenge: >90 days)	+1	□
Alternative: Time to onset from cessation of the drug/herb		
• ≤30 days (except for slowly metabolized chemicals: >30 days)	+1	□
2. Course of ALP after cessation of the drug/herb		
Percentage difference between ALP peak and ULN		
• Decrease ≥50% within 180 days	+2	□
• Decrease <50% within 180 days	+1	□
• No information, persistence, increase, or continued drug/herb use	0	□
3. Risk factors		
• Alcohol use current drinks/day: >2 for women, >3 for men)	+1	□
• Alcohol use (current drinks/day: ≤2 for women, ≤3 for men)	0	□
• Pregnancy	+1	□
• Age ≥ 55 years	+1	□
• Age < 55 years	0	□
4. Concomitant use of drug(s)/herb(s)		
• None or no information	0	□
• Concomitant drug/herb with incompatible time to onset	0	□
• Concomitant drug/herb with time to onset 5–90 days	−1	□
• Concomitant drug/herb known as hepatotoxin and with time to onset 5–90 days	−2	□
• Concomitant drug/herb with evidence for its role in this case (positive rechallenge or validated test)	−3	□
5. Search for alternative causes	Tick if negative	Tick if not done
Group I (7 causes)		
• HAV: Anti-HAV-IgM	□	□
• HBV: HBsAg, anti-HBc-IgM, HBV-DNA	□	□
• HCV: Anti-HCV, HCV-RNA	□	□
• HEV: Anti-HEV-IgM, anti-HEV-IgG, HEV-RNA	□	□
• Hepatobiliary sonography/Doppler/CT/MRC	□	□
• Alcoholism (AST/ALT ≥2)	□	□
• Acute recent hypotension history (particularly if underlying heart disease)	□	□
Group II (5 causes)		
• Complications of underlying disease(s) such as sepsis, metastatic malignancy, autoimmune hepatitis, chronic hepatitis B or C, primary biliary cholangitis or sclerosing cholangitis, genetic liver diseases	□	□

Table 9.3 (continued)

Suspected product:	Date:	
Items for cholestatic or mixed liver injury	Score	Result
• Infection suggested by PCR and titer change for		
• CMV (anti-CMV-IgM, anti-CMV-IgG)	□	□
• EBV (anti-EBV-IgM, anti-EBV-IgG)	□	□
• HSV (anti-HSV-IgM, anti-HSV-IgG)	□	□
• VZV (anti-VZV-IgM, anti-VZV-IgG)	□	□
Evaluation of groups I and II		
• All causes—groups I and II—reasonably ruled out	+2	□
• The 7 causes of group I ruled out	+1	□
• 6 or 5 causes of group I ruled out	0	□
• Less than 5 causes of group I ruled out	−2	□
• Alternative cause highly probable	−3	□
6. Previous hepatotoxicity of the drug/herb		
• Reaction labelled in the product characteristics	+2	□
• Reaction published but unlabelled	+1	□
• Reaction unknown	0	□
7. Response to unintentional reexposure		
• Doubling of ALP with the drug/herb alone, provided ALP below 2ULN before reexposure	+3	□
• Doubling of ALP with the drugs(s)/herbs(s) already given at the time of first reaction	+1	□
• Increase of ALP but less than ULN in the same conditions as for the first administration	−2	□
• Other situations	0	□
Total score		

The above items specifically refer to the cholestatic or mixed liver injury, adapted from a previous detailed report of the updated RUCAM [3]. Abbreviations: *ALT* alanine aminotransferase, *AST* aspartate aminotransferase, *CMV* cytomegalovirus, *CT* computer tomography, *DILI* drug induced liver injury, *EBV* Epstein Barr virus, *HAV* hepatitis A virus, *HBc* hepatitis B core, *HBsAg* hepatitis B antigen, *HBV* hepatitis B virus, *HCV* hepatitis C virus, *HEV* hepatitis E virus, *HSV* herpes simplex virus, *MRC* magnetic resonance cholangiography, *RUCAM* Roussel Uclaf Causality Assessment Method, *ULN* upper limit of the normal range, *VZV* Varicella zoster virus. Total score and resulting causality grading: ≤0, excluded; 1–2, unlikely; 3–5, possible; 6–8, probable; ≥9, highly probable

based DILI and HILI reports published worldwide by regulatory agencies, large medical centers, registries, and authors reporting case series, case reports, epidemiological studies, and clinical trials [3, 8]. RUCAM supports the contention that DILI requires a rigorous causality management for individual case evaluation, as expressed in encouraging and critical publications reviewing actual liver injury cases [5, 19], an approach highly appreciated and discussed in another commentary [20].

In addition to the many reports that professionally and successfully used RUCAM as referenced [3, 8], one thorough publication of DILI cases assessed by RUCAM merits further attention as a report of excellence [17]. As this study had been conceptualized prospectively, this ensured completeness of case data and high RUCAM-based causality gradings of highly probable (18%), and probable (70%), with lower gradings of possible (5%), unlikely or excluded (9%). The prospective use of RUCAM also facilitated early recognition of alternative causes in eight patients of the study cohort: acute hepatitis E virus (HEV) in three patients, autoimmune hepatitis in two patients, and hepatitis A and B, and sarcoidosis in one patient each [17]. Of note, HEV is a specific item in the updated RUCAM [3, 8, 9], a relevant diagnostic parameter rarely considered by other CAMs. In line with previous views [3, 8, 9], the results of the study under discussion also confirm that reliable causality data are achievable without the need of large, costly DILI networks, dependent on global introspection [17].

Issues of achieving the correct diagnosis in liver injury cases have a long history, with problems not confined to DILI [5–8, 13–18] but recently expanded to herb induced liver injury (HILI) that could account for 12–20% of acute liver injuries due to xenobiotics [5, 9, 18–20]. Indeed, the diagnosis of DILI and HILI cases is made difficult by confounding variables which include missing alternative causes, unverified diagnoses, and limited data quality [3–9, 19, 20].

9.7 Practical Example

A 64 year-old female patient with osteoarthritis of the hip was treated with diclofenac 50 mg tablets three times daily. After 85 days of treatment, she complained of dark urine, itching, jaundice, and epigastric pain, which led her to discontinue the medication. At hospital admission, increased serum activities were found: ALT 1832 U/L (normal <34), AST 1586 U/L (normal

<31), and ALP 168 U/L (normal <115); R value was 37, indicating a hepatocellular type of liver injury. Autoimmune parameters and viral hepatitis serology parameters were negative, as was abdominal ultrasound. Symptoms and jaundice resolved after four weeks months, and all liver tests were normal 3 months after onset. Causality was assessed prospectively with the updated RUCAM and its subscale for the hepatocellular injury (Table 9.2) [3] and revealed a highly probable causality for diclofenac, based on a final score of +10 achieved with the following items and scores out of the following seven categories:

1. Time to onset from the beginning of the drug, 5–90 days, **achieved score + 2**;
2. Course of ALT after cessation of the drug, percentage difference between ALT peak
   and ULN, decrease ≥50% within 8 days, **score + 3**;
3. Risk factor Age ≥ 55 years, **score + 1**;
4. Concomitant drug(s), none or no information, **score 0**;
5. Search for alternative causes, all causes—groups I and II—reasonably ruled out, **score + 2**;
6. Previous hepatotoxicity of the drug, reaction labelled in the product characteristics, **score + 2**;
7. Response to unintentional reexposure, other situations, **score 0**.

This case as example shows that the prospective use of RUCAM ensures completeness of data and helps achieve a high causality grading.

9.8 Conclusions

Idiosyncratic DILI is a rare, unpredictable event that affects susceptible users, and mimicks almost all liver diseases such as chronic hepatitis and nonalcoholic or alcoholic liver diseases with their high prevalence in the general population. Therefore, alternative causes often confound the DILI diagnosis and causes a delayed cessation of the suspected drug. International preference of assessing causality in cases of suspected DILI focuses on the use of RUCAM, an approach supported by many advantages of RUCAM as compared to other causality assessment methods. The clinician facing an elevated value of ALT or ALP should systematically consider a possible DILI not limited to the prescribed drugs but also to herbs and dietary supplements. These remedies are usually not reported by the patients and should always be subject to questions by the physician. Once a DILI is suspected the approach should always be the same one: is it a liver injury? Which type of liver injury? What are the products prescribed or not to the patients? Finally apply RUCAM product by product filling the form according to the type of the liver injury. The final score usually permits to identify the most likely drug. If not all the possible drugs should be discontinued unless they are indispensable. A discussion can subsequently conducted on the score found by RUCAM.

The future will certainly bring progress in several areas: diagnostic and prognostic biomarkers, improvement of causality assessment certainly based on RUCAM incorporating data and algorithms coming from the artificial intelligence and prevention of DILI in well identified susceptible patients.

Self Study

Questions

1. Which statement is true?
   (a) RUCAM is the worldwide most commonly used causality assessment method to establish or dismiss the diagnosis of DILI.
   (b) Pathogenesis of idiosyncratic DILI is best studied with animal models.
   (c) Idiosyncratic DILI is not foreseeable and not preventable.
   (d) Patients with idiosyncratic DILI may profit from a variety of antidotes.
2. Which statement/statements is/are true?
   (a) For the diagnosis of DILI, many alternative causes have to be excluded, since previous DILI cases often were not DILI but had to be attributed to other causes.
   (b) To describe the liver injury signature, a liver histology is required.
   (c) RUCAM represents an objective, quantitative diagnostic algorithm that uses defined key elements with individual scores.

Answers

1. Which statement is true?
   (a) CORRECT: The worldwide preferred method is RUCAM, which is highly appreciated by regulatory agencies, large clinical centers, pharmaceutical manufacturers and authors of DILI case reports. RUCAM received an update in 2016, and this updated version should be used for future DILI cases.
   (b) Human idiosyncratic DILI is not reproducible in animal models, which are therefore not suitable for characterizing this toxic liver disease in humans.
   (c) CORRECT: Since idiosyncratic DILI is not predictable, patients under a drug therapy should be advised to carefully watch out for possible clinical signs
   (d) such as dark-colored urine, itching, jaundice, and abdominal pain.
   (e) No antidotes are available for idiosyncratic DILI, N-Acetylcysteine is an antidote only available for intrinsic DILI by overdosed acetaminophen.

2. Which statement/statements is/are true?
   (a) CORRECT: Alternative causes are a problem in DILI cases and can be found by using RUCAM for general case evaluation and specific causality assessment.
   (b) DILI signature is based on serum activities of ALT and ALP rather than on liver histology obtained through invasive liver biopsy. ALT and ALP values clearly define DILI signature as hepatocellular liver injury or as cholestatic/mixed liver injury.
   (c) CORRECT: RUCAM is the preferred tool to assess causality of suspected DILI cases and cannot be replaced by any global introspection approach, which is, by definition, a subjective tool, lacking definition, transparency, and scoring system, and may lead to questionable results and conclusions.

References

1. Teschke R. Alcoholic steatohepatitis (ASH) and acute alcoholic hepatitis (AH): cascade of events, clinical features, and pharmacotherapy options. Exp Opin Pharmacother. 2018;19:779–93. https://doi.org/10.1080/14656566.2018.1465929.
2. Teschke R. Liver injury by carbon tetrachloride intoxication in 16 patients treated with forced ventilation to accelerate toxin removal via the lungs: a clinical report. Toxics. 2018;6:25. https://doi.org/10.3390/toxics6020025.
3. Danan G, Teschke R. RUCAM in drug and herb induced liver injury: the update. Int J Mol Sci. 2016;17:14. https://doi.org/10.3390/ijms17010014.
4. Björnsson ES. Hepatotoxicity by drugs: the most common implicated agents. Int J Mol Sci. 2016;17:224. https://doi.org/10.3390/ijms17020224.
5. Sarges P, Steinberg JM, Lewis JH. Drug-induced liver injury: highlights from a review of the 2015 literature. Drug Saf. 2016;39:561–75. https://doi.org/10.1007/s40264-016-0427-8.
6. Teschke R, Andrade R. Editorial: Drug-induced liver injury: expanding our knowledge by enlarging population analysis with prospective and scoring causality assessment. Gastroenterology. 2015;148:1271–3. https://doi.org/10.1053/j.gastro.2015.04.027.
7. Teschke R, Danan G. Review: drug induced liver injury with analysis of alternative causes as confounding variables. Br J Clin Pharmacol. 2018;84:1467–77.
8. Danan G, Teschke R. Drug-induced liver injury: why is the Roussel Uclaf Causality Assessment Method (RUCAM) still used 25 years after its launch? Drug Saf. 2018;41(8):735–43.
9. Teschke R, Danan G. Causality assessment methods in drug-induced liver injury. In: Chen M, Will Y, editors. Drug-induced liver toxicity (Chapter 27). James Kang Y, Casey D.C. Methods in pharmacology and toxicology. Springer protocols. Berlin: Springer Nature; 2018. p. 555–94. https://doi.org/10.1007/978-1-4939-7677-5_27.
10. Yoon E, Babar A, Choudhary M, Kutner M, Pyrsopoulos N. Acetaminophen-induced hepatotoxicity: a comprehensive update. J Clin Transl Hepatol. 2016;28:131–42. https://doi.org/10.14218/JCTH.2015.00052.
11. Iorga A, Dara L, Kaplowitz N. Drug-induced liver injury: cascade of events leading to cell death, apoptosis or necrosis. Int J Mol Sci. 2017;18:1018. Special issue. Molecular research on drug induced liver injury, guest editors R. Teschke and G. Danan.
12. Teschke R, Schulze J, Eickhoff A, Danan G. Drug induced liver injury: can biomarkers assist RUCAM in causality assessment? Int J Mol Sci. 2017;18:803. https://doi.org/10.3390/ijms18040803. Special issue: Molecular research on drug induced liver injury.
13. Aithal GP, Grove JI. Genome-wide association studies in drug-induced liver injury: step change in understanding the pathogenesis. Semin Liver Dis. 2015;35:421–31.
14. McEuen K, Borlak J, Tong W, Chen M. Drug lipophilicity and extent of metabolism are culprits of drug-induced liver injury. Int J Mol Sci. 2017;18:1335.
15. Teschke R, Danan G. Drug-induced liver injury: is chronic liver disease a risk factor and a clinical issue? Expert Opin Drug Metab Toxicol. 2017;13:425–38. https://doi.org/10.1080/17425255.2017.1252749.
16. Douros A, Bronder E, Andersohn F, Klimpel A, Thomae M, Sarganas G, Kreutz R, Garbe E. Drug-induced liver injury: results from the hospital-based Berlin case-control surveillance study. Br J Clin Pharmacol. 2014;79:988–99.
17. Rathi C, Pipaliya N, Patel R, Ingle M, Phadke A, Sawant P. Drug induced liver injury at a tertiary hospital in India: Etiology, clinical features and predictors of mortality. Ann Hepatol. 2017;16:442–50. with commentary: Teschke R, Danan G. (eds). Prospective Indian study of DILI with confirmed causality using the Roussel Uclaf Causality Assessment Method (RUCAM): a report of excellence. Ann Hepatol 2017;16:324–25
18. Zhu Y, Niu M, Chen J, Zou ZS, Ma ZJ, Liu SH, Wang RL, He TT, Song HB, Wang ZX, Pu SB, Ma X, Wang LF, Bai ZF, Zhao YL, Li YG, Wang JB, Xiao XB. Comparison between Chinese herbal medicine and Western medicine-induced liver injury of 1985 patients. J Gastroenterol Hepatol. 2016;31:1476–82. https://doi.org/10.1111/jgh.13323.
19. Shahbaz O, Mahajan S, Lewis JH. Highlights of drug- and herb-induced liver injury in the literature from 2016: how best to translate new information into clinical practice? Exp Opin Drug Metab Tox. 2017;13:935–51. Available at: https://doi.org/10.1080/17425255.2017.1362391. Accessed July 1, 2018.
20. Teschke R. Commentary Drug- and herb-induced liver injury in 2016 with highly appreciated critical comments: related or not, that is the question. Clin Diagn Pathol. 2018;2(1):1–2. https://doi.org/10.15761/CDP.1000122.

Further Reading

Lu RJ, Zhang Y, Tang FL, Zheng ZW, Fan ZD, Zhu SM, Qian XF, Liu NN. Clinical characteristics of drug-induced liver injury and related risk factors. Exp Ther Med. 2016;12:2606–16.

Teschke R, Danan G. Editorial: Molecular research on drug induced liver injury. Int J Mol Sci. 2018;19:216. https://doi.org/10.3390/ijms19010216.

Yu YC, Mao YM, Chen CW, Chen JJ, Chen J, Cong WM, Ding Y, Duan ZP, Fu QC, Guo XY, Hu P, Hu XQ, Jia JD, Lai RT, Li DL, Liu JX, Lu LG, Ma SW, Ma X, Nan YM, Ren H, Shen T, Wang H, Wang JY, Wang TL, Wang XJ, Wei L, Xi Q, Xi W, Yang CQ, Yang DL, Yu YY, Zeng MD, Zhang L, Zhao XY, Zhuang H. CSH guidelines for the diagnosis and treatment of drug-induced liver injury. Hepatol Int. 2017;11:221–41. https://doi.org/10.1007/s12072-017-9793-2.

Related Links/Journals/Book

Teschke R, Andrade RJ. Special issue "Drug, herb, and dietary supplement hepatotoxicity". Int J Mol Sci. 2016;17(9):1488. https://doi.org/10.3390/ijms17091488. Available at: http://www.mdpi.com/journal/ijms/special_issues/Hepatotoxicity. Last accessed July 1, 2018

Chen M, Will Y. Drug-induced liver toxicity. In: James Kang Y, Casey DC, editors. Methods in pharmacology and toxicology. Springer protocols. Berlin: Springer Nature; 2018. p. 555–94. https://doi.org/10.1007/978-1-4939-7677-5_27.

Acquired Metabolic Disorders

10

Ivanesa L. Pardo Lameda and Timothy R. Koch

Key Concepts

- A diagnosis of ornithine transcarbamylase deficiency must be considered early in individuals with suspected hepatic encephalopathy because rapid reduction in the production of nitrogenous waste and increased excretion of nitrogenous waste are required to prevent neurological damage.
- Exposure to multiple chemicals can alter the heme biosynthetic pathway in erythroid and nonerythroid tissues leading to increased levels of porphyrins in stool, urine, and plasma.
- Abnormal iron storage in hepatocytes, the pituitary, myocytes, keratinocytes, joints, and pancreatic beta-cells results from an autosomal recessive disorder that involves the HFE gene, as well as from excessive intake or absorption of oral iron, repeated blood transfusions in individuals with anemia, or chronic hepatitis C.
- Decreased alpha 1 antitrypsin protein levels can be identified in individuals with genetic mutations of the alpha 1 antitrypsin gene located on chromosome 14 or with Tropical Pulmonary Eosinophilia due to intestinal worm infestation.
- Excessive deposition of copper in the eyes, brain, and liver results from a mutation of the ATP7B gene located on chromosome 13, which alters the biosynthesis of the ATP7B protein and thus results in difficulty releasing copper from the liver.

I. L. Pardo Lameda
Center for Advanced Laparoscopic General & Bariatric Surgery, Washington, DC, USA

T. R. Koch (✉)
Center for Advanced Laparoscopic General & Bariatric Surgery, Washington, DC, USA

MedStar Washington Hospital Center and Georgetown University School of Medicine, Washington, DC, USA
e-mail: timothy.r.koch@medstar.net

10.1 Introduction

The liver is a complex and critically important organ involved in both the biosynthesis of as well as the metabolism of numerous biochemical products. Acquired metabolic liver disorders result from the loss of this hepatic homeostasis. The most common metabolic liver disorders are the spectrum of non-alcoholic fatty liver disease/non-alcoholic steatohepatitis (which are discussed in Chap. 24) and alcoholic liver disease (which is discussed in Chap. 25). The focus of this chapter is the potential origins for, diagnosis of, and treatment of acquired metabolic liver disorders, which include ornithine transcarbamylase deficiency, porphyria, hemochromatosis, and alpha 1 antitrypsin deficiency (see Table 10.1). This chapter also describes the important genetic metabolic liver disease, Wilson disease. This chapter is not intended to provide a description of the mainly pediatric hereditary metabolic liver disorders, which include congenital hyperbilirubinemias, glycogen storage diseases, and lipid storage diseases.

Table 10.1 Metabolic diseases of the liver

Disorder	Excessive product	Diagnosis
Ornithine transcarbamylase deficiency	Ammonia	Increased serum ammonia; Elevated urinary orotic acid
Porphyria (Cutanea Tarda)	Porphyrins	Increased urinary uroporphyrin & 7-carboxylate porphyrin
Hemochromatosis	Iron	Elevated serum ferritin or transferrin saturation; Genetic testing; MRI liver; Liver biopsy
Alpha 1 antitrypsin deficiency	Defective Alpha-1 Antitrypsin protein	Alpha 1 antitrypsin protein level; Alpha 1 antitrypsin Pi-typing; DNA variant testing
Wilson disease	Copper	Decreased serum copper and Ceruloplasmin; increased 24 h urinary copper

F. Radu-Ionita et al. (eds.), *Liver Diseases*, https://doi.org/10.1007/978-3-030-24432-3_10

10.2 Ornithine Transcarbamylase Deficiency

10.2.1 Brief Historical Overview

Ornithine Transcarbamylase (OTC) deficiency is the most common urea cycle disorder. It was first described in 1962 by Russel, affecting 1 in 8000 live births in the US [1], with a prevalence of 1:14,000–70,000. When the urea cycle is impaired, it fails to eliminate nitrogen waste, which then accumulates in the form of ammonia. Late onset disease has been diagnosed in 12% of patients with OTC deficiency [2]. The timing of presentation is variable due to X-chromosome inactivation seen in X-linked recessive traits, such as this one. Hyperammonemia, if left untreated, will manifest as neurological symptoms that may range from mild cognitive and psychomotor changes, to altered level of consciousness and coma [3]. These complications are often irreversible [4] and can carry a high mortality rate, especially if a diagnosis is made late (13–50%) [2, 5].

There have been multiple case reports in the literature describing hyperammonemia induced encephalopathy, coma and death. Usually, these patients have had a recent increased stress to their physiology like an injury or surgery; or have had an alteration to their diet, such as high protein diets like Atkins or bariatric surgery early postop diets [5]. After a thorough workup, these patients are eventually diagnosed with OTC deficiency, although sometimes too late.

10.2.2 Definition of the Disorder

The liver is the only site of the complete urea cycle (see Fig. 10.1). Ornithine Transcarbamylase (OTC) is an intra-mitochondrial enzyme that is responsible to convert carbamoylphosphate and ornithine into citrulline, primarily in hepatocytes. Decreases in the activity of OTC will impair the urea cycle in the removal of nitrogenous waste, which will translate into an accumulation of ammonia. Hyperammonemia will increase gamma amino butyric acid (GABA) activity, leading to neurological consequences [6].

OTC deficiency is an X-linked disorder. The OTC gene is located at band Xp21.1; and the mutation has over 150 variations, which is responsible for the different phenotypes of the disease. Most commonly, the disease presents in male newborns with a heterozygote gene. Heterozygous females may remain asymptomatic until they become acutely or chronically challenged by enough physiological stress [6]. The variety of symptoms in these patients will depend on the degree of X-chromosome inactivation in different tissues, and especially the liver. About 85% of female that carry the mutation will remain asymptomatic during their lifetime. The remainder of female carriers can have symptoms that may range from behavioral and learning disabilities to protein intolerance, cyclical vomiting, and episodes of hyperammonemic coma (Table 10.1).

Symptoms of hyperammonemia are usually neurological and range from mild cognitive and psychomotor

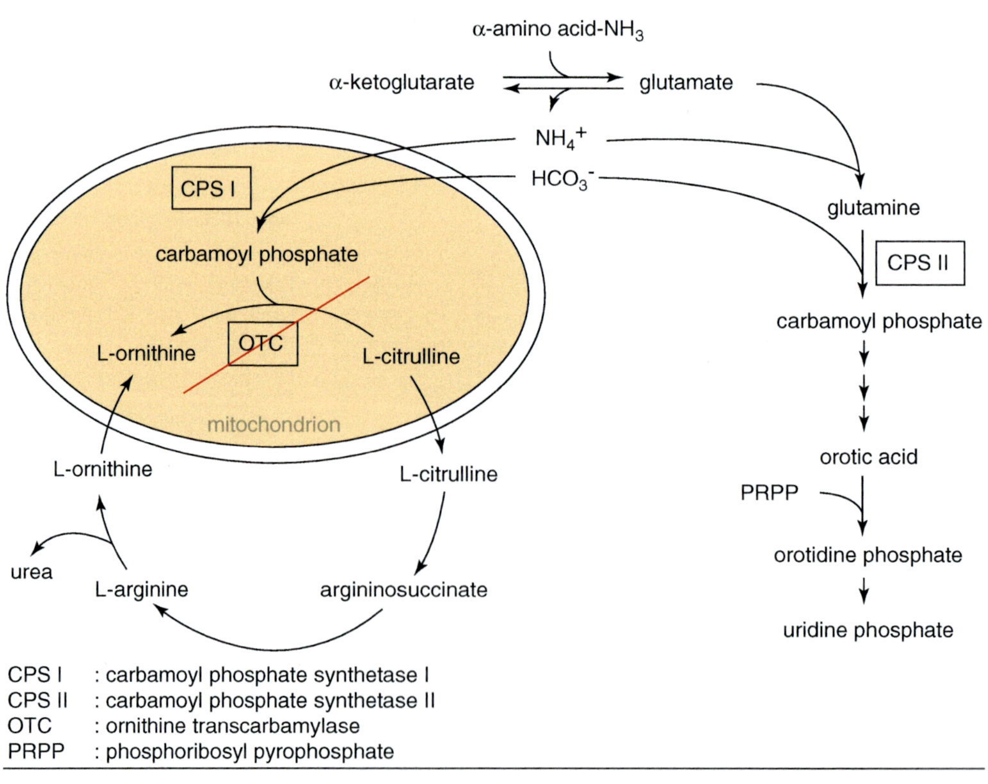

Fig. 10.1 Ornithine transcarbamylase (OTC) deficiency is the most common urea cycle disorder. Inadequate levels of the liver enzyme ornithine transcarbamylase leads to overproduction of ammonia. [Reproduced with the permission of Springer International Publishing from Hartung B, et al. Int J Legal Med (2016) 130: 783–785]

changes, to altered level of consciousness. An ammonia level > 200 micromol/L will cause cerebral edema, herniation and death [3]. An acute hyperammonemic episode may start with mild symptoms such as poor feeding, vomiting, and irritability; rapidly advancing to lethargy, tachypnea, hypoxemia, ataxia, seizures and coma. Patients will rapidly decompensate, and demise is imminent, if undiagnosed, and untreated.

10.2.3 Diagnosis

Patients with OTC deficiency present with an increase blood ammonia level as well as an increased urine orotic acid (as shown in Fig. 10.1), while liver function remains normal. The initial battery of labs to assist with diagnosis include: plasma ammonia, liver function test, arterial pH, lactate, glucose, electrolytes, anion gap, plasma amino acids, urine organic acids and urine orotic acid. In order to differentiate OTC deficiency from other urea cycle disorders, quantification of amino acids will be needed. In OTC deficiency, the following will be observed: low citrulline and arginine, and increased glutamine and alanine levels. A normal liver and kidney function will be preserved until hypoxia or shock develops.

Enzyme analysis (OTC activity) is possible to be performed on liver biopsy specimens, but this may be normal depending on the pattern of X-inactivation in the liver; and mutational analysis of OTC will only detect 70–80% of coding mutations (Table 10.2).

Other possible causes of hyperammonemia need to be excluded, such as: severe dehydration; liver failure; reactive hypoglycemia contributing to a catabolic state; precipitants of metabolic decompensations such as infection, injury or surgery; certain medications like valproic acid; as well as carnitine and zinc deficiency, which can interfere with OTC function [3].

The most important goal is to achieve a rapid diagnosis. This will prompt an immediate treatment plan and minimize the mortality risk.

Table 10.2 Treatment of metabolic diseases of the liver

Disorder	Suggested medical treatments[a]
Ornithine transcarbamylase deficiency	Low protein intake; IV dextrose and/or lipids; IV sodium benzoate; hemodialysis (if critically Ill)
Porphyria	Avoidance of triggers; glucose; panhematin; phlebotomy; hydroxychloroquine/chloroquine
Hemochromatosis	Phlebotomy; desferoxamine; avoid alcohol and iron supplements
Alpha 1 antitrypsin deficiency	Avoid alcohol; vaccinations against hepatitis A & hepatitis B; liver transplantation; antihelminthics
Wilson disease	Penicillamine; trientine; zinc acetate

[a]IV: Intravenous

10.2.4 Treatment

Rapid initiation of treatment is directed at preventing neurological damage. The pillars of treatment are to reverse catabolism, promote waste nitrogen excretion and treat any underlying precipitant (see Table 10.2).

Catabolism can be offset by the immediate discontinuation of protein intake while increasing carbohydrate and lipid intake. This can be accomplished with intravenous dextrose and lipids. A patient will require placement of a central venous line. Intravenous 10–25% dextrose is then initiated to provide 40% of the caloric needs of the patient, with IV intralipids provided for the remainder 60% of caloric needs. The daily caloric goal should exceed 80 kcal/kg/day.

Excretion of nitrogenous waste can be accomplished by the addition of ammonia scavengers, e.g. intravenous sodium benzoate and sodium phenylacetate (IV Ammonul®). The suggested dosage of IV Ammonul® is 55 mL/m^2 (prior to mixture with dextrose solution) given intravenously over 90 min, and then followed by the same dose as a 24-h intravenous infusion. Additionally, intravenous citrulline and arginine will help stimulate the urea cycle by pulling aspartate into it, thus increasing nitrogen clearance. Excretion of nitrogenous waste can also be accomplished by initiation of hemodialysis of critically ill patients who have Grade 3 hepatic encephalopathy (somnolence to semi-stupor) or Grade 4 hepatic encephalopathy (coma), using the West Haven Criteria.

Once the patient is stabilized, treatment can be transitioned to oral citrulline, benzoate, and/or phenylacetate. Plasma ammonia levels need to be monitored in these patients. Furthermore, it is essential that these patients receive nutritional counseling in order to ensure lifelong protein restriction. Anecdotal reports suggest that reversal of or a reduction in the length of intestinal bypass in individuals who have undergone prior bariatric surgery may result in improved clearance of nitrogenous waste. The use of long-term non-absorbable antibiotics, such as rifaximin, is unclear but it could be of theoretical benefit. Studies of the chronic or intermittent use of antibiotics are an important question to be further addressed.

10.3 Porphyria

10.3.1 Brief Historical Overview

Hippocrates is thought to have described porphyria (porphura in ancient Greek translates as "purple"). The role of porphyrin pigments in this disorder was described in 1871 by the German biochemist, Dr. Felix Hoppe-Seyer, while the term porphyria, to describe the clinical syndrome, has been ascribed to Dr. B.J Stokvis from work in 1889.

10.3.2 Definition of the Disorder

The heme biosynthetic pathway in erythroid and nonerythroid tissues is important in cellular metabolism. Porphyrias are genetic diseases and there are at least eight subtypes of porphyria caused by variants of this pathway resulting in defective enzymatic activity [7–9]. Production of porphyrins can be initiated by exposure to alcohol, chlorinated aromatic chemicals, hormones, antibiotics, and barbiturates [7].

The classic acquired porphyria is the development of porphyria cutanea tarda (Type 1) following exposure to Agent Orange (a mixture of two phenoxy herbicides: 2,4-dichlorophenoxyacetic acid and 2,4,5-trichlorophenoxyacetic acid, that also contained a trace of a toxic dioxin). Clinical features of this disorder include the development of blistering and thinning of areas of sun-exposed skin. This disease association was supported in 1993 in a report from the National Academy of Sciences (USA) entitled: Veterans and Agent Orange—Health Effects of Herbicides used in Vietnam. Other chemicals [10] that have been linked to development of porphyria cutanea tarda include hexachlorobenzene. In porphyria cutanea tarda, there are inadequate liver levels of the enzyme, uroporphyrinogen decarboxylase. Porphyria cutanea tarda is also associated with hepatic iron and with Hepatitis C.

10.3.3 Diagnosis

Increased levels of porphyrins can be measured in stool, urine, and plasma. Screening, which is performed while a patient has symptoms, can be performed by determination of a plasma total porphyrin measurement.

The diagnosis of porphyria cutanea tarda is supported by finding, in a 24 h urine collection, increased urinary uroporphyrin and 7-carboxylate porphyrin. Serum ferritin should be normal to moderately elevated in a patient with porphyria cutanea tarda (high levels of ferritin should raise the question of hemochromatosis).

10.3.4 Treatment

The initial treatment [8, 9] of porphyria is prevention, e.g. the avoidance of environmental exposures that can initiate production of porphyrins (alcohol, chlorinated aromatic chemicals, hormones, antibiotics, and barbiturates). For acute (genetic) porphyrins, oral sugar can be provided. Hospitalization should be considered as needed for symptomatic treatment of dyspnea, pain, vomiting, or dehydration. Symptoms in these individuals may improve with intravenous infusion of glucose. Serious symptoms may respond to infusions of Panhematin (Hemin) 1 to 4 mg/kg/day given intravenously over 10–15 min once daily for 3–14 days, based upon a patient's clinical signs and symptoms (see Table 10.2).

The initial treatment of porphyria cutanea tarda is also prevention, e.g. the avoidance of alcohol and avoiding exposure to estrogen. Patients with porphyria cutanea tarda and hemoglobin >12 g/dl often clinically respond to removal of hepatic iron via phlebotomy to remove 500 ml of whole blood once weekly (with a goal to remove a total of 5–6 units of whole blood). Alternative therapy [11] is the use of oral low dose chloroquine (125 mg twice a week) or hydroxychloroquine (100 mg twice a week). Medical Providers should consider obtaining periodic retinal examinations in those individuals receiving chloroquine or hydroxychloroquine.

Liver transplantation is beneficial for patients with end-stage liver disease caused by protoporphyrin, in which hepatotoxic and pigment loading of hepatocytes and bile canalicular sludging can lead to progressive cholestasis and subsequent cirrhosis.

10.4 Hemochromatosis

10.4.1 Brief Historical Overview

The term hemochromatosis [12] appears to have derived from a German Dr. von Recklinghausen who in 1889 demonstrated that there was iron in the liver, and bleeding into the liver was thought to be the cause of this pigment. In 1927, Dr. JH Sheldon in the Quarterly Journal of Medicine described the iron content of tissues in hemochromatosis. Dr. Sheldon then published a monograph in 1935 describing the clinical and pathological features of 311 cases of hemochromatosis evaluated over a 70 year period.

10.4.2 Definition of the Disorder

Hereditary hemochromatosis is an autosomal recessive disorder that involves the HFE gene, and causes abnormal iron storage as the result of association of HFE protein with the transferrin receptor in the duodenum. A change at residue 282 from the amino acid cysteine to the amino acid tyrosine (termed: C282Y where C is the abbreviation for cysteine and Y is the abbreviation for tyrosine) has been identified in about 85% of individuals with hereditary hemochromatosis. Approximately 0.3% of Caucasians are homozygous for the mutant allele. There is abnormal iron deposition in hepatocytes, as well as in the pituitary, myocytes, keratinocytes, joints, and pancreatic beta-cells.

Secondary or acquired hemochromatosis can result from excessive intake of oral iron, excessive absorption of iron (due to alcoholism), repeated blood transfusions in individuals with anemia (sickle-cell anemia, X-linked sideroblastic anemia, congenital dyserythropoietic anemia, the multiple types of thalassemia, pyruvate kinase deficiency, or hereditary spherocytosis), or chronic hepatitis C [13]. Individuals receive 200–250 mg of iron with each transfused unit of packed red blood cells.

10.4.3 Diagnosis

The classic description of an individual with hereditary hemochromatosis is presentation with liver enlargement or cirrhosis in combination with "bronze" skin color and diabetes mellitus. Individuals can present with symptoms/findings of arthropathy, cardiomyopathy, or hypogonadism, or they can simply present with cirrhosis. The diagnosis of hemochromatosis is supported by testing revealing elevated serum ferritin or elevated serum transferrin saturation. Genetic testing can be then performed to examine the HFE C282Y mutation. In the 15% of individuals without the HFE gene mutations, patients can be sent for magnetic resonance imaging of the liver or proceed to the historical "gold standard" for diagnosis, which is performance of a liver biopsy with iron quantification.

10.4.4 Treatment

The patient should be asked to avoid intake of all alcohol products [14]. Phlebotomy is the initial effective treatment for hereditary hemochromatosis and, if begun early in the course of this metabolic disease, can prevent the development of cirrhosis. The pretreatment hemoglobin should be >12 g/dl. Phlebotomy to remove 500 ml of whole blood once weekly is performed to produce a transferrin saturation of <50% or a serum ferritin of <50 ng/ml. For maintenance treatment, an individual may require phlebotomy to remove 500 ml every 3 months (see Table 10.2).

In patients with hereditary hemochromatosis, liver transplantation is indicated for treatment of individuals with decompensated cirrhosis or hepatocellular carcinoma.

Some individuals [15], especially those with acquired hemochromatosis induced by multiple blood transfusions, have been treated with an iron chelating agent, desferoxamine. Desferoxamine is given subcutaneously at a dose of 25–40 mg/kg, 5 days weekly. Serious renal, pulmonary, and neurological adverse effects have been reported at higher doses.

Initial treatment of other causes of secondary or acquired hemochromatosis is the avoidance of alcohol containing products and discontinuation of iron supplements. If it has been diagnosed, chronic hepatitis C can be treated with appropriate antiviral therapy.

10.5 Alpha 1 Antitrypsin Deficiency

10.5.1 Brief Historical Overview

In 1964, Dr. F. Kueppers and associates reported in the journal SCIENCE that alpha 1 antitrypsin deficiency appeared to be a genetic disease. Individuals who had both alleles of this genetic disorder had alpha 1 antitrypsin protein levels that were < 10% of normals and had pulmonary emphysema. By contrast, individuals who were heterozygous had alpha 1 antitrypsin levels that were 50–60% of normals and had no apparent pulmonary disease.

10.5.2 Definition of the Disorder

Over 200 genetic mutations of the alpha 1 antitrypsin gene located on chromosome 14 have been reported. Upon genetic testing for alpha 1 antitrypsin, three alleles have been described, M, S, and Z. In examining the Proteinase inhibitor (Pi) locus, normal individuals have the MM alleles, heterozygotes have an M allele and a Z allele, while the presence of the homozygote ZZ alleles leads to the more severe form of protein misfolding. Individuals who are PiSZ have an increased risk of liver or lung disease. Alpha 1 antitrypsin is a protease inhibitor that is mainly biosynthesized by hepatocytes. This protein protects tissues from proteolytic enzyme damage, and this benefit appears to be protective with regards to white blood cells that produce neutrophil elastase. This defect can lead to tissue damage involving connective tissue in the lung and liver. The worldwide estimate is that three million individuals have genetic alpha1 antitrypsin deficiency. These individuals have an increased risk of development of hepatocellular carcinoma [16].

There have been sporadic reports of acquired alpha 1 antitrypsin deficiency, especially in Tropical Pulmonary

Eosinophilia. In individuals with Tropical Pulmonary Eosinophilia due to intestinal worm infestation, low levels of the protein, alpha 1 antitrypsin, have been reported. These individuals have normal M1 or M2 alleles.

10.5.3 Diagnosis

Individuals may be seen for emphysema, chronic bronchitis, asthma, or chronic liver disease (which can occur at any age). A diagnosis of alpha 1 antitrypsin deficiency should be considered in individuals presenting with bronchiectasis, necrotizing panniculitis, or unexplained vasculitis. Screening for this disorder can include determination of alpha 1 antitrypsin protein level by Nephelometry. Isoelectric focusing can be performed for Pi-typing. DNA probes that are specific for two to four of the most common genetic variants are used to evaluate the DNA of the SERPINA1 (alpha 1 antitrypsin) gene.

10.5.4 Treatment

Patients should avoid consumption of alcohol containing products [17]. It has been suggested that affected individuals should maintain proper nutritional status, including being within the normal range of weight or body mass index (due to the relationship between excessive weight and nonalcoholic fatty liver disease). Individuals should receive both the Hepatitis A vaccine as well as the Hepatitis B vaccine (see Table 10.2). Alpha 1 antitrypsin deficiency-related liver disease cannot be treated with augmentation therapy (using alpha 1 antitrypsin protein purified from plasma of healthy humans). Liver transplantation is considered for those individuals with end-stage chronic liver disease.

Antihelminthics are used for treatment of individuals with Tropical Pulmonary Eosinophilia. This treatment has been shown to increase protein levels of alpha 1 antitrypsin.

10.6 Wilson Disease

10.6.1 Brief Historical Overview

In 1912, Dr. SAK Wilson submitted an M.D. dissertation to the University of Edinburgh Medical School that was entitled "Progressive Lenticular Degeneration". This work first reported an association between neurological disease and a liver disorder, and Dr. Wilson brought the term "extrapyramidal" into the medical literature.

10.6.2 Definition of the Disorder

There is no description of an acquired Wilson disease, such as due to a somatic gene mutation. The pathophysiology of the disorder termed "Acquired Hepatocerebral Degeneration" is not related to copper metabolism [18].

Worldwide, 1 in every 30,000 individuals has Wilson disease. The ATP7B gene is located on chromosome 13, and more than 500 described mutations can cause Wilson disease. This autosomal recessive genetic disorder is caused by a gene mutation that alters the biosynthesis of the ATP7B protein, resulting in difficulty releasing copper from the liver. This defect interferes with the normal clearance of copper via biliary excretion of copper. A minor amount of copper (estimates are 0.34 mg/day) is lost through hair loss, loss of skin cells, and sweat, and normal individuals thus maintain an estimated 100–150 mg of hepatic copper stores. In normal physiology, bile itself reduces copper absorption, suggesting that bile output from the liver can in part regulate the amount of copper that is absorbed.

In Wilson disease, there is subsequently excessive deposition of copper in the eyes, brain, and liver. The most common presentation is that of liver disease in an individual in their teenage years. A complex of neurological symptoms including difficulties with speech, difficulty swallowing, behavioral changes, tremors, stiffness of muscles, and poor coordination can result from the accumulation of copper in the central nervous system.

10.6.3 Diagnosis

The altered metabolism of copper in Wilson disease is supported by low serum or plasma levels of copper, low serum levels of the copper-related protein, ceruloplasmin, elevated 24-h urinary excretion of copper, slit lamp examination for Kayser-Fleischer (termed: K-F) rings in the cornea, cranial magnetic resonance imaging, and sequencing of the ATP7B gene. Screening family members of patients with Wilson disease can identify asymptomatic individuals [19].

10.6.4 Treatment

The primary treatment of Wilson disease is the use of chelating agents [20], e.g. penicillamine or trientine (in those individuals intolerant of penicillamine), to facilitate clearance of copper from the body ("decoppering the patient"), in combination with a low copper diet (see Table 10.2). The suggested treatment with penicillamine is to take by mouth 250 mg daily in the first week of treatment with incremental increases as tolerated every 4–7 days (by adding an additional 250 mg to the daily dose) with a goal of intake of up to 1.5 g daily. Individuals receiving penicillamine should also be given a daily oral supplement of 25–50 mg of Vitamin B6. Penicillamine is Pregnancy Category D (it can cause fetal harm), and mothers taking this drug should not nurse their baby. Penicillamine can cause potentially fatal adverse effects. This treatment requires periodic monitoring of complete blood count, liver function tests, 24 h urine copper excretion, and serum or plasma copper and ceruloplasmin. The goal is to demonstrate a daily urinary excretion of up to 1000 mcg of copper. After 3 months, adequate treatment would be supported by a decline in 24 h urinary copper excretion and by a decline in free copper in serum to <10 mcg/dl.

The suggested treatment with trientine is start at 750 mg/day taken by mouth in divided doses every 6–12 h within the first week, with a goal of increasing slowly to 1250 mg/day (but not to exceed 2 g/day). Trientine is Pregnancy Category: C (use with caution if benefits outweigh risks). Trientine has multiple reported adverse effects, and development of elevated body temperature can be a sign of hypersensitivity. This treatment requires periodic monitoring of 24 h urine copper excretion, liver function tests, and serum or plasma copper and ceruloplasmin. The goal is to demonstrate a daily urinary excretion of up to 1000 mcg of copper. After 3 months, adequate treatment would be supported by a decline in 24 h urinary copper excretion and by a decline in free copper in serum to <10 mcg/dl.

During treatment with chelating agents, neurological symptoms can worsen in patients with Wilson's disease. As one potential explanation, low vitamin E levels have been reported in individuals with Wilson disease, and vitamin E deficiency can lead to damage to central and peripheral nerves.

After decoppering by utilization of a chelating agent, chronic treatment with oral zinc acetate (200 mg of elemental zinc daily) has been approved by the United States Food & Drug Administration for maintenance therapy in individuals with Wilson disease [21]. This treatment may be more effective when combined with the chronic use of a low copper diet. This treatment requires periodic monitoring of liver function tests and serum or plasma copper, zinc, and ceruloplasmin.

Other agents that have been reported to be of potential benefit in subsets of individuals with Wilson disease include sodium dimercaptosuccinate, dimercaptosuccinic acid, and tetrathiomolybdate.

Individuals with Wilson disease who present with fulminant liver failure or are unresponsive to medical therapy should be evaluated for potential liver transplantation.

10.7 Conclusions and Future Perspectives

Late onset ornithine transcarbamylase deficiency is a very rare disorder, carrying lethal prognosis if an early diagnosis and treatment implementation is not undertaken. Most reports in the literature consist of case reports or small case series, some of them in susceptible patient population as is the bariatric surgery patient. More studies are required to identify altered expressions of ornithine transcarbamylase deficiency, and different phenotypes of the disorder, in order to better identify these patients.

In future work, pathophysiological mechanisms of disease remain an area of focus for clinical research in this field. Further studies of risks factors, potential environmental agents, and potential exposures are very important for preventing the development of acquired metabolic liver disorders, which include ornithine transcarbamylase deficiency, porphyria, hemochromatosis, and alpha 1 antitrypsin deficiency.

Self Study

Questions

1. Which statements are true?
   (a) Ornithine Transcarbamylase deficiency is the most common urea cycle disorder.
   (b) Hyperammonemia causes symptoms of peripheral neuropathy beginning with paresthesias of the extremities, progressing to numbness, and then to a constant burning sensation.
   (c) Patients with Ornithine Transcarbamylase deficiency present with a decreased urine orotic acid.
   (d) Initial treatment of ornithine transcarbamylase deficiency involves a reduction in the production of nitrogenous waste as well as increased excretion of nitrogenous waste.
2. Which statement is true?
   (a) Porphyrias result from a urea cycle disorder.
   (b) The development of blistering and thinning of areas of sun-exposed skin can result from exposure to a mixture of two phenoxy herbicides: 2,4-dichlorophenoxyacetic acid and 2,4,5-trichlorophenoxyacetic acid.
   (c) The avoidance of alcohol does not prevent development of porphyria cutanea tarda.
   (d) Individuals receiving chloroquine or hydroxychloroquine should undergo periodic examination of renal or kidney function.

3. Which statement is true?
   (a) Hereditary hemochromatosis is an autosomal dominant disorder that involves the HFE gene.
   (b) Symptoms/findings of hemochromatosis include liver enlargement, cirrhosis, "bronze" skin color, diabetes mellitus, arthropathy, cardiomyopathy, or hypogonadism.
   (c) In individuals without HFE gene mutations, computerized tomography imaging of the liver is generally useful for supporting a diagnosis of hemochromatosis.
   (d) Phlebotomy is the initial treatment for hereditary hemochromatosis and the pretreatment hemoglobin should be >10 g/dl with a serum ferritin of <50 ng/ml.
4. Which statements are true?
   (a) Alpha 1 antitrypsin is a protease inhibitor mainly biosynthesized by hepatocytes that protects tissues from proteolytic enzyme damage.
   (b) Upon genetic testing for alpha 1 antitrypsin, three alleles have been described, M, S, and Z.
   (c) There have been sporadic reports of acquired alpha 1 antitrypsin deficiency, especially in individuals with Tropical Pulmonary Eosinophilia and the homozygote ZZ alleles.
   (d) Alpha 1 antitrypsin deficiency-related liver disease is treated with augmentation therapy using alpha 1 antitrypsin protein purified from plasma of healthy humans.
5. What is the most effective initial treatment for Wilson Disease?
   (a) Low copper diet.
   (b) Oral zinc supplements.
   (c) Decoppering with penicillamine
   (d) Decoppering with trientine

Answers

1. Which statements are true?
   (a) Ornithine Transcarbamylase deficiency is the most common urea cycle disorder with a prevalence of 1:14,000–70,000.
   (b) Untreated hyperammonemia will manifest as neurological symptoms that may range from mild cognitive and psychomotor changes, to altered level of consciousness and coma.
   (c) Patients with Ornithine Transcarbamylase deficiency present with an increased urine orotic acid.
   (d) Ornithine transcarbamylase deficiency must be considered early in individuals with suspected hepatic encephalopathy because rapid reduction in the production of nitrogenous waste and increased excretion of nitrogenous waste are required to prevent neurological damage.
2. Which statement is true?
   (a) Porphyrias are the result of defective enzymatic activity in the heme biosynthetic pathway in erythroid and nonerythroid tissues.
   (b) The classic acquired porphyria is the development of porphyria cutanea tarda (Type 1) following exposure to Agent Orange (two phenoxy herbicides: 2,4-dichlorophenoxyacetic acid and 2,4,5-trichlorophenoxyacetic acid containing a trace of a toxic dioxin). Clinical features of this disorder include the development of blistering and thinning of areas of sun-exposed skin.
   (c) The initial treatment of porphyria cutanea tarda is prevention, e.g. the avoidance of alcohol and avoiding exposure to estrogen.
   (d) Medical Providers should consider obtaining periodic retinal examinations in those individuals receiving chloroquine or hydroxychloroquine. The protective effect of hydroxychloroquine in retarding renal damage occurrence in individuals with autoimmune disorders has been reported.
3. Which statement is true?
   (a) Hereditary hemochromatosis is an autosomal recessive disorder that involves the HFE gene, and causes abnormal iron storage as the result of association of HFE protein with the transferrin receptor in the duodenum.
   (b) The classic description of an individual with hereditary hemochromatosis is presentation with liver enlargement or cirrhosis in combination with "bronze" skin color and diabetes mellitus. Individuals can present with symptoms/findings of arthropathy, cardiomyopathy, or hypogonadism, or they can simply present with cirrhosis.
   (c) In the 15% of individuals without the HFE gene mutations, patients can be sent for magnetic resonance imaging of the liver or proceed to the historical "gold standard" for diagnosis, which is performance of a liver biopsy with iron quantification.
   (d) Phlebotomy is the initial effective treatment for hereditary hemochromatosis and, if begun early in the course of this metabolic disease, can prevent the development of cirrhosis. The pretreatment hemoglobin should be >12 g/dl. Phlebotomy to remove 500 ml of whole blood once weekly is performed to produce a transferrin saturation of <50% or a serum ferritin of <50 ng/ml.
4. Which statements are true?
   (a) Alpha 1 antitrypsin is a protease inhibitor that is mainly biosynthesized by hepatocytes. This protein protects tissues from proteolytic enzyme damage, and this benefit appears to be protective with regards to white blood cells that produce neutrophil elastase.

This defect can lead to tissue damage involving connective tissue in the lung and liver.

(b) Upon genetic testing for alpha 1 antitrypsin, three alleles have been described, M, S, and Z. In examining the Proteinase inhibitor (Pi) locus, normal individuals have the MM alleles, heterozygotes have an M allele and a Z allele, while the presence of the homozygote ZZ alleles leads to the more severe form of protein misfolding. Individuals who are PiSZ have an increased risk of liver or lung disease.

(c) There have been sporadic reports of acquired alpha 1 antitrypsin deficiency, especially in Tropical Pulmonary Eosinophilia. In individuals with Tropical Pulmonary Eosinophilia due to intestinal worm infestation, low levels of the protein, alpha 1 antitrypsin, have been reported. These individuals have normal M1 or M2 alleles.

(d) Alpha 1 antitrypsin deficiency-related liver disease cannot be treated with augmentation therapy (using alpha 1 antitrypsin protein purified from plasma of healthy humans).

5. What is the most effective initial treatment for Wilson Disease?

(a) A low copper diet is not effective for decoppering an individual with Wilson disease.

(b) The United States Food and Drug Administration did not approve zinc supplements for the initial decoppering of individuals with Wilson disease.

(c) Penicillamine is the preferred treatment for the initial decoppering of an individual with Wilson disease.

(d) Trientine is used for decoppering individuals with Wilson disease who are intolerant of penicillamine.

References

1. Häberle J, Boddaert N, Burlina A, Chakrapani A, Dixon M, Huemer M, Karall D, Martinelli D, Crespo PS, Santer R, Servais A, Valayannopoulos V, Linder M, Rubio V, Dionisi-Vici C. Suggested guidelines for the diagnosis and management of urea cycle disorders. Orphanet J Rare Dis. 2012;7:32.
2. Brassier A, Gobin S, Arnoux JB, Valayannopoulos V, Habarou F, Kossorotoff M, Servais A, Barbier V, Dubois S, Touati G, Barouki R, Lesage F, Dupic L, Bonnefont JP, Ottolenghi C, De Lonlay P. Long-term outcomes in ornithine transcarbamylase deficiency: a series of 90 patients. Orphanet J Rare Dis. 2015;10:58. https://doi.org/10.1186/s13023-015-0266-1.
3. Acharya G, Mehra S, Patel R, Frunza-Stefan S, Kaur H. Fatal non hepatic hyperammonemia in ICU setting: a rare but serious complication following bariatric surgery. Case Rep Crit Care. 2016;2016:8531591.
4. Becker D, Balcer L, Galetta S. The neurological complications of nutritional deficiency following bariatric surgery. J Obes. 2012;2012:608534. https://doi.org/10.1155/2012/608534.
5. Fenves A, Shchelochkov O, Mehta A. Hyperammonemic syndrome after Roux-en-Y gastric bypass. Obesity. 2015;23(4):746–9.
6. Kromas ML, Mousa OY, John S. Hyperammonemia-induced encephalopathy: a rare devastating complication of bariatric surgery. World J Hepatol. 2015;7(7):1007–11.
7. Bissell DM, Anderson KE, Bonkovsky HL. Porphyria. N Engl J Med. 2017;377(9):862–72.
8. Stein P, Badminton M, Barth J, Rees D, Stewart MF, British and Irish Porphyria Network. Best practice guidelines on clinical management of acute attacks of porphyria and their complications. Ann Clin Biochem. 2013;50(Pt 3):217–23.
9. Balwani M, Wang B, Anderson KE, Bloomer JR, Bissell DM, Bonkovsky HL, Phillips JD, Desnick RJ, Porphyrias Consortium of the Rare Diseases Clinical Research Network. Acute hepatic porphyrias: recommendations for evaluation and long-term management. Hepatology. 2017;66(4):1314–22.
10. Smith AG, Foster JR. The association between chemical-induced porphyria and hepatic cancer. Toxicol Res (Camb). 2018;7(4):647–63.
11. Salameh H, Sarairah H, Rizwan M, Kuo YF, Anderson KE, Singal AK. Relapse of porphyria cutanea tarda after treatment with phlebotomy or 4-aminoquinoline antimalarials: a meta-analysis. Br J Dermatol. 2018. https://doi.org/10.1111/bjd.16741.
12. Ulvik RJ. Hereditary haemochromatosis through 150 years. Tidsskr Nor Laegeforen. 2016;136(23–24):2017–21.
13. Zou D-M, Sun W-L. Relationship between hepatitis C virus infection and iron overload. Chin Med J. 2017;130(7):866–71.
14. Golfeyz S, Lewis S, Weisberg IS. Hemochromatosis: pathophysiology, evaluation, and management of hepatic iron overload with a focus on MRI. Expert Rev Gastroenterol Hepatol. 2018;12(8):767–78.
15. Rostoker G, Vaziri ND. Iatrogenic iron overload and its potential consequences in patients on hemodialysis. Presse Med. 2017;46(12 Pt 2):e312–28.
16. Townsend SA, Edgar RG, Ellis PR, Kantas D, Newsome PN, Turner AM. Systematic review: the natural history of alpha-1 antitrypsin deficiency, and associated liver disease. Aliment Pharmacol Ther. 2018;47(7):877–85.
17. Mitchell EL, Khan Z. Liver disease in alpha-1 antitrypsin deficiency: current approaches and future directions. Curr Pathobiol Rep. 2017;5(3):243–52.
18. Renjen PN, Khanna L, Rastogi R, Khan NI. Acquired hepatocerebral degeneration. BMJ Case Rep. 2013. https://doi.org/10.1136/bcr-2013-009387. pii: bcr2013009387.
19. Li H, Liu L, Li Y, He S, Liu Y, Li J, Tao R, Li W, Shang S. Familial screening of children with Wilson disease: necessity of screening in previous generation and screening methods. Medicine. 2018 Jul;97(27):e11405. https://doi.org/10.1097/MD.0000000000011405.
20. Ferenci P, Czlonkowska A, Stremmel W, Houwen R, Rosenberg W, Schilsky M, Jansen P, Moradpour D, the European Association for Study of Liver. EASL clinical practice guidelines: Wilson's disease. J Hepatol. 2012;56(3):671–85.
21. Santiago R, Gottrand F, Debray D, et al. Zinc therapy for Wilson disease in children in French pediatric centers. J Pediatr Gastroenterol Nutr. 2015;61(6):613–8.

Further Readings

Ornithine Transcarbamylase Deficiency

Russell A, Levin B, Oberholzer VG, Sinclair L. Hyperammonemia. A new instance of an inborn enzymatic defect of the biosynthesis of urea. Lancet. 1962;2(7258):699–700.

Chikwava K, Finegold D. Final diagnosis-partial ornithine transcarbamylase (OTC) deficiency. Case presentation at UPMC pathology: Case. p. 335.

Hu WT, Kantarci OH, Merritt JL, McGrann P, Dyck PJB, Lucchinetti CF, Tippmann-Peikert M. Ornithine transcarbamylase deficiency presenting as encephalopathy during adulthood following bariatric surgery. Arch Neurol. 2007;64(1):126–8.

Levy H, Picker J. New England Consortium of Metabolic Programs. Ornithine transcarbamylase deficiency (OTC deficiency).

Gyato K, Wray J, Huang ZJ, Yudkoff M, Batshaw M. Metabolic and Neuropsychological phenotype in women heterozygous for ornithine transcarbamylase deficiency. Ann Neurol. 2004;55:80–6.

Porphyria

Downey DC. Porphyria and chemicals. Med Hypotheses. 1999;53(2):166–71.

Jarrell JF, Gocmen A, Akyol D, Brant R. Hexachlorobenzene exposure and the proportion of male births in Turkey 1935-1990. Reprod Toxicol. 2002;16(1):65–70.

Hemochromatosis

Moyer TP, Highsmith WE, Smyrk TC, Gross JB Jr. Hereditary hemochromatosis: laboratory evaluation. Clin Chim Acta. 2011;412(17, 18):1485–92.

Gattermann N. The treatment of secondary hemochromatosis. Deutsches Ärzteblatt Int. 2009;106(30):499–504.

Bacon BR, Adams PC, Kowdley KV, Powell LW, Tavill AS. Diagnosis and management of hemochromatosis: 2011 practice guideline by the American Association for the Study of Liver Diseases. Hepatology. 2011;54(1):328–43.

Phlebotomy Guidelines: http://www.irondisorders.org/Websites/idi/files/Content/854256/Physician%20Chart%20phlebotomy%20detail2011.pdf

Alpha 1 Antitrypsin Deficiency

Ray D, Harikrishna S, Immanuel C, Victor L, Subramanyam S, Kumaraswami V. Acquired alpha 1-antitrypsin deficiency in tropical pulmonary eosinophilia. Indian J Med Res. 2011;134:79–82.

Vascular Disorders of the Liver

11

Vlad Damian Vintilă, Alexandra Maria Chitroceanu, and Ana-Maria Vintilă

Abbreviations

BCS	Budd-Chiari syndrome
HVOTO	Hepatic venous outflow tract
PVT	Portal vein thrombosis
SOS	Sinusoidal obstruction syndrome
VOD	Veno-occlusive disease
HHT	Hereditary haemorrhagic telangiectasia
Angio-MR	Magnetic resonance angiography
Angio-CT	Computed tomography angiography
TIPS	Transjugular intrahepatic portosystemic shunt

Key Concepts

- Vascular disorders of the liver are rare conditions, usually affecting young people, with high morbidity and mortality that can occur in the absence of a proper diagnosis and disease-specific management.
- An underlying systemic prothrombotic condition is found in patients with Budd-Chiari Syndrome and portal vein thrombosis
- Anticoagulation should be initiated without waiting in patients with Budd-Chiari Syndrome and acute portal vein thrombosis.
- Sinusoidal obstruction syndrome occurs as an iatrogenic complication of exposure to toxic agents for sinusoidal endothelium of the liver and hematopoietic bone marrow cells.
- Vascular malformations in hereditary haemorrhagic telangiectasia affect the liver extensively and evolve continuously from small telangiectasia to large arteriovenous malformations.

11.1 Introduction

The liver is a very vascular organ and at rest receives up to 25% of total cardiac output [1]. It is divided into eight independent segments, each segment having a separate hepatic artery and portal vein in the centre and hepatic veins in the periphery [2]. The microscopic units of the liver are known as hexagonal hepatic lobules, formed by radiating hepatocytes and many specialized capillaries known as sinusoids [2]. Every component of the hepatic vascular system (hepatic arteries, portal and hepatic veins, sinusoids, and lymphatics) can present a spectrum of variants and pathologic conditions. In the last years, international collaborations provided data-supported approaches, which allowed to increase knowledge and awareness in understanding and management of these conditions. Vascular disorders of the liver affect less than 5/10,000 patients and together comprise a number of rare conditions that can cause non-cirrhotic portal hypertension with high morbidity and mortality [3]. Moreover, they are usually diagnosed in young people, with a contrarily normal life expectancy if these conditions are timely diagnosed and managed properly [3]. Diagnosis is based on a high degree of clinical suspicion and usually

V. D. Vintilă (✉)
Carol Davila University of Medicine and Pharmacy, Bucharest, Romania

University of Medicine and Pharmacy, University Emergency Hospital, Bucharest, Romania

Department of Cardiology, Emergency University Hospital, Bucharest, Romania

A. M. Chitroceanu
Department of Cardiology, University and Emergency Hospital, Bucharest, Romania

A.-M. Vintilă
Carol Davila University of Medicine and Pharmacy, Bucharest, Romania

Department of Internal Medicine and Cardiology, Colţea Clinical Hospital, Bucharest, Romania

F. Radu-Ionita et al. (eds.), *Liver Diseases*, https://doi.org/10.1007/978-3-030-24432-3_11

confirmed by imaging. Doppler ultrasound, angio-MR, angio-CT provide information of similar accuracy depending of the type of vascular disorder and have the advantage of being non-invasive. Liver biopsy is excessive in most of the case and usually not recommended. Treatment depends on the type of vascular disorder, associated conditions and patient's clinical status. Given the rarity of some vascular disorders of the liver, not all will be discussed in this chapter. A spectrum of variants and diseases involving the hepatic venous outflow tract will be considered, notably Budd-Chiari Syndrome (BCS). Anomalies, and disease involving the portal vein such as acute portal vein thrombosis (PVT), chronic PVT, and cavernous transformation will be discussed. Sinusoidal obstruction syndrome (SOS) also reviewed. Congenital vascular malformations involving the liver are also explained, with an emphasis on hepatic vascular malformations in hereditary haemorrhagic telangiectasia (HHT) and congenital shunts.

11.2 Budd-Chiari Syndrome or Hepatic Venous Outflow Tract Obstruction

Budd-Chiari syndrome (BCS) known also as hepatic venous outflow tract obstruction (HVOTO) is define by an obstruction on the hepatic veins, at any level between small intrahepatic veins to the entrance of the inferior vena cava and right atrium, independent of the mechanism of obstruction, leading to an impaired hepatic venous drainage [3]. Cardiac disease, pericardial disease or sinusoidal obstruction syndrome (SOS) are excluded from this definition [3, 4]. BCS can be classified depending on the level of obstacle: small hepatic veins, inferior vena cava, and any combination thereof, having among these categories distinct presentation and geographical distribution [5].

Aetiology: According to the cause, BCS can be classified into primary or secondary. Primary BCS is the consequence of a primarily venous disease (thrombosis or phlebitis), and secondary BCS is the result of an external compression or invasion by a lesion originating outside the vein (benign or malignant tumour or infectious process) [3, 4].

An underlying systemic prothrombotic condition is found in up to 80% in patients with BCS [6]. However, the aetiology is often multifactorial. A combination of such conditions is present in nearly half, particularly in patients with heterozygous factor V Leiden or in patients taken oral contraceptives or pregnant women [7]. Antiphospholipid antibodies are responsible for 30% of BCS cases whereas lupus anticoagulant or anti-beta-2 glycoprotein 1 antibodies for 4–5% [3]. The aetiology of primarily BCS differ greatly among countries. In Europe, BCS is mostly secondary to thrombosis in hepatic veins, whereas in Asia, Behcet disease, membranous obstruction of the inferior vena cava are the most common aetiologies [8]. BCS has been related to myeloproliferative neoplasms in 35–50% cases in western countries, JAK2 mutation, V617F mutation account for 90% of them and CARL mutations in 2–5% [9].

The main primary tumours involving in secondary BCS are carcinoma: hepatocellular, renal and adrenal, primary hepatic hemangiosarcoma, epithelioid hemangioendothelioma, sarcoma of the inferior vena cava, right atrial myxoma, alveolar hydatid disease [10]. Infectious processes account for a small number of cases and most common are: amoebic and pyogenic abscess, polycystic liver disease [7]. Moreover, BCS may occur following trauma [7], hepatic resection or transplantation [11].

The local factor that develops thrombosis of the hepatic venous tract remains unidentified in most patients [4].

The diagnosis of the underlying cause (primary or secondary) of BCS has important implications for treatment. If left untreated, symptomatic BCS is lethal within a few days, to a few years [12].

Morphological changes: hepatic venous outflow tract obstruction induces venous wall inflammation, increased sinusoid pressure and portal hypertension. Centrilobular sinusoidal dilatation and congestion, liver cell loss and fibrosis are considered histopathological features for BCS [4]. However, these features are not specific, being also seen in heart failure, constrictive pericarditis and SOS [12]. Ultimately, a cirrhotic pattern develops, nodular regenerative hyperplasia, macroregenerative nodules being common in advanced cases [13]. These lead to fibrous enlargement of the portal tract, with portovenous and portoportal bridging fibrosis and thrombosis of intrahepatic portal veins [4, 13]. Because of the marked heterogeneous distribution of these lesions, liver biopsy is not recommended, the assessment of fibrosis proved irrelevant for prognosis [12].

Functional changes: The hepatic vein obstruction is predominantly due to the occlusion of at least two hepatic veins, but the occlusion is not synchronous, an acute clinical presentation coincides in most of the cases with the ultimate obstruction of an individual hepatic vein overlapping a chronic obstruction [12, 14]. It is associated with an obstruction of the IVC in approximately one third of patients, while isolated IVC obstruction is rare [14]. Hepatic vein occlusion causes elevated sinusoidal pressure, liver congestion and increased lymphatic filtration of interstitial fluid [15]. Increased sinusoidal pressure within proportions of the hepatic parenchyma with blood stasis induce portal hypertension and ascites, which is also increased by the impaired lymphatic drainage capability. Several mechanisms tend to preserve blood perfusion to the liver: increased arterial blood flow, redistribution of portal blood flow to the areas with preserved outflow and the development of venous collateral circulation (intrahepatic and extrahepatic) [13]. Although these mechanisms can prevent the development of clinical manifestations of liver disease, in the absence of treatment, irreversible liver abnormalities progressively develop to centrilobular fibrosis [4].

Diagnosis: Clinical presentation ranges from absence of symptoms to fulminant hepatic failure [16]. Asymptomatic BCS cases accounts for up to 20% of cases, and is often associated with the presence of large hepatic venous collaterals [3, 4]. Classical signs and symptoms include fever, abdominal pain, ascites, hepatomegaly, ankle swelling, gastrointestinal bleeding and hepatic encephalopathy [4, 17]. In a multicentre prospective study, ascites were present in 83% percent of patients with BCS, hepatomegaly in 67%, abdominal pain in 61% and gastrointestinal bleeding in 5% [18]. The course of these manifestations can be progressive or with periods of exacerbations and remissions. BCS can present a long insidious course, or a short period of prodrome followed by an accelerated falling course. In approximately 15% of cases portal venous obstruction is associated, suggesting a more severe form [17, 18].

Diagnosis is establish by confirming the hepatic venous outflow obstruction. Doppler ultrasound, angio-MR and angio-CT provide information of similar accuracy and have the advantages of being non-invasive or minimally invasive [3, 12]. Doppler ultrasound is the first line investigation and has a sensitivity of more than 75% but the awareness and expertise of the examiner are crucial [3].

Imaging findings classify BCS lesions as direct signs—visualization the obstacle and indirect signs (secondary to the venous obstruction)—intrahepatic or extrahepatic collateral circulation, perfusion abnormalities and anatomical changes to the liver, all resulting from portal hypertension [19]. The obstruction can present with several aspects, including short-length, extended narrowing of venous lumen, a complete obstruction simulating a membrane or a fibrous cord, with upstream dilatation [12, 19]. Venography is recommended if the diagnosis is uncertain and it is compulsory for percutaneous interventions [3]. Hepatic nodules can be seen using imaging in more than a half of patients with BCS, resulting from perfusion disturbances and being usually benign [3]. These nodules are usually small (<4 cm in diameter), multiple, hypervascularized and disseminated through the liver [20]. Although hepatocellular carcinoma in BCS account for 4% of the cases, currently there are no clear diagnosis criteria, a biopsy should be performed in selected cases (less or equal to three nodules, nodules >3 cm in diameter, heterogeneity or washed out on venous phase, patients with high levels of alphafetoprotein [20]. Secondary BCS related to an external compression or invasion is ruled out also by using the same radiological approaches [3]. Liver biopsy should only be taken into consideration in selected cases where the imaging has failed to demonstrate obstruction, due to the associated risk of bleeding that may delay the initiation of anticoagulation therapy [4]. To note that the assessment of fibrosis proved irrelevant for prognosis [4].

Treatment: In most cases, the underlying disorder causing BCS in unrecognized at presentation. Patients with BCS presenting with ascites and varices require the same treatment as cirrhotic patients [21].

Anticoagulant therapy should be initiated without waiting, as soon as possible and for an indefinite period of time in order to reduce the clot extensions and new thrombotic episodes [18]. Although ineffective on chronic liver disease, early anticoagulation has improved survival in patients with moderate BCS, probably by a preventive systemic effect in other sites on thrombosis [19]. Currently, there are no data regarding the use of Non-Vitamin K Antagonists, treatment with Warfarin or Acenocumarol should be consider for an indefinite period. Treatment for the underlying prothrombotic condition should be started in the same time.

The experience of thrombolysis is limited, and complications can be fatal [3].

Patients with focal or segmental obstruction of the hepatic venous outflow tract are eligible for percutaneous angioplasty, with or without stenting. Focal or segmental stenosis are present in 60% of patients with IVC obstruction, and 25–60% of those with hepatic vein obstruction [3]. These patients may benefit by percutaneous angioplasty of one HV, of the IVC or both [22]. The rationale for angioplasty is to re-establish the physiological drainage of portal and sinusoidal blood [22]. At present, less than 10% of patients with BCS are eligible for stenting (Fig. 11.1) [6, 23].

Patients who do not improve with medical and endoscopic treatment are proposed for transjugular intrahepatic portosystemic shunt (TIPS) [12]. The rationale for TIPS is to decompress the liver by transforming the portal vein into an outflow tract [12]. Patients are selected based on the extent of the vascular lesions, particularly patients with multitroncular HV obstructions with mall intrahepatic collaterals [24].

The minority of patients in which TIPS fails or those with fulminant hepatic failure are proposed for liver transplantation, the rationale being a complete correction of the hepatic consequences of vascular obstructions [12].

Prognosis: Without treatment, symptomatic BCS is lethal within a few days to a few years [12]. Current therapeutic strategies permits to achieve 5-year survival rates over 80% [6]. Child-Pugh score and its components have been found to be independent prognostic factors. Moreover, prognostic scores based on a combination of these factors have been developed [4]. These scores are useful for the assessment of transplant-free survival and clinical studies, but not for individual management [25]. At present, long term prognosis is determined by hepatocellular carcinoma or by complications of the underlying blood disease (leukaemia in patients with myeloproliferative disease) [12].

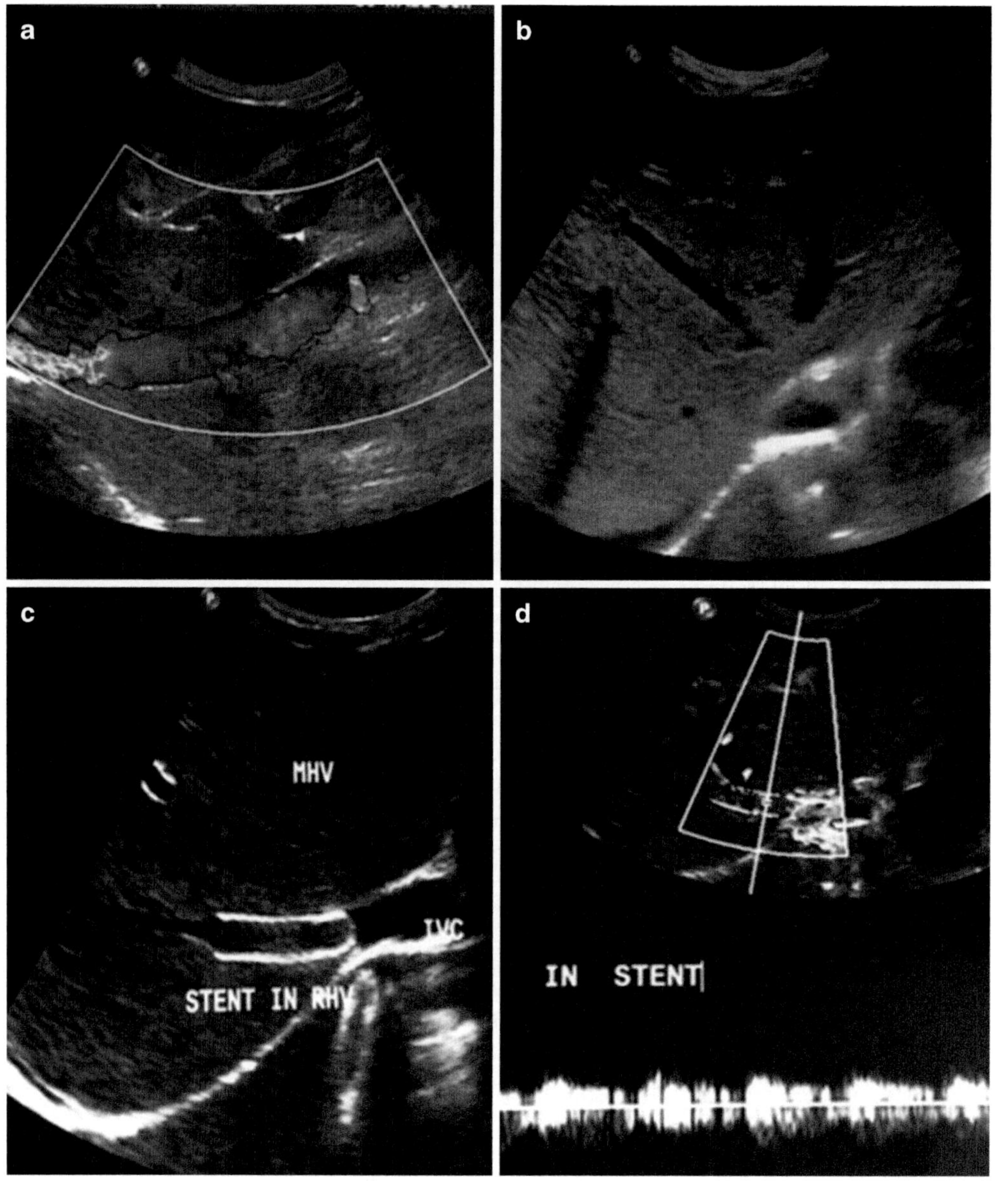

Fig. 11.1 (a) Pre-procedure sonography coupled with Doppler ultrasound showing a patent IVC. (b) Segmental narrowing of all hepatic veins in a case of BCS. This patient underwent right hepatic vein angioplasty and stenting and follow-up sonography (c) and Doppler (d) showed a patent stent. (Reproduced with permission from Das CJ, Soneja M, Tayal S, Chahal A, Srivastava S, Kumar A, Baruah U (2018) Role of radiological imaging and interventions in management of Budd-Chiari syndrome. Clin Radiol 73:610–624)

11.3 Portal Vein Thrombosis

Portal vein thrombosis (PVT): is characterised by an obstruction of the portal veins, and its branches, which include splenic, superior and inferior mesenteric veins [26]. Isolated splenic or superior mesenteric vein obstruction is included in the entity of **splanchnic vein obstruction** [12]. Obstruction may be complete or partial [3].

PVT is classified into acute or chronic [4]. Acute thrombosis refers to recent and symptomatic, while chronic thrombosis refers to long standing process. They represent successive stages of the same disease and share similar causes, differing in their management [4]. After acute thrombosis, in the absence of recanalization, portal lumen obliterates and a set of collateral portoportal veins develops to replace the portal vein [4, 12]. This term is called **portal cavernoma** or **cavernomatous transformation of the portal vein** and corresponds to a long-standing process [4, 12]. In children, cavernoma might result from a malformation [27]. PVT is responsible for up to 30% and 75% of cases of portal hypertension in adults and children, in developing countries [4].

Aetiology: Except from childhood portal cavernoma, a thrombus is the cause of the disease. PVT is caused by a combination of local and systemic factors. Local factors include cancer (any abdominal organ), cirrhosis (these two are the leading local risk factors) and intraabdominal infections (such as secondary peritonitis) [4]. PVT is common in patients with cirrhosis, more that 30% of liver transplant recipients have PVT at the time of transplant [28]. The risk of developing PVT associated with cirrhosis is correlated to the severity of liver disease and the presence of the inherited prothrombotic disorders [29]. Systemic factors refer to an inherited or acquired prothrombotic condition [3]. Usually, one or several systemic factors are identified, the most common being myeloproliferative disease (25–30%) and factor II Leiden (in 15%) [30]. The simultaneous presence of several prothrombotic causes in patients with PVT is more frequent than in general population [31]. Identification of a local risk factor does not exclude the possibility that a general risk factor is present [31]. In this section, we will focus on the non-cirrhotic, non-malignant portal thrombosis, cirrhotic PVT and malignant being discussed separately elsewhere.

Morphological changes: In patients with non-cirrhotic portal vein thrombosis, alterations in portal venous flow result in a spectrum of altered hepatic histology, ranging from large regenerative nodules to nodular regenerative hyperplasia without bridging fibrosis [32]. Unlike the central atrophy that is characteristic for cirrhosis, the central portion of the liver is relatively spared due to collateral portal venous flow developing over time [33]. However, peripheral liver cells apoptosis may occur, because collateral blood flow to subcapsular regions is insufficient [33]. Abnormal liver circulation result in a distorted architecture of the liver with micro- and macroscopic nodules of hyperplastic hepatocytes that are not surrounded by fibrous septae [34]. Nodular regenerative hyperplasia, as in BCS, must be differentiated from hepatocellular carcinoma [3].

Functional changes: Despite acute complete portal thrombosis, there is limited evidence for liver ischemia, because the immediate development of porto-portal collaterals, involving the porta hepatis and because the compensated increase in hepatic arterial blood flow [35]. Above the obstacle, ischemia does not develop because of the small tributaries to superior or inferior mesenteric veins [36]. Spontaneous recanalization is exceptional, and in a matter of weeks a portal cavernoma is formed by collateral veins which contribute to maintain the perfusion of portal blood to the liver [37]. Because they cannot reduce portal pressure, spleen enlargement and portosystemic collaterals develop [12]. Within a year gastroesophageal varices will be formed [12, 37]. Synchronous, liver architecture is compromised, with preserved blood perfusion to the central of the liver and hardship in the periphery, with increase in size of segments I and IV of the liver and atrophy of left liver lobe and peripheral parts of the right lobe [12]. However, frank liver dysfunction is absent, subtle signs being common, such as a decrease in coagulation factors levels and subclinical hepatic encephalopathy [38].

Diagnosis: Diagnosis of PVO is presently made in 50–70% of the cases in the acute setting [39]. Common symptoms of acute complete PVT include acute abdominal or lumbar pain, with moderated distended abdomen by ileus, without any other features of intestinal occlusion [37]. Partial thrombosis is associated with fewer symptoms, PVT being recognised only at the stage of cavernomatous transformation [3]. In patients with chronic PVT, the severity of portal hypertension typically contrasts with a mild or absent liver dysfunction (with normal levels of transaminases, alkaline phosphatase and gamma-glutamyl transferase) [4]. 50% of the patients present with ascites, but ascites emerge after a triggering event like bleeding or infection, and it is usually reversible [30]. Features of hypersplenism may be marked and bleeding related to portal hypertension is massive though better tolerated than patients with cirrhosis [12].

Acute PVT is rapidly diagnosed using noninvasive imaging. It shows thrombus occupying the lumen of the portal vein or its branches, with a poorly development of porto-portal collaterals [40], Doppler ultrasound, CT scan and MRI are almost equivalent, depending on the expertise of the operator [3, 4]. Standard abdominal echography reveals a hyperechogenic material in the lumen with distensions of the portal veins [4]. Doppler imaging allows to prove the absence of flow in part of the lumen [3, 4]. Because the mesenteric veins are difficult to visualize at echography, CT or MRI are more sensitive for assessment of thrombus extension [3, 4]. Thrombus is revealed by CT scan as a hyperattenuating material in the portal vein (Fig. 11.2a) [41, 42]. After contrast injection is revealed as a lack of luminal enhancement, with increased hepatic enhancement in the arterial phase and decreased hepatic enhancement in the portal phase [41]. If the thrombus is less than a week old, it appears as a hyperintense material on MRI T1-weighted sequences [40]. Portal cavernoma is seen as a lattice of serpiginous structures that enhance the portal phase of vascular contrast while the normal portal vein is not visible [12].

Treatment: Since the aim of the treatment between acute and chronic portal vein thrombosis differs, we will discuss them separately. The aim of the treatment of acute PVT is the recanalization of the obstructed veins and prevention of the extension of thrombosis to mesenteric veins followed by intestinal infarction and portal hypertension [3, 4].

For acute PVT, immediate initiation of anticoagulation prevents thrombus extension [30]. There have been no controlled studies of anticoagulation therapy in patients with acute PVT [4]. In a recent prospective study, intestinal infarction was a rare complication (2/95 patients) which require only limited intestinal resection, even if in 60% of the patients superior mesenteric vein was involved [30]. In the setting of intestinal infarction, emergency laparotomy should be performed [4]. Full recanalization of the portal vein was achieved in 40% of patients by 6 months of treatment, and did not occur in any of the patients beyond 6 months of treatment [30]. Also, high recanalization rates were observed after anticoagulation in post splenectomy PVT patients or for acute thrombosis involving the superior mesenteric vein [43]. Splenic vein thrombosis and ascites suggest failure in

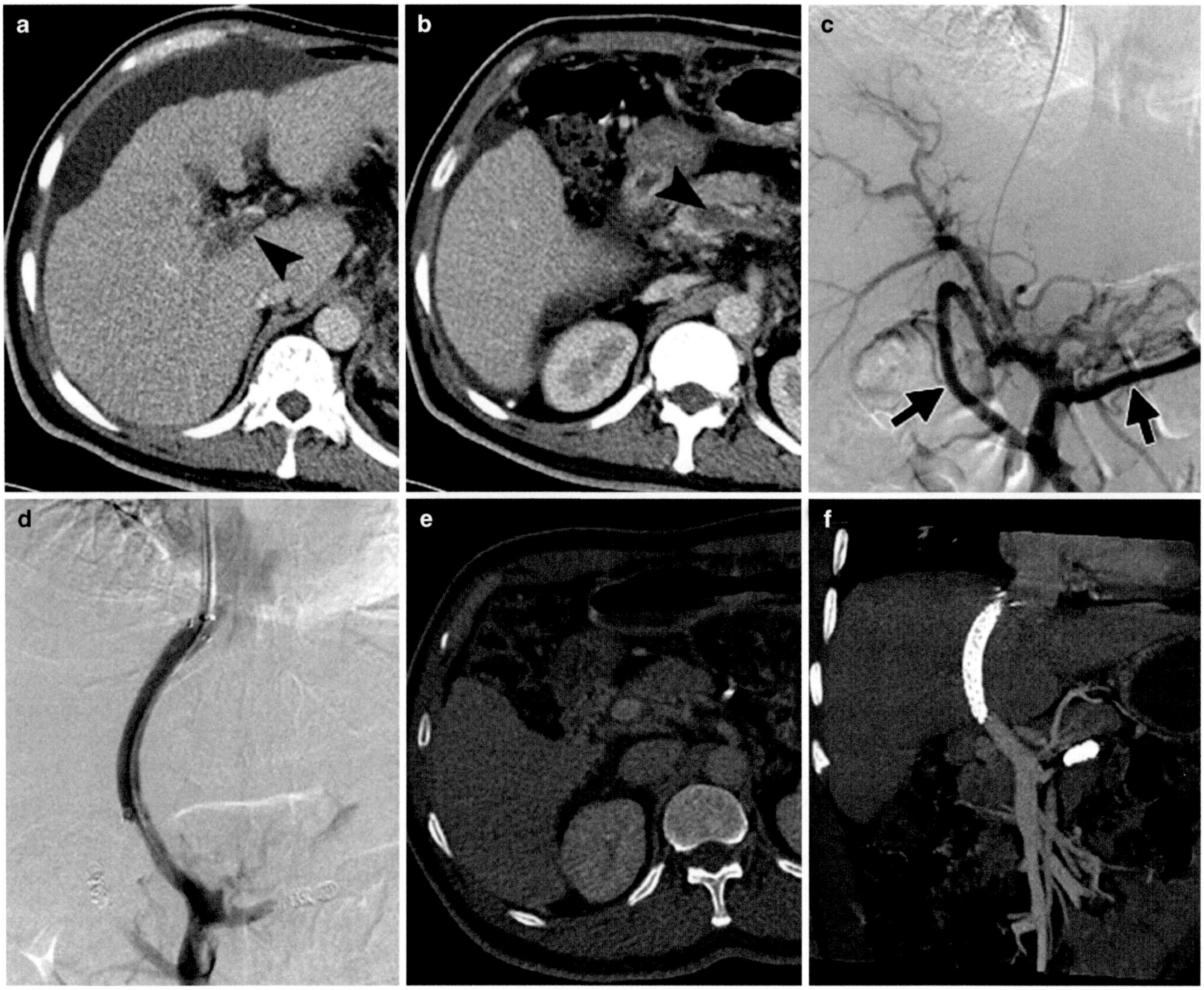

Fig. 11.2 (**a**, **b**) Contrast-enhanced CT scans show severe thrombosis (arrowhead) in the intrahepatic portal branches (**a**) and the main portal vein (**b**). (**c**) Direct portal venogram shows extensive thrombosis in the portal venous system, multiple collaterals (arrows), and hepatofugal flow. (**d**) One covered stent was deployed after the competing collaterals were embolized. Fifteen months after TIPS placement (**e**, **f**) CT scans show complete recanalization of the portal vein. (Reproduced with permission from Luo X et al. (2015) Advanced Cirrhosis Combined with Portal Vein Thrombosis: A Randomized Trial of TIPS versus Endoscopic Band Ligation Plus Propranolol for the Prevention of Recurrent Esophageal Variceal Bleeding. Radiology 276:286–293)

recanalization [30]. Spontaneous recanalization is infrequent in patients not receiving anticoagulation therapy [30]. The optimal duration of anticoagulation therapy has not been determined, however, according to a panel of international experts [3, 4], at least 3-month period should be considered, while permanent anticoagulation for patients with permanent prothrombotic conditions should be taken into consideration [43]. In most of the studies, anticoagulation was based on unfractionated heparin, LMWH or VKA targeting an INR between 2 and 3 [3].

The reported experience with thrombolytic therapy, systemic or in situ, is extremely limited [3, 4]. The reported recanalization rates have been similar to those achieved with anticoagulation alone, but with major procedure-related complications. A higher mortality rate was noted with approaches using transhepatic route [44]. Surgical thrombectomy has proved a benefit in 30% of the patients, but with a high recurrence rate when performed more than 30 days after the onset [45].

Current studies report that balloon angioplasty with or without stenting without thrombolysis or thrombectomy could be an alternative and save treatment for post-operative main portal vein and superior mesenteric vein thrombosis [46].

Data on TIPS are limited, beyond the technical challenge of the procedure, medium-term efficacy require further evaluation (Fig. 11.2b) [4, 42].

The aim of the treatment for chronic PVT is to prevent recurrent thrombosis, and the prevention and treatment of the associated complications, gastrointestinal bleeding and portal cholangiopathy [4]. At present there are no controlled studies regarding treatment of gastroesophageal varices in patient with chronic PVT. Some retrospective multivariate studies found that screening for gastroesophageal varices, beta-adrenergic blockers or endoscopic therapy reduces the risk of bleeding and by thus, improves survival [4]. In a number of uncontrolled surveys, endoscopic sclerotherapy has achieved eradication of varices and a reduction in bleeding rate [4].

The experience in splenectomy, devascularisation and TIPS insertion in patients with portal cavernoma is limited [47]. The prevention of recurrent thrombosis in chronic PVT requires also anticoagulation, with the same mentions as in acute PVT [3, 4]. To note that a recent retrospective study showed that warfarin had independently improved the survival of patients with chronic PVT, most of them having a risk factor for thrombosis [4]. Another retrospective analysis found a decreased incidence of gastrointestinal bleeding after starting anticoagulation therapy [4]. Patients with portal cholangiopathy usually present with jaundice and biliary symptoms. Insertion of a biliary prosthesis after endoscopic extraction of stones is a proved therapy and the lack of the recurrence after prosthesis removal was noted in almost half of patients [48]. Other techniques involve portosystemic shunting, bilio-enteric anastomosis, biliary surgery without portal decompression, but current data are limited [3, 4].

Prognosis: With the effective prevention and control of bleeding and thrombosis, the outcome is given by age and the course of the underlying disease [12].

The mortality of acute PVT is high due to late recognition of intestinal infarction, and portal hypertension developed with associated complications (variceal bleeding) [4]. Above half of the patients do not achieve recanalization and will develop gastroesophageal varices with a 2 year high probability of bleeding [37].

The outcome for treated patients with chronic PVT is currently good [4]. Mortality is related to the recurrent bleeding from portal hypertension, followed by recurrent thrombosis at splanchnic or extrasplanchnic sites. In a 5-year followed up period, less than 5% of patients with PVT died from classical complications [4].

11.4 Sinusoidal Obstruction Syndrome

Sinusoidal obstruction syndrome (SOS) is characterized by a loss of sinusoidal endothelium integrity with a consequent sinusoidal obstruction by outflow block [3]. Damaged sinusoids can be associated with a partial or complete occlusion of small hepatic veins, therefore being previously known as hepatic veno-occlusive disease (VOD) [49]. SOS is a primary circulatory disorder that can occur in the absence of central vein occlusion, the involvement of central vein being related to more severe disease [4]. Therefore the alternative term of SOS was considered in replacement of VOD.

Aetiology: SOS occurs as an iatrogenic complication of exposure to toxic agents for sinusoidal endothelium of the liver and hematopoietic bone marrow cells [3]. A large number of drugs and toxins have been associated with SOS: plant pyrrolizidine alkaloids, myeloablative regimens used in the setting of haematopoietic stem cell transplantation, chemotherapy for liver metastasis of colorectal cancer, thiopurine derivatives [50]. Other reported conditions are liver irradiation and platelet transfusion containing ABO-incompatible plasma [3]. Lately, an inherited condition combining VOD and immunodeficiency associated with mutations in Sp110, has been described. The acronym for this condition is VODI [51]. Although its mechanism is unknown, one possible explanation is an accompanying opportunistic viral infection affecting the endothelium of sinusoids or central vein [51].

Morphological changes: Despite of its multiple causes, patients with SOS present similar morphological changes [50]. Circulatory obstruction precedes liver dysfunction. According to the level of obstruction, various degrees of centrilobular hepatocellular necrosis may occur [3]. As a result, SOS lesions appear to have a patchy distribution [3]. It may also associate one or more other lesions such as centrilobular perisinusoidal and endovenular fibrosis, peliosis and nodular regenerative hyperplasia (Fig. 11.3) [3, 49, 50]. All of these changes seem to be related to SOS severity or represent late lesions [50].

Functional changes: SOS is a clinical diagnosis based on several common liver disease signs and symptoms: weight gain with or without ascites, hepatomegaly and jaundice [52]. However, patients can be asymptomatic or can present with features of portal hypertension or multiple organ dysfunction syndrome.

Diagnosis: Starting from the definition, the diagnosis of SOS expects a histologic examination of the liver [12]. Percutaneous liver biopsy is usually contraindicated by thrombocytopenia, coagulopathy or ascites [4]. Transjugular liver biopsy with hepatic venous pressure gradient is of major help in confirming SOS [3]. In patients receiving myeloablative regimens used in the context of haematopoietic stem cell transplantation, a hepatic venous pressure gradient >10 mmHg proved to have a specificity of 91% and a sensitivity of 52% for the diagnosis of SOS [3].

After excluding confiding situations, the diagnosis can be made based on a high index of clinical suspicion in a patient who has signs and symptoms of SOS and had received a therapy known to cause liver injury [3, 4]. Increased serum level of bilirubin is a sensitive but not specific marker [4]. The American Association for Study of Liver Disease

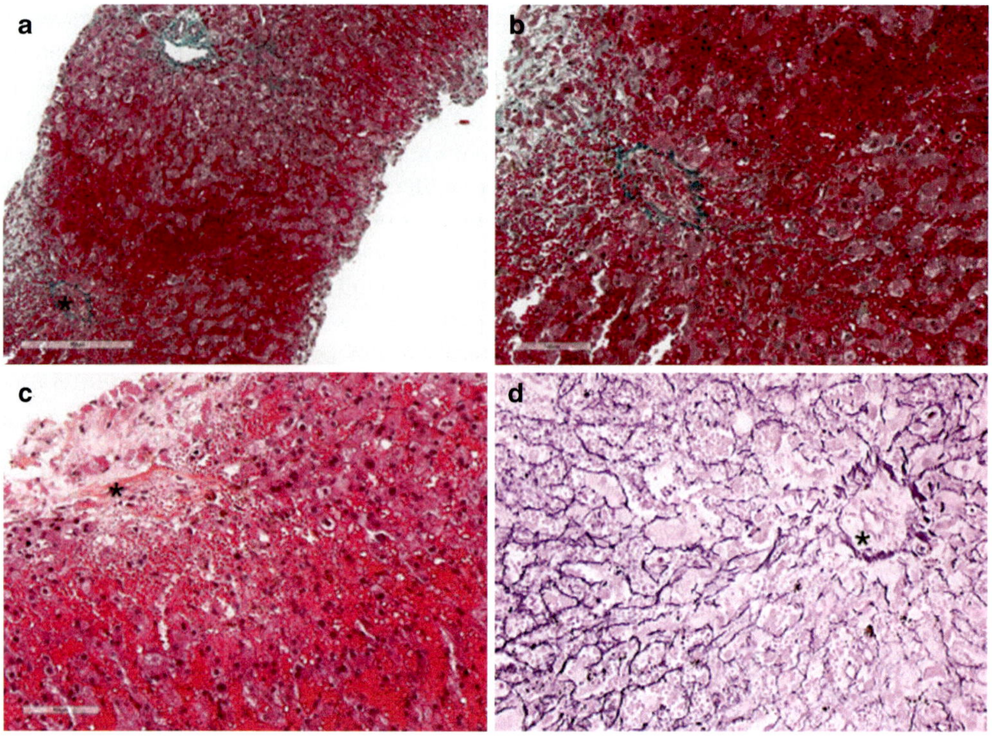

Fig. 11.3 Acute sinusoidal obstruction syndrome related to gemtuzumab use (Mylotarg) after haematopoietic stem cell transplantation (**a**, **b**) Masson trichrome, (**c** hematein eosin-safran; **d**: argentation stain): dilatation and congestion of sinusoids are limited to centrilobular zones around the terminal hepatic vein ∗; endothelial cells of veins and sinusoids are damaged, leading to a huge hematic deposition in Disse space and to hepatocyte necrosis around the central veins. (Reproduced from Valla D-C, Cazals-Hatem D. (2016) MINI REVIEW Sinusoidal obstruction syndrome, Clin Res Hepatol Gastroenterol 40:378–385)

(ASSLD) introduced clinical criteria for SOS diagnosis [4]. These criteria, known as Seattle or Baltimore criteria, present clinical features for diagnosis used for defining populations for research [3]. For example, the Seattle criteria were developed for patients receiving myeloablative regimens containing cyclophosphamide, clinical findings must occur within 20 days of transplantation [3]. These criteria does not apply in patients receiving regimens to cause late onset disease [3]. Their sensitivity and specificity are currently not well established, and their use in different settings of SOS aetiology have not been evaluated [3].

The diagnosis may be supported by imaging techniques, Doppler echocardiography showing signs of portal hypertension, liver and spleen enlargement; none of these findings are specific for SOS [53]. Reversal of flow in portal vein and monophasic flow in hepatic vein have been used to diagnose SOS, but lacks sensitivity [54]. Magnetic Resonance imaging may show patchy signal enhancement compatible with histologically severe SOS. Because of its associated toxicity, Computer Tomography is not recommended [4].

Treatment: Identifying patients at risk is useful in preventing SOS. In patients with pre-existing liver disease, previous history of SOS, recent treatment with gemtuzumab ozagamicin or myelofibrosis with extramedullary haematopoiesis, both European and American Guidelines recommend the use of chemotherapy regimens with lower liver toxicity, without cyclophosphamide [55]. At present, the only proved strategy to prevent or reduce the severity of sinusoidal changes and their clinical expression is reducing the intensity of chemotherapeutic regimen [49]. Prophylactic pharmacological strategies have not proved a reduction in overall risk of SOS or the risk of fatal SOS in randomized controlled trials [4]. The routine use of intravenous heparin or subcutaneous low-molecular weight heparin as prophylaxis for SOS, the use of ursodeoxycholate, prostaglandin E1, pentoxifylline or N-acetylcysteine are unproved prophylactic measures [4]. The prophylactic use of ursodeoxycholate reduces the frequency of jaundice and alanine aminotransferase levels, without any benefit in SOS [55].

Treatment of SOS depends on its clinical severity and is based mostly on supportive care with therapy of fluid overload, sepsis and organ failure [3]. Fluid overload should be managed with diuretics, paracentesis, hemofiltration, and haemodialysis [3].

Defibrotide, a mixture of the single-stranded oligodeoxyribonucleotides derived from depolymerisation of porcine intestinal mucosa DNA, proved a benefit for treatment of severe SOS both in adult and children patients [4]. Moreover, it has also demonstrated benefit for SOS prophylaxis in paediatric hematopoietic cell transplantation patients [4].

Heparin and thrombolytic therapy proved no positive effect [56].

TIPS and surgical shunting have been used in selective cases for symptoms relief, but proved no benefit in survival [57].

SOS is usually an iatrogenic complication caused by the therapy used for patients with malignancy [49]. Liver transplantation is limited by the underlying malignancy itself.

However, it may be considered in selected cases with a favourable prognosis [4].

Prognosis: The outcome of SOS lies upon the context and the magnitude of exposure to toxic agents [12]. Predictors of poor prognosis are the slope of bilirubin serum levels, weight gain, higher levels of alanine aminotransferase, higher hepatic venous pressure gradient and multiple organ failure [4].

11.5 Congenital Vascular Malformations Affecting the Liver

Congenital vascular malformations. Vascular malformations of the liver determine an abnormal intra or extrahepatic shunting of blood [4]. They comprise several entities based on the functional shunting. Shunting can develop between the hepatic artery to the portal vein (arterioportal shunt) or to the hepatic vein (arteriovenous shunt) or/and between the portal vein to the systemic circulation (portosystemic or portohepatic shunt) [4]. These types of congenital shunting can be isolated, although rare, and diagnosed in infants or children or may coexist in hereditary haemorrhagic telangiectasia with liver involvement [4]. Although in this chapter we will discuss only the congenital shunts, these shunts can also be acquired, associated with hepatocellular carcinoma and/ or cirrhosis, or after trauma (including liver biopsy, transhepatic cholangiography, or biliary surgery).

Hepatic vascular malformations in hereditary haemorrhagic telangiectasia (HHT).

HHT, or Rendu-Osler-Weber disease is a rare, genetic disorder with an autosomal dominant inheritance pattern, characterized by widespread cutaneous, mucosal, and visceral arteriovenous malformations involving the lung, brain and/or liver [3]. Most of patients present a mutation in one of two genes disease related: endoglin and activin A receptor type II-like 1, gene involved in transforming pathway of growth factor b (TGFb). Those dysfunctional gene are expressed predominantly on vascular endothelium [4].

Morphological changes: Vascular malformations in HHT affect the liver extensively, and evolve continuously from tiny telangiectasias to large arteriovenous malformations [58]. Due to a heterogeneous liver blood perfusion, nodular regenerative hyperplasia or focal nodular hyperplasia emerge, the latter having a 100-fold greater prevalence in HHT patients than in general population [59].

Functional changes: Three types of intrahepatic shunting may coexist (arterioportal, arteriovenous, and portosystemic) leading to different, concomitant or successively functional features: high output heart failure, portal hypertension, biliary disease, hepatic encephalopathy, or mesenteric ischemia [60]. High output heart failure is characterized by a hyperdynamic circulation developed through arteriohepatic and/or portohepatic shunting [61]. Portal hypertension emerge from arterioportal shunting and secondary portal fibrosis and/or regenerative hyperplasia [61]. Shunting can cause biliary ischemia which can result in bile duct necrosis and the extreme process of liver necrosis [61].

Diagnostic: Although HHT is a congenital disease, symptoms of liver vascular malformations appear predominantly in females around 30 years of age [4]. Only 8% of patients with liver vascular malformations on imaging are symptomatic [62]. High output heart failure represents the predominant clinical presentation, with exertional dyspnoea, ascites, oedema [4] and atrial fibrillation [63]. The next most common presentation is portal hypertension and the clinical picture includes ascites, varices and variceal bleeding due more often to gastrointestinal telangiectasias than to variceal bleeding [4, 63]. Patients can also present with anicteric cholestasis with or without cholangitis, encephalopathy, or mesenteric angina [3, 4, 63]. Biochemical changes are not specific, with a slight elevation of alkaline phosphatase and gamma glutamyl-transpeptidase, without any changes in the live synthetic function [60].

Currently, according to EASL Clinical Practice Guidelines, the diagnosis of HHT requires several criteria known as Curaçao criteria [3]. Diagnosis of HHT is suspected in a symptomatic patients with clinical features suggesting HHT and requires laboratory assessment and imaging methods such as abdominal Doppler Ultrasound and/or abdominal CT [62]. According to the Curaçao criteria, Doppler ultrasound can give a severity of grading (from 0+ to 4) which correlates with clinical outcome, and enables management and follow-up. Intrahepatic hypervascularization and enlarged hepatic artery seen on Doppler ultrasound or CT have the highest diagnostic accuracy [4, 64]. Moreover, because of the presence of nodular regenerative hyperplasia, the liver may appear nodular on imaging studies, and should be differentiated from cirrhosis. Liver biopsy in the diagnosis of liver vascular malformations in HHT is unnecessary [3, 4]. Genetic testing can be performed to establish the diagnosis in patients with diffuse liver vascular malformations who do not meet clinical diagnostic criteria for HHT [65]. Echocardiography can be performed to evaluate the hemodynamic impact [3]. Further tests (endoscopy, MR, angiography) may be performed in special cases, depending on the severity of liver vascular malformations [4].

Treatment: In asymptomatic HHT cases with or without liver involvement no treatment is recommended [3, 4]. In symptomatic HHT patients with liver involvement treatment is given by the type of clinical presentation [66]. Patients with high output heart failure should be managed according to heart failure guidelines, with salt retention, diuretics, beta blockers, angiotensin-converting enzyme inhibitors [3, 4]. Complications given by portal hypertension and encephalopathy should be treated as recommended in cirrhotic patients [3, 4]. Supportive care is also important, with blood transfusions or iron administration for anaemia, and treatment of the variceal bleeding [3].

In non-responders to initial medical treatment, peripheral embolization of liver vascular malformations is the most effective and repeatable trans-arterial treatment [65].

Liver transplantation is the only definitive curative option for liver vascular malformations in HHT [3, 4]. It is reserved for selected cases such as ischemic biliary necrosis, complicated portal hypertension and refractory heart failure [65].

Bevacizumab, an antibody to vascular endothelial growth factor (VEGF) has been shown to reduce the liver volume and ameliorate cardiac output after 3-month courses in patients with severe liver vascular malformations and high cardiac output [67]. However, further studies are needed before this therapy should be recommended.

Prognostic: Clinical outcome of liver vascular malformations in HHT correlates with their severity. In a recent cohort study with a median follow-up of 44 months, mortality related to hepatic vascular malformations occurred in 5% of patients, with incidence rates of complications and death 3.6 and 1.1 per person-years, respectively [63].

11.5.1 Isolated Congenital Liver Shunts

Congenital Arteriovenous (Hepatic artery to hepatic vein) malformations consists of discrete abnormalities with stable evolution and without change in dimensions [68]. These changes are very rare and usually present as a high-output heart failure in a neonate [4]. The diagnosis is based on MRI [68]. Initial treatment is pharmacological and the aim is reducing the symptoms of heart failure [4]. In non-responders to medical treatment, embolization and surgical resection should be considered [4].

Congenital Arterioportal (Hepatic artery to portal vein) malformations are very rare and cause portal hypertension manifested within the first year of life [4]. Clinical features include signs of portal hypertension, splenomegaly, and or variceal bleeding [4]. The diagnosis is based on Doppler ultrasound [68]. Treatment consists of embolization of the feeding artery with or without resection [4]. Liver transplantation should be considered in selected cases [4].

Congenital Portosystemic (Portal vein to systemic circulation) malformations are rare developmental anomalies secondary to abnormal development of the portal venous system [4]. They may be associated with other congenital anomalies [69]. They are divided into intrahepatic and extrahepatic shunts with common clinical features but different treatment [69]. Through the malformations the intestinal blood reaches the systemic circulation bypassing the liver. Due to the lack of metabolization of plasma ammonia, its serum increased level determines cognitive changes [4]. Symptoms include fatigue and mental retardation, with recurrent episodes of portosystemic encephalopathy [70]. Ascites and portal hypertension are not usually seen [4]. Diagnosis and classification is based on MRI [69]. Preoperative evaluation of portal vein by angiography is important, in order to determine portal vein patency, portal pressure and the type of portosystemic shunt [71]. Every shunt that persists after one year of life should be closed before complications emerge [69]. Symptomatic cases are immediately treated either by open surgery or laparoscopy with the intention of shunt ligaturation [69]. Endovascular embolization using periphery metal coils of the shunt is performed in selected centers [4]. The choice of surgical or endovascular approach is based upon patient's clinical condition, shunt anatomy and size and local expertise [69]. Liver transplantation may be the only treatment of extrahepatic or large intrahepatic multifocal shunts not suitable for embolization, or in cases of previous failed endovascular interventions [69]. To a standard therapeutic approach is not established.

11.6 Conclusions

Vascular disorders of the liver consist of multiple entities with different pathophysiology background, different clinical picture and different prognosis. As a general rule, therapy implies anticoagulant therapy, endovascular manoeuvres and surgical option. Thrombolysis shows no benefit, while increasing the risk of bleeding complications. TIPS is seldom recommended, while liver transplantation remains a final option for most of the patients with vascular disorders.

Self Study

Questions

1. Which of the following diseases are not treated with anticoagulants?
   A. Budd-Chiari Syndrome
   B. Acute Portal Vein Thrombosis
   C. Sinusoidal Obstruction Syndrome
   D. Chronic Portal Vein Thrombosis
   E. Splanchnic Vein Thrombosis
2. Which statement is true?
   A. In Haemorrhagic Hereditary Telangiectasia angio-MRI is the only imaging technique which can give a severity grading of liver vascular malformations which correlates with clinical outcome.
   B. The diagnosis of Sinusoidal Obstruction Syndrome is based on CT or liver biopsy.

C. Genetic testing can be made to establish the diagnosis in patients with Budd-Chiari Syndrome.
D. The diagnosis of Chronic Portal Vein Thrombosis requires angiography.
E. Liver transplantation is the only definitive curative option for liver vascular malformations in Haemorrhagic Hereditary Telangiectasia

Answers

1. Which of the following diseases are not treated with anticoagulants?
   Answer: C
2. Which statement is true?
   Answer: E.

References

1. Abdel-Misih SRZ, Bloomston M. Liver anatomy. Surg Clin North Am. 2010;90:643–53.
2. Elsayes KM, Shaaban AM, Rothan SM, Javadi S, Madrazo BL, Castillo RP, Casillas VJ, Menias CO. A comprehensive approach to hepatic vascular disease. Radiographics. 2017;37:813–36.
3. Clinical Practice Guidelines EASL. Vascular diseases of the liver. J Hepatol. 2016;64:179–202.
4. DeLeve LD, Valla D-C, Garcia-Tsao G. Vascular disorders of the liver. Hepatology. 2009;49:1729–64.
5. Ludwig j H e, db M, Jona v H. Classification of hepatic venous outflow obstruction: ambiguous terminology of the Budd-Chiari syndrome. Mayo Clin Proc. 1990;65:51–5.
6. Seijo S, Plessier A, Hoekstra J, et al. Good long-term outcome of Budd-Chiari syndrome with a step-wise management. Hepatology. 2013;57:1962–8.
7. Denninger M-H, Chaït Y, Casadevall N, Hillaire S, Guillin M-C, Bezeaud A, Erlinger S, Briere J, Valla D. Cause of portal or hepatic venous thrombosis in adults: the role of multiple concurrent factors. Hepatology. 2003;31:587–91.
8. Uskudar O, Akdogan M, Sasmaz N, Yilmaz S, Tola M, Sahin B. Etiology and portal vein thrombosis in Budd-Chiari syndrome. World J Gastroenterol. 2008;14:2858–62.
9. Poisson J, Plessier A, Kiladjian J-J, et al. Selective testing for calreticulin gene mutations in patients with splanchnic vein thrombosis: a prospective cohort study. J Hepatol. 2017;67:501–7.
10. Valla D-C. Hepatic venous outflow tract obstruction etiopathogenesis: Asia versus the West. J Gastroenterol Hepatol. 2004;19:S204–11.
11. Kubo T, Shibata T, Itoh K, Maetani Y, Isoda H, Hiraoka M, Egawa H, Tanaka K, Togashi K. Outcome of percutaneous transhepatic venoplasty for hepatic venous outflow obstruction after living donor liver transplantation. Radiology. 2006;239:285–90.
12. Valla D-C, Cazals-Hatem D. Vascular liver diseases on the clinical side: definitions and diagnosis, new concepts. Virchows Arch. 2018;473:3–13.
13. Cazals-Hatem D, Vilgrain V, Genin P, Denninger M-H, Durand F, Belghiti J, Valla D, Degott C. Arterial and portal circulation and parenchymal changes in Budd-Chiari syndrome: a study in 17 explanted livers. Hepatology. 2003;37:510–9.
14. Faraoun SA, Boudjella MEA, Debzi N, Afredj N, Guerrache Y, Benidir N, Bouzid C, Bentabak K, Soyer P, Bendib SE. Budd–Chiari syndrome: a prospective analysis of hepatic vein obstruction on ultrasonography, multidetector-row computed tomography and MR imaging. Abdom Imaging. 2015;40:1500–9.
15. Simonetto DA, Yang H, Yin M, et al. Chronic passive venous congestion drives hepatic fibrogenesis via sinusoidal thrombosis and mechanical forces. Hepatology. 2014;61:648–59.
16. Janssen HLA, Garcia-Pagan J-C, Elias E, Mentha G, Hadengue A, Valla D-C. Budd-Chiari syndrome: a review by an expert panel. J Hepatol. 2003;38:364–71.
17. Murad SD, Valla D-C, de Groen PC, Zeitoun G, Hopmans JAM, Haagsma EB, van Hoek B, Hansen BE, Rosendaal FR, Janssen HLA. Determinants of survival and the effect of portosystemic shunting in patients with Budd-Chiari syndrome. Hepatology. 2004;39:500–8.
18. Murad S, Plessier A, Hernandez-Guerra M, et al. Etiology, management, and outcome of the Budd-Chiari syndrome. Ann Intern Med. 2009;151:167–75.
19. Faraoun SA, Boudjella MEA, Debzi N, Benidir N, Afredj N, Guerrache Y, Bentabak K, Soyer P, Bendib SE. Budd-Chiari syndrome: an update on imaging features. Clin Imaging. 2016;40:637–46.
20. Moucari R, Rautou P-E, Cazals-Hatem D, et al. Hepatocellular carcinoma in Budd–Chiari syndrome: characteristics and risk factors. Gut. 2008;57:828 LP–835.
21. Valla D-C. The diagnosis and management of the Budd-Chiari syndrome: consensus and controversies. Hepatology. 2007;38:793–803.
22. Klein AS. Management of Budd-Chiari syndrome. Liver Transplant. 2006;12:S23–8.
23. Das CJ, Soneja M, Tayal S, Chahal A, Srivastava S, Kumar A, Baruah U. Role of radiological imaging and interventions in the management of Budd-Chiari syndrome. Clin Radiol. 2018;73:610–24.
24. Fu Y-F, Li Y, Cui Y-F, Wei N, Li D-C, Xu H. Percutaneous recanalization for combined-type Budd-Chiari syndrome: strategy and long-term outcome. Abdom Imaging. 2015;40:3240–7.
25. Rautou P-E, Moucari R, Escolano S, et al. Prognostic indices for Budd–Chiari syndrome: valid for clinical studies but insufficient for individual management. Am J Gastroenterol. 2009;104:1140.
26. Kinjo N, Kawanaka H, Akahoshi T, et al. Portal vein thrombosis in liver cirrhosis. World J Hepatol. 2014;6:64–71.
27. de Franchis R. Expanding consensus in portal hypertension. J Hepatol. 2015;63:743–52.
28. Stine JG, Shah PM, Cornella SL, Rudnick SR, Ghabril MS, Stukenborg GJ, Northup PG. Portal vein thrombosis, mortality and hepatic decompensation in patients with cirrhosis: a meta-analysis. World J Hepatol. 2015;7:2774–80.
29. Amitrano L, Anna Guardascione M, Brancaccio V, Margaglione M, Manguso F, Iannaccone L, Grandone E, Balzano A. Risk factors and clinical presentation of portal vein thrombosis in patients with liver cirrhosis. J Hepatol. 2004;40:736–41.
30. Plessier A, Darwish-Murad S, Hernandez-Guerra M, et al. Acute portal vein thrombosis unrelated to cirrhosis: a prospective multicenter follow-up study. Hepatology. 2009;51:210–8.
31. Janssen HLA, Meinardi JR, Vleggaar FP, et al. Factor V Leiden mutation, prothrombin gene mutation, and deficiencies in coagulation inhibitors associated with Budd-Chiari syndrome and portal vein thrombosis: results of a case-control study. Blood. 2000;96:2364–8.
32. Kobayashi S, Ng CS, Kazama T, Madoff DC, Faria SC, Vauthey JN, Charnsangavej C. Hemodynamic and morphologic changes after portal vein embolization: differential effects in central and peripheral zones in the liver on multiphasic computed tomography. J Comput Assist Tomogr. 2004;28
33. Tublin ME, Towbin AJ, Federle MP, Nalesnik MA. Altered liver morphology after portal vein thrombosis: not always cirrhosis. Dig Dis Sci. 2008;53:2784–8.
34. Nakanuma Y, Hoso M, Sasaki M, Terada T, Katayanagi K, Nonomura A, Kurumaya H, Harada A, Obata H. Histopathology of

the liver in non-cirrhotic portal hypertension of unknown aetiology. Histopathology. 2018;28:195–204.
35. Valla D-C, Condat B. Portal vein thrombosis in adults: pathophysiology, pathogenesis and management. J Hepatol. 2000;32:865–71.
36. Elkrief L, Corcos O, Bruno O, et al. Type 2 diabetes mellitus as a risk factor for intestinal resection in patients with superior mesenteric vein thrombosis. Liver Int. 2013;34:1314–21.
37. Turnes J, García–Pagán JC, González M, et al. Portal hypertension and related complications after acute portal vein thrombosis: impact of early anticoagulation. Clin Gastroenterol Hepatol. 2008;6:1412–7.
38. Sharma P, Sharma BC, Puri V, Sarin SK. Natural history of minimal hepatic encephalopathy in patients with extrahepatic portal vein obstruction. Am J Gastroenterol. 2009;104:885.
39. Rajani R, Björnsson E, Bergquist A, Danielsson Å, Gustavsson A, Grip O, Melin T, Sangfelt P, Wallerstedt S, Almer S. The epidemiology and clinical features of portal vein thrombosis: a multicentre study. Aliment Pharmacol Ther. 2010;32:1154–62.
40. Berzigotti A, García-Criado Á, Darnell A, García-Pagán J-C. Imaging in clinical decision-making for portal vein thrombosis. Nat Rev Gastroenterol Hepatol. 2014;11:308.
41. Bach AM, Hann LE, Brown KT, Getrajdman GI, Herman SK, Fong Y, Blumgart LH. Portal vein evaluation with US: comparison to angiography combined with CT arterial portography. Radiology. 1996;201:149–54.
42. Seedial SM, Mouli SK, Desai KR. Acute portal vein thrombosis: current trends in medical and endovascular management. Semin Interv Radiol. 2018;35:198–202.
43. Condat B, Pessione F, Helene Denninger M, Hillaire S, Valla D. Recent portal or mesenteric venous thrombosis: increased recognition and frequent recanalization on anticoagulant therapy. Hepatology. 2003;32:466–70.
44. Ferro C, Rossi UG, Bovio G, Dahamane M, Centanaro M. Transjugular intrahepatic portosystemic shunt, mechanical aspiration thrombectomy, and direct thrombolysis in the treatment of acute portal and superior mesenteric vein thrombosis. Cardiovasc Intervent Radiol. 2007;30:1070–4.
45. Sogaard KK, Astrup LB, Vilstrup H, Gronbaek H. Portal vein thrombosis; risk factors, clinical presentation and treatment. BMC Gastroenterol. 2007;7:34.
46. Cao G, Ko G-Y, Sung K-B, Yoon H-K, Il GD, Kim J-H. Treatment of postoperative main portal vein and superior mesenteric vein thrombosis with balloon angioplasty and/or stent placement. Acta Radiol. 2013;54:526–32.
47. Senzolo M, Tibbals J, Cholongitas E, Triantos CK, Burroughs AK, Patch D. Transjugular intrahepatic portosystemic shunt for portal vein thrombosis with and without cavernous transformation. Aliment Pharmacol Ther. 2006;23:767–75.
48. Harmanci O, Bayraktar Y. How can portal vein cavernous transformation cause chronic incomplete biliary obstruction? World J Gastroenterol. 2012;18:3375–8.
49. Valla D-C, Cazals-Hatem D. Sinusoidal obstruction syndrome. Clin Res Hepatol Gastroenterol. 2016;40:378–85.
50. Rubbia-Brandt L, Lauwers GY, Wang H, et al. Sinusoidal obstruction syndrome and nodular regenerative hyperplasia are frequent oxaliplatin-associated liver lesions and partially prevented by bevacizumab in patients with hepatic colorectal metastasis. Histopathology. 2010;56:430–9.
51. Marquardsen FA, Baldin F, Wunderer F, et al. Detection of Sp110 by flow cytometry and application to screening patients for veno-occlusive disease with immunodeficiency. J Clin Immunol. 2017;37:707–14.
52. Angliviel B, Benoist S, Penna C, El Hajjam M, Chagnon S, Julié C, Beauchet A, Rougier P, Nordlinger B. Impact of chemotherapy on the accuracy of computed tomography scan for the evaluation of colorectal liver metastases. Ann Surg Oncol. 2009;16:1247–53.
53. Slade JH, Alattar ML, Fogelman DR, et al. Portal hypertension associated with oxaliplatin administration: clinical manifestations of hepatic sinusoidal injury. Clin Colorectal Cancer. 2009;8:225–30.
54. Mahgerefteh SY, Sosna J, Bogot N, Shapira MY, Pappo O, Bloom AI. Radiologic imaging and intervention for gastrointestinal and hepatic complications of hematopoietic stem cell transplantation. Radiology. 2011;258:660–71.
55. Ruutu T, Eriksson B, Remes K, Juvonen E, Volin L, Remberger M, Parkkali T, Hägglund H, Ringdén O. Ursodeoxycholic acid for the prevention of hepatic complications in allogeneic stem cell transplantation. Blood. 2002;100:1977–83.
56. Imran H, Tleyjeh IM, Zirakzadeh A, Rodriguez V, Khan SP. Use of prophylactic anticoagulation and the risk of hepatic veno-occlusive disease in patients undergoing hematopoietic stem cell transplantation: a systematic review and meta-analysis. Bone Marrow Transplant. 2006;37:677.
57. Azoulay D, Castaing D, Lemoine A, Hargreaves GM, Bismuth H. Transjugular intrahepatic portosystemic shunt (TIPS) for severe veno-occlusive disease of the liver following bone marrow transplantation. Bone Marrow Transplant. 2000;25:987.
58. Song W, Zhao D, Li H, Ding J, He N, Chen Y. Liver findings in patients with hereditary hemorrhagic telangiectasia. Iran J Radiol. 2016;13:e31116.
59. Faughnan ME, Palda VA, Garcia-Tsao G, et al. International guidelines for the diagnosis and management of hereditary haemorrhagic telangiectasia. J Med Genet. 2011;48:73–87.
60. Garcia-Tsao G. Liver involvement in hereditary hemorrhagic telangiectasia (HHT). J Hepatol. 2007;46:499–507.
61. Blewitt RW, Brown CM, Wyatt JI. The pathology of acute hepatic disintegration in hereditary haemorrhagic telangiectasia. Histopathology. 2003;42:265–9.
62. Schelker RC, Barreiros AP, Hart C, Herr W, Jung E-M. Macro- and microcirculation patterns of intrahepatic blood flow changes in patients with hereditary hemorrhagic telangiectasia. World J Gastroenterol. 2017;23:486–95.
63. Buscarini E, Leandro G, Conte D, et al. Natural history and outcome of hepatic vascular malformations in a large cohort of patients with hereditary hemorrhagic telangiectasia. Dig Dis Sci. 2011;56:2166–78.
64. Wu JS, Saluja S, Garcia-Tsao G, Chong A, Henderson KJ, White RI. Liver involvement in hereditary hemorrhagic telangiectasia: CT and clinical findings do not correlate in symptomatic patients. Am J Roentgenol. 2006;187:W399–405.
65. Buscarini E, Plauchu H, Garcia Tsao G, et al. Liver involvement in hereditary hemorrhagic telangiectasia: consensus recommendations. Liver Int. 2006;26:1040–6.
66. Khalid SK, Garcia-Tsao G. Hepatic vascular malformations in hereditary hemorrhagic telangiectasia. Semin Liver Dis. 2008;28:247–58.
67. Dupuis-Girod S, Ginon I, Saurin J, et al. Bevacizumab in patients with hereditary hemorrhagic telangiectasia and severe hepatic vascular malformations and high cardiac output. JAMA. 2012;307:948–55.
68. Gallego C, Miralles M, Marín C, Muyor P, González G, García-Hidalgo E. Congenital hepatic shunts. Radiographics. 2004;24:755–72.
69. Papamichail M, Pizanias M, Heaton N. Congenital portosystemic venous shunt. Eur J Pediatr. 2018;177:285–94.
70. Kim MJ, Ko JS, Seo JK, Yang HR, Chang JY, Kim GB, Cheon J-E, Kim WS. Clinical features of congenital portosystemic shunt in children. Eur J Pediatr. 2012;171:395–400.
71. Murray CP, Yoo S-J, Babyn PS. Congenital extrahepatic portosystemic shunts. Pediatr Radiol. 2003;33:614–20.

12 Liver Ischaemia-Reperfusion Injury

Farid Froghi, Saied Froghi, and Brian R. Davidson

Key Concepts

- Ischaemia-reperfusion occurs due to a temporary cessation and restoration of blood flow to the liver.
- Liver IR injury develops as a result of a complex network of inflammation and endothelial activation resulting in cell death.
- Liver IR injury is common in liver surgery and transplantation and remains the main cause of morbidity and mortality.
- Several treatments have shown benefit in experimental IR, however none have been translated into routine clinical practise.
- Promising recent developments in pharmacological agents and machine perfusion of organs are currently being investigated.

12.1 Introduction

The absence of oxygen and nutrients during ischaemia affects all tissues with aerobic metabolism. Ischaemia of these tissues creates a condition which upon the restoration of circulation results in further inflammation and oxidative damage (reperfusion injury). Restoration of blood flow to an ischaemic organ is essential to prevent irreversible tissue injury, however reperfusion of the organ or tissues may result in a local and systemic inflammatory response augmenting tissue injury in excess of that produced by ischaemia alone. This process of organ damage with ischaemia being exacerbated by reperfusion is called ischaemia-reperfusion (IR) injury and is relevant to several disease processes where there is a temporary cessation followed by restoration of blood supply including liver surgery and transplantation. Regardless of the disease process, severity of IR injury depends on the length of ischaemic time as well as size and pre-ischaemic condition of the affected tissue. The liver is the largest solid organ in the body, hence liver IR injury can have profound local and systemic consequences, particularly in those with pre-existing liver disease.

Liver IR injury is common following liver surgery and transplantation and remains the main cause of morbidity and mortality.

12.1.1 Definitions

Ischaemia is a reduction or absence of blood supply to an organ resulting in a lack of oxygen and vital nutrients in tissues.

Warm ischaemia occurs with interruption of blood flow at body temperature (37 °C) and develops in situ during liver surgery, transplantation or systemic shock.

Cold ischaemia occurs during cold (4 °C) ex vivo organ preservation. Cold ischaemia is usually coupled with warm ischaemia during liver transplantation surgery.

Reperfusion is the restoration of blood supply to an ischaemic organ.

Ischaemia-reperfusion (IR) injury is the cellular damage after reperfusion of previously viable ischaemic tissues.

12.2 Aetiology

The liver has a dual blood supply from the hepatic artery (20%) and the portal vein (80%). A temporary reduction in blood supply to the liver causes IR injury. This can be due to a *systemic* reduction or *local* cessation and restoration of blood flow.

F. Froghi · S. Froghi · B. R. Davidson (✉)
UCL Division of Surgery and Interventional Science, University College London, London, UK

Department of Hepato-pancreatico-biliary Surgery, Royal Free Hospital, London, UK
e-mail: b.davidson@ucl.ac.uk

F. Radu-Ionita et al. (eds.), *Liver Diseases*, https://doi.org/10.1007/978-3-030-24432-3_12

- *Systemic* causes include severe hypotension and shock followed by resuscitation—the so called 'shock liver' that occurs in trauma and sepsis. Liver hypoperfusion can also occur in patients who recover from a cardiac arrest or undergo cardiopulmonary bypass.
- *Local* cessation and restoration of liver blood supply occurs with temporary 'inflow occlusion' applied to control bleeding in liver surgery and routinely occurs with liver transplantation during organ procurement until the donor organ is revascularised in the recipient. Portal vein resection and reconstruction during surgery for liver, biliary or pancreatic cancers may also involve temporary clamping of the portal vein and results in a degree of liver IR injury.

12.2.1 Liver Surgery

Liver resections are performed for primary or secondary tumours of the liver and carry a substantial risk of bleeding especially in patients with chronic liver disease. Significant blood loss is associated with increased transfusion requirements, tumour recurrence, complications and increased morbidity and mortality. Several methods of hepatic vascular control have been described in order to minimise blood loss during elective liver resection (Fig. 12.1). The simplest and most common method is inflow occlusion by applying a tape or vascular clamp across the hepatoduodenal ligament (Pringle manoeuvre). This occludes both the arterial and portal vein inflow to the liver and leads to a period of warm ischaemia (37 °C) to the liver parenchyma resulting in 'warm' IR injury when the temporary inflow occlusion is relieved. In major liver surgery, extensive mobilisation of the liver itself without inflow occlusion results in a significant reduction in hepatic oxygenation.

12.2.2 Liver Transplantation

Liver transplantation is performed as a curative procedure for patients with end-stage liver disease. IR injury occurs as a result of cellular damage during the retrieval surgery, organ preservation as well as the transplantation surgery itself. The current process of organ procurement involves both warm and cold ischaemia. Warm ischaemia occurs during the organ retrieval surgery where liver mobilisation and episodes of donor hypotension result in hypoperfusion of the liver. In non-heart beating donors, warm ischaemia occurs before the donor organs are flushed with cold preservation solution which leads to a severe ischaemic insult. Cold ischaemia starts during cold perfusion of the donor organ and continues in the setting of cold preservation. The donor liver also sustains a short period of warm ischaemia during implantation surgery as the vessels are anastomosed and the liver warms. Reperfusion injury then occurs once the liver is revascularised and blood flow is re-established in the recipient. This process is occasionally referred to as the 'preservation-reperfusion injury'.

12.3 Risk Factors

Identifying risk factors for IR injury are extremely important in patient selection for liver surgery and transplantation. The main factors are the donor or patient age, the duration of

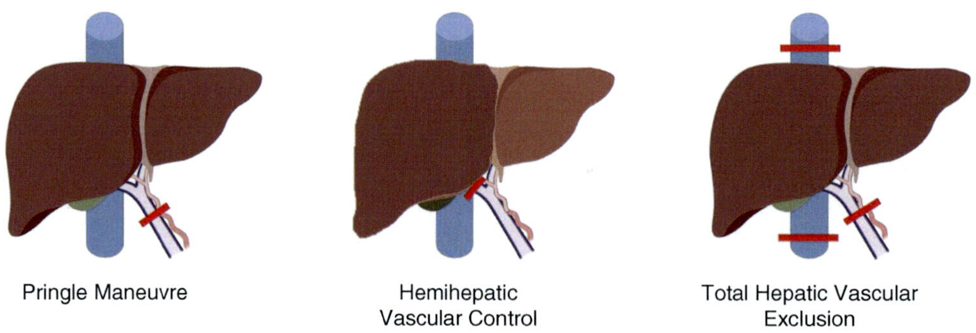

Fig. 12.1 Methods for vascular control in liver surgery. Pringle (1908) described the first method by total compression of the hepatoduodenal ligament at the foramen of Winslow with a tape or vascular clamp. This is the easiest and most common method for controlling hepatic inflow, which is also used for rapid control of traumatic bleeding from the liver. However, concomitant occlusion of oxygenated hepatic artery supply as well as portal blood flow, increasing the risk of liver ischaemic lesions and intestinal congestion. Hence, to maintain oxygenated arterial supply to the remnant liver, a selective occlusion of the portal vein only has been proposed. Bismuth and Makuuchi (1987), later described hemihepatic vascular occlusion to reduce visceral congestion and ischaemia to the remnant liver. This technique interrupts arterial and venous inflow to the right or left hemiliver avoiding both splanchnic blood stasis and remnant liver ischaemia. Although selective clamping can reduce bleeding during parenchymal transection, it requires portal vein and hepatic artery dissection which is time consuming and can itself be the source of bleeding. Total hepatic vascular exclusion of the liver involves concomitant occlusion of the inferior vena cava (IVC) as well as inflow occlusion at the portal triad. This technique, or variations thereof involving IVC occlusion is very rarely used in liver resections as it causes significant haemodynamic instability

organ ischaemia, presence or absence of liver steatosis and in transplantation whether the donor organ has been retrieved from a brain dead or cardiac death donor.

12.3.1 Liver Surgery

In liver surgery, prolonged hepatic inflow occlusion causes post-operative liver dysfunction. Elderly patients tolerate liver resection less than younger patients due to an impaired ability to eliminate free radicals and reduced response to growth factors in the process of liver regeneration after hepatectomy. Liver steatosis or pre-existing dysfunction reduce the ischaemic tolerance of the liver. These combined with extensive parenchymal resections increase the risk of IR injury to the small remnant liver and post-operative hepatic insufficiency.

12.3.2 Liver Transplantation

There is an acute shortage of organ donors for liver transplantation. Approximately, 15–20% of patients with end-stage liver disease die on the waiting list in the US and UK due to a shortage of organ donors. This is compounded by a worldwide reduction in the number of brain-dead donors (DBD) with improvements in neurosurgical care. In contrast there has been a rise in the use of non-heart beating donors (DCD) which sustain a greater ischaemic injury. Currently, around 20% of DBD donor livers are discarded due to the high risk of graft failure. The discard rate for DCD donors are as high as 70% [1] as they are associated with a higher degree of IR injury and ultimately reduced graft and patient survival.

To reduce the mortality on the transplant waiting list livers from older, steatotic donors with prolonged periods of warm and cold ischaemic times have been used for transplantation. These *extended criteria donors* are particularly susceptible to IR injury and are associated with a higher degree of primary non-function (PGN) and post-transplant biliary complications. Donor risk is discussed in more detail in the treatments section of this chapter.

12.4 Pathophysiology

A complex cellular and molecular network of hepatocytes, Kupffer cells, liver sinusoidal endothelial cells (LSEC), leukocytes and cytokines play a role in the pathogenesis of IR injury. In general, both warm and cold ischaemia share similar mechanisms of injury. Hepatocyte injury is a predominant feature of warm ischaemia, whilst endothelial cells are more susceptible to cold ischaemic injury. There are currently no proven treatments for liver IR injury. Understanding this complex network is essential in developing therapeutic strategies in prevention and treatment of IR injury. The following is a brief summary of the main events which are illustrated in Fig. 12.2.

12.4.1 Intracellular Events

Cellular acidosis occurs in the initial ischaemic period as a result of cellular hypoxia and a shift from aerobic to anaerobic respiration. This involves ATP depletion and accelerated glycolysis within mitochondria as well as lactic acid production. The initial reduction in pH has been shown to play an important protective role in the ischaemic period. However, increasing levels of intracellular toxic acidic metabolites affects pH-dependant cellular processes including cell signalling, electrolyte homeostasis (Na^+/K^+ ATPase pump and Ca^{2+}) and mitochondrial dysfunction which in turn leads to cellular swelling and hepatocyte damage. Upon reperfusion, the pH values return to normal which enhances pH-dependant activation of harmful enzymes such as proteases and phospholipidases leading to cellular and mitochondrial membrane damage and exacerbated injury to tissues. This phenomenon has been termed the *pH paradox*.

Intracellular Ca^{2+} overload occurs due to a failure of membrane pumps and release from endoplasmic reticulum Ca^{2+} stores. This along with failure of the Na/K^+ ATP pump leads to cell swelling. Ca^{2+} is taken up by the mitochondria to act as a buffer for the increase in cytosolic levels. This results in disruption of the mitochondrial electron transport chain, failure of ATP production and release of cytochrome C into the cytosol which triggers cell death. Important Ca^{2+} dependant enzymes involved in apoptosis such as calpains, protein kinase C and phospholipidase C are also activated.

ROS production and oxidative stress are the hallmark of liver IR injury pathogenesis. A combination of excess production of reactive oxygen/nitrogen species (ROS/RNS) as well as concomitant depletion of endogenous antioxidants lead to cellular injury. ATP depletion in the ischaemic phase leads to anaerobic respiration and an increase in ATP-degradation products such as adenosine, hypoxanthine and xanthine. At early reperfusion, the rate of oxygen delivery exceeds that of cellular activity returning to aerobic pathways. This results in the production of damaging oxygen free radicals (superoxides, hydrogen peroxide and reactive nitrogen species). This process is thought to occur via three main pathways: xanthine oxidase, NADPH oxidase and uncoupling of the mitochondrial electron transport chain. In the early phase of reperfusion Kupffer cells are thought to be the main source of ROS production with natural killer (NK) T cells and neutrophils being the main source in the later stages. The excess ROS causes direct damage to hepatocytes

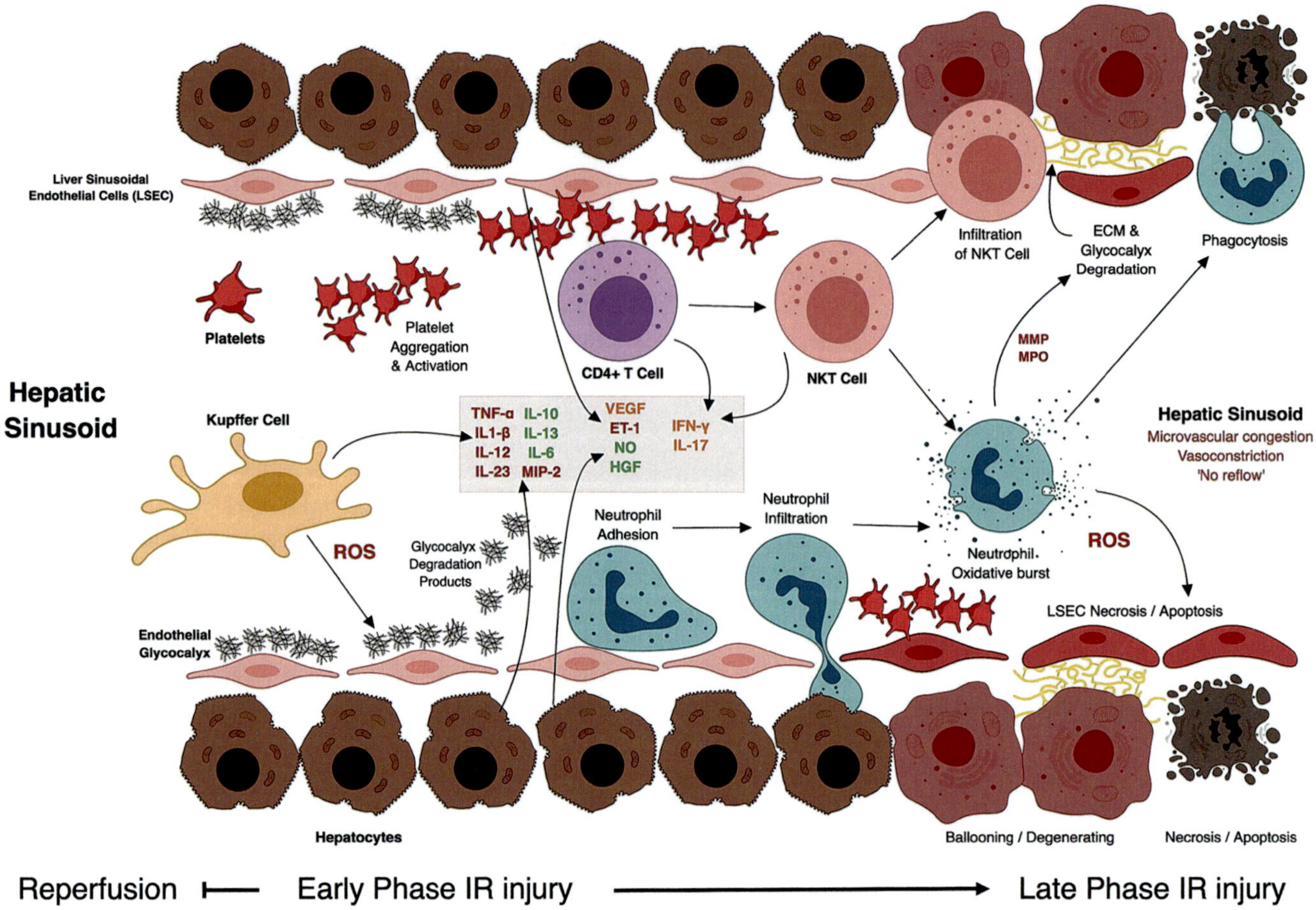

Fig. 12.2 Pathophysiology of hepatic ischaemia-reperfusion injury. In summary, the pathogenesis of liver IR involves an early and late phase initiated during ischaemia. The early phase of reperfusion is characterised by activation of complement cascade which in turn activates resident Kupffer cell (KC) and appearance of reactive oxygen species (ROS) and endothelial cell activation. As reperfusion progresses, the release of cytotoxic mediators leads to a substantial breakdown of the hepatic microcirculation and activation and recruitment of circulating inflammatory cells which compounds the damage already sustained during the ischaemic period causing apoptosis and necrosis of hepatocytes

and endothelial cells by acting on proteins, enzymes, nucleic acids, cytoskeleton and lipid peroxides leading to lipid peroxidation and mitochondrial dysfunction.

Mitochondrial dysfunction is initiated by a lack of oxygen which interrupts oxidative phosphorylation and ATP production. Lack of ATP disrupts mitochondrial electrolyte homeostasis which are essential for aerobic respiration. Furthermore, at reperfusion the mitochondria can be a source of toxic ROS production. Activated phospholipidase and protease enzymes cause direct damage to the mitochondria membrane leading to membrane instability and mitochondrial permeability transition. This leads to rapid influx of large molecular weight solutes through 'mitochondrial megachannels' causing swelling and initiating apoptotic pathways through cytochrome C release.

Cell death occurs in hepatocytes and LSECs through both apoptosis and necrosis. Cell necrosis refers to cell death in tissues due to disease or injury whereas apoptosis is an energy dependant activation of genes involved in programmed cell death. Whilst it is intuitive to think cellular injury in IR occurs exclusively due to necrosis, several in vivo and ex vivo studies of liver IR have shown activation of apoptotic pathways including caspase-3 and Bax.

12.4.2 Innate Immune Response

DAMPs are damage associated molecular patterns; 'danger signalling molecules' that can initiate and perpetuate a non-infectious inflammatory response. DAMPs are the normal constituents of cells and extracellular matrix which are either released as a result of cell death or expressed on the cell surface as a result of cellular injury. LSEC and hepatocyte cell death as a result of ischaemia releases cell fragments such as DNA material, histones and high-mobility group box 1 (HMGB1) into the circulation. DAMPs interact with pattern recognition receptors (PRR) such as Toll-like receptors (TLR) on Kupffer cells, dendritic cells, and neutrophils to initiate an inflammatory process. This inflammatory process arising from tissue injury allow destruction and removal of harmful tissue. There is increasing evidence for TLR4 activation in IR injury supporting evidence for antigen independent activation of CD4+ T cells [2].

Complement activation plays an important role in both local and remote IR injury acting directly via the formation of membrane attack complexes (MAC) and indirectly by cytokine and chemokine activation. The complement system is activated by one of three pathways: the antibody dependent classical pathway, the alternate pathway and the mannose binding lectin pathway. Whilst all three pathways are implicated in the development and enhancement of IR injury, the relative importance of each pathway is not clear. Complement enhances Kupffer cell activation and neutrophil recruitment to the liver.

12.4.3 Cellular Response

Kupffer Cells are the liver resident macrophages and form the earliest cellular response in liver ischaemic injury. Kupffer cells are activated during ischaemia and early stages of reperfusion via the complement system and become a powerful source of cytokine (TNF-alpha and IL-1β) and ROS production. This leads to LSEC activation and expression of adhesion molecules such as ICAM-1 and VCAM-1 which in turn enhance circulating leukocyte chemotaxis, adhesion and transmigration.

Neutrophils are recruited to the liver after reperfusion by a complex network of chemokines released from KCs and LSECs such as macrophage inflammatory protein-2 (MIP2). Neutrophils cause cellular injury by releasing matrix metalloproteases (MMP) and myeloperoxidases (MPO) which are potent oxidants. The neutrophil oxidative burst supersedes KCs as the main source of ROS production in the later stages of IR injury which causes direct damage to hepatocytes, LSECs and the extracellular matrix (ECM). A combination of ECM degradation and LSECs activation further promotes neutrophil adhesion and infiltration within the liver parenchyma.

CD4+ T cells are recruited to the liver after reperfusion and play an important role in the adaptive immune response to liver IR. There are several subsets of CD4+ T cells and depending on the subset can have a protective or harmful effect. Of note, natural killer (NK) T cells contribute to neutrophil activation via release of interferon gamma (IFNg) and IL-17. Knockout models of CD4+ T cells expressing αβ TCR can inhibit neutrophil recruitment and oxidative burst.

Platelets are activated and adhere to LSECs within minutes of reperfusion through interaction with adhesion molecules (ICAM-1, VCAM-1 and E-selectin) and ECM degradation products such as fibrinogen. Platelet adhesion and aggregation leads to reduced microcirculatory perfusion.

12.4.4 Inflammatory Mediators

Several proinflammatory and anti-inflammatory cytokines, chemokines and growth factors are produced by KCs, hepatocytes, LSECs, and leukocytes. The relevant important cytokines are listed in Table 12.1 and Fig. 12.1.

12.4.5 Microcirculatory Failure

A combination of platelet and leukocyte accumulation as well as direct damage to hepatocytes, LSECs and vasoconstriction in early reperfusion results in a reduction in sinusoidal diameter and reduced flow. Some areas even have no flow despite reperfusion of the liver—this is referred to as the 'no reflow' phenomenon.

- *Imbalance of vasoactive substances* important in liver blood flow regulation results in microvascular failure. Vasoconstriction occurs due to an excess of endothelin-1 (ET-1) production in early reperfusion secondary to KC activation. ET-1 is a powerful vasoconstrictor and excess levels result in micro and macrovascular reduction in blood flow to the liver. Nitric oxide (NO), released by vascular endothelial cells in response to shear stress, on the other hand is a vasodilator and promotes cell survival through inhibition of caspase activities. NO also regulates microcirculatory vascular tone and inhibits platelet aggregation. Other protective effects of NO include inhibition of proinflammatory cytokines and suppression of induced T cells. Therefore, a reduction of NO production would result in decreased microvascular perfusion.
- *Endothelial glycocalyx* (GXL) degradation has recently been implicated in liver IR. This is a thin and fragile layer of proteoglycans and glycosaminoglycans on the luminal surface of all blood vessels including the liver sinusoids. It plays an important role in vascular permeability, endothelial-leukocyte/platelet interaction (inflammation and coagulation) as well as mechanotransduction (NO production).

In hepatic IR, the glycocalyx layer is disintegrated, both in the liver sinusoids and systemic vasculature by direct damage from ROS and cytokines (TNF-α) as well as cleavage of its core proteins by enzymes released from LSECs and neutrophils (MMP and MPO). The endothelial GXL prevents macromolecule transit into the intersti-

Table 12.1 Key inflammatory cytokines in IR injury

Cytokines	Primary secretion	Actions	Mechanism
TNF-α	KCs, Hepatocytes, distant organs	Pro-inflammatory:	Direct liver injury through inducing production of epithelial neutrophil activating protein-78 (ENA-78) and ROS, activate nuclear factor (NF)-κB, mitogen-activated protein kinase and c-Jun N-terminal kinase (JNK). Upregulation of chemokines ICAM-1, VCAM-1 and P-selectin.
IL-1β	KCs and Hepatocytes	Pro-inflammatory:	Upregulation of leukocyte aggregation and adhesion by activating NF-κB and macrophage inflammatory protein (MIP)-2. Upregulation of NO synthesis through the protein kinase B (Akt), NF-κB, and inducible nitric oxide synthase (iNOS) pathways.
IL-12 and IL-23	KCs and Hepatocytes	Pro-inflammatory:	Stimulates CD4 T cells to produce IL-17, which enhances accumulation of neutrophils and aggravates liver damage. Increase TNF-α production by activating NF-κB and signal transducer and activator of transcription (STAT)-4.
IFN-γ	T cells and NKT cells	Dual function:	Enhancement or downregulation of neutrophil accumulation and activation in a dose-dependent manner.
VEGF	LSECs, KCs and Hepatocytes	Dual function:	Exogenous administration of VEGF protects the liver by upregulating iNOS production. However, IR injury activates VEGF receptor and Src tyrosine kinase and upregulates the expression of TNF-α, E-selectin, monocyte chemoattractant protein-1 (MCP-1) all of which result in the accumulation of intrahepatic T lymphocytes, macrophages and neutrophils, producing liver damage.
IL-6	KCs and Hepatocytes	Anti-inflammatory:	Promotes hepatocyte proliferation and reduces damage by upregulation of glutathione (GSH) expression, activation of STAT-3 and downregulation of oxidative stress markers.
IL-10 and IL-13	KCs and T lymphocytes	Anti-inflammatory:	Protective role mediated by upregulation of B-cell lymphoma (Bcl)-2/bcl-x, heme oxygenase (HO)-1, and downregulation of NF-κB, IL-2, IL-1β, MIP-2, IFN-γ, E-selectin, cytokine-induced neutrophil chemotaxin, and neutrophil aggregation.
HGF	Hepatocytes	Anti-inflammatory:	It can increase hepatocyte DNA synthesis, proliferation, and glutathione expression, inhibit cytokine-induced neutrophil chemotaxin and neutrophil permeability, and downregulate the expression of the oxidative stress marker ICAM-1 in sinusoidal endothelial cells, further reduces liver damage and promotes liver cell proliferation

VEGF vascular endothelial growth factor, *HGF* hepatocyte growth factor

tium and degradation leads to increased vascular permeability and tissue oedema. The consequences of systemic GXL injury are mainly as a result of increased vascular permeability which leads to acute lung injury and respiratory failure, proteinuria and renal failure, increased cardiac strain in the heart, bacterial translocation and intestinal ileus. Recent evidence has shown that GXL shedding is associated with ARDS and multiple organ failure in ICU patients [3].

Furthermore, GXL degradation augments the inflammatory response in two ways: first, the degraded products act as DAMPS in the circulation which leads to activation of innate immune responses. Second, the protective layer that is formed by the GXL reduces the leukocyte interaction with the adhesion molecules expressed on the endothelial surface acting as an 'immune camouflage'. With loss of endothelial GXL, there is an increased interaction of leukocytes with the cell surface adhesion molecules (ICAM-1 and VECAM-1) leading to an augmented inflammatory cell response. Similarly, platelet interactions with endothelial surface molecules such as von Willebrand Factor and P-Selectin are increased leading to activation of coagulation cascade (Fig. 12.2).

12.5 Clinical Manifestation

The consequences of liver IR can be divided into *local (direct)* injury to the liver or *systemic (remote)* injury to other organs.

12.5.1 Direct Injury to the Liver

Direct liver IR injury can manifest itself as derangement in liver function and if severe could lead to fulminant liver failure. The mildest form of hepatic IR injury can be seen as a post-operative rise in liver aminotransferase enzymes after liver surgery where a short period of inflow occlusion has been applied. More severe forms can lead to post-operative hepatic insufficiency and mortality after liver surgery.

In liver transplantation IR injury can result in early allograft dysfunction (10%) which may progress to primary non-function (2%) requiring re-transplantation. The problem is particularly common with use of marginal donors. Ischaemic cholangiopathy is a late complication presenting within 12 months of liver transplantation. The rate of biliary complications is higher in DCD (16–29%) than DBD

Table 12.2 Suzuki histological classification of the severity of liver ischaemia-reperfusion injury

Numerical assessment	Sinusoidal congestion	Vacuolisation/ ballooning	Necrosis
0	None	None	None
1	Minimal	Minimal	Single cell
2	Mild	Mild	<30%
3	Moderate	Moderate	30–60%
4	Severe	Severe	>60%

(3–17%) grafts. The relative increase in the incidence of post-transplant ischaemic cholangiopathy with the use of DCD and extended criteria donors is partly due to the increased severity of IR injury.

The extent of *local* liver IR injury is usually measured by a rise in aspartate/alanine transaminases (AST/ALT) and lactate dehydrogenase (LDH). Although the rise in transaminases correlate with the degree of IR injury, a specific cut-off for diagnosis of IR injury has not been established. This is primarily due to other factors affecting liver function post liver surgery and transplantation such as liver regeneration and graft rejection. Hence, peak transaminase levels in the first 7 post-operative days have been proposed for use in clinical trials of liver transplantation as a surrogate marker for IR injury severity and to predict graft and patient survival.

Liver biopsy can be used for a definitive diagnosis of IR injury by immunohistochemical grading using the Suzuki classification (Table 12.2). In this classification sinusoidal congestion, hepatocyte necrosis and ballooning degeneration are graded from 0 to 4. A liver biopsy is not routinely performed for establishing the diagnosis of IR injury as it carries a significant risk of bleeding and histological changes can take up to 4 h after reperfusion to become apparent.

12.5.2 Remote Injury to Other Organs

Systemic or *remote* IR injury occurs as a result of the spill over of the inflammatory process initiated in the liver into the systemic circulation and the effects are shared across aetiologies. Oxygen free radicals and activated leukocytes play a central role in the process of remote IR injury. In its most severe form, IR injury leads to the development of systemic inflammatory response syndrome (SIRS) through systemic release of inflammatory mediators and activation of leukocytes. A devastating consequence of this is multiple organ dysfunction syndrome (MODS); the progressive physiological failure of two or more independent organ systems requiring physiological support to maintain homeostasis. It is a documented consequence of prolonged hepatic inflow occlusion and is responsible for 30–40% of deaths in tertiary referral intensive care units.

12.5.2.1 Post-reperfusion Syndrome (PRS)

In liver transplantation, an early and significant event after reperfusion of the grafted liver is haemodynamic instability, hypotension and shock. This *post-reperfusion syndrome* is defined as an abrupt decrease in mean arterial pressure (MAP) greater than 30% below the baseline value, lasting for at least 1 min which occurs during the first 5 min of reperfusion of the graft liver. It occurs in 20% of patients and can be persistent (lasting more than 30 mins) or recurrent (reappearing within 30 min of resolution) and potentially lethal.

In the heart, arrhythmias such as ventricular fibrillation or tachycardia with or without ischaemia can occur in the early reperfusion phase. This is due to a sudden load of cold and acidotic blood coming from the reperfused liver causing coronary vasoconstriction and right heart strain. Significant electrolyte disturbances at reperfusion with increasing serum potassium and a reduction in calcium levels contribute to the development of cardiac arrhythmias. Prolonged hypotension at this stage leads to the development of acute kidney injury which is common after liver transplantation (>50%). Post-operative AKI is an independent risk factor for developing chronic kidney disease within 1-year post liver transplantation.

Furthermore, there is a sudden increase in pulmonary vascular resistance caused by pulmonary arteriolar vasoconstriction in response to a surge of inflammatory mediators. Acute lung injury (ALI) ensues due to neutrophil accumulation and increased pulmonary microvascular permeability which can progress to acute respiratory distress syndrome (ARDS) and respiratory failure requiring ventilatory support.

In the gut, prolonged portal vein clamping leads to venous congestion and oedema which causes a degree of bacterial translocation and increased inflammatory response. This is compounded by the fact that hepatic immune and detoxifying mechanisms that usually clear gut pathogens are hampered during reperfusion of the ischaemic liver.

Severe forms of PRS can lead to acute fibrinolysis and coagulopathy requiring antifibrinolytic treatment.

12.6 Prevention and Treatment

There is currently no accepted treatment for liver IR injury. Several pharmacological agents and surgical techniques have been beneficial in reducing markers of hepatocyte injury in experimental liver IR, however, they are yet to show clinical benefit in human trials. The following is an outline of current and future strategies which may be effective in reducing the detrimental effects of liver IR injury in liver surgery and transplantation.

12.6.1 Liver Surgery

12.6.1.1 Intermittent Clamping

Inflow occlusion or portal triad clamping (PTC) can be continuous or intermittent; alternating between short periods of inflow occlusion and reperfusion. Intermittent clamping (IC) increases parenchymal tolerance to ischaemia. Hence, prolonged continuous inflow occlusion rather than short intermittent periods results in greater degree of post-operative liver dysfunction. IC permits longer total ischaemia times for more complex resections. Alternating between 15 min of inflow occlusion and 5 min reperfusion cycles can be performed safely for up to 120 min total ischaemia time. There is a potential risk of increased blood loss during the periods of no inflow occlusion. However, these intervals provide an opportunity for the surgeon to check for haemostasis and control small bleeding areas from the cut surface of the liver. The optimal IC cycle times are not clear, although intermittent cycles of up to 30 min inflow occlusion have also been reported with no increase in morbidity, blood loss or liver dysfunction compared to 15 min cycles. IC is particularly beneficial in reducing post-operative liver dysfunction in patients with liver cirrhosis or steatosis.

12.6.1.2 Ischaemic Preconditioning (IPC)

Ischaemic preconditioning was first realised in canine models of myocardial infarction where brief periods of ischaemia followed by reperfusion was protective against further sustained ischaemia. The precise mechanism for ischaemic tolerance is not clear, but we know from experimental studies that this phenomenon exists in skeletal muscles, liver and the kidney [4]. In liver surgery, IPC involves a short period of ischaemia (10 min) and reperfusion (10 min) intraoperatively by portal triad clamping prior to parenchymal transection during which a longer continuous inflow occlusion is applied to minimise blood loss. It allows continuous ischaemia times of up to 40 min without significant liver dysfunction. However, the protective effect of IPC decreases with increasing age above 60 years old and compared to IC it is less effective in steatotic livers. Moreover, IPC may impair liver regeneration capacity and may not be tolerated by the small remnant liver in those with more complex and extensive liver resections increasing the risk of post-operative hepatic insufficiency.

12.6.1.3 Remote Ischaemic Preconditioning (RIPC)

In order to avoid direct ischaemic insult to the liver by inflow occlusion, remote ischaemic preconditioning (RIPC) has been used. RIPC involves preconditioning a remote organ prior to ischaemia of the target organ. It has been shown to be reduce warm IR injury to the liver in experimental studies. A recent pilot randomised trial of RIPC in patients undergoing major liver resection for colorectal liver metastasis used a tourniquet applied to the right thigh with 10 min cycles of inflation-deflation to induce IR injury to the leg for 60 min [5]. This was performed after general anaesthesia prior to skin incision. A reduction in post-operative transaminases and improved liver function was shown without the use of liver inflow occlusion. These results are promising but require validation in a larger trial addressing clinical outcomes.

12.6.1.4 Pharmacological Agents

Antioxidants are either free radical scavengers or inhibit specific pathways in ROS production. Allopurinol for example is a xanthine oxidase inhibitor which has a protective effect on the mitochondria through a reduction in oxidative stress and lipid peroxidation as well as increasing ATP levels. Vitamin E acts as a radical scavenger while α-lipoic acid has a transition metal resulting in chelation with ROS. *Melatonin* is an endogenous antioxidant produced by the pineal gland and is an important hormone in regulating the circadian rhythm. In experimental models of warm IR injury, melatonin administration reduced TNF-α and iNOS production. Although in experimental studies markers of cell injury are reduced with antioxidants, they have failed to show an improvement in clinical outcomes after liver resection in human clinical trials.

- *Anti-inflammatory* agents such as methylprednisolone has been extensively studied in warm IR in experimental studies. It reduces hepatocellular apoptosis and inflammatory mediator release as well as reducing post-operative transaminases. There is some evidence that methylprednisolone administration combined with intermittent inflow occlusion can reduce complications and length of hospital stay following liver surgery. However, routine use has been hampered with concerns of immune suppression and conflicting outcomes of clinical trials.

Pharmacological preconditioning with volatile anaesthetic agents such as sevoflurane or isoflurane 30 mins prior to warm ischaemia in liver resections reduces postoperative liver dysfunction, especially in those with liver steatosis [6]. Experimental evidence suggests the mechanism for hepatoprotection is through upregulation of the haem-oxygenase-1 pathway [7].

12.7 Liver Transplantation

Organ resuscitation is the process of improving the viability and function of marginal donor organs prior to transplantation with the primary aim of reducing the risk of IR injury and complications. Surgical and pharmacological interventions to reduce IR injury are eagerly pursued to optimise *high risk* donor livers for transplantation. This would potentially expand the donor pool leading to a reduction in waiting list deaths. Reducing the severity of IR injury would also lead to a reduction in complications associated with *low risk* donors. This process starts at organ donation and continues in the preservation and implantation in the recipient (Fig. 12.3.).

Identifying high risk donor livers is essential not only in matching organs with recipients but in the future may allow optimisation prior to transplantation. Several factors are associated with poor graft and patient survival in liver transplantation. The donor risk index (DRI) was developed to identify factors that would predict the risk of graft failure [8]. The DRI has been combined with preservation and recipient factors such as cold ischaemia times and model for end-stage liver disease (MELD) scores to better predict graft failure. However, the expansion of the donor pool to extended criteria donors as well as national allocation systems has hampered the widespread use of DRI in clinical practice.

With the advent of machine perfusion and opportunities for organ resuscitation during preservation, a new model of donor risk prediction has been developed in the United Kingdom. The UK DRI is based entirely on donor factors at organ retrieval prior to transport and preservation and aims to identify high risk organs that would benefit from resuscitation strategies [9, 10].

12.8 Donor Strategies

12.8.1 Donor Optimisation

Donor co-morbidities and damage sustained during the final illness of donors affect the quality of the donor liver. In DBD, this is compounded by the pathophysiological consequences of brain-stem death which is classically a triphasic process involving: first a Cushing's reflex of hypertension and bradycardia, followed by a massive release of catecholamines resulting in a transient hypertension, tachycardia and myocardial impairment. The final agonal phase is characterised by loss of sympathetic drive which results in a profound and refractory vasodilation, hypovolaemia and neurogenic pulmonary oedema. Other physiological derangements which may occur include diabetes insipidus, electrolyte abnormalities, disseminated intravascular coagulopathy and metabolic acidosis. In DBD donors, there is an opportunity for protect-

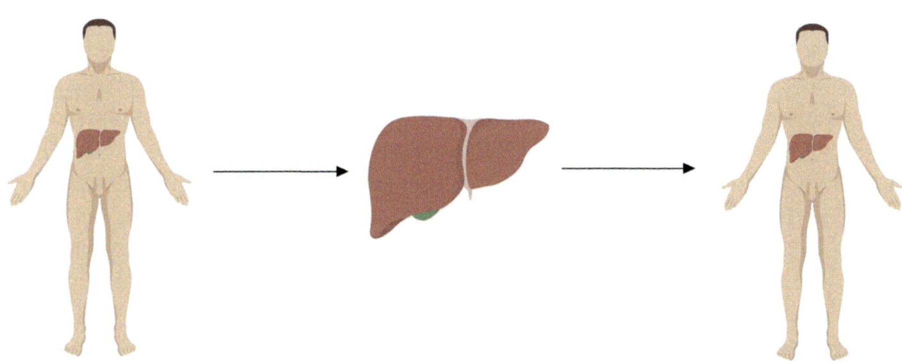

	Donor	Preservation	Recipient
Risk Factors	DBD vs. DCD Age Co-morbidities BMI / Steatosis	Warm ischaemia time Cold ischaemia time	Age MELD score Re-transplantation
Treatments	Donor optimisation Normothermic Regional Perfusion (NRP)	Preservation solutions Hypothermic machine perfusion (HMP) Normothermic machine perfusion (NMP) Pharmacological agents (e.g. oxygen, defatting agents)	Surgical techniques Ischaemic pre-conditioning Pharmacological agents (e.g. Antioxidants, NO donation, Endothelial protection)

Fig. 12.3 Summary of risk factors and treatment strategies for attenuating IR injury in liver transplantation. *DBD* donor after brain death, *DCD* donor after circulatory death, *BMI* body mass index, *MELD* model for end stage liver disease

ing the donor organs form these physiological changes as soon as a potential donor is identified. Physiological optimisation aims to improve the viability of the donor organs by correction of hypovolaemia, the use of vasopressin and weaning of epinephrine, ventilatory support after apnoea testing and methylprednisolone to attenuate systemic inflammation of brain-stem death. Such opportunity for optimisation does not exist in DCD donation due to time pressures in retrieving the organs and avoiding prolonged warm ischaemia.

12.8.2 Normothermic Regional Perfusion (NRP)

DCD donation involves a prolonged warm ischaemia time between withdrawal of organ support, progressive hypotension and hypoxia culminating in cardiac death. This causes liver injury which is then exacerbated by cold ischaemia when the abdominal organs are perfused with cold preservation solution. In the UK, this is of particular concern as legal requirements prevent cannulation and heparinisation of the donor for at least 5 min after confirmation of death [11, 12]. NRP has been developed to reduce hepatocellular damage caused by prolonged warm ischaemia and subsequent cold perfusion in controlled donations from DCD donors. This technique involves delivering oxygenated cold perfusion using an extracorporeal membrane oxygenation circuits (ECMO) to the abdominal organs in situ by cannulation of the iliac vessels and the abdominal aorta. Several reports have indicated the use of NRP in controlled DCD donation reduces the rates of delayed graft function and primary non-function, hepatic artery thrombosis as well as ischemic cholangiopathy in liver transplantation. The optimal duration of NRP is not known and varies significantly in these reports from 2 to 4 h. NRP has been combined with hypothermic machine perfusion to further improve the viability of organs retrieved from DCD donors [13].

12.9 Preservation and Resuscitation

12.9.1 Preservation Solutions

Preservation solutions have been designed to mitigate the cellular and molecular damage that occurs during ischaemia. They have a fundamental role in solid organ transplantation, enabling preservation and transportation of organs to recipient location over long distances. The various compositions largely consist of electrolytes, buffers, impermeants and metabolites (ROS scavengers and nutrients) [1]. There are different electrolyte compositions to reflect intra- or extra-cellular ratios of Na^+ and K^+ with added calcium, chloride and magnesium. Buffers (e.g. bicarbonate) counteract changes in pH whilst free radical scavengers (e.g. glutathione) reduce ROS formation. Impermeants such as colloids, mannitol and citrate have a high molecular weight and counteract passage of electrolytes and water across cell membranes thereby preventing cell swelling. Preservation solutions combined with cooling to reduce oxygen and metabolic demand improves organ viability ex vivo.

Static cold storage (SCS) involves rapid flushing of the organs in situ with preservation fluids and after retrieval surgery, the liver is submerged in a sterile bag containing the same solution and placed on ice for storage during transport. Owing to its convenience, low cost and effectiveness this method of organ preservation has been the standard method of transporting donor livers for decades. SCS remains the standard of care for liver preservation, however, it still leads to anaerobic respiration and cellular damage. Whilst this may be well tolerated by low-risk livers and lead to modest IR injury at implantation, in marginal livers it leads to an augmented IR injury and worse clinical outcomes. New developments in machine perfusion and pharmacological additives to resuscitate marginal livers will require a modification of preservation solutions in future [1].

12.9.2 Hypothermic Machine Perfusion (HMP)

Hypothermic perfusion of the donor organs can be employed with or without supplementary oxygenation. The concept of ex vivo machine perfusion has been studied for decades. The development of ideal perfusion circuits was hampered due to the technical expertise and costs associated with incorporating them in clinical practice compared to SCS and the difficulty of demonstrating clinical benefit. However, this topic has been revisited with great interest for improving graft viability in extended criteria and DCD donors.

Hypothermic oxygenated perfusion (HOPE) reduces metabolic activity and oxygen demand whilst supporting reduced aerobic activity with supplemental oxygen in the perfusion solution. Flow of the perfusion fluid helps remove toxic metabolites produced during ischaemia. Although flow triggers shear-dependant endothelial protective mechanism such as nitric oxide production, high flow pressures and prolonged perfusion cause injury to the pressure sensitive liver sinusoidal endothelial cells. An optimal perfusion pressure and duration is yet to be determined. HOPE can be delivered continuously throughout transportation which is expensive and is a logistical challenge requiring in transport perfusion and expertise. Furthermore, *continuous* HOPE may increase the risk of vascular endothelial damage through prolonged perfusion in transport. To overcome these challenges, *end-ischaemic* HOPE is applied for a short period prior to implantation at the recipient centre after SCS in transportation. Experimental evidence suggests that even short periods (1–2 h) of cold oxygenated perfusion as a 'rescue therapy' in DCD livers yields hepatocyte protection with improvements in bile flow through a reduction of necrosis, reduced platelet adhesion and enhanced ATP recovery [14]. End-ischaemic HOPE also reduces the inflammatory response through reduction of DAMPS, TLR activation and cytokine release and ultimately has a protective effect on hepatocyte viability and function [15].

Several clinical series of HOPE in humans have been reported with variations in perfusion technique (dual: hepatic artery and portal vein or single: portal vein only), solution and pressures as well as timings. The evidence for this technique is based on comparative cohorts which have an inherent risk of bias. Randomised controlled trials (RCTs) are required with statistical improvements in patient centred outcomes such as graft and patient survival, length of hospital stay, complications and quality of life. The first prospective RCT of end-ischaemic HOPE for extended criteria DBD donor livers is under way and the results are eagerly awaited [14].

12.9.3 Normothermic Machine Perfusion (NMP)

Normothermic machine perfusion (NRP) has been developed to maintain cellular metabolism and organ function in preservation. This requires a constant supply of nutrients and oxygenated perfusion at body temperature (37 °C). Several NMP circuits have been designed to incorporate pumps, a blood reservoir, a heat exchanger and an oxygenator. In murine models, NMP's protective effects have been demonstrated through reducing endothelial injury and replenishing ATP supplies as well as mitochondrial protection. In large animal models of liver preservation, NMP has been shown to improve bile production and reduce markers of hepatocellular injury as well as a reduction in platelet aggregation at reperfusion [16]. These results are encouraging but clinically relevant end points such as improved post-transplant survival are required. A potential benefit of ex vivo NMP is that it would allow assessment of liver function and viability prior to transplantation. The diagnostic accuracy of machine-based parameters and their ability to predict relevant clinical outcomes such as graft failure have not been proven in robust prospective observational studies.

A recently published phase 3 randomised control trial of NMP compared to SCS showed a significant reduction in peak post-transplant AST levels and a reduction in early allograft dysfunction but no improvement in any patient centred outcomes (mortality, morbidity, length of ITU and hospital stay) [17]. Improvements in the technology has allowed development of portable perfusion machines for NMP, nonetheless it still has the cost and logistical challenges that come with machine perfusion in transport which may hinder its applicability at a large scale. In order to mitigate for this, a feasibility trial for *end-ischaemic* NMP after SCS has recently been conducted and the results of this are awaited. NMP technology is promising and future developments will allow opportunities for pharmacological interventions in preservation with objective measures on liver function and viability prior to transplantation.

12.10 Recipient Strategies

12.10.1 Washout Techniques

The toxic metabolites, electrolytes and inflammatory mediators which accumulate within the liver during SCS are washed out into the systemic circulation once the graft is revascularised. This sudden cold, acidotic and toxic hit to the heart and lungs leads to development of haemodynamic instability and post-reperfusion syndrome. In order to minimise this surge, the liver is washed out and warmed prior to revascularisation using different washout techniques and solutions.

Washout can be performed using preservation solutions, crystalloids or colloids like human albumin solution, on bench or in situ prior to venous reperfusion, in antegrade or retrograde fashion, through the portal vein only or dual perfusion through portal vein and hepatic artery, with or without venting of the vena cava. Portal vein only flushing without vena cava venting has been shown to significantly reduce the incidence of haemodynamic instability [18]. Machine perfusion of livers has the potential to significantly reduce the incidence of PRS by avoiding build-up of toxic mediators. NMP significantly reduced the haemodynamic instability at reperfusion in a large animal model of liver transplantation compared to SCS livers [19].

12.10.2 Remote Ischaemic Preconditioning (RIPC)

Direct intraoperative ischaemic preconditioning of the liver by intermittent inflow occlusion in the recipient during transplantation is challenging. Besides the fact that the recipient liver is explanted, inflow occlusion of the recipient cirrhotic liver is poorly tolerated, and the risks of IPC against potential systemic benefits is not known. Direct IPC by portal triad clamping in the donor liver during retrieval surgery has been performed in DBD donors, however it risks prolonging retrieval time and reduce venous return to the heart causing haemodynamic instability. Hence, remote ischaemic preconditioning (RIPC) of the organ recipient has been proposed. In a recent feasibility trial, three 5 min cycles of lower limb IR was used as the stimulus on the recipient prior to implantation surgery which failed to demonstrate an improvement in short-term measures of IR injury [20]. This was perhaps due to the timings and duration of the RIPC protocol.

12.10.3 Pharmacological Agents

There is currently no pharmacological agent in routine clinical use for reducing IR injury. A number of experimental drugs have shown to be beneficial in reducing markers of severity in liver IR injury, however, none have conclusively shown clinical benefit. For a comprehensive review see Cannistra et al. [21]. Some of the main drugs and their mechanism of action are summarised below:

- *Antioxidants* have been extensively studied in experimental models of warm and cold liver IR given the central role of oxidative stress. Examples of antioxidants include α-tocopherol, ascorbic acid, melatonin, N-acetylcysteine, bucillamine, superoxide dismutase, allopurinol and hydrogen sulphide. However, there is currently no conclusive evidence from human trials in liver transplantation that they lead to reduced post-operative complications. *α-lipoic acid* (ALA) for example is a natural ROS scavenger found in some foods and endogenously synthesised in human mitochondria. A 600 mg perfusion of ALA prior to cold ischaemia reduced plasma DAMP levels and increased transcription of hypoxia-inducible factor-1 (HIF-1α) in a double blinded randomised trial of 40 donor livers. It may have also contributed to a reduction of post-reperfusion syndrome, however it did not improve graft function or reduce complications [20].
- *Antioxidant gene therapy* is a novel application of recombinant viral vectors to upregulate genes such as superoxide dismutase involved in ROS scavenging or those protective in ischaemia such as HIF-1α.
- *Nitric oxide* has an important protective role in liver IR injury and exogenous administration of NO by inhalation or NO donors such as sodium nitroprusside have been shown in murine models to improve hepatic blood flow and be cytoprotective. Shikonin, a Chinese herbal medicine has recently been shown to be protective in a murine model of warm hepatic IR through activation of the PI3k/Akt pathway which is important in eNOS production [20].
- *Endothelial glycocalyx* protection and prevention of local and systemic GXL disruption could potentially provide a unifying target to reduce the many direct and remote complications of hepatic IR injury. Donor graft steatosis is a major risk factor for graft failure in liver transplantation mainly due to reduced microcirculatory flow. Steatotic livers have a poor response to shear stress (mechanotransduction) and endothelial protection from stress damage is an important function of the GXL. This was as shown by reduced levels of eNOS activity and NO production as well as decreased Kruppel-like factor 2 (KLF2) expression in subnormothermic machine perfusion of steatotic livers compared to normal livers leading to a perturbed microcirculatory state [22]. In another study of steatotic liver preservation it was shown that GXL protection was associated with significantly reduced hepatocyte damage and higher NO production [23]. In the recipient, there is significant shedding of the GXL at reperfusion which may contribute to postoperative complications [24].

12.11 Future Perspectives

Hepatic IR injury remains the main cause of morbidity and mortality in liver surgery and transplantation. Despite over two decades of research in this area, therapeutic options to treat or prevent liver IR are limited. This is primarily due to the difficulties in translation of promising agents into human clinical studies. Recent advances in our understanding of the immunological responses and endothelial dysfunction in the pathogenesis of liver IR injury may pave the way for the development of new and more effective and targeted pharmacological agents. With the advent of machine perfusion, there is a great opportunity for re-conditioning or resuscitating marginal donors with the aim of increasing the donor pool and reducing waiting list deaths. These technologies are currently being evaluated in humans but determining the optimal perfusion conditions will require extensive clinical investigation.

Self Study

Questions

1. What is ischaemia-reperfusion injury?
2. What causes liver IR injury in liver surgery?
3. What is post-reperfusion syndrome in liver transplantation?
4. Name two strategies used to reduce IR injury in the liver donor.
5. List five donor and preservation risk factors associated with increasing IR injury and graft failure in liver transplantation.

Answers

1. Ischaemia-reperfusion injury is the cellular damage sustained upon reperfusion of previously viable ischaemic tissues.
2. Liver IR injury occurs due to mobilisation of the liver as well as temporary inflow occlusion (Pringle manoeuvre) used to reduce blood loss.
3. Post-reperfusion syndrome (PRS) refers to the haemodynamic instability that occurs at reperfusion of the graft. It is defined as an abrupt decrease in mean arterial pressure (MAP) greater than 30% below the baseline value, lasting for at least 1 min which occurs during the first 5 min of reperfusion of the graft liver.
4. Donor optimisation (for DBD) and Normothermic Regional Perfusion (for DCD)
5. Donor age, BMI, steatosis, DCD, cold and warm ischaemia times.

References

1. Fuller B, Froghi F, Davidson B. Organ preservation solutions: linking pharmacology to survival for the donor organ pathway. Curr Opin Organ Transplant. 2018;23:361–8.
2. Zhai Y, Petrowsky H, Hong JC, Busuttil RW, Kupiec-Weglinski JW. Ischaemia–reperfusion injury in liver transplantation—from bench to bedside. Nat Rev Gastroenterol Hepatol. 2013;10:79–89.
3. Murphy LS, Wickersham N, McNeil JB, Shaver CM, May AK, Bastarache JA, Ware LB. Endothelial glycocalyx degradation is more severe in patients with non-pulmonary sepsis compared to pulmonary sepsis and associates with risk of ARDS and other organ dysfunction. Ann Intensive Care. 2017;7:102.
4. Koti RS, Seifalian AM, Davidson BR. Protection of the liver by ischemic preconditioning: a review of mechanisms and clinical applications. Dig Surg. 2003;20:383–96.
5. Kanoria S, Robertson FP, Mehta NN, Fusai G, Sharma D, Davidson BR. Effect of remote ischaemic preconditioning on liver injury in patients undergoing major hepatectomy for colorectal liver metastasis: a pilot randomised controlled feasibility trial. World J Surg. 2017;41:1322–30.
6. Beck-Schimmer B, Breitenstein S, Urech S, De Conno E, Wittlinger M, Puhan M, Jochum W, Spahn DR, Graf R, Clavien P-A. A randomized controlled trial on pharmacological preconditioning in liver surgery using a volatile anesthetic. Ann Surg. 2008;248(6):909–18. https://doi.org/10.1097/SLA.0b013e31818f3dda.
7. Schmidt R, Tritschler E, Hoetzel A, Loop T, Humar M, Halverscheid L, Geiger KK, Pannen BHJ. Heme oxygenase-1 induction by the clinically used anesthetic isoflurane protects rat livers from ischemia/reperfusion injury. Ann Surg. 2007;245:931–42.
8. Feng S, Goodrich NP, Bragg-Gresham JL, Dykstra DM, Punch JD, DebRoy MA, Greenstein SM, Merion RM. Characteristics associated with liver graft failure: the concept of a donor risk index. Am J Transplant. 2006;6:783–90.
9. Collett D, Friend PJ, Watson CJE. Factors associated with short-and long-term liver graft survival in the United Kingdom: development of a UK donor liver index. Transplantation. 2017;101(4):786–92. https://doi.org/10.1097/TP.0000000000001576.
10. Schlegel A, Kalisvaart M, Scalera I, Laing RW, Mergental H, Mirza DF, Perera T, Isaac J, Dutkowski P, Muiesan P. The UK DCD risk score: a new proposal to define futility in donation-after-circulatory-death liver transplantation. J Hepatol. 2018;68:456–64.
11. Butler AJ, Randle LV, Watson CJE. Normothermic regional perfusion for donation after circulatory death without prior heparinization. Transplantation. 2014;97:1272–8.
12. Oniscu GC, Randle LV, Muiesan P, Butler AJ, Currie IS, Perera MTPR, Forsythe JL, Watson CJE. In situ normothermic regional perfusion for controlled donation after circulatory death—The United Kingdom experience. Am J Transplant. 2014;14:2846–54.
13. De Carlis L, De Carlis R, Lauterio A, Di Sandro S, Ferla F, Zanierato M. Sequential use of normothermic regional perfusion and hypothermic machine perfusion in donation after cardiac death liver transplantation with extended warm ischemia time. Transplantation. 2016;100:e101–2.
14. Czigany Z, Schöning W, Ulmer TF, et al. Hypothermic oxygenated machine perfusion (HOPE) for orthotopic liver transplantation of human liver allografts from extended criteria donors (ECD) in donation after brain death (DBD): a prospective multicentre randomised controlled trial (HOPE ECD-DBD). BMJ Open. 2017;7:e017558.
15. Westerkamp AC, Mahboub P, Meyer SL, Hottenrott M, Ottens PJ, Wiersema-Buist J, Gouw ASH, Lisman T, Leuvenink HGD, Porte RJ. End-ischemic machine perfusion reduces bile duct injury in donation after circulatory death rat donor livers independent of the machine perfusion temperature. Liver Transplant. 2015;21:1300–11.
16. Kollmann D, Linares I, Ganesh S, et al. Platelet aggregation contributing to reperfusion injury can be prevented by normothermic ex vivo liver perfusion prior to liver transplantation. J Hepatol. 2018;68:S69.
17. Nasralla D, Coussios CC, Mergental H, et al. A randomized trial of normothermic preservation in liver transplantation. Nature. 2018;557(7703):50–6.
18. Gruttadauria S, Cintorino D, Musumeci A, et al. Comparison of two different techniques of reperfusion in adult orthotopic liver transplantation. Clin Transpl. 2006;20:159–62.
19. Kettler K, Fontes P, Lopez R, Marsh W, Soltys K, van der Plaats A, et al. 52: post-reperfusion syndrome in liver transplantation the end of an era Crit Care Med. 2018;46.
20. Robertson FP, Goswami R, Wright GP, Imber C, Sharma D, Malago M, Fuller BJ, Davidson BR. Remote ischaemic preconditioning in orthotopic liver transplantation (RIPCOLT trial): a pilot randomized controlled feasibility study. HPB. 2017;19:757–67.
21. CannistrÃ M, Ruggiero M, Zullo A, Gallelli G, Serafini S, Maria M, Naso A, Grande R, Serra R, Nardo B. Hepatic ischemia reperfusion injury: a systematic review of literature and the role of current drugs and biomarkers. Int J Surg. 2016;33:S57–70.
22. Beijert I, Mert S, Huang V, Karimian N, Geerts S, Hafiz EOA, Markmann JF, Yeh H, Porte RJ, Uygun K. Endothelial dysfunction in steatotic human donor livers: a pilot study of the underlying mechanism during subnormothermic machine perfusion. Transplant Direct. 2018;4:e345.
23. Lopez A, Panisello-Rosello A, Castro-Benitez C, Adam R, Lopez A, Panisello-Rosello A, Castro-Benitez C, Adam R. Glycocalyx preservation and no production in fatty livers—the protective role of high molecular polyethylene glycol in cold ischemia injury. Int J Mol Sci. 2018;19:2375.
24. Schiefer J, Lebherz-Eichinger D, Erdoes G, Berlakovich G, Bacher A, Krenn CG, Faybik P. Alterations of endothelial glycocalyx during orthotopic liver transplantation in patients with end-stage liver disease. Transplantation. 2015;99:2118–23.

13 Autoimmune Hepatitis

Christos Liaskos, George Efthymiou,
and Dimitrios P. Bogdanos

Abbreviations

AIH	Autoimmune hepatitis
AMA	Anti-mitochondrial antibody
LC1	Liver cytosol type 1
LKM-1	Liver kidney microsomal type 1
p-ANCA	Perinuclear antineutrophil cytoplasmic antibodies
SMA	Smooth muscle antibody

Key Concepts
- Autoimmune hepatitis (AIH) is an autoimmune liver disease, which if is left untreated (without immunosuppression) leads to immune-mediated hepatocyte destruction, fibrosis/cirrhosis and liver failure
- The current diagnostic criteria require evidence of hyperglobulinaemia, detectable characteristic autoantibodies and histological evidence of immune-mediated destruction of hepatocytes (such as interface hepatitis)
- Clinical presentation and natural history of the disease greatly varies from acute, sub-acute to chronic disease, asymptomatic to full-blown liver disease affecting all ages, both genders and all ethnicities
- AIH must be considered as a cause of acute and/or chronic liver disease, in suspected cases with no other profound cause
- The goal of treatment in AIH is to induce and maintain complete remission
- The disease generally appears to be well controlled under corticosteroid treatment with or without combination treatment with azathioprine. Other treatment regimen can lead to disease remission in case of standard treatments fail

13.1 Introduction

Autoimmune hepatitis (AIH) is a relatively rare autoimmune liver disease of unknown aetiology. The disease is characterized by immune-mediated destruction of the hepatocytes and progressive inflammation and subsequent liver fibrosis leading to organ's failure, if the disease is left untreated. Genetic, epigenetic and immunological factors are considered important for the development of the disease.

13.2 Diagnostic Criteria

In an attempt to assist firm diagnosis, the International Autoimmune Hepatitis Group (IAIHG) of experts, established in early 1990s proposed a series of criteria that classified patients as "probable" or "definite" for autoimmune hepatitis. These criteria (Table 13.1), were revised in 1999 [1] and for long were used, mainly for research purposes, until the simplified criteria were developed and are currently a proper diagnostic tool used in routine practice.

The current diagnostic criteria [2] for the disease are well established and their simplified form (Table 13.2) which is used for clinical purposes includes: (a) elevated IgG levels (or total gamma globulins i.e. evidence of hyperglobulinaemia; (b) presence of disease related or characteristic autoantibodies; and (c) histological features of lymphocytic hepatitis. They also require absence of viral hepatitis, as this increases the chances the findings mentioned above to be due

C. Liaskos · G. Efthymiou · D. P. Bogdanos (✉)
Division of Rheumatology and Clinical Immunology, Faculty of Medicine, School of Health Sciences, University of Thessaly, Larissa, Greece
e-mail: bogdanos@med.uth.gr

F. Radu-Ionita et al. (eds.), *Liver Diseases*, https://doi.org/10.1007/978-3-030-24432-3_13

Table 13.1 1999 IAIHG revised diagnostic criteria of autoimmune hepatitis

Feature	Score
Female sex	+2
AP ÷ AST (or ALT)	
<1.5	+2
1.5–3.0	+0
>3.0	−2
Serum globulins or IgG above normal	
>2.0	+3
1.5–2.0	+2
1.0–1.5	+1
<1.0	0
ANA, SMA or LKM-1	
>1:80	+3
1:80	+2
1:40	+1
<1:40	0
AMA positive	−4
Hepatitis viral markers	
Positive	−3
Negative	+3
Drug history	
Positive	−4
Negative	+4
Average alcohol intake	
<25 g/day	+2
>60 g/day	−2
Liver histology	
Interface hepatitis	+3
Predominantly lymphoplasmacytic infiltrate	+1
Rosetting of liver cells	+1
None of the above	−5
Biliary changes	−3
Other changes	−3
Other autoimmune disease(s)	+2
Optional additional parameters:	
Seropositivity for other defined autoantibodies	+2
HLA DR3 or DR4	+1
Response to therapy:	
Complete	+2
Relapse	+3
Interpretation of aggregate scores	
Pre-treatment	
Definite AIH	>15
Probable AIH	10–15
Post-treatment	
Definite AIH	>17
Probable AIH	12–17

Abbreviations: *AIH* autoimmune hepatitis, *ALT* alanine aminotransferase, *AMA* anti-mitochondrial antibodies, *ANA* anti-nuclear antibodies, *AP* alkaline phosphatase, *AST* aspartate aminotransferase, *HLA* human leukocyte antigen, *IgG* immunoglobulin G, *LKM-1* liver-kidney microsomal antibodies, *SMA* smooth muscle antibodies

Table 13.2 Simplified diagnostic criteria of autoimmune hepatitis

Feature	Cut-off	Points
ANA/SMA	≥1:40	1
ANA/SMA	≥1:80	2[a]
or LKM-1	≥1:40	
or SLA	Positive	
IgG	>Upper normal limit	1
	>1.1 times the upper normal limit	2
Liver histology[b]	AIH compatible	1
	AIH typical	2
Absence of viral hepatitis	Yes	2
Interpretation of aggregate scores		
Definite AIH ≥7 points		
Probable AIH ≥6 points		

Abbreviations: *AIH* autoimmune hepatitis, *ANA* anti-neutrophil antibodies, *IgG* immunoglobulin G, *LKM1* liver-kidney microsomal antibodies, *SMA* smooth muscle antibodies, *SLA* soluble liver antigen

[a]Addition of points achieved for all autoantibodies (maximum = 2 points)

[b]Evidence of hepatitis is a necessary condition

to AIH alone. Unfortunately, the simplified criteria have low sensitivity for AIH patients with fulminant failure and paediatric AIH [2].

13.3 Autoantibody Serology

Based on the type of autoantibody present in the serum of the affected individual, the disease is classified in two types. Type 1 AIH is characterized by the presence of anti-smooth muscle antibodies (ASMA) and/or without anti-nuclear antibodies (ANA). Type 2 AIH is presented with positive anti-liver/anti-kidney microsomal-1 (anti-LMK1) antibodies and/or anti-liver cytosol (anti-LC) type 1 antibodies. Several other autoantibodies can be detectable in sera from patients with AIH, but these are either non-specific or not relevant with the disease [3–5] (Fig. 13.1).

13.4 Aetiology

There is no proved and specific evidence of the cause of the disease. The disease has a relatively strong genetic background and amongst various environmental factors, infectious triggers, mainly viral agents, have been considered relevant to its pathogenesis. Toxins and drugs are also implicated, as their potential to induce AIH-like disease in animals is well documented. Both innate and adaptive immunity is involved in disease's development and progression, as shown in animal models of the disease and studies conducted in humans.

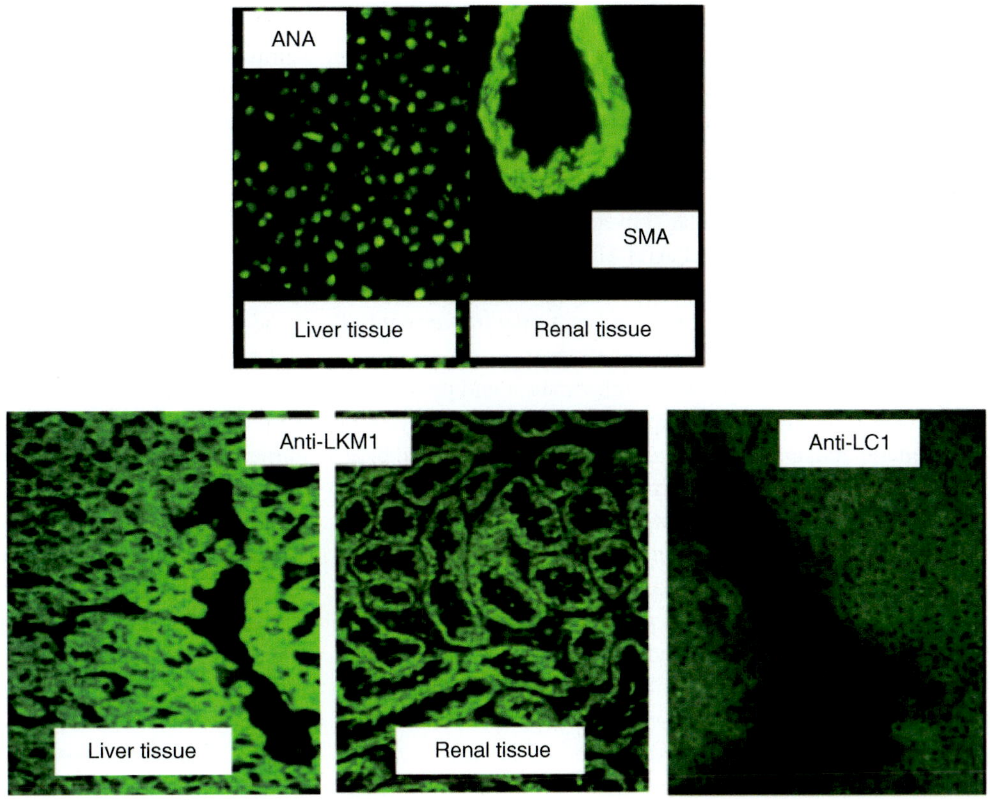

Fig. 13.1 Autoimmune hepatitis related autoantibodies. Anti-nuclear antibody (ANA), smooth muscle antibody (SMA), anti-liver kidney microsomal antibody (anti-LKM1) and anti-liver cytosol antibody (anti-LC1) by indirect immunofluorescence

13.5 Pathogenesis

The prevailing view is that AIH is a T-cell mediated (CD4 and CD8) autoimmune disease [6]. The disease develops under a state of breakdown of antigen-driven immunological tolerance in susceptible individuals with impaired immunoregulatory function [7]. Though the loss of tolerance has been attributed to be secondary to environmental triggers, such triggers (infectious and non-infectious) have not been isolated so far. Several infectious agents have been associated with AIH-1, AIH-2 or both (Fig. 13.2) and case studies, data from animal models, immunological or virological data have provided some support linking infection to AIH, but no solid evidence has been provided so far [8].

Viruses appear as more likely triggers compared to bacterial infections. Early studies linking hepatitis C virus infection with AIH-2 have been on the fact that 2–11% of patients with chronic hepatitis C virus infection had detectable anti-LKM-1 antibodies, the serological marker of AIH-2, which is present in 85% of the patients. Evidence of immunological cross-reactivity involving hepatitis C virus and cytochrome P4502D6, the autoantigenic target of anti-LKM1, has been

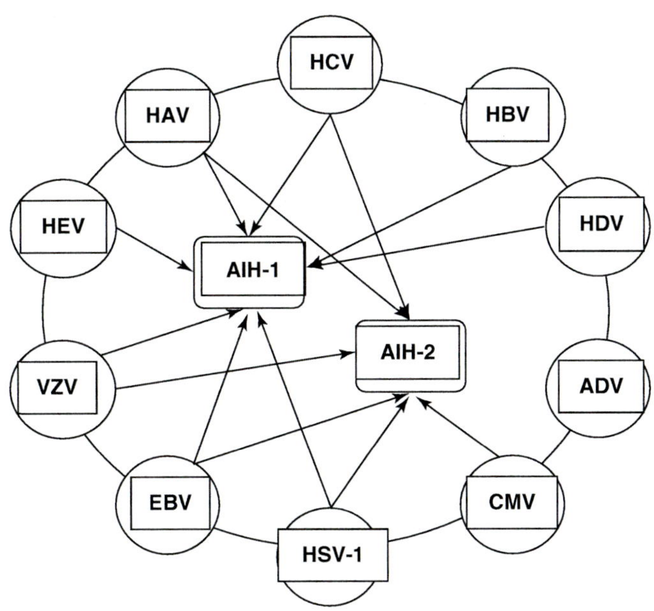

Fig. 13.2 Schematic representation of viral associations with autoimmune hepatitis. *HAV* hepatitis A virus, *HBV* hepatitis B virus, *HCV* hepatitis C virus, *HDV* hepatitis D virus, *ADV* adenovirus, *CMV* cytomegalovirus, *HSV-1* herpes simplex virus, *EBV* Epstein-Barr virus, *VZV* varicella zoster virus, *HEV* hepatitis E virus

obtained, further supporting the notion for a potential link. Animal models based on the viral/autoantigenic mimicking sequences have provided additional evidence. The murine model of concanavalin A-induced AIH shares several features with AIH and is the most widely used model to study the pathogenesis of AIH [9, 10]. Such models have appreciated the role of innate cellular subsets, such as those of iNKT cells in the development of AIH [11]. Fresh substantiation has also supported the notion that AIH patients (at least paediatric ones) are characterized by a functional impairment of their regulatory T cell (Treg) populations.

With the advance of biostatic information and processing of big data stemming from genetic studies, the role played by the genetic make-up of the affected individuals has been widely assessed. Genome wide association studies have established most of the susceptibility gene associations [12]. A female preponderance is unquestionable. HLA associations are also well documented for both types of the disease, depending on the ethnic background/origin of the affected individuals. Hence, established links with variations in the HLA locus on the short arm of chromosome 6 are repeatedly emerging. The associations, which appear to be the strongest, are within the genes encoding the HLA class II *DRB1* alleles. A Dutch GWAS, and its replication in German cohorts, revealed *DRB1*0301* and *DRB1*0401* as primary and secondary susceptibility genotypes. What is still a matter of debate is whether clinical features such as prognosis/outcome of the disease, extent of response to treatment and clinical phenotypes are associated with specific HLA alleles or not. Susceptibility to AIH-2 have been linked to alleles encoding the DR3 (*DRB1*0301*) and DR7 (*DRB1*0701*) molecules in the United Kingdom and Latin America. Such data are treated with caution, especially for AIH-2, the most rare form of AIH, due to the small number of analysed biological samples. In addition, data stemming from metanalyses question findings of individual studies, especially those relating AIH with non-HLA single nucleotide polymorphisms. A recent metanalysis has concluded that there no relation between (previously noted) IL-10, an immunoregulatory cytokine, promoter polymorphisms (in particular rs1800896, rs1800871, and rs1800872 polymorphisms) and AIH or other autoimmune liver diseases.

Associations outside the HLA locus involve *TNF-α*, *CTLA-4* gene promoters and *Fas* genes amongst others but data are not conclusive. Of interest are also the gene associations of the GWAS related to *CARD10* and *SH2B3* genes.

13.6 Natural History

The disease can affect all sexes, ages and ethnicities. The disease spectrum is highly heterogeneous. It can run an asymptomatic course, a very mild subclinical/clinical course, can have an acute/very acute course and at times rarely can lead to fulminant hepatic failure due to acute hepatitis. It can be the first manifestation of liver disease in infants as well as in very old people, without prior history of liver disease [13, 14].

The disease can be accompanied by general, non-specific symptoms such as fatigue and malaise, arthralgia and unexplained abdominal pain or jaundice. Symptoms and signs related to established cirrhosis, such as variceal haemorrhage, ascites and hepatic encephalopathy are not frequent these days due to the fact that patients are usually controlled under immunosuppression for very long.

As in other autoimmune disease, AIH may co-occur with other extrahepatic autoimmune diseases, such as autoimmune thyroiditis, autoimmune rheumatic diseases and celiac disease. Early days, the concept of overlap syndromes was used to describe patients with overlapping features of AIH and primary biliary cholangitis (formerly known as primary biliary cirrhosis) or that of AIH with primary sclerosing cholangitis. This terminology is not any more used, as the concept of overlap syndromes has been neglected.

13.7 Epidemiology

Study results largely vary, but according to European Association for the Study of Liver Disease (EASL) guidelines, the prevalence of AIH ranges from 15 to 25 cases per 100,000 inhabitants in Europe and is increasing in both women and men. This increase is not yet clear whether reflects increase in technological advancements (autoantibody diagnostics, imaging features of liver disease, regular checkups) and physicians' awareness of it relates to the true impact of an unknown yet triggering cause [13, 15–17].

The ethnic background largely affects the prevalence of the disease. One of the most notable features is that seen in Alaskan natives, who present a higher frequency of acute icteric disease at disease onset. A well-documented feature is seen in African-American patients, who appear to be more frequently cirrhotic, as well as that related to Mexican Mestizos, who are presented with cirrhosis. Whether such documentation related to true ethnic predispositions and the genetic make-up of the affected individuals or relate to socioeconomic reasons, such as that of lack of access to proper health care and subsequent delayed diagnosis is not yet established, as the data are still limited and proper studies have not been conducted so far.

13.7.1 Histopathological Features

The hallmark histologic feature of AIH is interface hepatitis. The specificity of this feature, however, is low as it can be seen in hepatitic forms of liver damage such as viral hepatitides. Most investigators support, with some exceptions, that there is no pathognomonic histopathological finding related to AIH and that those frequently found in patients with this disease are nonspecific [1, 18, 19].

Nevertheless, a firm diagnosis of the disease, as noted by the scoring of the simplified criteria cannot be established in the absence of liver biopsy assessment. Thus, all guidelines (American, European, Japanese and other) recommend that the diagnosis of AIH should not be made in the absence of a liver biopsy. In addition to interface hepatitis, emperipolesis and hepatic rosette formation have been considered AIH-related features of the disease and in their presence, the diagnosis is highly likely. A typical AIH histopathological picture is that of mononuclear inflammatory infiltrate mostly plasma cells, located principally in the portal tracts. This lymphocyte inflammation is that which most likely leads to piecemeal necrosis of hepatocytes and the destruction of limiting plate, also known as interface hepatitis, bridging fibrosis which connects the portal and central area of hepatocytes, regenerating nodules, and finally established cirrhosis and subsequent lever failure. The hepatitis form of histopathological features does not exclude the presence of cholangitis features and ductopenia in a proportion of patients with AIH.

The experience of the pathologist is essential for proper assessment and can be of great help for decision making. It needs to be reminded that liver biopsy is unquestionably the most trustworthy method for judging the gravity of the hepatocyte destruction, both in terms of grading and staging) [1].

Assessment of liver histology was a tool used in AIH to monitor therapeutic interventions. Assessments included quantitation of hepatic inflammation and staging of liver destruction. More recent attempts to use various indexes, such as that of the modified Hepatic Activity Index (mHAI) established for chronic viral hepatitis, has been used for staging of AIH with questionable results, mainly due to the fact that most scoring systems are based on viral hepatitis assessments and cannot be applied to AIH. The lack of applications of the diagnostic scoring in acute and severe AIH is another troubling issue, which is yet to be solved. The value of fibroscan and other non-invasive parameters for assessing the extent of fibrosis in AIH remains unclear. In several cases, patients may also have another liver disease. For example AIH and non-alcoholic liver disease or AIH and viral hepatitis or AIH and alcoholic liver disease. These co-existence challenges the extent by which liver biopsy can be of definite help and could assist firm diagnosis in patients with suspected AIH (on the top of the con-current liver disease of any other cause). This is also important for the understanding that, so far we have for the diagnostic assessment we follow in suspected cases.

13.7.2 Diagnostic Work Up

AIH must be considered as a cause of acute and chronic liver damage, with no profound cause. Differential diagnosis must include other causes of acute and mainly chronic liver disease including nonalcoholic hepatosteatosis (NASH), chronic viral hepatitis, Wilson disease, a1 anti-trypsin deficiency, drug-induced hepatitis and other. We must always have in our minds the possible diagnosis of other autoimmune liver diseases such as primary biliary cholangitis, and primary sclerosing cholangitis, as well as the fact that even in the case AIH is diagnosed this cannot exclude the co-occurrence of PBC or PSC. A multi-step approach is required to assist diagnosis. Symptomatology, clinical signs, laboratory tests, imaging features and histological assessment, if required, can confirm or dismiss disease's presence.

Noticeable elevation of serum transaminases (AST, ALT) and hyperglobulinaemia are commonly found while marked elevation of ALP is infrequent. Excluding cirrhotic patients, serum levels of AST, ALT, and IgG (especially in paediatric patients) mirror to some extent disease severity. Whether the same features also reflect at presentation instantaneous projection of future prognosis is to be questioned.

The serological immunological markers required for the diagnosis of AIH include those tested at the basis of autoantibody work-up [20]. None of the autoantibodies tested are sensitive enough, or specific enough to be used by themselves. ANA, SMA, and anti-LKM1 are tested by indirect immunofluorescence, which remains the gold standard for autoantibody assessment. The molecular targets of SMA, anti-LKM1 and anti-LC1 have been identified as filamentous actin, CYP2D6 and formimino-transferase cyclodeaminase, respectively. Molecular based assays such as ELISA and line/dot/blot assays are widely used for their proper detection in conjunction with, or as a reflex assay to indirect immunofluorescence. The diagnostic accuracy, specificity, and sensitivity of these markers vary depending on the method used and the cut offs established. Anti-soluble liver antigen (SLA) antibodies are also found in up to 15% of patients with AIH and as they cannot be recognized by indirect immunofluorescence, their testing solely relies on molecular assays [21]. The testing of these autoantibodies is only used for diagnostic purposes and with few exceptions, their repeated testing is not encouraged, as it does not assist management decisions. Atypical perinuclear antineutrophil cytoplasmic antibodies (pANCA) can also be associated with AIH, but their target remains unknown. The presence of anti-mitochondrial antibodies and PBC-specific ANAs point towards the diagnosis of PBC. Anti-SLA antibodies appear to be related with are with more severe disease, treatment failure, and higher relapse rate and their presence alarms physicians for proper patient monitoring [4].

13.8 Disease Treatment and Management

Physicians must be aware that currently treatment guidelines exist for the management of patients with AIH. AIH was probably the first liver disease for which an effective and efficient therapeutic interference was convincingly established, almost 50 years ago. The disease appears to be well controlled under corticosteroid treatment. Over the years and due to the large heterogeneity of the disease, treatment of AIH still remains a therapeutic challenge in a small percentage of the affected individuals. Therapeutic decisions take into account the diverse features of the disease and the evolving understanding of the pathogenesis of the disease, as this stems from studies in animals and on-going clinical trials of new drug regimen. What remains well defined is that if the disease is left untreated, individuals develop cirrhosis and subsequently die of liver failure few years after diagnosis, if liver transplantation is not an alternative option.

The aim of treatment is to achieve complete remission and to prevent subsequent evolution of the histologically-progressed liver destruction. This can only be accomplished if permanent (in most of the cases) maintenance therapy is introduced. A minor percentage of the patients can accomplish a sustained remission following treatment withdrawal.

Patients who require treatment are those who have:

1. Confluent necrosis on liver biopsy presented as piecemeal or bridging necrosis and multilobular necrosis in histopathological assessment,
2. Elevated AST levels at least 5 times the upper level of normal values (ULN), and
3. Increased γ-globulin levels at least >2 × ULN) had a very good prognosis if therapy with steroids was introduced.

Initiation of treatment could decrease or normalize liver function tests, improve symptomatology and histological features and ultimately elongate survival.

Still up to now, questionable remains the beneficial effect of steroid treatment in asymptomatic older patients with mild necroinflammatory activity. Untreated patients with mild disease have a significant 10-year survival rate of 60–90% [[180], [181]]. Hence, it is not of surprise, in view of the prolonged adverse reactions and relative contraindications of immunosuppression, that several physicians decide not to treat this sub-group of patients. In a handful of cases, spontaneous resolution of the disease has been described further questioning the necessity to treat such patients.

The current dogma, and most clinically relevant, for the management of the patients is that untreated AIH has an unsettled, fluctuating, unpredictable disease course. The majority of these asymptomatic patients or at least a substantial proportion of those become symptomatic during the course of their disease follow-up. This is clinically relevant because, those patients progressed towards compensated and subsequently de-compensated end-stage liver disease with liver failure. The development of hepatocellular carcinoma in a proportion of those cannot be left unnoticed, further highlighting the need to identify patients with milder disease, at early stages, who can be of benefit in order to avoid subclinical disease progression. The key steps towards that is the close monitoring of these patients of at least their ALT and/or IgG levels and the decision making if levels are increased or fluctuated over time. Such a decision most likely need to include performance of liver biopsy for the confirmation of the diagnosis and staging of the disease.

In symptomatic patients and patients with advanced fibrosis or cirrhosis, treatment should always be initiated as this represents a negative prognostic predictor. In addition, even in advanced fibrosis and cirrhosis substantial regression of scarring after successful treatment has been reported. In view of the progressive nature of AIH and the effectiveness of immunosuppressive therapy, the consensus group recommends that all patients with active disease should receive treatment.

Treatment related side effects should be counterbalanced to the risk of subclinical disease progression and evolution into symptomatic disease as well as the prospect of a complete and sustained response to treatment.

13.8.1 Standard Treatment

The goal of treatment in AIH is to induce and maintain complete remission i.e. suppression of the inflammatory activity and auto-aggression as this will prevent from progression to cirrhosis [22]. Several guidelines have been issued defining remission, include those testifying remission as defined by the accomplishment of transaminase levels beneath twice the UNL. Most recent guidelines necessitate remission to be defined via normal levels of transaminases, as well as bilirubin and IgG [23]. As it was expected, patients who fulfilled the old criteria for remission could still have histologically progressive disease. This proportion could be minimized (justifying the need for more strict criteria) when the new definition is applied, emphasizing the weight of attaining normal biochemical and serological indicators to avoid disease deterioration and progression.

It is now well established that use of corticosteroids leads to complete remission and subsequently improves mortality. Induction is usually consisted of high dose predniso(lo)ne as monotherapy or with azathioprine. The starting dose of steroids is 60 mg/day in adults and 1–2 mg/kg/day (up to 60 mg/day) in children in the absence of azathioprine [23]. A dose of 60 mg daily is given the first week followed by 40 mg in the second and 30 mg per day in weeks three and four. The maintenance dose of prednisone is 20 mg daily until the endpoint is reached. Tapering of prednisone is a necessity and discontinuation is an alternative in case of combination therapy with azathioprine. Patients are classified as in remission, relapse, or treatment failure based on their histological and laboratory response to steroids, and the presence or absence of clinical symptomatology. As histological remission delays by 3–6 months compared to biochemical remission, proper therapeutic intervention must be sustained in spite of the normalization of liver enzymes. EASL and AASLD do not have a consensus regarding combination treatment. AASLD states that a fixed dose of 50 mg/day or 1–2 mg/kg/day of azathioprine at the same time as steroids is required, while EASL recommends 1–2 mg/kg/day of azathioprine as a starting point 2 weeks after the introduction of steroids. EASL considers that prednisolone can be replaced by budesonide at a starting dose of 9 mg/day in order to achieve remission, especially in those patients who are expected to experience steroid related side effects [22].

Immunosuppressive therapy should be avoided in patients with pre-existing comorbidities. Budesonide is an alternative, as well as combination of budesonide and azathioprine which has been emerged as an alternative first-line therapy. In cases of inadequate or incomplete response, or azathioprine intolerance, mycophenolate mofetil, cyclosporine A, and tacrolimus can be introduced as alternative treatments.

Remission is achieved when the patient remains asymptomatic with normalization of transaminases, IgG, and absence of histological inflammation. Relapse is the norm upon discontinuation of any treatment and approximately half of the patients experience relapse within 6 months of discontinuation. The description of relapse is defined by elevation of AST (three times the UNL), the reappearance of histological and the re-appearance of histological features of the disease in the absence of treatment.

Prognosis largely depends on treatment. Several randomized, controlled trials have shown that untreated AIH patients have 5-year and 10-year survival rates of 50% and 10%, respectively. Up to 80% of patients will achieve remission, if treatment is based upon the issued guidelines, after the proposed duration of treatment. A considerable proportion of patients with require life-long immunosuppression [24].

Treatment failure occurs in 10% of patients that undergo monotherapy with steroids. Liver cirrhosis can develop in up to 40% of patients under treatment. The development of cirrhosis is associated with an incomplete response, treatment failure, and multiple relapses. Development of cirrhosis necessitates proper monitoring and esophageal varices surveillance and regular screening for the development of hepatocellular carcinoma as for other cirrhotic patients. Overall, management of liver cirrhosis in autoimmune hepatitis is similar regardless of aetiology. Finally, liver transplantation is considered the Standard of care can be that of liver transplantation in patients exhibiting fulminant hepatic failure or those who progress to end stage liver disease despite multiple lines of therapy [25].

Self Study

Questions

1. A 35-year old woman presents to the clinic with a 5-months history of malaise and vague abdominal pain. Liver biochemistry shows an increase in ALT/AST (× 3.5 ULN), increased IgG, but slight increase of gGT and ALP. Diagnostic work-up is excluding viral hepatitides, alcohol abuse, non-alcoholic steatohepatitis and Wilson's disease. She denies systematic use of any drugs. A suspicion of autoimmune hepatitis is made and the diagnostic work up includes liver autoantibody testing including:
   (a) Antinuclear antibodies
   (b) Smooth muscle autoantibodies
   (c) Anti-mitochondrial antibodies
   (d) All the above and increase IgG
   (e) All the above and liver biopsy
2. What is true about AIH?
   (a) The disease affects only young women
   (b) AIH is always responding to steroids
   (c) The disease can affect both sexes, at any age, all ethnicities
   (d) The patient always have detectable AIH-related autoantibodies by indirect immunofluorescence
3. What is the initial recommended treatment of choice for AIH?
   (a) Monotherapy with predniso(lo)ne
   (b) Combination of predniso(lo)ne and azathioprine
   (c) None of the above
   (d) A or B

Answers

1 A 35-year old woman presents to the clinic with a 5-months history of malaise and vague abdominal pain. Liver biochemistry shows an increase in ALT/AST (× 3.5 ULN), increased IgG, but slight increase of gGT and ALP. Diagnostic work-up is excluding viral hepatitides, alcohol abuse, non-alcoholic steatohepatitis and Wilson's disease. She denies systematic use of any drugs. A suspicion of autoimmune hepatitis is made and the diagnostic work up includes liver autoantibody testing including:
   (a) Patients with AIH can have detectable antinuclear antibodies but they can also be negative for those. Thus, a single test for ANA is not sufficient for proper diagnosis

(b) Patients with AIH can have detectable smooth muscle antibodies but they can also be negative for those. Thus, a single test for SMA is not sufficient for establishing diagnosis
(c) Combination of tests, including that of SMA, ANA and AMA can assist diagnosis of AIH or primary biliary cholangitis. In this case, primary biliary cholangitis cannot be excluded and testing of all three autoantibodies is necessary. However, simple testing cannot lead to firm diagnosis of AIH, as histological assessment is also required
(d) CORRECT. A combination of detectable disease-related autoantibody, increased IgG and histological features compatible with or confirmatory of AIH is establishing a definite diagnosis of AIH

2 What is true about AIH?
(a) The disease does not affect only young women. It can be present in women of any age, as well as in men, through there is a female predominance (3:1)
(b) The great majority of the cases respond to steroids but not all of them. Combination therapy with azathioprine or alternative treatments may be required to achieve remission
(c) CORRECT: The disease can affect both sexes, all ages and at variable prevalence is noted in all ethnicities
(d) Indirect immunofluorescence testing can be negative in up to 10–15% of AIH cases. Testing of autoantibodies not detectable by this technique such as anti-soluble liver antigen antibodies may be the only positive test and is required in 'seronegative' cases

3 What is the initial recommended treatment of choice for AIH?
(a) Standard treatment includes either monotherapy with predniso(lo)ne or combination of predniso(lo)ne with azathioprine. Several physicians start with monotherapy but other start with combination treatment to avoid long-lasting adverse effects of steroid therapy
(b) Standard treatment includes either monotherapy with predniso(lo)ne or combination of predniso(lo)ne with azathioprine
(c) Standard treatment includes either monotherapy with predniso(lo)ne or combination of predniso(lo)ne with azathioprine
(d) CORRECT: Standard treatment includes either monotherapy with predniso(lo)ne or combination of predniso(lo)ne with azathioprine

References

1. Alvarez F, Berg PA, Bianchi FB, Bianchi L, Burroughs AK, Cancado EL, et al. International Autoimmune Hepatitis Group Report: review of criteria for diagnosis of autoimmune hepatitis. J Hepatol. 1999;31(5):929–38.
2. Hennes EM, Zeniya M, Czaja AJ, Pares A, Dalekos GN, Krawitt EL, et al. Simplified criteria for the diagnosis of autoimmune hepatitis. Hepatology. 2008;48(1):169–76.
3. Vergani D, Alvarez F, Bianchi FB, Cancado EL, Mackay IR, Manns MP, et al. Liver autoimmune serology: a consensus statement from the committee for autoimmune serology of the International Autoimmune Hepatitis Group. J Hepatol. 2004;41(4):677–83.
4. Bogdanos DP, Invernizzi P, Mackay IR, Vergani D. Autoimmune liver serology: current diagnostic and clinical challenges. World J Gastroenterol. 2008;14(21):3374–87.
5. Wen L, Ma Y, Bogdanos DP, Wong FS, Demaine A, Mieli-Vergani G, et al. Pediatric autoimmune liver diseases: the molecular basis of humoral and cellular immunity. Curr Mol Med. 2001;1(3): 379–89.
6. Ma Y, Bogdanos DP, Hussain MJ, Underhill J, Bansal S, Longhi MS, et al. Polyclonal T-cell responses to cytochrome P450IID6 are associated with disease activity in autoimmune hepatitis type 2. Gastroenterology. 2006;130(3):868–82.
7. Vergani D, Longhi MS, Bogdanos DP, Ma Y, Mieli-Vergani G. Autoimmune hepatitis. Semin Immunopathol. 2009;31(3):421–35.
8. Hardtke-Wolenski M, Jaeckel E. Mouse models for experimental autoimmune hepatitis: limits and chances. Dig Dis. 2010; 28(1):70–9.
9. Ehser J, Holdener M, Christen S, Bayer M, Pfeilschifter JM, Hintermann E, et al. Molecular mimicry rather than identity breaks T-cell tolerance in the CYP2D6 mouse model for human autoimmune hepatitis. J Autoimmun. 2013;42:39–49.
10. Bogdanos DP, Lenzi M, Okamoto M, Rigopoulou EI, Muratori P, Ma Y, et al. Multiple viral/self immunological cross-reactivity in liver kidney microsomal antibody positive hepatitis C virus infected patients is associated with the possession of HLA B51. Int J Immunopathol Pharmacol. 2004;17(1):83–92.
11. Smyk DS, Mavropoulos A, Mieli-Vergani G, Vergani D, Lenzi M, Bogdanos DP. The role of invariant NKT in autoimmune liver disease: can vitamin D act as an immunomodulator? Can J Gastroenterol Hepatol. 2018;2018:8197937.
12. de Boer YS, van Gerven NM, Zwiers A, Verwer BJ, van Hoek B, van Erpecum KJ, et al. Genome-wide association study identifies variants associated with autoimmune hepatitis type 1. Gastroenterology. 2014;147(2):443–52 e5.
13. van Gerven NM, Verwer BJ, Witte BI, van Erpecum KJ, van Buuren HR, Maijers I, et al. Epidemiology and clinical characteristics of autoimmune hepatitis in the Netherlands. Scand J Gastroenterol. 2014;49(10):1245–54.
14. Gregorio GV, Portmann B, Reid F, Donaldson PT, Doherty DG, McCartney M, et al. Autoimmune hepatitis in childhood: a 20-year experience. Hepatology. 1997;25(3):541–7.
15. Boberg KM, Aadland E, Jahnsen J, Raknerud N, Stiris M, Bell H. Incidence and prevalence of primary biliary cirrhosis, primary sclerosing cholangitis, and autoimmune hepatitis in a Norwegian population. Scand J Gastroenterol. 1998;33(1):99–103.
16. Feld JJ, Heathcote EJ. Epidemiology of autoimmune liver disease. J Gastroenterol Hepatol. 2003;18(10):1118–28.

17. Werner M, Prytz H, Ohlsson B, Almer S, Bjornsson E, Bergquist A, et al. Epidemiology and the initial presentation of autoimmune hepatitis in Sweden: a nationwide study. Scand J Gastroenterol. 2008;43(10):1232–40.
18. Krawitt EL. Autoimmune hepatitis. N Engl J Med. 2006;354(1):54–66.
19. Czaja AJ, Carpenter HA. Autoimmune hepatitis with incidental histologic features of bile duct injury. Hepatology. 2001;34(4 Pt 1):659–65.
20. Bogdanos DP, Mieli-Vergani G, Vergani D. Autoantibodies and their antigens in autoimmune hepatitis. Semin Liver Dis. 2009;29(3):241–53.
21. Radzimski C, Probst C, Teegen B, Rentzsch K, Blocker IM, Dahnrich C, et al. Development of a recombinant cell-based indirect immunofluorescence assay for the determination of autoantibodies against soluble liver antigen in autoimmune hepatitis. Clin Dev Immunol. 2013;2013:572815.
22. European Association for the Study of the L. EASL Clinical Practice Guidelines: autoimmune hepatitis. J Hepatol. 2015;63(4):971–1004.
23. Manns MP, Czaja AJ, Gorham JD, Krawitt EL, Mieli-Vergani G, Vergani D, et al. Diagnosis and management of autoimmune hepatitis. Hepatology. 2010;51(6):2193–213.
24. van Gerven NM, Verwer BJ, Witte BI, van Hoek B, Coenraad MJ, van Erpecum KJ, et al. Relapse is almost universal after withdrawal of immunosuppressive medication in patients with autoimmune hepatitis in remission. J Hepatol. 2013;58(1):141–7.
25. Liberal R, Zen Y, Mieli-Vergani G, Vergani D. Liver transplantation and autoimmune liver diseases. Liver Transpl. 2013;19(10):1065–77.

Primary Sclerosing Cholangitis

14

Andreas L. Koutsoumpas, George Efthymiou, Maria G. Mytilinaiou, and Dimitrios P. Bogdanos

Abbreviations

AASLD	American Association for the Study of Liver Diseases
AIH	Autoimmune hepatitis
ALP	Alkaline phosphatase
ASC	Autoimmune sclerosing cholangitis
CCA	Cholangiocarcinoma
ERC	Endoscopic retrograde cholangiography
GP2	Zymogen granule glycoprotein 2
GWAS	Genome wide association studies
HLA	Human leukocyte antigen
IBD	Inflammatory bowel disease
IgG	Immunoglobulin G
MRC	Magnetic resonance cholangiography
MRI	Magnetic resonance imaging
OLT	Orthotopic liver transplantation
PBC	Primary biliary cholangitis
PSC	Primary sclerosing cholangitis
UC	Ulcerative colitis
UDCA	Ursodeoxycholic acid

Key Concepts

- Primary sclerosing cholangitis is a chronic progressive autoimmune cholestatic liver disease characterised by intrahepatic and extrahepatic bile duct destruction.
- Diagnosis of the disease is made upon evidence of cholestatic liver blood test elevation, characteristic endoscopic features of cholangiopathy and liver biopsy histological features compatible with primary sclerosing cholangitis.
- The hypotheses of the leaky gut and the importance of the gut–liver T-cell trafficking axis are largely used to explain the development of the disease and the frequent co-occurrence of inflammatory bowel diseases in genetically prone individuals with immunoregulatory deficiency.
- Currently, there is no drug or treatment able to prolong transplant-free survival in patients with PSC, but ursodeoxycholic acid in moderate doses is widely used.
- In PSC patients with dominant stricture, pruritus, and/or cholangitis, ERCP with endoscopic dilatation is endorsed to alleviate symptoms.

A. L. Koutsoumpas · G. Efthymiou · M. G. Mytilinaiou
D. P. Bogdanos (✉)
Division of Rheumatology and Clinical Immunology, Faculty of Medicine, School of Health Sciences, University of Thessaly, Larissa, Greece
e-mail: bogdanos@med.uth.gr

14.1 Introduction

Primary sclerosing cholangitis (PSC) is a chronic cholestatic liver disease characterized by immune-mediated inflammation and multifocal biliary strictures, leading to cirrhosis, portal hypertension and hepatic decompensation, the only curative option being that of liver transplantation [1, 2].

Disease recurrence post liver transplantation is a well-described feature [3]. Approximately two thirds of the affected patients have co-existent inflammatory bowel disease (IBD), a phenomenon, which acquires clinical and pathophysiological connotations. Contrariwise, just 3–5% of patients with IBD have PSC and this cannot be neglected.

The paradoxical predominance of males and the lack of efficient response to corticosteroids have positioned PSC for several years in the list of immune-mediated diseases with questionable 'autoimmune origin'. The presence of autoantibodies and the clonality of T-cell receptors supported for years the view that PSC is an autoimmune disease [4].

F. Radu-Ionita et al. (eds.), *Liver Diseases*, https://doi.org/10.1007/978-3-030-24432-3_14

Ulcerative colitis (UC) is the most prominent form of IBD that co-occurs with PSC, but Crohn's disease, as well as, indeterminate colitis is also present. Cholangiocarcinoma (CCA)—and colorectal cancer—are serious comorbidities of the disease. Recognition of the disease has started to emerge soon after the implementation of endoscopic retrograde cholangiography (ERC) and the appreciation of the increased prevalence of CCA in patients suffering from PSC [5].

Subsequent appreciation of the heterogeneous phenotypes of the disease and the thorough description of well-defined, but still enigmatic, entities such as those of small-duct PSC, immunoglobulin G (IgG)4-related PSC (or PSC with high IgG4 levels) and autoimmune hepatitis (AIH) with overlapping features have added more jigsaws on the puzzling portrait of this perplexing disease.

Typical cholestatic and histological features of PSC and normal bile ducts on cholangiography characterize small duct PSC. IgG4-positive PSC is considered a separate entity, most likely related to the sphere of the IgG4-related syndrome.

14.2 Diagnostic Criteria

Diagnosis of the disease is largely based on radiological evidence of cholangiopathy demonstrating multifocal intrahepatic and/or extrahepatic biliary strictures and segmental dilations and increased cholestatic biochemical profile, i.e. elevated serum alkaline phosphatase (ALP) levels that persist for more than 6 months [6].

Largely the diagnosis is established on the exclusion of known causes of secondary cholangitis. MRC is currently the preferred diagnostic tool of choice in order to establish a firm diagnosis, as both sensitivity and specificity are adequate. Of note, ALP can fluctuate over the course of the disease and the disease is not excluded by definition if ALP levels are normal or is normalized over time (and prior to treatment). Unprompted control of ALP levels may bear prognostic significance, as these patients seem to have better outcome [7].

Compatible features on liver biopsy, such as those of chronic cholangitis and periductal fibrosis, are considered equally important for the establishment of diagnosis, but in general, liver biopsy is considered only necessary for the diagnosis of overlap with AIH or small-duct primary sclerosing cholangitis. Thus, a young male with cholestasis, characteristic cholangiopathy and IBD at presentation practically does not require liver biopsy for placing a definite diagnosis. Nevertheless, when liver biopsy is performed, staging of the disease can be accomplished [8].

Therefore, it is not surprising that in the guidelines for the diagnosis and management of PSC issued by the American Association for the Study of Liver Diseases (AASLD), patients with cholestatic biochemical profile are recommended to undergo indirect (MRC) or direct cholangiography (ERC) for making the diagnosis of PSC. The guidelines recommend against routine liver biopsy for the diagnosis of PSC in patients with typical cholangiographic findings. Of note, in patients with a normal ERC or MRC, it is recommended a liver biopsy to diagnose small duct PSC while in patients with disproportionately elevated aminotransferases, the guidelines recommend performing a liver biopsy to diagnose or exclude overlap syndrome [2].

Non-invasive serum markers cannot yet be considered efficient for the evaluation of fibrosis related to PSC. Fibroscan or magnetic resonance elastography are useful tools for the assessment of fibrosis but studies are still needed to establish their potential application in PSC [6].

14.3 Epidemiology

There is a slight but notable male predominance (considering also the female preponderance of AIH and PBC), as approximately 60% of patients with PSC are male. The prevalence and incidence of the disease largely varies; the prevalence ranges from 0 to 16.2 cases per 100,000 people and the incidence from 0 to 1.3 per 100,000 people per year and primary sclerosing cholangitis are male (median age approx. 40 years) [9].

Several studies from northern Europe reported an increase of the incidence and the prevalence of the disease, but leave debatable whether these increases are true or related to increased awareness, and more efficient diagnostic work up (mainly due to the development and more frequent application of endoscopic ERC and MRC) [6].

14.4 Natural History

At the time of diagnosis, a patient may have end-stage liver disease with or without CCA. However, more than half of the patients with PSC are asymptomatic and their disease is unmasked when diagnostic work up reveals increased cholestatic liver-function tests and subsequent testing leads to a diagnosis of PSC [10].

Hepatomegaly and splenomegaly can be present as well as non-specific symptoms of fatigue, and abdominal pain. Pruritus and jaundice are observed in a proportion of the patients but are not predominant features of the disease at presentation [2].

Median survival rates greatly vary amongst studies. The disease is generally slow in progression and the median survival rate is approximately 20 years. This rate becomes shorter (around 13 years) if patients are followed up in transplantation centres, which arguably monitor patients with more severe disease, and subsequently worst outcome [11]. Ninety two percent of the patients from this population were receiving ursodeoxycholic acid (UCDA).

14.5 Serological Features

Increased IgM is noted in approximately 40% of PSC patients. Increased IgG in serum is found increased (1.5 times the upper limit of normal) in approximately 60% of patients with PSC.

Several attempts have been made and studies are still trying to establish a clear evidence of the presence of disease-related, antigen-specific autoantibodies. Antineutrophil cytoplasmic antibodies (ANCA) are present in the great majority of the patients, but their diagnostic relevance is not widely appreciated probably due to the lack of proper autoantigen recognition [12].

Several studies have attempted to identify PSC-specific autoantigenic targets. Fresh data suggested that IgA reactivity targeting zymogen granule glycoprotein 2 (GP2) is a mucosal target of antibodies in patients with PSC, and that their presence defines patients with more severe disease. IgG and IgA anti-GP2 antibody responses are also found in patients with IBD (predominantly Crohn's disease) and are associated with disease severity [13, 14]. A multicentre effort, including our centre, has shown that simultaneous detection of IgA antibodies against isoforms 1 and 4 yield a sensitivity of 66.0% and a specificity of 97.9% resulting in the best diagnostic performance. IgA positivity is significantly associated with the presence of cirrhosis in PSC and this may indicate that such an autoantibody could be used as marker for risk stratification [15].

Increase of aminotransferase levels is detected, but a sharp elevation points towards the presence of co-existent AIH and requires immediate attention for therapeutic purposes and prompt initiation of immunosuppression.

Bilirubin monitoring, leading to the appreciation that its levels increases over time could be an indication of progression of the disease characterized by stricture, or even development of CCA and is always considered alarming.

14.6 Imaging Features

Participation of both the intrahepatic and extrahepatic biliary tree is the norm, except of disease phenotypic permutations, which there understanding has emerged over the years. Strictures differ in length, diameter and location and occur in 45–58% of patients during follow up. Dominant strictures defined as stenoses with a diameter of ≤1.5 mm in the common bile duct or of ≤1 mm in the hepatic duct are found in up to 60% of patients during follow up and raise a suspicion of CCA. In view of that, the AASLD recommends initial management with endoscopic dilatation with or without stenting in PSC patients with dominant strictures and in case of a failed attempt recommends dilatation of the biliary tract by percutaneous cholangiography (with or without stenting). Also, on superimposed malignancy prior to endoscopic treatment for dominant strictures, performance of brush cytology and/or endoscopic biopsy is also advised.

14.7 Histopathological Features

Staging from 1 to 4 is widely used for PSC in routine practise, but permutations exist [2]. Liver biopsy findings include paucicellular non-suppurative cholangitis absent cholestasis, ductular proliferation, and peri-ductal fibrosis, which classically acquires an "onion skin" appearance. Ductopenia can be present or absent. Of note, the "onion skin" is relatively infrequent, and despite being pathognomonic, its lack does not exclude firm diagnosis [16].

All other histopathological features, such as fibro-obliterative cholangitis can occur on ductopenic rejection following liver transplantation, acquired immune deficiency syndrome cholangiopathy and IgG4-associated cholangiopathy, and this is why liver biopsy has not been considered a must for establishing or refuting a diagnosis.

14.8 Autoimmune Hepatitis in PSC

PSC-AIH overlap syndrome is observed in up to 5% of adult patients with PSC and can be developed several years after the original diagnosis of PSC [17]. Co-existence of PSC and AIH must be considered in cases of PSC who experience significant elevation of unexplained transaminasemia (3–5 times fold increase or higher the upper normal limit) and in patients with AIH with partial or no response to immunosuppressive treatment and profound cholestatic liver enzyme biochemistry profile. Autoimmune sclerosing cholangitis (ASC), is a distinct entity originally described in children and subsequently in adults. ASC is a form of sclerosing cholangitis with overlapping AIH features. It is the main cause of sclerosing cholangitis in children cases. ASC does not show male predominance but, similar to adult PSC, —though less profoundly—, co-exists with IBD in approximately half of the affected children. Serological features are indistinguishable to those of AIH, including the presence of AIH-related ANA and SMA and evidence of hyperglobulinaemia. More than half of the affected children respond well to a combination of steroids and ursodeoxycholic acid (UDCA). Those who do not respond will require liver transplantation and the recurrence of the disease is a well-recognized entity. Thus far, it is not clear whether ASC shares common underlying pathophysiological features with PSC or AIH.

14.9 Extrahepatic Manifestations

PSC is usually following the diagnosis of IBD by 5–10 years, the two diseases not necessarily being associated in terms of severity [18]. A provocative study has noted that the colon was affected in all patients with coexisting primary PSC and IBD, irrespectively of whether they had UC or CD; this further underlines the need for colonoscopy at diagnosis in every newly diagnosed PSC patient with no evidence of IBD [19]. That study reported pancolitis in 94% of PSC-UC and colitis in 96% of PSC-CD patients [19]. This colitis appears softer compared to that noted in patients with IBD alone. Such an assessment is also of importance for the surveillance of colon cancer, which is 4–5 times more frequent in PSC patients with IBD compared to IBD alone and 10 times higher compared to general population.

PSC is the most common cause of CCA in developed countries and one of the best-known risk factors for CCA. CCA in PSC is presented in 5–10% of PSC patients over their lifetime, with an overall risk of 0.5–1.5% per year [20].

Up to 25% of patients with PSC have gallstones. Their presence must be taken into account for prognostic reasons. The prevalence and risk factors for gallbladder neoplasia among patients with PSC undergoing orthotopic liver transplantation (OLT) has been the focus of prompt pathological analyses and high frequencies of inflammatory, metaplastic, and neoplastic changes have been noted in gallbladders of patients with PSC undergoing OLT, dysplasia being present in a remarkable 37% of patients and adenocarcinoma in 14% [21].

Prompt screening and monitoring includes testing of the serum tumour marker CA 19-9, which though is not a specific marker, can be useful if is elevated in patients with previously normal ALP levels, who are presented with jaundice, fever or weight loss. Ultrasonography, liver MRI or ERC are useful imaging tools for the prompt diagnosis of CCA and several clinicians advise their patients to undergo CA 19-9 testing and ultrasonographic evaluation at annual basis.

14.10 Pathogenesis

The pathogenesis of PSC is incompletely understood. The disease is considered autoimmune in nature, but several aspects of the disease are peculiar and do not fit with the ones currently found in other autoimmune liver disease, such as AIH and primary biliary cholangitis (PBC). Of relevance, PSC can co-exist with AIH but not with PBC, a finding that lacks convincing explanation.

In general, genetic, epigenetic, as well as environmental risk factors are considered important for the development and the progression of the disease over time [6]. Genome wide association studies (GWAS) and genetic studies involving siblings of patients with PSC with or without IBD have been supportive of the influence of the genetic make up of the patients. It appears that siblings of patients with PSC and IBD have 11-fold and 8-fold higher risk of developing PSC comparing to controls. Such an estimate reveals the same degree of heritability, which is noted in most autoimmune disorders. Up to now, several susceptibility loci for PSC have been recognized through GWAS. The human leukocyte antigen (HLA) complex embodies the strongest associations, pointing mainly towards HLA-DRB1s [22].

The same GWAS have identified more than 20 non-HLA susceptibility loci for PSC and 29 notable candidate genes within those loci: MMEL1, TNFRSF14, BCL2L11, CD28, CTLA4, CCL20, GPR35, MST1, FOXP1, NFKB1, IL2, IL21, BACH2, IL2RA, SIK2, CCDC88B, HDAC7, RFX4, RIC8B, SH2B3, ATXN2, CLEC16A, SOCS1, TCF4, CD226, PRKD2, STRN4, UBASH3A and PSMG1. Another 20 notable candidate genes are found within the nine suggestive risk loci, two of those, namely MST1 and HHEX, requiring special mention as they appear to be highly expressed in the liver [22]. Both affect cell proliferation and a specific deletion of MST1 plays a role in development of hepatocellular carcinoma, a feature also noted for HHEX. PSC has been considered a disease mainly established via lymphocyte trafficking between the gut and the liver and is of interest that MST1 plays role in leukocyte adhesion and chemotaxis affecting lymphocyte function-associated antigen-1.

Most studies make use of the close association of PSC with IBD to formulate hypothesis regarding disease's pathogenesis. In this context, it has been considered very likely that responsible for disease's development is the 'leaky gut', which is based on the hypothesis, supported by data provided by animal studies, that mucosal injury in patients suffering with IBD would lead to 'leakage' of bacterial products into the portal circulation and subsequent immune activation and inflammation targeting the biliary ducts [23].

Another hypothesis, not mutually exclusive of the previous one, is based on the appreciation of a gut–liver T-cell trafficking axis, which is the ultimate cause for biliary epithelial cell destruction and biliary inflammation. The paradoxical presence of PSC presence in patients with IBD after colectomy cannot be thoroughly explained by any of those theories.

Risk genes in the immune system are well documented including CTLA4 and FOXP1, genes important for immune regulation and associated with a vast number of autoimmune diseases. Most other risk genes for PSC are highly expressed in the immune system, underlying the autoimmune nature of the disease, or at least the important role played by the immune system in its development. Nevertheless, PSC risk genes also participate in apoptosis, autophagy, metabolism, cell growth and death [22].

Autoreactive lymphocytes against yet unidentified autoepitopes expressed in biliary epithelial cells are likely perpetuators of disease development. Innate immune cells, such as natural killer cells and natural killer T cells, have also been considered important for the perpetuation of the pathogenic pathways that lead to disease's induction, but their role is largely unknown. Provocative data are supporting the idea that at later stages of the disease, i.e. those following the initial immune insult superinfection may signify an essential element for disease evolution. Data from a single study showed that in patients with dominant stenosis and biliary Candida infection, survival free of liver transplantation was reduced in comparison to those with sterile bile in patients, the former developing more advanced disease [24]. Of note, the beneficial effect of vancomycin treatment in PSC has been reported, though in small series.

14.11 Medical Treatment

The most widely inspected drug in PSC is UDCA, a hydrophilic bile acid. Several studies have reported favourable effects with UDCA in patients with PSC, but others failed to replicate such findings.

Despite being effective in treating PBC, studies so far conducted in PSC have been inconclusive. Pilot studies in the early 1990s have shown improvement of the cholestatic biochemical profile and some have even showed histological improvement at a dosage of 10–15 mg/kg/day. Subsequent studies in North America indicated no improvement in liver histology and symptomatology but only in serum liver tests [25]. Higher doses were introduced to assess whether larger doses are essential for the enhancement of the bile acid pool in the setting of cholestasis, as this could theoretically increase the immunomodulatory potential of the drug; however, higher UDCA doses appear to be injurious [26].

A large study from the Scandinavian UDCA trial recruited 219 PSC patients for a period of 5 years using 17–23 mg/kg/day of UCDA. The data were somewhat surprising. The biochemical response was poor and that led authors to raise questions regarding the efficacy of UDCA or the adequate compliance of specific study populations. Despite the large number of patients and the lengthy period of assessment, only a trend towards better survival in the UDCA-treated group was noticed [27].

Because the evidence provided so far is not supportive, AASLD recommendations are against the use of UCDA as medical therapy of adult patients with PSC [2]. The European Association for the Study of Liver moves towards a similar vein, but using a smoother wording in the recommendations, stating "that the limited data base does not yet allow a specific recommendation for the general use of UDCA in PSC". However, at present clinicians are widely using UDCA for the treatment of PSC at moderate doses (15–20 mg/kg daily) [28]. Meta-analyses do not provide evidence of a reduced risk of cancer in UDCA-treated PSC patients [29].

Combination of UDCA and metronidazole does not slow down disease progression but improves biochemistry cholestatic profiles. UDCA together with fibrates have been used for patients who are resistant in terms of biochemical response to UDCA alone. The documented efficacy on liver blood tests of patients with PSC receiving drugs with anticholestatic properties such as peroxisome proliferator-activated receptor agonists and fibrates is promising but remains to be demonstrated in larger studies. The use of sirolimus is not evidence based. A recent pilot clinical trial of 10 patients with PSC, including nine with ulcerative colitis and one with Crohn's disease, who underwent faecal microbiota transplantation has been encouraging. No safety issues were raised and 30% of the patients showed a ≥50% decrease in ALP levels [30].

Patients with overlapping features of PSC and AIH are treated with steroids, but the use of corticosteroid use or other immunosuppressants is not recommended for treatment of PSC in the absence of overlapping AIH [31]. Other treatments that have been tested and are not proven beneficial are prednisolone, budesonide, colchicine, penicillamine, azathioprine, tacrolimus, methotrexate, mycophenolate mofetil, and biologic treatment with antitumor necrosis factor antibodies. Though they are not recommended, we must clarify that studies investigating their efficacy and safety profile are extremely limited and the obtained data are scarce to completely neglect them [28]. PSC patients with IgG4-related disease treated with immunosuppressive treatments show resolution of biliary structuring, sharp decrease of IgG4 concentrations and normalization of liver tests.

Surgical options for PSC include biliary reconstructive procedures like choledochoduodenostomy, choledochojejunostomy, and liver transplantation, which is the only curable treatment for patients with decompensated cirrhosis and 5-year survival rates of up to 80%.

Data from 3710 patients who had received transplants between 2001 and 2015 of the European Liver Transplant Registry indicate short-term and long-term survival in at 91% at 1 year, 82% at 5 years, and 74% at 10 years [28]. Early referral to a liver centre/transplant unit is key component of the successful handling of cirrhotic PSC patients. Indications for liver transplantation embrace a Model for End-Stage Liver Disease score of >14 [32]. A metanalysis demonstrates that colectomy before liver transplantation reduced the risk of recurrent PSC [33].

In conclusion, primary sclerosing cholangitis is a progressive immune-mediated cholestatic liver disease stamped by intrahepatic or extrahepatic stricturing, leading to fibrosis, cirrhosis and liver failure, if left without liver transplantation. Symptomatology at presentation largely varies from being asymptomatic to that noting itching, malaise, icterus and portal hypertension. The diagnosis is based on evidence of cholestatic liver biochemistry and bile duct stricturing on cholangiography. Approximately two thirds of patients have concomitant inflammatory bowel disease and colonoscopy screening and surveillance is required. The disease is associated with increased malignancy risk including cholangiocarcinoma and colon cancer. Genetic, environmental and immunological elements are important for the induction and the progression of the disease. No curative medical treatment currently exists but ursodeoxycholic acid is widely used for its treatment without evidence of improvement of transplant-free survival. Disease recurrence following liver transplantation can be noted.

Self Study

Questions

1. A 28-year-old male presents to his primary care physician because of a 6 weeks history of generalized fatigue, itching, and recent weight loss. His past medical history is notable for ulcerative colitis, treated with mesalamine. Abdominal examination, elicits mild tenderness to palpation in the right upper quadrant, but Murphy's sign is not present. Laboratory tests show elevated gamma-glutamyl-transpeptidase (GGT) and alkaline phosphatase. Endoscopic retrograde cholangiopancreatography (ERCP) reveals radiological features characteristic of PSC. Which of the following is likely to be FALSE:
   (a) Anti-mitochondrial antibodies are positive
   (b) Transaminases are always within the normal levels
   (c) Radiological evidence will never reveal dominant strictures
   (d) A, B and C
2. Factors that may increase the risk of primary sclerosing cholangitis DO NOT include:
   (a) Young age
   (b) Male gender
   (c) Evidence of inflammatory bowel disease
   (d) None of the above
3. Regarding primary sclerosing cholangitis the following is FALSE:
   (a) Most patients have inflammatory bowel disease
   (b) Liver biopsy is imperative in order to confirm diagnosis
   (c) Magnetic resonance cholangiography is the diagnostic modality of choice
   (d) A and C

Answers

1 A 28-year-old male presents to his primary care physician because of a 6 weeks history of generalized fatigue, itching, and recent weight loss. His past medical history is notable for ulcerative colitis, treated with mesalamine. Abdominal examination, elicits mild tenderness to palpation in the right upper quadrant, but Murphy's sign is not present. Laboratory tests show elevated gamma-glutamyl-transpeptidase (GGT) and alkaline phosphatase. Endoscopic retrograde cholangiopancreatography (ERCP) reveals radiological features characteristic of PSC. Which of the following is likely to be FALSE:
   (a) FALSE. Young age is a risk factor for primary sclerosing cholangitis, the disease mainly affecting Anti-mitochondrial antibodies are detectable in patients with primary sclerosing cholangitis (PBC), a disease with a remarkable female predominance. PBC and PSC do not overlap and true AMA cannot be detect in PSC patients There is Patients with AIH can have detectable antinuclear antibodies but they can also be negative for those. Thus, a single test for ANA is not sufficient for proper diagnosis
   (b) FALSE. Transaminases can be normal or high (usually mildly increased) in patients with PSC.
   (c) FALSE. Dominant strictures are seen in a considerable proportion of the patients. Their presence is highly suggestive of the disease. Their absence is not excluding diagnosis of PSC
   (d) CORRECT. All the above are FALSE statements for PSC

2 Factors that may increase the risk of primary sclerosing cholangitis DO NOT include:
   (a) FALSE. The disease is usually affecting young males, who may have concomitant inflammatory bowel disease
   (b) FALSE The disease affects both males and females but PSC has a male preponderance (2:1)
   (c) FALSE: Approximately two thirds of the affected patients have co-existent inflammatory bowel disease (IBD), a phenomenon, which acquires clinical and pathophysiological connotations. Contrariwise, just 3–5% of patients with IBD have PSC
   (d) CORRECT: all the above are risk factors for PSC 3.

3 Regarding primary sclerosing cholangitis the following is FALSE:
   (a) The statement that most patients have inflammatory bowel disease is true for primary sclerosing cholangitis
   (b) Liver biopsy is assisting the firm diagnosis of primary sclerosing cholangitis but is not a prerequisite for making diagnosis, especially in a young male with

ulcerative colitis and characteristic cholangiographic features
(c) Magnetic resonance cholangiography is indeed the diagnostic modality of choice
(d) CORRECT: both A and C are TRUE for PSC

References

1. Aadland E, Schrumpf E, Fausa O, Elgjo K, Heilo A, Aakhus T, et al. Primary sclerosing cholangitis: a long-term follow-up study. Scand J Gastroenterol. 1987;22(6):655–64.
2. Chapman R, Fevery J, Kalloo A, Nagorney DM, Boberg KM, Shneider B, et al. Diagnosis and management of primary sclerosing cholangitis. Hepatology. 2010;51(2):660–78.
3. Lerut J, Demetris AJ, Stieber AC, Marsh JW, Gordon RD, Esquivel CO, et al. Intrahepatic bile duct strictures after human orthotopic liver transplantation. Recurrence of primary sclerosing cholangitis or unusual presentation of allograft rejection? Transpl Int. 1988;1(3):127–30.
4. Thorpe ME, Scheuer PJ, Sherlock S. Primary sclerosing cholangitis, the biliary tree, and ulcerative colitis. Gut. 1967;8(5):435–48.
5. Wee A, Ludwig J, Coffey RJ Jr, LaRusso NF, Wiesner RH. Hepatobiliary carcinoma associated with primary sclerosing cholangitis and chronic ulcerative colitis. Hum Pathol. 1985;16(7):719–26.
6. Lazaridis KN, LaRusso NF. Primary sclerosing cholangitis. N Engl J Med. 2016;375(25):2501–2.
7. Al Mamari S, Djordjevic J, Halliday JS, Chapman RW. Improvement of serum alkaline phosphatase to <1.5 upper limit of normal predicts better outcome and reduced risk of cholangiocarcinoma in primary sclerosing cholangitis. J Hepatol. 2013;58(2):329–34.
8. Burak KW, Angulo P, Lindor KD. Is there a role for liver biopsy in primary sclerosing cholangitis? Am J Gastroenterol. 2003;98(5):1155–8.
9. Molodecky NA, Kareemi H, Parab R, Barkema HW, Quan H, Myers RP, et al. Incidence of primary sclerosing cholangitis: a systematic review and meta-analysis. Hepatology. 2011;53(5):1590–9.
10. Tischendorf JJ, Hecker H, Kruger M, Manns MP, Meier PN. Characterization, outcome, and prognosis in 273 patients with primary sclerosing cholangitis: a single center study. Am J Gastroenterol. 2007;102(1):107–14.
11. Boonstra K, Weersma RK, van Erpecum KJ, Rauws EA, Spanier BW, Poen AC, et al. Population-based epidemiology, malignancy risk, and outcome of primary sclerosing cholangitis. Hepatology. 2013;58(6):2045–55.
12. Angulo P, Peter JB, Gershwin ME, DeSotel CK, Shoenfeld Y, Ahmed AE, et al. Serum autoantibodies in patients with primary sclerosing cholangitis. J Hepatol. 2000;32(2):182–7.
13. Pavlidis P, Forbes A, Bogdanos DP. Anti-GP2 antibodies in inflammatory bowel disease patients with ileal pouch. J Crohns Colitis. 2013;7(11):e602–3.
14. Pavlidis P, Komorowski L, Teegen B, Liaskos C, Koutsoumpas AL, Smyk DS, et al. Diagnostic and clinical significance of Crohn's disease-specific pancreatic anti-GP2 and anti-CUZD1 antibodies. Clin Chem Lab Med. 2016;54(2):249–56.
15. Sowa M, Kolenda R, Baumgart DC, Pratschke J, Papp M, Tornai T, et al. Mucosal autoimmunity to cell-bound GP2 isoforms is a sensitive marker in PSC and associated with the clinical phenotype. Front Immunol. 2018;9:1959.
16. Ludwig J, Barham SS, LaRusso NF, Elveback LR, Wiesner RH, McCall JT. Morphologic features of chronic hepatitis associated with primary sclerosing cholangitis and chronic ulcerative colitis. Hepatology. 1981;1(6):632–40.
17. Gohlke F, Lohse AW, Dienes HP, Lohr H, Marker-Hermann E, Gerken G, et al. Evidence for an overlap syndrome of autoimmune hepatitis and primary sclerosing cholangitis. J Hepatol. 1996;24(6):699–705.
18. Loftus EV Jr, Sandborn WJ, Tremaine WJ, Mahoney DW, Zinsmeister AR, Offord KP, et al. Risk of colorectal neoplasia in patients with primary sclerosing cholangitis. Gastroenterology. 1996;110(2):432–40.
19. Boonstra K, van Erpecum KJ, van Nieuwkerk KM, Drenth JP, Poen AC, Witteman BJ, et al. Primary sclerosing cholangitis is associated with a distinct phenotype of inflammatory bowel disease. Inflamm Bowel Dis. 2012;18(12):2270–6.
20. Razumilava N, Gores GJ. Classification, diagnosis, and management of cholangiocarcinoma. Clin Gastroenterol Hepatol. 2013;11(1):13–21 e1. quiz e3-4
21. Lewis JT, Talwalkar JA, Rosen CB, Smyrk TC, Abraham SC. Prevalence and risk factors for gallbladder neoplasia in patients with primary sclerosing cholangitis: evidence for a metaplasia-dysplasia-carcinoma sequence. Am J Surg Pathol. 2007;31(6):907–13.
22. Jiang X, Karlsen TH. Genetics of primary sclerosing cholangitis and pathophysiological implications. Nat Rev Gastroenterol Hepatol. 2017;14(5):279–95.
23. Lichtman SN, Keku J, Clark RL, Schwab JH, Sartor RB. Biliary tract disease in rats with experimental small bowel bacterial overgrowth. Hepatology. 1991;13(4):766–72.
24. Rudolph G, Gotthardt D, Kloters-Plachky P, Kulaksiz H, Rost D, Stiehl A. Influence of dominant bile duct stenoses and biliary infections on outcome in primary sclerosing cholangitis. J Hepatol. 2009;51(1):149–55.
25. Lindor KD. Ursodiol for primary sclerosing cholangitis. Mayo Primary Sclerosing Cholangitis-Ursodeoxycholic Acid Study Group. N Engl J Med. 1997;336(10):691–5.
26. Lindor KD, Kowdley KV, Luketic VA, Harrison ME, McCashland T, Befeler AS, et al. High-dose ursodeoxycholic acid for the treatment of primary sclerosing cholangitis. Hepatology. 2009;50(3):808–14.
27. Olsson R, Boberg KM, de Muckadell OS, Lindgren S, Hultcrantz R, Folvik G, et al. High-dose ursodeoxycholic acid in primary sclerosing cholangitis: a 5-year multicenter, randomized, controlled study. Gastroenterology. 2005;129(5):1464–72.
28. Dyson JK, Beuers U, Jones DEJ, Lohse AW, Hudson M. Primary sclerosing cholangitis. Lancet. 2018;391(10139):2547–59.
29. Hansen JD, Kumar S, Lo WK, Poulsen DM, Halai UA, Tater KC. Ursodiol and colorectal cancer or dysplasia risk in primary sclerosing cholangitis and inflammatory bowel disease: a meta-analysis. Dig Dis Sci. 2013;58(11):3079–87.
30. Allegretti JR, Kassam Z, Carrellas M, Mullish BH, Marchesi JR, Pechlivanis A, et al. Fecal microbiota transplantation in patients with primary sclerosing cholangitis: a pilot clinical trial. Am J Gastroenterol. 2019;114(7):1071–9.
31. European Association for the Study of the L. EASL Clinical Practice Guidelines: management of cholestatic liver diseases. J Hepatol. 2009;51(2):237–67.
32. Kamath PS, Wiesner RH, Malinchoc M, Kremers W, Therneau TM, Kosberg CL, et al. A model to predict survival in patients with end-stage liver disease. Hepatology. 2001;33(2):464–70.
33. Steenstraten IC, Sebib Korkmaz K, Trivedi PJ, Inderson A, van Hoek B, Rodriguez Girondo MDM, et al. Systematic review with meta-analysis: risk factors for recurrent primary sclerosing cholangitis after liver transplantation. Aliment Pharmacol Ther. 2019;49(6):636–43.

Parasitic Liver Diseases

15

Yousry Hawash

Key Concepts
- Several parasites are involved in human liver diseases of distinct severities
- Owing to travel and immigration to endemic countries, sporadic cases have been frequently reported in non-endemic countries
- High level of clinical suspicion based on the patient's demographic, anamnestic, clinical data, and laboratory data is required for diagnosis.
- These diseases are incidental findings requiring no treatment in most of cases.
- The diseases tend to be aggressive and sometimes fatal in malnourished or immunosuppressed patients.
- Treatment is carried out using medical and/or surgical intervention.

15.1 Introduction

The human liver is frequently involved in infectious diseases, including the parasites-attributed, owing to its large size and its unique dual blood supply [1]. Parasitic liver diseases while relatively common in resource-poor countries, where parasites are endemic, are rare diagnosis in non-endemic countries. Nonetheless, sporadic cases of liver parasitosis have been reported and the number is rising in resource-rich countries secondary to frequent international travel, migration, and/or food trade [2]. Parasitic liver infections may be caused by a variety of parasites, summarized in Table 15.1.

Y. Hawash (✉)
Department of Medical and Molecular Parasitology, The National Liver Institute, Menoufia University, Menoufia, Egypt

The causative parasites can be divided into three main categories: those caused by protozoa, helminths (worms), and arthropods. Of these, the first two categories are by far the most common and will be the subject of this review.

Diseases can be a result of primary infection as in fascioliasis or as a part of systemic infections as in visceral leishmaniasis. Liver parasitosis in well-nourished and immunologically normal individuals, is an incidental finding, minimally symptomatic, and require no treatment. On the contrary, parasitic infections in patients those seen with depressed immunity, tend to be severe with adverse long-term

Table 15.1 A list of parasitic infections found associated with hepatobiliary diseases

List of parasitic infection (the causative parasite)
Helminthic infections:
Schistosomiasis (*Schistosoma* species)
Echinococcosis (*Echinococcus* species)
Clonorchiasis (*Clonorchis sinensis*)
Opisthorchiasis (*Opisthorchis felineus* and *O. viverrini*)
Fascioliasis (*Fasciola hepatica* and *F. gigantica*)
Ascariasis (*Ascaris lumbricoides* and *A. suum*)
Strongyloidiasis (*Strongyloides stercoralis*)
Capillariasis (*Capillaria hepatica*)
Toxocariasis (*Toxocara canis* and *T. cati*)
Enterobiasis (*Enterobius vermicularis*)
Fasciolopsiasis (*Fasciolopsis buski*)
Dicrocoeliasis (*Dicrocoelium dendriticum*)
Visceral pentastomiasis (*Linguatula serrata*)
Protozoan infections:
Amoebiasis (*Entamoeba histolytica*)
Giardiasis (*Giardia lamblia*)
Cryptosporidiosis (*Cryptosporidium* species)
Visceral Leishmaniasis (*Leishmania donovani* complex)
Malaria (*Plasmodium* species)
Toxoplasmosis (*Toxoplasma gondii*)
Trypanosomiasis (*Trypanosoma* species)
Babesiosis (*Babesia* species)

F. Radu-Ionita et al. (eds.), *Liver Diseases*, https://doi.org/10.1007/978-3-030-24432-3_15

consequences [3]. Diagnosis of parasitic liver diseases in most of cases is challenging because most of the causative infections are symptomless in its acute stage and even when hepatic injuries do occur, non-specific symptoms arise [4]. Thus, clinical suspicion based on the patient's demographic, anamnestic and clinical data, supported by an imaging or a laboratory test finding is mandatory for proper disease diagnosis and treatment. In this chapter, the clinically-relevant parasitic infections that have been found associated with liver diseases are considered, reviewed and discussed. We provide an updated outlook for each disease's etiology, pathogenesis, presentation and management.

15.1.1 Parasitic Liver Diseases: Helminths

Helminths or worms, are multicellular eukaryotic organisms capable to infect distinct mammalian hosts including humans. Helminths affecting the human liver are categorized into three major kinds: nematodes, trematodes, and cestodes. Helminths may inhabit the liver or gain access to it or its tributaries via the bile duct orifice or via the portal blood or through its capsule and sometimes the path to the liver is not known. Helminth infections are often associated with peripheral eosinophilia [5]. The human liver can be affected by a variety of helminths, illustrated in Fig. 15.1.

15.1.1.1 Schistosomiasis

Schistosomiasis is a neglected tropical disease attributed to five species of the genus *Schistosoma*, namely; *S. mansoni, S. japonicum, S. haematobium, S. mekongi,* and *S. intercalatum*. Schistosomiasis affects around 200 million people, mostly in Asia, Africa and the Americas [6]. The adult worms involved in intestinal schistosomiasis inhabit the mesenteric veins while that of urinary schistosomiasis reside the vesical plexus of veins. Upon sexual reproduction, eggs are released and shed with the patient's feces or urine to the environment based on the species. On reaching the fresh water, the eggs release miracidia that swim till reaching the species-specific snail intermediate hosts. Within the snail, sporocysts are produced and finally emerged as free-swimming cercaria. Cercariae infect human through skin penetration, losing tails, and became schistosomulae migrating until full maturity in the hepatic sinusoids. The mature adults leave the hepatic sinusoids to the more spacious, better oxygenated portal vein and copulate. Released ova penetrate the vascular wall to the rectal or vesical lumen, according to the species. The migrating juvenile and mature worm cause non-specific reactive hepatitis while eggs deposited in the liver parenchyma provoke an immune response with development of granulomas. The liver inflammation, produced, may lead to scarring, fibrosis and portal hypertension. Subsequently, portal hypertension may result in splenomegaly, ascites and

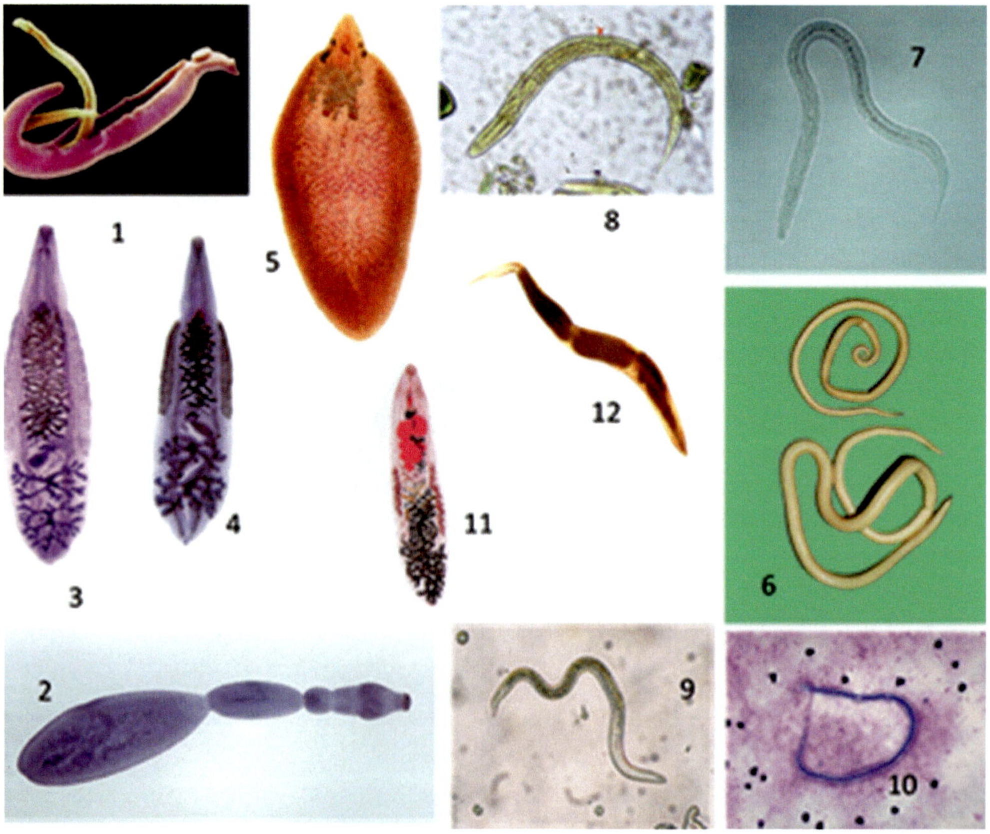

Fig. 15.1 A group of helminths found associated with human liver diseases. 1—Male and female *Schistosomes* in copula; 2—*Echinococcus granulosus* adult worm; 3—*Clonorchis sinensis* adult worm; 4—*Opisthorchis viverrini* adult worm; 5—*Fasciola hepatica* adult worms; 6—Male and female adults of *Ascaris lumbricoides*; 7—*Toxocara* adult worm; 8—*Strongyloides stercoralis* rhabditiform larva; 9—*Capillaria hepatica* adult worm; 10—Microfilaria in thick blood film; 11—*Dicrocoelium dendriticum* adult fluke; 12—*Enterobius vermicularis* adult female worm

esophageal varices. The initial infection is often asymptomatic but symptoms like itch or fever may be exhibited. Chronic phase with dysuria and/or hematuria in *S. haematobium* may develop.

Identification of the characteristic ova in stool or urine or tissues biopsies (rectal, vesical, hepatic) are the gold standard for diagnosis. Antibody detection tests in serum and antigen detection tests in urine are also available. Although it is not yet widely available, PCR-based molecular diagnosis was also tried [7]. Imaging studies, such as US, can demonstrate periportal fibrosis or other complications of chronic infection. Eosinophilia can be used as a crude marker of infection and successful treatment. Despite the fear of developing resistance toward it, praziquantel remains the drug of choice for treatment. The residual fibrotic lesions need no surgical correction but in certain instances subsequent complications may require surgical intervention.

15.1.2 Echinococcosis

Echinococcosis is a zoonotic infection caused by a cestode parasite of the genus *Echinococcus* [8]. Infection is generally contracted via contact with canine faeces. Two species in the genus *Echinococcus* are commonly involved: *Echinococcus granulosus* infection leads to the development of self-limiting and asymptomatic hydatid cysts, predominantly in the liver, and *Echinococcus multilocularis* causes cysts, mainly in the lung, but in this case the cysts are not self-limiting, and instead grow continuously, like a tumor.

The cystic hydatid disease is more common in regions where sheep are raised. Two separate life cycles of *Echinococcus granulosus* are recognized: a domestic and a sylvatic cycle. In the domestic cycle, the dog is the definitive host, whereas in the sylvatic cycle, the wild carnivores are the definitive hosts. The adult worms reside the small intestine of the dog and lay eggs that passed with the faeces to the environment. Man got infected through accidental ingestion of eggs contaminating hands, food or drinks. Inside the small intestine, the eggs release the oncosphere that penetrate the gut wall to the liver, lung or any other internal organs via the portal blood. Larvae encyst in the liver tissue forming fluid-filled cysts or hydatids. The cysts may be rupture (e. g. surgery, puncture), or damaged or got infected. Following rupture, dissemination of the floating scolices into the nearby cavity occur with secondary cysts formation. The release of hydatid fluid may cause a strong anaphylactic reaction and threaten the patient's life.

The clinical features of hydatidosis depend on the cyst site and size. Pain in the right upper quadrant, and hepatomegaly or a palpable epigastric or costal arch mass may be exhibited. Ruptured hydatid cysts into the biliary tract present with cholangitis. Apart from peripheral eosinophilia and an occasional increase in liver transaminases, laboratory findings are not particularly striking. Hydatid cyst may compress the bile ducts, cause cholestasis and mild jaundice. Imaging is a useful tool for confirming the diagnosis and exhibition of complications. Ultrasonography also helps in classifying the cysts stage. Serologic tests cannot substitute clinical or imaging investigations, but they can confirm the hydatid origin of a cyst. Treatment of liver hydatidosis varies, from surgical intervention to percutaneous drainage to medical therapy. Surgical removal of the cyst after albendazole treatment regimen, in conjunction with or without partial liver resection is the treatment of choice in majority of cases [9].

15.1.3 Clonorchiasis and Opisthorchiasis

Clonorchiasis is a parasitic disease caused by the Chinese liver fluke *Clonorchis sinensis* while opisthorchiasis is caused by one of two species *Opisthorchis viverrini* and *Opisthorchis felineus*. Both *Clonorchis sinensis* and *Opisthorchis viverrini* are endemic in East Asia, while *Opisthorchis felineus* presents in Asia as well as Europe [10]. The two flukes have a similar life cycle distributed in three different hosts: a mammalian host, a snail and a fish. In the definitive host, mature worms reside the biliary tree, feeding, moving and producing eggs that shed to the environment with the patient's stool. on reaching fresh water, the eggs are ingested by specific-species snails, where eggs hatch and release miracidia. The miracidia mature initially as sporocysts, then as rediae, and finally as cercariae. In the presence of an appropriate fish, cercariae invade the fish's skin and encyst as metacercariae in the fish muscle. Upon consumption of infected improperly-cooked fish, the metacercariae excyst and release larvae in the human duodenum, travel via the ampulla of Vater to the biliary tree.

The adult fluke repeatedly moves over the biliary epithelium, feeding and migrating resulting in mechanical tissue injuries. By time, these injuries become more evident and ulcerates. The fluke's eggs may become deposited in the periductal tissue through the ulcer and induce granulomatous inflammation around. In addition, the adult fluke secretes or excretes metabolic products, some of which are highly immunogenic, while the remaining may be toxic to or interact with the biliary epithelium. All these factors lead to dilatation of the bile ducts, chronic inflammation followed by adenomatous hyperplasia, and bile duct wall thickening. The heavy worm burden, inflammation and obstruction can lead to cholecystitis, cholangitis, hepatic abscess, pancreatitis and even cholangiocarcinoma [11].

Infections in their acute stage are usually asymptomatic. However, shortly after *C. sinensis* infection, urticaria, right upper quadrant abdominal pain and fever may develop. High-grade fever, arthralgia, lymphadenopathy and abdominal pain may occur. Chronic symptoms as abdominal pain and discomfort, weight loss and anorexia may be also exhibited. Hepatomegaly and right upper quadrant tenderness may be observed both in the acute and chronic phase.

Diagnosis of *Opistorchiidae* is usually carried out through identification of the characteristic eggs in patient's stool. Adult worms may occasionally be visualized moving with ultrasound examination of the biliary tract and gallbladder or identified in surgically- or endoscopically-obtained aspirate samples. Serological testing for *C. sinensis* IgG antibodies are also available. ELISA test for detection of *O. viverrini* antigens in urine, with adequate sensitivity is also present. Molecular detection of the parasite in stool have been tried for both genera with various sensitivities. Praziquantel, with cure rate of ≥80%, is the drug of choice for treatment.

15.1.4 Fascioliasis

Fascioliasis is a parasitic disease caused by flat fluke *Fasciola hepatica* and *Fasciola gigantica* [12]. The life cycle is like that of the liver flukes but does not have an intermediate fish host. Adult worms reside in the biliary tree producing eggs that embryonate in fresh water and release miracidia that invade snails. Stages of sporocysts, rediae and cercariae are developed in the snail. Cercariae encyst as metacercariae on the aquatic plants that transmit infection to humans if ingested raw. The metacercariae excyst in the duodenum, hatch to juvenile worms that invade the gut wall to the peritoneum. The immature worms penetrate the liver capsule and migrate via the parenchyma till the large biliary ducts where maturation into adult worms and oviposition occurs. During this journey, the juvenile flukes may reach to ectopic sites and may result in nodules or abscesses formation [13].

Inflammation, wall-thickening and/or dilatation of the gallbladder or bile ducts are the characteristic lesions produced by the adult fluke. Clinically, patients may present with right upper quadrant pain, fever and eosinophilia. During the acute stage, diagnosis is often made by serology. Eggs in aspirated bile, liver tissue, or stool can be detected after a certain period. The adult worm is occasionally identified in surgically or endoscopically obtained aspirates and seen as moving object in ultrasound imaging. The small hypodense nodules and linear tracks within the liver parenchyma secondary to migration of the juvenile worms can be seen with CT or MRI. Triclabendazole is used for treatment as the first choice and nitazoxanide as an alternative.

15.1.5 Ascariasis

Human ascariasis is typically attributed to roundworm *Ascaris lumbricoides*. However, *Ascaris suum*, the roundworm of pig, can also cause infection in humans. Ascariasis is the most frequent helminthiasis in man, around 25% of the world's population are infected, mostly children from poor communities [14]. Infection is acquired via ingestion of the mature eggs in food, drinks or soil. On reaching the duodenum, the eggs release larvae that migrate down to the small intestine. Larvae penetrate the gut wall and reach the lung through the bloodstream or lymphatics. Larvae mature in the lungs and make their way up the airway to the pharynx and are swallowed back to the duodenum and mature to an adult worm. The migrating larvae and/or adult worms can cause several diseases. Larvae can cause hepatitis, and/or liver abscesses, pneumonitis and/or pulmonary eosinophilia "Loffler's syndrome". The adult worm may migrate to the appendicular orifice closing it and causes appendicitis or reach the biliary tree and causes obstruction, cholecystitis, jaundice, pancreatitis, cholangitis, and liver abscess [15]. When the female penetrates deeply into the bile ducts, it lays eggs, which are carried into the liver parenchyma, leading to granulomatous hepatitis or liver abscess. Bacteria attaching to the migrating worm cuticle cause suppurative cholangitis. The eggs or parasite fragments in the bile ducts can become a nucleus to stones.

Ascariasis is often asymptomatic, but symptoms attributed to larval migration to the lung such as fever, cough and dyspnea or attributed to the migrating adults such as abdominal discomfort, nausea, and/or diarrhea may be present. Diagnosis is usually made through finding the characteristic eggs in faeces. Plain radiographs are helpful in diagnosis of intestinal obstruction and/or perforation, while ultrasound examination is useful in biliary and pancreatic ascariasis. Worm migration may be monitored by radiography. Worm can be occasionally detected and extracted with biopsy forceps while doing endoscopic retrograde cholangiopancreatography as a diagnostic procedure. Mebendazole and albendazole are used for treatment of non-complicated ascariasis. Treatment of Ascaris-induced complications may be conservative or occasionally requires surgical intervention.

15.1.6 Visceral Larva Migrans

Visceral larva migrans (VLM) is a clinical syndrome of eosinophilia, hepatomegaly and pneumonitis related to migration of certain nematode larvae to the human liver [16]. Larvae of *Toxocara* species and *Capillaria* are commonly-involved in VLM. To a lesser extent, larvae of *Ascaris* species, *Fasciola* species, hookworm and *Strongyloides* species are also incorporated. VLM attributed to microfilariae of different filariae species have been also reported.

Inside the liver, larvae that fail to reach maturity, induce eosinophilic infiltration and granuloma formation. Patients may complain of vague abdominal pain, fever and general weakness. Other symptoms like cough and dyspnea may be found if the lungs are involved. Nonetheless, most of cases are asymptomatic and incidentally diagnosed in the presence of eosinophilia and a high ELISA titer for the suspected nematode antigens. The liver pathology appears as a macroscopic nodule, rather than microscopic diffuse inflammation. Imaging series show solitary or plural nodules with irregular shape, ranging in diameter from 5 mm to 2 cm. Most infections are self-limiting, and only severe cases warrant treatment, With albendazole or mebendazole or ivermectin according to the causative nematode.

15.1.7 Hepatic Capillariasis

Hepatic capillariasis is a rare zoonotic infection with hepatic manifestations caused by a nematode parasite *Capillaria hepatica*. Despite its low prevalence, the infection can cause significant morbidity and mortality [17]. Infection occurs through accidental ingestion of the embryonated eggs contaminating food or drink. Upon ingestion of eggs, larvae hatch, penetrate the coecal wall reaching the liver via the portal blood and mature to adult worms. The larvae in the liver cause chronic focal inflammation and septal hepatic fibrosis. The adult worm deposits eggs in the parenchyma and initiate formation of necrotizing granulomatous inflammation. In the end stages, the eggs are seen with inflammation and fibrosis of liver parenchyma without adult worms. Patients usually present with persistent fever, hepatomegaly and eosinophilia. Other symptoms like vomiting, splenomegaly, pneumonitis, extreme weakness, constipation, abdominal distension, and sometimes ascites have been also reported. A definitive diagnosis can be only made by obtaining a liver biopsy. No effective treatment is yet known but drugs like thiabendazole, albendazole and ivermectin can be useful in some cases.

15.1.8 Ectopic Pinworm Infection

Enterobius vermicularis, also known as pinworm, is a common nematode worm infection, especially in children. Infection is initiated via ingestion of embryonated eggs contaminating hands, food or drinks. In the gut, larvae liberated from the eggs and mature to adult worm in the colon, where reproduction and oviposition happens. Perianal itching is a common manifestation in children while in adults, infection is usually asymptomatic. Migration of adults to perianal tissue and urogenital tract in females have been documented. However, the adult worm migration to the biliary tree or to the liver parenchyma, even in few cases, has been surprising findings as the mechanism of hepatic involvement is still unclear [18].

Hepatic hyalinized nodules with peripheral inflammation and central necrosis with worm's remnants have been described. Before the advent in the imaging methods, hepatic enterobiasis was an incidental intra-operative finding.

15.1.9 Strongyloidiasis

Strongyloidiasis is an opportunistic parasitic infection attributed to nematodes *Strongyloides stercoralis* and *S. fuelleborni*. The worm has unique life cycle alternating between free-living and parasitic cycles with autoinfection potentials [19]. The parasitic cycle is initiated by filariform larvae penetrating human skin. Then, larvae migrate via the bloodstream to the lungs, where they are eventually coughed up and swallowed. In the small intestine larvae molt twice and become adults. Females live threaded in the epithelial lining of the small intestine and produce eggs. Eggs release rhabditiform larvae that may be passed in the stool or cause autoinfection. The free-living adults mate and produce eggs. Rhabditiform larvae hatch, mature and eventually become infective filariform larvae. In autoinfection, the rhabditiform larvae become infective filariform larvae, which can penetrate either the intestinal mucosa or the perianal skin; in either case, the filariform larvae may disseminate throughout the body. Therefore, this parasite can persist and replicate within a host for decades.

Strongyloidiasis is often asymptomatic in well-nourished patients with normal immune status. Occasionally, patients may present with diarrhea, urticaria, and abdominal pain. In immunosuppressed individual, infections may take more aggressive form "hyperinfection syndrome", with more serious symptoms such as dyspnea and/or complications such as intestinal obstruction and gastrointestinal hemorrhage. An extension of hyperinfection syndrome is the disseminated form, in which the larvae spread to organs such as the liver, pancreas, heart, and brain [20].

Diagnosis is usually made through detection of the rhabditiform larvae in fecal sample or in tissue biopsy. A mild eosinophilia might be the only clinical finding during asymptomatic infection. PCR has long been successfully used as a method of identification, joined by luciferase immunoprecipitation systems in more recent years. Stool sample culture can be a more practical screening test in resource-poor areas. Serological tests are also available, but cross-reactivity with *Ascaris lumbricoides*, filariae, and schistosomes was reported. Albendazole and ivermectin have both been successfully used to in treatment. Because just a single worm could reinitiate hyperinfection syndrome, anti-helminthic application should continue until larvae cease to be detectable. The auto-infective cycle takes about 2 weeks to complete, so it would be wise to continue with treatment 2 weeks after negative stool samples.

15.1.10 Fasciolopsiasis

Liver involvement in *Fasciolopsis buski* infection is a very rare event but documented. Like *Fasciola* species, the life cycle of fasciolopsiasis requires two intermediate hosts; the fresh water snail and water vegetations. Human infection occurs via ingestion of water vegetations containing the infective metacercariae. Most cases of fasciolopsiasis are silent intestinal infections, but in heavy infection abdominal pain, diarrhea and malabsorption may be present. A patient suffered from polycystic liver disease have been reported [21]. Ultrasonography and CT scan abdomen showed multiple tiny cysts in both lobes of the liver and kidney. Abdominal pain, vomiting and persistent diarrhea were the associated symptoms. Pallor, jaundice, lower limb oedema and hepatosplenomegaly have been the associated signs. Iron deficiency anaemia, hypoalbuminemia, with *Fasciolopsis buski* eggs in stool were the laboratory test findings. The case has been successfully treated with praziquantel.

15.1.11 Dicrocoeliasis

Infection with *Dicrocoelium dendriticum* "the lancet liver fluke" in humans is very rare event. This liver fluke, which commonly infects ruminants, has a complex life cycle with two intermediate hosts; the land snail and the ant. Human infection occurs by accidental ingestion of the second intermediate host [22]. A patient suffered from recurrent acute cholecystitis whose Kato stool examination showed *Dicrocoelium dendriticum* eggs has been reported. The case has been successfully treated with Mirazid®.

15.1.12 Visceral pentastomiasis

Visceral pentastomiasis is a zoonotic disease caused mainly by the nymphs of *Linguatula serrata*, or *Armillifer armillatus*. Few sporadic cases have been reported. Like herbivores, man acquires the infection through accidental ingestion of the embryonated egg shed in respiratory secretions, saliva or faeces of the definitive hosts (*Linguatula serrata*; dogs or *Armillifer armillatus*; reptiles). Consumption of uncooked infested snake meat can also transmit infection. Upon reaching the gut, larvae hatch, penetrate the gut wall to the liver via the bloodstream. During migration, the larvae cause eosinophilic infiltration, granuloma formation, or eosinophilic abscess scattered throughout the liver parenchyma [23]. Most of the cases are asymptomatic and discovered only during surgery or autopsy. Generally, the diagnosis largely depends on parasitological and histopathologic examination.

15.2 Parasitic Liver Diseases: Protozoa

Protozoa are single-celled eukaryotic microorganisms. Protozoa may live intracellular or live extracellular such as *Entamoeba*. While intracellular protozoa like *Plasmodium* species reside the hepatocytes, other like *Leishmania* and *Toxoplasma* inhabit the reticuloendothelial cells. Liver involvement in protozoan infections are mostly in the form of disseminated systemic disease. Occasionally, intestinal protozoa like *Giardia*, and *Cryptosporidium* species migrate upward to the bile duct via its orifice causing diseases like cholecystitis and cholangitis. Unlike helminths, the liver involvement in protozoan infections are not associated with peripheral eosinophilia. The most common hepatic protozoal infections are demonstrated in Fig. 15.2.

15.2.1 Amoebiasis

Amoebiasis is parasitic disease attributed mainly to *Entamoeba histolytica*, a common enteric protozoon residing the colon. It is much more frequent in tropics and affects around 10% of the world's population. Amoebiasis is the third most common cause of parasite-related death worldwide [24]. The typical clinical feature of amoebiasis is the dysenteric form, but 90% of infected people are carriers. Extra-intestinal amoebiasis affect the liver and lung, especially in malnourished and immunocompromised patients. The amoeba present in two developmental forms: trophozoite and cyst. Infection is acquired via ingestion of infected cysts contaminating food or drinks. The cysts are acid resistant so can reach the small intestine, where the trophozoites excyst. Trophozoites travel to the colon, grow, and pass through the epithelium into the submucosa. Penetration into the mucosa causes necrosis and ulceration leading to dysentery. The trophozoites enter the colonic venous circulation to reach the liver, lung or the brain causing amoebic abscesses [25]. The abscess contains a viscous secretion, free of amoebae.

The clinical manifestations of the amoebic liver abscess vary according to its size, number and localization. Fever and right upper abdominal quadrant pain are two common symptoms. The pain may radiate to the right shoulder and increases with movement or coughing. The liver is usually large and tender. Diagnosis is confirmed via detection of the amoebic antigens, cysts, and/or trophozoites in patient stool. Imaging findings include a space-occupying lesion, sometimes indistinguishable from a pyogenic abscess. Amoebic culture and visualization of trophozoites can be done using the aspirate.

Amoebiasis are usually treated with metronidazole, tinidazole or chloroquine. For amoebic liver abscess, when the clinical response to medical treatment is unsatisfactory,

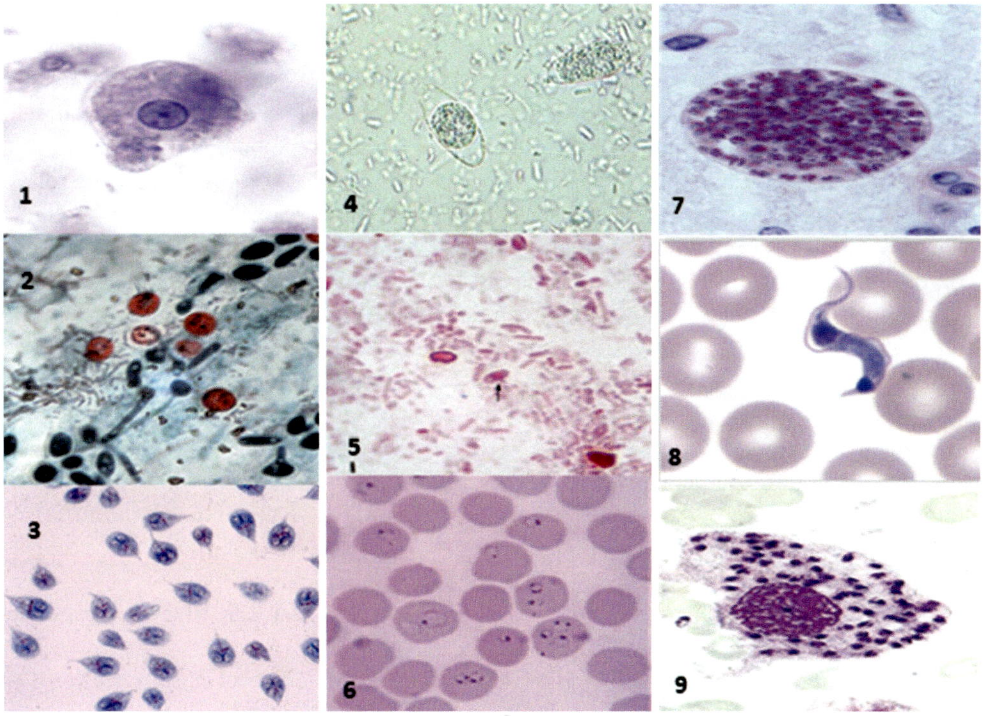

Fig. 15.2 A group of protozoa found associated with human liver diseases. 1—*Entamoeba histolytica* trophozoite stage; 2—*Cryptosporidium* oocysts in acid fast stained smear; 3—*Giardia lamblia* trophozoites; 4—*Cystoisospora belli*; 5—*Enterocytozoon bieneusi*; 6—*Plasmodium* species ring stage; 7—*Toxoplasma gondii* tissue cyst; 8—*Trypanosoma cruzi* trypomastigotes in blood film; 9—*Leishmania donovani* amastigotes in biopsy specimen

percutaneous aspiration/drainage can be used as a diagnostic or therapeutic tool and should be performed under imaging guidance.

15.2.2 Giardiasis

Giardiasis is a common intestinal infection caused by the flagellated protozoa, *Giardia lamblia*. Like *Entamoeba*, *Giardia* is present in one of two developmental stages: cyst and trophozoite forms. Man acquire infection via ingestion of cysts contaminating hands, food or drink. In the small intestine, excystation occurs, giving rise to the trophozoites, the tissue irritative developmental form. Responding to unknown stimuli, trophozoites may encyst in the ileum and are shed to the environment with stools [26].

Infection may pass unnoticed without symptoms or presents with diarrhea, vomiting, abdominal distension. The liver involvement with *Giardia* is a rare event; however, granulomatous hepatitis, cholangitis or biliary, and/or steatosis have been reported in uncontrolled HIV-positive patients [27]. Diagnosis of giardiasis requires detection of *Giardia* cysts or trophozoites in stool or duodenal aspirate. Tests based on identification of the parasite antigen or nucleic acids in faeces are also available. The extraintestinal complications such as gallbladder distension, ductal stricture or obstruction are diagnosed with radiological and endoscopic examinations. Metronidazole is the drug of choice used in treatment of intestinal giardiasis, but sometimes, surgical interventions may be needed for some biliary tree complications.

15.2.3 Cryptosporidiosis

Cryptosporidiosis is an intestinal infection caused by the protozoan parasite *Cryptosporidium*. Like giardiasis, the liver involvement in cryptosporidiosis is uncommon and occur in selected populations, such as immunocompromised individuals [28]. Infection transmission occurs through ingestion of oocysts developmental form contaminating hands, food or drink. Upon ingestion, the oocysts excyst and release sporozoites, the intracellular developmental disease producing developmental forms. Inside the enterocytes, the sporozoites mature and undergo asexual reproduction to produce merozoites that are released into the intestinal lumen. The merozoites can either infect other cells or mature into gametocytes, sexual reproductive stages. Fertilization occurs producing thin-walled infectious oocysts that passed to the environment awaiting ingestion by the next host. The parasite life cycle has great potentials for the occurrence of autoinfection, and persistent or overwhelming infections, especially in immunocompromised patients.

Infection may occur without symptoms or manifest itself as diarrheal illness. The diarrhea is self-limited in immunocompetent patient, but it is a major problem in immunocompromised patients causing chronic debilitating diarrhea. Biliary cryptosporidiosis is described in patients with low immunity, causing cholecystitis and sclerosing cholangitis. Two distinct pathological complications are described: papillary stenosis with extrahepatic ductal dilatation and sclerosing cholangitis or acalculous cholecystitis [29].

Besides diarrhea, pain in the right upper quadrant, nausea, vomiting and fever are common associated symptoms. Diagnosis is undertaken through identification of the parasite oocysts, antigen and or nucleic acid in patient faeces. The bile duct wall thickening, and/or the gallbladder dilatation are two radiological findings reported in biliary cryptosporidiosis. Papillary stenosis or ductal strictures are documented with endoscopic ultrasonography. There is no drug proved effective against cryptosporidiosis but drugs like nitazoxanide, paromomycin and azithromycin are tried with correction of the immunosuppression status of the patient in parallel. The pathological findings described in extraintestinal cryptosporidiosis has been also reported in immunosuppressed patients co-infected with one of the two enteric protozoa: the *Enterocytozoon bieneusi* and the *Cystoisospora belli* [30].

15.2.4 Malaria

Malaria is a common parasitic infection worldwide. It is estimated that 10% of the world's population are infected, and it causes one to two million deaths per year. Five *Plasmodium* species are encountered in malaria: *P. falciparum*, *P. vivax*, *P. malariae*, *P. ovale* and *P. Knowlesi*. Of these, the first two species are the most important owing to their high virulence [31]. Infection transmission usually occurs via skin bite with female *Anopheles* mosquito. However, malaria associated with blood transfusion, organ transplantation, and pregnancy have been also recognized. The parasite life cycle involves two hosts: man, and insect.

During a blood meal, an infected female mosquito inserts the sporozoites, the infective developmental form, into the dermal circulation. Sporozoites reach the hepatocytes, reside there and form schizonts, that rupture releasing merozoites. Importantly, in *P. vivax* and *P. ovale*, sporozoites persist inside the liver cells as dormant developmental form termed hypnozoites. These form is responsible for the occurrence of relapse in malaria. From the liver cells to the blood, the parasites undergo asexual multiplication in the erythrocytes. A number of parasites differentiate into sexual erythrocytic stages, gametocytes that have potentials to be ingested by an *Anopheles* mosquito during a blood meal. In the mosquito's stomach, fertilization occurs and as result, oocysts are produced, and ruptured releasing sporozoites into the mosquito's saliva.

Jaundice is a frequent sign in malaria, but, there is a wide variation in its reported incidence. It is mostly due to coexistent haemolysis, malnutrition and/or hepatocyte dysfunction. The cytoadherence of the parasitized red blood cells to the vascular and sinusoidal endothelium of the liver, causes hepatocellular dysfunction due to reduction in portal blood flow, anoxemia and intrahepatic cholestasis. In acute *falciparum* malaria, additional pathological changes have been described in terms of steatosis, focal hepatocyte swelling and necrosis and focal accumulation of histiocytes forming non-granulomatous lesions [32].

Diagnosis is made through identification of parasite trophozoites in thick or thin blood smears preceded with or without rapid detection test positive for parasite antigen in blood. Other methods like quantified buffy coat and PCR based detection tests have a role in epidemiological studies. Malarial hepatitis diagnosis is made on clinical evidence and confirmed by the appropriate laboratory tests of liver dysfunction. The ultrasound examination may find hepatomegaly with low echogenicity and thick gallbladder. Jaundice is indicative of severe malaria and, mandate intravenous antimalarial treatment.

15.2.5 Visceral Leishmaniasis

Visceral leishmaniasis (VL) is a severe parasitic infection caused by an intracellular flagellated protozoa of the genus *Leishmania*. The parasite present in two developmental forms: promastigotes and amastigotes. VL is an opportunistic infection and potentially fatal unless treated [33]. Transmission usually occur via skin bite by an infected female sandfly but can also occur via blood transfusion or organ transplantation. Upon the sand fly's bite, promastigotes, present in the insect saliva, are inserted into the skin, lose flagella, internalized by macrophages, and transformed into amastigotes. Within macrophages, the amastigotes multiply and proceed to infect other mononuclear cells via the blood and lymphatic circulation. Dissemination leads to bone marrow infiltration, hepatosplenomegaly and sometimes lymphadenopathy [34]. With a blood meal, the Sandfly got infected through ingesting infected cells containing amastigotes. In the fly's gut, the amastigotes are released, transformed into promastigotes into the fly's proboscis and became ready to initiate another cycle.

Patients with VL present with non-specific manifestations of persistent systemic infection: fever, fatigue, weakness, anorexia and weight loss. Anaemia, hepatomegaly, splenomegaly and adenopathy are additional features. Diagnosis in most of cases is laboratory-based. Pancytopenia and marked polyclonal hypergammaglobulinemia are valuable in diagnosis of clinically-suspected cases. Microscopic or molecular detection of amastigote in lymph nodes, bone marrow and/or spleen biopsies or cultured aspirates is confirmatory. A latex agglutination test detecting antigen in the urine has recently described with promising initial results. Treatment is usually carried out via intravenous liposomal amphotericin B.

15.2.6 Toxoplasmosis

Toxoplasmosis is a common infection caused by the protozoan parasite *Toxoplasma gondii*. The protozoon exists in three morphological forms: oocyst containing sporozoites, tissue cyst with bradyzoites, and proliferating tachyzoite form. The oocysts in cat's faeces can be accidentally ingested through contaminated hands, food or drink. The oocysts develop into tachyzoites that divide rapidly in the cells causing tissue destruction and infection spread. Tachyzoites in blood or body organs can be transferred to a new host through transfusion or organ transplantation. Moreover, pregnant woman can infect her fetus through the placenta. Eventually tachyzoites reside in muscle tissues and the CNS and convert to tissue cysts, bradyzoites. Ingestion of undercooked meat containing viable cysts is also a source of infection, should be considered [35].

Tachyzoites may disseminate to different organs including the liver during an acute primary infection or reactivation of a chronic latent infection, especially in immunocompromised host. Toxoplasmosis is a benign disease and often goes unnoticed in immunocompetent individuals. The liver involvement in toxoplasmosis manifests itself as giant cell hepatitis or non-specific reactive hepatitis [36]. Liver granulomas, cholestasis, cell necrosis and cirrhosis are occasionally described sequela. Diagnosis usually relies on serological tests for detection of antibody classes IgG and IgM in serum. Pyrimethamine alone or combined with sulfadiazine are frequently used therapeutic medications.

15.2.7 Babesiosis

Babesiosis is a parasitic infection caused by intracellular protozoa, *Babesia* [39]. Human infection is acquired via the skin bite of the deer tick, *Ixodes scapularis*. Five species of *Babesia* have been known to cause human infection: *Babesia microti*, *B. duncani*, *B. divergens*, and *B. venatorum*. Like malaria, transmission by blood transfusions and transplacental transmission have been also documented [40]. The clinical features and diagnosis are close to that of malaria. Babesiosis can cause acute liver failure particularly in patients who are at risk of severe infection. Patients with splenectomy, malignancy, HIV infection, or those on immunosuppressive therapy are at high risk for severe disease. Intravenous treatment with clindamycin, quinine and/or exchange transfusion is usually reserved for those patients presenting with severe parasitemia, severe anemia, pulmonary, liver, or renal impairment [41].

15.2.8 Chagas' Disease (Trypanosomiasis)

Chagas' disease is a neglected tropical disease caused by infection with protozoan parasite, *Trypanosoma cruzi* [37]. Chagas' disease is characterized with an intense inflammatory response in many tissues, including the liver. Infection is transmitted to humans by blood-sucking triatomine bugs and by transfusion. In the blood, the trypomastigotes invade host cells, particularly, macrophage, muscle and nerve cells. Acute disease normally presents as either facial edema and/or non-specific flu-like illness but can be more severe in immunosuppressed patients. The chronic phase is lifelong and often with cardiac complications. The liver affection takes the forms of centroacinar cell necrosis and inflammatory infiltration, especially in the portal fields [38].

15.3 Concluding Remarks and Future Directions

The causative parasites of liver disease in humans are diverse and remain an important health issue worldwide. The pathogenic changes leading to hepatic dysfunction in these parasitic infections are equally diverse. Although some parasitic diseases of the liver are less frequently reported, even in some endemic areas, practicians should recognize that travel, immigration and food trade make infection with parasites possible in any setting. A high index of clinical suspicion and detailed travel history are required for proper diagnosis of liver parasitosis, as are prompt notification and laboratory confirmation. The confirmation of parasitic infections is made by identification of parasites in properly selected specimens or in host tissues. Direct microscopic observation of parasitic diagnostic stages is the method of choice for diagnosis of numerous infections, namely, malaria, visceral leishmaniasis, babesiosis, and intestinal parasitic infections. However, due to the occult nature of many parasitic infections involved in liver diseases, microscopy is not always possible. Diseases such as amoebic liver abscess, echinococcosis, toxocariasis, toxoplasmosis, or capillariasis almost always require detection of species-specific antibodies in patient's serum before a diagnosis can be approved. In other infections, such as schistosomiasis, giardiasis, cryptosporidiosis and strongyloidiasis, parasites may be detected in feces or other biological specimens, but due to interrupted shedding or sampling limitations, direct detection of parasites is neither sensitive nor reliable. Most of parasitic infections that affect the human liver are benign and self-limiting in immunocompetent patients, however, infections such as visceral leishmaniasis, and strongyloidiasis may be severe enough to threaten life of some malnourished immunosuppressed individuals. Treatment is often done through medical and/or surgical interference. A deeper insight on the host-parasite interactions at the molecular level is required to identify the host-derived factors that influence parasite's entry, growth, and spread in human host. Such information could unravel the mechanisms by which the hepatocellular dysfunctions occur as a late sequel to parasite infections and could hopefully open novel therapeutic and/or preventive approaches to one terrible complication of parasitic infections.

Self Study

Questions

1. Which one of the followings is true regarding schistosomiasis?
   (a) The liver pathology is mainly attributed to the adult worm
   (b) The liver pathology is mainly attributed to the worm's eggs
   (c) Diagnosis is usually carried out through serology
   (d) Albendazole is the first drug of choice for treatment
2. Which of the followings is consistent with hydatidosis?
   (a) It is a zoonotic disease
   (b) Man is a definitive host
   (c) Stool analysis is diagnostic
   (d) Treatment is always surgical
3. Cholangiocarcinoma is a complication of which parasites?
   (a) *Clonorchis sinensis*
   (b) *Fasciola gigantica*
   (c) *Fasciola hepatic*
   (d) *Echinococcus granulosus*
4. Which one of the following is consistent with fascioliasis?
   (a) Opportunistic infections
   (b) Protozoan infections
   (c) Acquired via oral ingestion
   (d) Treated with albendazole
5. An adverse clinical outcome associated with ascariasis?
   (a) Liver cysts
   (b) Cholangiocarcinoma
   (c) Biliary obstruction
   (d) Visceral larva migrans
6. An appropriate first-line therapy for visceral larva migrans?
   (a) Albendazole
   (b) Ivermectin
   (c) Praziquantel
   (d) Azithromycin
7. Which one of the following does not describe hepatic capillariasis?
   (a) Infection is attributed to a trematode, *Capillaria hepatica*
   (b) The pathology is attributed to the larvae in the liver
   (c) The pathology is attributed to the adults in the coecum
   (d) A definitive diagnosis mandates a liver biopsy
8. Ingestion of ants can transmit which of the followings parasites?
   (a) Fasciolopsis buski
   (b) Enterobius vermicularis
   (c) Dicrocoelium dendriticum
   (d) Opisthorchis viverrini
9. Eating snake meat can transmit which of the following parasitic infections?
   (a) Hepatic filariasis
   (b) Hepatic schistosomiasis
   (c) Visceral larva migrans
   (d) Visceral pentastomiasis
10. Which one of the following protozoan infection commonly occurs in the liver?
   (a) Amoebic liver abscess
   (b) Hepatic malaria
   (c) Visceral leishmaniasis
   (d) Hepatic toxoplasmosis

Answers

1. Which one of the followings is true regarding schistosomiasis?
   The liver pathology is mainly attributed to the worm's eggs
2. Which of the followings is consistent with hydatidosis?
   It is a zoonotic disease
3. Cholangiocarcinoma is a complication of which parasites?
   Clonorchis sinensis
4. Which one of the following is consistent with fascioliasis?
   Acquired via oral ingestion
5. An adverse clinical outcome associated with ascariasis?
   Biliary obstruction
6. An appropriate first-line therapy for visceral larva migrans?
   Albendazole
7. Which one of the following does not describe hepatic capillariasis?
   The pathology is attributed to the adults in the coecum
8. Ingestion of ants can transmit which of the followings parasites?
   Dicrocoelium dendriticum

9. Eating snake meat can transmit which of the following parasites?
   Visceral pentastomiasis
10. The most protozoan infection in the liver?
   Amoebic liver abscess

References

1. Yoh NT, Wagener G. The splanchnic and systemic circulation in liver disease. In: Wagener G, editor. Liver anesthesiology and critical care medicine. 2018. p. 63–68. Cham: Springer.
2. Walker NF, Chiodini PL. Liver lesions in the returning traveller. Medicine. 2018;46(1):16–9.
3. Fishman JA. Infection in organ transplantation. Am J Transplant. 2017;17(4):856–79.
4. Chiodini PL, Godbole G. Parasitic infections of the liver and bile ducts. Surgery of the liver, bile ducts and pancreas in children. 2017; 12:5.
5. Kovalszki A, Weller PF. Eosinophils and eosinophilia. In: Clinical immunology. 5th ed. 2019. p. 349–61.
6. Colley DG, Bustinduy AL, Secor WE, King CH. Human schistosomiasis. The Lancet. 2014;383(9936):2253–64.
7. Weerakoon K, Gordon C, McManus D. DNA diagnostics for schistosomiasis control. Tropical Medicine and Infectious Disease. 2018;3(3):81.
8. Gottstein B, Beldi G. Echinococcosis. In: Infectious diseases. 4th ed. 2017. p. 1038 45).
9. Yang S, Zhao Y, McManus DP, Yang Y. Current research advance on Echinococcosis. In: Echinococcosis. 2017. InTech.
10. Zheng S, Zhu Y, Zhao Z, Wu Z, Okanurak K, Lv Z. Liver fluke infection and cholangiocarcinoma: a review. Parasitol Res. 2017;116(1):11–9.
11. Hughes T, O'Connor T, Techasen A, Namwat N, Loilome W, Andrews RH, Khuntikeo N, Yongvanit P, Sithithaworn P, Taylor-Robinson SD. Opisthorchiasis and cholangiocarcinoma in Southeast Asia: an unresolved problem. Int J General Med. 2017;10:227–37.
12. Mas-Coma S, Bargues MD, Valero MA. Human fascioliasis infection sources, their diversity, incidence factors, analytical methods and prevention measures. Parasitology. 2018:1–35.
13. Teke M, Önder H, Çiçek M, Hamidi C, Göya C, Çetinçakmak MG, Hattapoğlu S, Ülger BV. Sonographic findings of hepatobiliary fascioliasis accompanied by extrahepatic expansion and ectopic lesions. J Ultrasound Med. 2014;33(12):2105–11.
14. Deslyper G, Holland CV. Overview on Ascariasis in humans in South Asia. In: Singh SK, editor. Neglected tropical diseases-South Asia. Cham: Springer; 2017. p. 83–120.
15. Das AK. Hepatic and biliary ascariasis. J Global Infect Dis. 2014;6(2):65.
16. Gupta P, Sinha SK, Malik S, Dhaka N, Srinivasan R, Kochhar R. Hepatic visceral larva migrans: a diagnostic enigma. Trop Doct. 2018;48(4):345–7.
17. Yadav SC, Sathe PA, Ghodke RK. Hepatic capillariasis: A rare parasitic infection. Indian J Pathol Microbiol. 2016;59(1):124.
18. Furnée EJ, Spoto C, de Graaf MJ, Smakman N. Enterobius vermicularis infection of the liver in a patient with colorectal carcinoma with suspected liver metastasis. BMJ Case Rep. 2015;2015:bcr2015212271.
19. Nutman TB. Human infection with Strongyloides stercoralis and other related Strongyloides species. Parasitology. 2017; 144(3):263–73.
20. Ofori E, Ramai D, Khan A, Xiao P, Reddy M, Shahzad G. Hepatobiliary strongyloidiasis presenting as an ampullary lesion on esophagogastroduodenoscopy/endoscopic ultrasound. Gastroenterol Rep. 2018.
21. Jali SN, Padhi PK, Nageswar M, Tripathy DM, Meher LK, Naik DK. Fasciolopsiasis: a rare case report from a tertiary care hospital in south Odisha, India. Asian J Sci Technol. 2018;9(4): 7981–3.
22. Abd Ella OH, Mohammad AE. Dicrocoelium dendriticum infection in a patient with chronic Schistosomiasis haematobium. J Egypt Soc Parasitol. 2015;240(2496):1–4.
23. Latif BM, Muslim A, Chin HC. Human and animal pentastomiasis in Malaysia. J Tropic Life Sci. 2016;6(2):131–5.
24. Berger S. Amoebiasis: global status: 2018 edition. Los Angeles, CA: Gideon Informatics Inc; 2018.
25. Anesi JA, Gluckman S. Amebic liver abscess. Clin Liver Dis. 2015;6(2):41–3.
26. Einarsson E, Ma'ayeh S, Svärd SG. An up-date on Giardia and giardiasis. Curr Opin Microbiol. 2016;34:47–52.
27. Araki H, Shimizu S, Hayashi K, Yamada T, Kusakabe A, Kanie H, Mizuno Y, Kojima I, Saitou A, Nagao K, Suzuki Y. Acute acalculous cholecystitis caused by Giardia lamblia. Internal Med. 2017;56(13):1657–62.
28. Xiao L, Cama VA. Cryptosporidium and cryptosporidiosis. In Foodborne parasites. 2018. Cham: Springer; p. 73–117.
29. Gupta S, Johnson A, Meyrick S, Davies AP, Chalmers R. A case of hepato-biliary infection secondary to cryptosporidium in a patient on tacrolimus. JMM Case Rep. 2018;5(8):e005159.
30. Naseer M, Dailey FE, Alhareth Al Juboori SS, Tahan V. Epidemiology, determinants, and management of AIDS cholangiopathy: A review. World J Gastroenterol. 2018;24(7):767.
31. Flemming A. Malaria: hitting all stages of the parasite life cycle. Nat Rev Drug Discov. 2015;14(8):527.
32. Chandra S, Dhawale S, Chouhan A. Hepatic dysfunction in falciparum malaria. J Evol Med Dental Sci. 2015;4(2):184–92.
33. Chappuis F, Sundar S, Hailu A, Ghalib H, Rijal S, Peeling RW, Alvar J, Boelaert M. Visceral leishmaniasis: what are the needs for diagnosis, treatment and control? Nat Rev Microbiol. 2007;5(11 supp):S7.
34. Das S, Sarkar N, Chatterjee K, Aich B, Bhattacharya M. Portal hypertension and reactive hemophagocytosis in pediatric visceral leishmaniasis. Bangladesh J Med Sci. 2015;14(4):409–12.
35. Dubey JP. Toxoplasmosis of animals and humans. Boca Raton: CRC Press; 2016.
36. Choi EY, Lamps LW. Granulomas in the liver, with a focus on infectious causes. Surg Pathol Clinics. 2018;11(2):231–50.
37. Bern C. Chagas' disease. New Engl J Med. 2015;373(5):456–66.
38. Rodriguez-Guardado A, González ML, Rodriguez M, Flores-Chavez M, Boga JA, Gascon J. Trypanosoma cruzi infection in a Spanish liver transplant recipient. Clin Microbiol Infect. 2015;21(7):687–e1.
39. Vannier E, Krause PJ. Babesiosis in China, an emerging threat. Lancet Infect Dis. 2015;15(2):137–9.
40. Fang DC, McCullough J. Transfusion-transmitted Babesia microti. Transfus Med Rev. 2016;30(3):132–8.
41. Meissner EG, McGillicuddy JW, Squires J, Skipper D, Self S, Wray D, Moritz ED, Stramer SL, Nadig S. Across state lines: Fulminant Babesia microti infection in a liver transplant recipient. Transplant Infectious Disease. 2017 Oct;19(5):e12741.

Further Reading

Bogitsh BJ, Carter CE, Oeltmann TN. Human parasitology. New York: Academic Press; 2018.

Carnero PR, Mateo PH, Martín-Garre S, Pérez ÁG, Del Campo L. Unexpected hosts: imaging parasitic diseases. Insight Imag. 2017;8(1):101–25.

Chan AW, Quaglia A, Haugk B, Burt A. Nonviral infectious liver disease. In: Atlas of liver pathology. 2014; New York, NY: Springer. p. 105–117.
Dooley JS, Lok AS, Garcia-Tsao G, Pinzani M. Sherlock's diseases of the liver and biliary system. New York: John Wiley & Sons; 2018.
Dunn MA. Parasitic diseases. Schiff's Dis Liver. 2011;9:1017–33.
Hadžić N. Liver disease in immunodeficiencies. Liver Dis Child. 2014:370.
Jones D, Sturm E, Lohse AW. Access to care in rare liver diseases: new challenges and new opportunities. J Hepatol. 2017.
Lefkowitch JH. Scheuer's liver biopsy interpretation E-book. Oxford: Elsevier Health Sciences; 2015.
Sanford CA, Jong EC, Pottinger PS. The travel and tropical medicine manual E-Book. Oxford: Elsevier Health Sciences; 2016.
Wilcox CM, Mönkemüller KE. AIDS and the gastrointestinal tract. Philadelphia: GI/Liver Secrets Plus E-Book; 2014. p. 427.

16 Viral Hepatitis B

Dar-In Tai

Key Concepts

- HBV is a highly infectious, small, circular, incomplete double-stranded DNA virus.
- Chronic infection is common when patients are infected in the early stages of life.
- The course of chronic HBV infection is a trilogy, starting with immune tolerance, followed by immune clearance, and finally a residual phase.
- Immune tolerance is preventative against cytokine storm. It could be a survival strategy and is associated with genetic evolution during human migration.
- The severity and duration of liver inflammation determine the pathogenesis of liver cirrhosis and hepatocellular carcinoma.
- Most chronic HBV carriers terminate HBV replication and may achieve delayed HBsAg clearance several decades later.
- Current HBV-specific therapy may suppress viral replication but is unable to clear covalently closed circular DNA in the nucleus. Virologic relapse may reach 50% during the first year after treatment ends.
- New therapeutic strategies and agents are needed for eradication of chronic HBV infection.

16.1 Introduction

Hepatitis B virus (HBV) infection is a cause of chronic liver disease with a long medical history in humans. It was first discovered in 1963 by Baruch Samuel Blumberg (Nobel Prize for Medicine, 1976) when he performed double immunodiffusion assays using sera from aboriginal Australians. Many epidemiological studies soon identified HBV infection as a global chronic disease, with the highest prevalence rates in Asia and Africa. Before vaccination programs in these two continents, the prevalence of hepatitis B surface antigen (HBsAg) was generally above 15%. More than four billion people have been chronically infected with HBV worldwide. The WHO estimated that chronic hepatitis B resulted in 880,000 deaths from cirrhosis and hepatocellular carcinoma (HCC) in 2015.

D.-I. Tai (✉)
Liver Research Center, Chang Gung Memorial Hospital, Linkou Medical Center, Taoyuan City, Taiwan

16.2 HBV Genome

HBV is classified as part of the Hepadnaviridae family, which comprises small, hepatotropic DNA viruses that replicate through reverse transcription [1]. The complete HBV virion is a sphere with a diameter of 40–45 nm. HBV has a 3.2 kbp, circular, incomplete double-stranded DNA genome.

The viral genome encodes four overlapping open reading frames (ORFs: S, C, P, and X). The S ORF encodes the viral surface envelope proteins, which can be structurally and functionally divided into the pre-S1, pre-S2, and S regions. The core, or C, gene contains the pre-core and core regions that are expressed as the hepatitis B e antigen (HBeAg) and hepatitis B c antigen (HBcAg), respectively. The P and X ORFs encode HBV DNA polymerase and the hepatitis B x antigen (HBxAg).

Other important Hepadnaviridae *viruses* within this family are woodchuck hepatitis B *virus*, duck hepatitis *virus*, ground squirrel hepatitis B *virus*, tree squirrel hepatitis B virus, and heron hepatitis B virus.

16.3 HBV Genotypes

HBV co-diverged with modern human migration and evolved into eight genotypes (A–H) in various geographic locations. There is an interaction between human leukocyte antigen (HLA) and HBV genotype [2].

F. Radu-Ionita et al. (eds.), *Liver Diseases*, https://doi.org/10.1007/978-3-030-24432-3_16

The distribution of HBV genotypes is mainly A, D and E in Africa; A and D in Europe; D in south Asia; B and C in East Asian; and F, G and H in America [1]. In general, genotypes A and B have a shorter HBV replication stage and better infection outcome than genotypes C and D.

16.4 HBV Mutation

HBV genome is one of the most variable among DNA viruses. This is mainly related to the error-prone HBV DNA polymerase and its very high virion production. HBV genome mutations occur frequently during the immune clearance stage, vaccination, and anti-HBV therapy. There could be selection of viral strains based on the environmental stress to the virus. This is especially occurred in patients unable to suppress viral replication efficiently. HBV mutants can be found frequently in patients with HCC [3]. Some of these mutants may be related to hepatocarcinogenesis.

16.5 HBV Transmission

HBV primarily infects humans and chimpanzees. It is highly infectious, and most infections occur intra-family or in early childhood [4]. HBV may be transmitted to humans from contaminated food, water, needles, a wound, sexual contact, close contact, or through maternal-fetal exchanges.

HBV enters the host cell by binding with sodium taurocholate co-transporting polypeptide (NTCP) on the cell membrane [5]. NTCP is mainly expressed in hepatocytes, which is one of the main reasons for the hepatotropic effect of HBV. The discovery of this receptor has led to an increased number of studies on HBV replication. NTCP can be transfected into hepatoma cell lines and expressed on the cell membrane. Such NTCP-expressing HCC cell lines may be infected with HBV-contaminated serum. The HBV may replicate in the HCC cells and excrete complete virions into culture media. This replication model greatly supports the screening of therapeutic agents for HBV.

Once it enters the hepatocyte, the relaxed circular DNA (rcDNA) is released from the envelope protein. Through host DNA repair enzymes, the rcDNA is converted to covalently closed circular DNA (cccDNA) in the nucleus. The fundamental role of HBV cccDNA has served as an example for transcription of all viral RNAs, which are required to produce viral genomes and express viral proteins [1].

During active HBV replication, the HBV genome and its products rarely modulate the host's cellular gene transcription [6]. This behavior makes HBV replicate peacefully in hepatocytes without interfering with hepatocyte function and transaminase levels in the immune tolerance phase.

16.6 Acute Infection

Acute hepatitis may develop 2–3 months after an individual is infected with HBV. Serum sickness, urticaria, or arthralgia may occur preceding the elevation of transaminase levels. The symptoms of acute hepatitis vary from no significant symptoms to the development of jaundice and hepatic failure. Most cases of acute infection resolve several months later with the development of anti-hepatitis B surface antigens (anti-HBs). The spontaneously produced anti-HBs may produce life-long protection from HBV infection. In less than 1% of acute hepatitis B patients with jaundice, the disease may progress into fulminant hepatic failure. Disturbed consciousness occurs within 4–8 weeks after the appearance of jaundice [1].

Before the nucleos(t)ide analogues (NA) era, more than 80% of patients with fulminant hepatic failure did not survive. Liver transplantation was the only life-saving therapy. At present, artificial liver supporting system and NA therapy can be offered. NA therapy significantly decreases mortality and necessity for liver transplantation if therapy is started before deep jaundice appears [7]. The artificial liver supporting system could prolong wait times or delay the need for liver transplantation [8].

16.7 Chronic Infection

A patient with persistent HBsAg for more than 6 months is considered a chronic HBsAg carrier. HBV may replicate in hepatocytes without causing direct cytopathy or immune-related cytopathy. This type of chronic infection is related to age and transmission route. In East Asia, maternal to fetus (vertical) or perinatal infection results in an 80–90% persistent infection rate. This rate decreased to around 23% when infection occurred at preschool age, and decreased further to 2.3% when infection occurred at college student age [4]. In African, early termination of HBV replication would prevent maternal-fetal infection. Most chronic HBsAg carriers in Africa contract HBV infection in the early stage of life by horizontal transmission. There is an age-related immune tolerance phase in most mammals, which during infancy may decrease allergy and mortality among neonates. Unfortunately, this mechanism is prone to progress to chronic persistent infection of HBV.

Chronic infection begins with an immune tolerance phase, in which HBV is actively replicated in the liver without causing inflammation. The immune system does not recognize HBsAg or Hepatitis B e antigen (HBeAg), or may recognize them but not elicit a strong immune reaction. Through unknown mechanisms, this initially weak immune response becomes stronger with age. Within two to four decades, an immune clearance reaction will often develop to terminate HBV replication.

Our immune system is carefully orchestrated. Innate immunity, T and B cells, cell-mediated and antibody responses all contribute to HBV clearance.

Once this immune clearance reaction successfully suppresses HBV replication, HBsAg may persist without significant HBV replication in the residual phase. About 50% of HBsAg carriers will ultimately clear HBsAg at age 80 [9]. Those patients unable to clear HBV replication smoothly have an increased risk of chronic hepatitis, liver cirrhosis, and hepatocarcinogenesis [1, 4, 9, 10].

16.8 Genetic Factors Predisposing to Chronic Persistent Infection

Chronic HBV infection and HCC may be clustered in families. This prompted researchers to investigate genetic factors related to chronic HBV infection. In genome-wide association studies conducted with East Asian populations, HLA-DP and -DQ loci were identified to be associated with chronic persistent infection [11, 12]. However, these genetic polymorphisms are present in East Asians only (Fig. 16.1b). Therefore, such genetic risk factors do not play a role in the high prevalence of chronic HBV infection in Africa [13]. Age of infection may underlie the main mechanism for chronic persistent HBV infection in Africans as well as in other continents.

The high prevalence of persistent HBV infection-related HLA-DP and -DQ loci in East Asians probably evolved during human migration. A trend of decreased immune-related gene expression was found for the period shortly after human migration out of Africa (Fig. 16.1a). Higher expression genotypes for IL-28B, interferon lambda 4, complement factor B, and CD40 are more prevalent in Africans than in either Europeans or South Asians [13]. In addition, when human

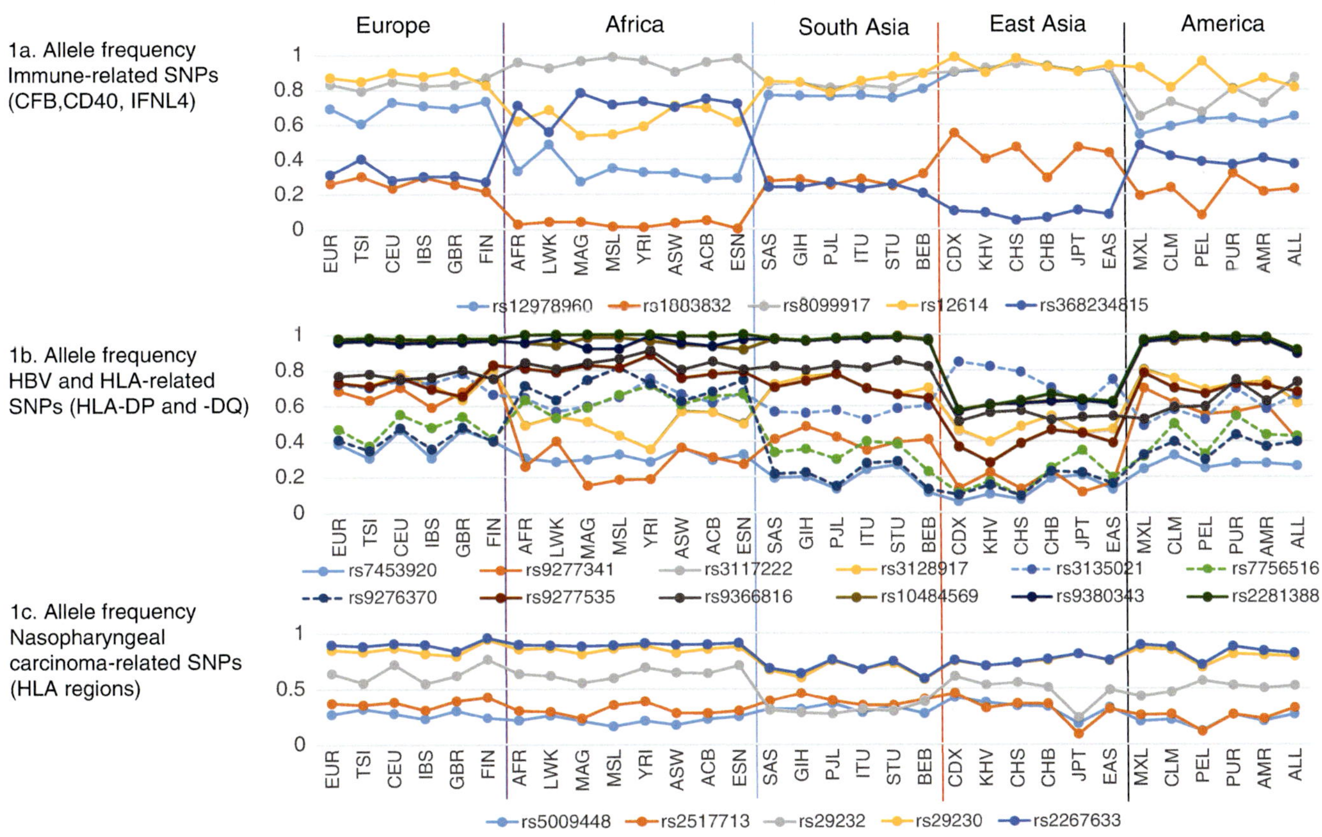

Fig. 16.1 Allele frequency of viral hepatitis- and NPC-related SNPs in different geographic groups. (**a**) Allele frequency of immune-related SNPs (CFB, CD40, and IFNL4). Significant allele type differences were found between African and European populations, and between African and South Asian populations, in all immune-related SNPs. (**b**) Allele frequency of HBV- and HLA-related SNPs (HLA-DP and -DQ). Significant allele differences were found between South and East Asian populations in 8 of 12 HLA-related SNPs, and between African and South Asian populations in 3 of 12 SNPs. (**c**) Allele frequencies of NPC-related SNPs (HLA regions). There was no significant difference among different populations in five NPC-related SNPs. Abbreviations: *ACB* African Ancestry from Barbados in the Caribbean, *AFR* Africa, total, *ALL* global, total, *AMR* America, total, *ASW* African ancestry in Southwest United States, *BEB* Bengali in Bangladesh, *CDX* Chinese Dai in Xishuangbanna, China, *CEU* Utah residents with ancestry from Northern and Western Europe, *CHB* Han Chinese in Beijing, China, *CHS* Han Chinese South, China, *CLM* Colombians in Medellin, Colombia, *EAS* East Asia, total, *ESN* Esan from Nigeria, *EUR* Europe, total, *FIN* Finnish in Finland, *GBR* British from England and Scotland, UK, *GIH* Gujarati Indians in Houston, TX, *IBS* Iberian populations in Spain, *ITU* Indian Telugu in the UK, *JPT* Japanese in Tokyo, Japan, *KHV* Kinh in Hochi Minh city, Vietnam, *LWK* Luhya in Webuye, Kenya, *MAG* Mandinka in Gambia, *MSL* Mende in Sierra Leone, *MXL* Mexican ancestry in Los Angeles, CA, *PEL* Peruvian in Lima, Peru, *PJL* Punjabi in Lahore, Pakistan, *PUR* Puerto Ricans in Puerto Rico, *SAS* South Asia, total, *STU* Sri Lankan Tamil in the UK, *TSI* Toscani in Italy, *YRI* Yoruba in Ibadan, Nigeria

migration reached the Indochina Peninsula, there was a sharp geography change from the flat land in Bangladesh to the mountainous and forested area of Chinese Dai. The latter environment in China and the Indochina Peninsula harbors a great diversity of plants and animals. Regions with higher plant and animal biodiversity often also feature an increased range and abundance of vector- or non-vector-borne diseases. Accordingly, the inhabitants of these areas should be able to handle an increased number of unfamiliar microorganisms. Those subjects who demonstrate direct and strong immune responses may die of cytokine storm in fulminant hepatitis, SARS, influenza, or other infections. Therefore, the persistent HBV infection-related single nucleotide polymorphisms (SNPs) on HLA-DP and -DQ loci could be an adaptive evolutionary response to the local environment.

16.9 Serological Diagnosis of HBV

The HBV genome encodes five proteins. The detection of HBsAg in sera and persistence for 6 months is a strong indication of chronic HBV infection. In the case of chronic hepatitis B under NA therapy, quantitative HBsAg level may have prognostic predict value [14]. The presence of hepatitis B core protein antibody (anti-HBc) is an evidence of nature HBV infection. High titer IgM class anti-HBc can be seen in acute hepatitis B. The presence of HBeAg in patients' serum is an indicator of the immune tolerance phase with active HBV replication. Most patients seropositive for both HBsAg and HBeAg antibody (anti-HBe) are in the residual stage. About 10% of these patients may still have a high serum titer of HBV DNA, which is usually associated with active HBV replication and liver inflammation [15].

The clearance of nuclear cccDNA is an important therapeutic end point. After HBV DNA is carefully digested, serum HBV RNA is assessed as a surrogate marker for cccDNA [16].

16.10 Immune Response

HBV is not directly cytopathic [6]. Most of the inflammation is induced by the immune clearance response. Immune tolerance is a survival strategy [13]. Excess immune response may induce fulminant hepatitis, while weak immune response may result in persistent HBV infection. Chronic HBV infection starts with an immune tolerance phase, followed by the immune clearance phase, and finally progresses to the residual phase.

During the immune tolerance phase, host immune cells are not completely unresponsive to HBV proteins. Selective B cell responses to viral proteins have been documented. Antibodies to HBsAg and HBeAg are generally absent. On the other hand, HBcAg, HBx or HBV DNA polymerase antibodies can be found.

Similar situations are identified in the T cell response. During the immune tolerance phase, HBsAg carriers show PMA (phorbol 12-myristate 13-acetate)/ionomycin-induced cytokine secretion similar to that of healthy controls. However, tumor necrosis factor-alpha and IL-22 levels are higher, and *chemokine* (*C-C* motif) ligand 3 (*CCL3*) levels are lower in HBsAg carriers at the immune tolerance phase than in healthy controls. In addition, programmed cell death protein 1 (PD-1) positive $CD4^+$ and $CD8^+$ T cells are both more frequent in the immune tolerance phase in HBsAg carriers than in healthy controls. IFN-ϒ-producing $CD3^+$ cells induced by HBV-specific peptides are present in HBsAg carriers in immune-tolerant, chronic active hepatitis, and inactive carrier stages. However, a stronger response can be seen in patients with chronic active hepatitis [17, 18].

While adaptive B and T cell responses are important in HBV immune clearance, how to induce a strong adaptive immune response in a patient with immune tolerance is still a mystery. We do not know why HBeAg positive patients in the immune tolerance phase gradually progress to the immune clearance phase. One explanation is that our innate immunity is continuously challenged by microorganisms and environmental substances. The strength of the innate immune response thus increases with age. Toll-like receptor (TLR)-mediated production of anti-inflammatory cytokines (e.g., IL-10) is high in pre-term infants, progressively declines over the first year of life, and is lowest in adults [19]. In contrast, the production of pro-inflammatory cytokines (e.g., IL-1β, TNF-α) gradually increases with age. This age-associated change and other unclear cofactors may orchestrate an immune clearance reaction once a break point is reached.

16.11 Fulminant Hepatic Failure

Either acute or chronic persistent HBV infection may induce fulminant hepatitis. HBV-specific $CD8^+$ T cell response plays a key role in viral clearance and disease pathogenesis. Other factors such as immune complex, complement activation, innate immunity, and ischemia may also contribute to massive hepatic necrosis and hepatic failure.

In the global HBV vaccination era, fulminant acute hepatic failure has become quite rare. Off-therapy and immune suppression-related HBV flares have become the main causes of fulminant hepatic failure. It has developed into an important concern in the treatment of chronic hepatitis B with cessation of NA therapy [20], and in patients receiving immune suppression or chemotherapy [21].

16.12 Chronic Hepatitis, Liver Cirrhosis and Massive Hepatic Necrosis

Persistent viral replication and intermittent inflammation in patients with chronic hepatitis B induces liver fibrosis [22]. Patients with severe flares usually have associated massive hepatic necrosis or so-called bridging hepatic necrosis. They may develop liver cirrhosis within several months (Fig. 16.2) [23]. This rapidly developed liver cirrhosis is quite different from chronic hepatitis C or other chronic liver diseases, which usually require decades to develop into liver cirrhosis. On the other hand, strong immune-related inflammation or long-term NA therapy might induce sustained viral suppression. In such cases, regression of liver fibrosis may be found. An example of this is shown in Fig. 16.2.

Liver cirrhosis is the major risk factor influencing survival in chronic persistent HBV infection [7, 8]. Non-invasive modalities for measurement of liver fibrosis have become an important indicator in screening policy and treatment planning.

Several fibrosis-detecting modalities had been developed. Fibrosis 4 (FIB 4, calculated from age, AST, ALT and platelet count), conventional ultrasound (US), and US-based elastography are the most popular modalities currently in use [24, 25]. They have different cutoff values under different etiologies, degrees of steatosis, and other confounding factors. How to use these modalities in suitable conditions should be considered carefully.

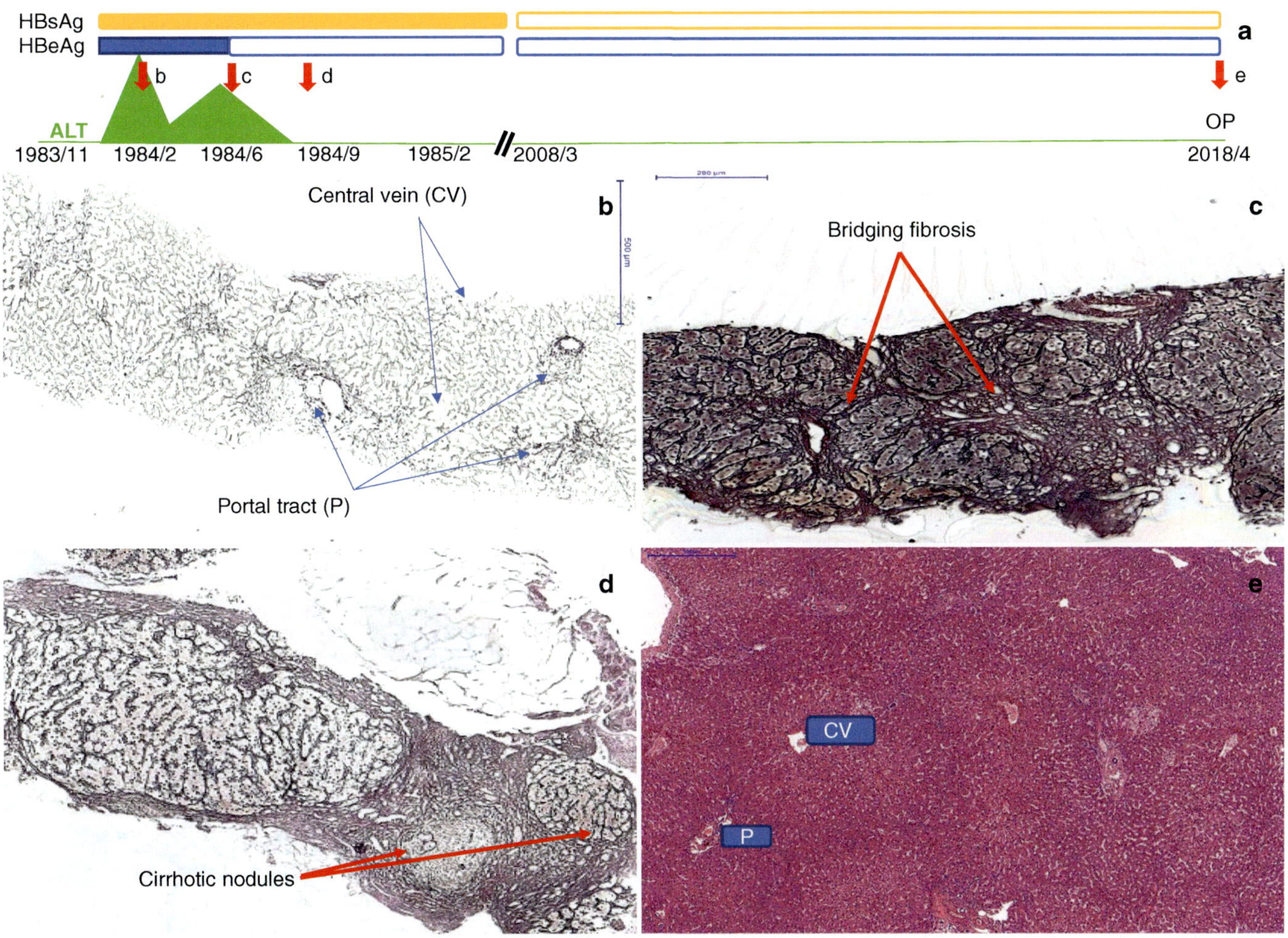

Fig. 16.2 A 22-year-old HBeAg positive female rapidly developed liver cirrhosis that spontaneously resolved 34 years later. (**a**) The clinical course and timing of four liver histology studies are shown; three biopsies were performed during a severe ALT flare-up as part of an Ara-A clinical trial. Viral replication was shut down and became persistent normal ALT after HBeAg seroconversion. She lost to followed-up and return with HBsAg clearance. The last biopsy was collected during a segmentectomy for a progressively enlarged angiomyolipoma which detected during periodic followed-up. (**b**) The initial silver-stained histology section revealed relatively normal reticulum architecture. (**c**) Four months later, severe bridging fibrosis was noted. (**d**) Well-recognized cirrhotic nodules were noted 7 months after the initial biopsy. (**e**) Thirty-four years after HBeAg seroconversion, hematoxylin and eosin staining of the non-tumor portion of the liver biopsy revealed a nearly normal liver with an Ishak fibrosis score of 1–2

16.13 Hepatocellular Carcinoma

Chronic HBV infection is associated with a high risk of liver cancer. Male gender, perinatal infection, old age, long HBV replication phase, HBV integration, liver cirrhosis, personal habits, aflatoxin, drug abuse [26], and environmental factors all contribute to HBV-related hepatocarcinogenesis. A combination of these processes results in an increased HCC risk [1, 4, 9, 10]. The HBV is capable of integration into the human genome, even during the immune tolerance phase. This phenomenon makes it possible for HCC to occur in patients with minimal fibrosis and no evidence of cirrhosis. This is quite different from cases of chronic HCV carriers, or patients with alcoholic or non-alcoholic liver cirrhosis, among which HCC usually develops if they have progressed to cirrhosis.

The molecular mechanisms of liver cancer are complicated and diverse, with different etiologies. Tumor protein p53 (TP53) oncosuppressor and catenin beta 1 (CTNNB1) oncogene are the most frequently mutated genes (31–37%) in HBV-related HCC [27].

Host genetic factors associated with HBV-related hepatocarcinogenesis had been researched intensively, but without reproducible results.

16.14 HBV Vaccination

A nationwide vaccination program has been conducted in Taiwan since 1984. A significant drop in HBsAg prevalence from more than 15% to less than 1% was reported. Maternal viral load greater than 10^8 copies/mL results in a 10% vaccination failure rate in the offspring. A short course of NA therapy starting at the last trimester and ending 1 month after delivery greatly reduced this failure rate [28].

To protect against infection, a course of vaccinations may be needed in adults without previous exposure to HBV. This is especially advisable in those planning travel from low endemic areas to high endemic areas. For those encountering used needles or other materials from HBsAg carriers, a dose of Hepatitis B immunoglobulin should be given as soon as possible followed by HBV vaccination.

16.15 Anti-HBV Therapy

While many drugs have been approved for treatment of chronic hepatitis B, complete virology response (CVR) rates were lower than 30% in most trials [1]. Therefore, according to the guidelines, only patients with elevated ALT level, HBV DNA greater than 10,000 copies/mL, or liver cirrhosis should be treated.

16.16 Pegylated Interferon Alpha (IFN-α) Therapy

For those with HBeAg-positive chronic hepatitis B, the first choice should be pegylated interferon-alpha (IFN-α) therapy for 1 year. This immune modulatory therapy requires weekly intramuscular injections for the duration of the treatment. The HBeAg seroconversion rate 6 months after completing 52 weeks of pegylated IFN-α therapy completion was around 32–36% [29]. IFN-α responders were generally patients with younger age, female gender, ALT elevation, low HBV DNA level, and genotype A or B. There is a relatively higher HBsAg clearance rate (around 5%) associated with IFN-α therapy compared to other anti-HBV therapy [1].

For those with HBeAg-negative chronic hepatitis B, pegylated IFN-α therapy for 1 year is still recommended. The sustained virologic response rate (SVR), as defined by HBV DNA <2000 IU/mL, 6 months after therapy was around 20% [30]. HBsAg seroconversion occurred in 3% of patients.

16.17 Nucleos(t)ide Analogues Therapy

The drug of choice for nucleos(t)ide analogues (NA) therapy in the CHB is entecavir (ETV) or tenofovir disoproxil fumarate (TDF). These drugs are highly effective HBV suppressors with low drug resistance. Drug resistance was a problem for first-generation NA therapy but has ceased to be so in the second generation. ETV (1.2%) and TDF (0%) had low 5-year drug resistance rates in treatment-naïve patients [1].

TDF is currently widely used in chronic hepatitis B, but will be replaced by tenofovir alafenamide fumarate, which has low renal and bone toxicity [31].

NAs are taken orally, have few side effects, and can effectively suppress HBV viral loads and liver inflammation. However, the HBeAg seroconversion rate is dependent on ethnicity and the duration of therapy. Among patients who received 4–5 years of ETV therapy, it was 15–38% in Asians and 55–58% in Europeans [1]. The difference could be related to disparate genetic backgrounds between East Asians and other populations [13]. When only Europeans studies were compared, the TDF (around 35%) had a lower HBeAg seroconversion rate than ETV. Whether a strong HBV suppression may evade immune surveillance remains to be determined through further evaluation.

The duration of NA therapy remains under debate. When NA therapy is stopped, HBV virologic and clinical relapse in the first year occurs with a likelihood of around 50% [32–34]. Some patients may develop a vigorous flare and proceed to hepatic failure [20]. Long-term treatment is required to maintain virologic control in patients with liver cirrhosis. For those patients without liver cirrhosis, stopping NA therapy after HBV DNA is undetectable for 1 year may be considered, and could promote HBsAg clearance.

16.18 Combination Therapy

Combination therapies of IFN-α and NAs have been studied with different strategies, but so far, none have been conclusively adapted for clinic use. Recently, sequential NA therapy followed by pegylated IFN-α therapy was found to produce a higher HBeAg seroconversion rate (14.9–44% versus 0–6.1%) than monotherapy [29]. In HBeAg negative patients, sequential NA followed by pegylated IFN-α had a higher HBsAg clearance rate (9–11%) than monotherapy (1–3%)

Combination therapy is more effective than monotherapy, but also increases treatment costs. Further studies will be needed to improve understanding of the immune clearance mechanism, develop new therapeutic strategies, and identify new anti-HBV specific agents in order to develop more efficient combination therapies.

16.19 Future Perspectives

Current anti-HBV therapies may suppress rather than eradicate HBV in patients with chronic hepatitis B. Further understanding of the mechanism of immune tolerance, as well as host and HBV interaction, and development of new therapeutic strategies are needed.

16.20 Conclusion

Chronic HBV infection is associated with timing of HBV infection and host genetic background. Such infection is characterized by an initial immune tolerance phase with high HBV replication, followed by an immune clearance phase, and finally a residual phase with low HBV replication. A significant decrease in chronic HBV infection has been achieved through a global HBV vaccination program in neonates. The survival of patients with chronic hepatitis B is also improving with the widespread use of NA therapy. These efforts have decreased fibrogenesis and hepatocarcinogenesis. However, two-thirds of patients relapse 3 years after the end of an NA therapy. There is still an urgent need for new therapeutic strategies, agents, and trials in chronic HBV infection.

Self Study

Questions

1. **Which statement is false?**
   (a) HBV is a highly infectious, small, circular, incomplete double stranded RNA virus.
   (b) Chronic infection is common when infected in the early stages of life.
   (c) The course of chronic HBV infection is a trilogy, starting with immune tolerance, followed by immune clearance, and finally a residual phase.
   (d) Immune tolerance is a survival strategy to avoid cytokine storm. It could be associated with genetic evolution during human migration.
2. **Which statement is true?**
   (a) The severity and duration of liver inflammation determine the development of liver cirrhosis and hepatocellular carcinoma.
   (b) Most chronic HBV carriers may terminate HBV replication, but are unable to achieve delayed HBsAg clearance even several decades later.
   (c) Current HBV-specific therapy may suppress viral replication and clear covalently closed circular DNA in the nucleus.
   (d) Clustering of chronic HBsAg infection in a family is related to HBV transmission, but not to genetic background.

Answers

1. **Which statement is false?**
   (a) HBV is a highly infectious, small, circular, incomplete double stranded <u>DNA</u> virus.
2. **Which statement is true?**
   (a) The severity and duration of liver inflammation determine the development of liver cirrhosis and hepatocellular carcinoma.
   (b) Most chronic HBV carriers may terminate HBV replication, <u>and at age 80, 50% of HBsAg carriers achieve delayed HBsAg clearance.</u>
   (c) Current HBV-specific therapy may suppress viral replication and <u>is unable to</u> clear covalently closed circular DNA in the nucleus.
   (d) Clustering of chronic HBsAg infection in a family is related to HBV transmission <u>and to inherited HLA-DP and -DQ loci</u>.

References

1. Liaw Y-F, Zoulim F, editors. Hepatitis B virus in human diseases. New York: Humana Press; 2016.
2. Wen J, Song C, Jiang D, Jin T, Dai J, Zhu L, et al. Hepatitis B virus genotype, mutations, human leukocyte antigen polymorphisms and their interactions in hepatocellular carcinoma: a multi-centre case-control study. Sci Rep. 2015;5:16489.
3. Lazarevic I. Clinical implications of hepatitis B virus mutations: recent advances. World J Gastroenterol. 2014;20:7653–64.
4. Beasley RP. Rocks along the road to the control of HBV and HCC. Ann Epidemiol. 2009;19(4):231–4.
5. Yan H, Zhong G, Xu G, He W, Jing Z, Gao Z, et al. Sodium taurocholate cotransporting polypeptide is a functional receptor for human hepatitis B and D virus. Elife. 2012;1:e00049.
6. Wieland S, Thimme R, Purcell RH, Chisari FV. Genomic analysis of the host response to hepatitis B virus infection. Proc Natl Acad Sci U S A. 2004;101:6669–74.
7. Liaw YF. Impact of therapy on the outcome of chronic hepatitis B. Liver Int. 2013;33(Suppl 1):111–5.
8. Bunchorntavakul C, Reddy KR. Acute liver failure. Clin Liver Dis. 2017;21:769–92.
9. Tai DI, Tsay PK, Chen WT, Chu CM, Liaw YF. Relative roles of HBsAg seroclearance and mortality in the decline of HBsAg prevalence with increasing age. Am J Gastroenterol. 2010;105:1102–9.
10. Tai DI, Lin SM, Sheen IS, Chu CM, Lin DY, Liaw YF. Long-term outcome of HBeAg-negative HBsAg carriers in relation to changes of alanine aminotransferase levels over time. Hepatology. 2009;49:1859–67.
11. Kamatani Y, Wattanapokayakit S, Ochi H, Kawaguchi T, Takahashi A, Hosono N, et al. A genome-wide association study identifies variants in the HLA-DP locus associated with chronic hepatitis B in Asians. Nat Genet. 2009;41:591–5.
12. Mbarek H, Ochi H, Urabe Y, Kumar V, Kubo M, Hosono N, et al. A genome-wide association study of chronic hepatitis B identified novel risk locus in a Japanese population. Hum Mol Genet. 2011;20:3884–92.
13. Tai DI, Jeng WJ, Lin CY. A global perspective on HBV-related SNPs and evolution during human migration. Hepatol Commun. 2017;1:1005–13.
14. Liaw YF. Clinical utility of HBV surface antigen quantification in HBV e antigen-negative chronic HBV infection. Nat Rev Gastroenterol Hepatol. 2019. https://doi.org/10.1038/s41575-019-0197-8.15.
15. World Health Organization. Guidelines on hepatitis B and C testing, Geneva. 2017. http://www.who.int/hepatitis/publications/guidelines-hepatitis-c-b-testing/en/. Accessed Feb 2017.
16. Li X, Zhao J, Yuan Q, Xia N. Detection of HBV covalently closed circular DNA. Viruses. 2017;9(6). pii: E139.
17. Kennedy PTF, Sandalova E, Jo J, Gill U, Ushiro-Lumb I, Tan AT, et al. Preserved T-cell function in children and young adults with immune-tolerant chronic hepatitis B. Gastroenterology. 2012;143(3):637–45.
18. Mason WS, Gill US, Litwin S, Zhou Y, Peri S, Pop O, et al. HBV DNA integration and clonal hepatocyte expansion in chronic hepatitis B patients considered immune tolerant. Gastroenterology. 2016;151:986–98.
19. Kollmann TR, Levy O, Montgomery RR, Goriely S. Innate immune function by Toll-like receptors: distinct responses in newborns and the elderly. Immunity. 2012;37:771–83.
20. Chang ML, Jeng WJ, Liaw YF. Clinical events after cessation of lamivudine therapy in patients recovered from hepatitis B flare with hepatic decompensation. Clin Gastroenterol Hepatol. 2015;13:979–86.
21. Mandala M, Fagiuoli S, Francisci D, Bruno R, Merelli B, Pasulo L, et al. Hepatitis B in immunosuppressed cancer patients: pathogenesis, incidence and prophylaxis. Crit Rev Oncol Hematol. 2013;87:12e27.
22. Liaw YF, Tai DI, Chu CM, Chen TJ. The development of cirrhosis in patients with chronic type B hepatitis: a prospective study. Hepatology. 1988;8:493–6.
23. Chen CJ, Tsay PK, Huang SF, Tsui PH, Yu WT, Hsu TH, et al. Effects of hepatic steatosis on non-invasive liver fibrosis measurements between hepatitis B and other etiologies. Appl. Sci. 2019;9:1961.
24. Lim JK, Flamm SL, Singh S, Falck-Ytter YT. Clinical Guidelines Committee of the American Gastroenterological Association. American Gastroenterological Association Institute guideline on the role of elastography in the evaluation of liver fibrosis. Gastroenterology. 2017;152:1536–43.
25. Shiha G, Ibrahim A, Helmy A, Sarin SK, Omata M, Kumar A, et al. Asian-Pacific Association for the Study of the Liver (APASL) consensus guidelines on invasive and non-invasive assessment of hepatic fibrosis: a 2016 update. Hepatol Int. 2017;11:1–30.
26. Ng AWT, Poon SL, Huang MN, Lim JQ, Boot A, Yu W, et al. Aristolochic acids and their derivatives are widely implicated in liver cancers in Taiwan and throughout Asia. Sci Transl Med. 2017;9(412) https://doi.org/10.1126/scitranslmed.aan6446.
27. Ahn SM, Jang SJ, Shim JH, Kim D, Hong SM, Sung CO, et al. Genomic portrait of resectable hepatocellular carcinomas: implications of RB1 and FGF19 aberrations for patient stratification. Hepatology. 2014;60:1972–82.
28. Chen HL, Lee CN, Chang CH, Ni YH, Shyu MK, Chen SM, et al. Taiwan Study Group for the Prevention of Mother-to-Infant Transmission of HBV (PreMIT Study); Taiwan Study Group for the Prevention of Mother-to-Infant Transmission of HBV PreMIT Study. Efficacy of maternal tenofovir disoproxil fumarate in interrupting mother-to-infant transmission of hepatitis B virus. Hepatology. 2015;62:375–86.
29. Woo ASJ, Kwok R, Ahmed T. Alpha-interferon treatment in hepatitis B. Ann Transl Med. 2017;5:159.
30. Marcellin P, Lau GK, Bonino F, Farci P, Hadziyannis S, Jin R, et al. Peginterferon alfa-2a alone, lamivudine alone, and the two in combination in patients with HBeAg-negative chronic hepatitis B. N Engl J Med. 2004;351:1206–17.
31. Agarwal K, Brunetto M, Seto WK, Lim YS, Fung S, Marcellin P, et al. 96 weeks treatment of tenofovir alafenamide vs. tenofovir disoproxil fumarate for hepatitis B virus infection. J Hepatol. 2018;68:672–81.
32. Jeng WJ, Chen YC, Sheen IS, Lin CL, Hu TH, Chien RN, et al. Clinical relapse after cessation of tenofovir therapy in hepatitis B e antigen-negative patients. Clin Gastroenterol Hepatol. 2016;14:1813–20.
33. Jeng WJ, Sheen IS, Chen YC, Hsu CW, Chien RN, Chu CM, et al. Off-therapy durability of response to entecavir therapy in hepatitis B e antigen-negative chronic hepatitis B patients. Hepatology. 2013;58:1888–96.
34. Chang ML, Liaw YF, Hadziyannis SJ. Systematic review: cessation of long-term nucleos(t)ide analogue therapy in patients with hepatitis B e antigen-negative chronic hepatitis B. Aliment Pharmacol Ther. 2015;42:243–57.

Viral Hepatitis C

17

Luigi Elio Adinolfi, Emanuele Durante Mangoni, Aldo Marrone, Rosa Zampino, and Luca Rinaldi

Key Concepts

- HCV is a small blood-borne RNA virus belonging to the genus Hepacivirus in the Flaviviridae family. Currently, 7 HCV genotypes, 84 subtypes and several quasispecies are recognized.
- HCV replication occurs primarily in the liver, but the virus infects and replicates into most human cells and tissues causing local and systemic inflammation, therefore is considered a systemic infection.
- HCV causes acute and chronic liver disease, cirrhosis and hepatocellular carcinoma as well as extrahepatic manifestations (cryoglobulinemia, diabetes, atherosclerosis, and lymphoproliferative, cardiovascular, neuropsychiatric and renal diseases).
- Liver steatosis and insulin resistance are features of HCV infection that accelerate liver disease progression and the development of hepatocellular carcinoma and extrahepatic manifestations.
- Direct-acting antivirals (DAAs) have been approved for HCV infection treatment with up to 98% cure rates, so HCV is largely treatable infection. In addition, DAAs are able to improve or reverse both hepatic and extrahepatic manifestations.

L. E. Adinolfi (✉) · A. Marrone · R. Zampino · L. Rinaldi
Department of Advanced Medical and Surgical Sciences, University of Campania "L. Vanvitelli", Naples, Italy
e-mail: luigielio.adinolfi@unicampania.it

E. D. Mangoni
Department of Precision Medicine, University of Campania "L. Vanvitelli", Naples, Italy

17.1 Introduction

The hepatitis C virus (HCV) is endemic all over the world and is a leading cause of liver disease and liver transplantation representing a significant public health problem. HCV is transmitted parenterally through contact with contaminated blood and most patients who acquire the infection are unable to spontaneously eliminate the virus, thereby developing a chronic infection that causes liver fibrosis and often evolves into cirrhosis and hepatocellular carcinoma (HCC). Although viral replication occurs primarily in the liver, HCV is able to infect and replicate into most human cells and tissues, causing local and systemic inflammation that plays a role in a wide range of extrahepatic manifestations, including lipid and glucose metabolic imbalances. Therefore, HCV infection is considered a systemic disease. Recently, direct-acting antivirals (DAAs) have been approved to treat HCV infection, which is now a largely treatable infection. In fact, DAAs are able to achieve HCV clearance in up to 98% of cases, improving or reversing both hepatic and extrahepatic manifestations.

17.2 Virology

HCV is a small, enveloped, positive-strand RNA virus. Comparison of HCV nucleotide sequences revealed the presence of genotypes, subtypes and quasispecies.

17.2.1 Taxonomic Classification and Genotypes

HCV has unique biological characteristics, ensuring its inclusion in the new genus Hepacivirus in the Flaviviridae family [1]. Due to the wide diversity of HCV strains, we currently recognize 7 genotypes and 84 subtypes, all of which can cause acute and chronic liver disease in humans.

F. Radu-Ionita et al. (eds.), *Liver Diseases*, https://doi.org/10.1007/978-3-030-24432-3_17

Genotype 1 is the most widespread worldwide, followed by genotypes 3, 4 and 2. The HCV genotypes may differ from one another in 25–33% of the entire genome sequence, while the subtypes are more closely related within each genotype showing a genetic diversity of 15–25%. Furthermore, the virus exists in each host as "quasispecies" a complex of genetic variants belonging to individual subtypes with similarities of nucleotide sequences ranging from 90% to 99% [2]. This genetic diversity underlies the ability of HCV to adapt to different compartments of the host, to evade the immune response and to persist chronically. Furthermore, the genetic variability of HCV is one of the main obstacles to the development of an effective active immunization strategy. Knowledge of HCV genotypes has epidemiological, pathophysiological and therapeutic implications.

17.2.2 Viral Structure

HCV consists of approximately 9.6 kb of single-stranded RNA molecule with positive polarity acting as messenger RNA for viral protein translation. Single-stranded genomic RNA encodes an open reading frame, translated into a single polyprotein from which ten viral proteins are generated (Fig. 17.1).

The HCV structural proteins—core E1 and E2 constitute the viral nucleocapsid and the envelope. The core protein consists of a positively charged domain implicated in RNA-binding and homo-oligomerization and a hydrophobic domain, involved in membrane, endoplasmic reticulum (ER) and mitochondria association. This subunit also mediates the intracellular binding of HCV to lipid droplets, one of the most relevant biological characteristics of this pathogen. The expression of the core protein in experimental animal liver cells is associated with steatosis and neoplastic transformation. E1 and E2 are extensively glycosylated proteins incorporated in the lipid double layer of the viral envelope in the form of a heterodimer and mediate the close extracellular association of HCV particles with lipoproteins and lipids [3]. E1 and E2 also possess highly variable domains that are largely responsible for escape from the host immune response, as well as conserved regions that mediate attachment and entry of viruses into target cells. Of note, E1 and E2 contain the epitopes of anti-HCV antibodies used for serological diagnosis.

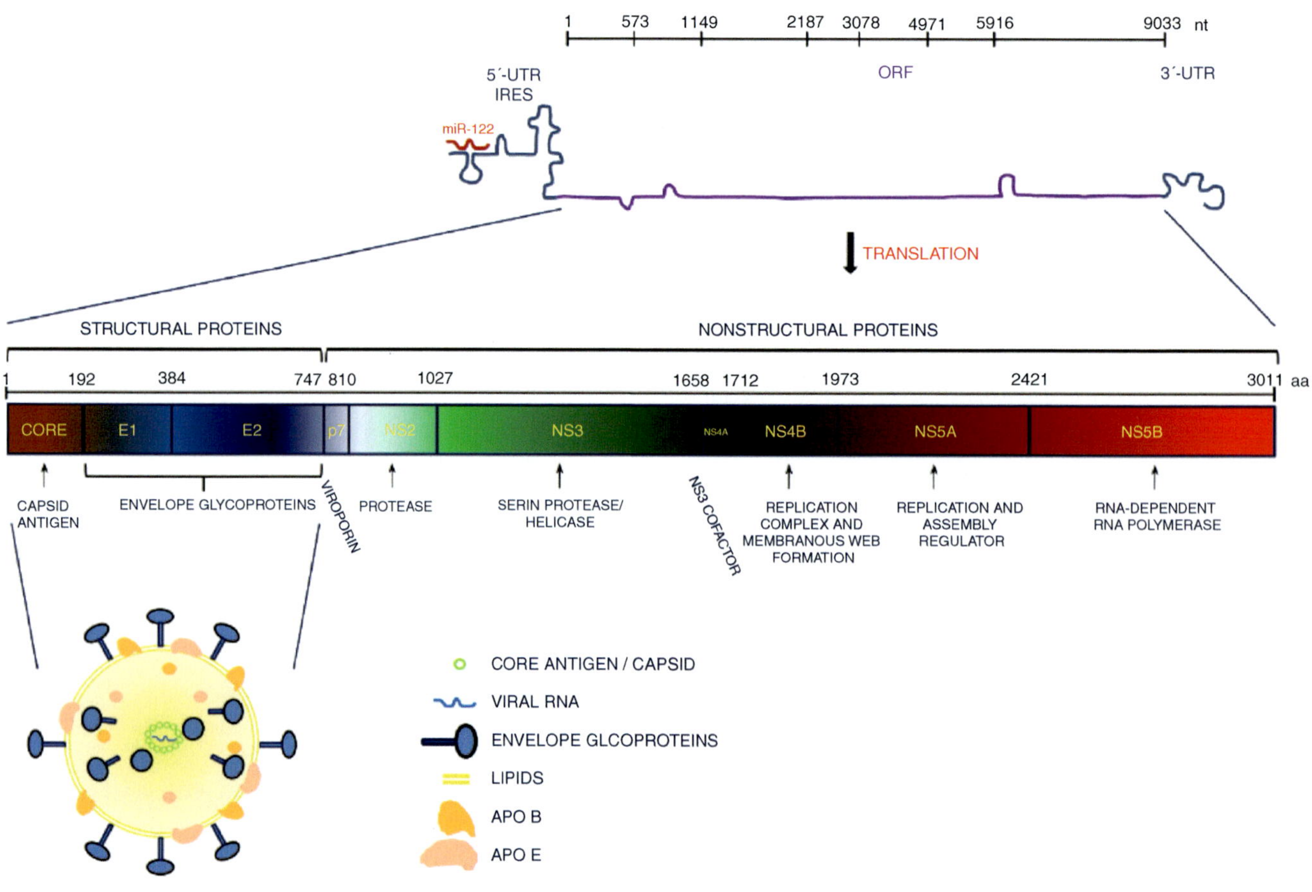

Fig. 17.1 The HCV genome

Non-structural (NS) proteins, expressed in HCV target cells, include p7, NS2, NS3, NS4A, NS4B, NS5A and NS5B, and modulate viral replication, assembly and virulence expression. Each of the NS proteins has multiple functions. The main role in the processing of the polyprotein and in the assembly of the virus is played by the heterodimeric complex of the NS3 and NS4A proteins, consisting of a serine protease and a RNA helicase. The NS3-NS4A also breaks down the proteins of the target cells involved in antiviral signaling, hindering e.g. induction of the type I interferon pathway. NS4B is an integral membrane protein involved in the generation of membranous web. NS5A plays an important role in HCV biology by contributing to replicase formation and virion assembly. The activity of the RNA-dependent viral RNA polymerase is exploited by NS5B. Most NS proteins gather in the cytoplasm in association with a membranous network rich in vesicles to form the replicase complex, where viral RNA synthesis occurs.

17.2.3 Viral Life Cycle

Persistence is the basis of the pathology of HCV and results from both virus-induced weakening of innate and adaptive host immune responses and a regulated viral replication so as to minimize the levels of intracellular viruses and the number of actually infected hepatocytes [4].

HCV is present in the extracellular compartment in close interaction with the lipoproteins, forming the so-called lipoviroparticles (LVP). This interaction is a strategy that HCV has developed to escape antibody neutralization and to entry in the cells. Incorporated into these lipid complexes, HCV binds easily to the low-density lipoprotein receptor (LDL-R) on hepatocytes. Numerous additional receptors are also needed to mediate the binding and internalization of HCV, including CD81, the class B type I high-density lipoprotein scavenger receptor, the claudin-1 and occluding tight-junction proteins and the Niemann-Pick C1-like 1 cholesterol absorption receptor. Thus, attachment and entry of HCV are only partially mediated by a direct interaction of the envelope glycoproteins to specific host membrane protein receptors and is strongly associated with lipoprotein-mediated attachment. These multiple receptors and entry factors are exploited in an orderly manner and account for HCV infectivity in primates and tropism for hepatocytes. Initially, LVP connect to the hepatocyte surface by glycosaminoglycans, LDL-R, and class B type I scavenger receptor. The latter activates cholesterol transfer, thus freeing up virus particles from the associated lipids and allowing the interaction of CD81 with its binding sites on HCV E2. The HCV particles bound to CD81 move laterally to tight junctions, interact with claudin-1 and occludin and are endocytosed through a clathrin-dependent mechanism [5]. Within endosomes, lipid transfer activities further modify LVP and binding with CD81 primes HCV E1 and E2 to trigger fusion between the viral envelope and endosomal membrane at low pH. This probably releases the HCV genome into the cytosol, where it binds to a hepatocyte-specific microRNA, miR-122 and to cellular ribosomes through the internal ribosomal entry site. Upon release into the cytosol, the RNA genome serves as a template for both translations and replication. HCV-RNA is also used for the synthesis of negative strands, which in turn function as templates for the new HCV-RNA positive strand. The HCV genome includes highly structured non-translated 5′- and 3′-regions that flank the open reading frame, which are involved in important functions including internal ribosomal entry and translation initiation. After the formation of the NS protein, the viral replicase complex, composed of NS3 to NS5B and the genomic RNA template, begins to express its function. NS5A plays a key role. It is a multifunctional phosphoprotein associated with intracellular membranes that binds RNA and activates NS5B, the RNA-dependent RNA polymerase of HCV. It has many interactions with various cellular factors, including cyclophilin A, phosphatidylinositol-4-kinase IIIa and apolipoprotein E, which are required for HCV replication. The enzyme that catalyzes the replication of viral RNA is NS5B, which shows a typical shape of a right hand with subdomains resembling fingers, thumb and palm, designing a circular catalytic site. The negative-strand RNA synthesis begins at the 3′ end of the viral genome, and is a rate limiting step, since the positive-strand RNAs are produced in much larger quantities [6]. HCV replication is enhanced by miR-122, a liver-specific micro-RNA that also regulates the expression of fatty acid and cholesterol metabolism genes. In addition to its role in RNA replication, NS5A is also essential for the assembly of HCV and seems to interact with the core protein linked to lipid droplets. The HCV that buds into the extracellular compartment exploits the complex cellular machine that works in series with its secretory compartment. During the transport of HCV particles through the secretory pathway and the Golgi apparatus, E1 and E2 are added to the complex HCV-RNA core protein and undergo post-translational changes, including the addition of mannose and glycans. HCV particles interact with the lipids an important pathophysiological aspects of HCV infection. The available data support a connection between the maturation of HCV particles and the secretion of hepatocyte lipoproteins [7]. HCV acquires its high lipid content during hepatocyte output, in a manner very similar to the maturation of very low-density lipoprotein (VLDL) particles. This process is modulated by the microsomal triglyceride transfer protein (MTP), a large protein that actively transports the lipids into the ER lumen and in this way promotes VLDL synthesis. In the ER, VLDL synthesis results from apoB100 and lipid association. Further lipidation of VLDL precursors containing apoB occurs in

Table 17.1 Prevalence, distribution and epidemiologic and clinical features of HCV genotypes

HCV genotypes	Estimated prevalence	Prevalent geographic distribution	Epidemiologic features	Main clinical correlates
1	49%	Worldwide, especially Europe and America	Older patients, nosocomial transmission. Subtype 1a associated with IVDA[a]	Progression to cirrhosis and HCC
2	11%	Sub-Saharan Africa, East Asia	Transfusion-transmission	Cryoglobulinemia
3	18%	South Asia, Latin America, Europe	Associated with IVDA	Viral induced steatosis, younger patients
4	17%	Africa, Middle East	Health-care related acquisition	No specific finding
5	2%	Sub-Saharan Africa	Sparse data	Sparse data
6	1.5%	Southeast Asia	Sparse data	Sparse data
Mixed	1.5%	South Asia, Caribbean	Sparse data	Sparse data

[a]Intra-venous drug abuser

Golgi to form mature VLDL particles and involves apoE- and apoC-containing microsome-associated lipid droplets. The same mechanisms appear to occur during the maturation of HCV particles. Indeed, inhibition of MTP activity suppresses the production of HCV virions. Interestingly, if lipid transfer driven by MTP is slow or insufficient, apoB100 undergoes misfolding and degradation, with a consequent reduction in the production of VLDL. It can therefore be hypothesized that HCV, exploiting MTP during the production of virions in infected hepatocytes, can secondarily affect the production of VLDL. These results, on the one hand, in the common hypolipidemia observed in chronic HCV infection and, on the other, in the accumulation of lipids inside the hepatocytes, causing hepatic steatosis.

By exploiting tight-junction proteins, HCV can spread from an infected hepatocyte to an uninfected neighboring cell, thus avoiding the extracellular pathway that would most likely be prone to antibody-mediated neutralization.

17.3 Epidemiology

HCV infection is universally distributed. In 2015, a global prevalence of 1% was estimated, with 71.1 million infected subjects and 1.75 million new cases of HCV infection per year [8, 9]. The prevalence of HCV increases with age reaching a peak between 55 and 64 years. The highest prevalence of HCV was observed in the eastern Mediterranean (2.3%) and in European regions (1.5%), in the other regions the prevalence varies from 0.5% to 1% [9]. The distribution of HCV infection is different in people of diverse countries, and can be concentrated in some groups (e.g., among people who use injectable drugs) and/or in the general population. Based on the dissemination of the HCV genotype, it has been suggested that sub-Saharan Africa and Southeast Asia may be the original geographic areas of the different HCV genotypes. The spreading of HCV genotypes varies by region. The HCV genotype 1 has the highest prevalence in most countries (United States, Europe, Australia and Japan); genotype 3 is common in South Asia and genotype 4 has the highest frequency in Egypt and North Africa. Table 17.1 shows the prevalence and distribution of HCV genotypes and the main associated epidemiological and clinical features [8, 9].

17.4 Transmission

HCV is a bloodborne virus that can be transmitted even with exposure to small amounts of blood. The common circumstances of transmission are the use of illicit drug injections, unsafe injection practices and medical treatments and blood transfusions or use of unscreened blood products. Therefore, the most common practices that can transmit the virus are: (a) inject drug use by sharing syringes and needles; (b) inadequate re-use or sterilization of medical equipment in health facilities; (c) transfusion of blood or unscreened blood products. Less commonly, transmission of HCV can occur through sexual intercourse and vertical transmission from an infected mother to the child upon delivery.

Hepatitis C is not transmitted through breast milk, food, water or common relational contact of daily life, such as embracing or kissing.

17.5 Diagnosis

The HCV virologic markers consist of enzyme immunoassays (EIAs) to detect anti-HCV antibodies and HCV core antigen and nucleic acid-based molecular assays to detect and quantify HCV RNA and to define HCV genotypes.

17.5.1 Anti-HCV Antibodies

The serological diagnosis is based on the detection of anti-HCV antibodies. Currently, regardless of the viral genotype, EIA assays, which use core antigens and recombinant antigens from the NS3, NS4 and NS5 regions, have a high sensitivity (97%) and specificity (99%). False positive results are possible in patients with autoimmune diseases and some infectious diseases such as mononucleosis and syphilis while false negative results may occur in immunosuppressed subjects such as those with HIV infection or hypogammaglobulinemia, in patients with solid organ transplantation and in patients on hemodialysis. The recombinant immune-blot assay, initially used as a confirmatory test, is currently considered obsolete. EIAs may be negative in the early phase of acute hepatitis C with a window period of more than 40 days. HCV-Ab positivity may persist in individuals with spontaneous or treatment-induced viral clearance [10]. Therefore, detection of anti-HCV antibodies does not document an active HCV infection that must be confirmed by the presence of serum HCV-RNA. Quantitative HCV core antigen tests are currently available. They can be a substitute test for HCV RNA where molecular biology is unavailable. The HCV core antigen may be detectable during the serological window period of the acute infection. A strong correlation between the level of HCV core antigen and viremia has been reported in patients with chronic hepatitis C [11]. However, the sensitivity of the HCV core antigen test is lower than the current HCV RNA assays.

17.5.2 Nucleic Acid Detection

The detection and quantification of HCV RNA are essential for the diagnosis of HCV infection. Real-time RT-PCR is currently the method of choice for measuring the level of HCV RNA in serum for its high and wide range of sensitivity (10–15 IU/mL up to 8 log IU/mL), the low risk of contamination and speed of execution. At least four RT-PCR assays are available considered comparable in their results. However, the accuracy of the viral load measurement may depend on the genotype. Currently, the Abbott Real Time HCV assay and the Roche Cobas TaqMan assay are considered to be the gold standard for the quantification of HCV RNA [12].

17.5.3 Genotyping

HCV genotyping is crucial for epidemiology and has contributed to a better understanding of different clinical manifestations. Determination of HCV genotype prior to initiation of treatment was necessary in the interferon era. However, the recent use of pan-genotypic DAAs should no longer require genotyping prior to therapy.

Commercial tests for genotyping and subtyping use genome sequencing of the core/E1, NS5B and 5′UTR regions.

17.5.4 Point of Care and Rapid Tests

The use of DAAs is increasing the interest in developing rapid and easy diagnostic tests (point of care, POCs) to achieve the WHO goal of global HCV elimination by 2030 [13]. The POC and dry blood spot (DBS) tests determine qualitative and/or quantitative viral antibodies and/or antigens. A recent rapid POC test showed a sensitivity of 98.6% and a 100% specificity in detecting HCV [14].

17.6 Clinical Manifestations

HCV infection has a wide spectrum of clinical manifestations ranging from acute and chronic hepatic and extrahepatic diseases, thus HCV is considered a multi-facet systemic disease. Figure 17.2 shows the main manifestations associated with chronic HCV infection.

Acute hepatitis C (AHC) is often asymptomatic and evolves towards chronic infection in 60–80% of cases. This in turn may slowly progress towards compensated cirrhosis and subsequently, decompensated cirrhosis. Cirrhotic patients develop HCC with an incidence of about 3% per year. Up to 70% of patients with chronic HCV infection develop extrahepatic manifestations that may be the first clinical sign of infection.

17.6.1 Acute Hepatitis

The incubation period varies between 2 weeks and 6 months, and is mostly between 6 and 9 weeks. AHC generally has mild clinical manifestations and often remains undiagnosed. In a minority of cases, symptoms such as jaundice, weakness, anorexia, malaise, dyspepsia and hepatomegaly may develop. An increase in serum alanine aminotransferase (ALT) level of at least ten times the normal value can often be observed. 20–40% of the symptomatic subjects with AHC spontaneously eliminate HCV-RNA. The average elimination time has been recently estimated at 16.5 weeks. Female sex, IL28B genotype and HCV genotype 1 are independent predictors of spontaneous clearance [15]. Fulminant hepatitis due to HCV has been reported in 5 every 1000 cases of AHC [16].

The diagnosis of AHC is often difficult due to the absence of acute serological markers. The presence of HCV RNA, anti-HCV seroconversion, the sudden increase in serum ALT values, and the recent exposure can help to perform the correct diagnosis. However, in the absence of these elements, the differential diagnosis with a reactivation of chronic hepatitis C (CHC) is difficult.

IgM anti-HCV antibodies can be detected both during the acute and chronic phases and therefore are not diagnostic.

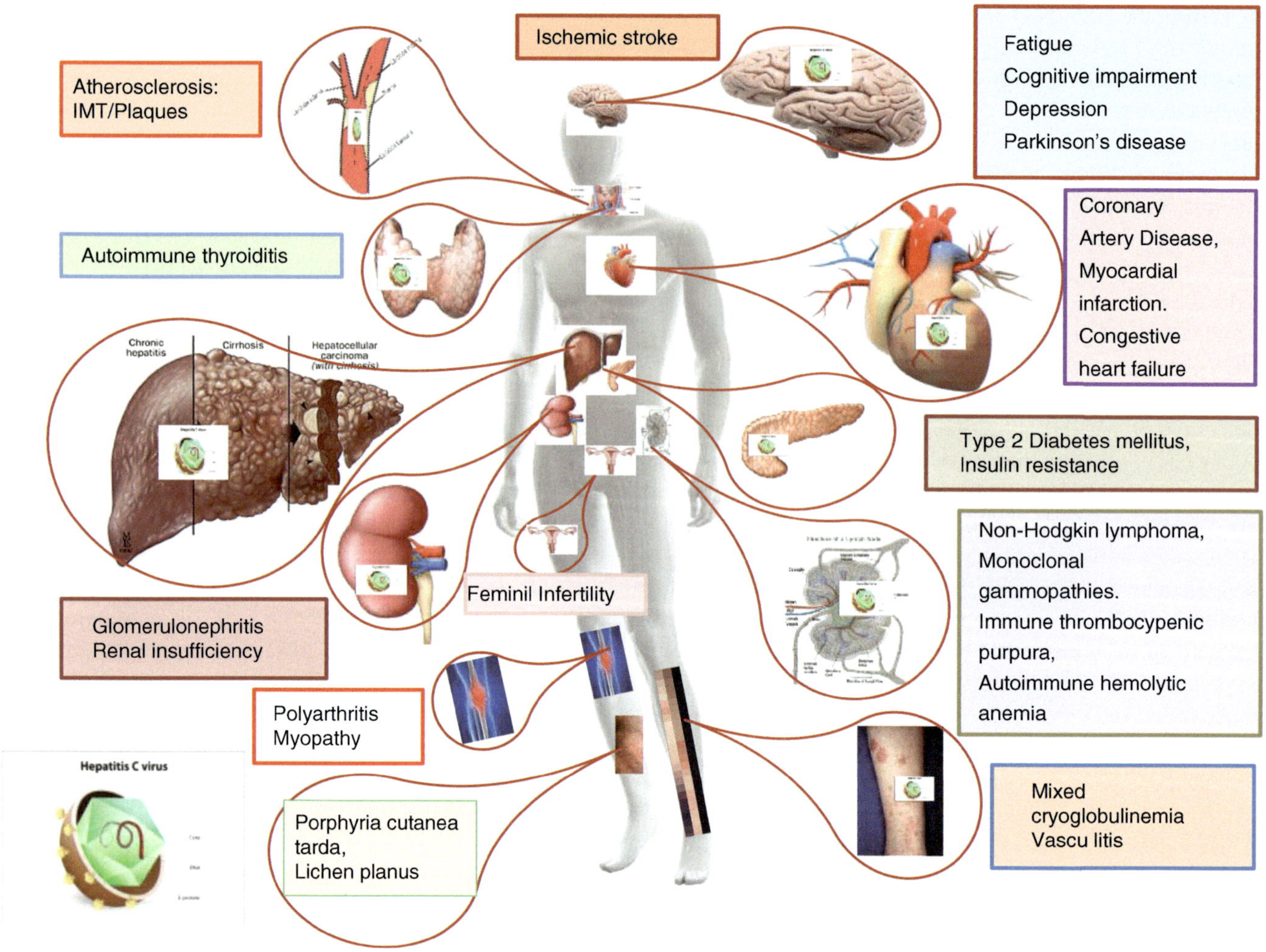

Fig. 17.2 Main hepatic and extrahepatic manifestations associated with HCV infection

Instead, the avidity test for anti-HCV IgG and IgM antibodies has recently proved to be able to make a correct diagnosis of AHC in 90% of cases [17].

17.6.2 Chronic Hepatitis

The infection is defined chronic after 6 months of HCV-RNA persistence. About 70% of infected patients show a chronic course with a slow progression of liver fibrosis toward the development of cirrhosis and its complications. CHC is generally asymptomatic or has mild and non-specific symptoms. Tiredness and malaise are the most frequent, but sometimes nausea, anorexia, myalgia, arthralgia and weight loss are possible. Hepatomegaly and splenomegaly are present in a high percentage of cases. Liver function tests are generally normal, with a mild increase in serum AST and ALT levels, although cases with persistently normal ALT are commonly observed.

Ultrasound scanning generally shows enlarged liver and/or spleen as for chronic hepatitis of other etiology, although a bright liver echo-pattern, expression of hepatic steatosis, is common in CHC. Liver biopsy and histological examination have been the gold standard in the evaluation of inflammation, fibrosis and steatosis in CHC. Currently, liver biopsy is reserved to select cases and fibrosis and disease progression are more commonly assessed using non-invasive methods including biomarkers (ARFI®, Aixplore®, Fibrotest®, FIB-4®, APRI®) and liver transient elastography (fibroscan®) [18].

17.6.3 Hepatic Steatosis

Liver steatosis is a distinctive feature of HCV infection. It is reported with an average prevalence of 55% and appears to be a final condition promoting virus survival. Viral and host factors contribute to the development of steatosis. In patients infected with HCV genotype 3, steatosis is directly related to viral load and is considered of viral origin being defined as "viral steatosis". In contrast, in patients with non-3 genotype infection, steatosis is mainly linked to host factors such as increased body mass index (BMI), obesity, visceral obesity, insulin resistance (IR) and type 2 diabetes mellitus (T2DM), thereby being designated "metabolic steatosis" [19].

The mechanisms by which HCV induces steatosis are complex and specific for genotype 3 (impaired MTP and peroxisome proliferator-activated receptor-α (PPAR-α), increased sterol regulatory element-binding proteins (SREBPs), reduced lipoprotein export B-oxidation, increased de novo lipogenesis, downregulation of PTEN gene expression, hyper-tumor necrosis factor-α (TNF-α), and hypoadiponectinemia) and non-3 genotypes (increased BMI and IR, hypoadiponectinemia, hyper-TNF-α, increased of reactive oxygen species (ROS), of suppressor of cytokine signaling (SOCS3), of free fatty acids (FFA), of FAS activity, and impaired fatty acid oxidation and increased oxidative stress) [19]. Steatosis induces liver and systemic inflammation and oxidative stress causing a more rapid progression of hepatic fibrosis and an increased risk of developing HCC, also contributes to the development of some extrahepatic manifestations, such as diabetes, metabolic syndrome and atherosclerosis [19]. Metabolic steatosis, but not viral steatosis, reduced the IFN response rate, whereas it does not affect the response rate to DAAs.

17.6.4 Cirrhosis

The initial signs of the evolution into liver cirrhosis (compensated cirrhosis) are hardly clinically identified and can be detected by histological examination or non-invasive tests. Compensated cirrhosis may be characterized by mild changes in laboratory parameters of liver function tests, such as decreased albumin and cholinesterase levels, increased bilirubin and prothrombin time, and a variable reduction in platelet counts. However, in most cases symptoms and liver function tests are not easily differentiated from those seen in chronic hepatitis.

Decompensated cirrhosis can occur in the natural history of the disease after a variable number of years. The clinical picture and complications are like those observed in cirrhosis from other etiologies (for more details see Chap. 23). Pruritus, dryness, palmar erythema, jaundice, *faetor hepaticus*, spider nevi, petechiae, excoriation due to itching, gynecomastia and testicular atrophy can be observed. In this phase of the disease the symptoms are related to impairment of the hepatic synthetic function and to the portal hypertension. The clinical manifestations include ascites, edema of the lower limbs, jaundice, the presence of esophageal varices and their bleeding with hematemesis or melena and hepatic encephalopathy. Clinical events such as infections, hyperglycemia, renal dysfunction, cardiovascular complications and neoplasms can trigger cirrhosis decompensation events.

17.6.4.1 Ascites

Ascites, defined as the pathological accumulation of fluid in the peritoneal cavity, is the consequence of the anatomical, pathophysiological and biochemical alterations that occur in patients with cirrhosis. Three theories on the formation of ascites have been proposed: underfilling, overflow and peripheral arterial vasodilatation (see Chap. 23). The appearance of ascites is a negative prognostic factor. The presence of ascites requires a chemical-physical, microbiological and cytological evaluation. Ascites therapy (see Chap. 23) is mainly medical and consists of non-pharmacological therapy and drug therapy. Non-pharmacological therapy consists of bed rest, reduction of fluid intake and avoiding the addition of salt to the diet. Drug therapy is mainly based on the use of diuretics such as anti-aldosterone agents and loop diuretics (see Chap. 23).

Ascites can become infected with intestinal bacteria causing spontaneous bacterial peritonitis (SBP), a condition associated with a high mortality rate. Diagnostic paracentesis is always required for diagnosis of SBP. The isolation of the causative microorganism from the ascitic fluid is obtained in a small number of cases. A neutrophil count in the ascitic fluid greater than 250 cells/ml is diagnostic of SBP. Antibiotic treatment must be promptly started to reduce mortality and include third-generation cephalosporin or fluoroquinolone for community-acquired infection and a carbapenem or piperacillin-tazobactam for nosocomial infections. SBP can trigger a hepato-renal syndrome (HRS) associated with high short- and medium-term mortality. The appearance of HRS must be intensively treated using predominantly splanchnic vasoconstrictors (terlipressin) and high doses of intravenous albumin.

17.6.4.2 Esophageal Varices

Portal hypertension causes the development of esophageal varices. In patients with liver cirrhosis with liver stiffness >20 kPa, assessed by transient elastography and platelet counts <150,000/mmc, it is necessary to perform an esophagogastroduodenoscopy (EGDS) to evaluate the presence and degree of varices [20]. Patients with medium to large varices should initiate prophylaxis with non-selective beta blockers (NSBB), propranolol or nadolol or carvedilol. Nitrated and anti-aldosterone agents may be also used. All these drugs can be used alone or in combination. In cases of varices veins with a high hemorrhagic risk, endoscopic ligation should be considered (see Chap. 23). In cases of varices with a high hemorrhagic risk, endoscopic ligation should be a good option. In suspected bleeding from esophageal varices, vasoactive drugs, such as terlipressin, somatostatin, octreotide, must be started rapidly. Furthermore, all measures must be taken to avoid hypovolemic shock. EGDS should be performed as soon as possible, in case of acute bleeding of acute esophageal variceal bleeding. In this case, ligation or sclerosis are important therapeutic options.

For secondary prevention of re-bleeding, treatment takes advantage of the NSBBs. In poorly responsive cases, a transjugular intrahepatic portosystemic shunt (TIPS) should be considered. Recently, the use of NSBB has been identified as a risk factor for portal vein thrombosis, due to the reduction of blood flow within the portal vein [21].

17.6.4.3 Hepatic Encephalopathy

Hepatic encephalopathy (HE), caused by severe liver failure and/or presence of porto-systemic shunts, is a brain alteration presenting a wide spectrum of neurological and/or psychiatric anomalies associated with a wide spectrum of clinical manifestations ranging from lowest expression that are clinical unapparent to severe clinical expression such as coma. Flapping tremor is an early sign of HE (see Chap. 63).

HE affects patients and their caregivers, because cognitive impairment makes difficult the management of these patients. The diagnosis requires the detection of signs suggestive of HE in a patient with severe liver insufficiency. The recognition of precipitating factors for HE (e.g., infection, bleeding, diuretic use, constipation, etc.) supports the diagnosis of HE and help to treat the condition.

Prevention of HE is carried out by non-absorbable disaccharides, such as lactulose or lactitol, and non-absorbable antibiotics (i.e. rifaximin at high dosage) or probiotics. Oral branched-chain amino acids can be used in chronic phase of HE, while intravenous L-ornithine L-aspartate are reserved to the acute phase.

17.7 HCC

The frequency of HCC in HCV infected patients ranges from 1% to 3% over 30 years, with an annual rate of 1–8% in the presence of cirrhosis [22]. The most important risk factors for HCC are viremia and liver steatosis [22]. Although the mechanisms involved in the development of HCC are not fully understood, a role is played by chronic inflammation, oxidative stress, insulin resistance, and endoplasmic reticulum stress. HCV structural and non-structural proteins and chronic infection are able to modulate signal pathways dysregulating cell cycle and cell metabolism, in a direct and indirect way. However, HCV does not integrate with host genome. Host genetic factors (i.e. PNPLA3 gene, CTNNB1 oncogene which encodes β-catenin protein, CDKN2A gene downregulated by HCV core protein to overcome hepatocyte senescence) can also contribute to the development of HCC [22].

Risk of HCC development is reduced, but it is not completely abolished, by antiviral treatment [23]. The presence of HCC reduces the rate of sustained virologic response (SVR) to DAAs.

Follow-up of cirrhotic patients every 6 months with US scan is fundamental for an early diagnosis of HCC lesions, even in the presence after SVR.

Patients cured for HCC with resection or ablation need to be treated with DAAs according with the recommendations for cirrhotic patients without HCC, showing similar rate of SVR than patients without HCC.

For patients with advanced HCC few therapeutic options are available. Sorafenib and Regorafenib slightly improve overall survival compared with placebo. More recently, programmed cell death protein 1 (PD1) immune check point inhibitor, as nivolumab and pembrolizumab have been evaluated in clinical trials with encouraging results in controlling small intrahepatic metastatic nodules and many other molecules are under evaluation.

17.8 Extrahepatic Manifestations

During chronic HCV infection, two-thirds of patients experienced extra-hepatic manifestations. Patients may develop one or more extrahepatic manifestations (Fig. 17.2) and these conditions are often the first and only clinical sign of infection [24]. Some of these conditions are common and well documented, while others are less frequent. Non-hepatic HCV-related conditions such as autoimmune or lymphoproliferative, cardiovascular, renal, metabolic and central nervous system diseases have been reported tightly associated with infection [24]. HCV infection was associated with a higher mortality rate for extrahepatic complications, while viral eradication significantly reduced the rate of extrahepatic deaths [25–27].

Extrahepatic manifestations may occur at any time during chronic HCV infection, therefore HCV patients should have a regular assessment for these complications during the initial visit and follow-up; conversely, patients with manifestations listed in Fig. 17.2 should be tested for HCV infection. Because of these associations, besides the liver, a thorough clinical and laboratory examination of an HCV-infected patient should cover hematologic, cardiologic, nephrologic, endocrinologic and rheumatologic signs and symptoms and a skin evaluation for findings of cryoglobulinemia, porphyria cutanea tarda and lichen planus.

17.8.1 Mixed Cryoglobulinemia

Mixed essential cryoglobulinemia (MC) is a lymphoproliferative disorder characterized by circulating serum immunocomplexes coupled to activated complement that precipitate into small and medium-sized blood vessels. More than 90% of patients with MC are infected with HCV and about half of HCV patients have cryoglobulins [24]. HCV infection is associated with types II and III MC. The data suggest a causal association between HCV infection and MC. Predisposing factors are female sex, age, advanced liver fibrosis [24]. The diagnosis of MC can be performed by leaving the serum at 4 °C for 7 days showing a typical visible cryoprecipitate which dissolves at 37 °C. Patients have low serum C4 levels and positive serum rheumatoid factor. Most of the cases of MC are asymptomatic. Manifestation and clinical signs depend on leukocytoclastic vasculitis with palpable purpura, neurological and renal damage, and arthralgia. Purpura often involves the legs and can leave brown spots on the skin after it resolves. Vasculitis can cause ischemic necrosis and cutaneous ulceration. Vasculitis may involve the vasa nervous, more frequently of peripheral nerves of the lower limbs causing asymmetric peripheral neuropathy predominantly sensory neuropathy, although it is possible to observe sensory motor neuropathy and multiplex mononeuritis. Arthralgia and myalgia are reported in over 70% of cases and often affect the proximal interphalangeal and metacarpophalangeal joints of hands, knees and ankles [24]. Renal involvement is one of the most serious complications of cryoglobulinemia. The membranoproliferative glomerulonephritis is the typical histological lesion observed in MC. Failure to treat can cause progressive renal failure [24].

The main therapeutic approach of MC should be focused on the eradication of HCV. The clinical improvement of MC is reported in most patients who have eliminated HCV by antiviral therapy. Patients with HCV-related glomerulonephritis should be treated with DAAs, in which SVR in a high proportion of cases leads to improvement of proteinuria and even full remission of glomerulonephritis [28]. In case of non-response or with advanced conditions, corticosteroid therapy and plasmapheresis may be alternative therapeutic options. Rituximab, a monoclonal anti-CD20 antibody, which causes B-cell depletion is an effective and safe treatment for MC. Rituximab is particularly indicated in patients who do not respond to antiviral therapy and in cases of severe vasculitis [25].

17.8.2 Lymphoproliferative Disorders

HCV has been widely associated with lymphoproliferative disorders and in particular non-Hodgkin lymphoma (NHL). It has been demonstrated that HCV infection leads to a two-fold increased the risk of development of NHL. Moreover, the mortality rate for NHL was two-times higher among HCV positive patients. About 10% of long-lasting HCV infection associated with mixed cryoglobulinemia type II evolve into NHL [29]. The pathogenic mechanisms are complex and involve direct effects of HCV during viral replication within B cells, which may activate proto-oncogenes (i.e., BCL2) and/or inhibition of apoptotic factors (i.e., p53, c-Myc), and indirect mechanisms such as continuous antigen stimulation and/or genetic aberration (i.e., t(14:18) translocation).

17.8.3 Cardiovascular Manifestations

Patients with HCV infection showed an increased risk of sub-clinical atherosclerosis, peripheral artery disease, heart failure and stroke, as well as increased cardiovascular mortality [30]. Several direct and indirect mechanisms have been hypothesized by which HCV can induce or facilitate the development of atherosclerosis. HCV has been shown to live and replicate in carotid plaques, supporting the hypothesis that HCV plays a direct pro-atherogenic role by inducing arterial inflammation. In addition, HCV infection causes hepatic and systemic inflammation and structural and non-structural HCV proteins play an important role in initiating and maintaining chronic inflammation that promotes atherosclerosis development [30]. HCV can also be involved in the development of atherosclerosis through the increase of pro-atherogenic chemokine and cytokine levels, increasing levels of oxidative stress and endothelial dysfunction. HCV also interferes with glucose and lipid metabolism, leading to IR, diabetes and hepatic steatosis which are known factors that induce atherosclerosis and increase the risk of cardiovascular disease [30]. HCV induces a chronic inflammatory vessel damage and instability of plaque. Such conditions significantly increased the risk of ischemic stroke in HCV patients. HCV clearance by interferon or DAAs has been shown to improve or reverse carotid atherosclerosis and reduce both cardiovascular events and mortality [27].

17.8.4 Neurologic and Psychiatric Diseases

Chronic HCV infection is associated with neuropsychiatric disorders in up to 50% of cases. Both the central and peripheral nervous system can be involved. Neurological conditions comprise encephalopathy, myelitis, encephalomyelitis, and cognitive impairment, whereas "brain fog", depression, anxiety, and fatigue are the main psychiatric disorders [31]. Moreover, HCV infection causes both motor and sensory peripheral neuropathy mostly associated with mixed cryoglobulinemia. The neuropsychiatric manifestations are independent of severity of the underlying chronic liver disease and hepatic encephalopathy. Direct and indirect mechanisms have been postulated [31]. The brain is a suitable site for HCV replication, in which the virus may directly exert neurotoxicity; other mechanisms proposed include the imbalance of the metabolic pathways of infected cells, alterations in the circuits, autoimmune disorders, and cerebral or systemic inflammation. A pathogenic role for HCV is also suggested by improvement of neurological and psychiatric symptoms in patients achieving a sustained virologic response following interferon treatment [31]; however, further studies are needed to evaluate the impact of treatment with DAAs on neuropsychiatric disorders associated with HCV.

17.8.5 Endocrine Diseases

HCV infection is strictly associated with an increased prevalence of IR and T2DM. IR has been reported in up to 70% in chronic HCV infection and this prevalence is higher than that observed in HBV infection and in the general population. IR is implicated in the development of hepatic steatosis and T2DM, which is shown with a higher prevalence in HCV patients than uninfected subjects [32]. It has been estimated that up to 33% of chronic HCV infected patients have T2DM. A two- to tenfold increase of T2DM has been reported in chronic HCV infection compared to liver diseases of other etiology. In particular, the prevalence of T2DM is two- to three-times higher in HCV than HBV infection. IR and T2DM accelerate the progression of liver fibrosis, the onset of HCC and some extrahepatic manifestations such as atherosclerosis and cardiovascular diseases [33].

HCV plays a direct role in the development of IR through the core protein. HCV genotypes 1 and 4 infected patients showed the highest prevalence of IR; in these genotypes, IR correlates with HCV RNA levels. Furthermore, HCV lives and replicates within pancreatic β-cells causing distress; in addition, HCV interferes with insulin signaling pathways, with host genetic and environmental factors inducing cytokine imbalance and liver steatosis [33].

IR or T2DM significantly reduced the rate of SVR to IFN, but not to DAAs. Current data show that HCV clearance by DAAs improves or reverses IR and fasting glucose levels, reduces glycated hemoglobin levels, induces a better control of T2DM and reduces the onset of de novo IR and T2DM [26, 34].

17.9 Natural History

Acute HCV infection is self-limiting in 20–30% of cases and in the other 70–80% the infections becomes chronic. The rate of chronicity can be affected by several factors such as age at time of infection, gender, ethnicity, and the presence of jaundice at the onset. Chronic HCV infection leads to a wide range of hepatic diseases, including chronic hepatitis, cirrhosis and HCC. A number of patients with cirrhosis remain stable and well compensated for years, while others develop complications of cirrhosis particularly related to portal hypertension (esophageal varices and hemorrhage, ascites and encephalopathy) and HCC.

The risk of developing cirrhosis within 20–30 years from the infection is estimate at 20–30%, although percentages are different in relation to the studied population.

The natural history of HCV is negatively influenced by various demographic, virologic, clinical and lifestyle factors. The duration of HCV infection, the male gender and ageing are the main risk factors for the progression of liver disease to cirrhosis and HCC; other factors include HCV genotype 3 infection, host genetic polymorphisms (PNPLA3, TGFB1), hepatic steatosis, IR, T2DM, obesity, alcohol use, daily use of marijuana and viral co-infection (HBV, HIV). The appearance of decompensated cirrhosis has a negative impact on natural history of the disease. The presence of ascites is associated with a 3-year mortality rate of 50%, while in the presence of a refractory ascites 1-year survival is 50%. Chronic HCV infection causes about 400,000 deaths each year, mainly due to cirrhosis and HCC [8, 9]. In this estimate, deaths due to extrahepatic manifestations of HCV are not considered. Due to the recent introduction of DAA therapeutic regimens the natural history of HCV infection has been revolutionized. DAAs have proven to be highly effective not only in inducing the elimination of HCV, but also in improving or reversing liver injury and many of the extrahepatic manifestations associated with HCV.

17.10 Treatment

As shown in Fig. 17.3, HCV therapy has been constantly evolving, resulting in a definitive cure for all cases of hepatitis C. The IFN has been a cornerstone of therapy for more than 20 years. Currently, the IFN-free DAA regimens allow the possibility of treatment to almost all the infected population including patients with advanced stages of the disease and with severe comorbidities (e.g., renal failure) always maintaining a high efficacy and an excellent tolerability profile.

These therapeutic regimens therefore represent the ideal weapon for achieving the ambitious WHO global hepatitis C virus eradication project by 2030 [9]. However, to ensure that the eradication can be achieved it is necessary to implement screening programs to identify HCV-infected populations and that access to therapy with DAAs is made possible on a large scale [35].

17.10.1 Objectives of Therapy

The goal should be to treat all HCV-positive patients for the purpose of eliminating HCV infection in order to improve

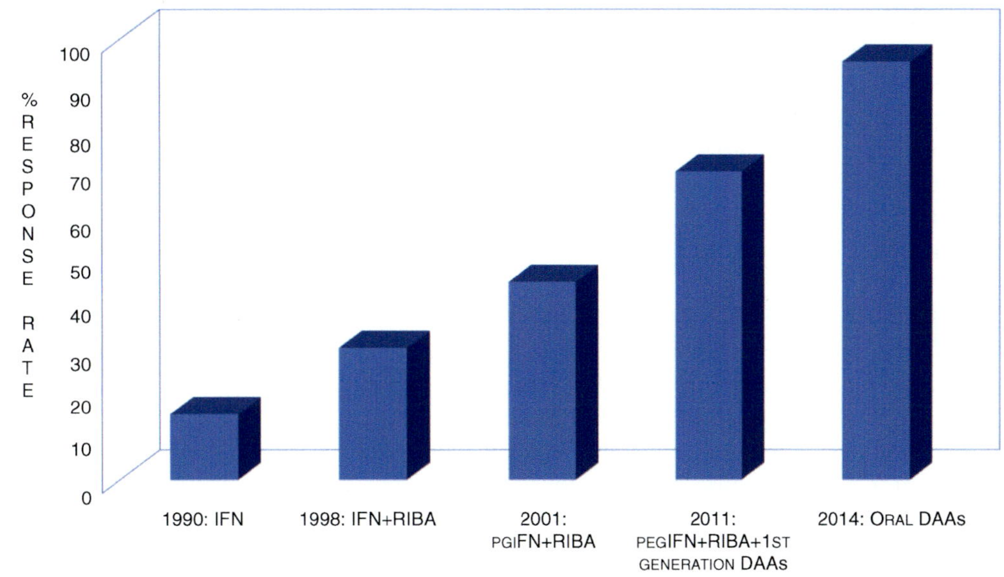

Fig. 17.3 Evolution of the treatment of chronic hepatitis C

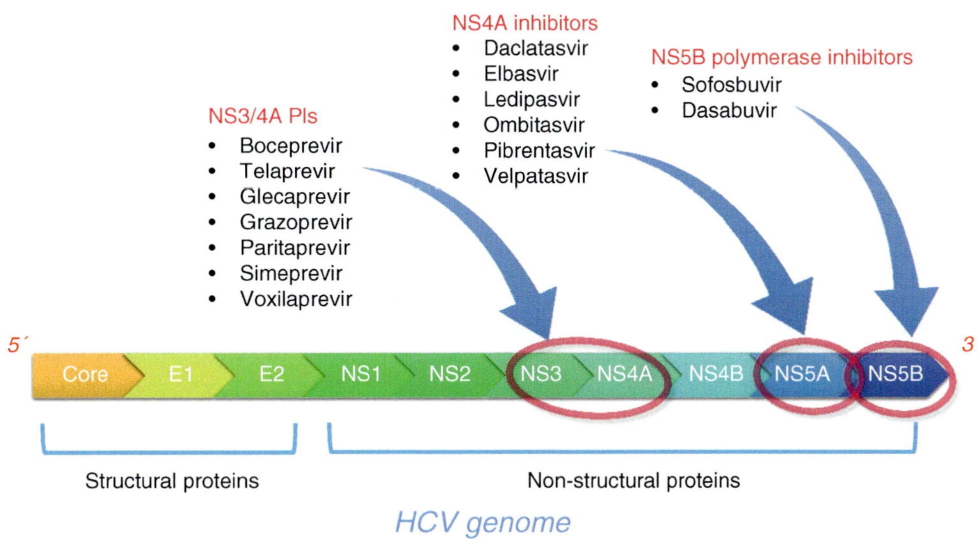

Fig. 17.4 DAAs molecular targets on HCV RNA structure

and prevent: (a) progression of liver injury and its complications; (b) extrahepatic manifestations; and (c) to reduce mortality; as well as to improve quality of life and prevent transmission of infection.

HCV RNA clearance 12 weeks after the end of DAA treatment is indicative of sustained virological response (SVR).

17.10.2 Direct Antiviral Drugs

DAAs act by inhibiting non-structural proteins and can be classified into three classes according to the target site: NS3/4A protease inhibitors (PI), NS5A inhibitors, NS5B RNA polymerase inhibitors (Fig. 17.4).

17.10.2.1 NS3/4A Protease Inhibitors

Boceprevir and Telaprevir were the first-generation drugs of this class, effective only towards genotype 1, with a low barrier to genetic resistance and therefore the need to use them in triple combination with pegIFN + RBV. For the development of resistance and for an extremely low tolerability profile, these drugs are no longer used. Second and third generation of NS3/4A inhibitors (e.g., Glecaprevir, Grazoprevir, Paritaprevir, Simeprevir, Voxilaprevir) have solved many of the problems associated with the use of first-generation drugs, showing a high barrier to genetic resistance, wide antiviral activity which include genotype 1 and 4, less significant activity on genotype 2, poorly effective on genotype 3, and few side effects. These features allow these drugs to be used in IFN-free association regimes and in a large number of patients.

17.10.2.2 NS5A Inhibitors

Inhibition of the NS5A enzyme has an important impact on viral replication at different stages of HCV life cycle. NS5A inhibitors (Daclatasvir, Elbasvir, Ledipasvir, Ombitasvir, Pibrentasvir, Velpatasvir) show a high antiviral activity towards all of the genotypes (pan-genotypic), but at the same time a relatively low genetic barrier, so it is necessary to combine these drugs with other DAAs.

17.10.2.3 NS5B RNA Polymerase Inhibitors

The NS5B protein is an RNA-dependent RNA polymerase capable of catalyzing the viral RNA synthesis and therefore represents a crucial phase of the HCV life cycle. Depending on the site of action, there are two different classes of RNA polymerase NS5B inhibitors. The nucleoside inhibitors (Sofosbuvir) act as a false polymerase substrate, which will be incorporated into the nascent RNA chain resulting in premature closure of the chain itself. Because the polymerase structure is highly conserved among all viral genotypes, Sofosbuvir has a pan-genotypic efficacy and a high genetic resistance barrier. Non-nucleoside NS5B inhibitors (Dasabuvir), on the other hand, act as allosteric inhibitors, binding outside the active site of the polymerase and causing conformational changes that inactivate the enzyme. Unlike Sofosbuvir, the range of non-nucleoside inhibitor activities is limited to genotype 1 and the genetic barrier is low.

17.10.3 DAA Therapeutic Regimens and Their Clinical Use

The use of combinations of drugs for the treatment of HCV is an inevitable strategy to prevent the onset of resistance. In fact, RNA polymerase in RNA viruses (such as HCV) is inherently error prone due to the absence of proofreading. Combined with an extremely high viral turnover, this error trend leads to a myriad of viral variants that coexist within a single host (quasispecies). Some of these variants seem intrinsically resistant to DAAs and would be rapidly selected in the case of monotherapy, thus becoming the predominant population in a short time, causing treatment to fail. Therefore, at present, a combination of two or more DAAs, with pre-established dosage is the base for the treatment of HCV infection. Therefore, each regimen requires a treatment protocol with a pre-established duration, with a selective action on specific genotypes or a pan-genotypic activity, depending on which combination of drugs has been selected (Table 17.2).

The drug combinations shown in Table 17.2 are remarkably effective, with an SVR of over 95% [36]. The duration of treatment with DAAs for HCV infection is relatively short and depending on the genotype and the absence or presence of cirrhosis and usually range from 8 to 24 weeks [36]. The duration of treatment is also influenced by the host's own parameters (e.g., stage of liver disease, naïve or experienced status for a previous IFN- or DAAs-based treatment). Advanced stages of disease (e.g., hepatic cirrhosis) and/or the status of experienced (e.g., previous treatment failure) generally require longer treatments and/or the use of RBV [36].

The tolerability profiles of second and third-generation DAAs is excellent. The most common side effects (asthenia, headache and itching) are generally mild and do not required discontinuation of treatment. Also, the presence of severe hepatic failure (Child-Pugh score B or C) or severe kidney failure (GFR <30 ml/min/1.73 m^2) cannot be considered an absolute contraindication to therapy, but influence the choice of therapeutic regimen to be adopted for a single case. For instance, Sofosbuvir is contraindicated in case of GFR <30 ml/min/1.73 m^2, whereas Glecaprevir/Pibrentasvir and Elbasvir/Grazoprevir combinations are contraindicated in case of cirrhosis in the Child-Pugh B-C score. Therefore, the high tolerability profile of DAAs and the possibility of choosing between different regimens in relation to patients' clinical condition makes these therapeutic regimens virtually possible for every HCV infected patient. To date, the only absolute contraindication is represented by the coexistence of a double organ failure, that is severe liver and kidney failure.

Table 17.2 DAA regimens approved for treatment of HCV infection in 2019

Drug	Activity	Concentration for tablet (mg)	Posology (n° of tablet/day)	Treatment duration (weeks)
Sofosbuvir	Pan-genotypic	400	One tablet	12–24 ± Ribavirin
Sofosbuvir/Velpatasvir	Pan-genotypic	400/100	One tablet	12–24 ± Ribavirin
Sofosbuvir/Velpatasvir/Voxilaprevir	Pan-genotypic	400/100/100	One tablet	12
Glecaprevir/Pibrentasvir	Pan-genotypic	100/40	Three tablets	8–12–16[a]
Grazoprevir/Elbasvir	Genotypes 1, 4	100/50	One tablet	12–16 ± Ribavirin
Paritaprevir/Ombitasvir/ Ritonavir + Dasabuvir	Genotypes 1, 4	75/12.5/50 250	Two tablets	12–24
Sofosbuvir/Ledipasvir	Genotype 1,3,4	400/90	One tablet	8–12–24 ± Ribavirin

[a]8 weeks in non-cirrhotic patients; 12 weeks in cirrhotic; 16 weeks in genotype 3

17.10.3.1 DAA Treatment and Drug-to-Drug Interaction

DAA therapy presents a challenge, the potential drug-drug interactions. The interaction risk assessment must be evaluated prior to starting therapy and before starting other medications during treatment. The DAAs pharmacological interactions are currently highly predictable and there are online websites that provide help in predicting potential drug-drug interactions (e.g., www.hep-druginteractions.org).

17.10.3.2 Post-Treatment Follow-Up

Patients with advanced fibrosis (F3) or cirrhosis who have achieved SVR should be monitored for HCC every 6 months by ultrasound. Patients with pre-treatment oesophageal varices should be periodically monitored by endoscopy.

17.11 Treatment of HCV Acute Hepatitis

AHC should be treated, similarly to those with chronic hepatitis, with a DAA regimen for 8 weeks. Considering that late recurrences have been reported, SVR should be evaluated 12- and 24-weeks post-treatment [36].

17.12 Treatment of Particular Patients with HCV

17.12.1 HBV and HIV Co-Infected

HBV-HCV coinfected patients should be treated with the same regimens used for HCV-infected patients.

In patients HIV-HCV coinfected drug-drug interaction is of particular importance, and special attention should be paid to anti-HIV drugs that are contraindicated, not recommended or that require dose adjustment with DAA regimens.

17.12.2 End-Stage Liver Disease

HCV patients with end-stage liver disease not suitable for DAA treatments, the therapeutic choice is liver transplantation. Recurrence of HCV after transplantation occurs universally, reducing the life expectancy of graft and patient survival. Post-transplant HCV recurrence should be considered as early as possible for DAA treatment.

17.12.3 Patients with Renal Insufficiency

Patients with mild to moderate renal impairment (GFR ≥30 ml/min) may be treated according to the general recommendations. Patients with GFR <30 ml/min and in haemodialysis can be treated with particular caution, sofosbuvir based-regimens should be avoided and these patients should be treated with a fixed regimen of glecaprevir/pibrentasvir for 8 or 12 weeks.

17.12.4 Non-hepatic Solid Organ Transplantation Patients

HCV patients on the waiting list for solid organ transplantation can be treated with DAAs according to the general recommendations. Similarly, organ transplant recipients should be treated considering the drug-to drug interaction.

17.12.5 Re-treatment of Non-SVR to DAA

A very small number of patients failed to achieve SVR with DAAs. In some case such failure is associated with the presence of resistance-associated substitutions (RASs) that confer reduced susceptibility to the corresponding classes of drugs. To optimize treatment, these patients must be screened for RASs before starting a new treatment.

17.13 Prevention of HCV Infection

There is currently no specific prophylaxis for HCV infection, nor is there any indication for antiviral therapies with DAAs as post-exposure prophylaxis without a documented HCV transmission [36]. Therefore, prevention is done through the correct application of the general rules of prophylaxis to prevent the spread of parenteral and sexually transmittable viruses.

The primary prevention interventions recommended by WHO are:

- hand washing and use of gloves;
- safe and appropriate use of health care injections;
- safe handling and disposal of sharps and waste;
- provision of comprehensive harm-reduction services to people who inject drugs including sterile injecting equipment;
- blood test donated blood for hepatitis B and C;
- training of health personnel;
- promotion of correct and consistent use of condoms.

WHO recommends anti-HCV antibodies screening for people who may be at increased risk of infection including:

- people who inject drugs;
- people who use intranasal drugs;
- recipients of infected blood products or invasive procedures in health-care facilities with inadequate infection control practices;
- children born to mothers infected with HCV;

- people with sexual partners who are HCV-infected;
- people with HIV infection;
- prisoners or previously incarcerated persons; and
- people who have had tattoos or piercings.

For people infected with HCV, WHO recommends:

- education and counselling on options for care and treatment;
- immunization with the hepatitis A and B vaccines to prevent coinfection;
- early and appropriate medical management including antiviral therapy if appropriate;
- regular monitoring for early diagnosis of chronic liver disease.

Glossary

AHC Acute hepatitis C
ALT Alanine aminotransferase
AST Aspartate aminotransferase
CHC Chronic hepatitis C
DAAs Direct-acting antivirals
DBS Dry blood spot
EGDS Esophagogastroduodenoscopy
EIA Enzyme immunoassays
ER Endoplasmic reticulum
HCC Hepatocellular carcinoma
HCV Hepatitis C virus
IR Insulin resistance
LVP Lipoviroparticles
MC Mixed cryoglobulinemia
MTP Microsomal triglyceride transfer protein
NS Non-structural proteins
NSBB Non-selective beta blockers
POC Point of care
SBP Spontaneous bacterial peritonitis
SVR Sustained virological response
T2DM Type 2 diabetes mellitus
TIPS Transjugular intrahepatic portosystemic shunt
VLDL Very low-density lipoprotein
WHO World Health Organization

Self Study

Questions

1. What is the basis of HCV persistence?
2. What is the relevance of HCV genotypes?
3. Is the detection of anti-HCV antibodies sufficient to diagnose HCV infection and start antiviral therapy with DAAs?
4. What is the role of anti-HCV IgM and the anti-HCV avidity test for the diagnosis of AHC?

Answers

1. HCV persists in the host because of its high genetic variability, allowing the escape of the virus from the immune system. Genetic variability is a consequence of the high rate of spontaneous mutations that accumulate within the HCV genome due of the lack of proofreading activity of the HCV RNA polymerase. By continuously modifying its antigens, HCV escapes immune response. Furthermore, the inclusion of HCV in lipoviroparticles also alters antiviral response. Finally, HCV is able to spread directly from infected to non-infected hepatocytes without passing through the extracellular compartment.
2. HCV genotypes are associated with peculiar epidemiological, pathophysiological and therapeutic characteristics. Genotype 1 is more common in older patients, often has nosocomial transmission and is associated with progression to cirrhosis and HCC. Genotype 2 is prevalent in Africa and East Asia and among younger subjects, it is often transmitted by transfusion and associated with cryoglobulinemia. Genotype 3 is closely associated with the use of illicit drugs in industrialized countries and causes a severe form of hepatic steatosis associated with hypocholesterolemia. Not all DAAs are effective against all HCV genotypes and treatment outcomes may differ according to the actual genotype.
3. The detection of anti-HCV antibodies is not sufficient to diagnose an active HCV infection, but it is necessary to highlight the presence of serum HCV-RNA, therefore, treatment with DAA should only be initiated in HCV RNA positive patients.
4. IgM antibodies are not diagnostic for AHC because they can be detected both during the acute and chronic stages of the disease. Instead, the avidity test of antibodies to the anti-HCV IgG and IgM anti-HCV antibodies makes a correct diagnosis of AHC in 90% of cases.

References

1. Smith DB, Bukh J, Kuiken C, Muerhoff AS, Rice CM, Stapleton JT, Simmonds P. Expanded classification of hepatitis C virus into 7 genotypes and 67 subtypes: updated criteria and genotype assignment web resource. Hepatology. 2014;59:318–27.
2. Petruzziello A, Marigliano S, Loquercio G, Cozzolino A, Cacciapuoti C. Global epidemiology of hepatitis C virus infection: an up-date of the distribution and circulation of hepatitis C virus genotypes. World J Gastroenterol. 2016;22:7824–40.
3. Catanese MT, Uryu K, Kopp M, Edwards TJ, Andrus L, Rice WJ, Silvestry M, Kuhn RJ, Rice CM. Ultrastructural analysis of hepatitis C virus particles. Proc Natl Acad Sci U S A. 2013;110:9505–10.
4. Li Y, Yamane D, Masaki T, Lemon SM. The Yin and Yang of hepatitis C: synthesis and decay of HCV RNA. Nat Rev Microbiol. 2015;13:544–58.
5. Lindenbach BD, Rice CM. The ins and outs of hepatitis C virus entry and assembly. Nat Rev Microbiol. 2013;11:688–700.

6. Paul D, Madan V, Bartenschlager R. Hepatitis C virus RNA replication and assembly: living on the fat of the land. Cell Host Microbe. 2014;16:569–79.
7. Scheel TKH, Rice CM. Understanding the hepatitis C virus life cycle paves the way for highly effective therapies. Nat Med. 2013;19:837–49.
8. Polaris Observatory HCV Collaborators. Global prevalence and genotype distribution of hepatitis C virus infection in 2015: a modelling study. Lancet Gastroenterol Hepatol. 2017;2:161–76.
9. WHO. Global Hepatitis report 2017. Hepatitis C, 18 July 2018. World Health Organization. http://www.who.int/iris/handle/10665/255016.
10. Kamili S, Drobeniuc J, Araujo AC, Hayden TM. Laboratory diagnostics for hepatitis C virus infection. Clin Infect Dis. 2012;55:S43–8.
11. Rockstroh JK, Feld JJ, Chevaliez S, Cheng K, Wedemeyer H, Sarrazin C, Maasoumy B, Herman C, Hackett J Jr, Cohen DE, Dawson GJ, Cloherty G, Pawlotsky JM. HCV core antigen as an alternate test to HCV RNA for assessment of virologic responses to all-oral, interferon-free treatment in HCV genotype 1 infected patients. J Virol Methods. 2017;245:14–8.
12. Ciotti M, D'Agostini C, Marrone A. Advances in the diagnosis and monitoring of hepatitis C virus infection. Gastroenterology Res. 2013;6:161–70.
13. Applegate TL, Fajardo E, Sacks JA. Hepatitis C virus diagnosis and the holy grail. Infect Dis Clin North Am. 2018;32:425–45.
14. Llibre A, Shimakawa Y, Mottez E, Ainsworth S, Buivan TP, Firth R, Harrison E, Rosenberg AR, Meritet JF, Fontanet A, Castan P, Madejón A, Laverick M, Glass A, Viana R, Pol S, McClure CP, Irving WL, Miele G, Albert ML, Duffy D. Development and clinical validation of the Genedrive point-of-care test for qualitative detection of hepatitis C virus. Gut. 2018. Apr 3. pii: gutjnl-2017-315783.
15. Grebely J, Page K, Sacks-Davis R, van der Loeff MS, Rice TM, Bruneau J, Morris MD, Hajarizadeh B, Amin J, Cox AL, Kim AY, McGovern BH, Schinkel J, George J, Shoukry NH, Lauer GM, Maher L, Lloyd AR, Hellard M, Dore GJ, Prins M, C3 Study Group. The effects of female sex, viral genotype, and IL28B genotype on spontaneous clearance of acute hepatitis C virus infection. Hepatology. 2014;59:109–20.
16. Spada E, Mele A, Mariano A, Zuccaro O, Tosti ME, SEIEVA collaborating group. Risk factors for and incidence of acute hepatitis C after the achievement of blood supply safety in Italy: results from the national surveillance system. J Med Virol. 2013;85:433–40.
17. Sagnelli E, Santantonio T, Coppola N, Fasano M, Pisaturo M, Sagnelli C. Acute hepatitis C: clinical and laboratory diagnosis, course of the disease, treatment. Infection. 2014;42:601–10.
18. Mendes LC, Stucchi RSB, Vigani AG. Diagnosis and staging of fibrosis in patients with chronic hepatitis C: comparison and critical overview of current strategies. Hepat Med. 2018;10:13–22.
19. Adinolfi LE, Rinaldi L, Guerrera B, Restivo L, Marrone A, Giordano M, Zampino R. NAFLD and NASH in HCV infection: prevalence and significance in hepatic and extrahepatic manifestations. Int J Mol Sci. 2016;17:803–15.
20. de Franchis R, on behalf of the Baveno VI Faculty. Expanding consensus in portal hypertension report of the Baveno VI consensus workshop: stratifying risk and individualizing care for portal hypertension. J Hepatol. 2015;63:743–52.
21. Zampino R, Lebano R, Coppola N, Macera M, Grandone A, Rinaldi L, De Sio I, Tufano A, Stornaiuolo G, Adinolfi LE, Durante-Mangoni E, Gaeta GB, Niglio A. The use of nonselective beta blockers is a risk factor for portal vein thrombosis in cirrhotic patients. Saudi J Gastroenterol. 2018;24:25–9.
22. Nevola R, Rinaldi L, Giordano M, Marrone A, Adinolfi LE. Mechanisms and clinical behavior of hepatocellular carcinoma in HBV and HCV infection and alcoholic and non-alcoholic fatty liver disease. Hepatoma Res. 2018;4:55.
23. Nault JC, Colombo M. Hepatocellular carcinoma and direct acting antiviral treatments: controversy after the revolution. J Hepatol. 2016;65:663–5.
24. Cacoub P, Comarmond C, Domont F, Savey L, Desbois AC, Saadoun D. Extrahepatic manifestations of chronic hepatitis C virus infection. Ther Adv Infect Dis. 2016;3:3–14.
25. Zignego AL, Ramos-Casals M, Ferri C, Saadoun D, Arcaini L, Roccatello D, Antonelli A, Desbois AC, Comarmond C, Gragnani L, Casato M, Lamprecht P, Mangia A, Tzioufas AG, Younossi ZM, Cacoub P, ISG-EHCV. International therapeutic guidelines for patients with HCV-related extrahepatic disorders. A multidisciplinary expert statement. Autoimmun Rev. 2017;16:523–41.
26. Adinolfi LE, Rinaldi L, Marrone A, Giordano M. The effect of sustained virological response by direct-acting antivirals on insulin resistance and diabetes mellitus in patients with chronic hepatitis C. Expert Rev Anti Infect Ther. 2018;16:595–7.
27. Petta S, Adinolfi LE, Fracanzani AL, Rini F, Caldarella R, Calvaruso V, Cammà C, Ciaccio M, Di Marco V, Grimaudo S, Licata A, Marrone A, Nevola R, Pipitone RM, Pinto A, Rinaldi L, Torres D, Tuttolomondo A, Valenti L, Fargion S, Craxì A. Hepatitis C virus eradication by direct-acting antiviral agents improves carotid atherosclerosis in patients with severe liver fibrosis. J Hepatol. 2018;69:18–24.
28. Cacoub P, Si Ahmed SN, Ferfar Y, Pol S, Thabut D, Hezode C, Alric L, Comarmond C, Ragab G, Quartuccio L, Hegazy M, Poynard T, Resche Rigon M, Saadoun D. Long-term efficacy of interferon-free antiviral treatment regimens in patients with hepatitis C virus-associated cryoglobulinemia vasculitis. Clin Gastroenterol Hepatol. 2019;17(3):518–26.
29. Mihăilă RG. Hepatitis C virus – associated B cell non-Hodgkin's lymphoma. World J Gastroenterol. 2016;22:6214–23.
30. Adinolfi LE, Zampino R, Restivo L, Lonardo A, Guerrera B, Marrone A, Nascimbeni F, Florio A, Loria P. Chronic hepatitis C virus infection and atherosclerosis: clinical impact and mechanisms. World J Gastroenterol. 2014;20:3410–7.
31. Adinolfi LE, Nevola R, Lus G, Restivo L, Guerrera B, Romano C, Zampino R, Rinaldi L, Sellitto A, Giordano M. Chronic hepatitis C virus infection and neurological and psychiatric disorders: an overview. World J Gastroentrol. 2015;21:2269–80.
32. Kralj D, Virović Jukić L, Stojsavljević S, Duvnjak M, Smolić M, Bilić Čurčić I. Hepatitis C virus, insulin resistance, and steatosis. J Clin Transl Hepatol. 2016;4:66–75.
33. Hammerstad SS, Grock SF, Lee HJ, Hasham A, Sundaram N, Tomer Y. Diabetes and hepatitis C: a two-way association. Front Endocrinol (Lausanne). 2015;6:134–53.
34. Adinolfi LE, Nevola R, Guerrera B, D'alterio G, Marrone A, Giordano M, Rinaldi L. Hepatitis C virus clearance by direct-acting antiviral treatments and impact on insulin resistance in chronic hepatitis C patients. J Gastroenterol Hepatol. 2018;33:1379–82.
35. Adinolfi LE, Guerrera B. All-oral interferon-free treatments: the end of hepatitis C virus story, the dream and the reality. World J Hepatol. 2015;7:2363–8.
36. European Association for the Study of the Liver. EASL recommendations on treatment of hepatitis C 2018. J Hepatol. 2018; https://doi.org/10.1016/j.jhep.2018.03.026.

18 Non-B, Non-C Viral Hepatitis

Hubert E. Blum

Key Concepts

- Worldwide, the hepatotropic non-B/non-C hepatitis viruses HAV, HDV and HEV are causes of acute and/or chronic liver diseases
- Acute HAV infection is usually a self-limited disease
- Diagnosis of acute hepatitis A is established by the detection of serum anti-HAV IgM that is followed by anti-HAV IgG that is associated with recovery and immunity against reinfection
- HDV infection is always associated with HBV infection

18.1 Introduction

In the 1940s, two distinct clinical forms of hepatitis were recognized: epidemic or infectious hepatitis, after the discovery of **hepatitis A virus (HAV)** in 1973 by R.H. Purcell and collaborators, designated as hepatitis A [1, 2], and serum hepatitis, after the discovery of hepatitis B virus (HBV) in 1960s by B. Blumberg and collaborators [3, 4] and by A.M. Prince [5, 6], designated as hepatitis B. In 1977 M. Rizzetto and collaborators discovered a novel antigen-antibody system that only occurs in association with hepatitis B [7]. This was later shown to be associated with a particle containing a low molecular weight, circular RNA genome encapsidated by HBV envelope proteins and designated as **hepatitis delta virus (HDV)** [8]. Further, in 1955 an enterically transmitted acute viral hepatitis was identified during an outbreak in New Delhi [9], initially termed ‚epidemic non-A, non-B hepatitis' and later **hepatitis E virus (HEV)** infection [10–14].

Worldwide, the hepatotropic non-B/non-C hepatitis viruses HAV, HDV and HEV are causes of acute or—for chronic hepatitis D or hepatitis E—chronic liver diseases (Fig. 18.1). They can present with a broad spectrum of clinical signs and symptoms, ranging from an asymptomatic carrier state to acute/fulminant hepatitis or—for chronic hepatitis D or hepatitis E—with the potential to progress to liver cirrhosis and its sequelae, including hepatocellular carcinoma (HCC). Thus, non-B/non-C viral hepatitis can be associated with significant morbidity and mortality and represents a global health care problem.

18.2 Epidemiology of Non-B/Non-C Viral Hepatitis

Based on the specific and sensitive detection of HAV, HCV and HEV infections, their epidemiology and global burden as well as their natural course could be studied in great detail. At the same time therapeutic and preventive strategies have been developed that should contribute to a reduced prevalence of these infections and their eventual elimination.

18.2.1 HAV Infection

HAV infection occurs worldwide and shows a distinct geographic distribution with a high prevalence in sub-Saharan-Africa, India, Pakistan and Afghanistan, an intermediate prevalence in Middle and South America, Northern Africa, the Middle East, Turkey, Iran, Kazakhstan and Mongolia, a low prevalence in Eastern Europe, Russia, China and Oceania and a very low prevalence in Western Europe, Scandinavia, North America and Australia (Fig. 18.2) [15]. Tens of millions of individuals worldwide become

H. E. Blum (✉)
Department of Medicine II, University Hospital Freiburg, Freiburg, Germany
e-mail: hubert.blum@uniklinik-freiburg.de

F. Radu-Ionita et al. (eds.), *Liver Diseases*, https://doi.org/10.1007/978-3-030-24432-3_18

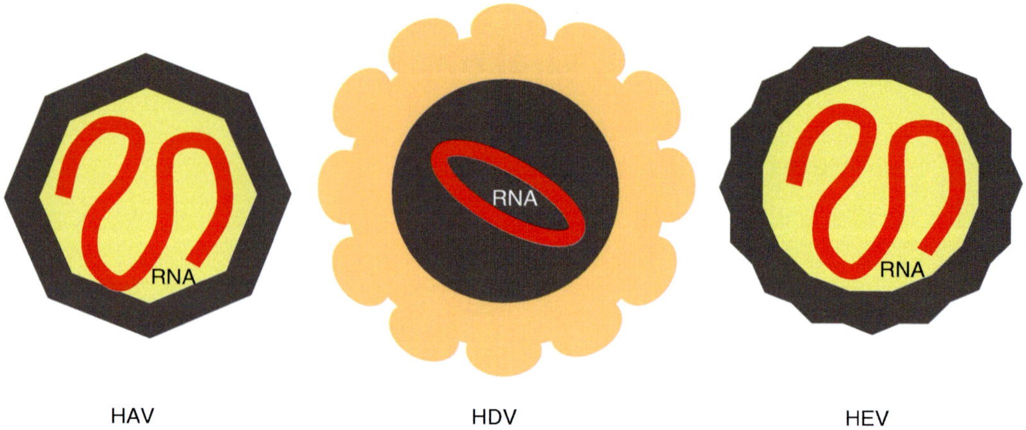

Fig. 18.1 Non-B/non-B hepatitis viruses HAV, HDV and HEV

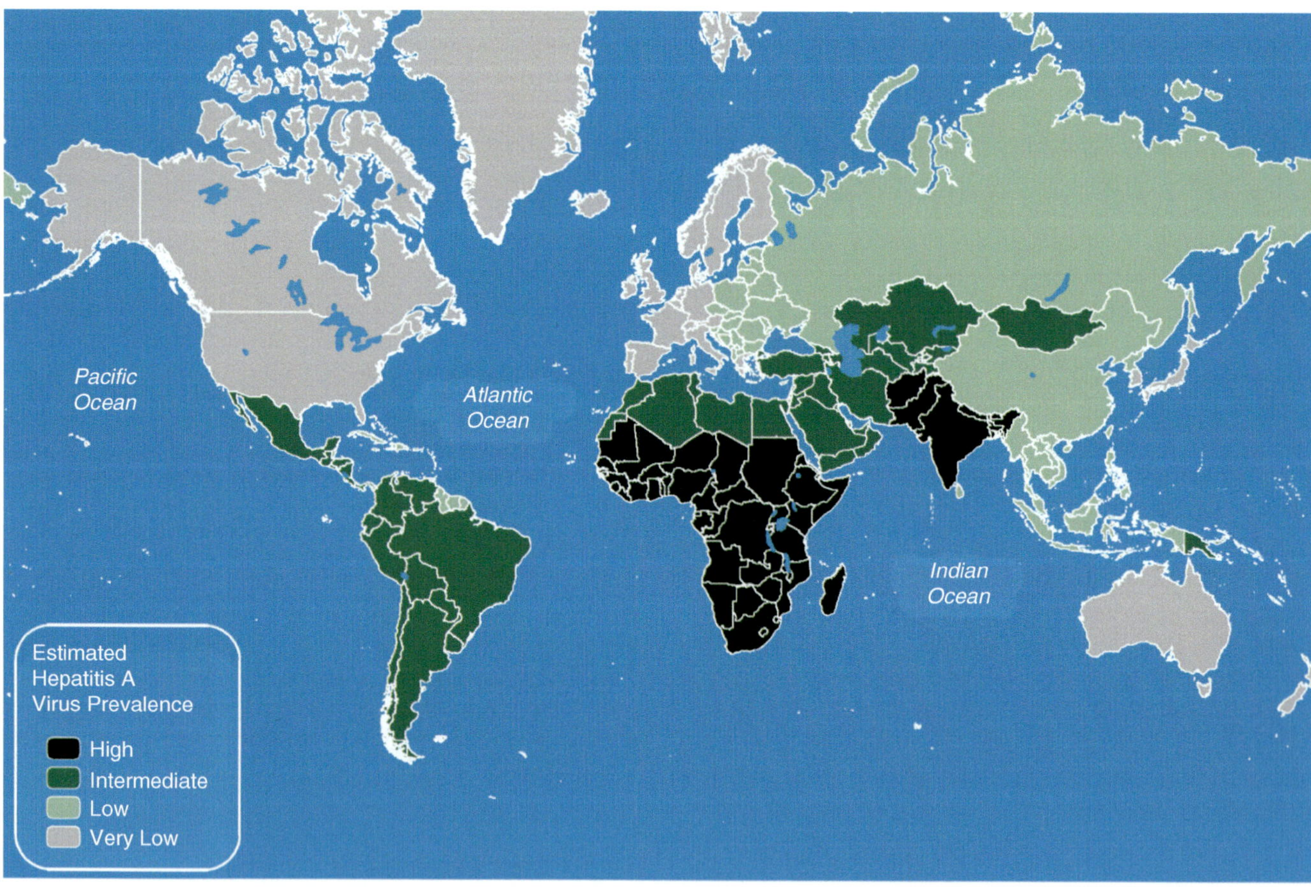

Fig. 18.2 Worldwide prevalence of HAV infection [15]

annually infected with HAV. The incidence strongly correlates with the socioeconomic indicators and with access to safe drinking water. Universal vaccination of children has been shown to significantly reduce the hepatitis A incidence rates [16] with an increasing anti-HAV seroprevalence between 1990 and 2005 in all age groups and geographic regions [15].

In the US, HAV infection has declined substantially since 1996 when vaccination has been recommended for individuals at risk [17–21]. In this context, acute hepatitis A has declined in the US by 92% between 1995 and 2007 from 12 cases to 1 case per 100,000 population [18, 20]. The major risk factor in the US now is international travel, mainly to Mexico and Central as well as South America.

18.2.2 HDV Infection

HDV infection is traditionally endemic in central Africa, the Amazon Basin, Eastern and Mediterranean Europe, the Middle East and parts of Asia. It occurs only in association with HBV. Data regarding the global burden of HDV infection are somewhat limited, however [22]. There are eight HDV genotypes; their geographic distribution and the worldwide prevalence of HDV infection is shown in Fig. 18.3 [23]. Longitudinal studies have shown a decrease in HDV prevalence in some endemic regions, such as Italy where in HBV infected individuals the prevalence of HDV infection has decreased from about 25% in 1983 to 8% in 1997 [24]. Similar trends were observed in Spain, Turkey and Taiwan, for example. On the other hand, epidemiological studies showed that HDV prevalence in HBV infected individuals remains in general <10% but is as high as 70% in some developing countries/areas such as Nigeria, Gabon, Iran, Pakistan, India, Takjikistan and Mongolia as well as the western Brazilian Amazon [23]. Further, in Northern Europe and the US HDV infection still is a health care problem. While HDV prevalence is stable in France, it increased in London/England from about 3% in the 1980s to about 9% in 2005 [25]. Also in Germany, after a decrease of anti-HDV prevalence from about 19% in 1992 to about 7% in 1997, since 1999 an increase to about 14% has been documented [26]. This increase is in part caused by migrants from regions with a high HDV prevalence or by still occurring clustered outbreaks, e.g., in Greenland [27] or Mongolia [28]. By comparison, in Italy the prevalence of anti-HDV in hepatitis B surface antigen (HBsAg)-positive patients consecutively reduced from 23% in 1987, to 14% in 1992 and to 8.7% in 1997 [29].

18.2.3 HEV Infection

The epidemiology of HEV infection, previously known as waterborne or enterically transmitted non-A, non-B hepatitis, is similar to that of HAV infection. The highest incidence of water-borne human HEV infection (genotypes 1 and 2) is found in Asia, Africa, the Middle East and Central America [30]. Waterborne outbreaks have occurred among others in South and Central Asia, tropical East Asia, Africa and Central America (Fig. 18.4) (http://www.cdc.gov/travel-static/yellowbook/2016/map 3-06.pdf).

Apart from fecally contaminated water, sporadic transmission of zoonotic HEV infection (HEV genotypes 3 or 4), has been demonstrated by consumption of certain meats (deer, wild boar, undercooked pig liver), blood transfusions [31] and solid organ transplantation [13, 14], termed 'autochthonous' HEV infection.

The burden of HEV infection in a given population is difficult to estimate. Rates of anti-HEV antibody positivity in the general population are lower in Europe and the US than in Africa and Asia (30–80%). Nevertheless, in a 1988–1994 survey of adult US citizens [32] anti-HEV prevalence was 21%, lower than anti-HAV (38%) but higher than anti-HBs (8.7%) or anti-HCV (2.0%). While the rates of HEV exposure in the United States appears to be declining [33], a sur-

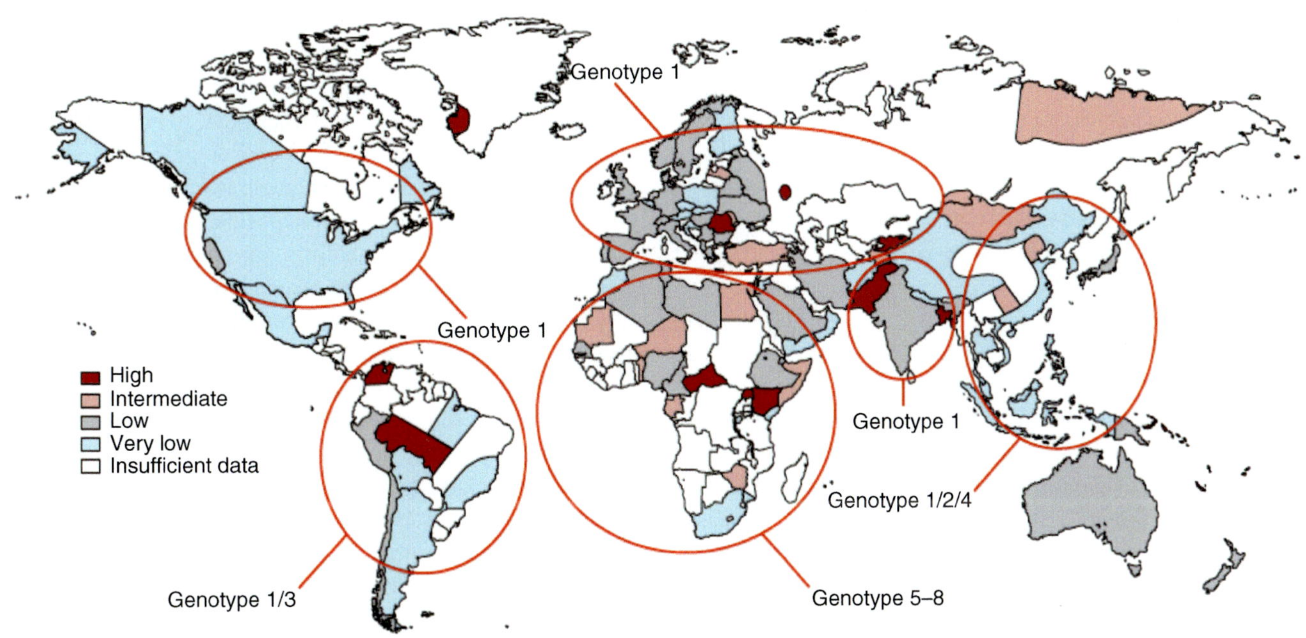

Fig. 18.3 Worldwide prevalence of HDV infection and geographic distribution of HDV genotypes [23]

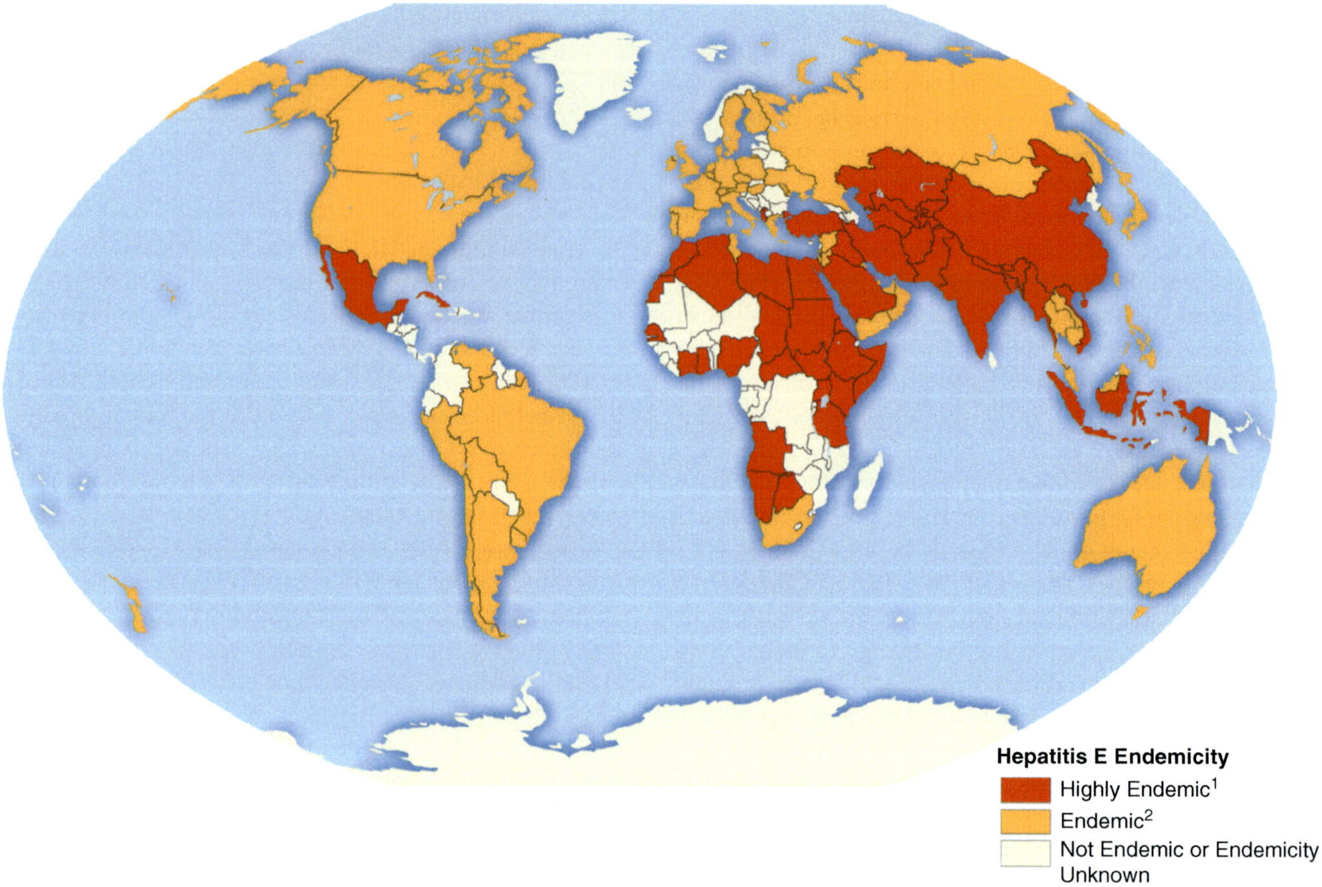

Fig. 18.4 Worldwide distribution of HEV infection (http://cdc.gov/travel-static/yellowbook/2016/map 3-06.pdf)

veillance analysis showed an increase of confirmed HEV cases in Europe between 2005 and 2015 (https://ecdc.europa.eu/en/publications-data/hepatitis-e-eueea-2005-2015).

Overall, the epidemiology of hepatitis E in developed countries is incompletely understood as is its mechanism of replication and species or cell specificity (Fig. 18.5).

18.3 Clinical Presentation and Management of Non-B/Non-C Viral Hepatitis

18.3.1 HAV Infection

Acute HAV infection (**World Health Organization. Global Alert and Response (GAR) Hepatitis A.** http://www.who.int/csr/disease/hepatitis/whocdscsredc2007/en/index4.html#estimated) is usually a self-limited disease. After an incubation period of 15–50 days more than 70% of patients complain of nausea, vomiting, anorexia, fever and abdominal pain, followed by jaundice and pruritus. Laboratory abnormalities include elevations of serum aminotransferases and bilirubin. Full clinical and biochemical recovery is observed within 2–3 months in 85% of patients and within 6 months in nearly all patients. Up to 10% of patients experience a relapse of symptoms during 6 months after acute illness. The duration of the relapse is usually less than 3 weeks but may last as long as 12 months. Multiple relapses with anti-HAV IgM h positivity have been reported.

Extrahepatic manifestations, such as arthralgia, leukocytoclastic vasculitis, glomerulonephritis, cryoglobulinemia, optic neuritis, transverse myelitis, thrombocytopenia, aplastic anemia and others, can be associated with acute hepatitis A. Cholestatic and relapsing hepatitis are special clinical presentations of acute hepatitis A (5–10%) that also resolve spontaneously. Rarely, hepatitis A may take a fulminant course or trigger the development of autoimmune hepatitis.

The diagnosis of acute hepatitis A is established by the detection anti-HAV IgM in serum that is followed by the development of anti-HAV IgG and clinical recovery from acute hepatitis and immunity against HAV reinfection.

In general, treatment consists of supportive care. There is no specific antiviral agent available. In the rare cases with a protracted cholestatic course associated with malaise and itching a predniso(lo)ne pulse therapy may be beneficial. In

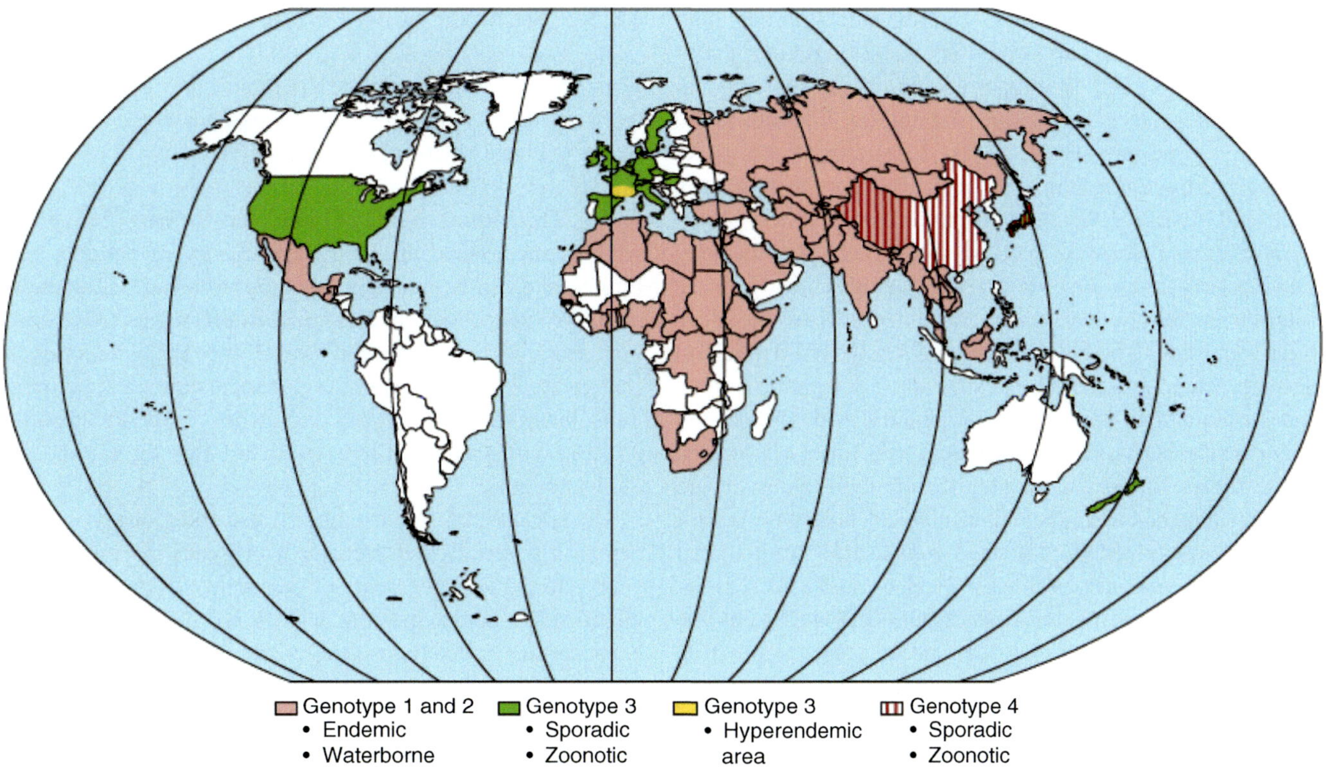

Fig. 18.5 Worldwide distribution of HEV genotypes [13]

the extremely rare fulminant course of hepatitis A liver transplantation should be considered. For the prevention of hepatitis A highly effective vaccines are commercially available, also in combination with a vaccine against hepatitis B. Further, for immediate protection against HAV infection a passive vaccine is available.

18.3.2 HDV Infection

HDV infection is caused by a defective RNA virus and is always associated with HBV infection either as HBV-HDV coinfection or as HDV superinfection of patients with preexisting HBV infection. Acute HBV-HDV is indistinguishable from classical acute HBV infection and is usually transient and self-limited. Among injection drug users, however, a high incidence of liver failure has been reported. HDV superinfection of chronically HBV-infected individuals may present as severe acute hepatitis in a previously unrecognized HBV carrier or as an exacerbation of a known chronic hepatitis B. HDV infection persists in almost all patients with suppression of HBV infection. The pathogenesis of HDV infection depends on HDV-associated factors, such as HDV genotype and the expression of specific HDAg species, on HBV-associated factors, such as HBV genotype and the levels of HBV replication as well as on host factors, such as the host immune response.

The treatment of chronic HDV infection remains one of the major challenges in the field of viral hepatitis [23], awaiting the development and implementation of novel therapeutic concepts. Since pegylated interferon alpha as monotherapy or in combination with adefovir for example rarely result in a sustained virological response [34, 35], several antiviral strategies are presently evaluated in clinical trials: pegylated interferon lambda, myrcludex, lonafarnib, ezetimibe, REP 2139 and 2165, respectively, GI-18000 and ALN-HDV. An HDV-specific vaccine is not available. Since HDV infection depends on the presence of HBV infection, HBV vaccines also prevent HDV infection. A HDV-specific vaccine does not exist.

18.3.3 HEV Infection

Today, HEV infection is one of the most common, yet least diagnosed etiologies of acute viral hepatitis, with distinct differences in transmission and outcomes in resource-rich and resource-limited areas. HEV usually causes a self-limited acute infection with acute hepatic failure developing in only a small proportion of patients. The incubation period ranges from 15–60 days. In the vast majority of patients the natural course is asymptomatic or mildly symptomatic. In symptomatic patients jaundice is accompanied with malaise, anorexia, nausea, vomiting, abdominal pain, fever and hepatomegaly. Less common symptoms are diarrhea, arthralgia, pruritus and a urticarial rash. Extrahepatic findings may include hematological abnormalities, acute thyreoiditis, glomerulonephritis and a broad spectrum of neurological abnormalities, such as aseptic meningitis, Guillain-Barre syndrome or peripheral neuropathy. Laboratory findings are elevated serum aminotransferases and bilirubin that normalize usually within 1–6 weeks after the onset of illness.

While the majority of patients clear HEV spontaneously some patients may develop a complicated course, such as acute liver failure, cholestatic hepatitis or chronic HEV Infection. About 0.5–4% of patients with acute HEV infection develop acute hepatic failure, especially in pregnant women and malnourished individuals or patients with preexisting liver disease, such as HCV-associated liver fibrosis/cirrhosis. Acute hepatic failure carries a high mortality if intensive care and liver transplantation are not available. Cholestatic hepatitis E is characterized by prolonged jaundice (>3 months) that resolves spontaneously with viral clearance and a decrease of anti-HEV IgM and an increase of anti-HEV IgG. Chronic HEV infection is empirically defined as presence of HEV RNA in serum or stool for longer than 6 months. It occurs almost exclusively in immunosuppressed patients (patients with HIV infection and patients after solid organ or bone marrow transplantation), infected with HEV genotype 3.

For most immunocompetent patients the management is supportive while immunocompromised patients may benefit from ribavirin or pegylated interferon alpha therapy [13, 36–38]. Two vaccines with long-term efficacy against HEV genotype 1 and 4 of >95% have been developed and evaluated in Nepal and China [39, 40].

18.4 Global Burden of Non-B/Non-C Viral Hepatitis

Viral hepatitis A, D and E are associated with significant morbidity and mortality, depending on the global, regional and national prevalence of these infections and the incidence of the associated liver diseases. In seminal studies, the global burden of disease (GBD) was determined by the systematic analysis of global and regional mortality from 235 causes of death for 20 age groups in 1990 and 2010 [41] as well as of disability-adjusted life years (DALYs) in patients with 291 diseases and injuries in 21 geographic regions in 1990, 2005 and 2010 [42]. In these studies deaths from acute hepatitis A and E were considered. Recently, the GBD study 2013 [43] shows a clear trend towards a reduction of the prevalence of hepatitis A and E.

The global and regional mortality from acute hepatitis A and E showed a significant overall increase between 1990 und 2010 [41]. By comparison, a recent follow-up study covering the years 1980–2016 [44] showed that the age-standardized death rate significantly decreased between 2006 and 2016.

18.5 Summary and Perspectives

Non-B/non-C viral hepatitis can be caused by the three hepatotropic viruses A, D and E. They can be detected by specific serological tests that can be complemented by the identification of the viral RNA genome in serum or stool (HAV and HEV). The natural course of acute non-B/non-C hepatitis is well characterized and is in the majority of patients self-limited and can be managed by supportive care. Exceptions are HDV superinfection of chronically HBV infected patients that usually take a chronic course and HEV infection in immunosuppressed patients, e.g., patients after a solid organ transplantation. In a minority of patients, acute viral hepatitis non-B, non-C can result in acute liver failure or a protracted clinical course.

Recent seminal studies showed that the global burden of hepatitis A and E is decreasing worldwide. In the coming years further improvements of our ability to prevent and to effectively manage patients with acute non-B/non-C viral hepatitis are expected, resulting in the control of these global infections and the eventual elimination of their associated morbidities and mortalities.

Acknowledgments *Conflict of interests*: The author declares no conflict of interest.

Financial disclosure: The author has no financing to disclose.

Self Study

Question

1. **Which statement is true**?
   (a) HAV infection occurs worldwide and shows a distinct geographic distribution with a high prevalence in Western Europe.
   (b) in acute HAV infection, after incubation period, patients complain of nausea, vomiting, anorexia, fever and abdominal pain.
   (c) HDV infection is not associated with HBV infection.
   (d) the majority of patients with HEV develop severe acute hepatic failure

Answer

1. **Which statement is true**?
   (a) HAV infection occurs worldwide and shows a distinct geographic distribution with a high prevalence in sub-Saharan-Africa, India, Pakistan and Afghanistan, and very low prevalence in Western Europe, Scandinavia, North America and Australia.

(b) **CORRECT**. In acute HAV infection, after an incubation period of 15–50 days, more than 70% of patients complain of nausea, vomiting, anorexia, fever and abdominal pain, followed by jaundice and pruritus.
(c) HDV infection is caused by a defective RNA virus and is always associated with HBV infection.
(d) the majority of patients clear HEV spontaneously some patients may develop a complicated course, such as acute liver failure, cholestatic hepatitis or chronic HEV Infection.

References

1. Feinstone SM, Kapikian AZ, Purceli RH. Hepatitis A: detection by immune electron microscopy of a viruslike antigen associated with acute illness. Science. 1973;182:1026–8.
2. Martin A, Lemon SM. Hepatitis A virus: from discovery to vaccines. Hepatology. 2006;43:S164–72.
3. Blumberg BS, Alter HJ, Visnich S. A "new" antigen in leukemia sera. JAMA. 1965;191:541–6.
4. Blumberg BS, Gerstley BJ, Hungerford DA, London WT, Sutnick AI. A serum antigen (Australia antigen) in Down's syndrome, leukemia, and hepatitis. Ann Intern Med. 1967;66:924–31.
5. Prince AM. An antigen detected in the blood during the incubation period of serum hepatitis. Proc Natl Acad Sci U S A. 1968;60:814–21.
6. Prince AM. Relation of Australia and SH antigens. Lancet. 1968;2:462–3.
7. Rizzetto M, Canese MG, Arico S, Crivelli O, Trepo C, Bonino F, Verme G. Immunofluorescence detection of new antigen-antibody system (delta/anti-delta) associated to hepatitis B virus in liver and in serum of HBsAg carriers. Gut. 1977;18:997–1003.
8. Rizzetto M, Hoyer B, Canese MG, Shih JW, Purcell RH, Gerin JL. Delta agent: association of delta antigen with hepatitis B surface antigen and RNA in serum of delta-infected chimpanzees. Proc Natl Acad Sci U S A. 1980;77:6124–8.
9. Gupta DN, Smetana HF. The histopathology of viral hepatitis as seen in the Delhi epidemic (1955–56). Indian J Med Res. 1957;45:101–13.
10. Balayan MS, Andjaparidze AG, Savinskaya SS, Ketiladze ES, Braginsky DM, Savinov AP, Poleschuk VF. Evidence for a virus in non-A, non-B hepatitis transmitted via the fecal-oral route. Intervirology. 1983;20:23–31.
11. Kane MA, Bradley DW, Shrestha SM, Maynard JE, Cook EH, Mishra RP, Joshi DD. Epidemic non-A, non-B hepatitis in Nepal. Recovery of a possible etiologic agent and transmission studies in marmosets. JAMA. 1984;252:3140–5.
12. Krawczynski K, Bradley DW. Enterically transmitted non-A, non-B hepatitis: identification of virus-associated antigen in experimentally infected cynomolgus macaques. J Infect Dis. 1989;159:1042–9.
13. Hoofnagle JH, Nelson KE, Purcell RH. Hepatitis E. N Engl J Med. 2012;367:1237–44.
14. Kamar N, Bendall R, Legrand-Abravanel F, Xia NS, Ijaz S, Izopet J, Dalton HR. Hepatitis E. Lancet. 2012;379:2477–88.
15. Jacobsen KH, Wiersma ST. Hepatitis A virus seroprevalence by age and world region, 1990 and 2005. Vaccine. 2010;28:6653–7.
16. Wasley A, Fiore A, Bell BP. Hepatitis A in the era of vaccination. Epidemiol Rev. 2006;28:101–11.
17. Wasley A, Samandari T, Bell BP. Incidence of hepatitis A in the United States in the era of vaccination. JAMA. 2005; 294:194–201.
18. Advisory Committee on Immunization P, Fiore AE, Wasley A, Bell BP. Prevention of hepatitis A through active or passive immunization: recommendations of the Advisory Committee on Immunization Practices (ACIP). MMWR Recomm Rep. 2006;55:1–23.
19. Wasley A, Grytdal S, Gallagher K. Centers for disease C, prevention. Surveillance for acute viral hepatitis—United States, 2006. MMWR Surveill Summ. 2008;57:1–24.
20. Daniels D, Grytdal S, Wasley A. Centers for disease C, prevention. Surveillance for acute viral hepatitis – United States, 2007. MMWR Surveill Summ. 2009;58:1–27.
21. Klevens RM, Miller JT, Iqbal K, Thomas A, Rizzo EM, Hanson H, Sweet K, et al. The evolving epidemiology of hepatitis a in the United States: incidence and molecular epidemiology from population-based surveillance, 2005–2007. Arch Intern Med. 2010;170:1811–8.
22. Rizzetto M, Ponzetto A, Forzani I. Hepatitis delta virus as a global health problem. Vaccine. 1990;8(Suppl):S10–4; discussion S21–13.
23. Hughes SA, Wedemeyer H, Harrison PM. Hepatitis delta virus. Lancet. 2011;378:73–85.
24. Gaeta GB, Stroffolini T, Chiaramonte M, Ascione T, Stornaiuolo G, Lobello S, Sagnelli E, et al. Chronic hepatitis D: a vanishing disease? An Italian multicenter study. Hepatology. 2000;32:824–7.
25. Cross TJ, Rizzi P, Horner M, Jolly A, Hussain MJ, Smith HM, Vergani D, et al. The increasing prevalence of hepatitis delta virus (HDV) infection in South London. J Med Virol. 2008;80:277–82.
26. Wedemeyer H, Heidrich B, Manns MP. Hepatitis D virus infection—not a vanishing disease in Europe! Hepatology. 2007;45:1331–2; author reply 1332–1333.
27. Borresen ML, Olsen OR, Ladefoged K, McMahon BJ, Hjuler T, Panum I, Simonetti J, et al. Hepatitis D outbreak among children in a hepatitis B hyper-endemic settlement in Greenland. J Viral Hepat. 2010;17:162–70.
28. Tsatsralt-Od B, Takahashi M, Endo K, Buyankhuu O, Baatarkhuu O, Nishizawa T, Okamoto H. Infection with hepatitis A, B, C, and delta viruses among patients with acute hepatitis in Mongolia. J Med Virol. 2006;78:542–50.
29. Gaeta GB, Stroffolini T, Smedile A, Niro G, Mele A. Hepatitis delta in Europe: vanishing or refreshing? Hepatology. 2007;46:1312–3.
30. Emerson SU, Purcell RH. Running like water—the omnipresence of hepatitis E. N Engl J Med. 2004;351:2367–8.
31. Stramer SL, Moritz ED, Foster GA, Ong E, Linnen JM, Hogema BM, Mak M, et al. Hepatitis E virus: seroprevalence and frequency of viral RNA detection among US blood donors. Transfusion. 2016;56:481–8.
32. Kuniholm MH, Purcell RH, McQuillan GM, Engle RE, Wasley A, Nelson KE. Epidemiology of hepatitis E virus in the United States: results from the Third National Health and Nutrition Examination Survey, 1988–1994. J Infect Dis. 2009;200:48–56.
33. Teshale EH, Denniston MM, Drobeniuc J, Kamili S, Teo CG, Holmberg SD. Decline in hepatitis E virus antibody prevalence in the United States from 1988–1994 to 2009–2010. J Infect Dis. 2015;211:366–73.
34. Niro GA, Ciancio A, Gaeta GB, Smedile A, Marrone A, Olivero A, Stanzione M, et al. Pegylated interferon alpha-2b as monotherapy or in combination with ribavirin in chronic hepatitis delta. Hepatology. 2006;44:713–20.
35. Castelnau C, Le Gal F, Ripault MP, Gordien E, Martinot-Peignoux M, Boyer N, Pham BN, et al. Efficacy of peginterferon alpha-2b in chronic hepatitis delta: relevance of quantitative RT-PCR for follow-up. Hepatology. 2006;44:728–35.
36. Peron JM, Abravanel F, Guillaume M, Gerolami R, Nana J, Anty R, Pariente A, et al. Treatment of autochthonous acute hepatitis E

with short-term ribavirin: a multicenter retrospective study. Liver Int. 2016;36:328–33.
37. Kamar N, Izopet J, Dalton HR. Chronic hepatitis e virus infection and treatment. J Clin Exp Hepatol. 2013;3:134–40.
38. I Mehrez M, Sa Fattah D, Aa Azeem N, A Saleh M, M Mostafa K. Hemochromatosis gene polymorphism as a predictor of sustained virological response to antiviral treatment in Egyptian chronic hepatitis C patients. Euroasian J Hepatogastroenterol. 2017;7:154–7.
39. Shrestha MP, Scott RM, Joshi DM, Mammen MP Jr, Thapa GB, Thapa N, Myint KS, et al. Safety and efficacy of a recombinant hepatitis E vaccine. N Engl J Med. 2007;356:895–903.
40. Zhu FC, Zhang J, Zhang XF, Zhou C, Wang ZZ, Huang SJ, Wang H, et al. Efficacy and safety of a recombinant hepatitis E vaccine in healthy adults: a large-scale, randomised, double-blind placebo-controlled, phase 3 trial. Lancet. 2010;376:895–902.
41. Lozano R, Naghavi M, Foreman K, Lim S, Shibuya K, Aboyans V, Abraham J, et al. Global and regional mortality from 235 causes of death for 20 age groups in 1990 and 2010: a systematic analysis for the Global Burden of Disease Study 2010. Lancet. 2012;380:2095–128.
42. Murray CJ, Vos T, Lozano R, Naghavi M, Flaxman AD, Michaud C, Ezzati M, et al. Disability-adjusted life years (DALYs) for 291 diseases and injuries in 21 regions, 1990–2010: a systematic analysis for the Global Burden Of Disease Study 2010. Lancet. 2012;380:2197–223.
43. Global Burden of Disease Study C. Global, regional, and national incidence, prevalence, and years lived with disability for 301 acute and chronic diseases and injuries in 188 countries, 1990–2013: a systematic analysis for the Global Burden of Disease Study 2013. Lancet. 2015;386:743–800.
44. Collaborators GBDCoD. Global, regional, and national age-sex specific mortality for 264 causes of death, 1980–2016: a systematic analysis for the Global Burden of Disease Study 2016. Lancet. 2017;390:1151–210.

The Microbiome in Liver Diseases

19

Hubert E. Blum

Key Concepts

- Emerging evidence points to a contribution of the microbiome to the pathogenesis of liver diseases including alcoholic liver disease, non-alcoholic fatty liver disease NAFLD, cholestatic liver diseases, liver cirrhosis and hepatocellular carcinoma (HCC), with special reference to bile acid metabolism
- the intestinal microbial community represents a microbial ecosystem consisting of trillion microbial cells with an aggregate 9.9 million microbial genes across the fecal microbiome

19.1 Introduction

The basic aspects of molecular and cell biology are not only integral part of biomedical research but are also translated into patient care. Several global consortia have been launched and in part been completed during the last decades. All of them continuously transform basic biomedical research and translate into medical applications and, after evaluation in randomized clinical trials, enter clinical practice with a tremendous potential to contribute to advances to the diagnosis, treatment and prevention of human diseases.

More than 15 years ago, the international human genome organization (HUGO) project established the complete sequence of the ca. three billion base pairs that make up the human genome [1, 2]. In order to utilize these data from the HUGO project for research as well as for clinical applications and to define the functions of newly identified genes, collectively termed 'functional genomics', strategies were developed to globally analyze genomic DNA sequences as well as their cell-, tissue- or organ-specific expression profile. Using chips, so-called 'microarrays', thousands or ten thousands of single-stranded DNA species, reverse transcribed RNA (cDNA) or oligonucleotides of known sequence can provide a global gene (genomics), gene expression (transcriptomics, proteomics) or metabolite (metabolomics) profile ('signature') that is characteristic for the disease of individual patients, including its natural course/prognosis and response to therapy.

In 2005 the international haplotype map (HapMap) project was initiated to identify, based on genome-wide association studies (GWAS) in ethnically different populations, single nucleotide polymorphisms (SNPs) and their association with specific human diseases and individual phenotypic characteristics, respectively [3, 4]. Through GWAS an increasing number of gene loci have been identified that are associated with individual (future) phenotypic traits, such as hair or eye color, height, body mass index and others as well as with the disposition to develop a specific disease [3, 4]. Further, genetic variants are associated with the individuals' response to drug treatment, e.g., to lithium [5]. Overall, GWAS allow an increasingly better understanding of disease pathogenesis and a more accurate assessment of the individual risk to develop a specific disease. Clinically, this may eventually translate into clinical advances in disease prevention, early diagnosis and therapy. It should be cautioned, however, that the contribution of a defined SNP to the risk assessment for a given disease must be weighed against established clinical parameters and needs to be carefully evaluated before entering clinical practice.

The human microbiome project (HMP) was established in 2007 as another global consortium [6–10]. The HMP and the 'Metagenomics of the Human Intestinal Tract (Meta-HiT) Consortium Europe' aim at the sequencing of all microbes (eukaryotes, archaea, bacteria, viruses) that inhabit specific body sites, such as the mouth, throat and airways, stomach and intestine, the urogenital system and the skin, respectively (Fig. 19.1a). Recent data demonstrate that specific compositions of the microbial community are associated with health and disease (Fig. 19.1b) [6–10]. These findings

H. E. Blum (✉)
Department of Medicine II, University Hospital Freiburg, Freiburg, Germany
e-mail: hubert.blum@uniklinik-freiburg.de

F. Radu-Ionita et al. (eds.), *Liver Diseases*, https://doi.org/10.1007/978-3-030-24432-3_19

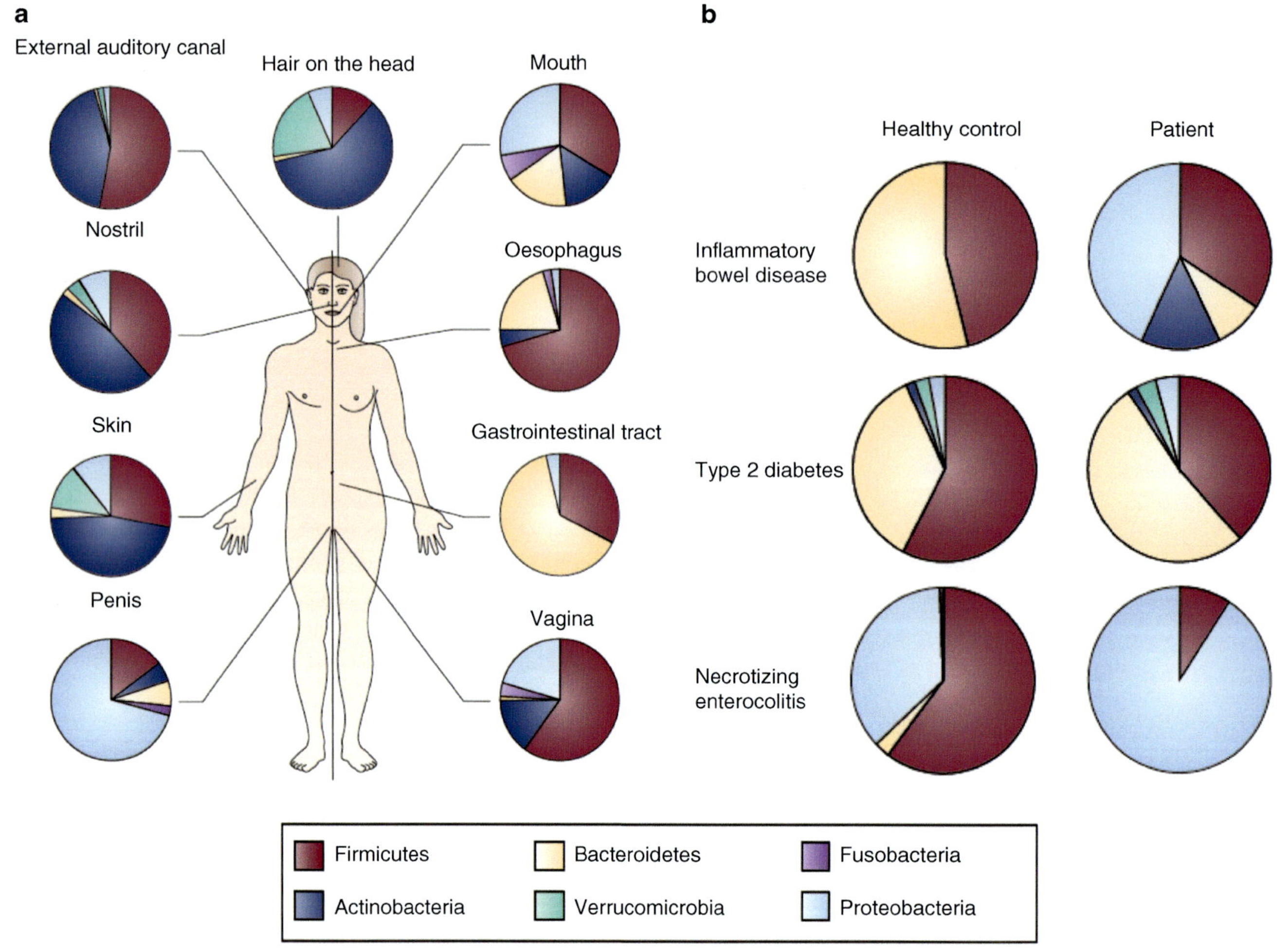

Fig. 19.1 (**a**) Different microbiomes in humans; (**b**) the intestinal microbiome in healthy individuals and patients [7]

suggest that the detailed characterization, function and variation of the microbial community will reveal important commensal host-microbe as well as microbe-microbe interactions with diagnostic, therapeutic and preventive implications [11, 12].

While the HMP has meanwhile developed into a major field of biomedical research, the intestinal microbial community in particular has turned out to play a major role in human health and disease pathogenesis as will be discussed in more detail below [13].

In recent years the intestinal microbial community has been studied in great detail. It represents a microbial ecosystem consisting of trillion microbial cells with an aggregate 9.9 million microbial genes across the fecal microbiome [14]. While until recently, the environment *in utero* has been considered sterile, DNA-based analyses identified bacterial species in maternal placenta, amniotic fluid and meconium. The colonization of the human gut begins at birth with a rapid expansion of bacterial diversity and is characterized by a successively changing composition that eventually becomes relatively stable in adulthood [15]. While the specific microbial species and subspecies and their proportions vary greatly from person to person the individual microbiome is unique and becomes more diverse in the elderly.

Important factors for the composition of the intestinal microbial community are endogenous and exogenous factors [16, 17]. Examples are mode of delivery of the neonates, diet (dietary supplements, breast-feeding, formula-feeding), xenobiotics, including antibiotics and other drugs [18–21]. Further, infections and exposure to environmental microbial agents are established risk factors for childhood diseases, such as obesity and allergy [22, 23]. Recent evidence further suggests that human genetic variation also influences the abundance of specific members of the intestinal microbial community [24].

Taken together, the emerging data suggest that the detailed characterization of the human intestinal microbiome, function and variation across different body sites will reveal important commensal host-microbe as well as microbe-, microbe interactions that may play a role in human health and disease.

Table 19.1 Functions of the intestinal microbial community in human health (examples)

	References
Host physiology	
Adaptive immunity	[25]
Autoimmunity	[26]
Innate immunity	[27]
Cell proliferation	[28]
Bone density	[20]
Vascularization	[29]
Neurological signalling	[30]
Biosynthesis	
Neurotransmitters	
Steroid hormones	
Vitamins	
Metabolism	
Dietary components	
Bile salts	
Drugs	
Xenobiotics	

Table 19.2 Disease associations with the intestinal microbial community (examples)

	References
Allergies/allergy protection	[23, 26, 40–42]
Atherosclerosis/thrombosis/cardiovascular diseases	[33–35, 43–46]
Cancer	[47–49]
Diabetes mellitus	[32, 50]
Immune-mediated inflammatory diseases	
– Inflammatory bowel diseases	[51–56]
– Multiple sclerosis	[57, 58]
– Rheumatoid arthritis	[59]
– Psoriasis	[60]
Kwashiorkor	[61, 62]
Liver diseases	[63, 64]
Metabolic syndrome/obesity	[31, 65–68]
Neurodevelopmental, psychiatric and neurodegenerative diseases	
– Autism	[36, 69]
– Depression	[36, 70]
– Alzheimer's disease, Parkinson's disease	[36, 38, 39, 71, 72]

In view of the numerous and diverse physiological functions of the intestinal microbiome in human health (Table 19.1) it is not surprising that it is also involved in gastrointestinal as well as non-gastrointestinal diseases, such as obesity/metabolic syndrome [13, 31, 32], and atherosclerosis/cardiovascular [33–35] as well as neurologic/psychiatric diseases [36–39], making it one of the most dynamic current topics in biomedical research (Table 19.2).

Global comparisons reveal a decrease of the gut microbiome diversity attributed to Western diet, life style practices, such as caesarian section, antibiotic use and formula-feeding of infants as well as sanitation of the living environment. While microbial diversity is decreasing, the prevalence of chronic inflammatory diseases such as inflammatory bowel disease (IBD), diabetes, obesity, allergies, asthma and others are on the rise in Western societies [73].

19.2 The Intestinal Microbiome in Liver Diseases

Considering that the liver receives about 75% of its blood supply from the intestine *via* the portal vein the liver is exposed to a wide range of nutrients, toxins as well as molecules from the intestinal microbiome. In this context, dysbiosis may be involved in the pathogenesis of liver diseases [63, 64]. Emerging evidence points to a contribution of the microbiome to the pathogenesis of different liver diseases and its complications, including alcoholic liver disease [74, 75], non-alcoholic fatty liver disease NAFLD [76], cholestatic liver diseases [77, 78], liver cirrhosis [79–81] and hepatocellular carcinoma (HCC), with special reference to bile acid metabolism [82–84].

In Western countries, alcoholic and NAFLD are major health problems that may progress to advanced fibrosis/cirrhosis and HCC [76, 85]. The pathogenesis involves a complex interaction of environmental factors, such as alcohol consumption/Western diet, obesity/type 2 diabetes mellitus/insulin resistance, genetic factors and changes in the intestinal microbiome. Dysbiosis of the intestinal microbiome [86], an imbalance between protective and harmful bacteria, and bacterial translocation due to an impairment of the intestinal barrier are considered key pathophysiological elements. In this context the salivary microbiome can reflect changes in the intestinal microbiome in patients with hepatic encephalopathy [87].

Central to pathogenesis-based therapeutic concepts in patients with NAFLD for example, are lifestyle changes (diet, exercise) that result in weight loss, reversal of steatosis, inflammation and even fibrosis. Manipulation of the intestinal microbiome by diet, probiotics or fecal transplantation may promote the growth of protective bacteria and an improved prognosis the individual's liver disease [85].

19.3 Summary and Perspectives

Basic biomedical research has made major advances in recent years and holds the promise to increasingly provide individual diagnostic, preventive as well as therapeutic options for patients with inherited or acquired, malignant or non-malignant diseases. Apart from an increasing number of host genetic susceptibility loci and environmental factors, the individual microbial community is central for the barrier between microbes and hosts. In particular, the intestinal microbial community is involved in a large number of normal biological functions in health as well as in numerous common, gastrointestinal and non-gastrointestinal diseases, including liver diseases. In recent years, the intestinal microbiome thus has become one of the most dynamic areas of biomedical research that holds an enormous potential for interventions regarding human diseases, including liver diseases.

Acknowledgments *Conflict of interests*: The author declares no conflict of interest.

Financial disclosure: The author has no financing to disclose.

Self Study

Question

1. **Which statement/statements is/are true**?
   (a) Dysbiosis of the intestinal microbiome is the imbalance between protective and harmful bacteria
   (b) Emerging evidence points to a contribution of the microbiome to the pathogenesis of different aspects liver diseases
   (c) human intestinal microbiome is also involved in gastrointestinal as well as non-gastrointestinal diseases, such as obesity/metabolic syndrome, and atherosclerosis/cardiovascular as well as neurologic/psychiatric diseases.
   (d) there is a decrease of human gut microbiome diversity attributed to Western diet, life style practices, such as caesarean section, antibiotic use and formula-feeding of infants as well as sanitation of the living environment.
   (e) while human gut microbiota is decreasing, the prevalence of chronic inflammatory diseases such as inflammatory bowel disease (IBD), diabetes, obesity, allergies, asthma and others are on the rise in Western societies

Answer

1. **Which statement/statements is/are true?**
   (a) **CORRECT**
   (b) **CORRECT**. Emerging evidence points to a contribution of the microbiome to the pathogenesis of different aspects liver diseases including alcoholic liver disease, non-alcoholic fatty liver disease NAFLD, cholestatic liver diseases, liver cirrhosis and hepatocellular carcinoma (HCC), with special reference to bile acid metabolism
   (c) **CORRECT**
   (d) **CORRECT**
   (e) **CORRECT**

References

1. Lander ES, Linton LM, Birren B, Nusbaum C, Zody MC, Baldwin J, Devon K, et al. Initial sequencing and analysis of the human genome. Nature. 2001;409:860–921.
2. Venter JC, Adams MD, Myers EW, Li PW, Mural RJ, Sutton GG, Smith HO, et al. The sequence of the human genome. Science. 2001;291:1304–51.
3. Manolio TA, Brooks LD, Collins FS. A HapMap harvest of insights into the genetics of common disease. J Clin Invest. 2008;118:1590–605.
4. Manolio TA, Collins FS. The HapMap and genome-wide association studies in diagnosis and therapy. Annu Rev Med. 2009;60:443–56.
5. Hou L, Heilbronner U, Degenhardt F, Adli M, Akiyama K, Akula N, Ardau R, et al. Genetic variants associated with response to lithium treatment in bipolar disorder: a genome-wide association study. Lancet. 2016;387(10023):1085–93.
6. Proctor LM. The human microbiome project in 2011 and beyond. Cell Host Microbe. 2011;10:287–91.
7. Spor A, Koren O, Ley R. Unravelling the effects of the environment and host genotype on the gut microbiome. Nat Rev Microbiol. 2011;9:279–90.
8. Human Microbiome Project C. Structure, function and diversity of the healthy human microbiome. Nature. 2012;486:207–14.
9. Human Microbiome Project C. A framework for human microbiome research. Nature. 2012;486:215–21.
10. Gevers D, Knight R, Petrosino JF, Huang K, McGuire AL, Birren BW, Nelson KE, et al. The Human Microbiome Project: a community resource for the healthy human microbiome. PLoS Biol. 2012;10:e1001377.
11. Morgan XC, Segata N, Huttenhower C. Biodiversity and functional genomics in the human microbiome. Trends Genet. 2013;29:51–8.
12. Rossen NG, Fuentes S, van der Spek MJ, Tijssen JG, Hartman JH, Duflou A, Lowenberg M, et al. Findings from a randomized controlled trial of fecal transplantation for patients with ulcerative colitis. Gastroenterology. 2015;149:110–8. e114
13. Lynch SV, Pedersen O. The human intestinal microbiome in health and disease. N Engl J Med. 2016;375:2369–79.
14. Li J, Jia H, Cai X, Zhong H, Feng Q, Sunagawa S, Arumugam M, et al. An integrated catalog of reference genes in the human gut microbiome. Nat Biotechnol. 2014;32:834–41.
15. Yatsunenko T, Rey FE, Manary MJ, Trehan I, Dominguez-Bello MG, Contreras M, Magris M, et al. Human gut microbiome viewed across age and geography. Nature. 2012;486:222–7.
16. Zhernakova A, Kurilshikov A, Bonder MJ, Tigchelaar EF, Schirmer M, Vatanen T, Mujagic Z, et al. Population-based metagenomics analysis reveals markers for gut microbiome composition and diversity. Science. 2016;352:565–9.
17. Falony G, Joossens M, Vieira-Silva S, Wang J, Darzi Y, Faust K, Kurilshikov A, et al. Population-level analysis of gut microbiome variation. Science. 2016;352:560–4.
18. De Filippo C, Cavalieri D, Di Paola M, Ramazzotti M, Poullet JB, Massart S, Collini S, et al. Impact of diet in shaping gut microbiota revealed by a comparative study in children from Europe and rural Africa. Proc Natl Acad Sci U S A. 2010;107:14691–6.
19. Trompette A, Gollwitzer ES, Yadava K, Sichelstiel AK, Sprenger N, Ngom-Bru C, Blanchard C, et al. Gut microbiota metabolism of dietary fiber influences allergic airway disease and hematopoiesis. Nat Med. 2014;20:159–66.
20. Cho I, Yamanishi S, Cox L, Methe BA, Zavadil J, Li K, Gao Z, et al. Antibiotics in early life alter the murine colonic microbiome and adiposity. Nature. 2012;488:621–6.
21. Maurice CF, Haiser HJ, Turnbaugh PJ. Xenobiotics shape the physiology and gene expression of the active human gut microbiome. Cell. 2013;152:39–50.

22. Fujimura KE, Demoor T, Rauch M, Faruqi AA, Jang S, Johnson CC, Boushey HA, et al. House dust exposure mediates gut microbiome Lactobacillus enrichment and airway immune defense against allergens and virus infection. Proc Natl Acad Sci U S A. 2014;111:805–10.
23. Fujimura KE, Sitarik AR, Havstad S, Lin DL, Levan S, Fadrosh D, Panzer AR, et al. Neonatal gut microbiota associates with childhood multisensitized atopy and T cell differentiation. Nat Med. 2016;22:1187–91.
24. Goodrich JK, Waters JL, Poole AC, Sutter JL, Koren O, Blekhman R, Beaumont M, et al. Human genetics shape the gut microbiome. Cell. 2014;159:789–99.
25. Honda K, Littman DR. The microbiota in adaptive immune homeostasis and disease. Nature. 2016;535:75–84.
26. Vatanen T, Kostic AD, d'Hennezel E, Siljander H, Franzosa EA, Yassour M, Kolde R, et al. Variation in microbiome LPS immunogenicity contributes to autoimmunity in humans. Cell. 2016;165:842–53.
27. Thaiss CA, Zmora N, Levy M, Elinav E. The microbiome and innate immunity. Nature. 2016;535:65–74.
28. Ijssennagger N, Belzer C, Hooiveld GJ, Dekker J, van Mil SW, Muller M, Kleerebezem M, et al. Gut microbiota facilitates dietary heme-induced epithelial hyperproliferation by opening the mucus barrier in colon. Proc Natl Acad Sci U S A. 2015;112:10038–43.
29. Reinhardt C, Bergentall M, Greiner TU, Schaffner F, Ostergren-Lunden G, Petersen LC, Ruf W, et al. Tissue factor and PAR1 promote microbiota-induced intestinal vascular remodelling. Nature. 2012;483:627–31.
30. Yano JM, Yu K, Donaldson GP, Shastri GG, Ann P, Ma L, Nagler CR, et al. Indigenous bacteria from the gut microbiota regulate host serotonin biosynthesis. Cell. 2015;161:264–76.
31. Ridaura VK, Faith JJ, Rey FE, Cheng J, Duncan AE, Kau AL, Griffin NW, et al. Gut microbiota from twins discordant for obesity modulate metabolism in mice. Science. 2013;341:1241214.
32. Pedersen HK, Gudmundsdottir V, Nielsen HB, Hyotylainen T, Nielsen T, Jensen BA, Forslund K, et al. Human gut microbes impact host serum metabolome and insulin sensitivity. Nature. 2016;535:376–81.
33. Koeth RA, Wang Z, Levison BS, Buffa JA, Org E, Sheehy BT, Britt EB, et al. Intestinal microbiota metabolism of L-carnitine, a nutrient in red meat, promotes atherosclerosis. Nat Med. 2013;19:576–85.
34. Zhu W, Gregory JC, Org E, Buffa JA, Gupta N, Wang Z, Li L, et al. Gut microbial metabolite TMAO enhances platelet hyperreactivity and thrombosis risk. Cell. 2016;165:111–24.
35. Wang Z, Roberts AB, Buffa JA, Levison BS, Zhu W, Org E, Gu X, et al. Non-lethal inhibition of gut microbial trimethylamine production for the treatment of atherosclerosis. Cell. 2015;163:1585–95.
36. Fung TC, Olson CA, Hsiao EY. Interactions between the microbiota, immune and nervous systems in health and disease. Nat Neurosci. 2017;20:145–55.
37. Sampson TR, Mazmanian SK. Control of brain development, function, and behavior by the microbiome. Cell Host Microbe. 2015;17:565–76.
38. Sampson TR, Debelius JW, Thron T, Janssen S, Shastri GG, Ilhan ZE, Challis C, et al. Gut microbiota regulate motor deficits and neuroinflammation in a model of Parkinson's disease. Cell. 2016;167:1469–80. e1412
39. Erny D, Hrabe de Angelis AL, Jaitin D, Wieghofer P, Staszewski O, David E, Keren-Shaul H, et al. Host microbiota constantly control maturation and function of microglia in the CNS. Nat Neurosci. 2015;18:965–77.
40. Ege MJ, Mayer M, Normand AC, Genuneit J, Cookson WO, Braun-Fahrlander C, Heederik D, et al. Exposure to environmental microorganisms and childhood asthma. N Engl J Med. 2011;364:701–9.
41. Lynch SV, Wood RA, Boushey H, Bacharier LB, Bloomberg GR, Kattan M, O'Connor GT, et al. Effects of early-life exposure to allergens and bacteria on recurrent wheeze and atopy in urban children. J Allergy Clin Immunol. 2014;134:593–601.e12.
42. Stein MM, Hrusch CL, Gozdz J, Igartua C, Pivniouk V, Murray SE, Ledford JG, et al. Innate immunity and asthma risk in Amish and Hutterite farm children. N Engl J Med. 2016;375:411–21.
43. Jonsson AL, Backhed F. Drug the bug! Cell. 2015;163:1565–6.
44. Tilg H. A gut feeling about thrombosis. N Engl J Med. 2016;374:2494–6.
45. Wang Z, Klipfell E, Bennett BJ, Koeth R, Levison BS, Dugar B, Feldstein AE, et al. Gut flora metabolism of phosphatidylcholine promotes cardiovascular disease. Nature. 2011;472:57–63.
46. Tang WH, Wang Z, Levison BS, Koeth RA, Britt EB, Fu X, Wu Y, et al. Intestinal microbial metabolism of phosphatidylcholine and cardiovascular risk. N Engl J Med. 2013;368:1575–84.
47. Feng Q, Liang S, Jia H, Stadlmayr A, Tang L, Lan Z, Zhang D, et al. Gut microbiome development along the colorectal adenoma-carcinoma sequence. Nat Commun. 2015;6:6528.
48. Sivan A, Corrales L, Hubert N, Williams JB, Aquino-Michaels K, Earley ZM, Benyamin FW, et al. Commensal Bifidobacterium promotes antitumor immunity and facilitates anti-PD-L1 efficacy. Science. 2015;350:1084–9.
49. Konishi H, Fujiya M, Tanaka H, Ueno N, Moriichi K, Sasajima J, Ikuta K, et al. Probiotic-derived ferrichrome inhibits colon cancer progression via JNK-mediated apoptosis. Nat Commun. 2016;7:12365.
50. Qin J, Li Y, Cai Z, Li S, Zhu J, Zhang F, Liang S, et al. A metagenome-wide association study of gut microbiota in type 2 diabetes. Nature. 2012;490:55–60.
51. Hall LJ, Walshaw J, Watson AJ. Gut microbiome in new-onset Crohn's disease. Gastroenterology. 2014;147:932–4.
52. Sha S, Xu B, Wang X, Zhang Y, Wang H, Kong X, Zhu H, et al. The biodiversity and composition of the dominant fecal microbiota in patients with inflammatory bowel disease. Diagn Microbiol Infect Dis. 2013;75:245–51.
53. Forbes JD, Van Domselaar G, Bernstein CN. Microbiome survey of the inflamed and noninflamed gut at different compartments within the gastrointestinal tract of inflammatory bowel disease patients. Inflamm Bowel Dis. 2016;22:817–25.
54. Forbes JD, Van Domselaar G, Bernstein CN. The gut microbiota in immune-mediated inflammatory diseases. Front Microbiol. 2016;7:1081.
55. Ramanan D, Bowcutt R, Lee SC, Tang MS, Kurtz ZD, Ding Y, Honda K, et al. Helminth infection promotes colonization resistance via type 2 immunity. Science. 2016;352:608–12.
56. Moschen AR, Gerner RR, Wang J, Klepsch V, Adolph TE, Reider SJ, Hackl H, et al. Lipocalin 2 protects from inflammation and tumorigenesis associated with gut microbiota alterations. Cell Host Microbe. 2016;19:455–69.
57. Cantarel BL, Waubant E, Chehoud C, Kuczynski J, DeSantis TZ, Warrington J, Venkatesan A, et al. Gut microbiota in multiple sclerosis: possible influence of immunomodulators. J Investig Med. 2015;63:729–34.
58. Jangi S, Gandhi R, Cox LM, Li N, von Glehn F, Yan R, Patel B, et al. Alterations of the human gut microbiome in multiple sclerosis. Nat Commun. 2016;7:12015.
59. Chen J, Wright K, Davis JM, Jeraldo P, Marietta EV, Murray J, Nelson H, et al. An expansion of rare lineage intestinal microbes characterizes rheumatoid arthritis. Genome Med. 2016;8:43.
60. Scher JU, Ubeda C, Artacho A, Attur M, Isaac S, Reddy SM, Marmon S, et al. Decreased bacterial diversity characterizes the altered gut microbiota in patients with psoriatic arthritis, resembling dysbiosis in inflammatory bowel disease. Arthritis Rheumatol. 2015;67:128–39.

61. Smith MI, Yatsunenko T, Manary MJ, Trehan I, Mkakosya R, Cheng J, Kau AL, et al. Gut microbiomes of Malawian twin pairs discordant for kwashiorkor. Science. 2013;339:548–54.
62. Subramanian S, Huq S, Yatsunenko T, Haque R, Mahfuz M, Alam MA, Benezra A, et al. Persistent gut microbiota immaturity in malnourished Bangladeshi children. Nature. 2014;510:417–21.
63. Haque TR, Barritt AS. Intestinal microbiota in liver disease. Best Pract Res Clin Gastroenterol. 2016;30:133–42.
64. Qin N, Yang F, Li A, Prifti E, Chen Y, Shao L, Guo J, et al. Alterations of the human gut microbiome in liver cirrhosis. Nature. 2014;513:59–64.
65. Turnbaugh PJ, Hamady M, Yatsunenko T, Cantarel BL, Duncan A, Ley RE, Sogin ML, et al. A core gut microbiome in obese and lean twins. Nature. 2009;457:480–4.
66. Shen J, Obin MS, Zhao L. The gut microbiota, obesity and insulin resistance. Mol Asp Med. 2013;34:39–58.
67. Mazidi M, Rezaie P, Kengne AP, Mobarhan MG, Ferns GA. Gut microbiome and metabolic syndrome. Diabetes Metab Syndr. 2016;10:S150–7.
68. Sonnenburg JL, Backhed F. Diet-microbiota interactions as moderators of human metabolism. Nature. 2016;535:56–64.
69. Choi GB, Yim YS, Wong H, Kim S, Kim H, Kim SV, Hoeffer CA, et al. The maternal interleukin-17a pathway in mice promotes autism-like phenotypes in offspring. Science. 2016;351:933–9.
70. Aizawa E, Tsuji H, Asahara T, Takahashi T, Teraishi T, Yoshida S, Ota M, et al. Possible association of Bifidobacterium and Lactobacillus in the gut microbiota of patients with major depressive disorder. J Affect Disord. 2016;202:254–7.
71. Bu XL, Yao XQ, Jiao SS, Zeng F, Liu YH, Xiang Y, Liang CR, et al. A study on the association between infectious burden and Alzheimer's disease. Eur J Neurol. 2015;22:1519–25.
72. Scheperjans F, Aho V, Pereira PA, Koskinen K, Paulin L, Pekkonen E, Haapaniemi E, et al. Gut microbiota are related to Parkinson's disease and clinical phenotype. Mov Disord. 2015;30:350–8.
73. Tasnim N, Abulizi N, Pither J, Hart MM, Gibson DL. Linking the gut microbial ecosystem with the environment: does gut health depend on where we live? Front Microbiol. 2017;8:1935.
74. Llopis M, Cassard AM, Wrzosek L, Boschat L, Bruneau A, Ferrere G, Puchois V, et al. Intestinal microbiota contributes to individual susceptibility to alcoholic liver disease. Gut. 2016;65:830–9.
75. Schnabl B. Liver capsule: mechanisms of alcoholic hepatitis. Hepatology. 2016;64:276.
76. Arab JP, Arrese M, Trauner M. Recent insights into the pathogenesis of nonalcoholic fatty liver disease. Annu Rev Pathol. 2018;13:321–50.
77. LaRusso NF, Tabibian JH, O'Hara SP. Role of the intestinal microbiome in cholestatic liver disease. Dig Dis. 2017;35:166–8.
78. Dyson JK, Beuers U, Jones DEJ, Lohse AW, Hudson M. Primary sclerosing cholangitis. Lancet. 2018;391:2547–59.
79. Tilg H, Cani PD, Mayer EA. Gut microbiome and liver diseases. Gut. 2016;65:2035–44.
80. Betrapally NS, Gillevet PM, Bajaj JS. Gut microbiome and liver disease. Transl Res. 2017;179:49–59.
81. Acharya C, Sahingur SE, Bajaj JS. Microbiota, cirrhosis, and the emerging oral-gut-liver axis. JCI Insight. 2017;2 https://doi.org/10.1172/jci.insight.94416.
82. Brenner DA, Paik YH, Schnabl B. Role of gut microbiota in liver disease. J Clin Gastroenterol. 2015;49(Suppl 1):S25–7.
83. Schramm C. Bile acids, the microbiome, immunity, and liver tumors. N Engl J Med. 2018;379:888–90.
84. Ma C, Han M, Heinrich B, Fu Q, Zhang Q, Sandhu M, Agdashian D, et al. Gut microbiome-mediated bile acid metabolism regulates liver cancer via NKT cells. Science. 2018;360 https://doi.org/10.1126/science.aan5931.
85. Woodhouse CA, Patel VC, Singanayagam A, Shawcross DL. Review article: the gut microbiome as a therapeutic target in the pathogenesis and treatment of chronic liver disease. Aliment Pharmacol Ther. 2018;47:192–202.
86. Boursier J, Mueller O, Barret M, Machado M, Fizanne L, Araujo-Perez F, Guy CD, et al. The severity of nonalcoholic fatty liver disease is associated with gut dysbiosis and shift in the metabolic function of the gut microbiota. Hepatology. 2016;63:764–75.
87. Bajaj JS, Betrapally NS, Hylemon PB, Heuman DM, Daita K, White MB, Unser A, et al. Salivary microbiota reflects changes in gut microbiota in cirrhosis with hepatic encephalopathy. Hepatology. 2015;62:1260–71.

Polycystic Liver Diseases

20

Carmen Fierbinteanu-Braticevici and
Alexandru Constantin Moldoveanu

Key Concepts

The imaging examinations and family history are currently the most useful in establishing the diagnosis. In cases when family history is unknown, and the imaging is suggestive for this disease, it is recommended that relatives should also be screened.

- While polycystic liver disease can be regarded as a hereditary disease, only about 20% of patients have been identified to have genetic mutations.
- It has been suggested that estrogens have an active role in the development and progression of hepatic cysts. Episodes of exposure to higher quantities of estrogens, including pregnancies, oral contraceptive therapy and post-menopause estrogen replacement therapy, have been linked to faster progression of polycystic liver disease.
- Evolution of the disease is benign for most patients, with little or no symptoms, but for some patients the compression effect caused by the cysts on adjacent structures can cause severe progressive symptoms and may require surgical or medical treatment.
- One of the most useful classifications is the Schnelldorfer's Classification, as it helps guide therapy.

20.1 Introduction

Polycystic liver disease (PLD) is a rare disease, manifesting with progressive bile duct enlargement and development of multiple cysts of various sizes in the liver. The disease is very frequently associated with polycystic kidney disease, but the disease can also be restricted to only the liver and has been suggested as a separate entity. Both the isolated polycystic liver disease and the in the case of polycystic kidney disease are inherited disorders, even though not all genes responsible have yet been identified. Evolution of the disease is benign for most patients, with little or no symptoms, but for some patients the compression effect caused by the cysts on adjacent structures can cause severe progressive symptoms and may require surgical or medical treatment.

20.2 Pathogenesis

Polycystic liver disease can be regarded as a hereditary disease, with either autosomal dominant transmission or autosomal recessive transmission. Only about 20% of patients have been identified to have one or more genetic mutations [1, 2]. The disease can be classified according to the genetic mutations known so far:

- Mutations of the PRKCSH gene on chromosome 19p13, which is involved in the development of the glucosidase 2 (the β subunit) [1].
- Mutations of the SEC63 gene on chromosome 6q21m which has a role in the protein translocation through the endoplasmic reticulum [3].
- Mutations of the ALG8 gene on chromosome 11p, which encodes the ALG6/ALG8 glucosyltransferase family [4].

C. Fierbinteanu-Braticevici (✉) · A. C. Moldoveanu
Department of Internal Medicine II and Gastroenterology - University Hospital Bucharest, "Carol Davila" University of Medicine and Pharmacy Bucharest, Bucharest, Romania

Department of Gastroenterology, University Hospital Bucharest, Bucharest, Romania

F. Radu-Ionita et al. (eds.), *Liver Diseases*, https://doi.org/10.1007/978-3-030-24432-3_20

- Mutations of the LRP5 gene on chromosome 11q13 which encodes the Low-density lipoprotein receptor-related protein 5 [5].
- Mutations of the SEC61B gene on chromosome 9q22 which encodes another protein translocator in the endoplasmic reticulum [4].

A different set of genetic mutations is associated with the combined polycystic kidney and liver disease, the most common being PKD1 which is found in most patients, encodes polycystin 1 and PKD2 which encodes polycystin 2. Both of these have autosomal dominant transmission. PKHD1, a gene that encodes fibrocystin, a protein involved in the development of bile duct architecture also causes polycystic kidney disease but has autosomal recessive transmission [6].

Mutations to the GANAB gene, on chromosome 11q12.3 can cause either isolated polycystic liver disease or liver disease associated with polycystic kidney disease.

Mutations of any of these genes will cause proliferation of biliary epithelial cells, through a number of signaling pathways, including the cAMP-mediated activation of mitogen activation protein kinase and extracellular regulated kinase (MAPK/ERK), the mammalian target of rapamycin mediated signaling cascade [7]. This will result in the formation of von Meyenburg's complexes which arise from the biliary tree but become separate entities as they become larger and accumulate more fluid.

20.3 Epidemiology

Prevalence of isolated polycystic liver disease is less than 0.01%, which is much lower compared to polycystic disease of both the liver and kidney where it is closer to 0.2% of the population. Around 80% of patients with kidney disease also present liver cysts, which implies that most cases of polycystic liver disease are associated with polycystic kidney disease, rather than being an isolated disease of the liver [8].

The disease affects both genders, but with a higher prevalence of symptomatic disease in the female gender [9]. It has been suggested that estrogens have an active role in the development and progression of hepatic cysts. Episodes of exposure to higher quantities of estrogens, including pregnancies, oral contraceptive therapy and post-menopause estrogen replacement therapy, have been linked to faster progression of polycystic liver disease [10].

20.4 Signs and Symptoms

Most patients with uncomplicated cysts are asymptomatic. Symptoms usually result from cyst compression on adjacent structures and can include abdominal discomfort or pain, reduced mobility and fatigue.

Compression of the cysts on the stomach and duodenum can cause or worsen symptoms of gastroesophageal reflux disease and can also include symptoms such as early satiety and postprandial fullness. Compression on the portal vein can cause symptoms of portal hypertension including collateral circulation, ascites [11], development of varices as well as variceal bleeding [12]. The cysts can also cause compression on the vena cava inferior [13] or of the suprahepatic veins, the latter establishing a Budd-Chiari syndrome, similar to the obstruction caused by thrombosis. Symptoms will include abdominal pain, hepatomegaly and transudate ascites. Compression of the bile ducts can cause jaundice and pruritus [8, 12, 14]. Other organs at risk of compression can also include the diaphragm and lungs resulting in dyspnea. A case of a large cyst compressing on the pancreas has also been described (Fig. 20.1) [13].

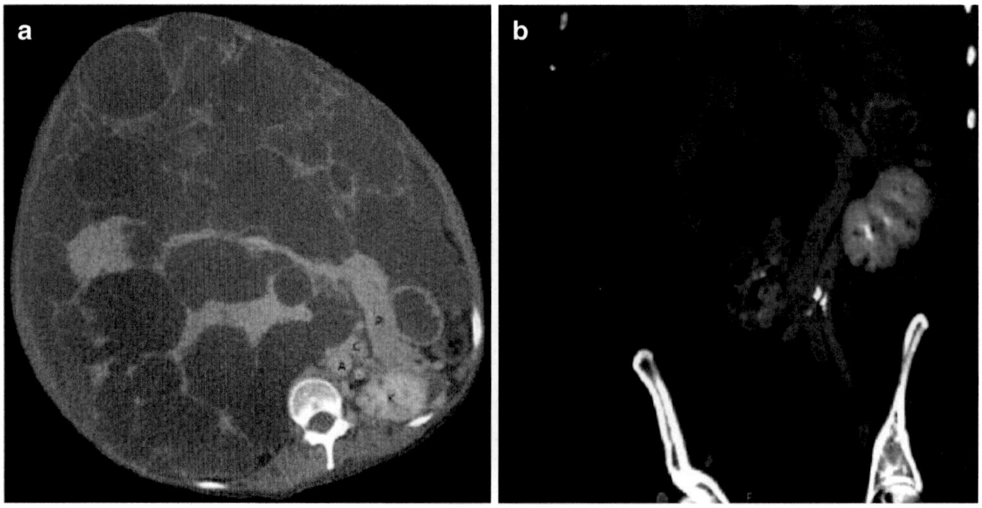

Fig. 20.1 (**a**) Axial section CT showing abdominal anatomy with kidney and pancreas in relation to liver. (**b**) Coronal plane CT venogram showing vena cava pushed on the left side of the aorta. (Reproduced from Serrano Rodriguez P et all., 2018)

20.5 Diagnosis

The imaging examinations and family history are currently the most useful in establishing the diagnosis. In cases when family history is unknown, and the imaging is suggestive for this disease, it is recommended that relatives should also be screened.

Laboratory tests will reveal increased cholestasis enzymes as well as increased transaminases if there is bile duct obstruction. Patients may present with elevated CA19-9 levels [15]. Other laboratory test abnormalities may also be present, depending on the compression effect on adjacent structures.

In abdominal ultrasound cysts appear as transonic, anechoic structures of various sizes, usually with cones of light. On computed tomography scans the cysts appear hypodense, have homogenous contents and a round and regular shape with no walls (Fig. 20.2). The structure does not become enhanced after contrast administration [16].

In magnetic resonance imaging the cysts appear to have a very low intensity on T1 images and a very high intensity on T2 images. Similar to computed tomography, they are homogenous. When complicated by hemorrhaging a high intensity signal is observed in both T1 and T2 imaging sequences. Magnetic resonance imaging is considered to have a better sensitivity for detecting complicated cysts [16].

20.6 Establishing Diagnosis

Establishing diagnosis has been somewhat of a challenge as there is no single test that can definitively establish diagnosis.

Isolated polycystic liver disease can be evaluated using the Reynolds criteria: a positive family history, lack of evidence for polycystic kidney disease and either at least one characteristic hepatic cyst (for patients under 40 years of age) or at least four characteristic hepatic cysts (for patients over 40 years of age) [17].

Others have suggested a simpler diagnostic algorithm, that allows establishing diagnosis with over 20 hepatic cysts in patients with no family history and over 4 hepatic cysts in patients with family history [18].

The evaluation of polycystic liver disease associated with kidney disease can be evaluated either through the Unified Ravine criteria or the Pei criteria.

The Unified Ravine criteria require positive family history and either at least three renal cysts (unilateral or bilateral, for patients between 15 and 39 years of age), at least two bilateral renal cysts (for patients between 40 and 59 years of age) or at least four bilateral renal cysts (for patients at least 60 years of age) [19].

The Pei Criteria for polycystic kidney disease were later developed from the Ravine Criteria to include cases with negative family history, allowing for diagnosis when the patient has more than ten bilateral renal cysts and upon the exclusion of any other causes causing cysts [19].

20.7 Differential Diagnosis

The differential diagnosis includes other pathologies that generate cysts or cyst-like structures and includes simple cysts, echinococcosis, cystadenoma, cystadenocarcinoma [20].

Simple hepatic cysts occur in 2–7% of the population, with a slight predilection towards the female gender. They appear on ultrasound as round anechoic lesions, with a thin or imperceptible wall, but a clearly defined back wall. They can present septa or debris in the interior. On computed tomography they appear homogenous and hypoattenuating, while on magnetic resonance they have an increased T2 signal. They are discovered on routine exams and do not usually cause symptoms.

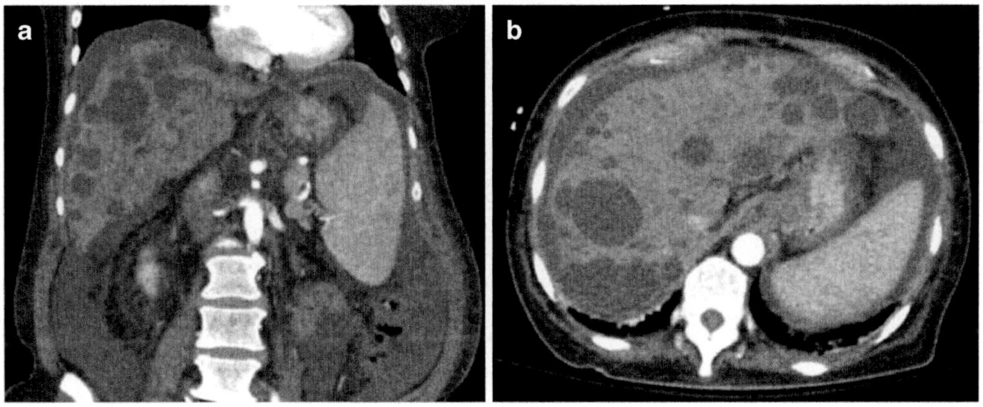

Fig. 20.2 Computed tomography of abdomen and pelvis (coronal and axial scans) showing polycystic liver disease along with evidence of portal hypertension in form of splenomegaly and ascites. (Reproduced from Khan MS et all, 2018)

Echinococcus granulosus and Echinococcus multilocularis are two species of tapeworm that can cause parasitosis in humans. On plain abdominal X-ray they can have curved or ring-shaped calcifications around the cysts (calcium deposits in the pericyst). Ultrasound and computed tomography can identify multiple septs and "daughter" cysts. Magnetic Resonance Imaging can reveal a high signal T2 and a low signal T1, can identify the septa and "daughter" cysts. The walls and septa become enhanced upon the administration of gadolinium contrast. Hepatic alveolar echinococcosis is a rarer manifestation of the infection with Echinococcus multilocularis and presents with large multiloculate necrotic masses without a fibrous capsule [21, 22].

Biliary cystadenoma is a benign cystic neoplasm of the liver and occurs in middle aged patients. It has a higher prevalence in women [23]. Rarely they can evolve towards becoming cystadenocarcinomas [23]. Biliary cystadenocarcinoma is a malign cystic neoplasm of the liver, with a rare incidence. Differentiating between cystadenoma and cystadenocarcinoma is difficult on imaging exams. On ultrasound they appear as one or more cysts, with anechoic contents (uncomplicated cysts) or with contents of various echogenicity (hemorrhaging or protein content). The walls can also contain calcifications and cast a cone of shadow. Computed tomography can identify similar characteristics, identifying recent hemorrhaging. Septa may become enhanced after administration of contrast substance.

Caroli disease is a rare malformation of the intrahepatic bile ducts which leads to the formation of cystic dilatations of the bile ducts. Ultrasound reveals intrahepatic anechoic cysts, with bundles of portal veins and hepatic arteries. More characteristically, there are dilated segments of the biliary radicles with no visible obstruction. Computed tomography, magnetic resonance imaging and magnetic resonance cholangiopancreatography, can improve diagnosis, the latter being proposed as the imaging test of choice [24]. While the differential diagnosis is usually clear, as polycystic liver disease does not present with dilatations that follow the duct radicles, the diagnosis can be sometimes more difficult because there are frequent associations with polycystic kidney disease [25].

20.8 Natural History and Complications

The natural history of the disease describes a continuous growth of the liver size of 0.9–3.2% on average per year, starting from Von Meyenburg complexes (multiple small cysts) and ending with severe disease (Fig. 20.3) [8].

Infection of the cysts can manifest with fever, pain and signs of septic shock. Diagnosis can be established using lab tests (high C reactive protein level and higher than previously CA19-9 levels) and imaging tests (wall thickening, heterogeneous debris inside the cyst), but diagnostic accuracy for both computed tomography as well as magnetic resonance imaging is low [2, 26].

Hemorrhaging of the cysts presents with acute pain in the right hypochondrium. Diagnosis can be established by ultrasound and magnetic resonance imaging [2, 16].

Cyst rupture manifests with severe pain. Diagnosis can be established by computed tomography scan. Depending on the severity of the rupture and hemodynamic complications, it can be treated either conservatively or surgically [27].

Abdominal wall hernias, paraumbilical and inguinal hernias appear to be more common in patients with polycystic liver diseases compared to patients with no liver or kidney diseases and can be explained by constant compression of the enlarged organs (liver and/or kidney).

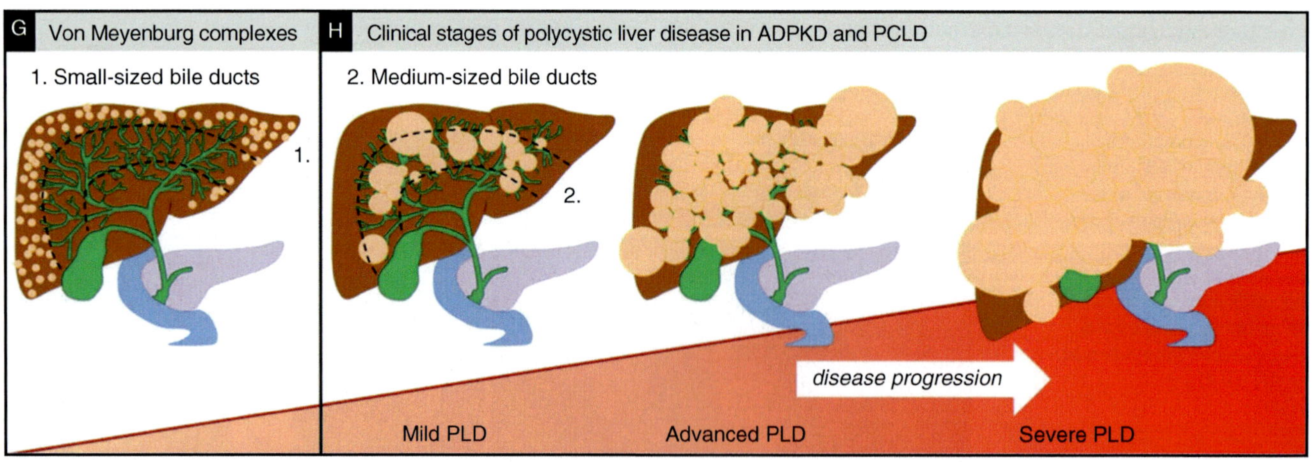

Fig. 20.3 Natural evolution of polycystic liver disease and autosomal dominant polycystic kidney disease. (Reproduced from Cnossen WR et all, 2014)

20.9 Classifications

One of the most commonly used classifications is the Schnelldorfer's Classification, as it helps guide therapy. Type A includes patients with either no or minimum symptoms, while types B, C and D include patients with moderate or severe symptoms. Type B refers to patients with large but few cysts that span an area of at least two sectors and present no venous obstruction. Type C includes patients with higher number of smaller cysts occupying areas of at least one sector and present no venous obstruction. Type D includes patients with any number and size of cysts but with symptoms of either portal vein or hepatic vein compression [28].

Another classification proposed to identify patients that are candidates for fenestration is the Gigot's Classification. Type I includes patients with fewer (less than 10) large (more than 10 cm in diameter) hepatic cysts, type II includes patients with diffuse cysts but with remaining areas of normal parenchyma, while type III includes patients with little remaining normal parenchyma. Patients classified as Gigot Type I are suitable candidates for fenestration [29].

20.10 Treatment

In Schnelldorfer's Type A, most patients are asymptomatic and require no treatment, aside from the avoidance of exposure to excess estrogen.

In Schnelldorfer's Type B, there are treatment options that consist in either removal of the fluid from the cysts, or the cyst altogether.

Removal of fluid can be done through percutaneous cyst aspiration. This method is preferred for large cysts that are accessible. It is, however, only a short term symptomatic solution, the recurrence rate being 80–100% in less than a year [30]. There is an option of injecting a sclerotizing agent such as alcohol, acidic solutions of tetracycline or minocycline, but this method has the same long-term rate of recurrence.

Another procedure is cyst fenestration (removal of a part of the cyst wall to allow drainage). The procedure can be performed laparoscopically or openly. A total of up to 2 L of fluid can be drained in a single session, but the procedure can be done in multiple sequential sessions. The cyst wall can then be treated by argon laser beam coagulation or electrocoagulation. The procedure will yield better results in the short term than aspiration, but most patients will still have recurrence at 24 months [31].

Cyst enucleation, which consists in the complete removal of the cyst, can be performed in isolated and few cysts. In areas with multiple small cysts, or large cysts with significant anatomical complications, a portion of the liver can also be removed. There are, however, higher risks associated with this procedure, including hemorrhage and bile leakage.

In Schnelldorfer's type C patients, partial hepatectomy with fenestration of remnant cysts is also an option.

Liver transplantation yields excellent results for most patients and presents the usual complications of this procedure (Figs. 20.4 and 20.5). It is recommended in all Schnelldorfer's type D patients.

In patients where the surgical risks are very high, alternative non-surgical therapies have been proposed.

Somatostatin analogues can proliferation of cholangiocytes through the reduction of various cytogenetic growth factors as well as vascular growth factors [32]. They can also reduce fluid secretion within the cysts. Results of trials with lanreotide have indicated a mild mean reduction of 2.9% in liver size with modest reduction in symptoms [33, 34]. Other studies have used long acting octreotide and demonstrated a 6–7% reduction in total liver volume [35].

Everolimus is an mTOR inhibitor that as given as an additional therapy to somatostatin analogs in one trial, but there was no additional decrease in liver size compared to somatostatin alone [36].

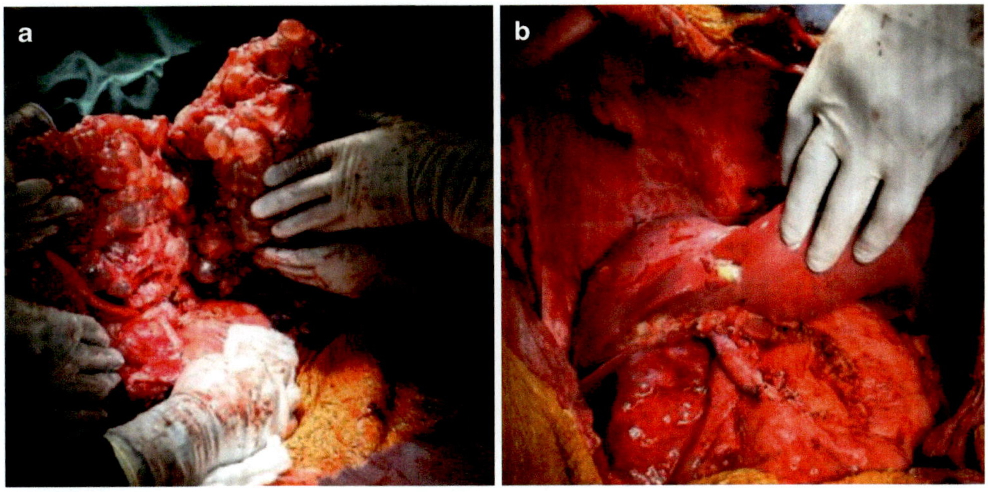

Fig. 20.4 (**a**) Intraoperative image of native liver. (**b**) Liver after reperfusion. (Reproduced form Serrano Rodriguez P et all, 2018)

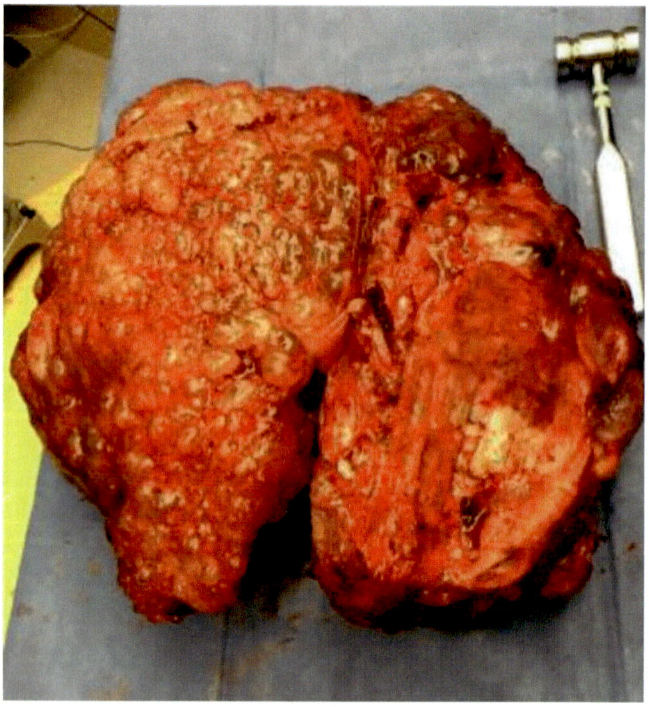

Fig. 20.5 Explanted liver with polycystic liver disease. (Reproduced form Serrano Rodriguez P et all, 2018)

Transarterial Embolization with N-butyl-2-cyanoacrylate and iodized oil was attempted and appears to be a safe and effective treatment [37, 38].

Self Study

Questions

1. Which statement regarding the diagnosis is true?
   (a) Polycystic liver disease is a hereditary disease and the genetic test is the definitive diagnosis.
   (b) All patients will present with abdominal pain.
   (c) Estrogens have a role in the progression of the disease.
   (d) Abdominal ultrasound is the most accurate test in diagnosing cyst hemorrhaging.
2. Which statement regarding the treatment is true?
   (a) Percutaneous cyst aspiration is a definitive treatment for most patients.
   (b) In Schnelldorfer's Type A patients, neither surgical nor medical therapy is needed.
   (c) Medical therapy is a viable alternative to surgery in all patients.
   (d) In cyst fenestration a total of 5 L of fluid can be extracted in a single session.

Answers

1. Which statement regarding the diagnosis is true?
   (a) While polycystic liver disease is a hereditary disease, only about 20% of patients will be identified to have a genetic mutation linked to the disease.
   (b) Most patients are completely asymptomatic. For symptomatic patients, pain is only one possible manifestation, as it depends on the location, size and relation to the adjacent structures of the cysts.
   (c) CORRECT ANSWER: Current studies suggest that the symptomatic disease is more prevalent in women and progression happens at a faster rate for women with multiple pregnancies and estrogen replacement therapy.
   (d) While abdominal ultrasound is extremely useful in screening patients and establishing diagnosis of the disease itself, for some complications, including hemorrhaging, magnetic resonance imaging is more accurate.
2. Which statement regarding the treatment is true?
   (a) Unfortunately, percutaneous cyst aspiration has a 80–100% recurrence rate.
   (b) CORRECT ANSWER: Only avoidance of estrogen-based products is needed in Schnelldorfer's Type A patients.
   (c) Medical therapy is only recommended in patients with unacceptable surgical risks. This is due to the relatively weak efficiency of the medical treatment compared to the surgical treatment.
   (d) Up to 2 L of fluid can be extracted in a single session. However, the patient can undergo multiple sessions in short succession if needed.

References

1. Li A, Davila S, Furu L, Qian Q, Tian X, Kamath PS, et al. Mutations in PRKCSH cause isolated autosomal dominant polycystic liver disease. Am J Hum Genet. 2003;72(3):691–703. https://doi.org/10.1086/368295.
2. Cnossen WR, Drenth JPH. Polycystic liver disease: an overview of pathogenesis, clinical manifestations and management. Orphanet J Rare Dis. 2014;9(1):69. https://doi.org/10.1186/1750-1172-9-69.
3. Davila S, Furu L, Gharavi AG, Tian X, Onoe T, Qian Q, et al. Mutations in SEC63 cause autosomal dominant polycystic liver disease. Nat Genet. 2004;36:575. https://doi.org/10.1038/ng1357.
4. Besse W, Dong K, Choi J, Punia S, Fedeles SV, Choi M, et al. Isolated polycystic liver disease genes define effectors of polycystin-1 function. J Clin Invest. 2017;127(5):1772–85. https://doi.org/10.1172/JCI90129.
5. Cnossen WR, te Morsche RHM, Hoischen A, Gilissen C, Chrispijn M, Venselaar H, et al. Whole-exome sequencing reveals LRP5 mutations and canonical Wnt signaling associated with hepatic cys-

togenesis. Proc Natl Acad Sci U S A. 2014;111(14):5343–8. https://doi.org/10.1073/pnas.1309438111.
6. Perugorria MJ, Masyuk TV, Marin JJ, Marzioni M, Bujanda L, LaRusso NF, et al. Polycystic liver diseases: advanced insights into the molecular mechanisms. Nat Rev Gastroenterol Hepatol. 2014;11(12):750–61. https://doi.org/10.1038/nrgastro.2014.155.
7. Qian Q. Isolated polycystic liver disease. Adv Chronic Kidney Dis. 2010;17(2):181–9. https://doi.org/10.1053/j.ackd.2009.12.005.
8. Abu-Wasel B, Walsh C, Keough V, Molinari M. Pathophysiology, epidemiology, classification and treatment options for polycystic liver diseases. World J Gastroenterol. 2013;19(35):5775–86. https://doi.org/10.3748/wjg.v19.i35.5775.
9. Leveille E, Drenth JP, UMC R, Bernts L. Polycystic Liver disease. National Organization for Rare Disorders (NORD). 2018.
10. Alvaro D, Mancino MG, Onori P, Franchitto A, Alpini G, Francis H, et al. Estrogens and the pathophysiology of the biliary tree. World J Gastroenterol. 2006;12(22):3537–45. https://doi.org/10.3748/wjg.v12.i22.3537.
11. Chauveau D, Grunfeld JP, Durand F, Belghiti J. Ascites in a polycystic patient. Nephrol Dial Transplant. 1997;12(1):228–30.
12. Khan MS, Khan Z, Javaid T, Akhtar J, Moustafa A, Lal A, et al. Isolated polycystic liver disease: an unusual cause of recurrent variceal bleed. Case Rep Gastrointest Med. 2018;2018:4. https://doi.org/10.1155/2018/2902709.
13. Al-Harthi A, Khan P, Al Marwani M. Polycystic liver disease with huge infected cyst displacing the pancreas, inferior vena cava and right kidney. Saudi J Med Med Sci. 2016;4(3):222–4. https://doi.org/10.4103/1658-631x.188259.
14. Van Keimpema L, De Koning DB, Van Hoek B, Van Den Berg AP, Van Oijen MG, De Man RA, et al. Patients with isolated polycystic liver disease referred to liver centres: clinical characterization of 137 cases. Liver Int. 2011;31(1):92–8. https://doi.org/10.1111/j.1478-3231.2010.02247.x.
15. Waanders E, van Keimpema L, Brouwer JT, van Oijen MG, Aerts R, Sweep FC, et al. Carbohydrate antigen 19-9 is extremely elevated in polycystic liver disease. Liver Int. 2009;29(9):1389–95. https://doi.org/10.1111/j.1478-3231.2009.02055.x.
16. Mortele KJ, Ros PR. Cystic focal liver lesions in the adult: differential CT and MR imaging features. Radiographics. 2001;21(4):895–910. https://doi.org/10.1148/radiographics.21.4.g01jl16895.
17. Reynolds DM, Falk CT, Li A, King BF, Kamath PS, Huston J 3rd, et al. Identification of a locus for autosomal dominant polycystic liver disease, on chromosome 19p13.2-13.1. Am J Hum Genet. 2000;67(6):1598–604. https://doi.org/10.1086/316904.
18. Temmerman F, Missiaen L, Bammens B, Laleman W, Cassiman D, Verslype C, et al. Systematic review: the pathophysiology and management of polycystic liver disease. Aliment Pharmacol Ther. 2011;34(7):702–13. https://doi.org/10.1111/j.1365-2036.2011.04783.x.
19. Pei Y, Obaji J, Dupuis A, Paterson AD, Magistroni R, Dicks E, et al. Unified criteria for ultrasonographic diagnosis of ADPKD. J Am Soc Nephrol. 2009;20(1):205–12. https://doi.org/10.1681/asn.2008050507.
20. Lantinga MA, Gevers TJG, Drenth JPH. Evaluation of hepatic cystic lesions. World J Gastroenterol. 2013;19(23):3543–54. https://doi.org/10.3748/wjg.v19.i23.3543.
21. Pedrosa I, Saiz A, Arrazola J, Ferreiros J, Pedrosa CS. Hydatid disease: radiologic and pathologic features and complications. Radiographics. 2000;20(3):795–817. https://doi.org/10.1148/radiographics.20.3.g00ma06795.
22. Kantarci M, Bayraktutan U, Karabulut N, Aydinli B, Ogul H, Yuce I, et al. Alveolar echinococcosis: spectrum of findings at cross-sectional imaging. Radiographics. 2012;32(7):2053–70. https://doi.org/10.1148/rg.327125708.
23. Levy AD, Murakata LA, Abbott RM, Rohrmann CA Jr. From the archives of the AFIP. Benign tumors and tumorlike lesions of the gallbladder and extrahepatic bile ducts: radiologic-pathologic correlation. Armed Forces Institute of Pathology. Radiographics. 2002;22(2):387–413. https://doi.org/10.1148/radiographics.22.2.g02mr08387.
24. Asselah T, Ernst O, Sergent G, L'Hermine C, Paris JC. Caroli's disease: a magnetic resonance cholangiopancreatography diagnosis. Am J Gastroenterol. 1998;93(1):109–10. https://doi.org/10.1111/j.1572-0241.1998.109_c.x.
25. Cabral Correia P, Morgado B. Caroli's disease as a cause of chronic epigastric abdominal pain: two case reports and a brief review of the literature. Cureus. 2017;9(9):e1701. https://doi.org/10.7759/cureus.1701.
26. Kanaan N, Goffin E, Pirson Y, Devuyst O, Hassoun Z. Carbohydrate antigen 19-9 as a diagnostic marker for hepatic cyst infection in autosomal dominant polycystic kidney disease. Am J Kidney Dis. 2010;55(5):916–22. https://doi.org/10.1053/j.ajkd.2009.12.023.
27. Akriviadis EA, Steindel H, Ralls P, Redeker AG. Spontaneous rupture of nonparasitic cyst of the liver. Gastroenterology. 1989;97(1):213–5.
28. Schnelldorfer T, Torres VE, Zakaria S, Rosen CB, Nagorney DM. Polycystic liver disease: a critical appraisal of hepatic resection, cyst fenestration, and liver transplantation. Ann Surg. 2009;250(1):112–8. https://doi.org/10.1097/SLA.0b013e3181ad83dc.
29. Gigot JF, Jadoul P, Que F, Van Beers BE, Etienne J, Horsmans Y, et al. Adult polycystic liver disease: is fenestration the most adequate operation for long-term management? Ann Surg. 1997;225(3):286–94.
30. Russell RT, Pinson CW. Surgical management of polycystic liver disease. World J Gastroenterol. 2007;13(38):5052–9.
31. Morgan DE, Lockhart ME, Canon CL, Holcombe MP, Bynon JS. Polycystic liver disease: multimodality imaging for complications and transplant evaluation. Radiographics. 2006;26(6):1655–68; quiz. https://doi.org/10.1148/rg.266065013.
32. Pyronnet S, Bousquet C, Najib S, Azar R, Laklai H, Susini C. Antitumor effects of somatostatin. Mol Cell Endocrinol. 2008;286(1–2):230–7. https://doi.org/10.1016/j.mce.2008.02.002.
33. van Keimpema L, Nevens F, Vanslembrouck R, van Oijen MG, Hoffmann AL, Dekker HM, et al. Lanreotide reduces the volume of polycystic liver: a randomized, double-blind, placebo-controlled trial. Gastroenterology. 2009;137(5):1661–8.e1-2. https://doi.org/10.1053/j.gastro.2009.07.052.
34. Khan S, Dennison A, Garcea G. Medical therapy for polycystic liver disease. Ann R Coll Surg Engl. 2016;98(1):18–23. https://doi.org/10.1308/rcsann.2016.0023.
35. Hogan MC, Masyuk TV, Page L, Holmes DR 3rd, Li X, Bergstralh EJ, et al. Somatostatin analog therapy for severe polycystic liver disease: results after 2 years. Nephrol Dial Transplant. 2012;27(9):3532–9. https://doi.org/10.1093/ndt/gfs152.
36. Chrispijn M, Gevers TJ, Hol JC, Monshouwer R, Dekker HM, Drenth JP. Everolimus does not further reduce polycystic liver volume when added to long acting octreotide: results from a randomized controlled trial. J Hepatol. 2013;59(1):153–9. https://doi.org/10.1016/j.jhep.2013.03.004.
37. Wang MQ, Duan F, Liu FY, Wang ZJ, Song P. Treatment of symptomatic polycystic liver disease: transcatheter super-selective hepatic arterial embolization using a mixture of NBCA and iodized oil. Abdom Imaging. 2013;38(3):465–73. https://doi.org/10.1007/s00261-012-9931-1.
38. Zhang JL, Yuan K, Wang MQ, Yan JY, Xin HN, Wang Y, et al. Transarterial embolization for treatment of symptomatic polycystic liver disease: more than 2-year follow-up. Chin Med J. 2017;130(16):1938–44. https://doi.org/10.4103/0366-6999.211882.

Hepato- and Porto-pulmonary Hypertension

21

Ioan Tiberiu Nanea and Gabriela Silvia Gheorghe

Key Concepts

1. **Porto-pulmonary hypertension (POPH)**
    - POPH represents the association between portal hypertension (PH), arterial pulmonary hypertension (PAH), increase of the pulmonary vascular resistance (PVR) > 240 dyne·s·cm^{-5} or >3 u Wood, normal capillary wedge pressure (PCWP) and normal left ventricular end diastolic pressure. PAH is defined by the increase of the resting mean pressure in pulmonary artery (mPAP) > 25 mmHg and increase of the mPAP during exercise >30 mmHg.
    - POPH is included in the first group of PAH, according to European Guidelines for the Diagnosis and Treatment of Pulmonary Hypertension classification.
    - POPH occurs more frequently in women with autoimmune hepatitis and primitive biliary cirrhosis
    - There are no relations between the occurrence of POPH and the severity of the hepatic disease, evaluated by Child-Pugh and MELD scores.
    - The occurrence of POPH is related to the hyperdynamic circulation in hepatic cirrhosis, the entry in the pulmonary circulation of the endotoxins, endothelin, thromboxane A_2 (TXA_2), interleukin 6 (IL-6), tumor necrosis alfa (TNF alfa), macrophages, and the reduced of the pulmonary level of nitric oxide (NO) and prostacyclin (PGI2).
    - The symptoms are non specific
    - The screening examination is transthoracic echocardiography (TTE)
    - The gold standard diagnostic test is right cardiac catheterization
    - Pulmonary vasodilator treatment is not always effective
    - In patients with moderate to severe POPH liver transplantation has no indication
2. **Hepato-pulmonary syndrome (HPS)**
    - HPS associates hepatic disease with increased O_2 alveolo-arterial gradient ($P(A\text{-}a)O_2$) above 15 mmHg, intrapulmonary capillary dilation, with or without hypoxemia
    - HPS occurs in patients with hepatic cirrhosis, chronic hepatitis, acute hepatic failure, PH of other causes like Budd-Chiari syndrome
    - The occurrence of HPS is not related to the severity of the hepatic disease evaluated by Child-Pugh and MELD scores.
    - The pulmonary pre capillary arterioles and the capillaries are dilated, there are pulmonary arterio-venous and porto-pulmonary anastomoses.
    - The pulmonary vasodilatation leads to the increase of the $P(A\text{-}a)O_2$ and hypoxemia in most cases.
    - Hypoxemia is worse in orthostatism. Orthodeoxia represents the decrease of the PaO_2 in orthostatism more than ≥4 mmHg or ≥5% from the value in recumbent position
    - Hypoxemia is improved by the administration of 100% O_2, unlike others diseases with intrapulmonary vascular shunts
    - Dyspnoea is worse in orthostatism and improves when lying down (platypnoea)

I. T. Nanea (✉) · G. S. Gheorghe
Carol Davila University of Medicine and Pharmacy, Bucharest, Romania

F. Radu-Ionita et al. (eds.), *Liver Diseases*, https://doi.org/10.1007/978-3-030-24432-3_21

- The symptoms are nonspecific. Some patients have orthodeoxia and platypnoea. There is an increased risk of stroke by paradoxical embolism.
- The screening test is the evaluation of the arterial gases with the measurement of $P(A\text{-}a)O_2$ in ambient air
- The gold standard tests are contrast-enhanced echocardiography and perfusion pulmonary scintigraphy with macro-aggregated albumin (>20 μm diameter) labelled with ^{99m}Tc (MAA scan).
- The treatment of HPS is hepatic transplant, in particular in patients in which administration of O_2 100% corrects hypoxemia

21.1 Introduction

Chronic liver diseases (CLD) and portal hypertension (PH) may be associated with severe pulmonary changes that alter prognosis and amend the therapeutic attitude: porto-pulmonary hypertension (POPH) and hepato-pulmonary syndrome (HPS). Both complications are particularly related to the presence of PH even in the absence of CLD. The pathophysiological mechanisms are different and it is unknown why some patients with hepatitis and/or PH develop one or another type of lung damage. There are rare cases in which both pulmonary complications can be associated. The onset of POPH and HPS implies a poor prognosis. Their therapeutic approach is different. Moderate to severe POPH is generally a contraindication for liver transplantation as it leads to a significant increase in mortality. HPS usually improves after liver transplantation.

21.2 Porto-Pulmonary Hypertension

21.2.1 Definition

POPH is defined as the association of PH with pulmonary arterial hypertension (PAH), assessed in turn through cardiac catheterization by increased mean pulmonary artery pressure (mPAP) > 25 mmHg at rest and >30 mmHg at exercise, pulmonary vascular resistance (PVR) > 240 dynes·s·cm^{-5} or ≥3 u Wood and pulmonary capillary wedge pressure (PCWP) or left ventricular end diastolic pressure (LVEDP) ≤ 15 mmHg [1]. POPH belongs to the first group of pulmonary hypertension, according to the classification of the European Guidelines for the Diagnosis and Treatment of Pulmonary Hypertension [2]. In patients with elevated PCWP, transpulmonary pressure gradient (TPG), calculated by the formula: mPAP-PCWP, was proposed as a diagnostic criterion for the POPH. In these patients, TPG > 12 mmHg indicates that PVR is increased [3].

21.2.2 Epidemiology

POPH occurs in approximately 1–2% of patients with PH and CLD and in 3–12.5% of liver transplant candidates [4]. It usually occurs in the fifth decade of life, after 4–7 years of evolution of PH [3]. 5.1% of PAH patients included in the REVEAL registry had POPH [3].

The risk factors for the appearance of POPH are female sex, autoimmune hepatitis and primitive biliary cirrhosis. Age, severity of hepatic impairment expressed by MELD and Child Pugh scores, serum bilirubin and INR value are not risk factors for POPH occurrence. Male sex, presence of ascites, hypoalbuminemia, C virus infection are negatively associated with the presence of POPH [5].

POPH development is independent of the cause of PH, although most patients have cirrhosis. POPH may occur in patients with portal vein thrombosis.

The classification of POPH is based on mPAP values.

- Mild POPH: mPAP 25–35 mmHg;
- Moderate POPH: mPAP 35–44 mmHg;
- Severe POPH: mPAP ≥45 mmHg;

Studies have shown that prognosis is worse as POPH is more severe.

21.2.3 Pathology

Anatomical changes in POPH occur in the precapillary lung vessels and are similar to those in idiopathic PAH. Muscle hypertrophy, endothelial proliferation, adventitial proliferation, plexiform lesions, in situ thrombosis, pulmonary arterioles micro aneurysms can be observed [3, 4].

21.2.4 Pathophysiology

Typically, 30–50% of patients with advanced CLD have increased cardiac output and decreased systemic vascular resistance and PVR. The cause of hyperdynamic circula-

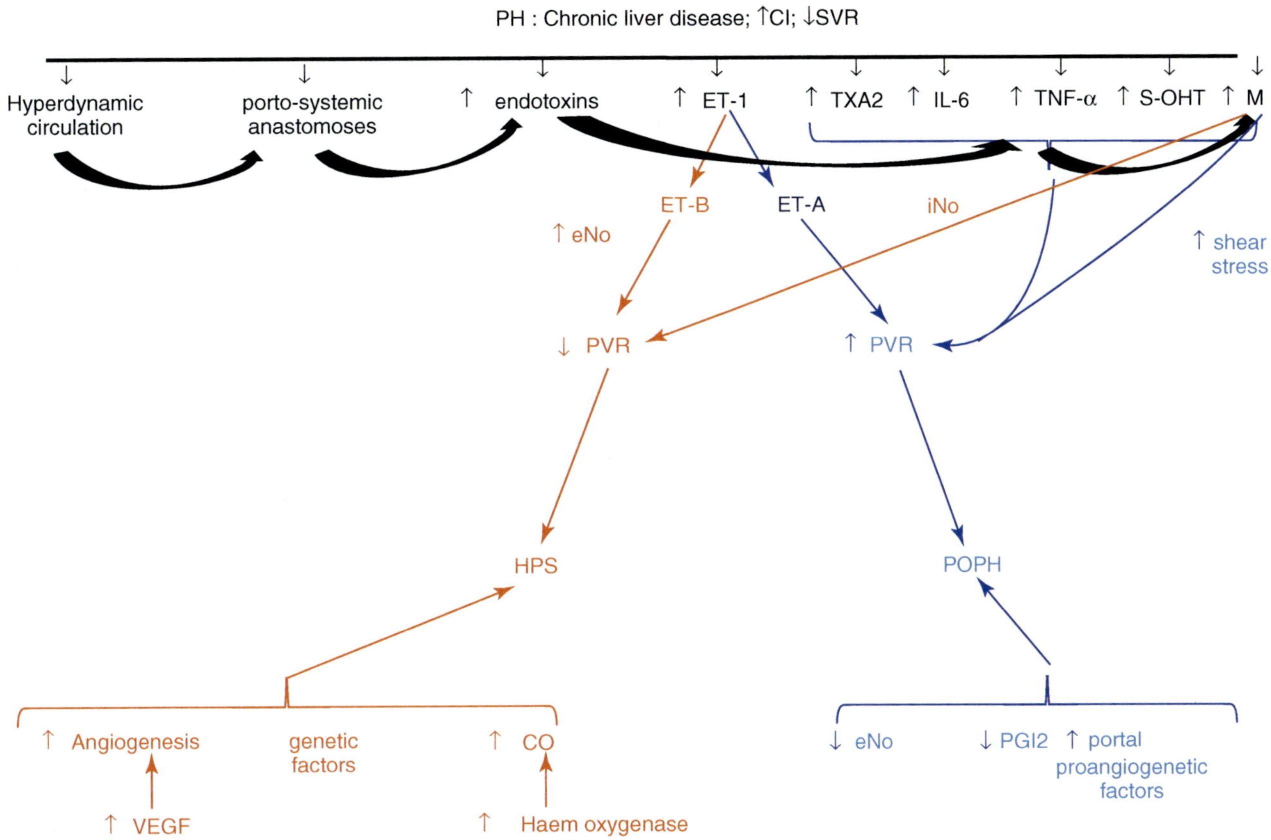

Fig. 21.1 Pathophysiology of the POPH and HPS-some hypothesis. *PH* pulmonary hypertension, *CI* cardiac index, *SVR* systemic vascular resistence, *ET-l* endothelin 1, *TXA2* thromboxane A2: *IL-6* interleukin 6, *TNF-α* transforming growth factor α, *5-OHT* serotonin. *M* macrophages, *ET-A* endothelin A receptors, *ET-B* endothelin B receptor, *eNO* endothelial nitric oxide, *iNO* inducible nitric oxide, *PVR* pulmonary vascular resistance, *HPS* hepato-pulmonary syndrome, *POPH* porto pulmonary hypertension, *PGI2* prostaglandin I_2, *VEGF* vascular endothelium growth factor; *Haem* Oxygenase microsomal enzyme that carries out the oxidation of haem and the production of CO, *CO* carbonic oxide The hyperdynamic circulation and the porto-systemic and porto-pulmonary anastomoses in PH and CLD determine the entry of the intestinal endotoxins in the pulmonary circulation that increase the production of the inflammatory substances and the accumulation of macrophages in the pulmonary vessels. ET-1 stimulates ET-A and determines vasoconstriction. Macrophages increase the pulmonary arterial parietal shear stress. There is a reduction of the eNO and an increase of the portal proangiogenetic factors. mPAP and PVR increase and the POPH occurs. In some patients, maybe depending of genetic factors, there is an increase of iNO because of the macrophages but also because of the ET-B stimulation by the ET-1. VEGF induces pulmonary angiogenesis. Haem oxygenase induces an increase of the pulmonary CO and vasodilatation. There is arteriolar and capillary dilation, PVR decreases and HPS occurs

tion appears to be stasis within splanchnic circulation and porto-systemic shunts that favor the penetration of vasodilator endotoxins and cytokines into circulation [1]. Increasing cardiac output may increase the pressure in the pulmonary artery [3]. The mild increase in mPAP without PVR increase is not included in POPH. The mechanism by which the pulmonary hyperdynamic circulation usually accompanied by reduced PVR produces increased PVR and POPH is not completely understood. There are several hypotheses (Fig. 21.1):

- Increased cardiac output in the pulmonary artery increases parietal shear stress and induces a variable vascular response, depending on individual cell factors. Patients with vasoconstriction and pulmonary vascular remodeling by proliferation of smooth muscle cells and vascular endothelial cells evolve to POPH. Patients experiencing pulmonary vasodilatation and PVR decrease develop HPS [1].
- Endotoxins in the gastrointestinal tract reach the pulmonary circulation where they determine accumulation of macrophages, that may contribute to the appearance of POPH [3].
- Porto-systemic shunts favor the entry into the inferior vena cava (IVC) and subsequently pulmonary circulation of vasoactive substances that are no longer inactivated in the liver, such as:

  - Endothelin 1, which has an increased blood level in patients with advanced liver disease and portal hypertension. Increased endothelin serum levels might reflect vascular parietal shear stress due to hyperdynamic circulation. It acts on ET_A receptors within the pulmonary arteries wall and produces vasoconstriction, vascular smooth muscle proliferation and intimal fibrosis. ET_B receptors, that under normal conditions determine vasodilatation become dysfunctional, inducing pulmonary vasoconstriction [3].
  - TXA2, IL-6, TNF alpha appear to be involved in the development of POPH [3].
  - Serotonin produced by the enterochromaffin cells of the intestinal wall gets into the lungs in large amounts through porto-caval shunts. PH-associated thrombocytopenia contributes to increased serotonin serum levels by limited storage within platelet granules [6]
- Pulmonary vascular endothelium has reduced levels of prostacyclin synthase in POPH [3]. Decrease in PGI_2 and NO levels reduces the vasodilatory capacity of pulmonary circulation. On the other hand, there is an increased production of NO in the pulmonary vessels in cirrhosis [6]

Other pathophysiology hypotheses were also discussed.

- Genetic factors have not been proven to be involved in the development of POPH. However, there are some studies showing that multiple single nucleotide polymorphism in the genes coding for estrogen receptor 1, aromatase, phosphodiesterase 5, angiopoietin 1, and calcium binding protein A4 are associated with the risk of developing POPH [7].
- There could be an imbalance between pro-angiogenic factors in the portal bloodstream and antiangiogenic factors produced by hepatocytes from type XVIII collagen and plasminogen: endostatin and angiostatin, respectively. Because of porto-caval shunts pro angiogenetic factors within portal blood are no longer annihilated by the hepatic anti angiogenetic factors and reach the lung [6]

Hemodynamic changes in PH and advanced cirrhosis, characterized by increased cardiac output and normal or low PVR values, determined some authors to propose PVR > 120 $dyn \cdot s \cdot cm^{-5}$ as a cut off point for the POPH diagnosis. Most authors, however, accept the value of 240 $dyn \cdot s \cdot cm^{-5}$ [3].

21.2.5 Clinical Manifestations

Clinical symptoms are not specific, being dominated by the manifestations of PH. PAH symptoms appear late in evolution: exertional dyspnea, precordial pain, palpitations, syncope. The patient may have edema in the lower limbs, ascites but most often these are due to CLD and PH. Physical examination may reveal signs of PAH and chronic cor pulmonale. Auscultation of the heart may find signs of PAH: accentuation and widened splitting of S2 within the pulmonary artery area, rarely diastolic murmur of pulmonary regurgitation. Hypertrophy and dilation of the right ventricle (RV) may result in the widening of heart dullness area, the occurrence of the Harzer sign (palpation of RV pulsations in the epigastrium), the systolic murmur at the base of the xiphoid appendix which is accentuated during post inspiratory apnea and suggests tricuspid regurgitation. Decompensation of RV leads to right ventricular protodiastolic gallop, jugular turgescence and contributes together with CLD and PH to hepatomegaly, lower limb edema and ascites. Transjugular intrahepatic portosystemic shunt (TIPS) can aggravate POPH by suddenly overloading venous circulation.

21.2.6 Workup

Biochemical tests acknowledge liver disease and assess its severity.

Pulmonary radiography is performed in order to exclude other respiratory conditions that can lead to PAH and chronic cor pulmonale. Later, it can show cardiomegaly due to RV enlargement and increased cross-sectional diameter of the heart and also signs of PAH.

The ECG is not sensitive. Right axial deviation, clockwise rotation, right atrial (RA) and ventricular (RV) hypertrophy, asserting the chronic cor pulmonale, may be noticed late in evolution.

Respiratory functional tests show no specific changes. Sometimes the reduction of the CO transfer coefficient, the increase of the alveolar-arterial difference in O_2 and restrictive ventilatory dysfunction may be noted. Measurement of NO in exhaled air shows elevated levels in liver cirrhosis with and without POPH and reduced levels in idiopathic PAH [6].

Arterial blood gas test shows moderate to severe hypoxemia, hypocapnia and respiratory alkalosis as a consequence of hyperventilation. Changes in blood gases in POPH are more important than in hepatic cirrhosis without PAH and in idiopathic PAH [6].

Pulmonary ventilation/perfusion scintigraphy is most often normal, with no mosaic appearance as in thromboembolic pulmonary hypertension [6].

Lung angio-CT does not provide any specific diagnostic features but it is useful for the differential diagnosis with thromboembolic PAH.

Echocardiography is the screening exam most useful in detecting POPH in patients with PH.

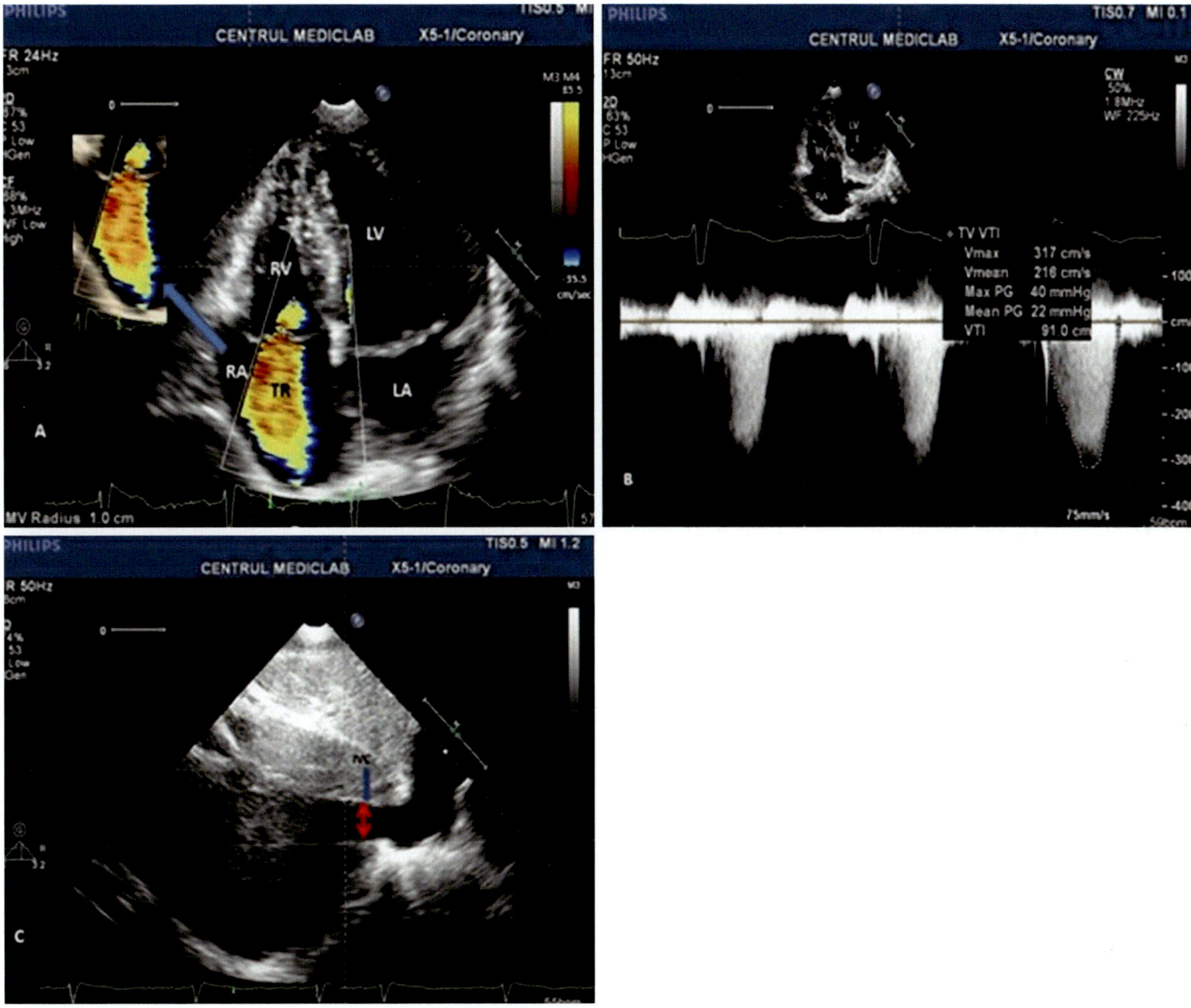

Fig. 21.2 Transthoracic echocardiographic evaluation of the sPAP (**a**) color Doppler tricuspid flow interrogation. Severe TR, with PISA (medallion). (**b**) continuous Doppler tricuspid flow interrogation. Maximal velocity of TR flow is 317 cm/s; maximal RV-RA gradient is 40 mmHg, according to the Bernoulli equation. (**c**) IVC diameter (2D evaluation) = 2 cm with <50% inspiratory collapse; sPAP = 40 + 10 mmHg. *RV* right ventricle, *RA* right atria, *LV* left ventricle, *LA* left atria, *IVC* inferior vena cava, *TR* tricuspid regurgitation, *sPAP* systolic pulmonary artery pressure, *PISA* proximal isvelocity surface area, *PG* pressure gradient

Pulmonary artery systolic pressure (sPAP) is determined by measuring the maximum velocity of the tricuspid regurgitation flow, applying the Bernoulli equation to determine the presumptive gradient between RV and RA and assessing the RA pressure through the diameter and inspiratory variations of IVC diameter (Fig. 21.2). PAH is defined by the increase in sPAP > 30 mmHg, with a positive predictive value of 59% and a negative predictive value of 100% [3]. sPAP over 50 mmHg denotes severe PAH with a positive predictive value of 74% and a negative predictive value of 97% [3] and requires cardiac catheterization.

mPAP can be determined by several formulas, using the pulmonary regurgitation signal (PR) or the acceleration time (AT) in the right ventricular outflow tract (RVOT). Using the peak PR velocity, mPAP can be approximated with the formula: mPAP = 4 (PR peak velocity)^2 + RA pressure. Using the end diastolic PR velocity, we can calculate the pulmonary artery diastolic pressure (dPAP) as 4 (end diastolic PR velocity)^2 + RA pressure. mPAP can be approximated by the formula mPAP = 2/3dPAP + 1/3sPAP. The normal value of AT in the RVOT is more than 100 ms while a value less than 100 ms is highly suggestive of PH. By this method mPAP is calculated as : mPAP = 90 − (0.62 × AT_{RVOT}).

In addition to sPAP and mPAP assessment, echocardiography is performed in order to **evaluate RV function** by measuring several parameters: TAPSE (abnormal limit < 1.7 cm), RV fractional area change (RVFAC) (abnormal limit < 35%), RV tissue Doppler S' velocity (abnormal limit < 10 cm/s). The RV size, volume and contractility can be more accurate assessed using 3D technique.

Echocardiography has become a mandatory test in PH patients and/or liver cirrhosis for POPH detection and for liver transplantation decision.

Right cardiac catheterization is the gold standard for the diagnosis of POPH. The increase of mPAP, PVR and normal values of PCWP are observed. The severity of POPH, essential for the indication of liver transplantation, can be assessed. Few studies suggest that POPH is less severe than idiopathic PAH. The NO vasodilatation test is usually negative and does not influence the therapeutic decision. Lack of NO response could be explained by endogenous NO production in POPH compared to idiopathic PAH [6].

Differential diagnosis stands for the other causes of PH classified according to the European Guidelines of Pulmonary Hypertension system [2]. Medical history, clinical examination and laboratory tests bring elements for differential diagnosis and cardiac catheterization identifies essential diagnostic features.

21.2.7 Pharmacological Treatment

- **Vasodilators** used in idiopathic PAH are less efficient in the treatment of POPH.
  - However, the vasodilatatory prostaglandin epoprostenol (PGI2) and its synthetic analogues iloprost and treprostinil, have been shown to be effective in the treatment of POPH. They also decrease the platelet aggregation. Epoprostenol i.v improves pulmonary hemodynamics but increases the incidence of ascites and splenomegaly. Its administration requires permanent central venous access and abrupt cessation of the infusion leads to rebound pulmonary vasoconstriction. Awdish et al. studied the efficiency of epoprostenol in 21 patients with POPH between 2002–2012. After 15.4 months of treatment there was an improvement in mPAP, PVR, cardiac index without deterioration of the liver tests [8]. However, the survival was not improved compared to patients without epoprostenol. The data are inconclusive for dermal or inhalatory administration. There are isolated data showing good results with iloprost iv or inhaled for 1 year [3, 6]. Oral treprostinil did not improve the exercise capacity in patients with PAH included in FREEDOM-C study [9].
  - Bosentan, an ET_A and ET_B endothelin receptor antagonist, causes hepatic cytolysis and can only be administered to patients with mild hepatic impairment, class A Child-Pugh. In these patients it can be administered over a long time following epoprostenol. It has the advantage of oral administration. There have been reports of clinical and hemodynamic improvement following bosentan administration for over 1 year [6]. Ambrisentan, a selective ET_A antagonist, is associated with liver toxicity. Macitentan is a dual antagonist of ET_A and ET_B approved for the treatment of the PAH [9], without studies in POPH. It could have an advantage over other endothelin receptor antagonists regarding the liver function which deteriorates in less patients on macitentan than in patients on placebo in SERPAHIN study [9].
  - Sildenafil and tadalafil, are type 5 phosphodiesterase blockers and can also be used in patients with advanced liver disease alone or associated with inhaled epoprostenol. Reichenberger et al. showed that treatment with sildenafil for 12 months increased exercise capacity and improved heart failure functional class throughout the follow-up period in 14 patients with moderate-to-severe POPH. Hemodynamic improvement occurred in the first 3 months of treatment (significant mPAP and PVR reduction) but was not sustained at 12 months [10]. In severe POPH sildenafil alone might not be efficient [3]
  - Riociguat is a soluble guanylyl cyclase (sGC) stimulator that increases cGMP syntheses and vasodilatation. It is approved for the treatment of group 1 PAH but there is little clinical experience in POPH [9]
  - Ca-channel blockers are not indicated because in POPH the NO pulmonary vasodilatation test is usually negative. In addition, Ca-channel blockers can produce mesenteric vasodilatation and may worsen PH [6].
- Beta blockers are not indicated in POPH but they can be used for PH or heart failure.
- Anticoagulants are contraindicated because of the coexistence of liver disease.
- Oxygen therapy is indicated if Pa O_2 < 60 mmHg at rest
- Loop and antialdosteronic diuretics are indicated for the treatment of hydrosaline retention and right heart decompensation.

21.2.8 Liver Transplantation in Patients with POPH

- Liver transplant is contraindicated in the presence of POPH with mPAP values >35 mmHg and PVR > 250 dyn s cm^{-5} [6]. After liver transplant, volume load increases in pulmonary circulation and POPH may worsen. Liver transplant can be performed in patients with mPAP < 35 mmHg at rest and PVR < 250 dyn s cm^{-5}, spontaneous or after vasodilator treatment. The transplant indication may be extended to patients with mPAP 35–50 mmHg if the PVR is <250 dyn s cm^{-5} and particularly <120 dyn s cm^{-5}. Very rarely POPH is improved after liver transplant and epoprostenol treatment can be reduced. POPH improvement after liver transplant occurs especially in patients with previously PVR <240 dyn s cm^{-5} [3]. However, the progression of POPH after liver transplant is also mentioned.

Surveillance of patients with POPH involves echocardiography once or twice a year. Patients with PH or liver cirrhosis without POPH should perform echocardiography once a year for the active detection of POPH, as its clinical manifestations are nonspecific and deferred.

21.2.9 Prognosis

The occurrence of PAH in patients with liver cirrhosis limits survival, but epidemiological data are different between different studies. **Survival at 5 years in patients with cirrhosis and mPAP > 50 mmHg is reported between 10% and 50%** [1]. Survival of patients with POPH seems inferior to those with idiopathic PH. Poor prognostic factors are reduced cardiac output and severe hepatic dysfunction. Swanson et al. showed in a group of 74 POPH patients followed between 1994–2007 that the 5-year mortality was 86% in untreated POPH patients, 55% in those with pharmacological treatment and 33% in those with pharmacological treatment and liver transplant. 54% of untreated patients died in the first year of diagnosis [11]. Perioperative mortality in POPH patients with liver transplant is on average 36% [12]. Perioperative mortality varies with the severity of POPH. Patients with moderate PAH (mPAP between 35–45 mmHg) have a perioperative mortality of approximately 50% following liver transplant. Almost all patients with severe POPH (mPAP>50 mmHg) die after liver transplantation [13].

21.3 Hepato Pulmonary Syndrome (HPS)

21.3.1 Definition

Hepato-pulmonary syndrome (HPS) associates CLD or PH with increased $P(A\text{-}a)O_2 \geq 15$ mmHg or >20 mmHg for patients >65 years old while breathing ambient air, hypoxemia ($PaO_2 < 80$ mmHg) and intrapulmonary vascular dilation demonstrated by contrast-enhanced echocardiography or lung perfusion scanning [3]. However, some patients do not have hypoxemia at least at the beginning of the disease. The concept was introduced in 1977 by Kennedy and Kudson [3].

21.3.2 Epidemiology

HPS has a prevalence of 1% in patients with CLD or PH but it increases to 30% in those proposed for hepatic transplantation [3]. Intra-pulmonary shunts or abnormalities of the oxygenation are more common, being cited in 5% of patients with cirrhosis and 25–65% of those with advanced hepatic disease proposed for hepatic transplantation [3]. It is generally manifested in the sixth decade of life.

21.3.3 Risk Factors

HPS is associated with hepatic cirrhosis and PH, but can also occur in patients with PH of another cause, especially Budd Chiari syndrome or in patients with chronic hepatitis, acute liver failure, hypoxic hepatitis. There are no correlations between the etiology of hepatitis, the sex of the patient and the prevalence of HPS. The severity of hepatic impairment assessed by Child Pugh and MELD scores is not correlated with the occurrence of HPS, although there is evidence that HPS is more common in patients with advanced hepatic disease.

21.3.4 Pathology

In HPS there is a pathological process of distal pulmonary vascular remodeling in the precapillary arterioles and pulmonary capillaries that dilate, producing pulmonary arterio-venous anastomoses that do not respect the alveolar-capillary units and porto-pulmonary anastomoses [6]. Vascular dilation is diffuse but more important within lower lobes. The arterio-venous anastomoses developed within the pleura were called "spider naevi".

21.3.5 Pathophysiology (Fig. 21.1)

HPS is characterized by pulmonary vasodilation which leads to an increase in the alveolar capillary gradient in O_2 and hypoxemia through several mechanisms:

- Ventilation-perfusion (V/Q) mismatch within the excessively perfused areas due to vasodilation
- The appearance of intrapulmonary shunts due to arterio-venous anastomoses.
- Reduction of O_2 diffusion due to increased distance between the alveoli and capillaries
- The transit time of the red blood cells through pulmonary capillaries is decreased due to hyperdynamic circulation typical for cirrhosis. This reduces contact time with the alveolar air and therefore the gas exchange [3].

The cause of pulmonary vasodilation is unclear and several hypotheses are discussed (Fig. 21.1).

- There is an increased production of endothelial NO (eNO) and inducible (iNO). Dysfunctional liver would excessively produce ET1 that reaches the lungs and stimulates the production of ET_B receptors within the pulmonary microcirculation. They stimulate the production of eNO.
- The mesenteric blood stasis due to PH allows the gram-negative intestinal bacteria to entry into blood stream. Endotoxemia stimulates the production of inflammatory mediators, like tumor necrosis factor alfa (TNF-α) and Haem-oxygenase that accumulates within the lung and attracts macrophages. These are seized within microcirculation and stimulate the production of iNO. Haem–oxygenase catalyzes the degradation of heme and produces carbon monoxide (CO) which acts as vasodilator and promoter of neovascular growth.
- Vascular endothelial growth factor (VEGF) is upregulated and increases the angiogenesis
- There is an increased levels of estrogen and progesterone in the context of liver failure
- There may be specific genetic pattern related to the polymorphisms in genes involved in the regulation of angiogenesis [14].

Arterial deoxygenation is more important in orthostatism, a phenomenon called orthodeoxia. The patient is dyspneic in orthostatism. Increasing perfusion in pulmonary bases in orthostatism accentuates the V/Q imbalance and shunt effect. Arterial oxygenation and dyspnea are relieved by recumbence, a phenomenon called platypnoea [1].

In HPS hypoxemia improves with 100% O_2 administration, in contrast to true intrapulmonary shunt [4].

Clinical manifestations are not specific. Symptoms are common with those of liver disease and PH. The patient experiences exertional dyspnea, physical asthenia and physical examination reveals vascular stars, clubbing, central cyanosis. Orthodeoxia and platypnoea are described as specific signs of HPS, but they are only present in some patients. HPS may coexist with other cardiac and lung diseases that can cause hypoxemia. The increase in stroke prevalence by paradoxical emboli was noted [3].

21.3.6 Workup

Laboratory tests assess the severity of liver disease and its overall impact.

Pulmonary radiography has no characteristic features. It is useful for differential diagnosis. Sometimes an increased interstitial pattern in the bases is described. Cardiomegaly occurs late by RV dilation.

High resolution computed tomography may highlight the early occurrence of pulmonary vessels dilation within the lung bases.

The ECG does not show specific features but may show late signs of RV and RA hypertrophy.

Respiratory function tests record CO transfer coefficient reduction and increased $P(A\text{-}a)O_2$ [3].

O_2 saturation (SaO_2) $\geq 96\%$ excludes $PaO_2 < 70$ mmHg with a sensitivity of 100% and a specificity of 88%. $SaO_2 < 95\%$ is not well correlated with PaO_2 that can vary ±10 mmHg in patients with cirrhosis for the same values of SaO_2.

Arterial blood gas analysis with the determination of $P(A\text{-}a)O_2$ performed during breathing in the ambient air is the screening test for the diagnosis of HPS [3]. Hypoxemia occurs and the $P(A\text{-}a)O_2$ increases above 15 mmHg. The increase in $P(A\text{-}a)O_2$ occurs early in HPS evolution and PaO_2 is the most important prognostic factor. Two other cut-off values have been proposed for $(Pa\text{-}Pa)O_2$: 20 mmHg and age correlated values, which would increase the negative predictive value of the diagnosis. The $P(A\text{-}a)O_2$ in relation to age can be calculated with the following formula: $P(A\text{-}a)O_2 = 10 + 0.43$ (age in years—20). PaO_2 level is a HPS severity classification criterion, although the patient is hyperventilated and PaO_2 underestimates the oxygenation deficiency.

Measurement of blood gases both in the supine and upright position can reveal the orthodeoxia, defined as a decrease in PaO2 of ≥4 mmHg or ≥5% of the supine value. However, the change in PaO_2 from supine to upright is not a screening test for the diagnosis of HPS [16]. Most patients have oxygen desaturation during sleep [16]. Inhaled 100% O_2 increases PaO_2.

Pulmonary perfusion scintigraphy using macro-aggregated albumin (diameter > 20 μm) marked with ^{99m}Tc (MAA scan) assesses pulmonary vasodilatation by measuring the proportion of macroaggregates that reach beyond the lung. Albumin macro aggregates are normally collected within the lung capillaries. If there are arteriolar-capillary vasodilation and arterio-venous anastomoses the pulmonary capillary barrier is surpassed and the macroaggregates get extrapulmonary, basically in the brain. The capture of >6% macroaggregates within the brain has a diagnostic specificity of nearly 100% [3, 15]. However, the method is not part of the mandatory diagnostic tests to be performed in the HPS. It is used in patients who associate chronic hypoxemic pulmonary parenchymal diseases.

21.3.7 Echocardiography

Classical transthoracic echocardiography does not offer specific elements. Dilation of right heart cavities can be highlighted, but cirrhosis not complicated with HPS may result in dilation of the right atrium due to hyperdynamic

Table 21.1 Quantitative classification of the intrapulmonary shunt

No shunt	No microbubbles
Stage 1	<30 microbubbles
Stage 2	30–100 microbubbles
Stage 3	>100 microbubbles

circulation. **The diagnostic technique of choice is contrast-enhanced echocardiography** used for detecting the cause of the right atrial dilation. In HPS microbubbles (≤90 μm in diameter) obtained after injection of 10 ml normal saline that has been hand-agitated pass lately from the right atrium into the left atrium after more than four heart cycles. In the atrial septal defect opacification of the left atrium occurs in the first three cycles after the right atrium opacification. The technique can also be applied during transesophageal echocardiography [3]. There is a quantitative classification of the intrapulmonary shunt using the number of microbubbles passing in the left ventricle during the contrast-enhanced echocardiography (Table 21.1) [16].

Contrast-enhanced echocardiography and MAA scan are the gold standard test for the diagnosis of HPS.

Pulmonary angiography may be normal or may reveal diffuse vascular dilation and arterio-venous anastomoses. Early vascular dilations have spidery appearance and advanced vascular dilations appear spongy. From angiographic point of view, HPS is classified as type I with normal angiography or diffuse vascular dilations and type II with arterio-venous anastomoses. Pulmonary angiography has no well-established role in diagnosis of HPS. Pulmonary angiography was proposed to be performed in patients with PaO_2 maintained <300 mmHg after breathing 100% O_2. These patients have pulmonary arterio-venous anastomoses and their hypoxemia usually does not improve after liver transplantation [3].

21.3.8 HPS Classification

HPS is classified according to PaO_2 level:

- **Mild $PaO_2 \geq 80$ mmHg**
- **Moderate PaO_2 60–80 mmHg**
- **Severe PaO_2 50–60 mmHg**
- **Very severe $PaO_2 < 50$ mmHg**

21.3.9 HPS Prognosis

Hypoxemia progresses on average by 5 mmHg/year. Progression may also occur in patients with stable liver disease. Mortality at 2.5 years is between 40–60%. There is a higher prevalence of stroke and paradoxical embolism.

Hypoxemia does not improve after liver transplant in patients with pulmonary arterio-venous anastomoses. The identification of these patients requires contrast enhanced echocardiography, pulmonary angiography and the calculation of the extrapulmonary shunt fraction. These patients may improve by performing pulmonary anastomoses embolization before liver transplant.

21.3.10 HPS Treatment

Hepatic transplantation is the treatment of choice in HPS. Immediately postoperatively hypoxia may worsen, causing high postoperative mortality in the past (16%) but in the recent years postoperative mortality decreased. Six months after the transplantation patients no longer need O_2 but HPS may recur later in patients with hepatic allograft becoming dysfunctional. Among the prognostic factors for postoperative mortality are:

- $PaO_2 \leq 50$ mmHg in room air with 67% predictive positive value and 93% negative predictive value,
- extrapulmonary shunt fraction>20% with 64% positive and negative 100% predictive value [17, 18].

21.3.11 Pharmacological Treatment

Methylene blue decreases the sGC stimulation by NO and the vasodilation and have some favorable results in small groups of patients by intravenous route of administration but is not currently used in practice [4, 16].

Octreotide is a somatostatin analog inhibiting the angiogenesis but does not improve the hypoxemia in HPS. Sorafenib inhibits tyrosine kinase receptor and the production of eNO and also inhibits VEGF dependent angiogenesis [16]. There are also therapeutic attempts with pentoxifylline as a anti TNF-α inhibitor, N(G)-nitro-L-arginine-methyl ester which is a nitric oxide synthetase inhibitor, the vasoconstrictor almitrine bismesylate or garlic.

21.3.12 Conclusions

POPH and HPS are infrequent complications of the PH associated or not with CLD. Their occurrence seems related to the hyperkinetic circulation and to the existence of porto-systemic anastomoses but their mechanisms are different and not fully understood.

In POPH there is pulmonary arterial vasoconstriction and pathological pulmonary vascular features similar to those in idiopathic PH. In HPS there is dilation of the pulmonary pre capillary arterioles and pulmonary capillaries, pulmonary

Table 21.2 Differences between POPH and HPS

	POPH	HPS
Definition	• mPAP > 25 mmHg resting; >30 mmHg during the exercise **AND** • PVR > 240 dyne·s·cm^{-5} or >3 u wood **AND** • PCWP or LVEDP ≤ 15 mmHg	• $P(A\text{-}a)O_2 \geq 15$ mmHg • $\pm PaO_2 < 80$ mmHg • Intrapulmonary vascular dilations
Pathological features	• Pulmonary arteries muscular hypertrophy • Endothelial proliferation • Adventiceal proliferation • Plexiform arterial lesions • In situ thrombosis • Microaneurysms in pulmonary arteries	• Arteriolar and capillary dilations • Pulmonary arterio-venous anastomosis • Porto-pulmonary anastomosis
Clinical features	• Non characteristic	• Non characteristic • Sometimes orthodeoxia; platypnoea • Stroke by paradoxical embolism
Screening tests	• TTE	• Arterial gases in ambient air with the determination of $P(A\text{-}a)O_2$
Gold standard test	• Right cardiac catheterization	• Contrast-enhanced echocardiography • MAA scan
Treatment	• Inconstant efficiency of the pulmonary vasodilation therapy • moderate or severe POPH is a contraindication for the hepatic transplantation	• Hepatic transplantation

POHP porto-pulmonary hypertension, *HPS* hepato-pulmonary syndrome, *TTE* transthoracic echocardiography, *mPAP* mean pulmonary arterial pressure, *PVR* pulmonary vascular resistance, *PCWP* pulmonary capillary wedge pressure, *LVEDP* left ventricular end diastolic pressures, *MAA* macro-aggregated albumin

arterio-venous anastomoses, increased $P(A\text{-}a)O_2$ and hypoxemia. The severity of the POPH depends on the level of increased mPAP. The severity of the HPS depends on the level of decreased PaO_2. The clinic is non specific in both POPH and HPS. Some patients with HPS have orthodeoxia, platypnoea and high risk of stroke by paradoxical embolism. The screening test for POPH is TTE and the gold standard is right cardiac catheterization. The screening test for HPS is the determination of the arterial gases in ambient air with the determination of $P(A\text{-}a)O_2$. Breathing 100% O_2 normalizes hypoxemia. The gold standard tests for HPS are contrast enhanced echocardiography and MAA scan. Both POPH and HPS are deleterious for the prognosis. The pulmonary vasodilation therapy is less efficient in POPH than in other forms of PH. Moderate or severe POPH is a contraindication for the hepatic transplantation. HPS improves after hepatic transplantation. (Table 21.2).

Self Study

Questions

1. A 57 years old woman with post necrotic hepatic cirrhosis and portal hypertension is admitted in the hospital for dyspnoea to minimal efforts. Electrocardiography: sinus tachycardia, right ventricular hypertrophy. Transthoracic echocardiography: right ventricular and right atrial dilation, mPAP 50 mmHg. Child Pugh score is B. Her treatment involves Propranolol 60 mg/day, Spironolactone 150 mg/day, Isodinitmononitrate 40 mg/day. What is the best therapeutic decision?
   (a) Including the patient on the liver transplant list
   (b) Sildenafil
   (c) Bosentan
   (d) Anticoagulation
   (e) Changing propranolol with bisoprolol

2. What is true about the hepato-pulmonary syndrome?
   (a) The prevalence in chronic liver disease is 50%
   (b) It occurs especially in patients with posthepatitis cirrhosis
   (c) Sildenafil is the most useful treatment
   (d) It improves after hepatic transplantation
   (e) The gold standard test for diagnosis is right cardiac catheterization

Answers

1. A 57 years old woman with post necrotic hepatic cirrhosis and portal hypertension is admitted in the hospital for dyspnoea to minimal efforts. Electrocardiography: sinus tachycardia, right ventricular hypertrophy. Transthoracic echocardiography: right ventricular and right atrial dilation, mPAP 50 mmHg. Child Pugh score is B. Her treatment involves Propranolol 60 mg/day, Spironolactone 150 mg/day, Isodinitmononitrate 40 mg/day. What is the best therapeutic decision?
   (b) Medium and severe POPH is a contraindication for the liver transplantation. Bosentan worsens the hepatic function. The anticoagulation increases the hemorrhagic risk in a patient with hepatic cirrhosis.

The non selective beta blockers are indicated in PH and not the selective one.

2. What is true about the hepato-pulmonary syndrome?
   (d) The prevalence of the HPS in chronic liver disease is 1% and 30% in those proposed for hepatic transplantation. It doesn't matter the etiology of the liver disease. Sildenafil can be used in POPH not in HPS. The gold standard test for diagnosis is MAA scan.

Future Perspectives

The effort must be do to better understand the pathophysiology of POPH and HPS. There is a possible genetic determination of the occurrence of the POPH and HPS. Future studies must bring additional data with regard to genetic status involved in POPH and HPS. The early diagnosis is very important for improving the treatment and therefore we need new methods.

References

1. Hoeper MM, Krowka MJ, Strassburg CP. Portopulmonary hypertension and hepatopulmonary syndrome. Lancet. 2004;363:1461–8.
2. The Joint Task Force for the Diagnosis and Treatment of Pulmonary Hypertension of the European Society of Cardiology (ESC) and the European Respiratory Society (ERS). 2015 ESC/ERS Guidelines for the diagnosis and treatment of pulmonary hypertension. Eur Heart J. 2016;37:67–119.
3. Porres-Aguilar M, Altamirano JT, Torre-Delgadillo A, Charlton MR, Rojo AD. Portopulmonary hypertension and hepatopulmonary syndrome: a clinician-oriented overview. Eur Respir Rev. 2012;21(125):223–33.
4. Bartolome SD, Krowka MJ. Pulmonary complications of intra-abdominal disease, part 13. In: Fishman's pulmonary diseases and disorders. 5th ed. New York: McGraw-Hill; 2015. p. 2496-1508, ISBN: 978-1-25-958912-6.
5. Kawut SM, Krowka MJ, Trotter JF, et al. Clinical risk factors for portopulmonary hypertension. Hepatology. 2008;48:196–203.
6. Chabot F, Gomez E, Boyer L, Kheir A, Le Pavec J, Sitbon O, Herve P. Hypertension portopulmonaire. Rev Mal Respir. 2006;23:629–41.
7. Roberts KE, Fallon MB, Krowka MJ, et al. Genetic risk factors for portopulmonary hypertension in patients with advanced liver disease. Am J Respir Crit Care Med. 2009;179:835–42.
8. Awdish RLA, Cajigas HR. Early initiation of prostacyclin in Portopulmonary hypertension: 10 years of a transplant center's experience. Lung. 2013;191(6):593–600.
9. DUBrock HM, Channick RN, Krowka MJ. What's new in the treatment of portopulmonary hypertension? Expert Rev Gastroenterol Hepatol. 2015;9:983–92. https://doi.org/10.1586/17474124.2015.1035647.
10. Reichenberger F, Voswinckel R, Steveling E, Enke B, Kreckel A, Olschewski H, Grimminger F, Seeger W, Ghofrani HA. Sildenafil treatment for portopulmonary hypertension. Eur Respir J. 2006;28:563–7.
11. Swanson K, Wiesner R, Nyeberg S, Rosen CB, Krowka MJ. Survival in portopulmonary hypertension: Mayo Clinic experience categorized by treatment subgroups. Am J Transplant. 2008;8:2445–53.
12. Mandal MS, Krowda MJ. Formation of national database on pulmonary hypertension and hepatopulmonary syndrome in chronic liver disease. Anesthesiology. 1997;87:450–1.
13. Wells JT, Runo JR, Lucey MR. Portopulmonary hypertension. Hepatology. 2008;48(1):13–5.
14. Roberts KE, Kawut SM, Krowka|| MJ, et al. Genetic risk factors for hepatopulmonary syndrome in patients with advanced liver disease. Gastroenterology. 2010;139(1):130–9.
15. Abrams GA, Nanda NC, Dubrovsky EV, et al. Use of macroaggregated albumin lung perfusion scan to diagnose hepatopulmonary syndrome: a new approach. Gastroenterology. 1998;114:305–10.
16. Soulaidopoulos S, Cholongitas E, Giannakoulas G, et al. Review article: Update on current and emergent data on hepatopulmonary syndrome. World J Gastroenterol. 2018;24(12):1285–98.
17. Arguedas MR, Abrams GA, Krowka MJ, Fallon MB. Prospective evaluation of outcomes and predictors of mortality in patients with hepatopulmonary syndrome undergoing liver transplantation. Hepatology. 2003;37(1):192–7.
18. Arguedas MR, Fallon MB. Hepatopulmonary syndrome. Curr Treat Options Gastroenterol. 2005;8(6):451–6.

Further Reading

DuBrock HM, Channick RN, Krowka MJ. What's new in the treatment of portopulmonary hypertension? Expert Rev Gastroenterol Hepatol. 2015;9(7):983–92. https://doi.org/10.1586/17474124.2015.1035647.

EASL Clinical Practice Guidelines. Liver transplantation. J Hepatol. 2016;64(2):433–85. https://doi.org/10.1016/j.jhep.2015.10.006.

Fritz JS, Fallon MB, Kawut SM. Pulmonary vascular complication of liver diseases. Am J Respir Crit Care Med. 2013;187(2):133–9.

Soulaidopoulos S, Cholongitas E, Giannakoulas G, et al. Review article: Update on current and emergent data on hepatopulmonary syndrome. World J Gastroenterol. 2018;24(12):1285–98.

Hepatic Abscesses

22

Bogdan Dorobanţu

Key Concepts
- Bacterial aetiology should be consider facing hepatic abscess
- Ascendant biliary contamination is the most common mechanism of HA
- Untreated pyogenic liver abscesses are fatal in 95–100% of cases
- Antibiotherapy associated with drainage or, in selected cases, liver resection is the main treatment
- In case of cryptogenic HA colonoscopy should be consider as colonic cancer can be involved

22.1 Definition

A hepatic abscess (HA) is a purulent collection, single or multiple, developed intrahepatically.

22.2 History

Hippocrates [1] (c. 400 BC) was among the first to recognize liver abscess as an entity, speculating even the importance of the features of the lesion fluid on disease prognosis. At the beginning of the nineteenth century Bright [2], later Fitz [3] and then Dieulafoy [4], suggested the pathogenic involvement of amoebas in the aetiology of liver abscesses, the first case of amoebaean abscess was documented by Osler in 1890. Ochsner and De Bakey [5, 6] described hepatic abscesses and their treatment at the end of the fourth decade of the nineteenth century; patient typology being represented by young males with abdominal diseases (the most common cause at the time being pylephlebitis secondary to appendicitis—Dieulafoy [4] introducing the term "foie appendiculaire").

22.3 Incidence

The incidence of liver abscesses has remained broadly unchanged over the last 60 years, with a prevalence of approximately 8–16 cases per 100,000 hospitalizations [7], but with changes seen in the age groups, shifting from decades 3–4 to decades 4–6, with increased incidence in patients over 60 years. At the same time, though incidence was known to be increased in men, at the moment the gap is closing (with the exception of amoebaean abscesses, in which case the ratio is 9–10: 1 ♂: ♀) [7].

22.4 Classification

Liver abscesses have been divided according to distribution of lesions, size, clinical features and type of treatment necessary, into macro- and microabscesses. Thus, liver macroabscesses are usually single or confluent, limited to a lobe of the liver (55% of cases present in the posterior segments of the right hemi-liver), with subacute symptoms and requiring drainage. Macroabscesses can be complicated by intraperitoneal fissure and secondary peritonitis, rupture into the pleural or pericardial cavity, rupture into a hollow organ.

B. Dorobanţu (✉)
"Carol Davila" University of Medicine and Pharmacy, Bucharest, Romania

"Dan Setlacec" Centre for General Surgery and Liver Transplantation, Fundeni Clinical Institute, Bucharest, Romania

F. Radu-Ionita et al. (eds.), *Liver Diseases*, https://doi.org/10.1007/978-3-030-24432-3_22

Microabscesses represent 35% of cases, are multiple, bilateral, with acute clinical forms and requiring medical treatment aimed at the primary lesion [8].

22.5 Aetiopathogeny

Liver abscesses may have bacterial aetiology (specific or nonspecific), fungal or amoebaean.

The vast majority of liver abscesses are caused by gastrointestinal flora (over 75%) with Escherichia coli being primarily incriminated (35–45%), followed by Klebsiella pneumoniae (more severe infection associated with the formation of gas bubbles, and more common in diabetic patients), and Staphylococcus aureus and group A streptococci in approximately 20–25% of cases [7].

The incidence of anaerobic microorganisms is lower (possibly due to technical difficulties in isolating them). The most common are Bacteroides fragilis, Fusobacterium spp. and Clostridium spp. By using appropriate micro bacteriological methods, abscesses determined by microaerophilic streptococci were also highlighted (S. milleri being extremely aggressive [9]). Introducing new microbiological methods showed significant decrease in the number of cryptogenic abscesses was reported (down to 13%, and up to 90% positive cultures).

Abscesses due to different Candida species occur mainly in liver transplant patients or in those receiving chemotherapy for leukaemia [10].

In the case of pyogenic abscesses several mechanisms have been described:

1. Ascendant biliary contamination the most common route of contamination, extrahepatic ductal obstruction (as a result of lithiasis, biliary or pancreatic cancer, or iatrogenic) and secondary cholangitis representing 30–50% of cases [11–14].

   In case of complete obstruction associated with increased pressure in the biliary tree the so-called "acute suppurative cholangitis" occurs, with miliary microabscesses, or single macroscopic abscesses if the obstruction is not complete. The same ascendant mechanism is incriminated in case of hepatic cysts contamination (hydatid or serous), and Caroli disease [15].
2. Haematogenous contamination via two dissemination routes: portal and arterial.

   In the first case, hepatic abscesses develop by suppurative thrombophlebitis of the portal vein secondary to appendicitis, diverticulitis, pancreatitis and infected haemorrhoids [6, 11, 12].

   Hepatic arterial infection can occur due to systemic bacteraemia (most commonly miliary microabscesses), to hepatic artery thrombosis after liver transplantation (more common in children) [16–18], or in hepatic artery therapeutic embolization (haemobilia, liver tumours) [19, 20]
3. Hepatic trauma (penetrative or non-penetrative) can be complicated by abscesses, by necrosis, haemorrhage and bile leak at their level, or iatrogenic following surgical manoeuvres [21] (hepatorrhaphies bringing the wound edges closer have been forbidden).
4. Direct contamination by propagation of a neighbouring infectious process (purulent cholecystitis, subphrenic abscess, perforation of the stomach or intestine) [22, 23]
5. Other mechanisms may include liver tumour necrosis, subsequent to biliary stents, liver biopsies, in the treatment of liver tumours by cryotherapy or radiofrequency ablation, or trans catheter chemoembolization via the hepatic artery [24–27]. There is also the possibility of 15–20% of cases developing abscesses without an obvious cause, which fall into the category of idiopathic liver abscesses—lately colonic lesions with mucosal defects were considered colonic causes of part of these abscess [28].

22.6 Diagnosis

22.6.1 Clinical Manifestations

Clinical diagnosis of liver abscesses is difficult because of nonspecific semiology, in many cases the only symptom being fever. Associated to fever one can register other nonspecific symptoms as well, such as fatigue, nausea, vomiting, abdominal pain, which dominate the clinical picture. Depending on the pathogen, specific symptoms may appear: jaundice for biliary obstruction (HA patients of biliary aetiology usually address the hospital sooner), heart failure syndrome in case of endocarditis. In general, microabscesses present acute symptoms, with fever, chills, profuse sweating, right upper quadrant pain, impaired general state to the extent of shock, liver failure. In case of macroabscesses the symptoms are subacute, lasting from several days to several weeks, with fever (90% of cases), vomiting (50–75%), night sweats, anorexia, and weight loss. Rarely, for abscesses ruptured into the abdomen, the clinical picture may become acute, with peritonitis and septic shock [12, 24, 29].

22.6.2 Imaging Explorations

Due to lack of specificity of symptoms, in most cases the diagnosis of HA is the prerogative of imaging methods, which as a result of the development of ultrasound and computed tomography in the '70s make it possible to establish an early diagnosis and even constitutes a method of treatment (percutaneous drainage guided by ultrasound or CT scan).

Ultrasound is the "front line" investigation and allows establishing a diagnosis to an accuracy of 85–95% (for lesions over 2 cm). CT scan and lately even FDG PET/CT (in metastatic liver disease) has the highest sensitivity (95–100%) for diagnosing HA larger than 0.5 cm and can detect the original focus [30].

Magnetic resonance imaging offers data comparable to ultrasound and CT, but is less accessible due to costs. Associated with the administration of a contrast agent (MRCP or angioMRI) it allows for obtaining fine details of the biliary tree and liver vascularization that can be useful, as well as differentiating abscesses under 3 mm from other lesions (haemangioma or metastasis) [31, 32].

Simple radiography can detect right lung atelectasis, elevation of the right hemidiaphragm or reactive pleural effusion, and in case of gas forming microorganism abscesses it can highlight air-fluid levels in the liver area [7].

22.6.3 Laboratory Tests

Biological tests are not specific and generally reflect inflammatory syndrome. In almost all cases of pyogenic abscesses, liver and blood tests are modified, leucocytosis being present in over 75% of cases (its absence does not exclude the diagnosis of HA) and anaemia being found in 50–65% of patients. In what concerns liver function tests, increased alkaline phosphatase was observed in 74% of patients and increased bilirubin in 40%. Blood cultures are positive in approximately 50% of cases [33].

22.6.4 Differential Diagnosis

The differential diagnosis is difficult to conduct due to often unspecific clinical manifestations, difficulty in the differential diagnosis of clinical hepatic abscesses with acute cholecystitis, cholangitis, subphrenic or subhepatic abscesses, liver tumors (entities that can determine in turn abscesses), hepatic hydatid cyst, in this context being understandable. Even in the presence of modern imaging methods, there are situations in which preoperative diagnosis of HAs is not easy to specify. Thus, suppurations with multiple microabscesses, with liver parenchyma carnification may take some pseudotumoral shapes that make them difficult to distinguish by imaging methods and even intraoperatively from abscessed tumours, and vice versa, lesions with clinical and imaging features suggestive of liver metastases having provided surprises after puncture biopsy or histopathology exam, the final diagnosis being that of multiple hepatic abscesses. The same diagnostic difficulties arise in the presence of necrotic tissue, blood clots or purulent macroabscesses.

22.7 Evolution

Untreated pyogenic liver abscesses are fatal in 95–100% of cases, death occurring due to subsequent rupture and/or sepsis. Spontaneous drainage often occurs into the peritoneum or pleural cavity, usually determining septic shock and death of the patient (they can rarely spontaneously drain externally or into the bowels—favourable prognosis). Prognostic factors are represented by age, number of abscesses and number of aetiological agents involved, along with the association of malignant lesions or other conditions of immunosuppression. In addition, hypoalbuminemia, hyperbilirubinemia and significant increase in blood level urea in turn appear as the main laboratory factors associated with a poor prognosis [7].

22.8 Treatment

Treatment of liver abscesses is different depending on the type and pathogenesis of the lesion, the biological status and age of the patient, addressing the cause of HA being always mandatory.

The main methods of treatment used in HA along with antibiotics and addressing the original cause are **drainage** (*percutaneous*—under ultrasound or CT guidance, and *surgical drainage*) or **liver resection**. The choice of method depends on the localization, size and multiplicity of the abscess in accordance with the biological state of the patient or the presence of an abdominal pathology that requires per primam surgical intervention (sometimes indicated in the combination of these methods).

In case of liver microabscesses (single or multiply disseminated) where drainage is impossible, treatment consists in *antibiotherapy*. Antibiotics may be administered in combination (e.g. betalactamines, aminoglycosides and metronidazole) or alone (broad-spectrum antibiotics) for a period that can vary between 3–12 weeks (some authors recommend 2 weeks iv administration followed by 4 weeks of oral administration) [7]. In case of limited hepatic area localization of microabscesses and antibiotic inefficiency, liver resection may be a therapeutic option (but with a poor prognosis).

Pyogenic macroabscesses benefit from **percutaneous drainage** under CT or ultrasound guidance as the treatment of choice, associated with antibiotherapy with a success rate of between 85–90% [34]. Most liquefied abscesses and even multiloculate ones can be drained through a single catheter, with eviction of content (and bacteriological sampling!). Subsequent to drainage, the remaining cavity should be followed-up by imaging methods to monitor its effectiveness. Complications of drainage can be represented by sepsis secondary to abscess handling, haemorrhage, pneumothorax,

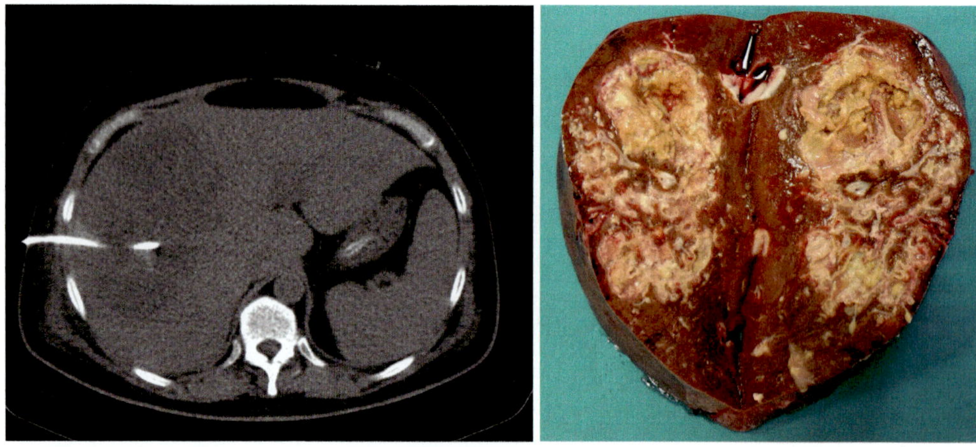

Fig. 22.1 Percutaneous drainage inefficiency followed by right hemiliver resection

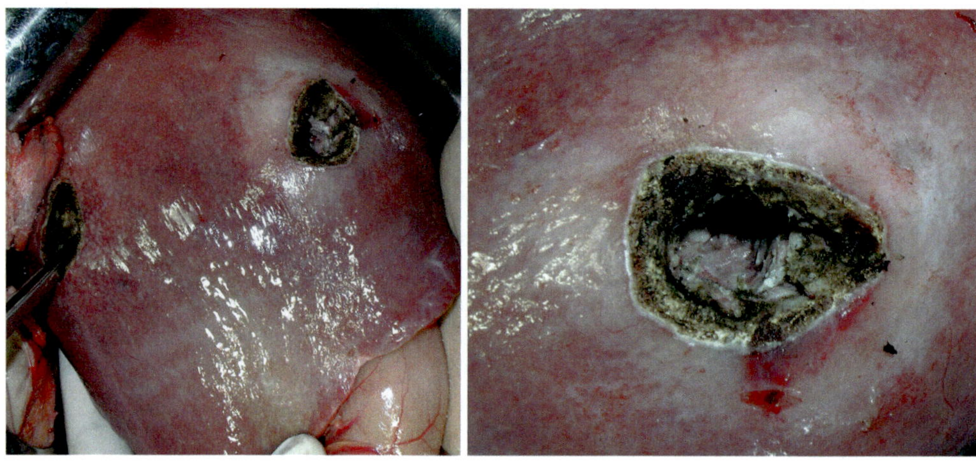

Fig. 22.2 Surgical drainage

empyema or catheter mispositioning with intraperitoneal contamination.

In case of percutaneous drainage inefficiency (10–30% of cases) by catheter placement deficiency, cavity compartmentalization, or viscosity of content, but especially in case of abscess developed by a malignant liver lesion or associated with chronic granulomatosis, surgical drainage is necessary and in the last two cases even liver resection [7] (Fig. 22.1).

Surgical drainage can be performed through open surgery by anterior transperitoneal approach (in most cases) (Fig. 22.2), but also by retroperitoneal approach preceded by resection of the 12th rib (solitary, single, large abscesses with posterior superior site). Laparoscopic approach is reserved for carefully selected cases (single abscess located in laparoscopically accessible segments) [35]. In all these cases, incision and evacuation of the abscess are followed by debridement and cavity lavage, followed by external drainage with declivitous placement of the drainage tubes. As with percutaneous drainage, bacteriological sampling is mandatory here as well, along with that of a fragment of the abscess wall for histological examination (to exclude an abscessed tumour). Another advantage of open approach is represented by intraoperative ultrasound, which can locate abscesses at liver parenchyma level.

Some authors recommend endoscopic papillosphincterotomy (ERCP) followed by extraction of calculi and placement of a naso-biliary catheter that allows antibiotic lavage for HA secondary to suppurative cholangitis caused by lithiasis [36].

Liver resection addresses well codified cases, when the clinical-biological condition of the patient allows it and presenting multiple abscesses in a limited area, or abscesses affecting a whole hemi-liver [37] (Fig. 22.1), and, as already mentioned, when there is a suspicion of abscessed liver tumour or liver abscesses associated with chronic granulomatous disease. Postoperative complications (14.8% of cases) may include bleeding or biliary leakage from the externally drained cavity or from the liver cutting surface, or late biliary fistula or abscess recurrence [31].

Mortality in case of hepatic abscesses has remained significant, but with a remarkable positive development following the appearance of antibiotics and diagnostic and imaging drainage methods, with a decrease in mortality from 60–80%

(before the '70s) to 7–11% currently [31]. Negative prognostic factors are represented by disseminated abscesses and sepsis at presentation, advanced age, presence of pre-existing liver diseases, or malignant liver tumours. In this context, in the case of single treatment with antibiotics mortality is about 50% [38].

22.9 Amoebaean Abscesses

Worldwide Entamoeba histolytica infestation is 10%, with an incidence of 15–30% in tropical areas. Amoebaean liver abscesses affect mainly men (9–10: 1) [29], and the most affected age groups include decades 3–5 (lately there is an increase in children under 3 years) [7]. The term abscess is not particularly appropriate for these lesions because their content is brown, pasty, amicrobial and lacking neutrophils, lesions being characterized by three microscopic zones: a central coagulation necrosis area, a middle area of parenchymal destruction, and a peripheral area in which amoebas are found next to healthy tissue.

Amoebiasis occurs after the ingestion of E. histolytica cysts, the trophozoites released in the intestine enter the portal circulation and cause liver infarction, with necrosis and abscess formation; in 90% of cases macroabscesses are formed in the right hepatic lobe at dome level or lower, in juxtaposition with the hepatic colonic angle.

Clinically, it manifests by subacute evolution of several weeks or months, with fever and pain in the right upper quadrant; while hepatomegaly is almost ubiquitous, jaundice is quite rare.

Anaemia and leucocytosis are the most common biological changes, but leucocytosis is predominant in acute stages and anaemia in long evolution. Indirect haemagglutination test is positive in 90% of cases. The diagnosis is established in one third of cases through parasitological exam of the aspirated content, and by histological examination in case of surgical treatment [39].

From an **imaging** point of view, ULTRASOUND EXAM is the main diagnostic method, accuracy and reliability of the method reaching up to 100%. Suggestive images are represented by round or oval formations, hypoechogenic-homogeneous. Ultrasound also appears as the main method of monitoring the dynamic evolution, highlighting changes in size, echogenicity, or number regarding the lesions. Return to a normal ultrasound aspect of the affected parenchyma spans over a period of months or even years.

CONTRAST AGENT CT SCAN also appears useful in diagnosis, an abscess being viewed as an area with low density, thin edges and adjacent thickened liver area. Lately some authors tends to identify and quantify the differentially abundant membrane proteins by comparing the membrane proteins of virulent and avirulent variants of E. histolytica, as Entamoeba histolytica membrane proteins are important players toward the pathogenesis of amoebiasis [40–43].

Amoebaean abscess complications are superinfection in 22% of cases and pleuropulmonary complications with diaphragm effraction and establishment of a pleural empyema in 20% of cases, sometimes discharged through vomica. In 6–9% of cases abscess rupture in the peritoneal cavity or in the abdominal viscera occurs (the most dangerous situation is represented by an abscess extended to the left liver lobe rupturing in the pericardium). This feature is explained by the fact that the amoebaean abscess is bordered by a thin capsule of granulation tissue, showing poor resistance to increased pressure and being the main cause of a spontaneous rupture.

First intent **treatment** is medical, with anti-amoebaean agents: metronidazole (750 mg ∗ 3/day for 7–14 days) or emetine, dehydroemetine, or chloroquine. If after 48 h from treatment initiation symptomatology does not improve, a superinfection or diagnostic error should be suspicioned, in both cases drainage representing the alternative to medical treatment [7]. Also, in case of complications such as ruptures, fissures, perforation, as well as percutaneous drainage insufficiency, surgical treatment (evacuation and external drainage of the cavity) is indicated, being however associated with a higher morbidity rate and longer hospital stay [44]; nevertheless, the minimally invasive approach has proven better results in selected cases [35, 45].

Self Study

Questions

1. Regarding pyogenic liver abscesses, one of following is true:
   (a) have an 80% mortality if untreated.
   (b) usually involves Clostridium spp.
   (c) the main treatment consist in antibiotherapy with drainage.
   (d) have the highest incidence in tropical areas.
2. Which statement/statements is/are true?
   (a) Amoebian HA is the most frequent worldwide
   (b) TACE used in liver tumors can determine HA
   (c) HAT following liver transplantation is one cause of HA
   (d) b, c
   (e) a, c

Answers

1. Regarding pyogenic liver abscesses, one of following is true:
   (a) have a 95–100% mortality if untreated.
   (b) usually involves gastrointestinal flora (over 75%) with Escherichia coli being primarily incriminated (35–45%), followed by Klebsiella pneumoniae.
   (c) the main treatment consist in antibiotherapy with drainage. CORRECT
   (d) amoebian HA have the highest incidence in tropical areas.
2. Which statement/statements is/are true?
   (a) Amoebian HA is the most frequent in tropical areas
   (b) TACE used in liver tumors can determine HA
   (c) HAT following liver transplantation is one cause of HA
   (d) b, c CORRECT
   (e) a, c

References

1. Hippocrate. The genuine works of hippocrates. Translated from the Greek with a preliminary discourse and annotations by F. Adams, vol. I and II. New York: William Wood; 1886, pp 57, 266
2. Bright R. Observations on jaundice. Guys Hosp Rep. 1836;1:630.
3. Fitz HR. Perforating inflammation of the vermiform appendix. Am J Med Sci. 1886;92:321.
4. Dieulafoy. Le foie appendiculaire: Abces du foie conscutifs a l'appendicite. Semin Med (Paris). 1898;18:449.
5. Ochsner A, DeBakey M. Diagnosis and treatment of amoebic abscess of the liver: a study based on 4,484 collected and personal cases. Am J Dig Dis. 1935;2:47.
6. Ochsner A, DeBakey M, Murray S. Pyogenic abscess of the liver. Am J Surg. 1938;40:292.
7. Meyers WC, Kim RD. Pyogenic and amebic liver abscess. In: Sabiston textbook of surgery. Philadelphia: W. B. Saunders Company; 2001. p. 390.
8. Tasbakan MI, Erdem HA, Pullukcu H, Yamazhan T, Sipahi OR, Tasbakan MS, Ceylan N, Yilmaz F, Arda B, Ulusoy S. Isolated hepatic sarcoidosis mimicking liver microabscesses: a case report. Ir J Med Sci. 2014;183(3):503–5.
9. Corredoira J, Casariego E, Moreno C, Villanueva L, Lopez, Varela J, Rodriguez A, Alonso P, Coira A. Prospective study of Streptococcus milleri hepatic abscess. Eur J Clin Microbiol Infect Dis. 1998;17(8):556–60.
10. Annunziata GM, Blackstone M, Hart J, Piper J, Baker AL. Candida (Torulopsis glabrata) liver abscesses eight years after orthotopic liver transplantation. J Clin Gastroenterol. 1997;24(3):176–9.
11. Chou FF, Sheen-Chen SM, Chen YS, Chen MC, Chen FC, Tai DI. Prognostic factors for pyogenic abscess of the liver. J Am Coll Surg. 1994;179(6):727–32.
12. Chu KM, Fan ST, Lai EC, Lo CM, Wong J. Pyogenic liver abscess. An audit of experience over the past decade. Arch Surg. 1996;131(2):148–52.
13. Origuchi N, Kimura W, Sawabe M, Muto T, Esaki Y. The development of a pancreatic abscess, suppurative pylethrombosis, and multiple hepatic abscesses after a pancreatojejunostomy for chronic pancreatitis: report of a case. Surg Today. 1999;29(4):358–60.
14. Popa G, Popescu I. Characteristics of cholangitic hepatic abscesses. Rev Chir Oncol Radiol O R L Oftalmol Stomatol Chir. 1985;34(3):189–98.
15. Abu ZM, El Eibiedy G, Abu-El-Einien A, Gad El-Hak N, Abd El-Wahab M, Azzat F. Surgical treatment of hepatic hydatid cysts. Hepato-Gastroenterol. 1998;45(23):1802–6.
16. Altemeier WA, Schowengerdt CG, Whiteley DH. Abscesses of the liver: surgical considerations. Arch Surg. 1970;101(2):258–66.
17. Lamps LW, Pinson CW, Raiford DS, Shyr Y, Scott MA, Washington MK. The significance of microabscesses in liver transplant biopsies: a clinicopathological study. Hepatology. 1998;28(6):1532–7.
18. Rabkin JM, Orloff SL, Corless CL, Benner KG, Flora KD, Rosen HR, Keller FS, Barton RE, Lakin PC, Petersen BD, Saxon RR, Olyaei AJ. Hepatic allograft abscess with hepatic arterial thrombosis. Am J Surg. 1998;175(5):354–9.
19. Hanazaki K, Kajikawa S, Horigome N, Shiohara E, Haba Y, Kuroda T, Iida F. Gas-forming liver abscess after transcatheter arterial embolization for hepatocellular carcinoma: report of a case. Surg Today. 1993;23(8):747–9.
20. Hashimoto T, Mitani T, Nakamura H, Hori S, Kozuka T, Kobayashi Y, Nakata A, Tsujimura T. Fatal septic complication of transcatheter chemoembolization for hepatocellular carcinoma. Cardiovasc Intervent Radiol. 1993;16(5):325–7.
21. Setlacec D, Apreotesei C. Therapeutic attitude in some clinical forms of hepatic trauma. Rev Chir Oncol Radiol O R L Oftalmol Stomatol Chir. 1979;28(5):327–34.
22. Broome CJ, Peck RJ. Hepatic abscess complicating foreign body perforation of the gastric antrum: an ultrasound diagnosis. Clin Radiol. 2000;55(3):242–3.
23. Horii K, Yamazaki O, Matsuyama M, Higaki I, Kawai S, Sakaue Y. Successful treatment of a hepatic abscess that formed secondary to fish bone penetration by percutaneous transhepatic removal of the foreign body: report of a case. Surg Today. 1999;29(9):922–6.
24. de Baere T, Roche A, Amenabar JM, Lagrange C, Ducreux M, Rougier P, Elias D, Lasser P, Patriarche C. Liver abscess formation after local treatment of liver tumors. Hepatology. 1996;23(6):1436–40.
25. Reed RA, Teitelbaum GP, Daniels JR, Pentecost MJ, Katz MD. Prevalence of infection following hepatic chemoembolization with cross-linked collagen with administration of prophylactic antibiotics. J Vasc Interv Radiol. 1994;5(2):367–71.
26. Wong E, Khardori N, Carrasco CH, Wallace S, Patt Y, Bodey GP. Infectious complications of hepatic artery catheterization procedures in patients with cancer. Rev Infect Dis. 1991;13(4):583–6.
27. Jia Z, Tu J, Cao C, Wang W, Zhou W, Ji J, Li M. Liver abscess following transarterial chemoembolization for the treatment of hepatocellular carcinoma: a retrospective analysis of 23 cases. J Cancer Res Ther. 2018;14(Suppl):S628–33.
28. Jeong SW, Jang JY, Lee TH, Kim HG, Hong SW, Park SH, Kim SG, Cheon YK, Kim YS, Cho YD, Kim JO, Kim BS, Lee EJ, Kim TH. Cryptogenic pyogenic liver abscess as the herald of colon cancer. J Gastroenterol Hepatol. 2012;27(2):248–55.
29. Frey CF, Zhu Y, Suzuki M, Isaji S. Liver abscesses. Surg Clin North Am. 1989;69(2):259–71.
30. Cavailloles FA, Mure A, Nasser H, Lecapitaine AL, Granier F. Multiple liver amoebic abscesses detected on FDG PET/CT. Clin Nucl Med. 2014;39(1):79–80.
31. Grigoroiu M, Ionescu M, Brasoveanu V, Hrehoret D, Boeti P, Popescu I. Pyogenic liver abscess. Chirurgia (Bucur). 2000;95(6):511–21.

32. Halvorsen RA Jr, Foster WL Jr, Wilkinson RH Jr, Silverman PM, Thompson WM. Hepatic abscess: sensitivity of imaging tests and clinical findings. Gastrointest Radiol. 1988;13(2):135–41.
33. Ciurea S. Abcesele hepatice. In: "Chirurgia ficatului" sub redactia lui Popescu I., Ed. 2004, p 357.
34. vanSonnenberg E, Ferrucci JT Jr, Mueller PR, Wittenberg J, Simeone JF. Percutaneous drainage of abscesses and fluid collections: technique, results, and applications. Radiology. 1982;142(1):1–10.
35. Yanaga K, Kitano S, Hashizume M, Ohta M, Matsumata T, Sugimachi K. Laparoscopic drainage of pyogenic liver abscess. Br J Surg. 1994;81(7):1022.
36. Dull JS, Topa L, Balgha V, Pap A. Non-surgical treatment of biliary liver abscesses: efficacy of endoscopic drainage and local antibiotic lavage with nasobiliary catheter. Gastrointest Endosc. 2000;51(1):55–9.
37. Schwartz SI. Hepatic resection for multiple abscesses. J Am Coll Surg. 1999;189(5):530.
38. SIS Chwartz. Liver. In: Schwartz: principles of surgery. New York: The McGraw-Hill Companies, Inc.; 1999. p. 1397.
39. Oancea T, Cojocea V, Singer D, Ciocirlie D, Codoreanu I. Amebic abscess of the liver. Rev Chir Oncol Radiol O R L Oftalmol Stomatol Chir. 1985;34(3):229–35.
40. Yee LN, Olivos-Garcia A, Teck KL, Noordin R, Qingsong L, Othman N. Entamoeba histolytica: quantitative proteomics analysis reveals putative virulence-associated differentially abundant membrane proteins. Am J Trop Med Hyg. 2018;99(6):1518–29.
41. Ujang J, Sani AAA, Lim BH, Noordin R, Othman N. Analysis of Entamoeba histolytica membrane proteome using three extraction methods. Proteomics. 2018;18:e1700397.
42. Saidin S, Yunus MH, Othman N, Lim YA, Mohamed Z, Zakaria NZ, Noordin R. Development and initial evaluation of a lateral flow dipstick test for antigen detection of Entamoeba histolytica in stool sample. Pathog Glob Health. 2017;111(3):128–36.
43. Othman N, Mohamed Z, Yahya MM, Leow VM, Lim BH, Noordin R. Entamoeba histolytica antigenic protein detected in pus aspirates from patients with amoebic liver abscess. Exp Parasitol. 2013;134(4):504–10.
44. Juvara I, Panaitescu D, Vereanu I, Radu C. An autochthonous case of amebic hepatic abscess with pleural dissemination. Rev Ig Bacteriol Virusol Parazitol Epidemiol Pneumoftiziol Bacteriol Virusol Parazitol Epidemiol. 1976;21(1):55–61.
45. Telich-Tarriba JE, Parrao-Alcantara IJ, Montes-Hernandez JM, Vega-Perez J. Drainage of amoebic liver abscess by single incision laparoscopic surgery. Report of a case. Cir Cir. 2015;83(4):329–33.

Liver Cirrhosis

23

Feifei Hou, Ran Wang, Bing Han, Zhaohui Bai, Yingying Li, and Xingshun Qi

Key Concepts

- Liver cirrhosis is the end stage of chronic liver diseases with an increasing morbidity worldwide.
- Complications, such as ascites, spontaneous bacterial peritonitis, hepatic encephalopathy, acute variceal bleeding, and hepatorenal syndrome, had a significantly negative effect on the prognosis of cirrhotic patients.
- Management aims at preventing the progression of liver cirrhosis and the development of decompensation events.
- Liver transplantation is the most effective curative treatment for liver cirrhosis.
- Child-Pugh and MELD scores are important tools for predicting the prognosis of liver cirrhosis.

23.1 Introduction

Liver cirrhosis is the end stage of various chronic liver diseases, which is the 13th leading cause of death worldwide with increasing mortality rates in the last decades. Histologically, it is characterized by nodular regeneration, extinction of hepatic parenchyma, collapse of hepatic tissues, and distortion of hepatic vessels. Clinically, patients with liver cirrhosis manifested as liver dysfunction and portal hypertension related complications, such as ascites, jaundice, variceal bleeding, and encephalopathy. In this chapter, we reviewed the current knowledge regarding epidemiology, etiology, pathology, clinical presentations, laboratory tests, imaging, diagnosis, staging, management, and prognostic assessment of liver cirrhosis.

23.2 Epidemiology

There is an increasing trend in the morbidity of liver cirrhosis in the world. In the United Kingdom, the morbidity of liver cirrhosis increased from 12.05 to 16.99 per 100,000 person years from 1992 to 2001. In Southern Sweden involving a population of 1.17 million, a total of 1317 patients with liver cirrhosis were identified from 2001 to 2011. The annual incidence of liver cirrhosis was estimated at 14.1/100,000. In China, the incidence of cirrhosis was about 17/100,000.

23.3 Etiology

23.3.1 Viral Hepatitis

Chronic hepatitis secondary to hepatitis B and C virus infections should be a major cause of liver fibrosis and cirrhosis. Hepatitis C virus infection is more common in more developed countries; by contrast, hepatitis B virus infection is dominant in Africa and most parts of Asia. It is estimated that 2–10% of patients with chronic hepatitis B

Feifei Hou and Ran Wang are the co-first authors.

F. Hou · R. Wang · B. Han · Z. Bai · Y. Li · X. Qi (✉)
Liver Cirrhosis Study Group, Department of Gastroenterology, General Hospital of Shenyang Military Area, Shenyang, China

F. Radu-Ionita et al. (eds.), *Liver Diseases*, https://doi.org/10.1007/978-3-030-24432-3_23

virus infection develop cirrhosis every year. Additionally, hepatitis A and E virus infections hardly progress into liver cirrhosis.

23.3.2 Alcoholic Liver Disease

Alcoholic toxicity can lead to hepatic tissue damage, and then develop liver steatosis and cirrhosis. In Europe, chronic alcohol use is the most common cause of liver cirrhosis.

23.3.3 Non-alcoholic Fatty Liver Disease

Non-alcoholic fatty liver disease refers to excessive fat accumulation in the liver after excluding alcohol and other definitive liver damage factors. It is often accompanied with obesity, diabetes, insulin resistance, hypertriglyceridemia, and cardiovascular diseases.

23.3.4 Cholestasis

Primary or secondary cholestasis can increase the concentrations of bile acids and bilirubin, thereby destroying hepatocytes and leading to the development of liver cirrhosis.

23.3.5 Circulation Disorders

Chronic right heart failure, constrictive pericarditis, hepatic venous outflow obstruction syndrome, and sinusoidal obstruction syndrome can cause long-term liver congestion and hypoxia, thereby resulting in necrosis and fibrosis in the central lobe of the liver.

23.3.6 Drugs and Industrial Poisons

Prolonged or repeated exposure to medications associated with liver injury (i.e., acetaminophen, methyldopa, etc.) or industrial toxicants (i.e., carbon tetrachloride, phosphorus, and arsenic) can evolve into cirrhosis.

23.3.7 Others

Genetic and metabolic diseases (i.e., hemochromatosis, Wilson's disease, antitrypsin deficiency, etc.), autoimmune liver diseases (i.e., primary biliary cirrhosis, primary sclerosing cholangitis, autoimmune hepatitis), and parasites (i.e., schistosomiasis, etc.) are also the possible causes of liver cirrhosis.

23.4 Pathology

Transition from chronic liver disease to liver fibrosis mainly involves inflammation, activation of hepatic stellate cells with ensuing fibrogenesis, angiogenesis, and parenchymal extinction lesions caused by vascular occlusion. Hepatic fibrosis is reversible at early stage, but is often irreversible when pseudo-lobule develops excessively with fibrous septum.

23.5 Clinical Stages and Presentations

Generally, liver cirrhosis is clinically divided into compensated and decompensated stages. Compensation stage is often asymptomatic with normal liver function or mildly abnormal hepatic enzyme. It is further classified into compensated cirrhosis without and with gastroesophageal varices. Classically, patients with mild portal hypertension (i.e., hepatic venous pressure gradient >5 mmHg and <10 mmHg) have no varices, but those with clinically significant portal hypertension (i.e., hepatic venous pressure gradient >10 mmHg and <12 mmHg) often have a higher risk of developing varices and decompensation. Upper gastrointestinal endoscopy is the golden diagnostic method of gastroesophageal varices. Recently, many non-invasive methods have been employed, such as liver and spleen stiffness, platelets count, and some liver fibrosis indexes. Decompensation events traditionally include ascites, variceal bleeding, hepatic encephalopathy, and jaundice. Infection and occlusive portal vein thrombosis are also considered as novel markers for clinical decompensation.

Ascites is the most common decompensation event in patients with cirrhosis. Common clinical presentations of ascites include abdominal distension, abdominal pain, and even frog-like abdomen and umbilical hernia. Dyspnea and palpitation may occur when the diaphragm is raised by a large amount of ascites. Major pathogenesis of ascites include sodium and water retention, hypoproteinemia, decreased effective arterial blood volume due to activation of sympathetic nervous system and renin-angiotensin-aldosterone system, retardation of lymphatic flow, and portal hypertension. According to the amount of fluid in the abdominal cavity, the grade of ascites is classified into mild, moderate, and large or gross ascites. Refractory ascites refers to the recurrence of ascites for at least three times during a

12-month period in spite of dietary sodium restriction and adequate diuretic dosage.

Spontaneous bacterial peritonitis is frequently complicated in patients with ascites. Spontaneous bacterial peritonitis is diagnosed if the ascitic polymorphonuclear leucocyte count is beyond 250/mm^3. Major pathogenic bacteria are Gram-negative bacilli, such as *E. coli*, Klebsiella pneumoniae, and other Enterobacteriaceae. Some Gram-positive bacteria, such as d Streptococci and Staphylococci, are involved in 23–40% of patients with spontaneous bacterial peritonitis. Clinical presentations are low-grade fever, anorexia, rapid growth of ascites, and peritoneal irritation. Average mortality rate is about 30%.

Hepatic hydrothorax is defined as a large amount of transudative pleural effusion in cirrhotic patients after excluding primary cardiopulmonary or malignant diseases. Common clinical presentations include dyspnea, shortness of breath, coughing, and chest pain. Patients with hepatic hydrothorax usually have a high percentage of ascites and Child-Pugh class B-C. Sodium restriction diet and diuretics cannot control the clinical manifestations.

Hepatorenal syndrome, which mainly manifests as oliguria, anuria, and azotemia, refers to the occurrence of renal dysfunction or failure in advanced cirrhosis without any obvious organic kidney disease or use of nephrotoxic-drugs. It is associated with hypovolaemia after gastrointestinal bleeding, paracentesis or diuretics or severe sepsis. Traditionally, hepatorenal syndrome is divided into two types. Type 1 hepatorenal syndrome is associated with rapid deterioration of renal function, usually occurring in severe sepsis. Prognosis of type 1 hepatorenal syndrome is poor with a 3-month survival rate of 15%. Type 2 hepatorenal syndrome refers to a steady and moderate functional renal failure, commonly occurring in cirrhosis with refractory ascites.

Hepatic encephalopathy is the most common cause of death in liver cirrhosis with a 1-year survival rate of about 36%. Common causes of hepatic encephalopathy include acute liver failure, portosystemic shunting, and gastrointestinal bleeding. According to the Spectrum of Neuro-cognitive Impairment in Cirrhosis (SONIC) classification criteria, hepatic encephalopathy is divided into two types. Covert hepatic encephalopathy is defined if a cirrhotic patient has neuropsychological and/or neurophysiological abnormalities but no disorientation or asterixis. Covert hepatic encephalopathy occurs in 20–80% of patients with liver cirrhosis. Overt hepatic encephalopathy is defined if a patient has obvious clinical signs of hepatic encephalopathy, which may present with directional and computational impairments, asterixis, drowsiness, and even coma. The prevalence of overt hepatic encephalopathy is 10–14% at the time of diagnosis of cirrhosis, 16–21% in patients with decompensated cirrhosis, and 10–50% in patients treated with transjugular intrahepatic portosystemic shunt.

Hepato-pulmonary syndrome is a rare complication of liver cirrhosis due to porto-pulmonary hypertension and portal hypertension. Dyspnea, cyanosis, and clubbing are common clinical presentations of hepato-pulmonary syndrome due to pulmonary vasodilation and dysfunction of arterial oxygen synthesis.

Cirrhotic cardiomyopathy is characterized by chronic cardiac dysfunction in cirrhosis patients without any known cardiac disease. It often manifests as reduced cardiac contractility with systolic and diastolic dysfunction and presence of electrophysiological abnormalities. Clinically, increased levels of pro-brain natriuretic peptide and troponin T and QT interval prolongation are frequently observed in cirrhosis.

Portal vein thrombosis refers to the formation of thrombus within the intrahepatic and/or extrahepatic portal vein, splenic vein, and superior mesenteric vein. Patients with portal vein thrombosis can present with severe abdominal pain, intestinal necrosis, and gastrointestinal bleeding. Risk factors for portal vein thrombosis include reduced portal vein flow velocity, worse liver function, thrombophilia, splenectomy, and other surgical procedures. Recently, use of non-selective beta-blockers is also considered as a major risk factor for portal vein thrombosis.

Sarcopenia, which is characterized by skeletal muscle mass depletion and muscle dysfunction, a hallmark sign of malnutrition in cirrhotic patients with a morbidity of 40–70%. Sarcopenia is associated with decreased hepatic synthetic function, clearance of ammonia, and increased systemic inflammation and muscle breakdown. Sarcopenia has a significantly negative effect among cirrhotic patients on the prognosis and quality of life.

Hepatocellular carcinoma is the fifth most common type of cancer and the second leading cause of cancer-related death worldwide. Liver cirrhosis is present in most (>80%) of hepatocellular carcinoma cases. Hepatocellular carcinoma has several specific epidemiologic features, including dynamic temporal trends, marked variations among geographic regions, racial groups, and gender, and presence of potentially preventable risk factors. Currently, the most effective curative treatment for hepatocellular carcinoma is liver transplantation, but its wide application is limited by the shortage of liver grafts and the possibility of tumor recurrence. Other major treatments include hepatic resection, local ablation, transarterial chemoembolization, molecular targeted drugs, and best supportive care. Prognosis of hepatocellular carcinoma largely depends on the severity of liver dysfunction, tumor stage at diagnosis, and patient access to radical treatment.

23.6 Laboratory Tests

Routine blood tests are usually normal in compensated cirrhosis. By contrast, in decompensated cirrhosis, due to the occurrence of gastrointestinal bleeding and hypersplenism, white blood cell, red blood cell, and platelet count will be below the normal range. Liver function tests used to evaluate the prognosis of cirrhosis and its complications mainly include serum transaminase, bilirubin, albumin, and prothrombin time.

23.7 Imaging

Ultrasonography is the first-line choice for diagnosis of liver cirrhosis, followed by computed tomography and magnetic resonance scans. Classical imaging features of liver cirrhosis include an imbalance in the ratio of right hepatic lobe to left hepatic lobe, hepatic fissure widening, and uneven or rough liver surface (Figs. 23.1 and 23.2). Doppler ultrasonography and contrast-enhanced CT and MRI scans are useful to observe the presence of portosystemic collaterals, portal vein flow velocity, and portal vein thrombosis. Transient elastography, which is employed for the measurement of tissue elasticity, is one of the most frequent methods for non-invasive assessment of liver fibrosis. Liver biopsy is the gold standard test for the diagnosis of cirrhosis, but is potentially invasive.

23.8 Diagnosis

Clinically, the diagnosis of liver cirrhosis is not difficult. Several major diagnostic criteria are as follows.

- Previous history of chronic liver diseases and possible etiology of cirrhosis, such as viral hepatitis, alcohol abuse, chronic drug abuse, and family history of liver diseases.
- Major clinical manifestations of liver dysfunction and portal hypertension.
- Major liver dysfunction tests, such as decreased albumin, elevated bilirubin, and prolonged prothrombin time.
- Ultrasonography and contrast-enhanced CT and MRI findings suggesting the characteristics of liver cirrhosis.
- Liver histology, if inconclusive.

23.9 Treatment

Treatment of cirrhosis should aim at interrupting or reversing fibrosis. However, antifibrotic drugs are often insufficient to reverse fibrosis consistently or improve outcomes in cirrhotic patients. Treatment of compensated stage directs at preventing from the progression into decompensation stage, and that of decompensated stage focuses on preventing the development of complications of cirrhosis.

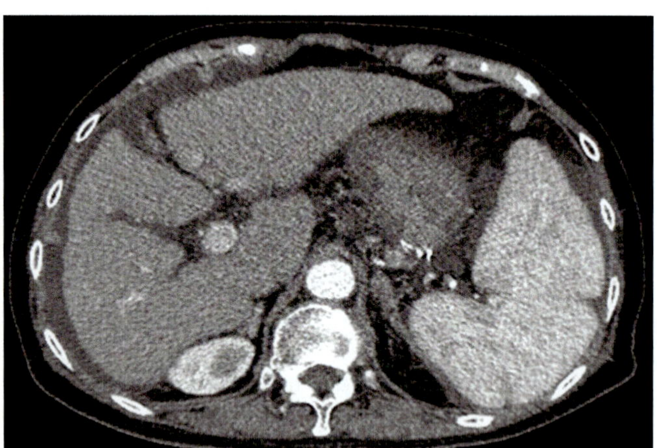

Fig. 23.1 Contrast-enhanced CT scan in a patient with liver cirrhosis showing an imbalance in the ratio of right to left hepatic lobe, splenomegaly, mild ascites around the liver and spleen, and uneven liver surface

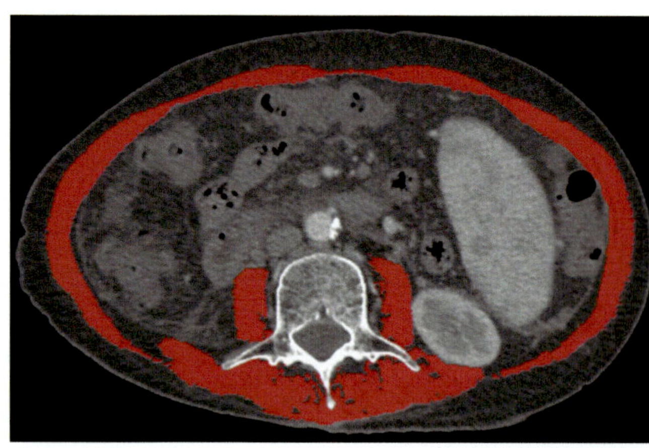

Fig. 23.2 CT scan in a patient with sarcopenia. Skeletal muscle is colored in red using Slice-O-Matic software. Skeletal muscle area at the third lumbar is used to calculate the SMI (skeletal muscle area index). Sarcopenia is diagnosed according to the criteria that SMI $\leq$52.4 cm^2/m^2 in males and $\leq$38.5 cm^2/m^2 in females

23.9.1 Antiviral Treatment

Viral replication activity is one of the most important risk factors for cirrhosis progression. Patients with hepatitis B virus related decompensated cirrhosis should be immediately receive antiviral treatment with nucleos(t)ide analogues, irrespective of hepatitis B virus DNA replication level. The first-line nucleos(t)ide analogues for chronic hepatitis C virus infection include entecavir, tenofovir, and tenofovir alafenamide, which are generally safe in patients with decompensated cirrhosis. Treatment with tenofovir for 5 years slow down the progression of hepatitis B virus related cirrhosis. Selection of antiviral drugs for patients with hepatitis C virus related cirrhosis should depend on hepatitis C virus genotype/subtype and severity of liver dysfunction. Antiviral drugs in such patients include IFN-free or ribavirin-free sofosbuvir, ledipasvir, velpatasvir and voxilaprevir. Because IFN could cause liver failure, it is disabled in patients with decompensated cirrhosis.

23.9.2 Ascites

Cirrhotic patients with mild or moderate ascites should be advised to reduce their sodium intake and to avoid foods with a high salt content. Dietary sodium restriction to 88 mmol per day is recommended. Spironolactone can be used alone or in combination with furosemide. The starting dose can be 100 mg of spironolactone and 40 mg of furosemide. Depending on the treatment response (weight loss of >1.5 kg/week), the dose can be increased in a stepwise fashion until a maximum dose of 400 mg of spironolactone and 160 mg of furosemide every day. Refractory ascites can be treated by large-volume paracentesis with albumin administration, transjugular intrahepatic portosystemic shunt, and liver transplantation. Once a diagnosis of spontaneous bacterial peritonitis has been made, antibiotics should be initiated immediately.

23.9.3 Variceal Bleeding

General principles for treatment of acute variceal bleeding include blood transfusion, vasoactive drugs, prophylactic antibiotics, endoscopic therapy, transjugular intrahepatic portosystemic shunt, and surgical shunt. Vasoactive drugs, mainly including terlipressin, somatostatin, and octreotide, can effectively reduce portal pressure, thereby controlling acute bleeding events. Empirical broad spectrum antibiotics have been shown to reduce bacterial infection, rebleeding, and mortality. Endoscopic therapy mainly includes band ligation, sclerotherapy, and glue injection. Evidence suggests that variceal band ligation is superior to sclerotherapy in terms of complications, re-bleeding, and variceal eradication. Early transjugular intrahepatic portosystemic shunt should be considered in patients at high risk of treatment failure after initial endoscopic and pharmacological therapy. Surgical shunt has been largely replaced by minimally invasive transjugular intrahepatic portosystemic shunt. Non-selective beta-blockers or endoscopic band ligation has been recommended for the primary prophylaxis of variceal bleeding in patients with cirrhosis who have high-risk varices. Notably, non-selective beta-blockers may be ineffective for preventing the growth of small varices and lead to drug-related adverse effects. Non-selective beta-blockers combined with endoscopic band ligation is the first-line choice for the secondary prophylaxis of variceal bleeding. Traditional non-selective beta-blockers include propranolol and nadolol. Carvedilol is more effective than propranolol in reducing hepatic venous pressure gradient.

23.9.4 Hepatic Encephalopathy

Primary therapy of hepatic encephalopathy is the resolution of precipitating factors, such as infection, gastrointestinal bleeding, dehydration, constipation, electrolyte disturbance, and drug abuse. Gut-based therapies (lactulose and rifaximin) and extra-luminal therapies (L-ornithine L-aspartate) are used for the management of hepatic encephalopathy. Clinical effectiveness and safety of albumin for the treatment of hepatic encephalopathy is under debate. Transjugular intrahepatic portosystemic shunt is a major precipitant of hepatic encephalopathy, and shunt reduction or occlusion may be required for the management of hepatic encephalopathy.

23.9.5 Hepatorenal Syndrome

Primary therapy of hepatorenal syndrome is also the resolution of precipitating factors, such as refractory ascites, spontaneous bacterial peritonitis, and massive gastrointestinal bleeding. Because splanchnic vasodilation leads to a reduction in the effective circulatory volume, vasoconstrictors are the first-line choice of therapy for hepatorenal syndrome. Currently, terlipressin combined albumin is the preferred treatment modality, which can improve the renal function and survival and serve as a bridge to liver transplantation. Recent evidence also suggests a potential survival benefit of transjugular intrahepatic portosystemic shunt in cirrhotic patients with hepatorenal syndrome, but hepatic encephalopathy and shunt dysfunction should be noted. Liver transplantation is a curative therapeutic option for hepatorenal syndrome.

23.10 Prognosis

Mortality rate is heterogeneous among countries and periods (Table 23.1). The mortality rate of cirrhosis in 187 countries was 22% during the 30-year period between January 1998 and December 2010. In Greece and Southern England, the 10-year mortality rate was 44% and 43%, respectively. Prognosis of cirrhosis is related to the etiology, degree of liver dysfunction, and complications. Child-Pugh score and model for end-stage liver disease (MELD) score are two important prognostic indexes. Child-Pugh score includes ascites, hepatic encephalopathy, total bilirubin, albumin, and international normalized ratio. MELD score includes total bilirubin, albumin, and creatinine. MELD score has been employed for determining the priority of liver transplantation in cirrhotic patients.

Table 23.1 Mortality rate of liver cirrhosis

First author (year)	Country	Period	Total pts.	Mortality rate
Nilsson (2016)	Southern Sweden	2001–2010	1317	10 years: 68.5%
John (2015)	Southern Brazil		527	5 years: 27% 10 years: 43%
D'Amico (2014)	Italy	1981–2006	494	25 years: 76.9%
Mokdad (2014)	187 countries	1980–2010	676,000	30 years: 22%
Samonakis (2014)	Greece	1991–2008	522	9 years: 44.3%
Jepsen (2008)	Danish	1995–2006	14,976	5 years: 62.5% 10 years: 78.5%
Roberts (2005)	Southern England	1968–1999	8192	35 years: 27.5%

Self Study

Questions

1. Which statement is correct?
   (a) Compensation stage is often symptomatic with abnormal liver function.
   (b) Hepatitis C virus infection is common in developed countries, but hepatitis B virus infection is common in most parts of Asia.
   (c) Type 2 hepatorenal syndrome is associated with rapid deterioration of renal function, commonly occurring in cirrhosis with refractory ascites.
   (d) Transjugular intrahepatic portosystemic shunt should be considered in the management of refractory ascites, acute variceal bleeding, hepatic encephalopathy, and hepatorenal syndrome.
2. Which statement/statements is/are true?
   (a) Decompensation events of liver cirrhosis include gastroesophageal varices, ascites, spontaneous bacterial peritonitis, hepatic hydrothorax, hepatorenal syndrome, hepatic encephalopathy, hepatopulmonary syndrome, and hepatocellular carcinoma.
   (b) Covert hepatic encephalopathy is common in cirrhotic patients.
   (c) Risk factors for portal vein thrombosis include reduced portal vein flow velocity, worse liver function, thrombophilia, splenectomy, and use of nonselective beta-blockers.
   (d) Contrast-enhanced CT and MRI scans are the gold standard tests for the diagnosis of cirrhosis.

Answers

1. Which statement is correct?
   (a) Compensation stage is often symptomatic with abnormal liver function. (Compensation stage is often asymptomatic with normal or mildly abnormal liver function.)
   (b) Hepatitis C virus infection is common in developed countries, but hepatitis B virus infection is common in most parts of Asia.—Correct—Hepatitis C virus infection is common in developed countries; hepatitis B virus infection is common in Africa and most parts of Asia.
   (c) Type 2 hepatorenal syndrome is associated with rapid deterioration of renal function, commonly occurring in cirrhosis with refractory ascites. (Type 1 hepatorenal syndrome is associated with rapid deterioration of renal function.)

(d) Transjugular intrahepatic portosystemic shunt should be considered in the management of refractory ascites, acute variceal bleeding, hepatic encephalopathy, and hepatorenal syndrome. (Transjugular intrahepatic portosystemic shunt is a major precipitant of hepatic encephalopathy, but not a choice of treatment for hepatic encephalopathy.)

2. Which statement/statements is/are true?

(a) Decompensation events of liver cirrhosis include gastroesophageal varices, ascites, spontaneous bacterial peritonitis, hepatic hydrothorax, hepatorenal syndrome, hepatic encephalopathy, hepatopulmonary syndrome, and hepatocellular carcinoma. (Compensation stage is often asymptomatic; however, patients with compensated liver cirrhosis can develop gastroesophageal varices and hepatocellular carcinoma.)

(b) Covert hepatic encephalopathy is common in cirrhotic patients.—Correct—Covert hepatic encephalopathy is common in cirrhotic patients.

(c) Risk factors for portal vein thrombosis include reduced portal vein flow velocity, worse liver function, thrombophilia, splenectomy, and use of non-selective beta-blockers.—Correct—Risk factors for portal vein thrombosis include reduced portal vein flow velocity, worse liver function, thrombophilia, splenectomy, and use of non-selective beta-blockers.

(d) Contrast-enhanced CT and MRI scans are the gold standard tests for the diagnosis of cirrhosis. (Liver biopsy is the gold standard test for the diagnosis of cirrhosis, but is potentially invasive.)

24 Primary Biliary Cholangitis

Eirini I. Rigopoulou

Key Concepts

- Primary biliary cholangitis (PBC) is a chronic autoimmune disease characterized by cholestasis due to destruction of small intrahepatic bile ducts progressing to fibrosis and liver failure in a proportion of patients.
- Antimitochondrial antibodies and PBC-specific antinuclear antibodies are considered disease specific and are essential for the diagnosis of PBC.
- Clinical presentation and disease progression is heterogeneous among PBC patients.
- Ursodeoxycholic acid (UDCA) has significantly improved the natural history of PBC, as shown by better transplant-free survival, though a proportion of patients don't respond to UDCA.
- Treatment strategies should be individualized based on patient's stratification risk as assessed by biochemical response to UDCA and other prognostic models.

24.1 Introduction

Primary biliary cholangitis (PBC) is a chronic autoimmune cholestatic liver disease characterized by the presence of antimitochondrial antibodies (AMA) and progressive destruction of small intrahepatic bile ducts, evolving in a proportion of patients to progressive fibrosis and subsequently leading to cirrhosis and hepatic failure [1].

Since 1851, when the first case of PBC was described, our knowledge on epidemiology and underlying pathophysiological mechanisms has evolved enormously. Consequently, new molecules have been exploited as treatment modalities for the disease. In fact, even the change in the disease's nomenclature in 2014 from Primary biliary cirrhosis, used since 1950, to Primary biliary cholangitis characteristically reflects physicians and patients changing perception on the disease's natural history during the last decades [2].

24.2 Epidemiology of PBC

Over the last few decades, a number of epidemiological studies have substantially changed the geoepidemiology of PBC, pointing towards an increased prevalence and incidence of the disease [3–6].

The first epidemiological attempt in 1974 by Hamlyn and Sherlock was a mortality survey in the region of England and Wales [7]. During this time PBC was considered a rare disease, with a predetermined fatal outcome in most patients and without effective treatment that could alter its course [7]. Geoepidemiology of PBC has evolved significantly during the last 40 years, pointing towards an increase in prevalence and incidence of the disease. Geoepidemiology of PBC is characterized by vast differences amongst geographical regions, indicating the disease to be most prevalent in North America and North Europe (Table 24.1). Accordingly, in the western world, where the disease has been mostly studied, the incidence and prevalence rates range from 3.3 to 32 per million person-years and 19 to 402 per million respectively [3–6]. Still, high prevalence rates have been also reported in South Europe, as was the case of Central Greece with prevalence rates 582 per million [6]. Hong-Kong and

E. I. Rigopoulou (✉)
Department of Internal Medicine, Faculty of Medicine, School of Health Sciences, University of Thessaly, Larissa, Greece
e-mail: eirigopoulou@med.uth.gr

F. Radu-Ionita et al. (eds.), *Liver Diseases*, https://doi.org/10.1007/978-3-030-24432-3_24

Table 24.1 Population-based studies on incidence and prevalence of PBC world wide

Region	Period	Patients (n)	Incidence (million/year)	Prevalence (/million)	Sex ratio (M:F)
Sheffield, UK	1977–1979	34	5.8	54	1:16
Western Europe	1977–1981	569	4	23	1:10
Orebro, Sweden	1976–1983	18	14	128	1:3.5
North Sweden	1973–1982	111	13.3	151	1:7.5
Denmark	1981–1985	233	9	–	1:3.2
Newcastle, UK	1965–1987	411	19.8	128	1:9.2
Victoria, Australia	1990–1991	84	–	19.1	1:11
Estonia	1973–1992	69	3.9	27	1:22
Oslo, Norway	1986–1995	21	16.2	146	1:3.2
Newcastle, UK	1987–1994	770	32	335	1:12
Ontario, Canada	1986–1988	225	3.3	22.4	1:13
Olmsted County, USA	1975–1995	46	27	402	1:6.4
Finland	1988–1999	545	17	180	1:6
Denmark	1977–2001	666	–	120	–
Sabadell, Spain	1990–2002	87	17.2	195	1:28
Alberta, Canada	1996–2002	137	30.3	227	1:5
Victoria, Australia	1990–2002	249	–	51	1:9
Iceland	1991–2000 2001–2010	168	20 25	383	1:4.6
South Israel	1990–1999 2000–2010	138	10 20	255	1:16
Crete, Greece	1990–2010	245	20.9	365	1:7.2
Holland	2000–2008	992	11	132	1:7.6
Central Greece	2000–2015	432	–	582	1:6.4
Hong Kong, China	2000–2015	1016	8.4	56.4	1:4
South Korea	2009–2013	2431	8.6	47.5	1:6.2

Data extracted from various studies (Refs. [1, 3–9])

South China have the lowest prevalence rates reported so far (56.4 and 47.5 per million respectively) [8, 9].

Significant predominance of women is also another characteristic feature of PBC with average reported female to male ratio of 10:1. Still, over the years several epidemiological studies have exhibited variations in gender ratios (Table 24.1).

Such a rise in PBC incidence and prevalence is considered multifactorial. Increased disease awareness in conjunction with advances in PBC diagnosis, the biggest being the discovery of AMA in 1965 by Barbara Doniah, have lead to increased disease diagnosis and mostly at earlier stages. The use of ursodeoxycholic acid (UDCA), as standard of care in PBC patients has also contributed towards the reported increase in disease's prevalence.

Still, it is disputed whether differences in geoepidemiology of PBC exist or have resulted from regional disparities in physician's expertise or patient's accessibility to healthcare facilities. Studies from Newcastle in late 90s have set some standards towards improvement of case-finding and case-ascertainment methodology, which has lead through the years to more accurate estimation of the epidemiology of disease [3, 4].

24.3 Pathogenesis of PBC

PBC is considered an archetype autoimmune disease based on the following features: the presence of AMA, the overwhelming predominance of women and the increased percentage of patients with other autoimmune diseases.

Even though its pathogenesis is still unfolding, accumulating evidence over the years indicates that immune-mediated biliary injury, ensuing from loss of immune tolerance, is robustly linked to genetic and environmental factors [10–12].

24.3.1 Genetic Factors

A genetic basis of the diseases is strongly supported by higher disease rates between family members. In fact, in a small series, monozygotic twins had much higher concordance rates compared to dizygotic twins (63% vs 0%) [13]. Analogously, first-degree relatives carry a high risk for expressing AMA and developing PBC; the relative risk of PBC among siblings was calculated around 10 [11]. In fact, female first-degree relatives of PBC patients have a greater prevalence of AMA compared to males. Indicative of a genetic background of PBC is the increased risk of other autoimmune conditions in PBC patients and their family members.

During the last decade, the application of genome-wide technology in large PBC cohorts has assisted the exploration of the disease genetics. Several genome-wide association studies (GWAS) in European, North American, Japanese and Chinese populations have demonstrated the HLA class II domain to exert the strongest association with PBC susceptibility across ethnicities [11, 14]. In detail, HLA DRB1*07,*08 alleles have been associated with increased susceptibility to PBC, while HLA DR*11,*12,*13 and *15 confer disease protection [11, 14]. Still, the importance of these HLA haplotypes is underscored by the fact that the minority of PBC patients carries them, suggesting other candidate genes and environmental factors to relate to PBC pathogenesis.

Up to the present GWAS have identified a significant number of non-HLA loci as risk factors for PBC, though with discrepant results between ethnicities. Most recognized loci are involved in mechanisms implicated in immune responses that are interrelated, including IL-12 production, T and B cell activation and IFN-γ production.

Non-HLA loci having reached significance in GWAS were different between Caucasian and Asian patients with PBC [14]. In PBC patients of European ancestry genetic variants at interleukin 12A and IL12R B2 have been linked with the disease, while such associations haven't been reported in Asian patients. Additional risk loci were interferon regulatory factor 5 (IRF5), transporin 3 (TNPO3) and transcriptor factor Spi-B (SPIB). Another GWAS reported TNFSF15 and POU2AF1 genes to confer susceptibility to PBC in Japanese patients, while TNFSF15 reached the highest association amongst other genes with PBC in a Han population. These genes might be implicated in pathogenetic mechanisms in PBC, though differences between populations most probably indicate, that other genes acting either as risks or protectively have not been recognized yet. In addition, most of GWAS hits don't affect protein-coding sequences and were difficult to associate with a molecular function, rendering their interpretation as key players in PBC pathogenesis rather complicating. In conclusion, GWAS were not as promising as initially thought towards elucidating genetics contribution to PBC pathogenesis.

24.3.2 Epigenetics

Emerging data during the last decade on epigenetics has assisted in better understanding some aspects of PBC pathogenesis, including female preponderance and discordant results in monozygotic twins and siblings. Epigenetics refer to inheritable genetic alterations that don't affect nucleotide sequence or chromosome structure and relate to their function [14, 15].

Most studies on PBC conducted so far have focused on the role of DNA methylation profiles of X chromosome and on small and noncoding RNA, with particular emphasis on microRNAs. An initial study on three pairs of monozygotic twins and eight pairs of sisters discordant for PBC have exhibited particular epigenetic differences mostly related to X chromosome, which is in agreement with the female predominance of the disease. Most of these genes are implicated in cellular pathways, as the downregulation of Th2 cytokines. A subsequent study reported demethylation of CXCR3 in CD4+ T cells, which inversely correlated with CXCR3 expression levels in CD4+ T cells from early-stage PBC patients. Considering that CXCR3 promoter is regulating differentiation and recruitment of Th1 cells, hypomethylation of the CXCR3 promoter could promote disease progression in PBC patients [15].

Several studies on the possible contribution of miRNAs in PBC implied their potential availability as novel biomarkers for the disease. One study, so far, has provided strong evidence on the role of miRNAs in biliary epithelial cells (BEC) damage in PBC patients, through disrupting the "bicarbonate umbrella" that protects them. In detail, miR-506 was reported to prevent the translation of anion exchanger 2 (AE2) mRNA, which regulates HC03- secretion from BECs, contributing to their damage [16].

Acknowledging the importance of epigenetics as a link between genetics and environment in PBC, continuing research should aim at shedding more light on its implication in disease development and prognosis.

24.3.3 Environmental Factors

Time and space clustering of PBC unrelated cases have pointed early days towards contribution of environmental triggers in breaking immunological tolerance and initiating the disease process [17]. Up to the time of this writing a significant amount of environmental exposures, including infectious agents, chemical xenobiotics, pollutants and cosmetics have been reported [17].

In four large epidemiological studies from UK, USA and continental Europe several factors were highlighted as potential risk factors for PBC development. All studies agree that recurrent urinary tract infections and cigarette smoking are more frequent among PBC patients than controls.

Molecular mimicry is the main pathogenic mechanism proposed by which infectious agents trigger autoimmune responses. *Escherichia coli has* been the most extensively studied agent so far, which is in line with reported increased frequency of UTIs in PBC patients [17–19]. Subsequent experimental studies have demonstrated T and B cell cross-reactivity involving *Escherichia coli* and mitochondrial antigens [18, 19]. Amongst other agents implicated as cross—active agents in PBC are *Mycobacterium gordonae*, *Novosphingobium aromaticivorans*, *Klebsiella pneumonia*, *Staphylococcus aureus*, *Proteus mirabilis*. Viruses have been also suggested to be involved in PBC pathogenesis, including a human retrovirus, Epstein-Barr and cytomegalovirus.

Xenobiotics are chemicals that function either by altering self or forming complexes with self proteins, which may result in induction of cross-reactive immune responses against antigenic epitopes, as are mitochondrial antigens in the case of PBC [20]. Further research has identified 2-nonynoic acid, a xenobiotic found in cosmetics, as potential trigger in PBC. This is in line with female predominance in PBC and data arising from two major epidemiological studies report increased association with nail polish and hair dyes in affected patients. Environmental toxins, such as benzene, have also been recognized as potential xenobiotic triggers of PBC, as indicated by the observations that PBC prevalence was increased in areas near contaminated water reservoirs, or near superfund toxic waste sites [17].

Akin to other autoimmune diseases, smoking has been also significantly associated with PBC in several studies from UK and the USA, as tobacco contained chemicals are suggested to decrease immunological tolerance.

24.3.4 The Role of AMA, T Cells and BECs in the Pathogenesis of PBC

In 1987 the lipoylated domains of the 2-oxoacid dehydrogenase (2-OADC) family of the mitochondrial respiratory chain have been identified as molecular targets of AMA in PBC. Amongst them, major autoantigens are the E2 subunit of pyruvate dehydrogenase complex (PDC-E2), the E2 subunit of 2-oxoglutarate dehydrogenase (OADCE2) complex, the E2 subunit of branched-chain 2-oxo acid dehydrogenase (BCOADC-E2) complex. Less common are the dihydrolipoamide dehydrogenase (E3)-binding protein (E3BP) and the E1a and E1b subunits of pyruvate dehydrogenase complex (PDC-E1a and PDC-E1b). A ExDKA motif with a lipoic acid attached to K at position 173 is essential for antigen recognition and is included in all immunodominant epitopes [1, 10].

Following this major breakthrough, several studies have tried to elucidate mechanisms being involved in loss of tolerance to 2-OADC components located specifically on the inner mitochondrial surface of BECs. The autoimmune attack responsible for progressive destruction of bile ducts in PBC is characterized by a multi-lineage loss of tolerance against major AMA epitopes. In detail, CD4+ and CD8+ T cells reactive against PDC-E2 complex are prominent in the periphery as well in the liver of PBC patients. Of note, B cells share overlapping immunodominant epitopes with CD4+ and CD8+ T cells [10].

Analogously, Natural killer (NK) cells secreting proinflammatory cytokines were found in high concentrations in the liver of PBC patients indicating that innate immune responses play a critical role in initiating and also maintaining autoreactive T-cells and in this manner are essential for disease progression [1, 10]. Studies investigating the role of CD4+CD25+ T regulatory cells (Treg cells) in the pathogenesis of PBC have demonstrated low numbers of such cells, which play a key role in central tolerance. Recently, Treg cells from PBC patients were shown to exhibit increased sensitivity to low dose IL-12, driving them towards Th1 polarization with reduced suppressive activity [21].

Still, there is a longstanding discussion on the mechanisms that underline BECs damage in PBC, bearing in mind that PDC-E2, which is the target of the autoimmune attack, is an ubiquitous protein present in mitochondria of all nucleated cells and is not confined to BECs exclusively. A number of seminal studies have proposed a scenario, where during apoptosis small BECs are able to translocate immunologically intact PDC-E2 to apoptotic bodies and form an antigenic epitope, which has been named apotope. This biliary apotope, in collaboration with macrophages from PBC patients and AMA can trigger locally a burst of pro-inflammatory cytokines leading to inflammatory infiltrate and surrounding apoptosis in PBC [12].

24.4 Clinical Presentation

In the initial descriptions of PBC, the majority of patients were jaundiced at diagnosis, indicating advanced disease stages. Nowadays, the clinical spectrum of PBC encompasses different phenotypes with a considerable proportion of patients (40–60%) being diagnosed at earlier disease stages, when patients are asymptomatic [1, 6, 22]. This is believed to be mainly the consequence of increased disease awareness and more frequent use of noninvasive diagnostic methods, including liver function tests and AMA testing for screening and diagnostic purposes respectively.

Symptomatic disease has been proven to develop in 36–89% of asymptomatic patients over a period of 5–17 years. Characteristic but not specific symptoms of the disease are fatigue and pruritus. Fatigue is reported in a large fraction of patients (up to 80%) with varying intensity and vast fluctuations. It affects drastically quality of life and even though it doesn't relate to PBCs stage or activity, it has been associated with increased mortality. Several mechanisms have been proposed to be implicated in fatigue's generation. Even the etiology of fatigue is still vague, it is believed to have a central and a peripheral component. The central component is mainly characterized by sleep disturbance and cognitive dysfunction and possible relates to inflammatory changes mediated by entry of inflammatory cells from the liver to the central nervous system. The peripheral component is characterized by loss of energy and inability to perform every day physical activity. These abnormalities have been associated with a decline in muscle dysfunction, related to excessive lactic acid accumulation. It is hypothesized that this might be the consequence of mitochondrial dysfunction due to excessive anaerobic metabolism in these PBC patients [23].

Pruritus is the second most common symptom in PBC patients (up to 70%). Except for cholestasis, that impairs the excretion of pruritogenic compounds, such as bile salts, histamine, progesterones, oestrogens and serotonin, a central component of pruritus has also been suggested based on opioidergic activity reported in cholestatic patients [23].

Osteoporosis is present in approximately 30% of PBC patients and is associated with duration and severity of underlying liver disease. In this context, osteoporosis is reported in up to 44% in patients awaiting liver transplantation. The etiology is multifactorial, including presence of cholestasis [1].

Hypercholesterolaemia, which is evident in the majority of PBC patients, is related to the presence of cholestasis. It's not associated with increased atherosclerotic risk and doesn't need treatment unless other parameters that relate to increased cardiovascular risks exist [1].

Other autoimmune diseases coexist in 35–55% of PBC patients, including Sjögren syndrome, autoimmune thyroid disease, rheumatoid arthritis, scleroderma or CREST syndrome and inflammatory bowel disease [1].

Patients in advanced PBC stages can have symptoms related to portal hypertension, including hemorrhage due to esophageal varices, ascites and hepatic encephalopathy. Of note, esophageal varices can be a feature of early stage PBC in a small proportion of patients.

24.5 Diagnosis

During evaluation of a patient with persistent cholestasis, it is mandatory to perform initially a liver ultrasound to exclude the presence of focal liver lesions and dilatation of the intra- and extrahepatic bile ducts [24, 25].

24.5.1 Biochemical Findings

The typical biochemical profile of a patient with PBC consists of increased alkaline phosphatase (ALP) levels with or without increase of g-glutamyl-transpeptidase (gGT) and milder elevation of alanine aminotransferase (ALT) and aspartate aminotransferase (AST). ALP correlates with the degree of ductopenia in non-cirrhotic patients. Increase in bilirubin levels is a characteristic of advanced stage and relates to severity of ductopenia and biliary piecemeal necrosis [24, 25].

Patients with PBC often present with increased levels of serum IgM. In cases where elevation of IgG occurs, the possibility of PBC-autoimmune hepatitis (AIH) variant must be further assessed, as this carries worst prognosis and needs alternative treatment regiments.

24.5.2 Autoantibodies

The cornerstone of PBC diagnosis is the detection of AMA, which are disease specific.

AMA are detected in over 90% of PBC patients and can precede the appearance of cholestasis and symptoms by many years.

Indirect immunofluorescence using Hep2 cells or rat liver, kidney and stomach cryostat sections as the substrate is the gold standard for AMA diagnosis. Typically, AMA exhibit a fine granular cytoplasmic staining of both distal and proximal renal tubules along with staining of gastric parietal cells and hepatocytes. AMA are considered positive when detected at a titre greater than 1 /40 [24–26].

Complementary to IIF, enzyme-linked immunosorbent assays (ELISAs) should be used in patients found to be AMA positive. An ELISA containing a recombinant fusion protein (MIT3), which includes the three immunodominant AMA targets (PDC-E2, BCOADC-E2 and OGDC-E2), has demonstrated improved performance over IIFL, being able to unmask 30–50% of AMA negative patients evaluated by IIFL. Additionally, immunoblotting can be used as a tool to identify and characterize the individual molecular targets visualized as bands, i.e. PDC-E2 at 74 kDa, BCOADC-E2 at 52 kDa and OGDC-E2 at 48 kDa [24–26].

AMA negative patients with high suspicion for PBC should be tested for PBC-specific ANA, which are considered not sensitive, though disease specific. PBC-specific ANA are reported in up to 50% of PBC patients and display two distinct immunofluorescence patterns: a multiple nuclear dot (MND) and a perinuclear/rim-like (RLM) pattern. The MND pattern, characterized by the presence of 3–20 dots throughout the nucleus, is generated by reactivity against sp100 and promyelocytic leukemia (PML) that usually co-occur. The RLM pattern exhibits a characteristic punctuated pattern of the nuclear surface, each representing a nuclear complex. The RLM pattern is generated by reactivity to nuclear pore complexes (NPC), which are supramolecular structures mediating nucleocytoplasmic transport. Most recognized ANA targets in PBC patients with RLM pattern are gp210, nucleoporin p62 and lamin B receptor [24–26].

The identification of PBC-specific molecular targets has facilitated the detection of these antibodies, as ELISAs and immunoblot assays have been established based on the use of recombinant antigens. Considering that the interpretation of IIF patterns might be often complex especially in people not familiar with the technique, these molecular based methods can overcome this and contribute to PBC diagnosis since they are sensitive and non-observer dependent.

In terms of prognosis, several studies have reported an association between presence of anti-sp100 and anti-gp210 with unfavorable disease course, as illustrated by worst biochemical and histological disease, faster disease progression and poorer outcome [27].

Overall, the diagnosis of PBC can be established based on the presence of cholestasis and the detection of AMA and/or PBC-specific ANA, which are specific for the disease. Performance of liver biopsy is not considered essential for PBC diagnosis any longer. According to the latest clinical practice guidelines for the management of patients with PBC a liver biopsy should be performed when autoantibodies are negative and when co-existence of other liver diseases is suspected, i.e. autoimmune hepatitis, non-alcoholic steatohepatitis, or liver involvement in the context of a systemic illness [24, 25].

24.5.3 Histology

The characteristic histological picture of PBC is that of chronic, non-suppurative lymphocytic inflammation surrounding the interlobular and septal bile ducts alongside with granuloma formation leading to cholestasis. During advanced stages bile duct loss (ductopenia) occurs and fibrosis progresses leading to cirrhosis. During the last 50 years two histological scoring systems (Scheuer and Ludwig) have been widely used to assess liver histology in PBC. Both divide histological changes in four stages [24, 25]. In both systems the four different stages are distinguished from each other on the basis of combinations of portal and periportal inflammation, ductular inflammation and fibrosis. Still, both scores have considerable drawbacks and render them not sufficient enough for the reliable assessment of liver histology. This mainly relates to the fact that PBC has a patchy distribution and often all four stages can be represented in a single sample. In addition, both systems fail to assess independently histological features considered to have prognostic value, including lymphocytic interface hepatitis, fibrosis and ductopenia [24, 25]. Another histologic feature of PBC is nodular regenerative hyperplasia, which may contribute to development of portal hypertension in the absence of cirrhosis.

Recently two novel scoring systems have been proposed for the evaluation of liver histology in PBC. Prognostic values like interface hepatitis, bile duct loss and fibrosis are evaluated separately and limited data show adequate interobserver and intra-observer reproducibility. Additional data are needed to address their prognostic relevance in larger number of PBC patients [24, 25].

24.5.4 Non-invasive Methods for Monitoring Disease Stage

Liver stiffness measurement (LSM) estimated by transient elastography (TE, Fibroscan) has been proven to be a highly accurate method for identification of PBC patients with severe fibrosis and cirrhosis. A number of studies report a higher diagnostic accuracy of TE compared to APRI score, ELF score, and hyaluronic acid level, while all of them have established ability on predicting clinical outcomes. Specifically, a study encompassing 103 PBC patients has shown LSM $\geq$9.6 kPa to be associated with a fivefold increase in the risk of liver decompensation, liver transplantation or death [28]. An increase of $\geq$2.1 kPa/year during longitudinal evaluation of TE has been also reported to have prognostic value. In addition, non response to UDCA treatment has been linked with worsening of LSM [24, 25, 28].

Accordingly LSM has been suggested as a tool to risk stratify PBC patients, while its incorporation in prognostic scores to predict patient's outcomes is anticipated. Even though the use of TE is increasing, LSM prognostic cut-off levels in determining low vs high risk patients as well as intervals for applicability of TE need to be determined.

24.6 Natural History of PBC and Treatment

24.6.1 Natural History of PBC in the Pre-UDCA Era

In the pre-UDCA era, PBC was regarded as a gradual progressive disease with no uniform pattern of evolution and impaired outcome compared to the general population [1, 24, 25, 29]. In this context, the natural history of PBC is schematically divided in four phases. The first is a long preclinical phase, where AMA are detected in serum without biochemical or clinical features of the disease. According to a recent population-based study one out of six AMA positive individuals are going to develop abnormal liver function tests during a 5-year period. Though in study of 29 untreated PBC patients time up to development of cholestasis varied from 1 to 19 years.

During the second phase, liver enzymes gradually increase, whereas patients remain asymptomatic. Characteristic of the third phase is the development of symptoms. Several studies have reported development of symptoms in 36–86% of patients during a period of 5–17 years [29]. Even though asymptomatic patients tend to have longer survival compared to symptomatic patients, they have impaired prognosis associated with non-liver related deaths. The fourth phase is characterized by symptoms of decompensated disease and inevitable evolution to death unless liver transplantation is offered to the patients. In line with this, a follow up study of 225 patients under ineffective treatment, estimated the histological progression per stage to be 1.5 years [30].

24.6.2 Natural History and Treatment of PBC

Treatment of PBC should involve a multidisciplinary patient approach including medications to delay disease progression, management of disease-related symptoms and careful surveying of patients according to disease stage [24, 25].

24.6.2.1 Medications to Delay Disease Progression

UDCA

The natural history of PBC has changed considerably over the last 50 years and this relates mainly to earlier diagnosis and use of UDCA. From early 1990s up to 2016, UDCA, a hydrophilic endogenous bile acid, was the only approved treatment for PBC.

Research over the last decades has indicated multiple sites and mechanisms of UDCA action. In detail, UDCA enriches and expands the bile acid pool, which results in less toxic bile composition. Additionally, UDCA enhances secretion of bile acids ameliorating hepatocyte damage, apoptosis and necrosis and thus diminishing inflammation and fibrosis. Analogously, UDCA enriched bile is less toxic to cholangiocytes. UDCA has been also shown to enhance the impaired expression of AE2 in PBC patients, resulting in restoration of secretin-induced HCO_3^- secretion. UDCA has been also proposed to have immunomodulatory properties as demonstrated by reduction of IFN-γ mediated by elevated glucocorticoid receptor in liver lymphocytes and independent of IL-12/18 [31].

UDCA is the initial recommended option for PBC patients and further treatment choices should be guided by the initial drug response [24, 25]. At a dose of 13–15 mg/kg/day, UDCA is generally well tolerated with no severe side effects. Occasionally, abdominal discomfort, flatulence or even diarrhea is reported, though usually transient during the initial period of administration.

Accumulating evidence over the years has proven that UDCA at a dose of 13–15 mg/kg/day offers advantage in terms of improved survival in PBC patients, especially those at stage I/II of the disease, who will demonstrate biochemical response.

Several studies have shown that progression of PBC to cirrhosis in patients under UDCA treatment depends on the pre-treatment disease stage. In a study of 183 non-cirrhotic, UDCA treated PBC patients the median time for developing cirrhosis from stage I, II and III was 25, 20 and 4 years respectively. These results suggest that those who benefit the most from UDCA treatment are patients with early disease stages [32]. In addition, administration of UDCA at early stages of PBC is associated with survival similar to the general population.

A recent multicenter study including 4805 PBC patients from 17 centers across Europe and North America spanning a 44-year period (1970–2014) has shown that in recent decades patients are diagnosed at older age, though at earlier biochemical and histological disease stages [33]. Accordingly, the authors demonstrated increased response to UDCA in this population, while for the first time provided evidence for lower decompensation rates and higher 10-year transplant –free survival in PBC patients [33].

Several studies, though, have shown non-response to UDCA treatment in up to 40% of patients. Inadequate response to treatment has been associated with rapid disease progression and higher risk of liver-related death or transplantation.

In the era of precision medicine it is of outmost importance to use indices to accurately prognosticate patients on high risk for adverse outcomes and need for aggressive treatment and close monitoring. In general such a strategy facilitates better allocation of health care resources tailored to each patient, while simultaneously improves delivery with less costs [34].

In line with these, one of the treatment priorities in PBC is the stratification of patients into low and high risk for development of complications of end stage live disease [24, 25, 34]. A major step forward was achieved in 2006, when biochemical response to UDCA treatment, defined as normalization or 40% decrease in alkaline phosphatase values after 1 year of treatment, was shown to be a strong predictor of long-term outcome of PBC [35]. These findings paved the way during the following period for the development of several prognostic models based on treatment response (Table 24.2) [24, 25, 29, 34]. The majority of these models agree that certain decrease or normalization of alkaline phosphatase after 12 month UDCA treatment is a robust prognostic indicator of favorable outcome. It is generally accepted that the preferred prediction model should include bilirubin and alkaline phosphatase. Nowadays Paris I/II criteria are considered the most accurate dichotomous models to predict 12-month response to UDCA (Table 24.2) [24, 25, 29, 34].

Still, these binary models cannot provide individualized prediction of prognosis for PBC patients. In 2015 and 2016, two continuous models, the GLOBE score and the UK-PBC score respectively, were developed in order to provide more accurate information on the prognosis of PBC patients. Both models use simple biochemical indices to assess biochemi-

Table 24.2 Criteria—prognostic scoring systems for defining biochemical non-response to ursodeoxycholic acid treatment and prognosis in primary biliary cholangitis

	Definition of treatment non-response	Time of assessment (months)
Binary criteria		
Barcelona	Decrease in ALP ≤ 40% and ALP ≥ 1× ULN	12
Paris I	ALP ≥ 3× ULN or AST ≥ 2 ULN or bilirubin>1 mg/dl	12
Rotterdam	Bilirubin ≥1× ULN and/or albumin <1× ULN	12
Toronto	ALP > 1.67× ULN	24
Paris II	ALP ≥ 1.5× ULN or AST ≥ 1.5 ULN or bilirubin>1 mg/dl	12
Ehime	Decrease in γ GT ≤ 70% and γ GT ≥ 1× ULN	6
Lammers	ALP > 2× ULN and/or bilirubin >1× ULN	12
Continuous scoring systems		
GLOBE score	Bilirubin, ALP, albumin and platelet count at 12 months Age at diagnosis	12
UK-PBC score	Bilirubin, ALP and AST (or ALT) at 12 months Albumin and platelet count at baseline	12

cal response to UDCA treatment and also parameters that are surrogate markers of disease stage and disease activity [24, 25, 29, 34]. In this way, both models combine prediction of treatment response and disease severity and estimate risk of liver-related death or liver transplantation free survival at specific time points in the future up to 15 years. In this way, both scores outperform Paris I criteria in terms of risk estimation of death or liver transplantation.

Even though these models need to be validated in larger populations and different ethnic groups, both of them have been proposed by recently published clinical practice guidelines as tools for selection of patients for second-line treatment in every day clinical praxis or in clinical trials [24, 25].

In the future a lot of effort should be put in establishing factors that could predict prognosis prior to starting treatment. In this way, high risk patients could be treated initially with a combination of drugs and be under strict monitoring in specialized liver clinics, while low risk patients could be treated with UDCA and be integrated in a primary care follow up. Along this line, in a recent paper a new model was introduced and validated for the prediction of pre-treatment UDCA response. In this model the authors incorporated factors that were associated with inadequate UDCA response, including high alkaline phosphatase concentration, higher total bilirubin concentration, lower aminotransferase concentration, younger age, longer interval from diagnosis to the start of UDCA treatment and worsening of alkaline phosphatase concentration from diagnosis [36]. Future research should aim at validating these models in larger populations and focus on their implementation in clinical practice. In summary, assessment of treatment response after 12 months of UDCA is mandatory in order to identify patients at risk of progression and individually explore further therapeutic options and follow up measures.

Obeticholic Acid

Obeticholic acid (OCA) has been approved by FDA in 2016 and is now recommended by the latest EASL, BASL and AASLD guidelines either as combination with UDCA in patients with inadequate response to UDCA or as monotherapy in patients intolerant to UDCA [24, 25]. OCA belongs to the family of farnesoid X receptor (FXR) agonists. FXRs are nuclear receptors highly expressed in the liver and intestine, where enterohepatic circulation of bile acids takes place. They regulate bile acid synthesis, secretion, transport and detoxification, while also exerting anti-inflammatory effects via induction of fibroblast growth factor (FGF)-19 expression. In detail, FXR agonists lower intrahepatic bile acid concentration by suppressing cholesterol 7a-hydroxylase, which is the rate-limiting step for the production of bile acids and by promoting transport of bile acids out of the hepatocytes.

OCA is a synthetic by-product of chenodeoxycholic acid with increased potency and thus considered a strong FXR agonist. Three studies up to the present have shown significant improvement in alkaline phosphatase and bilirubin when OCA was administered either as add-on treatment to UDCA or as monotherapy [24, 25, 37]. Initial recommended dose of OCA is 5 mg/day with a dose titration to 10 mg depending on tolerability at 6 months. One of the major drawbacks of OCA treatment is exacerbation of pruritus, which is dose-dependent. This was proven to be successfully managed by dose titration of the drug, as already stated, or addition of other drugs with anti-pruritic action, like rifampicin which leads to lower frequency of obeticholic acid discontinuation. In addition, OCA treatment was associated with alterations in lipid metabolism, as shown by a significant decrease of high-density lipoprotein cholesterol and an increase of low-density lipoprotein. The potential consequences of these changes on cardiovascular risk need to be addressed in future studies with long-term follow up. In addition, long-term survival benefit of PBC patients under combination of UDCA and OCA or OCA monotherapy needs to be assessed in the future.

Other Treatment Modalities

Over the previous years various trials have assessed the efficacy of different agents in patients with PBC. Though, none has gained approval for the treatment of PBC so far.

Fibrates, largely known for their established role in the treatment of hypertriglyceridemia, have been shown to activate peroxisome proliferator-activated receptors (PPAR). Different fibrates exhibit different specificities for the three PPAR isoforms (α, β/γ and δ) and in this way result in different effects.

Existing data originate from trials of fenofibrate, a selective PPARa-agonist in PBC and benzafibrate, a non-selective PPAR-agonist. Various pilot studies, where fibrates were used in addition to UDCA, had shown improvement in liver biochemistry, though were small in size. A recent multicenter French study has demonstrated beneficial effects after 2 year add-on treatment of benzafibrate to UDCA in patients with inadequate response to UDCA, as defined by the Paris II criteria [38]. In the combination group, two third of patients showed normalization of alkaline phosphatase and one third achieved complete normalization of many biochemical parameters, including alkaline phosphatase, bilirubin, albumin and aminotransferases, while also significant improvement in liver stiffness measurements was noted. In addition, pruritus improved remarkably in this group. Trials with other PPARs agonists, including seladelpar, a selective PPARδ-agonist and elafibranor, a dual PPARα/δ-agonist, are under way.

Budesonide is a highly effective steroid, the first that was used as a second-line treatment for PBC. Budesonide is a highly potent steroid with lower risk of systemic side effects compared to classic steroids that is due to its ability to first pass the liver by 90%, while only 10% reaches the systemic circulation. *In vitro* studies have shown a synergistic affect between budesonide and UDCA in upregulating AE2 expression. In view of conflicting results from various trials so far and of its steroid-related side effects especially in patients with decompensated cirrhosis, budesonide hasn't gained further interest as candidate treatment tool in PBC.

Over the years, results from the use of immunosuppressive treatment (methotrexate, colchicine, azathioprine, cyclosporine, mycophenolate mofetil) mainly as add-on to UDCA were rather disappointing.

A variety of trials with agents targeting the toxic effects of bile acid, biologic agents targeting cytokines and other immune pathways possibly involved in the pathogenesis of the disease are under way.

Briefly, agents aiming at bile acid depletion have gained interest. In detail, the effect of a fibroblast growth factor-19, which modulates bile acid synthesis by interaction with FGF receptor 4 has being explored. Analogously, inhibition of bile acid reabsorption in terminal ileum with antagonists of apical sodium-dependent bile acid transporter is also under investigation. Moreover improvement of bicarbonate secretion in response to bile acid exposure is being tested as this results in altering hydrophobicity of bile acid and cytotoxic cytokine release and regulates the circulating bile acid pool.

Considering the active involvement of T and B cells in the pathogenesis of BECs damage in PBC, targeting of these cells or co-stimulatory molecules that might induce their action has been a rational strategy. Accordingly, a number of clinical trials are completed or are still ongoing.

Evolving knowledge on the pathogenetic mechanisms of PBC will aid in identifying novel unknown targets for pharmacological intervention.

Liver Transplantation

Up to the present liver transplantation has been the most effective treatment for end-stage liver disease of various etiologies. Improvement of transplant-free survival over the years resulted in a decline of PBC as an indication for transplantation. Indications for transplantation in PBC patients include end-stage liver disease and intractable pruritus [24, 25].

In general, patient survival after liver transplantation is better in PBC compared to other etiologies. In detail, 5-year patient and graft survival has been reported to be 82–90% and 81–82% respectively [39]. Reported frequencies of PBC recurrence in the liver graft show a wide range between studies (17–46%), depending on different criteria used for the definition of PBC recurrence.

Indicative histological changes are essential for the diagnosis of PBC. Though, in these cases histology might often be confused with allograft rejection. Amongst various parameters, tacrolimus as immunosuppressant is considered a risk factor for PBC recurrence, while cyclosporine and preemptive use of UDCA has been suggested to have protective role [39].

24.6.2.2 Active Management of Disease-Related Symptoms

Management of symptoms in PBC often needs special attention and individualized treatment. Disease-specific symptoms, like pruritus and fatigue can frequently cause significant quality of life impairment and treatment often is complex [23].

There is no recommended treatment for fatigue, which is a frequent symptom in PBC patients leading to severe quality of life impairment in a proportion of them. Taking into account the multifactorial nature of fatigue in PBC, a structured approach could be beneficial for the patients, including assessment of fatigue's severity using standardized tools (i.e. PBC-40 questionnaire), exclusion and treatment of confounding factors (hypothyroidism, anemia) and support of patients through implementation of different copying strategies [23–25]. Up to the present no disease-specific management (UDCA, OCA), nor fatigue-oriented regiments (serotonin reuptake inhibitors, modafinil) were proven to reduce fatigue. In a recent meta-analysis, liver transplantation was suggested to offer some improvement in terms of fatigue, though without eradicating it.

Pruritus, another debilitating symptom affecting a significant proportion of PBC patients remains often difficult to manage. Current guidelines recommend a structured approach, where other causes of pruritus must be excluded (i.e. bile duct obstruction). Life style modifications such as use of skin moisturizers, avoiding hot water during baths, may soothe pruritus [23–25].

First-line treatment for pruritus are non-absorbable resins, like cholestyramine and newer formulations (colesevelam and colestipol), that bind bile acids and have shown to alleviate pruritus. Major drawbacks are the fact that they should be taken far from other drugs to avoid interference with their intestinal absorption and also the common appearance of side effects, like bloating, constipation and/or diarrhea.

Second-line treatment for pruritus is rifampicin (150–300 mg/day), a pregnane X receptor agonist, that has been used for treatment of cholestatic pruritus and its effect has been proven in placebo randomized clinical trials. Given potential side effects from rifampicin use (hepatotoxicity and hemolysis) a strict follow up is mandatory during treatment. Other drugs that have been administered in cases of non responsiveness to the abovementioned remedies are oral opiate antagonists (naltrexone and nalmefene) and selective serotonin reuptake inhibitors (SSRIs; e.g. sertraline) and gabapentin. All the above should be administered with caution due to their side effects. Severe intractable pruritus is rarely an indication for liver transplantation [23–25].

24.7 Variant Syndromes of PBC

A small proportion of PBC patients can manifest as variants of the disease. Amongst them are the AMA negative PBC, PBC-AIH variant and the premature ductopenic variant. Recognition of these cases is of paramount importance, since they usually have different prognosis and require different treatment strategies. Up to the present difficulties in managing these patients relates to the rarity of these entities, the lack of appropriate definitions and limited data on treatment modalities and response [24, 25, 40].

24.7.1 AMA Negative PBC

Patients being both AMA and PBC-specific ANA negative are scarce. In such cases where there is high suspicion of PBC based on the presence of cholestasis and other compatible clinical features, a liver biopsy must be performed to confirm the diagnosis. These patients have similar natural course, response to UDCA treatment and long term prognosis to those being AMA and/or PBC-specific ANA positive.

24.7.2 PBC-AIH Variant

Around 10% of PBC patients present with clinical and laboratory characteristics of AIH either simultaneously or during the natural course of the disease. The term PBC-AIH variant has been lately proposed by EASL as more suitable for this group of patients.

Criteria established for the diagnosis of AIH, including the revised and the simplified criteria should not be applied for the diagnosis of PBC-AIH variants [40]. Currently the Paris criteria proposed in 1998 are being used for the diagnosis of such cases in everyday clinical practice. According to these criteria, for the diagnosis of variant PBC-AIH, the presence of at least two out the three criteria for each disease is required. In detail, the criteria for PBC include: (1) increase of ALP $\geq$ x2 upper normal limit (ULN) or gGT $\geq$ x5 ULN, (2) presence of AMA and (3) existence of florid bile duct lesions and criteria for AIH include: (1) increase of ALT $\geq$ x5 ULN; (2) increase of serum IgG levels $\geq$x2 ULN or presence of SMA and (3) moderate or severe interface hepatitis in the liver biopsy.

However, recently the EASL clinical practice guidelines for AIH suggested considering patients for treatment at lower cut-off levels for IgG and ALT [40]. Bearing in mind these uncertainties, scientific societies consider the performance of a liver biopsy mandatory. In this way decision of further management should be guided based to the presence of histological characteristics of AIH, including interface hepatitis, lymphoplasmacytic infiltrates, hepatocellular rosette formation etc.. Additionally, non-response to UDCA treatment in conjunction with increased serum aminotransferases and IgG should be another indication for a liver biopsy, as this could indicate coexistence of AIH.

According to existing guidelines for PBC, these patients should receive immunosuppressive treatment (steroids alone or combined with azathioprine) [24, 25, 40].

24.7.3 Premature Ductopenic Variant

This is a rare PBC variant characterized by rapidly progressive cholestasis, jaundice and severe pruritus, while on histology extensive bile duct loss is evident without considerable fibrosis. These patients don't respond to UDCA and will eventually need a liver transplant.

24.8 Staging and Surveying of PBC Patients

Accurate staging and surveying of liver disease is also essential for risk stratification of PBC patients [24, 25]. Accumulating evidence indicate that except for advanced stage and non-response to UDCA treatment, other markers indicating poor prognosis of PBC patients are younger age at diagnosis, male sex, presence of PBC-specific ANA and increased bilirubin levels [1, 24–28]. It is advisable to manage these high-risk patients in specialist centers.

As mentioned previously, TE is currently the preferred tool for disease staging compare to histology. Still, in cases where a liver biopsy is performed, histological features like the degree of lymphopenic interface hepatitis and bile ductopenia are considered bad prognostic indicators for disease progression.

Surveying of liver disease is recommended in all PBC patients using liver biochemistry (bilirubin, albumin, ALP), platelets and TE measurements [24, 25]. A liver ultrasound is mandatory as surveillance for hepatocellular carcinoma in cirrhotic patients [24, 25].

24.9 Conclusion/Summary

Significant progress has been achieved in various fields of PBC research during the last decades. PBC patients are a heterogeneous population in terms of disease presentation and progression and response to treatment. During the last decade studies based on large PBC cohorts have facilitated the identification of prognostic factors and assisted the risk stratification of patients according to their demographic, clinical characteristics and response to UDCA treatment.

Advances in the era of PBC therapeutics are evolving, including the recent approval of obeticholic acid and investigation of a large spectrum of drugs and targeted therapies. The future of treatment in PBC could be the combination of agents in non-responders to UDCA or those considered of high risk of disease progression at initial evaluation.

Self Study

Questions

1. A 55-year old woman presents to the clinic with a 6-month history of progressively deteriorating pruritus and fatigue. Liver biochemistry shows an increase in ALP (×2.5 ULN) and slight increase of gGT and ALT. She denies alcohol drinking and systematic use of any drugs. On clinical examination she has palmar erythema and enlarged liver. Liver and bile duct ultrasound show hepatomegaly, with no liver lesions or bile duct dilatation. What is the test that you are going to order next for this patient?
   (a) Antinuclear antibodies
   (b) Antimitochondrial antibodies
   (c) Serum IgM
   (d) Liver biopsy
2. What is not true about PBC?
   (a) PBC affects predominantly men
   (b) PBC patients often have increased cholesterol levels
   (c) Hashimoto's thyroiditis co-exist in a significant proportion of patients
   (d) Antinuclear antibodies displaying a multiple nuclear dot and a perinuclear/rim-like pattern in indirect immunofluorescence are considered specific for PBC
3. What is the initial recommended treatment of choice in PBC?
   (a) Budenofalk
   (b) Ursodeoxycholic acid
   (c) Azathioprine
   (d) Fibrates

Answers

1. A 55-year old woman presents to the clinic with a 6-month history of progressively deteriorating pruritus and fatigue. Liver biochemistry shows an increase in ALP (×2.5 ULN) and slight increase of gGT and ALT. She denies alcohol drinking and systematic use of any drugs. On clinical examination she has palmar erythema and enlarged liver. Liver and bile duct ultrasound show hepatomegaly, with no liver lesions or bile duct dilatation. What is the test that you are going to order next for this patient?
   (a) Antinuclear antibodies can be positive in PBC and some of them are regarded as disease-specific. However, this is not the first test to be ordered in cases of high suspicion of PBC
   (b) CORRECT ANSWER. In patients with cholestasis and other clinical features suggestive of the PBC, the diagnosis can be established based on the detection of antimitochondrial antibodies (titre > 1/40), which are present in over 90% of patients and are considered disease specific.
   (c) Serum IgM is often elevated in PBC patients and can aid in establishing the diagnosis in atypical cases. Though serum IgM is not a criterion for PBC diagnosis.
   (d) Liver biopsy is not necessary in typical PBC cases with presence of cholestasis and antimitochondrial antibodies.
2. What is not true about PBC?
   (a) CORRECT ANSWER. PBC affects predominantly women. Average reported female to male ratio are 10:1
   (b) Hypercholesterolemia is a frequent feature in PBC patients

   (c) Hashimoto's thyroiditis is one of the most frequent autoimmune diseases that co-exist in PBC patients
   (d) Antinuclear antibodies displaying a multiple nuclear dot and a perinuclear/rim-like pattern in indirect immunofluorescence are considered specific for PBC and are present in up to 50% of PBC patients depending from the method used.
3. What is the initial recommended treatment of choice in PBC?
   (a) Budenofalk is not a licensed drug for PBC and cannot be recommended
   (b) CORRECT ANSWER. Ursodeoxycholic acid is recommended by scientific societies as first-line treatment for all patients with PBC that usually continues for life.
   (c) Azathioprine doesn't belong to the armamentarium of PBC. It can be administered in conjunction with steroids in variant PBC-AIH cases.
   (d) Fibrates are being studied in PBC as add-on treatment to UDCA in non-responders to UDCA. Up to the present they are non-licensed for PBC treatment.

References

1. Carey EJ, Ali AH, Lindor KD. Primary biliary cirrhosis. Lancet. 2015;386(10003):1565–75.
2. Beuers U, Gershwin ME, Gish RG, Invernizzi P, Jones DE, Lindor K, et al. Changing nomenclature for PBC: from 'cirrhosis' to 'cholangitis'. J Hepatol. 2015;63(5):1285–7.
3. Boonstra K, Beuers U, Ponsioen CY. Epidemiology of primary sclerosing cholangitis and primary biliary cirrhosis: a systematic review. J Hepatol. 2012;56(5):1181–8.
4. James OF, Bhopal R, Howel D, Gray J, Burt AD, Metcalf JV. Primary biliary cirrhosis once rare, now common in the United Kingdom? Hepatology. 1999;30(2):390–4.
5. Kim WR, Lindor KD, Locke GR 3rd, Therneau TM, Homburger HA, Batts KP, et al. Epidemiology and natural history of primary biliary cirrhosis in a US community. Gastroenterology. 2000;119(6):1631–6.
6. Gatselis NK, Zachou K, Lygoura V, Azariadis K, Arvaniti P, Spyrou E, et al. Geoepidemiology, clinical manifestations and outcome of primary biliary cholangitis in Greece. Eur J Intern Med. 2017;42:81–8.
7. Hamlyn AN, Sherlock S. The epidemiology of primary biliary cirrhosis: a survey of mortality in England and Wales. Gut. 1974;15(6):473–9.
8. Cheung KS, Seto WK, Fung J, Lai CL, Yuen MF. Epidemiology and natural history of primary biliary cholangitis in the Chinese: a territory-based study in Hong Kong between 2000 and 2015. Clin Transl Gastroenterol. 2017;8(8):e116.
9. Kim KA, Ki M, Choi HY, Kim BH, Jang ES, Jeong SH. Population-based epidemiology of primary biliary cirrhosis in South Korea. Aliment Pharmacol Ther. 2016;43(1):154–62.
10. Hirschfield GM, Gershwin ME. The immunobiology and pathophysiology of primary biliary cirrhosis. Annu Rev Pathol. 2013;8:303–30.
11. Webb GJ, Siminovitch KA, Hirschfield GM. The immunogenetics of primary biliary cirrhosis: a comprehensive review. J Autoimmun. 2015;64:42–52.
12. Lleo A, Maroni L, Glaser S, Alpini G, Marzioni M. Role of cholangiocytes in primary biliary cirrhosis. Semin Liver Dis. 2014;34(3):273–84.
13. Selmi C, Mayo MJ, Bach N, Ishibashi H, Invernizzi P, Gish RG, et al. Primary biliary cirrhosis in monozygotic and dizygotic twins: genetics, epigenetics, and environment. Gastroenterology. 2004;127(2):485–92.
14. Tanaka A, Leung PSC, Gershwin ME. The genetics and epigenetics of primary biliary cholangitis. Clin Liver Dis. 2018;22(3):443–55.
15. Joshita S, Umemura T, Tanaka E, Ota M. Genetics and epigenetics in the pathogenesis of primary biliary cholangitis. Clin J Gastroenterol. 2018;11(1):11–8.
16. Banales JM, Sáez E, Uriz M, Sarvide S, Urribarri AD, Splinter P, et al. Up-regulation of microRNA 506 leads to decreased Cl^-/HCO_3^- anion exchanger 2 expression in biliary epithelium of patients with primary biliary cirrhosis. Hepatology. 2012;56(2):687–97.
17. Smyk D, Rigopoulou EI, Baum H, Burroughs AK, Vergani D, Bogdanos DP. Autoimmunity and environment: am I at risk? Clin Rev Allergy Immunol. 2012;42(2):199–212.
18. Shimoda S, Nakamura M, Ishibashi H, Kawano A, Kamihira T, Sakamoto N, et al. Molecular mimicry of mitochondrial and nuclear autoantigens in primary biliary cirrhosis. Gastroenterology. 2003;124(7):1915–25.
19. Bogdanos DP, Baum H, Grasso A, Okamoto M, Butler P, Ma Y, et al. Microbial mimics are major targets of crossreactivity with human pyruvate dehydrogenase in primary biliary cirrhosis. J Hepatol. 2004;40(1):31–9.
20. Tanaka T, Zhang W, Sun Y, Shuai Z, Chida AS, Kenny TP, et al. Autoreactive monoclonal antibodies from patients with primary biliary cholangitis recognize environmental xenobiotics. Hepatology. 2017;66(3):885–95.
21. Liaskou E, Patel SR, Webb G, Bagkou Dimakou D, Akiror S, Krishna M, et al. Increased sensitivity of Treg cells from patients with PBC to low dose IL-12 drives their differentiation into IFN-γ secreting cells. J Autoimmun. 2018;94:143–55.
22. Prince MI, Chetwynd A, Craig WL, Metcalf JV, James OF. Asymptomatic primary biliary cirrhosis: clinical features, prognosis, and symptom progression in a large population based cohort. Gut. 2004;53(6):865–70.
23. Khanna A, Leighton J, Lee Wong L, Jones DE. Symptoms of PBC—pathophysiology and management. Best Pract Res Clin Gastroenterol. 2018;34–35:41–7.
24. EASL Clinical Practice Guidelines. The diagnosis and management of patients with primary biliary cholangitis. J Hepatol. 2017;67(1):145–72.
25. Hirschfield GM, Dyson JK, Alexander GJM, Chapman MH, Collier J, Hübscher S, et al. The British Society of Gastroenterology/UK-PBC primary biliary cholangitis treatment and management guidelines. Gut. 2018;67(9):1568–94.
26. Rigopoulou EI, Dalekos GN. Molecular diagnostics of primary biliary cirrhosis. Expert Opin Med Diagn. 2008;2(6):621–34.
27. Rigopoulou EI, Davies ET, Pares A, Zachou K, Liaskos C, Bogdanos DP, et al. Prevalence and clinical significance of isotype specific antinuclear antibodies in primary biliary cirrhosis. Gut. 2005;54(4):528–32.
28. Corpechot C. Utility of noninvasive markers of fibrosis in cholestatic liver diseases. Clin Liver Dis. 2016;20(1):143–58.
29. Goel A, Kim WR. Natural history of primary biliary cholangitis in the ursodeoxycholic acid era: role of scoring systems. Clin Liver Dis. 2018;22(3):563–78.
30. Locke GR 3rd, Therneau TM, Ludwig J, Dickson ER, Lindor KD. Time course of histological progression in primary biliary cirrhosis. Hepatology. 1996;23(1):52–6.

31. Beuers U. Drug insight: mechanisms and sites of action of ursodeoxycholic acid in cholestasis. Nat Clin Pract Gastroenterol Hepatol. 2006;3(6):318–28.
32. Corpechot C, Carrat F, Poupon R, Poupon RE. Primary biliary cirrhosis: incidence and predictive factors of cirrhosis development in ursodiol-treated patients. Gastroenterology. 2002;122(3):652–8.
33. Murillo Perez CF, Goet JC, Lammers WJ, Gulamhusein A, van Buuren HR, Ponsioen CY, et al. GLOBAL PBC Study Group. Milder disease stage in patients with primary biliary cholangitis over a 44-year period: a changing natural history. Hepatology. 2018;67(5):1920–30.
34. Bossen L, Gerussi A, Lygoura V, Mells GF, Carbone M, Invernizzi P. Support of precision medicine through risk-stratification in autoimmune liver diseases – histology, scoring systems, and non-invasive markers. Autoimmun Rev. 2018;17(9):854–65.
35. Parés A, Caballería L, Rodés J. Excellent long-term survival in patients with primary biliary cirrhosis and biochemical response to ursodeoxycholic acid. Gastroenterology. 2006;130(3):715–20.
36. Carbone M, Nardi A, Flack S, Carpino G, Varvaropoulou N, Gavrila C, et al. Italian PBC Study Group and the UK–PBC Consortium. Pretreatment prediction of response to ursodeoxycholic acid in primary biliary cholangitis: development and validation of the UDCA Response Score. Lancet Gastroenterol Hepatol. 2018;3(9):626–34.
37. Nevens F, Andreone P, Mazzella G, Strasser SI, Bowlus C, Invernizzi P, et al. POISE Study Group. A placebo-controlled trial of obeticholic acid in primary biliary cholangitis. N Engl J Med. 2016;375(7):631–43.
38. Corpechot C, Chazouillères O, Rousseau A, Le Gruyer A, Habersetzer F, Mathurin P, et al. A placebo-controlled trial of bezafibrate in primary biliary cholangitis. N Engl J Med. 2018;378(23):2171–81.
39. Montano-Loza AJ, Bhanji RA, Wasilenko S, Mason AL. Systematic review: recurrent autoimmune liver diseases after liver transplantation. Aliment Pharmacol Ther. 2017;45(4):485–500.
40. EASL Clinical Practice Guidelines. Autoimmune hepatitis. J Hepatol. 2015;63(4):971–1004.

The Paucity of Interlobular Bile Ducts 25

Consolato M. Sergi

Key Concepts
- The remodeling of interlobular bile ducts starts in the perinatal liver.
- Reduction of the number of interlobular bile ducts may be observed from the neonatal age through adult life.
- Watson syndrome (arterio-hepatic dysplasia) is one of the most known genetic syndromes in pediatrics.

25.1 Introduction

The remodeling interlobular bile ducts (IBDs) is a fascinating interplay in the perinatal liver. The bile flows from the bile canaliculus of two adjacent hepatocytes through the Hering's canals into the IBDs, which are in the portal triads between the hepatic lobules. The IBDs will transfer the bile to segmental bile ducts and major bile ducts, which confluence into the right and left major bile ducts and, finally, to the common bile duct. The *ductus choledochus*, i.e., the common bile duct after joining of the *ductus cysticus* of the gallbladder, discharges at the duodenal papilla. The proper remodeling of the primitive (embryonic) ductal plate of the liver is on the basis of the formation of IBDs. Ductules or also known as cholangioles have a diameter of fewer than 20 μm, while IBDs of septal location has a diameter of 200–400 μm. Segmental interlobular bile ducts draining into hepatic ducts have a diameter of 400–800 μm [1]. In this chapter, the paucity of IBDs (PIBD) is explained into three paragraphs, including the cholangiocyte structure, the remodeling of the primitive ductal plate of the liver, and the clinical and genetic syndromes associated with the lack or paucity of the interlobular bile ducts.

C. M. Sergi (✉)
Department of Laboratory Medicine and Pathology, University of Alberta, Edmonton, AB, Canada

Stollery Children's Hospital, Edmonton, AB, Canada
e-mail: sergi@ualberta.ca

25.2 Cholangiocyte

Cholangiocytes account for 3–5% of the liver cell populations [1]. The cholangiocyte is critical in the biliary system for its receptors and transmembrane carriers. Refining of the bile by the cholangiocytes is key in this process. Cholangiocyte bile contributes to about 40% of the total biliary bile initially produced by the hepatocytes and secreted into the canalicular system of the hepatocytes. Interestingly, the use of immunohistochemistry has added an available tool for the study of the canalicular network in this process. A polyclonal antibody against carcinoembryonic antigen (CEA) provides a useful picture of this network that was formerly identified by transmission and scanning electron microscopy. In the cholangiocytes, crucial components are the Cl^- exchanger (i.e., cystic fibrosis transmembrane conductance regulator or CFTR), which is a 3′,5′-cyclic adenosine monophosphate (cAMP) activated channel, and the Cl^-/HCO^- exchanger. The hormone secretin binds to a receptor on the basolateral domain of cholangiocytes and stimulates the activity of CFTR on the apical domain through cAMP machinery. The chloride anions located in the lumen are exchanged with intracellular bicarbonate anions resulting in cholangiocyte secretion. The resulting consequent change of the bile is unique because it is more mature and prone to the secretory system targeting the gallbladder and the gastrointestinal lumen for digestion and absorption of fats and fat-soluble vitamins. Fetal liver organ cultures have demonstrated bile acid synthesis in liver conjugates and bile acid conjugation and secretion as early as the 12 weeks' gestation and bile acids can be isolated from gallbladder and liver in 14–16-week-old fetuses [2–4].

25.3 Ductal Plate Remodeling of the Liver

The understanding of the development of the intrahepatic biliary system is probably crucial to interpreting the categories of neonatal and infantile cholangiopathies adequately, mainly if infants are preterm or small for gestational age

F. Radu-Ionita et al. (eds.), *Liver Diseases*, https://doi.org/10.1007/978-3-030-24432-3_25

[5–8]. The study of the literature reveals that there are three major theories about the development of the intrahepatic biliary system. The first theory sustains that the intrahepatic biliary tree is solely derived from ingrowth of the epithelium of the extrahepatic bile ducts [9]. A second theory suggests that the whole intrahepatic bile-draining system develops from hepatocyte precursor cells [10]. A third theory combines elements of both first two indicating a melting of two different epithelial structures [11]. Currently, most embryologists and hepatology investigators favor the second theory, which is based on light microscopic, immunohistochemical, and ultrastructural investigations [7, 12–14].

At the third post-ovulation week, the liver primordium begins with endodermal cells sprouting from the cranial portion of the primitive foregut and growing towards a mesoderm growing progressively in the direction of the *plexus vitellinus* of the embryo. In the other direction, caudally, the anlage of the extrahepatic biliary system takes place [7]. The ductular reaction, which is observed after sub-massive/massive liver necrosis in fulminant hepatitis wires the physical presence of common progenitor cells that can differentiate in biliary epithelium along the portal vein branches. At the 6th–9th post-ovulation week, progenitor cells of the hilum cells in connection with the mesenchyme adjacent the portal vein form first mono- and later double-layered epithelial cell cords with a slit-like lumen ("stage of the ductal plate"). This proto-structure is the fundamental intrahepatic biliary structure, which is also called "ductal plate". From 12 gestational weeks on, a continuous and progressive remodeling of the ductal plate occurs. In a detailed morphometric study performed on migrating biliary structures, it has been identified that most of the peripheral bilaminar structures increasingly disappear [7]. However, very few parts of this first intrahepatic biliary bilaminar proto-structure dilate and progressively migrate toward an open center of spatiotemporal balance of the portal tract. These peripherally located tubular structures are remodeling structures and represent the immature form of the definitive fully-functional IBDs. The transformation of the primitive ductal plate into mature and bile-draining IBDs is accompanied by the expression of keratins, formerly called cytokeratins. They are specific intermediate filaments of the cytoskeleton, which is a central framework of the hepatocytes and cholangiocytes [7, 13]. The epithelial cells designated to form the IBDs express CK-7 and CK-19 in addition to CK-8 and CK-18 by immunohistochemistry. The latter two keratins are also positive in normal adult hepatocytes. Apart from the immunohistochemistry and visual recognition of these structures, there is a potential advantage in examining the microstructure of the liver under the lens if we deploy computer-aided techniques in morphometry accurately using a computer-based image morphometry algorithm with piecewise polynomial interpolation analysis [15, 16]. The need for measurement arises from our reflection that some of the decisions that we make in our daily routine may be poorly reproducible. The incorporation of central processing units (CPUs) to morphometry has opened the possibility of better evaluating structural remodeling during the ontogenesis. In the liver, quantification of biliary structures and their maturation may be useful in the evaluation of the intrahepatic biliary system in neonatal and infantile cholangiopathies [5]. Previously, three stages have been identified, including the stage of the ductal plate, the stage of the remodeling "ductal plate", and the stage of the remodeled IBDs [8]. Setting a stringent definition of the IBD is paramount. This duct should not be muddled with neo-cholangioles or neo-ductules. The immunostaining for CK7 is an advance in the laboratory to identify even minute or hypoplastic bile duct radicles that might well be missed in routinely stained sections. The IBD is a well-defined epithelial structure with cubic epithelium. It must be round or nearly round, harboring a well-developed lumen, and devoid of vacuolation, hyperchromasia or apoptosis [8]. The IBD must be convoyed by a portal arteriole, which is located typically (over 90% of the cases) within three arteriolar diameters of distance. This notion of valid IBD remains crucial [17]. The IBDs do not show any degree of flattening, which may advocate for bile ductular proliferation [17]. In all biopsies, an arteriolar to portal tract may need to be calculated to justify the absence of the IBDs. An elastic Van Gieson or a Movat pentachrome stain, which was originally developed in 1955 by Henry Zoltan Movat (1923–1995), a Romanian-Canadian Pathologist in Toronto, may also be very useful. Two or more of these stages may be present in the same liver specimen. We found that the surface and the perimeter of the portal tracts, the longest axis of the migrating peripheral tubular structures, and the maturation of bile ducts follow a process continuous and active up to term, but they slow down between the 20th and the 32nd week of gestation, when intraportal granulopoiesis of the liver is active [7]. Previously, we also showed that the lack of IBDs in infants aged less than 12 months is an adverse prognostic factor [5]. This data is independent of the etiology of the neonatal liver disease. Further, this data has been supported by the expression of polyductin or fibrocystin, the gene product of the autosomal recessive polycystic kidney disease (ARPKD) [18]. Ductal plate malformation may be quite unpredictable and can occur in infantile cholangiopathies. It represents overall a common way to indicate a disorder of the orthologous development of the intrahepatic biliary system in which the apoptosis may play a major role [6, 8, 19]. The rapid advances in the investigation of the cilia morphology and the comprehensive review of the cellular and molecular pathophysiology of bile secretion have led to a better knowledge of the pathophysiology of cholangiopathy and structural cell damage [19].

25.4 The Paucity of Interlobular Bile Ducts

The role of liver biopsy in identifying an abnormality of the development of the intrahepatic biliary system in neonatology is crucial and correlates with the development of the hepatic hematopoiesis. This data is hugely influential for the prognosis in infants presenting with liver disease and to identify "immaturity" in the developing biliary tract rather than scarcity of an adequate intrahepatic biliary system [7]. A scarcity or paucity of IBDs (PIBD) is defined as a reduction in the number of IBDs [20, 21]. The lesion produced from this reduction in the number of IBDs may be observed from the neonatal age through adult life. According to Hadchouel [20], the first case of absence of intrahepatic bile ducts in childhood was reported as "congenital dysplasia of the interlobular bile ducts" in a child with cirrhosis and extensive skin xanthomata by MacMahon and Thannhauser in 1952 [22]. At that time, the term PIBD was not existing but mirrored the description of "hypoplasia of intrahepatic bile ducts" or "intrahepatic biliary atresia" as suggested by Witzleben 30 years later [23]. The term PIBD seems now worldwide accepted, although some authors prefer PILBD (paucity of the interlobular bile ducts) [12]. Non-syndromic PIBD constitutes probably the most frequent diagnosis in newborns and infants with conjugated hyperbilirubinemia in the first 4 weeks of life being more frequently observed than biliary atresia [5, 24]. Although it is only descriptive and does not imply any mechanism of physiopathology, it is readily accepted by both clinicians and pathologists. The magic number may be not correct until the liver is mature. Alagille described an IBD/PT ratio of 0.9–1.8 as the norm for children suggesting that 0.5 may be the cut-off for a scarcity of interlobular bile ducts [25]. In 1989, a higher value was proposed by Kahn et al. [26]. These authors found that a mean IBD/PT ratio equal to or greater than 0.9 may be seen after 35 weeks of gestation. The use of standardized textbooks of perinatal pathology with tables specific for the population under examination is crucial. In my experience, some variation may be the norm under the lens [27]. A re-approach to the normal value of IBD/PT ratio in newborns may be critical in investigating preterm neonates or small newborns for gestational age undergoing weeks-long stays at Neonatal Intensive Care Units (NICUs) [7, 28]. Costa et al. [28] found a smaller value of IBD/PT ratio (0.66) in comparison to those found by Alagille. Sergi et al. [7] computed an embryologic nomogram for the IBD system and emphasized that a diagnosis of PIBD should be made with extreme caution at neonatal age. In any case, it has been stressed that it is paramount always to consider the gestational age of the newborn and probably the number of weeks spent in NICUs. The maturation of the IBD system is paramount. In addition to IBD/PT ratio, Sergi et al. [7] found data related to bile duct maturity in counting all biliary cells (single cells, mono- and double-layered ductal plate, peripheral tubular structures, and remodeled bile ducts) [9]. This parameter was a constant index useful for the evaluation of the degree of maturity of the IBD system. Sergi et al. [7] showed a clear linear increase with gestational age (r^2: 50.908, $P < 0.0001$). The normal breakdown of the ductal plate results in a gradual remodeling of the primitive double-walled epithelial cylinder of bile duct type [5–9, 18]. The decrease of IBDs may be present since birth or can occur later because of a developmental abnormality, genetic syndromes (e.g., Alagille syndrome), or because of destruction (necro-inflammatory or autoimmune) such as in biliary atresia and sclerosing cholangitis, respectively. The histopathology identified in the liver may be either the main feature in the definition of the disease such as Alagille syndrome or part of a disease characterized by other features such as alpha-1-antitrypsin deficiency (AATD) [29]. The usual definition worldwide recognized for PIBD is a significantly decreased or substantial decreased ratio of the number of interlobular bile ducts to the number of portal tracts. If this ratio is below 0.5, the diagnosis of PIBD is robust. Apart from the prematurity, the confidence in this statement may be challenged if the newborn if the conditions of the adequacy of the liver biopsy are not reached. It would be important receiving at least ten complete portal areas for the histopathologic examination. However, in practice, it is rare to obtain a long core of liver tissue from premature babies or even newborns. In my experience in multiple centers and universities in my career, I would be happy if a needle core biopsy from the liver in this age group may reveal at least six well-formed portal tracts. If adequacy is not reached, the procedure to obtain an open wedge biopsy should be considered [30]. Further, challenges can arise from marked biliary ductular proliferation, fibrosis grade III/IV, and frank cirrhosis. It is key to remember that using connective staining, "true" or "genuine" IBDs may disclose a silhouette on the cross-section that may be subtle on hematoxylin and eosin staining. The pathologist should also screen the liver biopsy for a few indicators or clues that may help to address the underlying pathology of the liver disease other than PIBD. The presence of eosinophilic, PAS-positive and diastase resistant globules in a periportal location may suggest alpha-1-antitrypsin deficiency, which is an endoplasmic reticulum storage disorder [29, 31–33]. The absence of peroxisomes may suggest Zellweger syndrome, which is characterized by a reduction or lack of functional peroxisomes in the cells of a proband [20, 34–36]. Giant cells are a form of a reparative process of the liver lobules but are a prevalent finding in pediatric cholestasis. There is a universal agreement that the diagnosis of "giant cell hepatitis" should be accepted only when other causes have been carefully excluded. The presence of intralobular foamy cells would point to metabolic disorders and need to be investigated properly by transmission electron microscopy differentiating them from small round blue cell tumors [37–40]. In case of a prolonged obstruction, some bile duct loss can be present and should not be mistaken as PIBD, unless some dysmorphic features or non-syndromic clues are identified. Witzleben's three pathogenetic theories for PIBD include a complete or partial failure of the IBDs to form, an adequate formation of the IBDs that went to destruction (e.g., necro-inflammatory), and atrophy of the IBDs [23]. Syndromic

PIBD can occur in Alagille syndrome [41] and Williams-Beuren syndrome [42, 43]. In both Alagille and Williams-Beuren syndrome, a cardiovascular polytopic field defect may be disturbed present. Thus, it is reasonable that the decrease of the total number of portal tracts in the liver of these subjects is due to an injury to the primitive vascular anlage of the liver at the time of the embryonic ductal plate. The failure in the normal development of these blood vessels may damage the organization and stereological representation of the intrahepatic biliary system. Bloom and Shiojiri suggested that the branching of the portal veins influence the ontogenesis of the intrahepatic biliary system [43, 44] directly. Nosologically, the destructive theory finds its correlates in graft versus host disease (GVHD) of the liver, chronic rejection of the orthotopic liver transplantation, and in the setting of sclerosing cholangitis. Finally, atrophy of the intrahepatic biliary system may occur in the case of marginalized and unused interlobular bile ducts in the setting of chronic intrahepatic cholestasis. The disorders associated with bile duct paucity are shown in Table 25.1. The syndromic group comprises mainly the Alagille and Williams-Beuren syndrome, while the non-syndromic group comprises disorders without a genetic background. The idiopathic group would include the isolated defect of PIBD exclusively without additional elements addressing a more precise diagnosis. The list is far to be complete, and some genetic conditions will be included in the future once we screen the intrahepatic biliary system properly by light microscopy, electron microscopy, and molecular biology. In some literature, it has been recommended that the diagnosis of PIBD or vanishing bile duct syndrome needs to be made only when all portal tracts are devoid of bile ducts [44], but some other authors continue to advocate for the diagnosis of PIBD when the ratio IBD/PT is less than 0.5 [45]. Probably, the term PIBD should not be used if there is a complete loss of IBDs and Snover's interpretation may be labeled as "*a*-cholangia" (Greek: αχολαγγείοί) or non-ducts.

Table 25.1 PIBD associated disorders

Syndromic PIBD: Alagille syndrome, Williams-Beuren syndrome, Ivemark syndrome, Zellweger syndrome (cerebrohepatorenal syndrome), and major karyotype abnormalities (monosomy 45, X0, trisomy 17–18, trisomy 21)
Non-Syndromic PIBD: Alpha-1-antitrypsin deficiency (AATD), cystic fibrosis, virus-related PIBD, sclerosing cholangitis, chronic allograft rejection of the liver, GvHD of the liver, hypopituitarism, progressive intrahepatic familial cholestasis (PFIC), maternal use of progesterone during pregnancy, Norwegian cholestasis, hemophagocytic lymphohistiocytosis, congenital pancreatic hypoplasia, and renal microcystic disease
Idiopathic PIBD: Syndromic PIBD conditions include Alagille syndrome, Williams-Beuren syndrome, Ivemark syndrome, Zellweger syndrome (cerebrohepatorenal syndrome), major karyotype abnormalities (monosomy 45, X0, trisomy 17–18, trisomy 21). The consideration of clinical dysmorphology and auxologic criteria should prompt the pathologist to address the correct review of syndromic PIBD that are not limited to the first syndrome identified by Watson and Alagille. The category of syndromic PIBD should be broadened including the several genetic syndromes described with PIBD, and that can be recognized in clinics or the pediatric ambulatory

25.5 Alagille Syndrome (AGS)

This syndrome, which is also known as Watson syndrome or arterio-hepatic dysplasia, is one of the most known genetic syndromes in pediatrics and is associated with five major features in its complete form [46, 47]. In 1973, Watson and Miller reported nine cases of familial pulmonary valvular stenosis accompanied by neonatal liver disease [46]. Two years later, Alagille et al. identified the neonatal liver disease [47]. AGS includes the lack of interlobular bile ducts (PIBD) (Fig. 25.1a, b), pulmonary artery stenosis, butterfly-like vertebrae, posterior ocular embryotoxon, and a peculiar face characterized by a prominent forehead, deep-set eyes, mild hypertelorism, straight nose, and small pointed chin [48]. The incomplete forms of this syndrome are also quite frequent. Other organs may be involved with characteristics involving kidney, ear, pancreas, intestine among others and the heart may show from a ventricular septal defect to tetralogy of Fallot. There is an autosomal dominant inheritance with highly variable expressivity and nearly complete penetrance. The frequency is about 1:70,000–100,000 live newborns, but about 2/3 of the AGS patients are sporadic cases. Clinically, the liver involvement causes generalized jaundice, pruritus, xanthomas, and there are hyperbilirubinemia and hypercholesterolemia other than the increase of other cholestasis parameters (γ-glutamyl-transpeptidase and alkaline phosphatase). The cardiovascular defects identified so far are pulmonary stenosis, coarctation of the aorta, ventricular or atrial septal defects, tetralogy of Fallot, *patent ductus arteriosus*, *truncus arteriosus (communis)*, and a right hypoplastic ventricle. The non-cardiac vascular defects identified are a middle aortic syndrome, arterial hypoplasia (hepatic, renal, carotid, celiac), hypoplastic portal vein branch, and intracranial vascular anomalies including Moyamoya disease, which is a progressive cerebrovascular disorder. A skeleton X-ray survey may disclose spina bifida, an abnormal progression of interpedicular distances, shortening of distal phalanges and metacarpal bones, and clinodactyly other than the classic butterfly-like vertebrae. The ocular involvement includes posterior embryotoxon, which is a thin grey-white, arcuate ridge on the inner surface of the cornea detectable with slit-lamp bio-microscopy. Moreover, there may be retinal pigmentation, iris strands, cataract, glaucoma, optic disc drusen, and fundus hypopigmentation. Three non-specific symptoms have also been included and

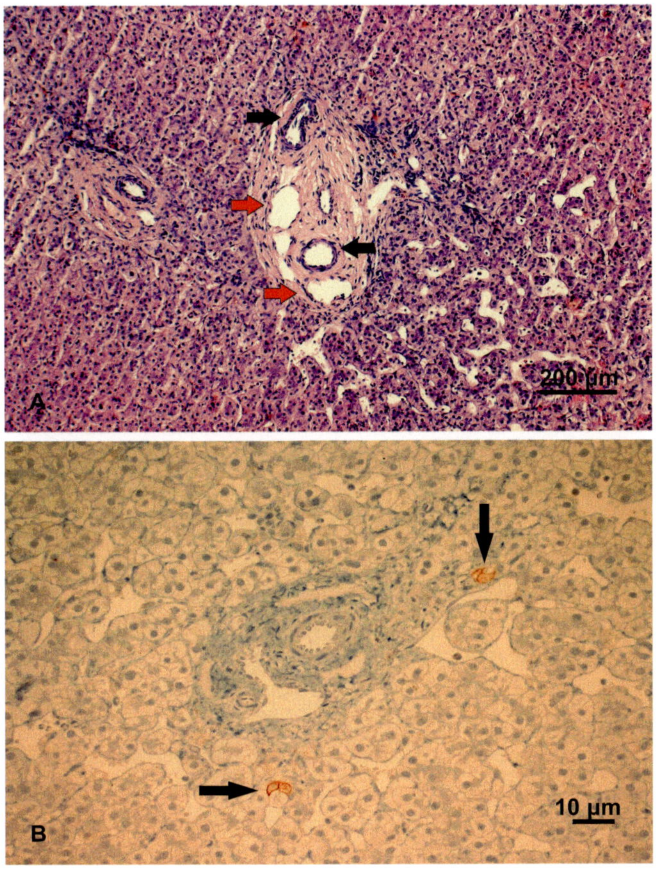

Fig. 25.1 (**a**) Liver histology of a patient with Alagille syndrome harboring a JAG1 mutation. In the center of the microphotograph there is a portal tract with two cross sections of a portal artery (black arrows) and two cross sections of a portal vein (red arrows). There is no evidence of an interlobular bile duct (Hematoxylin Eosin staining, 100× original magnification, bar = 200 μm). (**b**) Liver histology of the same patient with Alagille syndrome harboring a JAG1 mutation. In the center of the microphotograph there is no evidence of an interlobular bile duct using a monoclonal antibody against cytokeratin 7 (anti-CK7), which highlights the biliary epithelium. At the periphery of the portal tract, in the hepatic lobules, some hepatocytes show some focal expression (black arrows) (Immunohistochemistry, Avidin-Biotin Complex, 200× original magnification, bar = 10 μm)

are myopia, strabismus, and blindness. The involvement of the urinary system may disclose mesangial-lipidosis and tubular dysfunction of the kidney, tubulointerstitial nephritis, renal hypoplasia, renal agenesis, horseshoe kidney, and renal cystic change, suggesting an involvement in the group of the hepato-renal fibrocystic syndrome [19]. The ear may show temporal bone abnormalities, chronic otitis media, and deafness. The examination of the upper and lower respiratory system may show a high-pitched voice (larynx) and tracheal and bronchial stenosis (lung). The gastrointestinal tract may demonstrate small bowel atresia/stenosis and exocrine/endocrine pancreatic insufficiency. In children with AGS, growth retardation is well known, but the lack of mental retardation is never debated. Cytogenetically, 3–7% of patients with AGS have deletions of part or totality of the *JAG1* gene located in 20p12.1–11.23. The *JAG1* gene contains 26 exons and codes for a glycosylated transmembrane protein of 1218 amino acids. JAG1 functions as a ligand of the Notch membrane receptors. It has been detected that 95% of mutations are intragenic. These mutations are situated in the part of the *JAG1* gene encoding extracellular and transmembrane domains of the protein. Genetic changes include point mutations or small deletions/insertions, leading to frame-shift mutations, premature stop codons, splice site mutations, and missense mutations. In about 5% of patients, there are deletions of part or totality of the *JAG1* in 20p, and occasionally, translocations involving this gene have been reported: del(20p), del(20)(p12.3–p11.23), del(20)(p13–p12.2), del(20) (p11.2), ins(7;20), t(2;20). In very few patients, no mutation is identified in the DNA of the 26 exons and exon boundaries of *JAG1* ("atypical" AGS). Other than *JAG1* gene mutations, mutations of the *NOTCH2* gene can also cause AGS. NOTCH2 is a member of the Notch family of receptors. The ligation of molecules (ligands) to the NOTCH2 receptor is crucial for the development of cells useful for the development of the heart, liver, kidneys, bones, and other structures in a developing embryo. Notch2 signaling is also involved in immune system function, tissue repair, and bone remodeling after birth. In about half of patients with AGS, there is a genetic mutation, which occurs as a new change ("de novo") without being inherited from either parent. In patients with AGS, there is a risk, although modest, to develop hepatocellular carcinoma, but the prognosis relies on the PIBD and the extension of the cardiovascular and renal defects [5]. Liver transplantation is performed in about 25% of the patients affected with AGS, but a limiting factor may be the "early start AGS" cases with infants aged 5 months or even younger. In this situation, very few centers can perform liver transplantation, and this data may be important to communicate promptly to the family. Nevertheless, the diagnosis of PIBD may be difficult to assess early in life. In this setting, ductular proliferation with some portal fibrosis may be identified. It is paramount to be adherent to the morphologic criteria of the interlobular bile duct to avoid potential mistakes. Occasionally, an inflammation-free concentric periductular fibrosis may be noted, and differential diagnosis with sclerosing cholangitis needs to be made, and an intrahepatic cholangiogram may be crucial.

25.6 Williams-Beuren Syndrome (WBS)

WBS includes supravalvular aortic stenosis and multiple peripheral pulmonary arterial stenoses in individuals showing an elfin face, mental and growth deficiency, dental malformation, and infantile hypercalcemia. There is an autosomal dominant inherited contiguous gene deletion pattern involving genes from chromosome band 7q11.23, including *CLDN4*, *elastin*, and *LIM-kinase1*. Three regions are known for this syndrome. WBSCR8 (Williams-Beuren syndrome chromosome region 8 protein) of *CLDN4* (Claudin-4) gene, WBSCR17 (Williams-Beuren syndrome chromosome region 17) of *WBSCR17* (Williams-Beuren syndrome chromosome region 17), and WBSCR28 (Williams-Beuren syndrome chromosome region 28) of *WBSCR28* (Williams-Beuren syndrome chromosome region 28). Characteristically, *CLDN4* changes have been implicated in WBS [49]. The CLDN4 protein belongs to the claudin family. It contains 209 amino acids, four putative transmembrane segments, and directly interacts with TJP1/ZO-1, TJP2/ZO-2 and TJP3/ZO-3 playing an essential function as integral membrane protein and tight junction component for the obliteration of the intercellular space. PIBD has been reported in a 6-weeks-old newborn with WBS presenting with neonatal conjugated hyperbilirubinemia [50].

25.7 Ivemark Syndrome (IS)

Ivemark syndrome or heterotaxy syndrome (IS) is a rare embryological disorder with cardiac and extracardiac abnormalities. This syndrome results from failure of development of the left-right asymmetry of organs. The sequential segmental analysis of cardiac dissection and the understating of the development of the cardiac structures are crucial to understanding the unusual left-right asymmetry fully. IS may include dextrocardia, transposition of the great vessels with concordant atrioventricular connection and discordant atrioventricular connection, total anomalous pulmonary venous drainage, right atrial and right pulmonary isomerism, midline liver, asplenia, intestinal malrotation, and vena cava anomalies. Lateralization defects (e.g., *Situs Inversus*, asplenia or polysplenia) are defects of a primary developmental field, and extracardiac abnormalities are synchronic defects in the primary developmental field and not causally independent malformations. PIBD has been observed in a few patients [51–55].

25.8 Zellweger Syndrome

The *PEX-1* gene is a gene encoding information able to provide instructions to build the peroxisomal biogenesis factor 1 (PEX1p), which is a protein belonging to the group of peroxins. Peroxins are essential in the formation and normal functioning of the peroxisomes, which are subcellular structures that contain enzymes needed to break down fatty acids and toxic compounds. PEX1-related Zellweger syndrome spectrum (ZSS) occurs 1 in 50,000 births worldwide annually. It is an inherited group of disorders that includes Zellweger syndrome (ZS), neonatal adrenoleukodystrophy (NALD), and infantile Refsum disease (IRD). The diagnosis of ZSS is established in a proband with suggestive clinical and biochemical findings accompanied by the identification of biallelic pathogenic variants in one of the 13 PEX genes. ZSS clinical findings include hypotonia, poor feeding, brain defects, seizures, renal cysts, hepatomegaly, hepatic dysfunction with cholestasis, and bony stippling in newborns. The face is quite flat and shows a large anterior fontanel, split sutures, a prominent high forehead with a flattened occiput, up-slanting palpebral fissures, and a broad nasal bridge with epicanthal folds and hypoplastic supraorbital ridges. Older infants and children may show developmental delays with or without hypotonia, failure to thrive, hearing loss, vision impairment, liver dysfunction, adrenal dysfunction, leukodystrophy, peripheral neuropathy, and ataxia [56]. Biochemically, screening assays may evidence elevated plasma concentrations of C26:0 and C26:1, high ratios of C24/C22 and C26/C22, increased levels of phytanic acid and/or pristanic acid, reduced amounts of C16 and C18 plasmalogens, increased level of pipecolic acid in both plasma & urine, and increased concentrations of C27 bile acid intermediates trihydroxycholestanoic (THCA) and dihydroxycholestanoic (DHCA) [56]. A defect in peroxisome formation causes the symptoms of PEX1-related ZSS. Zellweger syndrome or cerebrohepatorenal syndrome remains the most severe prototypical member of the peroxisome biogenesis disorders (PBDs). PIBD may be recognized in ZS, and a careful genetic screening with genetic counseling may be appropriate [57–59].

25.9 Major Karyotype Abnormalities

There are only a few reports of an association between PIBD and chromosomal abnormalities, but the relationship is uncertain. PIBD has been reported in monosomy 45, X0 (Turner syndrome) [60, 61], trisomy 17–18 [62], and trisomy 21 [63]. Since all conceptuses with such karyotype may be viable, it must be stressed how critical is the evaluation of dysmorphological signs and the karyotype in any child with PIBD.

Non-Syndromic PIBD conditions include alpha-1-antitrypsin deficiency (AATD), cystic fibrosis, virus-related PIBD, sclerosing cholangitis, chronic allograft rejection of the liver, GvHD of the liver, progressive intrahepatic familial cholestasis (PFIC), hypopituitarism, maternal use of progesterone during pregnancy, Norwegian, hemophagocytic lymphohistiocytosis, congenital pancreatic hypoplasia, and renal microcystic disease.

25.10 Alpha-1-Antitrypsin Deficiency

Alpha-1 antitrypsin deficiency (AATD) is an autosomal recessive inherited disease with an increased risk for chronic obstructive pulmonary disease in adults, liver disease in children and adults, panniculitis of the soft tissue, and c-ANCA positive vasculitis. C-ANCA (PR3-ANCA, or cytoplasmic antineutrophil cytoplasmic antibodies) are a type of autoantibody with diffusely granular, cytoplasmic staining pattern under immunofluorescence microscopy. Liver disease in adulthood with cirrhosis may occur in the absence of a history of neonatal or childhood liver disease. In any case, there is an increased risk for hepatocellular carcinoma (HCC) in individuals with AATD [29, 33]. Some diseases have been controversially associated with AATD [31, 32]. The diagnosis of AATD is based on the low/very low concentration in serum of AAT by nephelometry or radial immunodiffusion or any other suitable biochemical technique and polyacrylamide gel isoelectric focusing (IEF) electrophoresis of serum in a gradient between pH 4 and 5 of the protein (SERPINA1) with determination of the protease inhibitor (PI) typing. The IEF relies on the migration patterns, whose isoforms are assigned an alphabetic letter. In IEF, the normal AAT protein (Pi∗MM) migrates in the middle of the isoelectric field, while the most frequent variant (Z) migrates most slowly [29]. PIBD may occur in newborns and infants with AATD [5, 64–67]. If two normal proteins are present the migration bands are called M (Pi∗MM), while the most frequent genetic variation of AAT is the Z variant (Pi∗ZZ in case of a homozygous individual or Pi∗MZ or Pi∗#Z in case of a heterozygous individual with a normal M band or with an abnormal secondary band (e.g., S variant, which will be Pi∗SZ). Normal migration patterns and deficiency of AAT would result in an M-like variant (e.g., M-Malton) [29, 33, 68]. Normal serum levels are 20–53 μmol/L (~100–220 mg/dL) by nephelometry, while AATD individuals are less than 50 mg/dL. However, since AAT is an acute phase reactant, AAT may increase even in patients with AATD. The following conditions need to be taken not account in case an AATD is suspected. These conditions include acute inflammation, cancer, and liver disease, pregnancy, estrogen therapy, and after blood transfusions or intravenous augmentation therapy. AATD is characterized by periportal eosinophilic globules, which are PAS positive and diastase resistant and stained with a monoclonal antibody against AAT by immunohistochemistry. During cholestasis in infants with AATD, three morphological patterns can be encountered, including (1) minor cell injury with cholestasis and no fibrosis, (2) fibrosis or cirrhosis with biliary duct proliferation, and (3) PIBD [20].

25.11 Cystic Fibrosis

Cystic fibrosis or mucoviscidosis is the most common lethal genetic disease in the USA of whites with an incidence of 1:2000–4500 newborns and a carrier rate of 1 in 20. The most common mutation is ΔF508 (more adequately designated as CFTRΔF508) of a protein that regulates chloride ion transport on chromosome 7 and is detected in about two-thirds of the individuals affected with cystic fibrosis. The protein is the product of the cystic fibrosis transmembrane conductance regulator (*CFTR*) gene. The occurrence of CFTRΔF508 is represented by deletion of three nucleotides spanning positions 507 and 508 of the CFTR gene, which results in the loss of a single codon for the amino acid phenylalanine. The abnormal CFTR lacking this phenylalanine residue cannot fold properly and cannot be excreted outside of the endoplasmic reticulum for further processing. Individuals with such genetic mutation experience reduced Cl^- in secretions, thicker respiratory secretions, respiratory infections, meconium ileus, liver disease, exocrine pancreatic insufficiency, and infertility. Liver disease is found in about 1/10 of patients with *CFTR* genetic mutations, although the exact rate may be higher than considered in the early studies [69–71]. Liver disease is characterized by elevated liver enzymes, steatosis, focal biliary cirrhosis, cirrhosis, and cholangiopathy [72, 73]. Liver disease may present as neonatal cholestasis, and PIBD may be a prominent feature. A more severe phenotype seems to be present in children with cystic fibrosis-related liver disease [74, 75].

25.12 Virus-Related PIBD

Other causes of non-syndromic PIBD include **viral diseases**. A viral insult to the interlobular bile ducts, especially in the perinatal age, may be catastrophic, specifically now that some vaccination protocols are missing in some countries [76]. Such a phenomenon has been described for ***cytomegalovirus*** (CMV), ***rubella***, ***reovirus 3***, ***parvovirus B19***, and ***hepatitis B virus*** (HBV). CMV induces an essential and high relevant damage to the biliary epithelial cells during perinatal life [77, 78]. The disappearance of interlobular bile ducts in allograft liver rejection may suggest some immunologic similarities in the PIBD-associated CMV neonatal infection [79]. PIBD has been reported on two occasions linked to rubella virus infection [20, 80]. Reovirus 3 is controversially discussed in the literature, although an exciting animal model has identified that the administration of rhesus rotavirus-type A to newborn Balb/c mice provokes an inflammatory obstruction of the biliary ducts, which resembles human biliary atresia [81, 82]. The role of parvovirus B19 is intriguing and has been suggested in two occasions as well [83, 84], while HBV in one case report [85]. HBsAg (also known as the Australia antigen) is the surface antigen of the HBV and indicates current hepatitis B infection. Intrahepatic duct damage has also been observed in children with Kawasaki disease [86].

25.13 Sclerosing Cholangitis

Neonatal and primary sclerosing cholangitis of children and adults are vanishing bile duct syndromes with ductopenia and are part of the non-syndromic PIBD group, which are under intense molecular investigation [87]. Primary sclerosing cholangitis (PSC) is a chronic cholestatic with the progressive fibro-sclerotic inflammatory disease of the liver and extrahepatic biliary tract. PSC is associated with inflammatory bowel disease (IBD), particularly ulcerative colitis (UC) in 80% of patients and causes multifocal strictures and segmental dilatations of the intrahepatic and extrahepatic biliary system. Neonatal sclerosing cholangitis (NSC) is a rare infantile nonsurgical correctable cholangiopathy first reported in eight children presenting with jaundice, hepatosplenomegaly, pale stools, and high serum γ-glutamyltransferase (GGT) activity [88]. Six out of the 13 infants with NSC, who have been investigated at the King's College Hospital, London, United Kingdom, showed mutations in the *DCDC2* gene, which encodes doublecortin domain-containing protein 2 (DCDC2) [89]. In four patients, there were homozygous changes (two frameshifts, two stop codon) and two patients showed compound heterozygous changes (two frameshifts, one stop codon) with all mutations predicting a truncated protein. The liver biopsy of NSC is similar to biliary atresia (BA), although a cholangiogram will show dilation of the extrahepatic bile ducts in NSC, while a cholangiogram would point to an obliteration of the extrahepatic biliary system in BA. In a typical patient with NSC, the liver biopsy shows varying degrees of portal tract fibrosis without edema and bile duct proliferation with occasional bile plugs and optional persistence of the ductal plate. Later, the biopsy may show PIBD in a background of portal tract fibrosis. Focally, the characteristic concentric periductal lamellar fibrosis may be identified. Also, disarray and atrophy of ductal epithelium can occur. Although biliary hamartomata (von Meyenburg complexes) are not seen, an ectasia of large ducts in some patients suggesting Caroli-disease–like changes may be encountered. The *DCDC2* gene is highly expressed in the central nervous system, and other organs including the liver throughout fetal and adult life and have been identified as a candidate gene for dyslexia. DCDC2 contains two doublecortin domains, which are microtubule-binding modifiers acting in the cytoskeleton. Microtubules are primarily involved in the structure of the cytoskeleton, in the movement and division of the cell, and intracellular transport. DCDC2 has the potential to interfere with tubulin binding, microtubule polymerization, and the development of a normal ciliary structure [89, 90].

Non-syndromic PIBD includes **GVHD** of the liver and chronic allograft rejection of the organ. An important therapeutic option for a variety of diseases is the allogeneic hematopoietic cell transplantation (HCT). Currently, GVHD remains the most frequent and challenging complication following allogeneic HCT. The principal target organs in patients with acute GVHD are the skin, gastrointestinal tract, and liver. Chronic GVHD remains the dominant cause of non-relapse mortality in patients surviving longer than 24 months after allogeneic hematopoietic cell transplantation. Chronic GVHD influences both quality of life and long-term outcomes negatively [78]. Despite advances in clinical practice and our knowledge in basic sciences of the autoimmune processes, the incidence and severity of chronic GVHD have regrettably increased over the last decade. The critical characteristics of chronic GVHD are cholestatic or hepatic GVHD (inflammatory or phase 1), autoimmune hepatitis (immunologic dysregulation or phase 2), and advanced liver GVHD with periportal fibrosis, ductopenia (fibrosis/sclerosis or phase 3) [91]. In acute GVHD, bile duct injury is slight or moderate and patchy in distribution. In chronic GVHD with liver injury, bile duct damage is more severe and results in PIBD with loss of more than 50% of interlobular biliary ducts. Chronic PIBD may fail to progress to frank cirrhosis because the inflammatory infiltrate is mostly absent. Currently, a re-transplantation seems to be the only option.

In **Liver Allograft Rejection**, cholestasis and injury of interlobular bile ducts occur both in acute and chronic rejection. There are mild, moderate, and severe rejection features involving the interlobular bile ducts with both Birmingham score and the Rejection Activity Index (RAI) score. The biliary changes include vacuolation, loss of polarity, flattening of the cuboidal cells and are associated with foci of liver cells necrosis and lymphocytic infiltration both in portal areas and lobules. The diagnostic criteria for acute rejection consist of a mixed portal inflammatory infiltrate, bile duct damage, and endothelialitis. There is no prognostic significance of the bile duct injury in acute rejection. Conversely, the bile duct injury with loss of bile ducts is a salient feature of chronic rejection. Initially, the liver biopsy of an ongoing chronic rejection shows florid periductal inflammation with progressive ductopenia. Subsequently, PIBD is associated with fibrosis and vascular obliteration and specific subendothelial foamy cells associated with an abridged number of hepatic arterial radicles supporting the hypothesis that obliterative arteriopathy may be the underlying pathogenic mechanism [92]. Recently, a timeline review of chronic allograft rejection has been proposed emphasizing the role of arteriole loss in addition to ductopenia [93]. In the chronic rejection evaluation, at least two findings should be present for diagnosis [94]. The early chronic rejection relies on bile duct loss in less than half of portal tracts and loss of arterioles in less than one-fourth of portal tracts. Moreover, zone 3 necrosis with mild centrilobular/perivenular fibrosis of the terminal hepatic venules, foam cell deposition and intimal inflammation of the large perihilar hepatic artery, and foam cell deposition and inflammation of the large perihilar bile ducts are seen. In late chronic rejection, there may be ductopenia in more than half of portal tracts, while the loss of arterioles is seen in more than one-fourth of portal tracts. Also, there are bridging fibrosis and focal obliteration of venules, luminal narrowing with foam cells and fibro-intimal proliferation of the large perihilar hepatic artery, and cholestasis and moderate/severe foam cell deposition of the large perihilar bile ducts [94].

PIBD may also be encountered in some other conditions such as **progressive intrahepatic familial cholestasis** (PFIC), **hypopituitarism**, **maternal use of progesterone during pregnancy**, **Norwegian cholestasis**, **hemophagocytic lymphohistiocytosis**, **congenital pancreatic hypoplasia**, and **renal microcystic disease** [30]. In PFIC, which is the most known differential diagnosis in the non-syndromic group above cited, there are three known types (PFIC1, PFIC2, and PFIC3) with each type harboring a different genetic cause. The hepatic uptake of bile salts, organic anions and cations are regulated by the sodium-dependent taurocholate cotransporter protein (NTCP), organic anion transporters (OATP1–2), and organic cation transporters (OCT1) at the basolateral membrane of the hepatocyte. These transporters are not directly ATP-dependent for their function. ATP-dependent function is mostly vital for transporters mediating the secretion from liver to bile (ATP-binding cassette proteins or ABC) with several members including the P-glycoprotein (MDR), the multidrug resistance proteins (MRPs), the cystic fibrosis transmembrane regulator, the transporter associated with antigen presentation (TAP) proteins and a peroxisomal long-chain fatty acid transporter. Three proteins are at the basis of PFIC 1–3. Mutations in the ATP8B1, ABCB11, and ABCB4 genes can cause PFIC, which is inherited with an autosomal recessive pattern [95]. The preferred nomenclature for the three PFIC disorders is a FIC1 deficiency, BSEP deficiency, and MDR3 deficiency. *ATP8B1* mutations cause PFIC1 because ATP8B1 gene provides instructions for making a protein that helps to maintain an appropriate balance of bile acids with bile acid accumulation, cell damage, and subsequent liver disease. It is uncertain how ATP8B1 mutations affect short stature, deafness, and other signs and symptoms of PFIC1. PFIC2 is linked to modifications of the *ABCB11* gene, which encodes for a protein called the bile salt export pump (BSEP), which promotes the export of bile salts out of liver cells. Genetic mutations in the ABCB11 result in the accumulation of bile salts in liver cells with consequent cell damage and liver disease. Finally, *ABCB4* mutations cause PFIC3. The ABCB4 gene provides instructions for building a protein that moves phospholipids across cell membranes. The lack of proper binding of phospholipids to bile acids determines cell damage due to the toxicity of the bile acids leading to liver disease [96]. The histopathology of PFIC is also different according to the typing and PIBD has been described in PFIC [97–99]. In PFIC1, the examination of the liver shows canalicular cholestasis with periportal biliary metaplasia of hepatocytes in a virtual absence of true ductular proliferation. In PFIC2, the histology is similar, but there is more disordered architecture than PFIC1. There is more pronounced lobular fibrosis, portal fibrosis, and inflammation with more prominent hepatocellular necrosis and giant-cell transformation in PFIC2 than in PFIC1. In PFIC3, there is portal fibrosis and true ductular proliferation accompanied by a mixed inflammatory infiltrate with occasional cholestasis and giant-cell transformation of hepatocytes. Cholestasis may be isolated or associated with other organ involvement in the presence of more specific conditions [30]. The mechanism underlying the other diseases is uncertain and is under intense investigation.

25.14 Conclusion

Since the original report of the first syndromic PIBD, there is a growing understanding that PIBD may be the most frequent non-surgically correctable infantile cholangiopathy. The syndromic group should include Williams-Beuren syndrome, Zellweger syndrome, and major karyotype abnormalities in addition to the Alagille syndrome. The non-syndromic PIBD has been described in association with numerous defects or abnormalities: metabolic (such as AATD) or viral diseases (e.g., CMV, rubella), altered bile acid metabolism, and cystic fibrosis. Finally, the third group of idiopathic PIBD warrants a separate identity which may group new diseases waiting for a more detailed grouping in syndromic or non-syndromic. In most of the PIBD patient, the prognosis is, in general, severe and liver transplantation is requested. The use of new genetic tools (e.g., CRISPR-Cas9) may open the root for alternative options in the future.

Self Study

Questions

1. **What are the three main stages of the development of the intrahepatic biliary system?**
   (a) Protohepatic structure, Hepatic structure, Post-hepatic structure
   (b) Ductal plate, Remodeling Ductal Plate, Remodeled Bile Ducts

(c) Remodeling Ductal Plate, Remodeled Bile Ducts, Remodeled Neoductules
(d) Protocholangioles, Neocholangioles, Interlobular Bile Ducts
(e) Ductal Plate, Remodeled Bile Ducts, Interlobular Bile Ducts

2. **Which two genes are mostly involved in Alagille syndrome?**
(a) JAG1 and CFTR
(b) PKHD1 and PKD2
(c) CFTR and JAG1
(d) PKHD1 and NOTCH2
(e) JAG1 and NOTCH2

3. **Which function does play the dominant gene of Primary Sclerosing Cholangitis?**
(a) Tubulin polymerization and centrosome assembly
(b) Centrosome assembly and chromatid structure of the cell cycle
(c) Tubulin binding and microtubule polymerization
(d) Keratin-binding and microtubule polymerization
(e) Cilia formation and centrosome assembly

Answers

1. **What are the three main stages of the development of the intrahepatic biliary system?**
(a) Protohepatic structure, Hepatic structure, Post-hepatic structure
(b) **Ductal plate, Remodeling Ductal Plate, Remodeled Bile Ducts (CORRECT)**
(c) Remodeling Ductal Plate, Remodeled Bile Ducts, Remodeled Neoductules
(d) Protocholangioles, Neocholangioles, Interlobular Bile Ducts
(e) Ductal Plate, Remodeled Bile Ducts, Interlobular Bile Ducts

2. **Which two genes are mostly involved in Alagille syndrome?**
(a) JAG1 and CFTR
(b) PKHD1 and PKD2
(c) CFTR and JAG1
(d) PKHD1 and NOTCH2
(e) **JAG1 and NOTCH2 (CORRECT)**

3. **Which function does play the dominant gene of Primary Sclerosing Cholangitis?**
(a) Tubulin polymerization and centrosome assembly
(b) Centrosome assembly and chromatid structure of the cell cycle
(c) **Tubulin binding and microtubule polymerization (CORRECT)**
(d) Keratin-binding and microtubule polymerization
(e) Cilia formation and centrosome assembly

References

1. Roberts SK, Ludwig J, Larusso NF. The pathobiology of biliary epithelia. Gastroenterology. 1997;112(1):269–79.
2. Bongiovanni AM. Bile acid content of gallbladder of infants, children and adults. J Clin Endocrinol Metab. 1965;25:678–85.
3. deBelle RC, Blacklow NR, Baylan M, Little JM, Lester R. Bile acid conjugation in fetal hepatic organ cultures. Am J Phys. 1976;231(4):1124–8.
4. Danielsson H, Rutter WJ. The metabolism of bile acids in the developing rat liver. Biochemistry. 1968;7(1):346–52.
5. Sergi C, Benstz J, Feist D, Nutzenadel W, Otto HF, Hofmann WJ. Bile duct to portal space ratio and ductal plate remnants in liver disease of infants aged less than 1 year. Pathology. 2008;40(3):260–7.
6. Sergi C, Adam S, Kahl P, Otto HF. Study of the malformation of ductal plate of the liver in Meckel syndrome and review of other syndromes presenting with this anomaly. Pediatr Dev Pathol. 2000;3(6):568–83.
7. Sergi C, Adam S, Kahl P, Otto HF. The remodeling of the primitive human biliary system. Early Hum Dev. 2000;58(3):167–78.
8. Sergi C, Kahl P, Otto HF. Contribution of apoptosis and apoptosis-related proteins to the malformation of the primitive intrahepatic biliary system in Meckel syndrome. Am J Pathol. 2000;156(5):1589–98.
9. Hammar JA. Uber die erste Entstehung der nicht kapillaren intrahepatischen Gallengange beim Menschen. Z Mikrosk Anat Forsch. 1926;5:59–89.
10. Desmet VJ. Embryology of the liver and intrahepatic biliary tract, and an overview of malformations of the bile duct. In: Bircher J, Benhamou JP, McIntyre N, Rizzetto M, Rhodes J, editors. The Oxford textbook of clinical hepatology. 2nd ed. Oxford: Oxford University Press; 1999. p. 51–61.
11. Roskams T, Desmet V. Embryology of extra- and intrahepatic bile ducts, the ductal plate. Anat Rec (Hoboken). 2008;291(6):628–35.
12. Desmet VJ, van Eyken P, Roskams T. Histopathology of vanishing bile duct diseases. Adv Clin Pathol. 1998;2(2):87–99.
13. Desmet VJ. The amazing universe of hepatic microstructure. Hepatology. 2009;50(2):333–44.
14. Desmet VJ. Congenital diseases of intrahepatic bile ducts: variations on the theme "ductal plate malformation". Hepatology. 1992;16(4):1069–83.
15. Hamilton PW, Allen DC. Morphometry in histopathology. J Pathol. 1995;175(4):369–79.
16. Amella C, Cappello F, Kahl P, Fritsch H, Lozanoff S, Sergi C. Spatial and temporal dynamics of innervation during the development of fetal human pancreas. Neuroscience. 2008;154(4):1477–87.
17. Snover DC. Biopsy diagnosis of liver disease. Netherlands: Wolters Kluwer; 1991, 300p.
18. Dorn L, Menezes LF, Mikuz G, Otto HF, Onuchic LF, Sergi C. Immunohistochemical detection of polyductin and co-localization with liver progenitor cell markers during normal and abnormal development of the intrahepatic biliary system and in adult hepatobiliary carcinomas. J Cell Mol Med. 2009;13(7):1279–90.
19. Johnson CA, Gissen P, Sergi C. Molecular pathology and genetics of congenital hepatorenal fibrocystic syndromes. J Med Genet. 2003;40(5):311–9.
20. Hadchouel M. Paucity of interlobular bile ducts. Semin Diagn Pathol. 1992;9(1):24–30.
21. Hadchouel M, Hugon RN, Gautier M. Reduced ratio of portal tracts to paucity of intrahepatic bile ducts. Arch Pathol Lab Med. 1978;102(8):402.
22. MacMahon HE, Thannhauser SJ. Congenital dysplasia of the interlobular bile ducts with extensive skin xanthomata; congenital acholangic biliary cirrhosis. Gastroenterology. 1952;21(4):488–506.
23. Witzleben CL. Bile duct paucity ("intrahepatic atresia"). Perspect Pediatr Pathol. 1982;7:185–201.

24. Kahn E. Paucity of interlobular bile ducts. Arteriohepatic dysplasia and nonsyndromic duct paucity. Perspect Pediatr Pathol. 1991;14:168–215.
25. Alagille D. Intrahepatic biliary atresia (hepatic ductular hypoplasia). In: Berenberg SR, editor. Liver diseases in infancy and childhood. Dordrecht: Martinus Nijhoff; 1976. p. 129–42.
26. Kahn E, Markowitz J, Aiges H, Daum F. Human ontogeny of the bile duct to portal space ratio. Hepatology. 1989;10(1):21–3.
27. Vogel M. Atlas der morphologischen Plazentadiagnostik. Berlin: Springer; 1996, 263p.
28. Costa AM, Pegado CS, Porto LC. Quantification of the intrahepatic biliary tree during human fetal development. Anat Rec. 1998;251(3):297–302.
29. Fabbretti G, Sergi C, Consalez G, Faa G, Brisigotti M, Romeo G, et al. Genetic variants of alpha-1-antitrypsin (AAT). Liver. 1992;12(4 Pt 2):296–301.
30. Sergi C, Bahitham W, Al-Bahrani R. Bile duct paucity in infancy. In: Mizuguchi Y, editor. Liver biopsy in modern medicine. London, UK: IntechOpen; 2011. p. 205–304.
31. Fargion S, Bissoli F, Fracanzani AL, Suigo E, Sergi C, Taioli E, et al. No association between genetic hemochromatosis and alpha1-antitrypsin deficiency. Hepatology. 1996;24(5):1161–4.
32. Fargion S, Sergi C, Bissoli F, Fracanzani AL, Suigo E, Carazzone A, et al. Lack of association between porphyria cutanea tarda and alpha 1-antitrypsin deficiency. Eur J Gastroenterol Hepatol. 1996;8(4):387–91.
33. Sergi C, Consalez GG, Fabbretti G, Brisigotti M, Faa G, Costa V, et al. Immunohistochemical and genetic characterization of the M Cagliari alpha-1-antitrypsin molecule (M-like alpha-1-antitrypsin deficiency). Lab Investig. 1994;70(1):130–3.
34. Warren M, Mierau G, Wartchow EP, Shimada H, Yano S. Histologic and ultrastructural features in early and advanced phases of Zellweger spectrum disorder (infantile Refsum disease). Ultrastruct Pathol. 2018;42(3):220–7.
35. Depreter M, Espeel M, Roels F. Human peroxisomal disorders. Microsc Res Tech. 2003;61(2):203–23.
36. Espeel M, Roels F, Giros M, Mandel H, Peltier A, Poggi F, et al. Immunolocalization of a 43 kDa peroxisomal membrane protein in the liver of patients with generalized peroxisomal disorders. Eur J Cell Biol. 1995;67(4):319–27.
37. Khan A, Sergi C. Sialidosis: a review of morphology and molecular biology of a rare pediatric disorder. Diagnostics (Basel). 2018;8(2) https://doi.org/10.3390/diagnostics8020029.
38. Sergi C, Penzel R, Uhl J, Zoubaa S, Dietrich H, Decker N, et al. Prenatal diagnosis and fetal pathology in a Turkish family harboring a novel nonsense mutation in the lysosomal alpha-N-acetylneuraminidase (sialidase) gene. Hum Genet. 2001;109(4):421–8.
39. Sergi C, Beedgen B, Kopitz J, Zilow E, Zoubaa S, Otto HF, et al. Refractory congenital ascites as a manifestation of neonatal sialidosis: clinical, biochemical and morphological studies in a newborn Syrian male infant. Am J Perinatol. 1999;16(3):133–41.
40. Sergi C. Transmission electron microscopy of pediatric small round blue cell tumors. In: Méndez-Vilas A, editor. Microscopy science: last approaches on educational programs and applied research. Spain: Formatex Research Center; 2018.
41. Crosnier C, Lykavieris P, Meunier-Rotival M, Hadchouel M. Alagille syndrome. The widening spectrum of arteriohepatic dysplasia. Clin Liver Dis. 2000;4(4):765–78.
42. Duque Lasio ML, Kozel BA. Elastin-driven genetic diseases. Matrix Biol. 2018;71–72:144–60.
43. Sakhuja P, Whyte H, Kamath B, Martin N, Chitayat D. Williams syndrome presenting with findings consistent with Alagille syndrome. Clin Case Rep. 2015;3(1):24–8.
44. Snover DC. Problems in the interpretation of liver biopsies after liver transplantation. Am J Surg Pathol. 1989;13(Suppl 1):31–8.
45. Demetris AJ, Jaffe R, Starzl TE. A review of adult and pediatric post-transplant liver pathology. Pathol Annu. 1987;22(Pt 2):347–86.
46. Watson GH, Miller V. Arteriohepatic dysplasia: familial pulmonary arterial stenosis with neonatal liver disease. Arch Dis Child. 1973;48(6):459–66.
47. Alagille D, Odievre M, Gautier M, Dommergues JP. Hepatic ductular hypoplasia associated with characteristic facies, vertebral malformations, retarded physical, mental, and sexual development, and cardiac murmur. J Pediatr. 1975;86(1):63–71.
48. Meunier-Rotival M, Hadchouel M. Alagille syndrome (AGS). Atlas Genet Cytogenet Oncol Haematol [Internet]. 21 Oct 2005, 2007. Available from: http://AtlasGeneticsOncology.org/Kprones/AlagilleID10090.html.
49. Ripka S, Gress TM. CLDN4 (claudin-4). Atlas Genet Cytogenet Oncol Haematol [Internet]. 12 Oct 2006, 2018; 10(2):77–8. Available from: http://AtlasGeneticsOncology.org/Genes/CLDN4ID42975ch7q11.html.
50. O'Reilly K, Ahmed SF, Murday V, McGrogan P. Biliary hypoplasia in Williams syndrome. Arch Dis Child. 2006;91(5):420–1.
51. Copelovitch L, O'Brien MM, Guttenberg M, Otto EA, Kaplan BS. Renal-hepatic-pancreatic dysplasia: a sibship with skeletal and central nervous system anomalies and NPHP3 mutation. Am J Med Genet A. 2013;161A(7):1743–9.
52. Villeneuve J, Pelluard-Nehme F, Combe C, Carles D, Chaponnier C, Ripoche J, et al. Immunohistochemical study of the phenotypic change of the mesenchymal cells during portal tract maturation in normal and fibrous (ductal plate malformation) fetal liver. Comp Hepatol. 2009;8:5.
53. Awasthi A, Das A, Srinivasan R, Joshi K. Morphological and immunohistochemical analysis of ductal plate malformation: correlation with fetal liver. Histopathology. 2004;45(3):260–7.
54. Devriendt K, Dooms L, Proesmans W, de Zegher F, Desmet V, Eggermont E. Paucity of intrahepatic bile ducts, solitary kidney and atrophic pancreas with diabetes mellitus: atypical Alagille syndrome? Eur J Pediatr. 1996;155(2):87–90.
55. Bernstein J, Chandra M, Creswell J, Kahn E, Malouf NN, McVicar M, et al. Renal-hepatic-pancreatic dysplasia: a syndrome reconsidered. Am J Med Genet. 1987;26(2):391–403.
56. Steinberg SJ, Raymond GV, Braverman NE, Moser AB. Zellweger spectrum disorder. In: Adam MP, Ardinger HH, Pagon RA, Wallace SE, Bean LJH, Stephens K, et al., editors. GeneReviews® [Internet]. Seattle, WA: University of Washington, Seattle; 1993.
57. Eyssen H, Eggermont E, van Eldere J, Jaeken J, Parmentier G, Janssen G. Bile acid abnormalities and the diagnosis of cerebro-hepato-renal syndrome (Zellweger syndrome). Acta Paediatr Scand. 1985;74(4):539–44.
58. Hanson RF, Isenberg JN, Williams GC, Hachey D, Szczepanik P, Klein PD, et al. The metabolism of 3alpha, 7alpha, 12alpha-trihydorxy-5beta-cholestan-26-oic acid in two siblings with cholestasis due to intrahepatic bile duct anomalies. An apparent inborn error of cholic acid synthesis. J Clin Invest. 1975;56(3):577–87.
59. Setchell KD, Street JM. Inborn errors of bile acid synthesis. Semin Liver Dis. 1987;7(2):85–99.
60. Gardner LI. Letter: Intrahepatic bile stasis in 45,X Turner's syndrome. N Engl J Med. 1974;290(7):406.
61. Molland EA, Purcell M. Biliary atresia and the Dandy-Walker anomaly in a neonate with 45,X Turner's syndrome. J Pathol. 1975;115(4):227–30.
62. Alpert LI, Strauss L, Hirschhorn K. Neonatal hepatitis and biliary atresia associated with trisomy 17-18 syndrome. N Engl J Med. 1969;280(1):16–20.
63. Puri P, Guiney EJ. Intrahepatic biliary atresia in Down's syndrome. J Pediatr Surg. 1975;10(3):423–4.
64. Alagille D. Alpha-1-antitrypsin deficiency. Hepatology. 1984;4(1 Suppl):11S–4S.
65. Dorney SF, Hassall EG, Arbuckle SM, Vargas JH, Berquist WE. SZ phenotype alpha-1-antitrypsin deficiency with paucity of the interlobular bile ducts. Aust Paediatr J. 1987;23(1):55–6.

66. Filipponi F, Soubrane O, Labrousse F, Devictor D, Bernard O, Valayer J, et al. Liver transplantation for end-stage liver disease associated with alpha-1-antitrypsin deficiency in children: pretransplant natural history, timing and results of transplantation. J Hepatol. 1994;20(1):72–8.
67. Malone M, Mieli-Vergani G, Mowat AP, Portmann B. The fetal liver in PiZZ alpha-1-antitrypsin deficiency: a report of five cases. Pediatr Pathol. 1989;9(6):623–31.
68. Spada F, Candiano G, Sergi C, Ghiggeri GM, Callea F, Gusmano R. Purification of alpha-1-antitrypsin monomer by preparative electrophoresis. J Clin Pathol. 1994;47(7):661–3.
69. Debray D, Narkewicz MR, Bodewes F, Colombo C, Housset C, de Jonge HR, et al. Cystic fibrosis-related liver disease: research challenges and future perspectives. J Pediatr Gastroenterol Nutr. 2017;65(4):443–8.
70. Staufer K, Halilbasic E, Trauner M, Kazemi-Shirazi L. Cystic fibrosis related liver disease—another black box in hepatology. Int J Mol Sci. 2014;15(8):13529–49.
71. Costa PC, Barreto CC, Pereira L, Lobo ML, Costa MA, Lopes AI. Cystic fibrosis-related liver disease: a single-center experience. Pediatr Rep. 2011;3(3):e21.
72. Kamal N, Surana P, Koh C. Liver disease in patients with cystic fibrosis. Curr Opin Gastroenterol. 2018;34(3):146–51.
73. Furuya KN, Roberts EA, Canny GJ, Phillips MJ. Neonatal hepatitis syndrome with paucity of interlobular bile ducts in cystic fibrosis. J Pediatr Gastroenterol Nutr. 1991;12(1):127–30.
74. Colombo C, Battezzati PM, Crosignani A, Morabito A, Costantini D, Padoan R, et al. Liver disease in cystic fibrosis: a prospective study on incidence, risk factors, and outcome. Hepatology. 2002;36(6):1374–82.
75. Rowland M, Gallagher C, Gallagher CG, Laoide RO, Canny G, Broderick AM, et al. Outcome in patients with cystic fibrosis liver disease. J Cyst Fibros. 2015;14(1):120–6.
76. Leung AK, Hon KL, Leong KF, Sergi CM. Measles: a disease often forgotten but not gone. Hong Kong Med J. 2018;24:512–20.
77. Kage M, Kosai K, Kojiro M, Nakamura Y, Fukuda S. Infantile cholestasis due to cytomegalovirus infection of the liver. A possible cause of paucity of interlobular bile ducts. Arch Pathol Lab Med. 1993;117(9):942–4.
78. Stern H, Tucker SM. Cytomegalovirus infection in the newborn and in early childhood. Three atypical cases. Lancet. 1965;2(7425):1268–71.
79. O'Grady JG, Alexander GJ, Sutherland S, Donaldson PT, Harvey F, Portmann B, et al. Cytomegalovirus infection and donor/recipient HLA antigens: interdependent co-factors in pathogenesis of vanishing bile-duct syndrome after liver transplantation. Lancet. 1988;2(8606):302–5.
80. Strauss L, Bernstein J. Neonatal hepatitis in congenital rubella. A histopathological study. Arch Pathol. 1968;86(3):317–27.
81. Huang YH, Shih HH, Tiao MM, Huang CC, Kuo KC, Huang FC, et al. Toll-like receptor 7 agonist induces hypoplasia of the biliary system in a neonatal mouse model. J Microbiol Immunol Infect. 2018;51(2):166–73.
82. Hertel PM, Estes MK. Rotavirus and biliary atresia: can causation be proven? Curr Opin Gastroenterol. 2012;28(1):10–7.
83. Hicks J, Barrish J, Zhu SH. Neonatal syncytial giant cell hepatitis with paramyxoviral-like inclusions. Ultrastruct Pathol. 2001;25(1):65–71.
84. Perrini S, Guidi B, Torelli P, Forte A. Parvovirus B19 associated acute cholestatic hepatitis. Pediatr Med Chir. 2014;36(5–6):102.
85. Ferrante L, Rubaltelli FF. Intrahepatic biliary atresia associated with the presence of Australia-antigen. Padiatr Padol. 1971;6(3):225–9.
86. Bader-Meunier B, Hadchouel M, Fabre M, Arnoud MD, Dommergues JP. Intrahepatic bile duct damage in children with Kawasaki disease. J Pediatr. 1992;120(5):750–2.
87. Tam PKH, Yiu RS, Lendahl U, Andersson ER. Cholangiopathies – towards a molecular understanding. EBioMedicine. 2018;35:381–93.
88. Amedee-Manesme O, Bernard O, Brunelle F, Hadchouel M, Polonovski C, Baudon JJ, et al. Sclerosing cholangitis with neonatal onset. J Pediatr. 1987;111(2):225–9.
89. Grammatikopoulos T, Sambrotta M, Strautnieks S, Foskett P, Knisely AS, Wagner B, et al. Mutations in DCDC2 (doublecortin domain containing protein 2) in neonatal sclerosing cholangitis. J Hepatol. 2016;65(6):1179–87.
90. Yu TW, Mochida GH, Tischfield DJ, Sgaier SK, Flores-Sarnat L, Sergi CM, et al. Mutations in WDR62, encoding a centrosome-associated protein, cause microcephaly with simplified gyri and abnormal cortical architecture. Nat Genet. 2010;42(11):1015–20.
91. Cooke KR, Luznik L, Sarantopoulos S, Hakim FT, Jagasia M, Fowler DH, et al. The biology of chronic graft-versus-host disease: a task force report from the National Institutes of Health consensus development project on criteria for clinical trials in chronic graft-versus-host disease. Biol Blood Marrow Transplant. 2017;23(2):211–34.
92. Oguma S, Belle S, Starzl TE, Demetris AJ. A histometric analysis of chronically rejected human liver allografts: insights into the mechanisms of bile duct loss: direct immunologic and ischemic factors. Hepatology. 1989;9(2):204–9.
93. Byrnes K, Oshima K. Liver transplant pathology: a timeline based approach and review. Diagn Histopathol. 2018;24:508–13. https://doi.org/10.1016/j.mpdhp.2018.09.002.
94. Demetris AJ, Bellamy C, Hubscher SG, O'Leary J, Randhawa PS, Feng S, et al. 2016 comprehensive update of the Banff working group on liver allograft pathology: introduction of antibody-mediated rejection. Am J Transplant. 2016;16(10):2816–35.
95. NLM. Progressive Familial Intrahepatic Cholestasis. 9 Oct 2018. In: Genetics home reference [Internet]. Lister Hill National Center for Biomedical Communications, National Library of Medicine (US), National Institutes of Health, Department of Health & Human Services. Available from: https://ghr.nlm.nih.gov/condition/progressive-familial-intrahepatic-cholestasis.
96. Oude Elferink RP, Kremer AE, Martens JJ, Beuers UH. The molecular mechanism of cholestatic pruritus. Dig Dis. 2011;29(1):66–71.
97. Mirza R, Abbas Z, Luck NH, Azam SM, Aziz S, Hassan SM, et al. Progressive familial intrahepatic cholestasis. J Coll Physicians Surg Pak. 2006;16(10):673–5.
98. Yehezkely-Schildkraut V, Munichor M, Mandel H, Berkowitz D, Hartman C, Eshach-Adiv O, et al. Nonsyndromic paucity of interlobular bile ducts: report of 10 patients. J Pediatr Gastroenterol Nutr. 2003;37(5):546–9.
99. Jacquemin E. Progressive familial intrahepatic cholestasis. Clin Res Hepatol Gastroenterol. 2012;36(Suppl 1):S26–35.

Nonalcoholic Fatty Liver Disease: A Wide Spectrum Disease

26

Natalia Rosso and Stefano Bellentani

Key Concepts
- NAFLD is a major cause of chronic liver disease, and its estimated global prevalence is 24%
- NAFLD is expected to become in few years the most frequent cause for the indication of liver transplantation
- The increasing worldwide incidence of NAFLD is tightly associated with the booming of obesity and Type 2 Diabetes Mellitus
- NAFLD is not only referred to adults but is the most common cause of liver disease also in the pediatric population
- It is a wide spectrum progressive disease that affects several organs
- To date, the proposed nutraceutical and pharmaceutical treatments have not yet provided solid results

26.1 Introduction

In 1980, Ludwig et al. [1] used the term Nonalcoholic Fatty Liver Disease (NAFLD) to describe a panel of liver injuries similar to alcoholic hepatitis that occurred in absence of relevant alcohol consumption or other known causes of chronic liver disease (HCV, HBV, drugs, etc.).

Nowadays NAFLD has emerged as a major cause of chronic liver disease. Particularly, NASH is increasing as an etiology for end-stage liver disease as well as for hepatocellular carcinoma (HCC)-related liver transplantation and is expected to surpass hepatitis C for this indication in the next years. NAFLD is strongly related to insulin resistance (IR) and is associated to clinical conditions such as overweight or obesity, type 2 diabetes mellitus (T2DM), hypertension, hypertriglyceridemia and low HDL-cholesterol (all of which constitute essential elements in the spectrum of metabolic syndrome (MS)). Overweight and obesity global epidemic burdens in both developed and developing countries. Such is the magnitude of the problem that the World Health Organization (WHO) has introduced the term "Globesity" to define the phenomenon. This booming of obesity is in parallel with the increasing incidence of NAFLD and NASH.

NAFLD is not only referred to adults, but there is now growing evidence indicating that NAFLD is the most common cause of liver disease also in the pediatric population. This worrisome trend is a mirror of the spread of hypercaloric diets and sedentary life habits among children and adolescents. Thus, its incidence in this young population represents the major threat to the upcoming years.

To date, there is no consensus concerning an effective pharmacological treatment for NASH, and the only currently recommended treatment is based on lifestyle modifications (diet and physical activity). However, the lack of compliance is still the main obstacle to overcome. Nowadays, drug interventions consist of the association of several drugs as an attempt to reverse the co-morbidities of the MetS.

Interestingly, it worth to be mentioned that NAFLD, although at a lower prevalence, might occur also in nonobese subjects (the so-called "lean" NAFLD) suggesting that other genetic factors different from obesity might play a determinant role in the onset of this disorder. Despite the significant role that NAFLD has on health care systems worldwide and more than 200 clinical trials ongoing around the world, NAFLD and NASH still remain without any approved therapy.

In this chapter, readers will find information about the most recent data regarding the epidemiology, associated risk factors, pathogenesis, available experimental models, diagnosis and the available treatment options for NAFLD.

N. Rosso (✉)
Fondazione Italiana Fegato, Basovizza, Trieste, Italy
e-mail: natalia.rosso@fegato.it

S. Bellentani (✉)
Clinica Santa Chiara SA, Locarno, Switzerland
e-mail: s.bellentani@clinicasantachiara.ch

F. Radu-Ionita et al. (eds.), *Liver Diseases*, https://doi.org/10.1007/978-3-030-24432-3_26

Definition
Currently, NAFLD is considered a wide spectrum disease that includes two phenotypes: nonalcoholic fatty liver (NAFL) and nonalcoholic steatohepatitis (NASH). While NAFL is considered a relatively benign and reversible condition, characterized by the deposition of intracellular lipid droplets within the hepatocytes (simple steatosis) without obvious cellular injury, NASH is a more aggressive disease characterized by cellular injury, inflammatory infiltrates and possible progression to fibrosis or cirrhosis.

NAFL and NASH are still negative definitions: a patient is classified as having NAFL/NASH when the amount of alcohol drank per day is lower than 20–30 g (140 g per week), and all the other causes of liver diseases (HBV, HCV, Drug-induced, biliary disease, autoimmune liver disease, etc.) have been excluded. As we proposed recently [2] it is probably time to reach an overall consensus throughout all the scientific community to change the nomenclature, and go from a negative to a positive definition of NAFLD/NASH, naming them "Metabolic-Associated Fatty Liver (MAFL) and Metabolic-Associated SteatoHepatitis (MASH)."

26.2 Epidemiology

26.2.1 Prevalence and Incidence of NAFL/NASH

NAFLD is currently the main cause of alteration of transaminases and GGT and the second indication of liver transplantation among adults, but also in children and adolescent, in the Western world [3].

According to the most updated data, the NAFLD global prevalence in the adult general population is estimated to be 25%, with a wide range marked by age, sex, region of origin, and ethnicity. The highest prevalence was recorded in the Middle East (32%), South America (31%) and Asia (27%) while the lowest was reported in Africa (14%). Europe and North America stand at intermediate values (20–30%). Europe and North America stand at intermediate values (20–30%) [4]. Among individuals with NAFLD, the global prevalence of NASH, diagnosed by liver biopsy, varies between 20% and 50%, with greater frequency and severity in men than in women, although the protective role of women is reduced in the post-menopausal phase. The prevalence of NAFLD rises significantly in the risk groups and reaches 94% in obese patients (BMI > 30 kg/m^2), 40–70% of patients with Type 2 Diabetes Mellitus (T2DM) or Metabolic Syndrome (MS), and 50% of the dyslipidemic subjects. A number of complications of MS (cardiovascular disease, obstructive sleep apnea [OSA]) are highly prevalent in patients with NAFLD. On the other hand, NAFLD is an independent predictor for cardiovascular disease and cardiovascular mortality, and in turn, cardiovascular mortality is the most common cause of death among patients with NAFLD and NASH.

Also, OSA, another complication of MS, is highly prevalent in NAFLD, and these patients are three times as likely to have NASH compared with patients without OSA.

The most dramatic epidemiological data concern the pediatric population, in which obesity and MS are in progressive global increase, particularly marked in Europe and USA [5] where the estimates are reaching US numbers (6.9%, three times higher in the period 2007–2010 than that in the period 1988–1994).

The diagnosis of NASH, which is the variant of NAFLD that can progress to NASH-cirrhosis and NASH-Hepatocellular Carcinoma (HCC), requires histological confirmation, therefore, the prevalence of NASH in the general population can only be estimated from a few biopsy series. This prevalence rate ranges between 1.5% and 6.45%.

Finally, it is important to recognize that NAFLD and NASH can occur in the absence of obesity. Although NAFLD is more common in obese individuals, the prevalence rate of NAFLD in lean individuals in the United States is about 7%, whereas prevalence rates in rural areas of some Asian countries can be as high as 25–30%.

The incidence of NAFLD and NASH from the general population is lacking, and it could be only estimated. Thus, the incidence reported to date, usually varies across the world, ranging from 28.01 per 1000 to 52.34 per 1000 person-years.

26.2.2 Natural History and Risk Factors for NAFL and NASH

NAFLD is a disease with different rates of progression among individuals and different clinical manifestations. This highly variable natural history reflects the diverse but convergent impacts of the environment, the intestinal microbiome that could influence the presence or absence of fatty liver, the glucose and lipid metabolism, other co-morbidities and genetic factors.

The natural history of NAFLD has been recently deeply investigated and designed by various recent studies. NASH is the predominant type of NAFLD that can progress, in about 10–15% of patients to cirrhosis. This progression is non-linear and, in fact, some patients with NASH, even those with fibrosis, may spontaneously regress. Although most patients with the non-NASH type of NAFLD do not progress, a few actually do progress to NASH and even cirrhosis.

However, cardiovascular mortality is the most common cause of death among patients with NAFLD and NASH. Liver-related complications are quite common in these patients and liver-related mortality is among the top three causes of death.

The presence of MS in an individual is the strongest risk factor for NAFLD. The association between both of them may be bidirectional, particularly with respect to diabetes and hypertension, meaning that not only does MS increase the risk of NAFLD, but also NAFLD may enhance several co-morbidities of MS. Indeed, NAFLD is now considered the hepatic manifestation of MS. Among the features of MS, T2DM has the clearest biologic link to the progression of NAFLD. Up to 75% of individuals with T2DM have NAFLD and among them, the prevalence of NASH and advanced fibrosis is higher compared with those non-diabetics with NAFLD as reported above. Likewise, it has been reported that 50% of patients with hypertension have NAFLD, and at the same time, NAFLD has been associated with changes in arterial stiffness, myocardial re-modeling, kidney disease, and heart failure. In line with this, it has been also reported that hypertension is strongly associated with the progression of hepatic fibrosis.

Finally NASH could progress not only to cirrhosis but in almost 40% of the cases directly to HCC [6]. NASH is now among the top three indications for liver transplantation in the United States due to decompensated liver disease and is the most rapidly growing cause of HCC worldwide [4].

26.2.3 Genetic and Epigenetic Factors

Genome-wide association studies have identified novel loci associated with disease severity phenotypes in NAFLD. To date, nonsynonymous SNPs in two genes: patatin-like phospholipase domain-containing-3 (*PNPLA3*) and trans-membrane 6 superfamily member 2 (*TM6SF2*) have been associated with NAFLD. The Ile148Met (rs738409) variant of *PNPLA3*, which takes part in lipid transformation, is now recognized as the major common genetic determinant of NAFLD and it is associated with progression to NASH [7, 8]. In addition, the rs58542926 C>T genetic variant of *TM6SF2* (which encodes the E167K aminoacidic substitution and determines neutral fat accumulation in the liver) has been reported to confer a susceptibility to NASH and fibrosis. Among the emerging newly discovered risk loci, variants near the genes encoding for membrane-bound O-acyltransferase domain-containing 7 (*MBOAT7*) and transmembrane channel-like 4 (*TMC4*) have been shown to be associated with the development and severity of NAFLD in patients of European descent [9]. Similarly, within the Latino population in South America, the *TM6SF2* Glu167Lys, and *PNPL3* Ile148Met protein variants seem to confer susceptibility to progressive NASH [10]. More recently a new genome-wide association study revealed a splice variant (rs72613567:TA) in *HSD17B13*, a gene that encodes the hepatic lipid droplet protein 17β-hydroxysteroid dehydrogenase type 13 [11]. This splice variant yields a truncated, nonfunctional protein that attenuates hepatocyte injury in patients with fatty liver (reduced ALT and AST) implying that *HSD17B13* normally promotes hepatocellular damage. Lately, hereditable mechanisms different from those encoded within the nucleotide sequence of genes are emerging. Epigenetic factors might also be a mechanism through which environmental exposures exert a heritable effect on disease risk, especially the remodeling of DNA methylation at key fibrosis modifiers genes. Differential abundance of serum microRNAs in monozygotic and dizygotic twins explain the discordance of NAFLD in genetically identical twins [12].

26.2.4 Environmental Factors

The most relevant environmental factors that have an important role to predispose individuals to NAFLD are dietary habits, physical activity, and socioeconomic factors. Individuals with NAFLD usually have unhealthy eating habits (eating processed food and/or foods with a high content of fat, salt, sugar or corn syrup) and eat more frequently at restaurants. Nutritional assessment of patients with NAFLD have further documented an increased consumption of low-nutrient, high-sodium and high-fat foods, especially diets high in meat-derive fats and lower amounts of fresh fruits. Subjects with fatty liver have also very low physical activity levels and increased sitting times compared with healthy individuals.

26.2.5 Lean NAFLD

Initially, lean NAFLD was described in Asian populations in absence of obesity, but more recently has been reported that NAFLD can develop also in 10–20% of lean Americans and Europeans [3]. Lean NAFLD encompasses a heterogeneous spectrum of disease arising from different etiologies such as increased visceral adiposity, high fructose and fat intake, genetic factors, congenital defects of metabolism, endocrine disorders, drug-related causes, jejunoileal bypass, starvation or total parental nutrition. A large proportion of lean NAFLD cases belong to a subgroup that comprises individuals who are non-obese, frequently sedentary, and with impaired insulin sensitivity, increased cardiovascular risk and increased liver lipid levels. Lean NAFLD usually presents fewer comorbidities, for this reason, is commonly believed that this subgroup would follow a relatively benign clinical course. However, NASH prevalence in obese and nonobese has been reported to be similar [13]. Moreover, the presence of advanced fibrosis in nonobese NASH patients is similar to the observed in obese subjects suggesting that once an individual has been diagnosed with NASH obesity might not be the main driver of fibrosis progression. Genetic factors might be involved in the risk of lean NAFLD, however, the presence of NASH in these patients was not explained by mutations in genes that influence either insulin resistance (*ENPP1* and *IRS1* polymorphisms) or the severity of steatosis (*PNPL3* and *TM6SF2* polymorphisms).

26.3 Pathogenesis

For several years the "two hits theory", proposed by Day in 1998, was accepted to explain NAFLD pathogenesis. In this theory, the "*first hit*" was defined by the accumulation of lipids in hepatocytes due to an altered intrahepatic lipid metabolism, and the "*second hit*" was represented by other related factors that led to hepatocyte injury, inflammation, and fibrosis. However, due to the complexity of the molecular pathways involved in this process, this view is now considered old-fashioned. In 2010, Tilg and Moschen proposed the "*Multiparallel hits Hypothesis*", a more complex and global theory to explain the pathogenesis of NAFLD. In this model, the adipose tissue and gut-related factors play a key role in the initiation of hepatic inflammation, suggesting that simple steatosis and NASH might be two different disorders and pointing to new non-hepatic players involved in the onset and progression of NAFLD. Evidence from patients that have undergone serial liver biopsies over an interval of several years demonstrates that the progression of NAFLD from simple steatosis to NASH and fibrosis is not linear and, probably, it is more dynamic than previously thought. Moreover, pathogenic drivers are not likely to be identical among all patients. Thus, both the mechanisms leading to disease and their clinical manifestations are highly heterogeneous.

In an attempt to define the pathogenic drivers that have been suggested to be involved in the onset of NAFL and NASH, is useful to keep in mind that the normal capacity of the liver to handle the primary metabolic energy substrates (carbohydrates and fatty acids (FA)) is largely overwhelmed. Thus, the accumulation of toxic lipid induces hepatocellular injury and death leading to fibrogenesis and genomic instability that predispose to cirrhosis and hepatocellular carcinoma. When FA are either supplied in excess or their disposal is impaired, they may serve as substrate for the generation of lipotoxic species that provoke endoplasmic reticulum (ER) stress and cell injury.

Under normal conditions, FA are delivered to the liver from blood following lipolysis of triacylglycerol (TAG) in white adipose tissue (WAT). Sequential TAG hydrolysis form diacylglycerol (DAG) and subsequently monoacylglycerol (MAG), which is hydrolyzed again to release the final FA and glycerol. The liberation of FA from TAG is also important to supply substrate for hepatic synthesis of very-low-density-lipoproteins (VLDL) (Fig. 26.1a). Impairment of WAT lipolysis inhibits the subsequent hepatic VLDL synthesis. Obesity is associated with an increase in basal lipolysis, due to an impaired sensitivity to the antilipolytic effects of insulin, resulting in excessive delivery of FA to the liver. The second source of FA is their hepatic synthesis from glucose and fructose by the *de novo lipogenesis* (DNL). Whereas the introduction of glucose into the DNL pathway is highly regulated, nearly all the fructose is removed from the portal blood by the liver, where it is committed to DNL without regulation. The consumption of sugar-sweetened beverages that contain either sucrose (which is converted to fructose and glucose in the gut) or a mixture of fructose and glucose is epidemiologically associated with fat accumulation in the liver and with NASH. Once FA reach the liver, they are non-covalently bound to fatty acid-binding protein-1 (FABP-1) and primarily metabolized either by mitochondrial β-oxidation or through esterification to form triglycerides (TG). TG not exported into the blood from the liver as VLDL, form lipid droplets in hepatocytes (the main feature of NAFL). Esterification of FA as neutral TG is generally considered as an adaptive protective response to a supply of FA that exceeds the metabolic capacity. However, recent studies suggest that this excess of TG, rather than a marker of metabolic abnormalities, may also play a causative role [14, 15]. The moiety of the intracellular fat has distinct toxic effects and the presence of the intermediate products seem to have a more deleterious effect on liver cells. Alterations in lipid metabolism lead to the accumulation of intermediate products such as DAG and phospholipids (sphingolipids and ceramides), and these compounds account for the fatty acid-induced toxicity and for the hepatic IR. Altered cholesterol homeostasis and hepatic free cholesterol (FC) accumulation have been also proposed as a trigger for the pathogenesis of NASH. Most probably, FC accumulates within the ER membrane impairing its fluidity. The resulting stiffening of the ER membrane leads to an impaired activity triggering the ER stress and eventual Unfolded Protein Response, cell apoptosis via JNK signaling and to the release of RE Ca^{+2} stores. Adjacent mitochondria readily take up the released Ca^{+2}, and the acute Ca^{+2} overload results in changes in mitochondrial potential and the opening of the permeability transition pore ensuing a potent cellular cell signal.

IR is recognized as another key factor linking MS and NAFLD and contributing to its pathogenesis. IR is characterized by reduced glucose disposal in nonhepatic tissues. As mentioned before IR promotes a higher lipolysis of WAT with the consequent mobilization of FA from this tissue to the liver. Ectopic fat accumulation within the liver, especially those lipid intermediates (such as DAG) further inhibits the insulin receptor and its downstream signaling and thus promote hepatic IR. Furthermore, impaired lipid oxidation and the subsequent increase of the hepatic lipid content lead to increase the hepatic IR. Expansion of the WAT, especially the visceral adipose tissue (VAT), promotes the release of deleterious cytokines that induce a chronic inflammatory status. Thus, inflammation is considered the major risk of obesity and it is associated with WAT dysfunction. Adipose tissue of obese subjects presents an increased number of macrophages, and they might account for much of the adipose tissue inflammatory cytokine secretion. In NAFLD, adipose tissue contributes to the systemic production of tumor necrosis factor α (TNF-α). TNF-α binds to its receptor and activates downstream inflammatory signaling pathways including OKK, mTOR or JNK. In turn, these effectors recruit downstream molecules, respectively nuclear factor-kappa b (NFκB), S6 kinase (S6K) and activator protein-1 (AP-1), which inhibit IRS phosphorylation, subsequently impairing insulin signaling in the liver. IR is also associated with an alteration in the adipokines profile (IL6, MCP1, adiponectin) which play a pivotal role in the initiation and perpetuation of the pathological events related with NAFLD.

More recently, the role of gut microbiota in the development of NAFLD has drawn the attention of the scientific society. The human intestinal tract contains highly diverse and dense gut microbiota that plays crucial roles in intestinal physiology such as the digestion of food (otherwise indigestible), the protection of mucosal surfaces and crosstalk with the immune system of the host. Among the trillions of

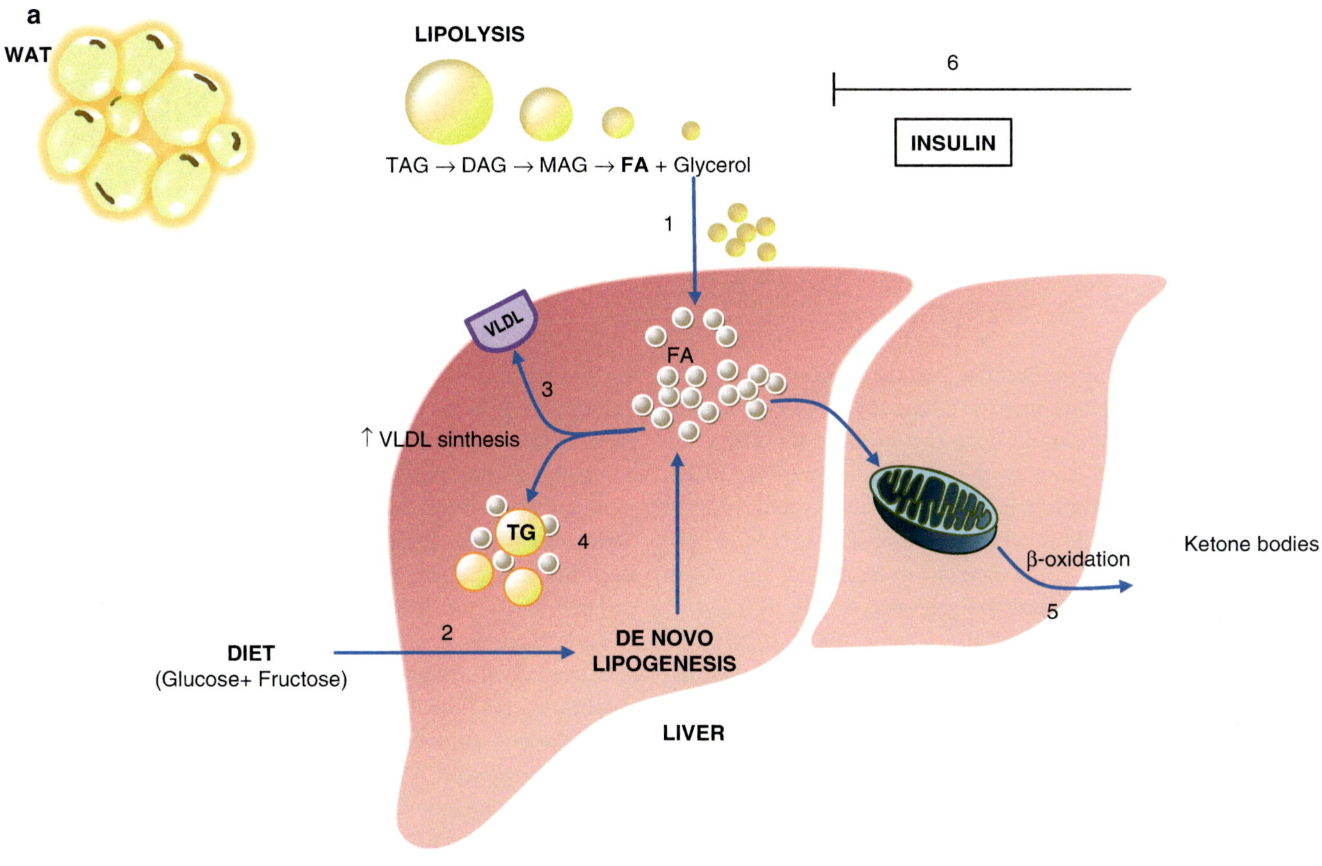

Fig. 26.1 (**a**) – *Hepatic fatty acids (FA) supply during normal conditions.* (1) Following the lipolysis of TAG in WAT FA are delivered to the liver from the blood. (2) FA can be synthesized in the liver (de novo lipogenesis) from the Glucose and Fructose contained in the diet. Once within the liver FA can follow different processes (3) can be exported as VLDL, metabolized by (4) esterification into neutral TG or (5) mitochondrial β-oxidation. The regulation of this process is highly regulated by (6) Insulin that has an important antilipolytic effect in WAT. (**b**) *Dysregulation in hepatic FA supply during NAFLD.* The normal process (described in **a**) are represented in blue, whereas the pathological-associated processes are evidenced in red. (1) Insulin resistance (IR), is associated with (2) an increased basal lipolysis in the WAT resulting in (3) an excessive delivery of FA to the liver. On the other side consumption of sugar-enriched diets promotes (4) an active hepatic FA synthesis (de novo lipogenesis). Impairment of WAT lipolysis (5) inhibits VLDL synthesis, and thus (6) increasing the TG intrahepatic pool. (7) Mitochondrial Dysfunction leads to impaired β-oxidation and the subsequent oxidative damage. (8) Accumulation of intermediate FA products (DAG, phospholipids, ceramides) account for the FA-induced toxicity triggering inflammation, profibrotic stimuli and (9) hepatic insulin resistance. (10) Expansion of WAT promotes the release of deleterious cytokines that induce a chronic inflammatory status that further compromise the hepatic functionality. (11) Dysbiosis induces and enhanced gut permeability (leaky gut) with the subsequent bacteria/LPS translocation to the blood contributing to the hepatic inflammation

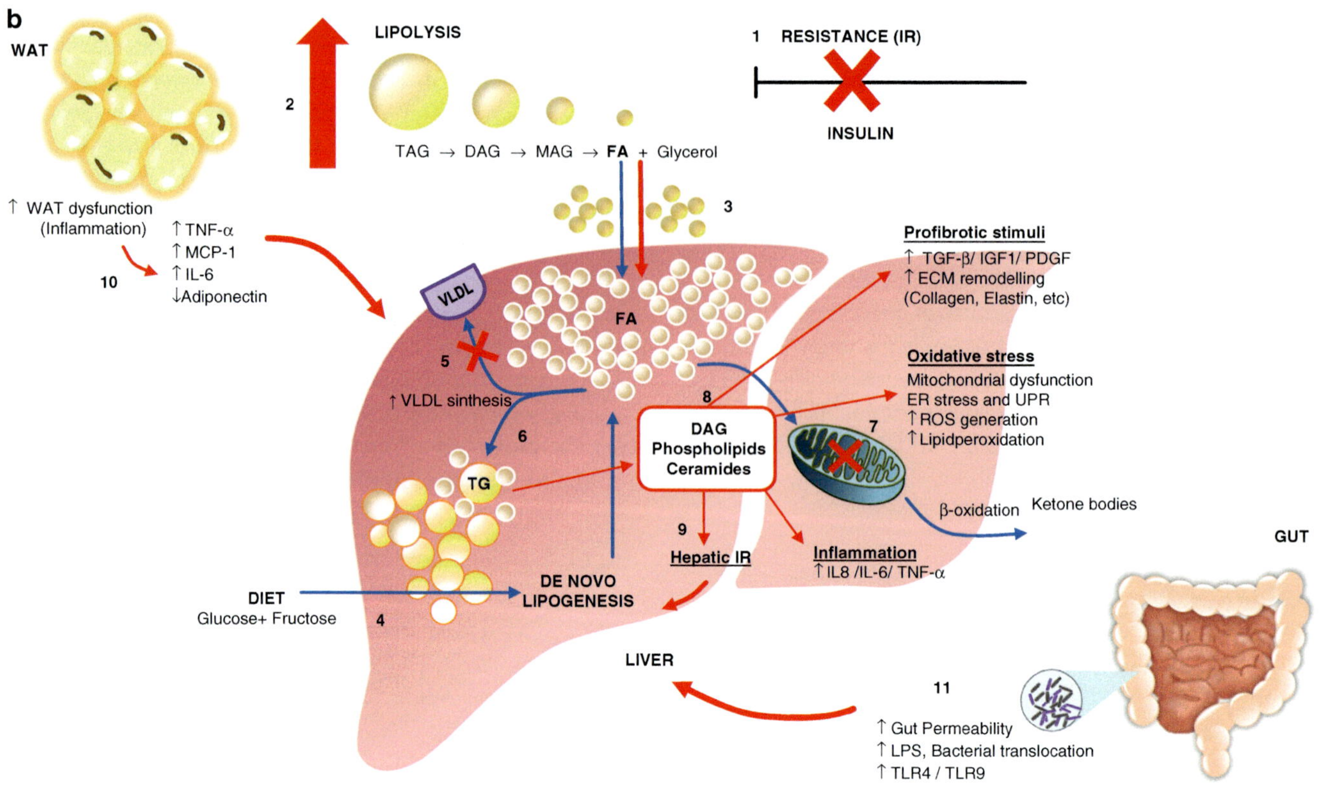

Fig. 26.1 (continued)

microbes that live in the human gut, the *Bacteroidetes* and the *Firmicutes* phyla are the two dominant groups of beneficial bacteria. Recently it has been shown that gut microbiota actively participates also in the pathogenesis of NAFLD. Differential gut microbiota composition (also called dysbiosis) has been reported in subjects with NAFL or NASH versus healthy controls. Specifically, it has been found an inverse association between the presence of NASH and the percentage of *Bacteroidetes* [16]. The increase of intrahepatic fat can be regulated by gut microbiota through mechanisms that regulate: (1) the appetite signaling; (2) the increased energy extraction from the diet; (3) the expression of genes involved in *DNL* and β-oxidation or (4) Inflammation-driven steatosis. Thus, hepatocellular inflammation may be secondary to alterations in the intestinal permeability (due to disruption of cellular tight-junctions) and subsequent translocation of either intact bacteria or microbial cell components (such as lipopolysaccharide [LPS] derived from the cell wall of gram-negative bacteria) to the circulation (the so-called "leaky-gut").

The worsening of the liver condition from NAFL to NASH is determined by the initiation of the fibrotic response. Fibrosis is a physiological intrinsic response to a persistent liver injury that leads to a wound-healing process to mitigate the damage. However, if the noxious stimuli become chronic the fibrotic process can lead to scar formation, compromising the normal liver architecture and disrupting the normal vasculature leading to the associated complications such as portal hypertension, liver failure, and hepatocellular carcinoma. Understanding the regulation of the initiation, progression, and perpetuation of fibrosis is of utmost importance especially for the development of therapeutic alternatives. Both humans and experimental studies have identified several cellular factors that play a determinant role in liver fibrogenesis. Hepatic stellate cells (HSC) are the main regulators of the extracellular matrix (ECM) production, under normal conditions, HSC have a quiescent phenotype and constitute 1/3 of the non-parenchymal cell population (storing the 85% of hepatic vitamin A). Upon noxious stimuli triggered by damaged hepatocytes, these cells become myofibroblasts (activated HSC) and undergo several phenotypic and functional changes. During the initial fibrogenic process, there is a cross-talk between injured hepatocytes and myofibroblasts which is further stimulated in a paracrine mode by the infiltrated leukocytes (macrophages and neutrophils) and the activated KC. Once activated myofibroblasts increase the proliferative rate and present a dysregulation of gene expression profile, particularly those involved in extracellular matrix (ECM) turnover, such as tissue inhibitors of metalloproteinases (TIMPs), matrix metalloproteinases (MMPs), collagen type I alpha I (Col1A1) and heat shock protein 47 (HSP47). Recent studies reviewed by Alegre and colleagues

[17] support the novel concept that hepatocyte cell death induces the release of extracellular danger signals and the further activation of a sterile inflammatory response (in absence of infection). This process can initiate the intrahepatic self-perpetuating noxious loop which is central to the development of liver fibrosis. The authors also reviewed in detail the role of inflammasomes as a novel key component of this loop. After activation of inflammasome caspase-1 activates IL-1β that is an important proinflammatory cytokine with diverse biological activities and is implicated in multiple diseases. Indeed, several pieces of evidence point toward the IL-1 pathway as an important mediator of the transition from liver injury to the onset of liver fibrogenesis and fibrosis. The mitochondrial-derived reactive oxygen species (ROS) are other important activators of the inflammasome that contribute to chronic liver disease. Altogether, these data indicate that fibrosis is a convergent final step of a complex series of different upstream processes.

26.4 Experimental Models

Several experimental models have been characterized in the field of translational research in an attempt to reproduce the molecular mechanisms involved in the onset of NAFL and the progression of NASH to be used as preclinical models. *In vitro* systems have provided useful and detailed information about the cellular response to the fatty acid overload. The currently available *in vitro* models cover a wide spectrum of variables, spanning from a simple cell culture or co-cultures (of two or more cells) exposed to different lipid mixtures, to more sophisticated 3D systems. In this section will be described the most common models used in research.

The most widely used model is the 2D monolayer culture, where cells are seeded in a stiff and flat polystyrene dishes. *In vitro* cultures of hepatocytes and HSC have been historically based on preparations of primary isolated cells from rat's liver. However, for the prediction of drug toxicity or to test drug-induced fibrosis in humans, the use of primary human hepatocytes or nonparenchymal cells is preferred since liver toxicity in humans shows poor correlation with animal studies. The yield of hepatocyte's isolation from human donors is scarce; the procedure is highly variable among preparations and depends on the etiology of the donor's liver. Induced pluripotent stem cells (iPSCs) represent an option as a source of hepatocytes since can be derived from nearly any cell type, including easily accessible cells like those from blood or skin. Since, iPSC-derived hepatocytes, in general, do not recapitulate the fully mature hepatocyte phenotype, hepatic cell lines became the most widely used alternative. Cell lines are readily available, easy to handle, phenotypically stable, low cost and have (almost) unlimited lifespan. The use of co-culture systems, such as hepatocytes and HSC, represents a valid platform for the study of cell cross-talk during fibrogenesis in the context of NAFLD. In fact, several studies have shown a superior correlation in *vivo* cellular phenotype by employing co-cultures rather than monoculture system. These 2D systems, have been proven to be valid for the assessment of cellular behavior but have limitations in maintaining the characteristics observed in the normal liver 3D microenvironment. The morphology, cellular heterogeneity and spatial organization maintained within 3D culture system allow the preservation of natural adhesion between cells, interaction between cells and extracellular matrix, and key cellular signaling pathways. Among these 3D culture systems (extensively reviewed here [18, 19]) can be mentioned different models with different characteristics: **(1) Spheroid models/organoids** that is a useful system for the study of complex signaling cascade between different cell types during liver disease); **(2) Microphysiological systems/Organ on chips** are perfused models where the regulation of the oxygen is highly controlled. These systems are used to reproduce the tissue-specific oxygen and nutrient gradients in order to satisfy the tissue-specific metabolic request; **(3) Precision-cut liver slices** are the systems that closely reflect the *in vivo* situation with maintaining the intact hepatic architecture and cellular heterogeneity; **(4) Cell sheet stacking** is a unique scaffold-free tissue-engineering approach where several layers of cell sheets can be assembled together in order to build more complex 3D structures; **(5) Scaffold/matrix-based 3D cultures** these platforms consist in reseeding cells in 3D scaffolds that can be made of synthetic materials to guarantee the preservation of the extracellular matrix molecules and to improve cell attachment and differentiation. In spite of all aforementioned advantages, all these 3D systems are not always easy to handle, and the experimental set-up has not been well standardized yet, thus limiting their use among different laboratories.

During the last years, *in vivo* models have played a vital role in the elucidation of the pathophysiological mechanisms of NAFLD; however, translation of the results to human scenario has repeatedly failed. The complexity of the pathophysiology involved in NAFLD progression is difficult to be fully reproduced in animals. Moreover, the differences both anatomically and physiologically between rodents and humans must not be disregarded. An ideal animal model must reproduce, as close as possible, the several criteria in order to be considered representative of human disease. Unfortunately, to date, none of the available models fulfills all these requirements and the choice of the best model relies on the selection of the model that better suits your needs.

Several models have been characterized (Table 26.1) based on the effect of the diet in the induction of NAFLD (reviewed elsewhere [20]), such as **(1) Methionine and choline-deficient (MCD)** diets (both essential nutrients)

Table 26.1 Summary of the available animal models used in the study of NAFLD

Models	Obesity	Insulin resistance	Dyslipidemia	Steatosis	NASH	Fibrosis	Use
Diet induced							
MCD	×	×	×	Yes	Yes	Yes	Study of intrahepatic events related with NASH
CDAA	×	×	Yes	Yes	Yes	Yes	
High cholesterol and cholate (Ath)	×	×	Yes	Yes	Yes	Yes	Study of atherosclerosis
High fructose	Yes	Yes	Yes	Yes	×	×	T2DM model
HFD	Yes	Yes	Yes	Yes	Yes	Minimal	Useful for the study of NAFL and the initial stages of NASH
Chemically induced							
Streptozotocin + HFD	X	Yes	–	Yes	Yes	Yes	Good model for the study of T2DM
CCl_4	×	×	×	Yes	Yes	Yes	Good fibrosis model
Genetically modified							
Ob/ob	Yes	Yes	×	Yes	×	×	Good model for the study of T2DM
Db/db	Yes	Yes	×	Yes	×	×	
Fa/fa	Yes	Yes	×	Yes	×	×	
Foz/Foz	Yes						
SREBP-1c	×	Yes		Yes	Yes	Yes	
$ApoE^{-/-}$	Yes	Yes	Yes				Models to explore cardiovascular morbidity and MetS in NASH
$Ldlr^{-/-}$	Yes	Yes	Yes				

results in impaired β-oxidation, impaired production of VLDL particles and hepatic VLDL secretion leading to steatosis, cell death, oxidative stress and changes in adipokines and cytokines. However, the animals do not exhibit any other metabolic features that are seen in human NAFLD, including obesity, peripheral IR, and dyslipidemia. On the contrary, the MCD diet induces weight loss. **(2) Semisynthetic choline-deficient L-amino acid-defined (CDAA)** diet is similar to MCD, but in CDAA diet proteins are substituted with an equivalent and corresponding mixture of L-amino acids. These animals develop s slightly more severe NASH albeit on marginally longer period. Animals fed with CDAA diet show a significant increase in body weight (but not obese), plasma TG and total cholesterol levels. **(3) Atherogenic diet (Ath)** the diet contains a relatively high dose of cholesterol (1–1.25%) and cholic acid (0.5%), a mixture that promotes the development of atherosclerosis. Ath diet induces steatosis, inflammation, hepatocellular ballooning, and fibrosis. Additionally, it induces increased levels of ALT, total cholesterol, and TG. However, Ath diet by itself does not induce obesity nor IR. This model is useful for the study of atherosclerosis but fails in reproducing the metabolic disorders related to NAFLD. **(4) High Fructose diet**: excessive fructose intake has been linked to the development and increased severity of NAFLD. Fructose supplementation in drinking water, in both rats and mice, induces simple steatosis (with no features of NASH); increase in body weight, TG, and glucose. **(5) High-Fat Diet (HFD) and its variations**: the HFD brings about a phenotype similar to the human disease characterized by obesity, IR, and hyperlipidemia. The excess of lipid supply directly via intake and via increased lipolysis leads to TG accumulation within the liver with the subsequent NASH development, even if this diet induces minimal fibrosis even after extended experimental periods.

Models induced by chemicals have been also characterized. The most widely used models are: **(1) Streptozotocin-induced diabetes** is a well-known experimental model of T2DM, achieved by the administration of a low dose of streptozotocin shortly after birth which results in a chemical inflammation and destruction of the pancreatic islets. When combined with HFD, it can be used as a model for NAFLD. The combination of these two approaches results in simple steatosis, NASH with inflammatory foci and ballooning and progressive pericellular fibrosis. It has been also reported a progressive increase in transaminases and fasting glucose, and the presence of multiple hepatocellular carcinoma. **(2) Carbon Tetrachloride (CCl_4)** is a compound commonly used for inducing liver damage. CCl_4 induces an oxidative stress response in the liver, which leads to the accumulation of lipid and protein peroxidation products and to a strong necrotic response. Most importantly, CCl_4 induces a dose-dependent fibrosis, but not obesity nor IR. Thus CCl_4, by itself, it is not a NAFLD model and this is the reason why it is used in combination with other dietary models.

An additional group of animal models is those related with genetic models of NAFLD (reviewed here [17]), briefly: **(1) Models of T2DM**: Lep^{ob}/Lep^{ob} (*ob/ob*) mice display a spontaneous mutation in the leptin gene, with a consequent leptin deficiency. These animals are hyperphagic, inactive, extremely obese and present IR. They present also mild to severe steatosis, even if ballooning and lobular inflammation (and thus NASH) are absent. However, these animals are resistant to hepatic fibrosis. Thus, for the development of NASH, these models need to be associated with the aforementioned diet/chemical models (MCD or HFD). Likewise, $Lepr^{db}/Lepr^{db}$ (*db/db*) mice present a mutation in leptin receptor gene rendering it nonfunctional. Consequently, these animals present a similar phenotype to that ob/ob mice, though normal to high leptin levels. Analogous mutation is also present in rats the $Lepr^{fa}/Lepr^{fa}$ (*fa/fa*, also known as Zucker rats). Both *db/db* and *fa/fa* animals do not spontaneously develop NASH and an additional stimulus is required. Another mutation associated with T2DM is the *Alms*1 gene (*foz/foz*) which is involved in the hypothalamic control of satiety. These animals present also hyperphagia, increased body weight, T2DM but for the development of NASH and fibrosis combination with other models is required. Sterol regulatory element binding protein (*SREBP*)-1c transgenic mice, which present an overexpression of this protein in adipose tissue, show IR secondary to impaired adipose differentiation leading to severe hepatic steatosis with the histological features of steatohepatitis with perivenular and pericellular fibrosis. **(2) Models of atherosclerosis**: deficiency in Apolipoprotein ($ApoE^{-/-}$) and lipoprotein receptor ($Ldlr^{-/-}$) predispose mice to develop hypercholesterolemia, atherosclerosis, and obesity. However, also in this case, for the development of NASH combination with HFD is required.

In spite of the promising results, substantial objections remain: (1) long-term exposure is required for observing the pathological phenotype; (2) the pathophysiological mechanisms not always coincide with human NAFLD; (3) the models have been characterized only in male adult animals excluding the application of this approach to the female and the pediatric populations. Therefore these models should be used with caution and their use should be limited to clearly defined liver-specific research goals. Limitations of each one of the models must be recognized to avoid misleading conclusions. In summary, due to the complex, multidirectional pathophysiology involved in NAFLD, the perfect animal model representing the complete spectrum of the disease in a workable time frame does not exist.

In conclusion, the complexity in the field of NAFLD is not limited to its pathophysiology, but also to the development of valid platforms for the discovery of therapeutic agents.

26.5 Diagnosis

NAFLD is commonly silent with no clinical manifestations nor specific symptoms, thus the diagnosis of the disease is often based on exclusion criteria. Although NAFL or NASH can be strongly suspected in an individual on the basis of imaging and clinical features (such as the presence of metabolic comorbidities and abnormal lab tests), liver biopsy remains the gold standard for the definitive diagnosis of NASH. Patients with only NAFL have a low risk of adverse consequences and progression to cirrhosis/HCC or non-liver associated adverse outcomes such as cardiovascular disease and malignancy. On the contrary, the presence of NASH increases the risks of liver and possibly non-liver-related outcomes compared to those patients with NAFL alone. The risk of liver-related mortality in NAFLD grows exponentially as the stage of fibrosis increases [21]. The identification of subjects at risk for NAFL and NASH is imprecise, and although there is significant on-going work, good and precise non-invasive markers for the diagnosis of NASH is still to be identified [22].

26.5.1 Diagnosis of NAFLD

NAFLD is now considered the hepatic manifestation of the MS. The majority of individuals with NAFLD are asymptomatic or paucisymptomatic (asthenia, abdominal pain at the upper quadrant). The need for a generalized screening and surveillance of NAFLD is still questionable mainly due to the high direct and indirect costs of diagnostic tests, the low predictive value of surrogate markers of hepatic injury (transaminases and non-invasive tests), and finally the risks of liver biopsy and lack of effective treatments. However, it is desirable that the progressive form of NAFLD (NASH), particularly when associated with advanced fibrosis, is correctly identified in patients at risk (age > 50 years, DM2 or MS). The anamnesis represents a crucial step in the clinical evaluation of the patient and must be oriented towards the presence of familiarity and comorbidity, stigmata of MS, determination of the glucose and lipid profiles. The serology markers of hepatic synthesis (total bilirubin, albumin, prothrombin time, creatinine), the platelet count, predictive of portal hypertension, a moderate increase in ALT (aminotransferase), GGT (γ-glutamyltranspeptidase) levels, with an AST/ALT ratio typically <1 are all biochemical markers that could help in the diagnosis of NASH, but they are all unspecific. Hyperferritinemia is also frequent, as markers of chronic inflammatory state induced by insulin resistance. In non-diabetic subjects, insulin sensitivity assessment using surrogate indices of insulin resistance, such as Homeostatic Model of Insulin Resistance Index (HOMA-IR) derived from blood glucose and insulin levels could be useful to identify patients at high risk of development of DM2. Finally, a genetic characterization by assessing the gene correlated to NASH could be useful in young and lean patients with juvenile NAFLD. Abdominal ultrasound is still the simplest and most widespread method of detecting hepatic steatosis.

Quantification of liver fat could be done either with fibroscan CAP (controlled attenuation parameter), which consists of a non-invasive measurement proportional to the attenuation of the ultrasound beam that undergoes through the liver parenchyma, or with magnetic resonance (MR) which is now able to quantify limited amounts of intra-hepatocyte triglycerides and has the ability to sample large parenchymal volumes. However, its use is limited by high costs.

26.5.2 Diagnosis of NASH and Fibrosis

The goal of the diagnostic procedure is the identification, among individuals with NAFLD, of the patients with NASH. Measurement of the severity of necro-inflammation (grading) and fibrosis (staging) is standardized in histopathological classification systems, such as NAS CRN score and the most recent SAF score, useful in the diagnostic and follow-up phase. To date, the demonstration of histological improvement is a fundamental requirement for the approval of a pharmacological treatment, required by the European Medicines Agency and the Food and Drug Administration (FDA). In particular, since the FDA does not recognize an indication of treatment in simple steatosis (NAFL), it is believed that therapy should have a histological effect in terms of NASH improvement. The reason for this approach is currently based on data demonstrating a risk of end-stage progression of liver disease that exists only in patients with NASH. Although histology represents the only reliable diagnostic method, the high costs and the non-negligible risk of complications limit its use on a large scale. In recent years, non-invasive biomarkers of hepatic injury for the selection of high-risk subjects, and validated predictive scores of fibrosis have been developed. The main ones are NAFLD Fibrosis score (NFS), FIB-4, BARD, FibroTest, FibroMeter, Enhanced Liver Fibrosis test (ELF), APRI. NFS, based on the combination of age, BMI, fasting glycemia or DMT2, platelet count, albumin and AST/ALT ratio.

Another non-invasive technique for the quantification of fibrosis is hepatic elastography, although the diagnostic accuracy has been widely validated in patients with HCV chronic hepatitis, but not in patients with NAFLD. Potential limitations consist of poor sensitivity in mild forms of fibrosis and technical difficulty in detecting and interpreting data in obese patients. MRI has obtained encouraging results in the quantification of steatosis and fibrosis recently.

26.6 Treatment

Although there has been steady progress in clarifying the pathogenesis of NAFLD/NASH, or in identifying the therapeutic targets and advancing drug development, and more than 200 clinical trials testing new drugs are ongoing worldwide, no drugs have yet been approved and registered specifically for the treatment of NASH.

The first line treatment, recommended in all patients with NAFLD and also aimed at the reduction of cardiovascular risk, is change in lifestyle (increase in physical activity and reducing weight by changing eating habits) It has been shown that a 7–10% reduction of the initial weight induces an improvement in both the levels of liver enzymes and in liver histology.

Drug therapy aimed at the treatment of concomitant metabolic disorders (lipid-lowering, anti-hypertensive and anti-diabetic) is recommended in all patients with NAFLD, in order to prevent and contain extra-hepatic co-morbidities. Insulin-sensitizing agents.

The thiazolidinedione (TZD) possess, among the drugs currently in use, the strongest pathogenetic rationale to be used in NASH. The other widely used clinical drug in the diabetic field, metformin, is not recommended as a specific therapy for NASH due to a lack of evidence of histological improvement resulting from its use.

The GFT505, PPARα/PPARδ agonist, has recently shown promising effects through the induction of hepatic oxidative metabolism and the inhibition of lipolysis and endogenous glucose synthesis. Already in use in the diabetic population, GLP-1 receptor agonists (glucagon-like peptide 1), a physiologically produced post-prandial hormone with glucose modulatory action, such as liraglutide, represent another promising treatment perspective in patients with NASH. Other regulators of metabolic homeostasis have been identified in bile acids. Obeticholic acid (OCA), a synthetic agonist of FXR (Farnesoid X Receptor) promotes the improvement of insulin-sensitivities, by reducing lipogenesis and increasing the oxidation of fatty acids, and a reduction of fibrosis at histology level.

Anti-oxidant agents, including vitamin E, could also induce a reduction of necroinflammation and ballooning degeneration.

Antifibrotic agents, such as simtuzumab, or bariatric surgery seem to be promising in improving insulin sensitivity, glycemic response and in reducing steatohepatitis and fibrosis.

26.7 Conclusions

NAFLD is becoming the most important and prevalent chronic liver disease in Western countries, but its incidence is increasing in emerging countries, making this disease a public health problem. The significant progress achieved in the understanding of the pathogenesis of NAFLD have allowed the identification of novel molecular pathways as targets for the development of new therapeutic approaches. Nevertheless, many objectives are still to be pursued, among them the most urgent are: the discovery and validation of new non-invasive markers and the definition of specific therapies for NASH and fibrosis. Also, genetics will play a key role, and the ultimate goal will be to define the genotype/phenotype of the individual patient with NAFLD and possibly identify those patients who could progress to cirrhosis and HCC. New therapeutical molecules will also be tested soon in long-term studies to demonstrate an effective benefit in terms of efficacy and lack of side effects. It is plausible that no single therapy will reverse NASH in all patients, but a combined therapy and tailored pharmacotherapy would represent a valid strategy to be used in the future.

Self Study

Questions

1. Which statement is true?
   (a) NAFLD/NASH treatment is nowadays based only on lifestyle changes, but it is enough to reach at least a reduction of 10% of the body weight to obtain a normalization of liver enzymes.
   (b) The diagnosis of NASH could be reached with non-invasive diagnostic markers.
   (c) The average prevalence of NAFLD worldwide is 35%.
   (d) Metformin, the most prescribed oral antidiabetic drugs, cannot be used in patients with NASH.
2. Which statement is true?
   (a) Lean NAFLD has a relatively benign clinical course with lower risk than NAFLD in obese subjects.
   (b) Among the experimental models, the *in vitro* systems are the best alternatives to reproduce the events involved in the progression of the disease.
   (c) *In vivo* models have played a vital role in the elucidation of the pathophysiological mechanisms of NAFLD; and there is wide variety of animal models to study this disease mimicking the human scenario.
   (d) The multifactorial nature of NAFLD hampers the progression in the field of pathophysiology and treatment.

Answers

1. Which statement is true?
   (a) **CORRECT ANSWER**: There are more than 200 clinical trials ongoing which explore different molecules belonging to different family of drugs, but still no drugs are approved to be used in the market worldwide.
   (b) The only possibility to make diagnosis of NASH is to perform liver biopsy, which remains still the gold standard for the diagnosis of NASH.
   (c) The real prevalence of NAFLD in the general population is ranging between 25% to 30% and could varies according to ethnicity, aged, sex, and the presence of co-morbidities such as type 2 diabetes mellitus, obesity, hypercholesterolemia, hypertension, etc.
   (d) All the drugs that are currently used in patients with type 2 diabetes mellitus and NAFLD/NASH should be continued even in the presence of NASH.
2. Which statement is true?
   (a) Lean NAFLD usually presents fewer comorbidities, for this reason, is commonly believed that this subgroup would follow a relatively benign clinical course. However, NASH prevalence in obese and nonobese has been reported to be similar. Moreover, the presence of advanced fibrosis in nonobese NASH patients is similar to the observed in obese subjects.
   (b) The currently available *in vitro* models cover a wide spectrum of variables, spanning from a simple cell culture or co-cultures (of two or more cells) exposed to different lipid mixtures, to more sophisticated 3D systems. However none of this experimental systems fulfil the all the events involved in the progression of the disease.
   (c) Due to the complex, multidirectional pathophysiology involved in NAFLD, the perfect animal model representing the complete spectrum of the disease in a workable time frame does not exist and translation of the results to human scenario has repeatedly failed.
   (d) **CORRECT ANSWER**: The complexity in the field of NAFLD is not limited to its pathophysiology, but also to the development of valid platforms for the discovery of therapeutic agents.

References

1. Ludwig J, Viggiano TR, McGill DB, Oh BJ. Nonalcoholic steatohepatitis: Mayo Clinic experiences with a hitherto unnamed disease. Mayo Clin Proc. 1980;55:434–8.
2. Bellentani S, Tiribelli C. Is it time to change NAFLD and NASH nomenclature? Lancet Gastroenterol Hepatol. 2017;2:547–8.
3. Younossi Z, Anstee QM, Marietti M, Hardy T, Henry L, Eslam M, et al. Global burden of NAFLD and NASH: trends, predictions, risk factors and prevention. Nat Rev Gastroenterol Hepatol. 2018;15(1):11–20.
4. Younossi ZM, Henry L, Bush H, Mishra A. Clinical and economic burden of nonalcoholic fatty liver disease and nonalcoholic steatohepatitis. Clin Liver Dis. 2018;22:1–10.
5. Welsh JA, Karpen S, Vos MB. Increasing prevalence of nonalcoholic fatty liver disease among United States adolescents, 1988–1994 to 2007–2010. J Pediatr. 2013;162:496–500.e1.
6. Piscaglia F, Svegliati-Baroni G, Barchetti A, Pecorelli A, Marinelli S, Tiribelli C, et al. Clinical patterns of hepatocellular carcinoma

in nonalcoholic fatty liver disease: a multicenter prospective study. Hepatology. 2016;63:827–38.

7. Romeo S, Kozlitina J, Xing C, Pertsemlidis A, Cox D, Pennacchio LA, et al. Genetic variation in PNPLA3 confers susceptibility to nonalcoholic fatty liver disease. Nat Genet. 2008;40:1461–5.
8. Valenti L, Al-Serri A, Daly AK, Galmozzi E, Rametta R, Dongiovanni P, et al. Homozygosity for the patatin-like phospholipase-3/adiponutrin I148M polymorphism influences liver fibrosis in patients with nonalcoholic fatty liver disease. Hepatology. 2010;51:1209–17.
9. Mancina RM, Dongiovanni P, Petta S, Pingitore P, Meroni M, Rametta R, et al. The MBOAT7-TMC4 variant rs641738 increases risk of nonalcoholic fatty liver disease in individuals of European descent. Gastroenterology. 2016;150:1219–1230.e6.
10. Anstee QM, Seth D, Day CP. Genetic factors that affect risk of alcoholic and nonalcoholic fatty liver disease. Gastroenterology. 2016;150:1728–1744.e7.
11. Abul-Husn NS, Cheng X, Li AH, Xin Y, Schurmann C, Stevis P, et al. A protein-truncating HSD17B13 variant and protection from chronic liver disease. N Engl J Med. 2018;378:1096–106.
12. Zarrinpar A, Gupta S, Maurya MR, Subramaniam S, Loomba R. Serum microRNAs explain discordance of non-alcoholic fatty liver disease in monozygotic and dizygotic twins: a prospective study. Gut. 2016;65:1546–54.
13. Leung JC-F, Loong TC-W, Wei JL, Wong GL-H, Chan AW-H, Choi PC-L, et al. Histological severity and clinical outcomes of nonalcoholic fatty liver disease in nonobese patients. Hepatology. 2017;65:54–64.
14. Samuel VT, Shulman GI. The pathogenesis of insulin resistance: integrating signaling pathways and substrate flux. J Clin Invest. 2016;126:12–22.
15. Yki-Järvinen H. Nutritional modulation of non-alcoholic fatty liver disease and insulin resistance. Nutrients. 2015;7:9127–38.
16. Mouzaki M, Comelli EM, Arendt BM, Bonengel J, Fung SK, Fischer SE, et al. Intestinal microbiota in patients with nonalcoholic fatty liver disease. Hepatology. 2013;58:120–7.
17. Alegre F, Pelegrin P, Feldstein AE. Inflammasomes in liver fibrosis. Semin Liver Dis. 2017;37:119–27.
18. Mazza G, Al-Akkad W, Rombouts K. Engineering in vitro models of hepatofibrogenesis. Adv Drug Deliv Rev. 2017;121:147–57.
19. van Grunsven LA. 3D in vitro models of liver fibrosis. Adv Drug Deliv Rev. 2017;121:133–46.
20. Van Herck MA, Vonghia L, Francque SM. Animal models of nonalcoholic fatty liver disease—a starter's guide. Nutrients. 2017;9 https://doi.org/10.3390/nu9101072.
21. Angulo P, Kleiner DE, Dam-Larsen S, Adams LA, Bjornsson ES, Charatcharoenwitthaya P, et al. Liver fibrosis, but no other histologic features, is associated with long-term outcomes of patients with nonalcoholic fatty liver disease. Gastroenterology. 2015;149:389–397.e10.
22. Chalasani N, Younossi Z, Lavine JE, Diehl AM, Brunt EM, Cusi K, et al. The diagnosis and management of non-alcoholic fatty liver disease: practice guideline by the American Association for the Study of Liver Diseases, American College of Gastroenterology, and the American Gastroenterological Association. Hepatology. 2012;55:2005–23.

Related Published Articles

Araújo AR, Rosso N, Bedogni G, Tiribelli C, Bellentani S. Global epidemiology of NAFLD/NASH: what we need in the future. Liver Int. 2018;38(Suppl 1):47–51.

Barbero-Becerra VJ, Giraudi PJ, Chávez-Tapia NC, Uribe M, Tiribelli C, Rosso N. The interplay between hepatic stellate cells and hepatocytes in an in vitro model of NASH. Toxicol In Vitro. 2015;29(7):1753–8. https://doi.org/10.1016/j.tiv.2015.07.010. PMID: 26187275.

Chavez-Tapia NC, Rosso N, Tiribelli C. In vitro models for the study of non-alcoholic fatty liver disease. Curr Med Chem. 2011;18(7):1079–84.

Giraudi PJ, Barbero Becerra VJ, Marin V, Chavez-Tapia NC, Tiribelli C, Rosso N. The importance of the interaction between hepatocyte and hepatic stellate cells in fibrogenesis induced by fatty accumulation. Exp Mol Pathol. 2014;98(1):85–92. https://doi.org/10.1016/j.yexmp.2014.12.006.

Marin V, Rosso N, Dal Ben M, Raseni A, Boschelle M, Degrassi C, et al. An animal model for the juvenile non-alcoholic fatty liver disease and non-alcoholic steatohepatitis. PLoS One. 2016;11(7):e0158817.

Alcoholic Liver Disease

27

Vatsalya Vatsalya and Hamza Zahid Hassan

Key Concepts

- Heavy and prolonged alcohol intake causes alcoholic liver disease
- Alcoholic liver disease is a progressive and multifaceted form of liver disease
- Multiple pathological pathways are involved in the development of alcoholic liver disease
- Known biomarkers of ALD have shown limited efficiency in identifying progression and severity
- There are no FDA approved treatments for alcoholic liver disease

27.1 Introduction

Heavy and chronic alcohol intake causes alcoholic liver disease (ALD) and the associated mortality risk [1]. Roughly 10–20% of heavy drinking alcoholics would develop some form of advanced ALD. ALD is the most common form of chronic liver disease worldwide. Some of the important newly-emerging markers of drinking patterns and total alcohol intake derived from the timeline followback assessment are heavy drinking days (HDD), total drinks (TD), number of drinking days (NDD) and average heavy drinking per drinking day (AvgDPD) that are closely associated with the onset of ALD [2]. Spectrum of ALD includes alcoholic fatty liver (AFL), alcoholic hepatitis (AH), alcoholic cirrhosis (AC) and hepatocellular carcinoma [3]. There are various risk factors and modifiers of ALD, some of the important ones are sex, genetics, race and ethnicity, underlying comorbid liver conditions, obesity, malnutrition and drug-induced liver injury, metabolic changes including iron overload, and nicotine abuse [4].

ALD is a multifactorial disease process and it also exhibits complications in several other organ systems [5]. Systemic protective mechanisms against alcoholic liver disease grow weaker with the progression and severity of ALD. Various metabolic dysregulations result in the development of AFL. Among them genetics/epigenetics changes, nutrition, oxidative stress, endoplasmic reticulum (ER) stress and gut-derived liver injury and inflammation are primary contributors of ALD by affecting liver cells and liver stellate cells (HSCs). Many of these factors are interlinked and show further exacerbation of ALD when congregated together. With varied form of diagnosis of ALD, these factors seem to lead in one or several conditions and explain the pathology better when evaluated together. Due to the complex natural history and staging of ALD, efforts to develop unique biomarkers for individual stages and diagnosis have not been thoroughly established yet. In this chapter, we discuss the recent advancements in the understanding of the major mechanisms and their involvement in the progression and severity of ALD with special emphasis on the onset of ALD.

V. Vatsalya (✉)
Division of Gastroenterology, Hepatology, and Nutrition, Department of Medicine, University of Louisville, Louisville, KY, USA

Robley Rex VA Medical Center, Louisville, KY, USA
e-mail: v0vats01@louisville.edu

H. Z. Hassan
Division of Gastroenterology, Hepatology, and Nutrition, Department of Medicine, University of Louisville, Louisville, KY, USA

F. Radu-Ionita et al. (eds.), *Liver Diseases*, https://doi.org/10.1007/978-3-030-24432-3_27

27.2 Malnutrition and Metabolic Dysfunction

Alcoholic liver disease is associated with malnutrition and nutritional dysregulation, especially with heavy and chronic alcohol consumption [6]. The most detailed reports on the association of malnutrition in ALD was from the Veterans Health Administration (VA) Cooperative Studies Program in patients having AH. All AH patient had some degree of malnutrition; and almost 50% of patients' energy intake was derived from alcohol. Although total calorie intake was frequently adequate, consumption of protein and critical micronutrients was often deficient. Importantly, the extent of malnutrition has been linked to the severity of alcoholic liver disease.

Recent studies have shown the role of alterations in nutritional status of dietary micro- and macro-nutrients in the onset and progression of ALD. Polyunsaturated fatty acids of ω-3 (anti-inflammatory) and ω-6 (pro-inflammatory) origin play an essential role in the pathogenesis of ALD. Onset of ALD in heavy drinking alcohol use disorder (AUD) patients showed decreases in ω-3, and increases in ω-6 fatty acids specially in the female sex [2]. Unsaturated fat enriched in linoleic acid (LA) in particular, likely promotes alcohol-induced liver damage. This is particularly concerning since dietary intake of LA has more than doubled over the past century, making it the most significant percentage of dietary unsaturated fatty acid consumed. Until recently, the mechanism of LA and alcohol interaction resulting in liver injury was not fully understood. LA is enzymatically changed by 12/15-lipoxygenase (12/15-LO) to bioactive oxidation products (OXLAMs) and non-enzymatically via free radical-mediated oxidation response to oxidative stress. Both the increased substrate availability (LA) and increased 12/15-LO activity contribute to an increase in the OXLAM production that subsequently contributes in the development of ALD [7]. Gut permeability and hepatic mitochondrial dysfunction are also affected by the OXLAMs.

Zinc is an important dietary supplement that is involved in various metabolic pathways of liver and also used as a therapy for alcoholic liver disease, primarily as a medication for alcoholic cirrhosis [8]. Serum zinc levels are lower in compensated ALD patients and get further decreased in patients with portal systemic encephalopathy, which can be corrected with long-term zinc supplementation. Hypozincemia (serum zinc level < 71 μg/dl) is observed in about 40% heavy alcohol drinking individuals that occurs due to poor intake and absorption, increased excretion, and alterations in zinc transporters, especially ZIP14. Hypozincemia is closely associated with the markers of alcohol drinking, heavy drinking days past 90 days (HDD90) and lifetime drinking history (LTDH); liver injury characterized by AST/ALT ratio; and acute inflammation (CRP shows a J-shaped response) supporting its role in the onset and progression of ALD [9]. In comorbid conditions of HIV infection in AD patients, an underlying proinflammatory response due to zinc deficiency and elevated LA likely exacerbates liver injury [10]. There are other nutritional elements that have been studied with mixed responses. Interaction of homocysteine and SAMe did not show much relevance either with the progression or severity of ALD. Lowering of magnesium, and increases in uric acid are emerging pathological biomarkers of the progression of ALD. It seems that high LA and hypozincemia are two important markers of nutritional alterations involved in the onset and progression of ALD.

27.3 Oxidative Stress

Reactive oxidants are produced from various systemic pathways and neutralized by anti-oxidant chemical species. Pro-oxidative agents that participate in liver injury/inflammation are singlet oxygen molecules, hydrogen peroxide, superoxide anions, and hydroxyl radicals. Under the influence of pathological triggers such as heavy alcohol intake, a surplus of pro-oxidative species accumulate and results in oxidative stress damaging the cellular macromolecules. Alcohol is metabolized by three major systems in the liver: rate limiting alcohol dehydrogenase (ADH) in the cytosol, cytochrome P450 2E1 (CYP2E1) in smooth endoplasmic reticulum (via microsomal ethanol P450 oxidases [MEOS]), and catalase in peroxisomes (such as H_2O_2). Table 27.1 describes the generation of these reactive oxygen species (ROS) and their target pathways. Reactive oxygen species (ROS) result in a wide array of pathological effects including depletion of ATP and nicotinamide dinucleotide, DNA damage, destruction of membranes via lipid peroxidation, release of pro-inflammatory cytokines, and abnormal protein stability [11].

By-products of PUFA peroxidation such as 4-hydroxynonenal (HNE) and malondialdehyde (MDA) initiate pro-inflammation pathways via cytokine synthesis and neutrophil chemotaxis. ROS and lipid peroxidation by-

Table 27.1 Generation of reactive oxides and mechanisms of inflammation in alcoholic liver disease

Generation of reactive species	Pathways/Mechanisms of action
• Mitochondrial electron transport chain • Cytochrome P450 2E1 • B oxidation • Increased NADH:NAD ratio • Increased $NADP^+$	• ATP and NAD depletion • DNA and protein damage • Glutathione depletion • Hepatic stellate activation • Release of inflammatory cytokines

products can lead to fibrosis by activating hepatic stellate cells, which synthesize collagen and promotes the inflammatory response. In addition, patients might also show ultrastructural mitochondrial abnormalities including megamitochondria and deletion of specific mitochondrial genome. Impaired mitochondrial respiratory chain (MRC) activity in the mitochondria results in the formation of superoxide anions and hydrogen peroxide. The surplus of fatty acids in the cytosol increases fatty acid oxidation in peroxisomes and the endoplasmic reticulum (ER). Initial reaction in peroxisomal β-oxidation is catalyzed by acyl-CoA oxidase (AOX) forming H_2O_2 (hydrogen peroxide) through electron transfer to the oxygen molecule. Microsomal oxidation is catalyzed by cytochrome P450 (CYP) enzymes 2E1, 4A10, and 4A14, which forms ROS through the flavoprotein-mediated donation of electrons to molecular oxygen [12].

Through the mechanism of progression, any additional changes may be sufficient to initiate the transition from hepatic steatosis to hepatic inflammation. This multifactorial approach would explain the disparity in manifestations and degree of severity in the ALD patients with similar heavy alcohol consumption. Alcohol metabolism generates acrolein, a severely toxic and reactive toxin that is a critical component in alcohol-induced liver disease [13]. Oxidative stress activates AMP-activated protein kinase (AMPK) signaling system, which has emerged in recent years as a kinase that controls the redox-state and mitochondrial function. Sterol regulatory element-binding protein (SREBP)-1c expression is reduced by activated AMPK. The cumulative result of AMPK activation is Acetyl-CoA build-up, decreased malonyl-CoA concentrations, and increased CPT-1 activity that increases fatty acid oxidation [14]. Kupffer cells (KCs) play a crucial mediating role in the initiation of liver inflammation as ultrastructural mitochondrial abnormalities in ALD [15]. When activated, Kupffer cells release M1 Kupffer cell-derived mediators that contribute significantly to hepatic inflammation.

27.4 Genetics/Epigenetics

While environmental factors have been well established in ALD, the genetic aspect of ALD was established in the last couple of decades. Excessive alcohol consumption leads to chronic ALD in a small proportion of heavy drinkers. The biological mechanisms that could explain this differential progression are yet understudied. One study on monozygotic twins provided explanation for about 50% of the variability in the progression of ALD due to the genetics [16]. Clinical phenotypes examined in most of the recent studies demonstrate substantial heterogeneity and variability, necessitating large samples and smaller effect sizes for genetic influences. Such research areas identifying subgroups of patients with a high genetic susceptibility to ALD can alter the current treatment guidelines of patients with ALD. As a result, there has been an increasing interest in examining the quantitative endophenotypes for gene-association in alcohol related diseases including ALD.

Patatin-like phospholipase encoding 3 gene sequence is associated with inflammatory changes in both ALD and Non-alcoholic fatty liver disease (NAFLD) [17]. Alcohol dehydrogenase 2 (ADH2) gene polymorphism seen uniquely among the Asian population has a significant bearing on the development of ALD. Several variants of ADH, especially the ADH2∗2 allele can change the rate of alcohol metabolism in the liver by altering the level of toxic metabolic products such as acetaldehyde [18]. Another genetic predisposition involved in the development of ALD is the genetic polymorphism of Cytochrome P4502E1, which is another primary enzyme of alcohol catabolism apart from the classic pathway of alcohol dehydrogenase. One case-control study compared the effects of alcohol consumption in patients with hemochromatosis (C282Y mutation in the HFE gene). Patients with hemochromatosis who consumed more than 60 mg of alcohol per day are nine times more likely to develop cirrhosis.

Based on the "second hit" or "multiple hits" theory, patients are predisposed to progressive ALD when a combination of gene and environmental interactions exists. Many molecular pathways of epigenetic mechanisms can be dysregulated by prolonged and unremitting alcohol intake leading to the development and progression of ALD. Identical DNA sequences could have variations in their genetic expression due to the epigenetic causes. The inherited variability that changes the expression of genes without altering the DNA sequences could be aided through various biochemical responses namely histone modifications, DNA methylation, and RNA-associated silencing by small non-coding RNAs. Distinct groups of genes contribute in the pathogenesis during the different stages of the ALD. Environmental factors interact with suspected genes to modify their degree of expression and participation in the pathogenesis (Fig. 27.1). Alterations from the normal physiological course of development, differentiation and tissue-specific gene expression could lead to modified target gene expression. Consequentially such epigenetic modifications in ALD could show manifestations as compromised immune conditions, age-sex dependent changes, and oncological events.

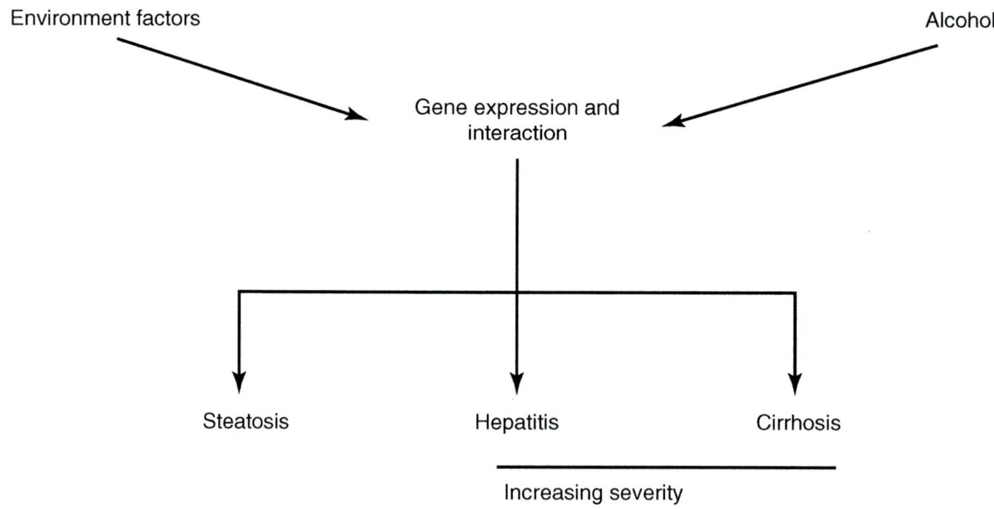

Fig. 27.1 Gene-environment interactions that determine the individual susceptibility to the different forms of alcoholic liver disease

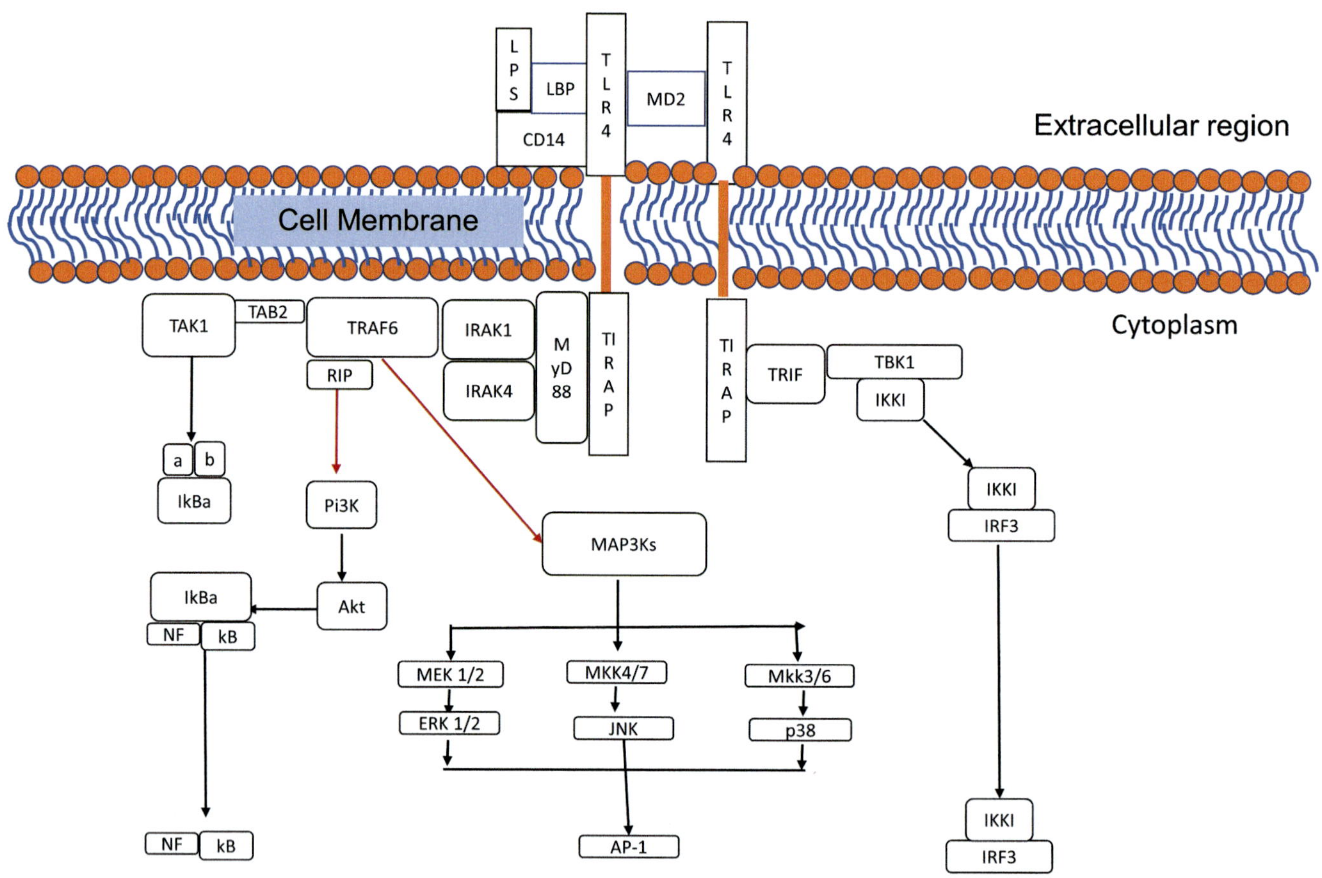

Fig. 27.2 Signaling pathway of Toll-like receptors. Red lines represent unknown pathway

27.5 Gut Permeability and Endotoxemia

The imbalance between the gut microbiome and gut permeability is one of the underlying causes of hepatic injury that subsequently initiates ALD. Alcohol and its catabolic derivative acetaldehyde disrupt the tight junction proteins and increase gut permeability that results in endotoxins passing through the gut membrane and entering the bloodstream. Factors that increase the risk of endotoxemia include gram-negative bacterial overgrowth in the intestine, increased intestinal permeability, and impaired hepatic clearance of endotoxin. Endotoxins reaching macrophages and other candidate immune cell types, stimulate the production of TNF-α and other proinflammatory cytokines via Toll-like receptor (TLR-4) signaling (Fig. 27.2) [19]. TLR-4 activation results in liver injury both by endotoxemia as well as via immune response and cell infiltration in the liver. As a result, endotoxins not only play a significant role in the hepatosteatosis and liver inflammation but also in hepatic fibrosis. Other activators of the TLR-4 receptor include bacterial peptidoglycan and flagellin.

Chronic alcohol consumption is also involved in the upregulation of hepatic TLRs, further sensitizing hepatocytes to inflammation and injury induced by gut-derived bacterial byproducts. TLRs also depend on other co-receptors for full ligand sensitivity, such as lipopolysaccharide (LPS), which requires Lymphocyte Antigen-96 (MD2). CD14 (Cluster of Differentiation 14) and LPS-Binding Proteins (LBP) are known to facilitate the presentation of LPS to MD-2, which stimulates the pathways of TIRF (TIR-domain-containing adapter-inducing interferon) and TRAM (TLR Adaptor Molecule). Several single nucleotide polymorphisms (SNPs) of the TLR4 in humans have been identified, which show increased susceptibility to gram-negative bacterial infections.

Gut microbiome plays a significant role in the prevention of gut barrier dysfunction; and loss/change of gut flora is associated with endotoxemia and liver injury/fibrosis of ALD. Heavy alcohol intake results in a time-dependent decline in the normal flora of both Bacteroidetes and Firmicute origin; and a significant increase in pathogenic species Actinobacteria and Proteobacteria that are associated with endotoxemia include Vibrio, Escherichia, Salmonella, and Helicobacter. Endotoxin levels and hepatic inflammation are a consequence of the transition of the gram-negative bacteria in response to chronic alcohol consumption.

Some of the primary factors that alter intestinal microbiome are gastric pH, gut motility, bile salts, immunological defense factors, antibiotic use, colonic pH, and competitive response of micro-organisms for nutrients against the intestinal binding sites. The altered luminal environment leads to modifications in the microbial flora by supporting the growth of pathological organisms and inhibiting the growth of normal healthy flora. In patients with heavy chronic alcohol abuse, bacterial colonies of Alcaligenes are generally significantly higher when compared to individuals maintaining alcohol-abstinence or social drinking habits. Increased luminal pH is a significant contributing factor in the alcohol-induced changes in the intestinal microbiota. Binge drinking causes a rapid increase in the serum endotoxin level and bacterial DNA that remains elevated for several hours after alcohol intake, and is significantly higher in patients with elevated liver enzyme levels [20]. Importantly, alcohol even in the absence of LPS can activate TLR4 signaling pathways.

27.6 Treatment of Alcoholic Liver Disease

Abstinence is the one of the most effective management of ALD; acamprosate or naltrexone combined with counseling could likely decrease alcohol consumption thus prevent progression of ALD. However, patients with ALD are still at risk of developing cirrhosis regardless of abstinence with history of chornic drinking. Steroids, nutritional supplementation, or aggressive enteral feeding are some of the medical management strategies that are used for alcoholic hepatitis, however they do not show any substantial improvement in short term survival. A time-dose dependent therapy of prednisolone (40 mg/day for 4 weeks then tapered over 2–4 weeks, or stopped as per the clinical indications) is considered partially effective in short term survival with an effect in the subgroup of patients with hepatic encephalopathy and/or a MDF score ≥32. Zinc supplementation is being used as a therapy for alcoholic cirrhosis, however clear interventional efficacy is understudied. Anticytokine therapy for a host of cytokines including TNFα, IL1β are also being used as another treatment option. IL1β antagonist, anakinra; and TNFα inhibitor, pentoxifylline have shown considerable reduction in mortality rate among AH patients in recent clinical trials. Combination therapy of anakinra, pentoxifylline and zinc has indicated better efficacy than steroidal therapy in a large clinical trial on AH. Recently Granulocyte-colony stimulating factor (G-CSF) has gained interest for the treatment of AH. It is a glycoprotein produced by macrophages, immune cells and endothelium that stimulates bone marrow to synthesize granulocytes and stem cells. Lastly, ALD remains the second most common indication for liver transplantation (LT) for chronic liver disease primarily in cirrhosis or acute over chronic ALD conditions.

27.7 Conclusion/Summary

Alcoholic liver disease is a multifactorial pathological process that manifests itself with varying degree of severity, and presentation by the classification of diagnosis. Molecular pathways that are involved in the development of alcohol-associated liver injury are extensively interlinked. Dysregulation in these mechanisms, either unaccompanied or along with others (as multi-pathway response) contributes to the pathological progression of ALD. Recent research focusing on the onset of pathology has provided much needed advancement and advantage in the understanding of the pathology that is involved in the progression and severity of late stage ALD diagnosis. Modifying effects of genetics and epigenetics, immune regulation, host gut microflora, and alcohol pharmacokinetics are major factors that are involved in the onset and progression of alcohol-related liver diseases.

Self Study

Questions

1. Which fatty acid among the following polyunsaturated fatty acids is involved in the pro-inflammatory response?
   (a) Docosahexaenoic acid
   (b) Eicosapentaenoic acid
   (c) Linoleic Acid
   (d) A-Linoleic Acid
2. What is the mechanism that activates AMP-activated protein kinase?
   (a) Oxidative stress
   (b) β-Oxidation by acyl-CoA oxidase
   (c) TLR-4 signaling
   (d) TNF-α production
3. Which gene variant among the following can change the rate of metabolism of alcohol in the liver?
   (a) ADH1B
   (b) ADH2
   (c) ADH3
   (d) ADH2∗2

Answers

1. Which fatty acid among the following polyunsaturated fatty acids is involved in the pro-inflammatory response?
   (c) Linoleic Acid
2. What is the mechanism that activates AMP-activated protein kinase?
   (a) Oxidative stress
3. Which gene variant among the following can change the rate of metabolism of alcohol in the liver?
   (d) ADH2∗2

References

1. Singal AK, Bataller R, Ahn J, Kamath PS, Shah VH. ACG Clinical Guideline: alcoholic liver disease. Am J Gastroenterol. 2018;113(2):175.
2. Vatsalya V, Song M, Schwandt ML, Cave MC, Barve SS, George DT, et al. Effects of sex, drinking history, and omega-3 and omega-6 fatty acids dysregulation on the onset of liver injury in very heavy drinking alcohol-dependent patients. Alcohol Clin Exp Res. 2016;40(10):2085–93.
3. Seitz HK, Bataller R, Cortez-Pinto H, Gao B, Gual A, Lackner C, et al. Alcoholic liver disease. Nat Rev Dis Primers. 2018;4(1):16.
4. Marsano LS, Vatsalya V, Hassan A, McClain CJ. Clinical features, disease modifiers, and natural history of alcoholic liver disease. In: Alcoholic and non-alcoholic fatty liver disease. New York: Springer; 2016. p. 165–82.
5. Vatsalya V, Bin Liaquat H, Ghosh K, Prakash Mokshagundam S, J McClain C. A review on the sex differences in organ and system pathology with alcohol drinking. Curr Drug Abuse Rev. 2016;9(2):87–92.
6. Kharbanda KK, Ronis MJ, Shearn CT, Petersen DR, Zakhari S, Warner DR, et al. Role of nutrition in alcoholic liver disease: summary of the symposium at the ESBRA 2017 congress. Biomolecules. 2018;8(2):16.
7. Warner DR, Liu H, Miller ME, Ramsden CE, Gao B, Feldstein AE, et al. Dietary linoleic acid and its oxidized metabolites exacerbate liver injury caused by ethanol via induction of hepatic proinflammatory response in mice. Am J Pathol. 2017;187(10):2232–45.
8. McClain C, Vatsalya V, Cave M. Role of zinc in the development/progression of alcoholic liver disease. Curr Treat Options Gastroenterol. 2017;15(2):285–95.
9. Vatsalya V, Kong M, Cave MC, Liu N, Schwandt ML, George DT, et al. Association of serum zinc with markers of liver injury in very heavy drinking alcohol dependent patients. J Nutr Biochem. 2018;59:49–55.
10. Vatsalya V, Cave M, Barve S, Ramchandani VA, McClain CJ, editors. Role of serum zinc and polyunsaturated fatty acids in the exacerbation of liver injury in treatment naive HIV-infected alcohol dependent patients. Hepatology. Hoboken, NJ: Wiley; 2017.
11. Moghe A, Ghare S, Lamoreau B, Mohammad M, Barve S, McClain C, et al. Molecular mechanisms of acrolein toxicity: relevance to human disease. Toxicol Sci. 2015;143(2):242–55.
12. Lu Y, Cederbaum AI. Cytochrome P450s and alcoholic liver disease. Curr Pharm Des. 2018;24(14):1502–17.
13. Vatsalya V, Kong M, Gobejishvili L, Chen W-Y, Srivastava S, Barve S, et al. Urinary acrolein metabolite levels in severe acute alcoholic hepatitis patients. Am J Physiol Gastrointest Liver Physiol. 2019;316(1):G115–22.
14. Browning JD, Horton JD. Molecular mediators of hepatic steatosis and liver injury. J Clin Invest. 2004;114(2):147–52.
15. Zeng T, Zhang C-L, Xiao M, Yang R, Xie K-Q. Critical roles of Kupffer cells in the pathogenesis of alcoholic liver disease: from basic science to clinical trials. Front Immunol. 2016;7:538.
16. Loomba R, Schork N, Chen C-H, Bettencourt R, Bhatt A, Ang B, et al. Heritability of hepatic fibrosis and steatosis based on a prospective twin study. Gastroenterology. 2015;149(7):1784–93.
17. Stickel F, Hampe J. Genetic determinants of alcoholic liver disease. Gut. 2012;61(1):150–9.
18. He L, Deng T, Luo HS. Genetic polymorphism in alcohol dehydrogenase 2 (ADH2) gene and alcoholic liver cirrhosis risk. Int J Clin Exp Med. 2015;8(5):7786–93.
19. Szabo G. Gut–liver axis in alcoholic liver disease. Gastroenterology. 2015;148(1):30–6.
20. Bala S, Marcos M, Gattu A, Catalano D, Szabo G. Acute binge drinking increases serum endotoxin and bacterial DNA levels in healthy individuals. PLoS One. 2014;9(5):e96864.

Further Reading and Additional Resources

Adachi Y, Moore LE, Bradford BU, Gao W, Thurman RG. Antibiotics prevent liver injury in rats following long-term exposure to ethanol. Gastroenterology. 1995;108(1):218–24.

Beier JI, Arteel GE, McClain CJ. Advances in alcoholic liver disease. Curr Gastroenterol Rep. 2011;13(1):56–64. https://doi.org/10.1007/s11894-010-0157-5.

Bezkorovainy A. Probiotics: determinants of survival and growth in the gut. Am J Clin Nutr. 2001;73(2 Suppl):399S–405S.

Blasbalg TL, Hibbeln JR, Ramsden CE, Majchrzak SF, Rawlings RR. Changes in consumption of omega-3 and omega-6 fatty acids in the United States during the twentieth century. Am J Clin Nutr. 2011;93(5):950–62. https://doi.org/10.3945/ajcn.110.006643.

Broitman SA, Gottlieb LS, Zamcheck N. Influence of neomycin and ingested endotoxin in the pathogenesis of choline deficiency cirrhosis in the adult rat. J Exp Med. 1964;119:633–42.

Browning JD, Horton JD. Molecular mediators of hepatic steatosis and liver injury. J Clin Invest. 2004;114(2):147–52. https://doi.org/10.1172/jci200422422.

Browning JD, Horton JD. Molecular mediators of hepatic steatosis and liver injury. J Clin Invest. 2004;114(2):147–52. https://doi.org/10.1172/JCI22422.
Cederbaum AI, Lu Y, Wu D. Role of oxidative stress in alcohol-induced liver injury. Arch Toxicol. 2009;83(6):519–48. https://doi.org/10.1007/s00204-009-0432-0.
Chapman RW, Morgan MY, Laulicht M, Hoffbrand AV, Sherlock S. Hepatic iron stores and markers of iron overload in alcoholics and patients with idiopathic hemochromatosis. Dig Dis Sci. 1982;27(10):909–16.
Das SK, Vasudevan DM. Alcohol-induced oxidative stress. Life Sci. 2007;81(3):177–87. https://doi.org/10.1016/j.lfs.2007.05.005.
Donohue TM Jr, Tuma DJ, Sorrell MF. Binding of metabolically derived acetaldehyde to hepatic proteins in vitro. Lab Investig. 1983;49(2):226–9.
Fletcher LM, Powell LW. Hemochromatosis and alcoholic liver disease. Alcohol. 2003;30(2):131–6.
Fooks LJ, Gibson GR. Probiotics as modulators of the gut flora. Br J Nutr. 2002;88(Suppl 1):S39–49. https://doi.org/10.1079/BJN2002628.
Fu S, Yang L, Li P, Hofmann O, Dicker L, Hide W, et al. Aberrant lipid metabolism disrupts calcium homeostasis causing liver endoplasmic reticulum stress in obesity. Nature. 2011;473(7348):528–31. https://doi.org/10.1038/nature09968.
Gabuzda GJ. Hepatic coma: clinical considerations, pathogenesis, and management. Adv Intern Med. 1962;11:11–73.
Gao B, Seki E, Brenner DA, Friedman S, Cohen JI, Nagy L, et al. Innate immunity in alcoholic liver disease. Am J Physiol Gastrointest Liver Physiol. 2011;300(4):G516–25. https://doi.org/10.1152/ajpgi.00537.2010.
Gustot T, Lemmers A, Moreno C, Nagy N, Quertinmont E, Nicaise C, et al. Differential liver sensitization to toll-like receptor pathways in mice with alcoholic fatty liver. Hepatology. 2006;43(5):989–1000. https://doi.org/10.1002/hep.21138.
He L, Deng T, Luo HS. Genetic polymorphism in alcohol dehydrogenase 2 (ADH2) gene and alcoholic liver cirrhosis risk. Int J Clin Exp Med. 2015;8(5):7786–93.
Honchel R, Ray MB, Marsano L, Cohen D, Lee E, Shedlofsky S, McClain CJ. Tumor necrosis factor in alcohol enhanced endotoxin liver injury. Alcohol Clin Exp Res. 1992;16(4):665–9.
Iimuro Y, Gallucci RM, Luster MI, Kono H, Thurman RG. Antibodies to tumor necrosis factor alfa attenuate hepatic necrosis and inflammation caused by chronic exposure to ethanol in the rat. Hepatology. 1997;26(6):1530–7. https://doi.org/10.1002/hep.510260621.
Ji C. Dissection of endoplasmic reticulum stress signaling in alcoholic and non-alcoholic liver injury. J Gastroenterol Hepatol. 2008;23(Suppl 1):S16–24. https://doi.org/10.1111/j.1440-1746.2007.05276.x.
Ji C. Mechanisms of alcohol-induced endoplasmic reticulum stress and organ injuries. Biochem Res Int. 2012; https://doi.org/10.1155/2012/216450.
Ji C, Kaplowitz N. Betaine decreases hyperhomocysteinemia, endoplasmic reticulum stress, and liver injury in alcohol-fed mice. Gastroenterology. 2003;124(5):1488–99.
Keshavarzian A, Choudhary S, Holmes EW, Yong S, Banan A, Jakate S, Fields JZ. Preventing gut leakiness by oats supplementation ameliorates alcohol-induced liver damage in rats. J Pharmacol Exp Ther. 2001;299(2):442–8.
Khoruts A, Stahnke L, McClain CJ, Logan G, Allen JI. Circulating tumor necrosis factor, interleukin-1, and interleukin-6 concentrations in chronic alcoholic patients. Hepatology. 1991;13(2):267–76.
Luckey TD, Reyniers JA, Gyorgy P, Forbes M. Germfree animals and liver necrosis. Ann N Y Acad Sci. 1954;57(6):932–5.
Madigan MT. Chapter 12: Prokaryotic diversity: the bacteria chapter. In: Martinko JM, editor. Brock biology of microorganisms. 11th ed. Upper Saddle River, NJ: Pearson Prentice Hall; 2006.
Malhi H, Kaufman RJ. Endoplasmic reticulum stress in liver disease. J Hepatol. 2011;54(4):795–809. https://doi.org/10.1016/j.jhep.2010.11.005.
Mandrekar P. Epigenetic regulation in alcoholic liver disease. World J Gastroenterol: WJG. 2011;17(20):2456.
McClain CJ, Cohen DA. Increased tumor necrosis factor production by monocytes in alcoholic hepatitis. Hepatology. 1989;9(3):349–51.
McClain CJ, Zieve L. Portal-systemic encephalopathy: recognition and variations. In: Davidson CS, editor. Problems in liver diseases. New York: Stratton Intercontinental Medical Book Corp.; 1979. p. 162–72.
McClain CJ, Barve SS, Barve A, Marsano L. Alcoholic liver disease and malnutrition. Alcohol Clin Exp Res. 2011;35(5):815–20. https://doi.org/10.1111/j.1530-0277.2010.01405.x.
McClain CJ, Song Z, Barve SS, Hill DB, Deaciuc I. Recent advances in alcoholic liver disease. IV. Dysregulated cytokine metabolism in alcoholic liver disease. Am J Physiol Gastrointest Liver Physiol. 2004;287(3):G497–502. https://doi.org/10.1152/ajpgi.00171.2004.
Mendenhall CL, Anderson S, Weesner RE, Goldberg SJ, Crolic KA. Protein-calorie malnutrition associated with alcoholic hepatitis. Veterans Administration Cooperative Study Group on Alcoholic Hepatitis. Am J Med. 1984;76(2):211–22.
Mendenhall CL, Moritz TE, Roselle GA, Morgan TR, Nemchausky BA, Tamburro CH, et al. Protein-energy malnutrition in severe alcoholic hepatitis: diagnosis and response to treatment. The VA Cooperative Study Group #275. JPEN J Parenter Enteral Nutr. 1995;19(4):258–65.
Mendenhall CL, Tosch T, Weesner RE, Garcia-Pont P, Goldberg SJ, Kiernan T, et al. VA cooperative study on alcoholic hepatitis. II: Prognostic significance of protein-calorie malnutrition. Am J Clin Nutr. 1986;43(2):213–8.
Mendenhall C, Roselle GA, Gartside P, Moritz T. Relationship of protein calorie malnutrition to alcoholic liver disease: a reexamination of data from two Veterans Administration Cooperative Studies. Alcohol Clin Exp Res. 1995;19(3):635–41.
Nanji AA, French SW. Dietary linoleic acid is required for the development of experimentally induced alcoholic liver injury. Life Sci. 1989;44(3):223–7.
Nanji AA, Jokelainen K, Tipoe GL, Rahemtulla A, Dannenberg AJ. Dietary saturated fatty acids reverse inflammatory and fibrotic changes in rat liver despite continued ethanol administration. J Pharmacol Exp Ther. 2001;299(2):638–44.
Nanji AA, Khettry U, Sadrzadeh SM. Lactobacillus feeding reduces endotoxemia and severity of experimental alcoholic liver (disease). Proc Soc Exp Biol Med. 1994;205(3):243–7.
Nanji AA, Yang EK, Fogt F, Sadrzadeh SM, Dannenberg AJ. Medium chain triglycerides and vitamin E reduce the severity of established experimental alcoholic liver disease. J Pharmacol Exp Ther. 1996;277(3):1694–700.
Nolan JP. The contribution of gut-derived endotoxins to liver injury. Yale J Biol Med. 1979;52(1):127–33.
Purohit V, Bode JC, Bode C, Brenner DA, Choudhry MA, Hamilton F, et al. Alcohol, intestinal bacterial growth, intestinal permeability to endotoxin, and medical consequences: summary of a symposium. Alcohol. 2008;42(5):349–61. https://doi.org/10.1016/j.alcohol.2008.03.131.
Rutenburg AM, Sonnenblick E, Koven I, Aprahamian HA, Reiner L, Fine J. The role of intestinal bacteria in the development of dietary cirrhosis in rats. J Exp Med. 1957;106(1):1–14.
Sakhuja P. Pathology of alcoholic liver disease, can it be differentiated from nonalcoholic steatohepatitis? World J Gastroenterol. 2014;20(44):16474–9. https://doi.org/10.3748/wjg.v20.i44.16474.
Setshedi M, Wands JR, Monte SM. Acetaldehyde adducts in alcoholic liver disease. Oxidative Med Cell Longev. 2010;3(3):178–85. https://doi.org/10.4161/oxim.3.3.12288.
Siebler J, Galle PR, Weber MM. The gut-liver-axis: endotoxemia, inflammation, insulin resistance, and NASH. J Hepatol. 2008;48(6):1032–4. https://doi.org/10.1016/j.jhep.2008.03.007.
Stickel F, Hampe J. Genetic determinants of alcoholic liver disease. Gut. 2012;61(1):150–9. https://doi.org/10.1136/gutjnl-2011-301239.

Szabo G, Bala S. Alcoholic liver disease and the gut-liver axis. World J Gastroenterol. 2010;16(11):1321–9.

Tsutsumi M, Takada A, Wang JS. Genetic polymorphisms of cytochrome P4502E1 related to the development of the alcoholic liver disease. Gastroenterology. 1994;107(5):1430–5.

Warner DR, Liu H, Miller ME, Ramsden CE, Gao B, Feldstein AE, et al. Dietary linoleic acid and its oxidized metabolites exacerbate liver injury caused by ethanol via induction of hepatic proinflammatory response in mice. Am J Pathol. 2017;187(10):2232–45. https://doi.org/10.1016/j.ajpath.2017.06.008.

Zeng T, Zhang CL, Xiao M, Yang R, Xie KQ. Critical roles of Kupffer cells in the pathogenesis of alcoholic liver disease: from basic science to clinical trials. Front Immunol. 2016;7 https://doi.org/10.3389/fimmu.2016.00538.

Zhao HY, Wang HJ, Lu Z, Xu SZ. Intestinal microflora in patients with liver cirrhosis. Chin J Dig Dis. 2004;5(2):64–7.

Zieve L. Pathogenesis of hepatic coma. Arch Intern Med. 1966;118(3):211–23.

Liver Disease in Pregnancy

28

Sheila Eswaran and Nancy Reau

Key Concepts
- Understand normal liver function during pregnancy
- Categorize liver diseases related to pregnancy based on trimester
- Recognize liver diseases unrelated to a pregnant state occurring during pregnancy
- Identify maternal and fetal outcomes related to liver disease during pregnancy

28.1 Introduction

Diagnosis and management of liver disease in women who are pregnant can be challenging. The management starts with an assessment to determine if the patient has pre-existing or coincidental liver disease not related to pregnancy verses liver disease related to pregnancy. Consideration of both the expectant mother and fetus are paramount in the approach to treatment.

28.2 Normal Pregnancy

During pregnancy, total blood volume and cardiac output increases. Hemodilution leads to decrease in hematocrit and albumin levels. Absolute hepatic blood flow remains unchanged, but the percentage of cardiac output to the liver decrease [1].

There is an increase in serum concentration of coagulation factors, which limit bleeding during delivery but are associated with an increased risk of thromboembolism during pregnancy and the post-partum period [1, 2].

Alkaline phosphatase (AP) is elevated due to placental AP (Table 28.1: Normal laboratory testing during pregnancy). Serum aspartate transaminase (AST) activity, alanine transaminase (ALT) activity and total bile acid concentrations do not normally differ between pregnant and nonpregnant women. Total and free bilirubin concentrations were significantly lower during all three trimesters, as was conjugated bilirubin during the second and third trimesters. Serum gamma-glutamyl transpeptidase (GGT) activity is lower in the second and third trimesters. Serum 5′-nucleotidase activity is slightly higher in the second and third trimesters [3]. Any elevations of transaminases and bilirubin require evaluation.

Elevated alpha-fetoprotein (AFP) serum levels are associated with hepatocellular carcinoma. AFP is a plasma protein

Table 28.1 Normal physiology and laboratory testing during pregnancy

Changes in pregnancy	
Cardiac output	↑
Total blood volume	↑
Hematocrit	↓
Albumin	↓
Coagulation factors	↑
Alkaline phosphatase	↑
AST and ALT	↔
Total bile acids	↔
Total bilirubin	↓
Conjugated bilirubin	↓
GGT	↓
5′ Nucleotidase	↓
Alpha-fetoprotein	↑

S. Eswaran (✉) · N. Reau
Rush University Medical Center, Chicago, IL, USA
e-mail: Sheila_Eswaran@rush.edu; Nancy_reau@rush.edu

F. Radu-Ionita et al. (eds.), *Liver Diseases*, https://doi.org/10.1007/978-3-030-24432-3_28

produced by the embryonic yolk sac and the fetal liver [4]. During pregnancy AFP levels in serum, amniotic fluid, and urine start to rise from about 14th week of gestation up until about 32 weeks gestation. Between week 15 and 20 weeks, serum levels usually range between 10 and 150 ng/mL. AFP is used as a screening test for congenital disabilities, chromosomal abnormalities during pregnancy.

28.3 Pre-existing or Coincidental Liver Disease During Pregnancy

28.3.1 Acute Viral Hepatitis

Patients with acute viral hepatitis may be asymptomatic or present with malaise, fatigue, anorexia, jaundice or abdominal pain. In cases of fulminant hepatitis, signs of coagulopathy and encephalopathy may be present. Pregnant women presenting with acute hepatitis should be tested for hepatitis HAV, HBV, HEV and HSV. Treatment of acute hepatitis is generally supportive and patients should be monitored for progression of hepatic dysfunction (Table 28.1).

Patients with hepatitis A or E, clinical manifestations usually are related temporally to recent travel to an endemic area or exposure to an infected person. Hepatitis B, C, or D are transmitted after parenteral exposure to contaminated blood or sexual contact with an infected partner [5].

Although HAV has been associated with preterm labor and premature rupture of membranes; this has been reported to have no significant impact on maternal or fetal outcomes [6]. Vertical transmission of HAV is rare but there are reports of outbreaks within neonatal care units. CDC recommends HAV immunoglobulin treatment for the neonate if the maternal HAV infection occurs within 2 weeks of delivery.

For patients in which HEV is suspected, early diagnosis is important to anticipate and prepare for possible progression to acute liver failure and need for liver transplantation evaluation [7].

28.3.2 Herpes Simplex Virus

Herpes simplex virus is a common sexually transmitted infection that can lead to hepatitis in immunocompromised individuals. Pregnant women who contract HSV in the second or third trimester are at risk for fulminant liver failure potentially explained by a suppressed immune system in the 27–33 weeks of gestation secondary to hemodilution [8, 9]. Acute HSV hepatitis can present with aminotransferases >500, fever, coagulopathy, encephalopathy, leukopenia, thrombocytopenia and renal failure [10]. HSV hepatitis is difficult to diagnose and has a mortality rate up to 74%. Although HSV DNA PCR has a higher sensitivity and specificity than HSV antibodies, a liver biopsy may be required for the diagnosis of HSV hepatitis. Maternal infection should be treated with acyclovir at 36 weeks of pregnancy [11]. Liver transplant should be considered in severe cases.

28.3.3 Hepatitis B

Pregnancy is generally well-tolerated by women with chronic hepatitis B infection who do not have advanced liver disease. Antepartum testing for hepatitis flare is recommended. The two indications for antiviral therapy are (1) the same as those for patients who are not pregnant, determined by HBV DNA levels, HBeAg status, and the activity or stage of liver disease and (2) for women with high viral load to prevent mother to child transmission (MTCT) in combination with passive and active immune prophylaxis [12].

Because high maternal viremia is correlated with the highest risk for transmission of HBV in pregnancy, treatment should be offered to pregnant women who have a high viral load greater than 10^6 and started preferably 6–8 weeks before delivery to allow enough time for HBV DNA levels to decline [13].

None of the HBV agents is approved by the US Food and Drug Administration for use in pregnancy All are rated pregnancy category C, except for tenofovir and telbivudine, which are category B (Table 28.2). Tenofovir alafenamide (TAF) is a phosphonamide prodrug of tenofovir that is more stable in plasma with lower circulating levels of tenofovir. Given the improved safety of TAF on bone mineral density and renal function, TAF is likely reasonable option. There are ongoing studies to determine safety the profile for TAF in both pregnant women and the newborns.

Mother to child transmission of hepatitis B is 70–90% for HBeAg+ mothers and 10–40% for HBeAg-mothers. Hepatitis B immunoglobulin and hepatitis B vaccination administered with in 12 h after the birth of infants of HBsAg-positive mothers, followed by two additional doses of vaccine within 6–12 months, prevents transmission in approximately 95%.

There is insufficient data to determine a reduced transmission rate of hepatitis B with cesarean section. Therefore a change in the mode of delivery for HBV-infected women is not recommended. Breastfeeding does not appear to increase the risk of transmission. Infants who received HBIG and the first dose of vaccine at birth can be breastfed as long as they complete the course of vaccination.

The end point of antiviral therapy for hepatitis B used to reduce risk of MTCT is typically immediately in the postpartum period unless treatment continuation is otherwise indicated for the benefit of the mother. Discontinuation of therapy requires careful monitoring because of the potential for HBV flares upon antiviral therapy withdrawal.

Table 28.2 Medication safety in the treatment of liver disease in pregnancy

Drug	FDA pregnancy category	Recommendations for pregnancy
Tenofovir disoproxil fumarate	B	First line due to safety and favorable resistance profile
Tenofovir alafenamide	C	No pregnancy data, probably safe
Telbivudine	B	Low risk
Adefovir	C	Minimal data: no teratogenicity
Entecavir	C	Not recommended unless benefit outweighs risk
Lamivudine	C	Low risk
Interferon	C	Not recommended: treatment deferred until after delivery
Ribavirin[a]	X	Contraindicated: severe fetal neurotoxicity
Cyclosporine	C	Safest of immune suppressants
Mycophenolate mofetil	D	Not recommended
Sirolimus	C	Not recommended
Tacrolimus	C	Use if mother's health mandates
Antithymocyte globulin	C	No pregnancy data
OKT3 (Muromonab-CD3)	C	No pregnancy data
Corticosteroids	C	Low risk; possible increased risk: cleft palate, adrenal insufficiency, premature rupture of membranes
Azathioprine	D	Data in IBD, transplant literature suggest low risk
Nadolol	C: first trimester	Prolonged half-life, use alternative; risk of intrauterine growth retardation in second/third trimesters
	D: second/third trimesters	
Propranolol	C: first trimester	Fetal bradycardia, intrauterine growth retardation in second/third trimesters
	D: second/third trimesters	
Penicillamine	D	Significant embryopathy; if required, reduce dose to 250 mg/day 6 weeks before delivery
Trientine	C	Limited human data: alternative to penicillamine
Ursodiol	B	Low risk: used in intrahepatic cholestasis of pregnancy

[a]Safety of direct-acting antivirals (DAAs) in pregnancy is unknown
[b]Contrast agent for ERCP

28.3.4 Hepatitis C

The incidence of HCV vertical transmission is 5–15%. A higher transmission rate is associated with HIV co-infection, high HCV viral load, prolonged rupture of membranes and the performance of obstetric procedures such as amniocentesis and fetal scalp monitoring. When possible, invasive obstetric procedures should be avoided in women with HCV. Factors not associated with the vertical transmission of HCV include viral genotype, the mode of delivery and breast-feeding. Pregnant women infected with HCV are not advised to have cesarean delivery to reduce transmission, unless indicated for other reasons.

Pregnancy related risk in women with chronic hepatitis C is not increased as long as patient does not have cirrhosis. Ideally, HCV should be eradicated pre-pregnancy. Treatment during pregnancy is not urgent and can be deferred until after delivery.

There is no evidence of an association between breast feeding and risk for transmission, but should be avoided when the potential risk for exposure is higher, such as when there are cracked nipples or skin breakdown.

28.3.5 Other Chronic Liver Diseases

The approach to chronic liver disease such as autoimmune hepatitis, primary biliary cirrhosis, Wilson disease is a balance between managing the effects of the liver disease to maternal and fetal health while minimizing deleterious effect of medications used for treatment. For example, AIH is associated with intrapartum flare risk and fetal prematurity and loss [14]. In addition, medication for AIH such as azathioprine is a pregnancy category D drug [15].

Providers should be aware that the FDA instituted the Pregnancy and Lactation Labeling Final Rule in 2014, which replaces pregnancy categories A, B, C, D and X with a narrative summary of the risk of prescription drug and biological products in pregnancy, lactation, and for females and males of reproductive potential. This system was designed to give patients and healthcare providers more evidenced based descriptive information to make risk assessments. Table 28.2 lists medication safety in the treatment of liver disease during pregnancy. These factors must be addressed in the management of chronic liver disease in pregnancy [16].

28.3.6 Benign Liver Lesion

Benign liver lesions are often asymptomatic and detected incidentally on imaging. When identified by ultrasound, an MRI or tagged RBC scan may be helpful to best characterize the lesion. A liver biopsy is rarely necessary to make a diagnosis.

If an adenoma is detected in a woman of childbearing age, the patient should be counseled on the risk of growth during pregnancy due to hormonal stimulation. Surgical resection or radiologic intervention should be considered for large adenomas (>5 cm) prior to pregnancy [17, 18]. Cases of ruptured hepatic adenoma during gestation have been described with a reported 59% maternal and 62% fetal mortality [19].

Reports of hemangiomas growing in size during pregnancy [20] are rare and routine follow up is recommended. Focal nodular hyperplasia is not impacted by hormonal changes or pregnancy [21].

Pregnancy is not contraindicated in patients with a hemangioma, FNH or adenoma <5 cm.

28.4 Liver Diseases Specific to Pregnancy

There are several causes of liver damage that are unique to pregnancy and should be considered in approach to a pregnant women with liver disease.

28.4.1 Hyperemesis Gravidarum

Nausea with or without vomiting is common in early pregnancy, however hyperemesis gravidarum, severe vomiting resulting in dehydration and weight loss, can occur. The incidence is 0.3–3% of pregnancies [22, 23] and typically presents in the first trimester with resolution by 20 weeks of gestation (Fig. 28.1: Liver Diseases). Elevated liver tests occurs in nearly 50% of patients who require hospitalization for HG [24]. Thought to be due to impaired mitochondrial fatty acid oxidation [25]. Aminotransferases are typically less than 300 U/L. Jaundice and synthetic dysfunction is rare [23]. Risk factors are molar pregnancy, multiple gestations [23] and a history of HG.

Although maternal complications of HG are rare, Wernicke's encephalopathy caused by vitamin B1 deficiency and death has been reported related to splenic avulsion, esophageal rupture and pneumothorax from forceful vomiting [23, 26–29]. One report also suggests higher depression and anxiety scale scores in women with the condition [30].

There is no difference in gestational age at birth or birth weight as long as pre pregnancy weight was normal and there is "catch-up" weight gain later in pregnancy. In addition, there is no significant association of hyperemesis gravidarum with congenital anomalies [31, 32].

Symptomatic treatment for nausea and vomiting in addition to reversal of electrolyte disturbances and dehydration is recommended [23, 33].

28.4.2 Intrahepatic Cholestasis of Pregnancy

The incidence of intrahepatic cholestasis (IHCP) of pregnancy is reported to be between 0.3% [34], and 5.6% [35, 36].

IHCP is due to cholestatic effect of reproductive hormones in susceptible women with genetically altered biliary transport proteins [37]. Primary bile acids, cholic and chenodeoxycholic acids, are normally conjugated with glycine or taurine before being secreted into the bile. High levels of cholic and chenodeoxycholic acid are detected in patients with IHCP.

Risk factors include multiple gestations, in vitro fertilization treatment, women older than 35 years of age and prior pregnancies with IHCP [38, 39]. IHCP is associated with hepatitis C, fatty liver and gall stone disease [40].

The classic presentation is in late second or third trimester with pruritus, typically of the palms and soles, abnormal liver function, and elevated serum bile acid levels which resolves with delivery. In the most cases, liver transaminases will also be elevated usually less than two times the upper limit of normal, but may rarely reach values greater than 1000 U/L. This may occur before or after the rise in serum bile acids. Jaundice is uncommon. Total bilirubin concentrations are elevated in 25% of cases, although levels rarely exceed 6 mg/dL.

While maternal outcomes are excellent, bile acids cross the placenta and can accumulate in the fetus. Complications related to IHCP occur when bile active level are over 40 μmol/L. There is an increased risks of meconium-stained amniotic fluid, preterm delivery and fetal death [41, 42]. Fetal death may be related to the sudden development of a fetal arrhythmia or vasospasm of the placental chorionic surface vessels induced by high levels of bile acids. Due to the

Fig. 28.1 Liver diseases in pregnancy based on trimester

First Trimester Week 0-12	Second Trimester Week 13-26	Third Trimester Week 27-40
Hyperemesis Gravidarum		
	Intrahepatic Cholestasis of Pregnancy	
	Preeclampsia/Eclampsia	
	HELLP	
		Acute Fatty Liver of Pregnancy
Pre-existing or coincidental liver disease		

risk of uterine death after 37 weeks gestation, delivery after 37 weeks is recommended [43].

Ursodeoxycholic acid at 10–15 mg/kg/day is recommended to reduce circulating bile acids, fetal complications and maternal pruritus [44, 45]. It is well tolerated and has no fetal toxicity.

28.4.3 Preeclampsia/Eclampsia

Preeclampsia is characterized by the new onset of hypertension and proteinuria, or hypertension and significant end-organ dysfunction with or without proteinuria, which occurs in the late second or third trimester [46]. In 2013, the American College of Obstetricians and Gynecologists removed proteinuria as an essential criterion for diagnosis when end organ damage is present with hypertension. Preeclampsia is caused by placental and maternal vascular dysfunction and resolves after delivery. Eclampsia refers to the development of grand mal seizures in a woman with preeclampsia. Worldwide, preeclampsia occurs in 4.6% of pregnancies [47]. Risk factors for preeclampsia are a past history of preeclampsia, pre-gestational diabetes, chronic hypertension, multiple gestational pregnancies, first pregnancies and family history of preeclampsia.

Liver involvement in severe preeclampsia presents as persistent right upper quadrant or epigastric pain due to hepatomegaly stretching the Glisson's capsule [48] or serum transaminase concentration ≥2 times upper limit of normal from hepatic vascular constriction [46].

Women with preeclampsia and elevated liver tests have a lower gestational age at delivery, infants with lower birth weights and fetal death [49]. However the magnitude of elevations more strongly correlate with maternal outcomes rather than fetal outcomes [50]. For the expectant mother, preeclampsia can be a progressive disease, worsening until delivery. Worldwide, 10–15% of direct maternal deaths are associated with preeclampsia and eclampsia [51] due to end organ failure.

In patients with severe preeclampsia, delivery is indicated. Rarely for select cases an expectant approach may be advised before 34 weeks of gestation with corticosteroids to provide time for further fetal growth [52].

28.4.4 Acute Fatty Liver of Pregnancy

The incidence of acute fatty liver of pregnancy (AFLP) is 1 in 7000–20,000 pregnancies. Maternal liver failure occurs due to direct hepatocyte damage from abnormal maternal-fetal fatty acid metabolism by products [53]. Approximately 20% of AFLP is associated with fetal long-chain 3-hydroxyacyl CoA dehydrogenase (LCHAD) deficiency, specifically G1528C mutation.

For pregnant women, AFLP typically presents in the third trimester and rarely in the second trimesters and post partum. Risk factors include prior AFLP, multiple gestation pregnancies, other hypertensive diseases of pregnancy and low BMI.

Presenting symptoms are those of progressive liver failure, malaise, abdominal pain, encephalopathy, with elevated bilirubin and aminotransferases 5–10 times the upper limit of normal, but not exceeding 500 IU/L.

Imaging with US, CT or MRI may reveal fatty appearing liver parenchyma. The Swansea criteria, which include symptoms (vomiting, abdominal pain, polydipsia/polyuria, encephalopathy), laboratory findings (bilirubin, hypoglycemia leukocytosis, elevated transaminases, ammonia, uric acid, acute kidney injury, coagulopathy) and imaging (ascites or brighter liver on ultrasound) are a diagnostic model for AFLP [54]. Liver biopsy is reserved for cases in which the diagnosis is uncertain. Microvesicular fatty infiltration of the hepatocytes seen on biopsy is diagnostic

Treatment hinges on delivery regardless of gestational age and supportive care in a critical care setting at a transplant center to management the complications of acute liver failure including potential cerebral edema, hypoglycemia, infections, renal dysfunction and bleeding. If hepatic function continues to decline, patients should be evaluated for liver transplantation.

Children born to mothers with AFLP should undergo genetic testing for LCHAD deficiency. Manifestations of this disease in children are peripheral neuropathy, retinopathy and hypoglycemia. Early diagnosis of LCHAD deficiency in the newborn can be life-saving

28.4.5 HELLP

HELLP syndrome is defined as hemolytic anemia, increased liver enzymes, and low platelets. Ten to twenty percent of women with severe preeclampsia/eclampsia and 0.1–0.2% of overall pregnancies develop HELLP. Patients present with hemolytic anemia, platelet count <100,000 cells/μL, total bilirubin >1.2 mg/dL, aminotransferases >2 times upper limit of normal during the third trimester and less commonly late second trimester or early post partum. The pathophysiology appears to be related with abnormal placenta formation followed by a systemic inflammatory response. Some hypothesize that HELLP is a severe form of preeclampsia, however it is important to note that HELLP may occur in the absence of hypertension or proteinuria. Risk factors include history of hypertensive disease of pregnancy, advanced maternal age, nulliparous and multiparty [55].

Maternal complications include disseminated intravascular coagulation (DIC), abruptio placentae, acute renal failure, pulmonary edema and retinal detachment [56, 57]. Hepatic infarction presenting with fever and abdominal pain and hepatic rupture presenting with abdominal swelling or shock can also occur [58]. These hepatic complications required supportive management and severe cases may require surgery, percutaneous or transvascular embolization or liver transplantation [59, 60]. HELLP is associated with a 1% risk of maternal death and a perinatal death rate of 7.4–20.4% depending on gestational age [61].

For pregnancies ≥34 and <23 weeks of gestation, delivery is recommended. For pregnancies ≥23 and <34 weeks of gestation in which maternal and fetal status are reassuring, corticosteroids for fetal pulmonary maturation is given followed by delivery [62, 63]. Although, initial data supported the use of dexamethasone for the management of HELLP, larger more recent data concludes no improvement in infant or maternal morbidity or morality [64–67].

Platelet transfusion is indicated with active bleeding, platelet count less than 20,000 cells/μL or platelet count is less than 40,000 cells/μL for delivery. Vaginal delivery is preferred, but cesarean section can be performed for usual obstetric indications.

28.4.6 Hepatic Venous Outflow Obstruction (Budd Chiari)

Pregnant women are at risk for hepatic vein thrombosis due to blood volume expansion, hypoproteinemia, the rise in pressure of the gravid uterus on the IVC and other intraabdominal vessels. In addition, pregnancy exacerbates other hypercoagulable states such as antiphospholipid syndrome, factor V Leiden and protein S deficiency. Patients with Budd Chiari may present with abdominal pain and may be complicated by gastrointestinal hemorrhage or progression to acute liver failure. Multidisciplinary management includes potential radiologic approaches (TIPS and angioplasty) and anticoagulation. Successful liver transplantation has been described.

28.5 Special Liver Related Considerations in Pregnancy

In the evaluation and management of pregnant women with liver disease there are recommendations that should be considered to ensure maternal and fetal safety.

28.5.1 Imaging

Ultrasonography in pregnancy is not associated with adverse maternal or fetal outcomes; and therefore is the imaging modality of choice in the initial evaluation of liver disease. There is a weak association between exposure to ultrasonography and non-right handedness in boys [68, 69]. There are limited data on the use of ultrasound contrast agents in pregnancy [70].

Generally, computed tomography (CT) and magnetic resonance imaging (MRI) are often utilized for better evaluation of deep soft tissue structures. Because MRI does not use ionizing radiation it is favored over CT. There are no precautions or contraindications for MRI specific to the pregnant woman.

The only prospective study evaluating the effects gadolinium administration reported no adverse perinatal or neonatal outcomes among 26 pregnant women who received gadolinium in the first trimester [71]. More recently a large retrospective study revealed exposure to MRI without contrast during the first trimester of pregnancy did not increase the risk of harm to the fetus or in early childhood compared with no exposure. However, gadolinium MRI at any time during pregnancy was associated with an increased risk of rheumatologic, inflammatory or infiltrative skin conditions and for stillbirth or neonatal death [72]. Therefore, gadolinium should be limited to situations in which there is a clear benefit.

The effects of CT ionizing radiation are, most likely, a result of break in biomolecular bonds of cellular DNA. The risk during pregnancy to a fetus depends not only on the radiation dose received but also on the gestational age at which it occurred [73]. Extremely high-dose exposure, in excess of 1 Gy (1000 mGy), is associated with fetal growth restriction, microcephaly and death [68]. However, these dose levels are not used in diagnostic imaging. For example an abdominal CT, a 10–50 mGy examination, leads to 1.3–35 mGy fetal exposure. Radiation exposure from CT procedures can be limited using low-exposure techniques that are adequate for diagnosis.

Oral contrast agents are not absorbed by the patient and do not cause real or theoretical harm. The addition of intravenous contrast media to CT enhances soft tissues and vascular structures. Although iodinated contrast media can cross the placenta and either enter the fetal circulation or pass directly into the amniotic fluid, animal studies have reported no teratogenic or mutagenic effects from its use. Prior theoretical concerns about the potential adverse effects of free iodide on the fetal thyroid gland have not been borne out in human studies [74].

Despite this lack of known harm, it generally is recommended that contrast only be used if absolutely required to obtain additional diagnostic information that will affect the care of the fetus or woman during the pregnancy.

Use of CT and associated contrast material should not be withheld if clinically indicated, but a thorough discussion of risks and benefits should take place. However, MRI should be considered as a safer alternative to CT imaging during pregnancy in cases in which they are equivalent for the diagnosis in question.

28.5.2 Liver Biopsy

Liver biopsy during pregnancy is uncommon. If required, a transjugular approach is safe, apart from a moderately increased risk of preterm birth (relative risk 2.6) and small for gestational age (relative risk 5.2) [75]. There is low radiation exposure (1–5 mGy) [76] and iodinated contrast exposure (12.5 mL) [77].

28.5.3 Endoscopy/ERCP/EUS/Sedation

Specific indications for endoscopy in a pregnant women with liver disease includes surveillance for varices, acute variceal bleeding and biliary disease.

The fetus is particularly sensitive to maternal hypoxia and hypotension, either of which can cause hypoxia leading to fetal demise. Maternal over sedation resulting in hypoventilation or hypotension or maternal positioning precipitating inferior vena cava compression by the gravid uterus can lead to decreased uterine blood flow and fetal hypoxia. Other risks to the fetus include teratogenesis (from medications given to the mother and/or ionizing radiation exposure) and premature birth [78, 79].

However, procedures are justified when there is a strong indication and failure to perform the procedure could expose the fetus and/or mother to harm [79]. Timing of non emergent endoscopy is most safe in the second trimester after organogenesis in the first trimester.

Endoscopic procedure requires a preoperative consultation with an obstetrician to help determine risk and timing of the procedure. The decision to monitor fetal heart rate should be individualized and depends on gestational age. Endoscopy should be postponed to second trimester whenever possible. For patients with liver disease, propofol (category B) at the lowest effective dose administered by anesthesiologist is recommended as it is a short-acting anesthetic agent with a short recovery period [80]. The patient should be placed in left pelvic tilt or left lateral position to avoid vena cava or aortic compression.

Alternatives to prophylactic endoscopic therapy for varices are nonselective β-blockers, but the safety of β-blockers is controversial because of reports of premature labor, fetal growth restriction, neonatal apnea, bradycardia and hypoglycemia. In addition, nonselective β-blockers may effect myometrial relaxation of the gravid uterus, which is a β_2-receptor-mediated process. The pregnant patient should be informed about the possible benefits and adverse effects of β-blockers during pregnancy [81]. Propranolol is category C, but there is experience with the use in pregnancy to treat maternal hypertension [82].

For an active variceal bleed, vasoactive drugs that are used to achieve hemostasis are contraindicated during pregnancy because these drugs (vasopressin and terlipressin) may induce labor or fetal malformations. Prophylactic or urgent endoscopic injection sclerotherapy (EIS) and endoscopic band ligation (EBL) are safe procedures during pregnancy [83–85].

When hemostasis is not achieved endoscopically in cirrhotic patients, an emergency transjugular intrahepatic portosystemic shunt (TIPSS) is indicated, but data about pregnant cirrhotic women are limited [86, 87]. Placement is associated with radiation exposure to the patient and fetus because the procedure usually requires prolonged fluoroscopy. There are reported cases of TIPSS placement in pregnancy in which the fetal dose of radiation was 5.2 mSv to 2.1 mGy.

28.5.4 ERCP

Pregnancy is associated with an increased risk of gallstone formation due to increased estrogen levels and may be complicated by common bile duct (CBD) stones, cholangitis or pancreatitis which are associated with poor fetal outcomes without intervention. The incidence of cholelithiasis in pregnant women is 3.5%. Patients may develop laboratory tests indicating a biliary complication. After an initial abdominal ultrasound, an ERCP may be performed during pregnancy when therapeutic intervention is intended. The major concerns regarding ERCP during pregnancy is the radiation exposure to the fetus and the risk of the procedure on the outcome of pregnancy [79, 81].

During ERCP, radiation exposure to the fetus may increase the risk of intrauterine fetal death, malformations, growth and development abnormalities, mutations and cancer. Therefore, these risks should be discussed with the pregnant patient and her family before ERCP. To minimize radiation exposure to the uterus, lead shielding should be used. However the majority of the fetal radiation dose occurs as a result of radiation scatter within the pregnant patient. The most effective method to reduce radiation-associated risk is to limit fluoroscopy time and overall radiation exposure. In addition, a 2-step procedure for ERCP has been proposed with (1) biliary sphincterotomy and stenting without fluoroscopy and (2) definitive ERCP with stone extraction after delivery [88, 89]. With these interventions, fetal exposure can be well below the 1Gy level considered to be of concern for radiation-induced teratogenesis.

Endoscopic ultrasonography may reduce unnecessary interventions in patients who have a low or moderate probability of developing CBD stones and it is a safe alternative to fluoroscopy for the evaluation of biliary disorders during pregnancy [90].

28.6 Cirrhosis and Portal Hypertension

Women with cirrhosis have a reduced fertility due to hormonal dysfunction leading to anovulation [91, 92]. The estimated frequency of cirrhosis of 1 per 3333 pregnancies Pregnancy in women with cirrhosis and portal hypertension have increase in prematurity, spontaneous abortions and maternal-fetal mortality [91, 93, 94] Women with noncirrhotic portal hypertension have normal frequency of fertility and a lower incidence of variceal bleeding during pregnancy.

Variceal bleeding is most serious compilation of portal hypertension during pregnancy. Esophageal variceal bleeding has been reported in 18–32% of pregnant women with cirrhosis and in up to 50% of those with known portal hypertension. Among those with preexisting varices, up to 78% will have gastrointestinal bleeding during pregnancy, with a mortality rate of 18–50% [92, 95, 96]. Management of variceal bleeding is outlined in the endoscopy section above.

Due to increased splenic blood flow with both pregnancy and portal hypertension, patients also have an increased risk of splenic artery aneurysm rupture. Twenty percent of all splenic artery aneurysm ruptures occur during pregnancy, most commonly in the third trimester. Management includes emergency splenectomy, trans catheter embolization of the aneurysm or stent-graft placement [98, 97–99].

Vaginal delivery with early placement of an epidural is recommended to allow the infant to descend with uterine contractions alone. In addition, a short second stage of labor and the use of low forceps or vacuum extraction have been advocated. A cesarean section should be considered if repeated Valsalva maneuvers are required, but is associated with a risk of bleeding complications at the surgical site due to portal hypertension [98, 100].

28.7 Liver Transplant

After transplant, resumption of normal reproductive function occurs in 50–75% of premenopausal women. Pregnancies have been reported as early as 1 month after liver transplantation [101–104].

Calcineurin inhibitors (cyclosporine and tacrolimus), prednisone, and azathioprine are generally considered safe [105]. Mycophenolate mofetil is teratogenic and should no be used during pregnancy. There is currently not enough safety data for sirolimus, everolimus and belatacept in pregnant women, therefore the use of these medications can not be recommended.

Patients should be monitored for pregnancy-induced hypertension, preeclampsia, acute cellular rejection and renal impairment. Data suggests that pregnancies occurring within 1-year post transplant may have an increased incidence of prematurity, low birth weight, and acute cellular rejection compared to those occurring later than 1 year [106].

28.8 Conclusion

Pregnancy alone can lead to normal or pathologic changes in hepatic function. In addition, coincident acute or chronic liver diseases can present at any time. When approaching a pregnant women with liver disease, a thoughtful multidisciplinary approach is necessary to consider the health of the fetus and mother.

Self Study

Questions

1. Twenty-seven year old female with cirrhosis due to autoimmune hepatitis presents 5 weeks pregnant. What do you recommend?
   (a) Discontinue azathioprine, start mycophenolate mofetil
   (b) Upper endoscopy for variceal surveillance third trimester
   (c) Upper endoscopy for variceal surveillance second trimester
   (d) Confirm diagnosis of cirrhosis and check portal pressures with transjugular liver biopsy to determine risk of liver related complications
   (e) AFP for hepatocellular carcinoma surveillance because she is at risk for liver cancer
2. Thirty-one year old female 32 weeks pregnant with history of preeclampsia presents with abdominal pain and confusion.
   Labs reveal:
   AST 450 IU/L
   Bilirubin 1.2 mg/dL
   Glucose 60 mg/dL
   Platelets 205
   Creatinine 2.0 mg/dL
   Prothrombin time 18 s
   Ammonia 100 μmol/L
   Which is true?
   1. An expectant approach is recommended before 34 weeks of gestation allowing for fetal pulmonary maturity
   2. Peripheral smear will show hemolysis
   3. Cerebral edema with herniation can occur
   4. Liver biopsy is necessary to make the diagnosis

Answers

1. What do you recommend?
   (a) Discontinue azathioprine, start mycophenolate mofetil. INCORRECT Mycophenolate mofetil is teratogenic and is contraindicated in pregnancy. Table 28.2.
   (b) Upper endoscopy for variceal surveillance third trimester. INCORRECT Endoscopy should occur in the second trimester whenever possible.
   (c) Upper endoscopy for variceal surveillance second trimester. CORRECT Timing of non emergent endoscopy is most safe in the second trimester after organogenesis in the first trimester.
   (d) Confirm diagnosis of cirrhosis and check portal pressures with transjugular liver biopsy to determine risk of liver related complications. INCORRECT Liver biopsy is relatively high risk and will not change management.
   (e) AFP for hepatocellular carcinoma surveillance because she is at risk for liver cancer. INCORRECT Alpha-fetoprotein (AFP) is elevated during normal pregnancy and should not be used for hepatocellular carcinoma surveillance in pregnancy.

2. Which is true?
   1. An expectant approach is recommended before 34 weeks of gestation allowing for fetal pulmonary maturity. INCORRECT Treatment of Acute Fatty Liver of Pregnancy hinges on delivery regardless of gestational age
   2. Peripheral smear will show hemolysis. INCORRECT Hemolysis occurs in HELLP syndrome
   3. Cerebral edema with herniation can occur. CORRECT Complications of AFLP include acute liver failure leading to cerebral edema, hypoglycemia, infections, renal dysfunction and bleeding
   4. Liver biopsy is necessary to make the diagnosis. INCORRECT The Swansea criteria are a diagnostic model for AFLP with liver biopsy is reserved only for cases in which the diagnosis is uncertain

References

Normal Pregnancy

1. Bremme KA. Haemostatic changes in pregnancy. Best Pract Res Clin Haematol. 2003;16(2):153–68.
2. Hellgren M. Hemostasis during normal pregnancy and puerperium. Semin Thromb Hemost. 2003;29(2):125–30.
3. Bacq Y, Zarka O, Bréchot JF, Mariotte N, Vol S, Tichet J, Weill J. Liver function tests in normal pregnancy: a prospective study of 103 pregnant women and 103 matched controls. Hepatology. 1996;23(5):1030–4.
4. Committee Opinion No ACOG. 640: cell-free DNA screening for fetal aneuploidy. Obstet Gynecol. 2015;126:e31–7.

Pre-existing or Coincidental Liver Disease During Pregnancy

5. CDC (2008) MMWR 39:1–26. http://www.cdc.gov/mmwr
6. Elinav E, Ben-Dov IZ, Shapira Y, et al. Acute hepatitis A infection in pregnancy is associated with high rates of gestational complications and preterm labor. Gastroenterology. 2006;130:1129–34.
7. Patra S, Kumar A, Trivedi SS, et al. Maternal and fetal outcomes in pregnant women with acute hepatitis E virus infection. Ann Intern Med. 2007;147:28–33.
8. Noor A, Panwala A, Forouhar F, Wu GY. Hepatitis caused by herpes viruses: a review. J Dig Dis. 2018;19(8):446–55.
9. Kaufman B, Gandhi SA, Louie E, Rizzi R, Illei P. Herpes simplex virus hepatitis: case report and review. Clin Infect Dis. 1997;24(3):334–8.
10. Norvell JP, Blei AT, Jovanovic BD, Levitsky J. Herpes simplex virus hepatitis: an analysis of the published literature and institutional cases. Liver Transpl. 2007;13(10):1428–34.
11. ACOG Committee on Practice Bulletins. ACOG Practice Bulletin. Clinical management guidelines for obstetrician-gynecologists. No. 82 June 2007. Management of herpes in pregnancy. Obstet Gynecol. 2007;109(6):1489–98.
12. Pan CQ, Duan ZP, Bhamidimarri KR, et al. An algorithm for risk assessment and intervention of mother to child transmission of hepatitis B virus. Clin J Gastroenterol Hepatol. 2012;10:452–9.
13. Jaffe A, Brown RS Jr. A review of antiviral use for the treatment of chronic hepatitis B virus infection in pregnant women. Gastroenterol Hepatol (N Y). 2017;13(3):154–63.
14. Schramm C, Herkel J, Beuers U, et al. Pregnancy in autoimmune hepatitis: outcome and risk factors. Am J Gastroenterol. 2006;101:556–60.
15. Lamers MM, van Oijen MG, Pronk M, et al. Treatment options for autoimmune hepatitis: a systematic review of randomized controlled trials. J Hepatol. 2010;53:191–8.
16. Mahadevan U, Kane S. American gastroenterological association institute technical review on the use of gastrointestinal medications in pregnancy. Gastroenterology. 2006;131(1):283–311. Review
17. Marrero JA, Ahn J, Rajender-Reddy K, American College of Gastroenterology. ACG clinical guideline: the diagnosis and management of focal liver lesions. Am J Gastroenterol. 2014;109(9):1328–47.
18. Shaked O, Siegelman ES, Olthoff K, Reddy KR. Biologic and clinical features of benign solid and cystic lesions of the liver. Clin Gastroenterol Hepatol. 2011;9(7):547–562.e1–4.
19. Bis KA, Waxman B. Rupture of the liver associated with pregnancy: a review of the literature and report of 2 cases. Obstet Gynecol Surv. 1976;31(11):763.
20. Saegusa T, Ito K, Oba N, et al. Enlargement of multiple cavernous hemangioma of the liver in association with pregnancy. Intern Med. 1995;34:207–11.
21. Rifai K, Mix H, Potthoff A, et al. No evidence of substantial growth progression of complications of large focal nodular hyperplasia during pregnancy. Scand J Gastroenterol. 2013;48:88–92.

Liver Diseases Specific to Pregnancy

22. Einarson TR, Piwko C, Koren G. Quantifying the global rates of nausea and vomiting of pregnancy: a meta-analysis. J Popul Ther Clin Pharmacol. 2013;20(2):e171–83.

23. Committee on Practice Bulletins-Obstetrics. ACOG practice bulletin no. 189: nausea and vomiting of pregnancy. Obstet Gynecol. 2018;131(1):e15–30.
24. Abell TL, Riely CA. Hyperemesis gravidarum. Gastroenterol Clin N Am. 1992;21(4):835–49. Review
25. Outlaw WM, Ibdah JA. Impaired fatty acid oxidation as a cause of liver disease associated with hyperemesis gravidarum. Med Hypotheses. 2005;65(6):1150–3.
26. Di Gangi S, Gizzo S, Patrelli TS, Saccardi C, D'Antona D, Nardelli GB. Wernicke's encephalopathy complicating hyperemesis gravidarum: from the background to the present. J Matern Fetal Neonatal Med. 2012;25:1499–504.
27. Eroglu A, Kurkcuoglu C, Karaoglanoglu N, Tekinbas C, Cesur M. Spontaneous esophageal rupture following severe vomiting in pregnancy. Dis Esophagus. 2002;15:242–3.
28. Liang SG, Ooka F, Santo A, Kaibara M. Pneumomediastinum following esophageal rupture associated with hyperemesis gravidarum. J Obstet Gynaecol Res. 2002;28:172–5.
29. Nguyen N, Deitel M, Lacy E. Splenic avulsion in a pregnant patient with vomiting. Can J Surg. 1995;38:464–5.
30. Mitchell-Jones N, Gallos I, Farren J, Tobias A, Bottomley C, Bourne T. Psychological morbidity associated with hyperemesis gravidarum: a systematic review and meta-analysis. BJOG. 2017;124(1):20–30.
31. Tsang IS, Katz VL, Wells SD. Maternal and fetal outcomes in hyperemesis gravidarum. Int J Gynaecol Obstet. 1996;55(3):231–5.
32. Hallak M, Tsalamandris K, Dombrowski MP, Isada NB, Pryde PG, Evans MI. Hyperemesis gravidarum. Effects on fetal outcome. J Reprod Med. 1996;41(11):871–4.
33. Bottomley C, Bourne T. Management strategies for hyperemesis. Best Pract Res Clin Obstet Gynaecol. 2009;23(4):549–64.
34. Laifer SA, Stiller RJ, Siddiqui DS, Dunston-Boone G, Whetham JC. Ursodeoxycholic acid for the treatment of intrahepatic cholestasis of pregnancy. J Matern Fetal Med. 2001;10(2):131–5.
35. Lee RH, Goodwin TM, Greenspoon J, Incerpi M. The prevalence of intrahepatic cholestasis of pregnancy in a primarily Latina Los Angeles population. J Perinatol. 2006;26(9):527–32.
36. Reyes H, Gonzalez MC, Ribalta J, Aburto H, Matus C, Schramm G, Katz R, Medina E. Prevalence of intrahepatic cholestasis of pregnancy in Chile. Ann Intern Med. 1978;88(4):487–93.
37. Jacquemin E, Cresteil D, Manouvrier S, Boute O, Hadchouel M. Heterozygous non-sense mutation of the MDR3 gene in familial intrahepatic cholestasis of pregnancy. Lancet. 1999;353(9148):210–1.
38. Floreani A, Gervasi MT. New insights on intrahepatic cholestasis of pregnancy. Clin Liver Dis. 2016;20(1):177–89.
39. Marschall HU, Wikström Shemer E, Ludvigsson JF, Stephansson O. Intrahepatic cholestasis of pregnancy and associated hepatobiliary disease: a population-based cohort study. Hepatology. 2013;58(4):1385–91.
40. Ropponen A, Sund R, Riikonen S, Ylikorkala O, Aittomäki K. Intrahepatic cholestasis of pregnancy as an indicator of liver and biliary diseases: a population-based study. Hepatology. 2006;43(4):723–8.
41. Garcia-Flores J, Canamares M, Cruceyra M, et al. Clinical value of maternal bile acid quantification in intrahepatic cholestasis of pregnancy as an adverse perinatal outcome predictor. Gynecol Obstet Invest. 2015;79:222–8.
42. Geenes V, Chappell LC, Seed PT, et al. Association of severe intrahepatic cholestasis of pregnancy with adverse pregnancy outcomes: a prospective population-based case-control study. Hepatology. 2014;59:1482–91.
43. Puljic A, Kim E, Page J, Esakoff T, Shaffer B, LaCoursiere DY, Caughey AB. The risk of infant and fetal death by each additional week of expectant management in intrahepatic cholestasis of pregnancy by gestational age. Am J Obstet Gynecol. 2015;212(5):667.e1–5.
44. Bacq Y, Sentilhes L, Reyes HB, Glantz A, Kondrackiene J, Binder T, Nicastri PL, Locatelli A, Floreani A, Hernandez I, Di Martino V. Efficacy of ursodeoxycholic acid in treating intrahepatic cholestasis of pregnancy: a meta-analysis. Gastroenterology. 2012;143(6):1492–501.
45. Gurung V, Middleton P, Milan SJ, Hague W, Thornton JG. Interventions for treating cholestasis in pregnancy. Cochrane Database Syst Rev. 2013;6:CD000493.
46. American College of Obstetricians and Gynecologists; Task Force on Hypertension in Pregnancy. Hypertension in pregnancy. Report of the American College of Obstetricians and Gynecologists' Task Force on Hypertension in Pregnancy. Obstet Gynecol. 2013;122(5):1122–31.
47. Abalos E, Cuesta C, Grosso AL, Chou D, Say L. Global and regional estimates of preeclampsia and eclampsia: a systematic review. Eur J Obstet Gynecol Reprod Biol. 2013;170(1):1–7.
48. Walters BN. Preeclamptic angina—a pathognomonic symptom of preeclampsia. Hypertens Pregnancy. 2011;30(2):117–24.
49. Kozic JR, Benton SJ, Hutcheon JA, et al. Abnormal liver function tests as predictors of adverse maternal outcomes in women with preeclampsia. J Obstet Gynaecol Can. 2011;33:995–1004.
50. Thangaratinam S, Koopmans CM, Iyengar S, et al. TIPPS (Tests in Prediction of Preeclampsia's Severity) Review Group. Accuracy of liver function tests for predicting adverse maternal and fetal outcomes in women with preeclampsia: a systematic review. Acta Obstet Gynecol Scand. 2011;90:574–85.
51. Duley L. The global impact of pre-eclampsia and eclampsia. Semin Perinatol. 2009;33(3):130–7.
52. Churchill D, Duley L, Thornton JG, et al. Interventionist versus expectant care for severe pre- eclampsia between 24 and 34 weeks' gestation. Cochrane Database Syst Rev. 2013;7:CD003106.
53. Ibdah JA, Bennett MJ, Rinaldo P, Zhao Y, Gibson B, Sims HF, Strauss AW. A fetal fatty-acid oxidation disorder as a cause of liver disease in pregnant women. N Engl J Med. 1999;340(22):1723–31.
54. Knight M, Nelson-Piercy C, Kurinczuk JJ, Spark P, Brocklehurst P, UK Obstetric Surveillance System. A prospective national study of acute fatty liver of pregnancy in the UK. Gut. 2008;57(7):951–6.
55. Fitzpatrick KE, Hinshaw K, Kurinczuk JJ, et al. Risk factors, management, and outcomes of hemolysis, elevated liver enzymes, and low platelets syndrome and elevated liver enzymes, low platelets syndrome. Obstet Gynecol. 2014;123:618–27.
56. Erkılınç S, Eyi EGY. Factors contributing to adverse maternal outcomes in patients with HELLP syndrome. J Matern Fetal Neonatal Med. 2018;31(21):2870–6.
57. Theilen LH, Fraser A, Hollingshaus MS, Schliep KC, Varner MW, Smith KR, Esplin MS. All-cause and cause-specific mortality after hypertensive disease of pregnancy. Obstet Gynecol. 2016;128(2):238–44.
58. Guo Q, Yang Z, Guo J, Zhang L, Gao L, Zhou B, Shi Q. Hepatic infarction induced by HELLP syndrome: a case report and review of the literature. BMC Pregnancy Childbirth. 2018;18(1):191.
59. Gutovich JM, Van Allan RJ. Hepatic artery embolization for hepatic rupture in HELLP syndrome. J Vasc Interv Radiol. 2016;27(12):1931–3.
60. Zarrinpar A, Farmer DG, Ghobrial RM, et al. Liver transplantation for HELLP syndrome. Am Surg. 2007;73:1013.
61. Sibai BM, Ramadan MK, Usta I, Salama M, Mercer BM, Friedman SA. Maternal morbidity and mortality in 442 pregnancies with hemolysis, elevated liver enzymes, and low platelets (HELLP syndrome). Am J Obstet Gynecol. 1993;169(4):1000.
62. Barnhart L. HELLP syndrome and the effects on the neonate. Neonatal Netw. 2015;34(5):269–73.
63. Cavaignac-Vitalis M, Vidal F, Simon-Toulza C, Boulot P, Guerby P, Chantalat E, Parant O. Conservative versus active management

in HELLP syndrome: results from a cohort study. J Matern Fetal Neonatal Med. 2017;21:1–7.
64. Martin JN Jr, Rose CH, Briery CM. Understanding and managing HELLP syndrome: the integral role of aggressive glucocorticoids for mother and child. Am J Obstet Gynecol. 2006;195(4):914–34.
65. Martin JN Jr, Owens MY, Keiser SD, et al. Standardized Mississippi Protocol treatment of 190 patients with HELLP syndrome: slowing disease progression and preventing new major maternal morbidity. Hypertens Pregnancy. 2012;31:79–90.
66. Woudstra DM, Chandra S, Hofmeyr GJ, et al. Corticosteroids for HELLP (hemolysis, elevated liver enzymes, low platelets) syndrome in pregnancy. Cochrane Database Syst Rev. 2010;2010:CD008148.
67. Fonseca JE, Méndez F, Cataño C, Arias F. Dexamethasone treatment does not improve the outcome of women with HELLP syndrome: a double-blind, placebo-controlled, randomized clinical trial. Am J Obstet Gynecol. 2005;193(5):1591–8.

Special liver Related Considerations in Pregnancy

68. Committee on Obstetric Practice. Committee opinion no. 723: guidelines for diagnostic imaging during pregnancy and lactation. Obstet Gynecol. 2017;130(4):e210–6.
69. Torloni MR, Vedmedovska N, Merialdi M, Betrán AP, Allen T, González R, Platt LD, ISUOG-WHO Fetal Growth Study Group. Safety of ultrasonography in pregnancy: WHO systematic review of the literature and meta-analysis. Ultrasound Obstet Gynecol. 2009;33(5):599–608.
70. Claudon M, Dietrich CF, Choi BI, Cosgrove DO, Kudo M, Nolsøe CP, Piscaglia F, Wilson SR, Barr RG, Chammas MC, Chaubal NG, Chen MH, Clevert DA, Correas JM, Ding H, Forsberg F, Fowlkes JB, Gibson RN, Goldberg BB, Lassau N, Leen EL, Mattrey RF, Moriyasu F, Solbiati L, Weskott HP, Xu HX, World Federation for Ultrasound in Medicine; European Federation of Societies for Ultrasound. Guidelines and good clinical practice recommendations for Contrast Enhanced Ultrasound (CEUS) in the liver - update 2012: a WFUMB-EFSUMB initiative in cooperation with representatives of AFSUMB, AIUM, ASUM, FLAUS and ICUS ultrasound. Med Biol. 2013;39(2):187–210.
71. De Santis M, Straface G, Cavaliere AF, Carducci B, Caruso A. Gadolinium periconceptional exposure: pregnancy and neonatal outcome. Acta Obstet Gynecol Scand. 2007;86:99–101.
72. Ray JG, Vermeulen MJ, Bharatha A, Montanera WJ, Park AL. Association between MRI exposure during pregnancy and fetal and childhood outcomes. JAMA. 2016;316(9):952–61.
73. Holt R, Abramowicz JS. Quality and safety of obstetric practices using new modalities- ultrasound, MR, and CT. Clin Obstet Gynecol. 2017;60(3):546–61.
74. Kochupillai N, Pandav CS, Godbole MM, Mehta M, Ahuja MM. Iodine deficiency and neonatal hypothyroidism. Bull World Health Organ. 1986;64(4):547–51.
75. Ludvigsson JF, Marschall HU, Hagström H, Höijer J, Stephansson O. Pregnancy outcome in women undergoing liver biopsy during pregnancy: a nationwide population-based cohort study. Hepatology. 2018;68(2):625–33.
76. Mammen T, Keshava SN, Eapen CE, Raghuram L, Moses V, Gopi K, Babu NS, Ramachandran J, Kurien G. Transjugular liver biopsy: a retrospective analysis of 601 cases. J Vasc Interv Radiol. 2008;19(3):351–8.
77. Hari A, Nair HK, De Gottardi A, Baumgartner I, Dufour JF, Berzigotti A. Diagnostic hepatic haemodynamic techniques: safety and radiation exposure. Liver Int. 2017;37(1):148–54.
78. Cappell MS. Risks versus benefits of gastrointestinal endoscopy during pregnancy. Nat Rev Gastroenterol Hepatol. 2011;8(11):610–34.
79. ASGE Standard of Practice Committee, Shergill AK, Ben-Menachem T, Chandrasekhara V, Chathadi K, Decker GA, Evans JA, Early DS, Fanelli RD, Fisher DA, Foley KQ, Fukami N, Hwang JH, Jain R, Jue TL, Khan KM, Lightdale J, Pasha SF, Sharaf RN, Dominitz JA, Cash BD. Guidelines for endoscopy in pregnant and lactating women. Gastrointest Endosc. 2012;76(1):18–24.
80. Qadeer MA, Vargo JJ, Khandwala F, Lopez R, Zuccaro G. Propofol versus traditional sedative agents for gastrointestinal endoscopy: a meta-analysis. Clin Gastroenterol Hepatol. 2005;3(11):1049–56.
81. Savas N. Gastrointestinal endoscopy in pregnancy. World J Gastroenterol. 2014;20(41):15241–52.
82. Tan J, Surti B, Saab S. Pregnancy and cirrhosis. Liver Transpl. 2008;14(8):1081–91.
83. Starkel P, Horsmans Y, Geubel A. Endoscopic band ligation: a safe technique to control bleeding esophageal varices in pregnancy. Gastrointest Endosc. 1998;48:212–4.
84. Iwase H, Morise K, Kawase T, Horiuchi Y. Endoscopic injection sclerotherapy for esophageal varices during pregnancy. J Clin Gastroenterol. 1994;18:80–3.
85. Ghidirim G, Mishin I, Dolghii A, Lupashcu A. Prophylactic endoscopic band ligation of esophageal varices during pregnancy. J Gastrointestin Liver Dis. 2008;17:236–7.
86. Lodato F, Cappelli A, Montagnani M, Colecchia A, Festi D, Azzaroli F, Compagnone G, Cecinato P, Golfieri R, Mazzella G. Transjugular intrahepatic portosystemic shunt: a case report of rescue management of unrestrainable variceal bleeding in a pregnant woman. Dig Liver Dis. 2008;40:387–90.
87. Wildberger JE, Vorwerk D, Winograd R, Stargardt A, Busch N, Gunther RW. New TIPS placement in pregnancy in recurrent esophageal varices hemorrhage—assessment of fetal radiation exposure. Rofo. 1998;169:429–43.
88. Sharma SS, Maharshi S. Two stage endoscopic approach for management of choledocholithiasis during pregnancy. J Gastrointestin Liver Dis. 2008;17:183–5.
89. Shelton J, Linder JD, Rivera-Alsina ME, Tarnasky PR. Commitment, confirmation, and clearance: new techniques for nonradiation ERCP during pregnancy (with videos). Gastrointest Endosc. 2008;67:364–8.
90. Roumieu F, Ponchon T, Audra P, Gaucherand P. Acute pancreatitis in pregnancy: place of the different explorations (magnetic resonance cholangiopancreatography, endoscopic ultrasonography) and their therapeutic consequences. Eur J Obstet Gynecol Reprod Biol. 2008;140:141–2.

Cirrhosis and Portal Hypertension

91. Shaheen AA, Myers RP. The outcomes of pregnancy in patients with cirrhosis: a population-based study. Liver Int. 2010;30(2):275–8.
92. Russell MA, Craigo SD. Cirrhosis and portal hypertension in pregnancy. Semin Perinatol. 1998;22:156–65.
93. Rasheed SM, Abdel Monem AM, Abd Ellah AH, et al. Prognosis and determinants of pregnancy outcome among patients with post-hepatitis liver cirrhosis. Int J Gynaecol Obstet. 2013;121:247–51.
94. Palatnik A, Rinella ME. Medical and obstetric complications among pregnant women with liver cirrhosis. Obstet Gynecol. 2017;129(6):1118–23.
95. Britton RC. Pregnancy and esophageal varices. Am J Surg. 1982;143:421–5.
96. Pajor A, Lehoczky D. Pregnancy and extrahepatic portal hypertension. Gynecol Obstet Investig. 1990;30:193–7.
97. Hillemanns P, Knitza R, Müller-Höcker J. Rupture of splenic artery aneurysm in a pregnant patient with portal hypertension. Am J Obstet Gynecol. 1996;174(5):1665.

98. Benjaminov FS, Heathcote J. Liver disease in pregnancy. Am J Gastroenterol. 2004;99:2479–88.
99. Pasha SF, Gloviczki P, Stanson AW, Kamath PS. Splanchnic artery aneurysms. Mayo Clin Proc. 2007;82:472–9.
100. Heriot JA, Steven CM, Sattin RS. Elective forceps delivery and extradural anaesthesia in a primigravida with portal hypertension and oesophageal varices. Br J Anaesth. 1996;76:325–7.
101. Cundy TF, O'Grady JG, Williams R. Recovery of menstruation and pregnancy after liver transplantation. Gut. 1990;31:337–8.
102. Douglas NC, Shah M, Sauer MV. Fertility and reproductive disorders in female solid organ transplant recipients. Semin Perinatol. 2007;31(6):332–8.. Review. Erratum in: Semin Perinatol 2008;32(1):67
103. Mass K, Quint EH, Punch MR, et al. Gynecological and reproductive function after liver transplantation. Transplantation. 1996;62:476–9.
104. de Koning ND, Haagsma EB. Normalization of menstrual pattern after liver transplantation: consequences for contraception. Digestion. 1990;46:239–41.
105. Sarkar M, Bramham K, Moritz MJ, Coscia L. Reproductive health in women following abdominal organ transplant. Am J Transplant. 2018;18(5):1068–76.
106. Christopher V, Al-Chalabi T, Richardson PD, et al. Pregnancy outcome after liver transplantation: a single-center experience of 71 pregnancies in 45 recipients. Liver Transpl. 2006;12:1138–43.

Cirrhotic Cardiomyopathy

29

Roxana Cristina Rimbas, Alexandra Maria Chitroceanu, and Dragos Vinereanu

Key Concepts

- Cirrhotic cardiomyopathy is defined as an abnormal cardiac function at rest and an impaired contractile responsiveness to stress in patients with liver cirrhosis.
- Heart failure secondary to cirrhotic cardiomyopathy is the most common cause of death in patients who undergo liver transplantation.
- An altered diastolic function with a subclinical systolic dysfunction are the mainstay in patients with cirrhotic cardiomyopathy.
- New echocardiographic methods and cardiac magnetic resonance might refine criteria for cirrhotic cardiomyopathy definition.
- Electrophysiological abnormalities with prolonged QT interval, chronotropic dysfunction, and electromechanical dyssynchrony are supportive criteria.
- Treatment is nonspecific and the only effective treatment seems to be liver transplantation.

R. C. Rimbas (✉) · D. Vinereanu
University of Medicine and Pharmacy Carol Davila, Bucharest, Romania

Cardiology Department, University and Emergency Hospital, Bucharest, Romania

A. M. Chitroceanu
University of Medicine and Pharmacy Carol Davila, Bucharest, Romania

29.1 Introduction

Liver cirrhosis (LC) is the final spectrum of several aggressions to the liver, with high impact to public healthcare, being an important cause of mortality worldwide (Hoyert and Xu 2011). Access to liver transplantation (LT) has improved the prognosis of LC [1]. However, cardiac dysfunction has emerged as a leading cause of mortality after LT (Madhwal et al. 2012). Therefore, most recent LT guidelines stated that a comprehensive pretransplant cardiac evaluation is highly required (McCaughan 2012).

Patients with LC develop a progressive impairment in their cardiac function during the course of their illness, a condition described more than 60 years ago named **cirrhotic cardiomyopathy (CCM)** (Kowalski and Abelmann 1953; Murray et al. 1958). Both authors defined a hyperdynamic state in patients with LC characterized by high cardiac output (CO), and low systemic vascular resistance (SVR). Cardiac function abnormalities consisting in impaired ventricular performance to different stressful stimuli are clinically not apparent at rest, because of the low SVR. Recent data support the concept of a specific heart disease, an intrinsic myocardial dysfunction generated by different substances, correlated with the severity of liver dysfunction. However, the most updated pre-LT evaluation guideline provides only an algorithm for the evaluation of major cardiovascular diseases, without giving any clear recommendations regarding CCM [1].

In this chapter we provide an overview of CCM, its definition, complex pathogenic mechanisms, old and new diagnostic tests, prognosis, and management strategies.

F. Radu-Ionita et al. (eds.), *Liver Diseases*, https://doi.org/10.1007/978-3-030-24432-3_29

29.2 Definition

Although first introduced more than 6 decades ago, the term **cirrhotic cardiomyopathy** was defined as a new clinical phenotype in 2005 by an international expert consensus committee at the World Congress of Gastroenterology in Montreal, Canada. CCM was defined as a ***chronic cardiac dysfunction*** in patients with LC, ***in the absence of cardiac disease***, regardless of the aetiology of cirrhosis [2]. Cardiac dysfunction is usually ***asymptomatic at rest***, and it is manifested as a **suboptimal ventricular responsiveness at time of increased demand** [2]. However, subclinical structural and functional disease is present, recognized as **altered diastolic relaxation with electrophysiological abnormalities** (Madhwal et al. 2012). Specific diagnostic criteria for the recognition of CCM, as they were provided by an international expert consensus committee are described in Fig. 29.1.

CCM includes a variety of structural myocardial changes, systolic and diastolic dysfunction, chronotropic incompetence, and electrophysiological abnormalities, in the context of a presumed augmented vascular function (Kazankov et al. 2011; Ripoll et al. 2011; Zardi et al. 2010). Of note, all actual definition criteria are based mostly on conventional echocardiography, which identifies only the late stages of cardiac dysfunction ([3, 4] Kazankov et al. 2011; Ripoll et al. 2011; Zardi et al. 2010; Møller and Henriksen 2010; Dowsley et al. 2012). Recently, many studies designed to characterize the intrinsic myocardial properties in LC, by using the new imaging methods Tissue Doppler Imaging (TDI) and speckle-tracking echocardiography (STE) tried to better define this entity ([3–7] Alexopoulou et al. 2012). These new imaging modalities might be essential to detect subclinical cardiac dysfunction, and to better define it, in presumed high preload conditions. However, the exact role of these new methods in the diagnosis and prognosis of CCM is still controversial. Moreover, serum levels of natriuretic peptide and troponin I are reported to be elevated in LC patients, but the role of these markers in the diagnosis and prognosis of CCM is also not well established [6–8].

29.3 Epidemiology

The prevalence of CCM remains unknown because the disease is asymptomatic at rest and remains well tolerated for months to years [9]. It is unmasked as left ventricular (LV) dysfunction in conditions of increased demand for CO such us exercise, drugs, haemorrhage, infections or surgery (Wong 2009). Its frequency seems to be from 3% to 23.4% [10]. However, it is also possible to identify myocardial dysfunc-

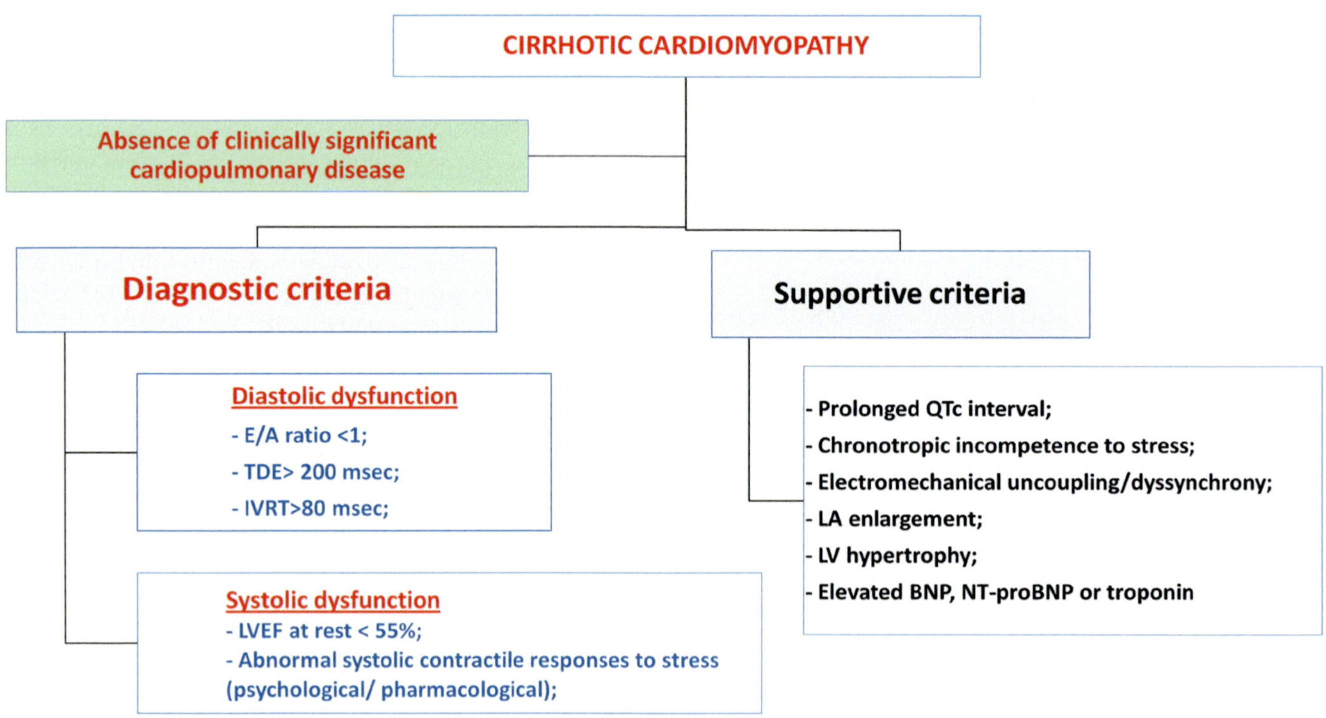

Fig. 29.1 Diagnostic criteria for Cirrhotic Cardiomyopathy according to the World Congress of Gastroenterology in Montreal Canada. E = peak velocity blood flow in early diastole; A = peak velocity blood flow in late diastole; E/A ratio = the ratio of peak velocity blood flow in early diastole to peak velocity blood flow in late diastole; TDE = E-wave deceleration time; IVRT = isovolumetric relaxation time; LV = left ventricle; LA = left atrium; LVEF = left ventricular ejection fraction; QTc = corrected QT interval; BNP = brain natriuretic peptide; NT-proBNP: N-terminal prohormone of brain natriuretic peptide

tion in up to 50% of LC patients (Henriksen et al. 2003). At present, the real prevalence of CCM is difficult to be estimated because of the lack of sensitivity of diagnostic tests to identify CCM at early stages. Moreover, in compensated stages of the LC, heart involvement is latent, and without a stress method CCM cannot be unmasked. Furthermore, worldwide LC has a huge geographical variability, depending on the aetiological factors such as chronic alcoholism, viral hepatitis B and C, autoimmune liver disease (Wong 2009).

29.4 Pathophysiology

CCM Cirrhotic cardiomyopathy is a complex and multifactorial disease, and involves interaction of multiple cellular, neuronal and humoral signalling pathways [11]. These include altered cardiomyocyte membrane physiology, ion channels defects, diminished β-adrenergic receptor signalling pathways, elevated sympathetic nervous tone, and over activity of vasodilator pathways such as nitric oxide, carbon monoxide and endocannabinoid system (Liu et al. 2006; Bolognesi et al. 2007; Baik et al. 2007). CCM has no direct genetic predisposition (Baik et al. 2007).

Liver insufficiency and increasing of the intrahepatic vascular resistance with development of the porto-systemic collateral vessels, leads to accumulation of high plasma levels of **inflammatory and vasoactive molecules**, such as endothelins, glucagon, tumor necrosis factor α (TNFα), IL1, IL6, TGFβ, adrenomedullin, calcitonin gene-related peptide, carbon monoxide, endocannabinoids, nitric oxide, prostacyclin and natriuretic peptide, that might be involved in CCM pathogenesis ([11, 12] Liu et al. 2006; Bolognesi et al. 2007; Baik et al. 2007; Chayanupatkul et al. 2014).

All key mediators involved in the CCM pathogenesis and their main mechanisms that generate cardiac systolic and diastolic dysfunction, and also electrophysiological abnormalities are summarized in Table 29.1. The key of understanding the pathophysiology of CCM lies in the ***hyperdynamic circulation*** with a compensatory increased in CO, due to a reduced SVR (Liu et al. 2006; Bonz et al. 2003). Cardiac contraction is affected especially in stressful conditions [11]. Before ascites formation, there is an ***expansion of the blood volume***, with a redistribution to the splanchnic territory as liver failure progresses ([11–13] Chayanupatkul et al. 2014). Despite an absolute increase in blood volume, there is an important **peripheral arterial vasodilatation**, which activates the renin-angiotensin-aldosterone (RAAS) and autonomic nervous system. This leads to an activation of sodium and water retention, which becomes more apparent as LC worsens (Wong 2009). Advanced liver disease is associated with important changes in SVR (Yang and Lin 2012). With the progression of cirrhosis, arterial compliance is increased, as a result of reduction in thickness of the vessel walls, as well as a decreased vascular tone, secondary to nitric oxide overproduction ([12] Liu et al. 2006; Bolognesi et al. 2007).

The hyperdynamic circulation is dependent on cardiac reserve (heart inotropism and chronotropism), and at initially phases CO is preserved at rest. Progression of the LC generates systolic myocardial dysfunction due to the increased blood volume. Simultaneously, there is a diastolic myocardial dysfunction due to myocardial hypertrophy, rigidity and subendothelial oedema ([11–14] Bolognesi et al. 2007; Baik et al. 2007; Chayanupatkul et al. 2014).

Heart cell contractility is mainly determined by stimulating β-adrenergic receptor system. In experimental studies in rats, cardiomyocyte membrane isolated from rats with LC presented multiple defects in β-adrenergic signalling pathway and lipid composition, leading to alter fluidity of the membrane. This interferes with the function of the proteins located in the membrane, such as calcium channels and β-adrenergic receptors (Ma et al. 1996). One of the main mechanisms of impaired cardiac contractility in response to stress is overproduction of nitric oxide that inhibit cardiomyocyte contractility ([11] Chayanupatkul et al. 2014). Moreover, endocannabinoids production is increased due to hemodynamic overload, and these substances are known to have a negative inotropic effect ([13] Bonz et al. 2003; Chayanupatkul et al. 2014; Garcia-Estan et al. 2002).

In summary, all inflammatory, pro-fibrotic, pro-apoptotic, and vasoactive molecules generated by liver insufficiency and increased intrahepatic vascular resistance lead to systolic and diastolic dysfunction, in the context of a peripheral arterial vasodilatation and high cardiac output (Fig. 29.2).

29.5 Diagnostic Tests

Most of the patients with stable liver disease are asymptomatic in the initial stages of CCM, with no apparent functional limitations, although they have subclinical structural cardiac disease [11, 15]. It is well known that LC patients have a reduced ventricular afterload. This extreme peripheral vasodilation is the natural way of "auto treating" the patient and preventing the development of overt congestive heart failure in these patients. LT is by far the most important challenge in cardiac function in LC patients, because there are significant fluctuations in preload and afterload during the immediate perioperative period and several days after transplantation (Torregrosa et al. 2005). Fifty percentage of LC patients undergoing LT show signs of cardiac dysfunction within the first postoperative week [16]. In this light, a complete and correct pre transplant evaluation of the cardiac function is mandatory.

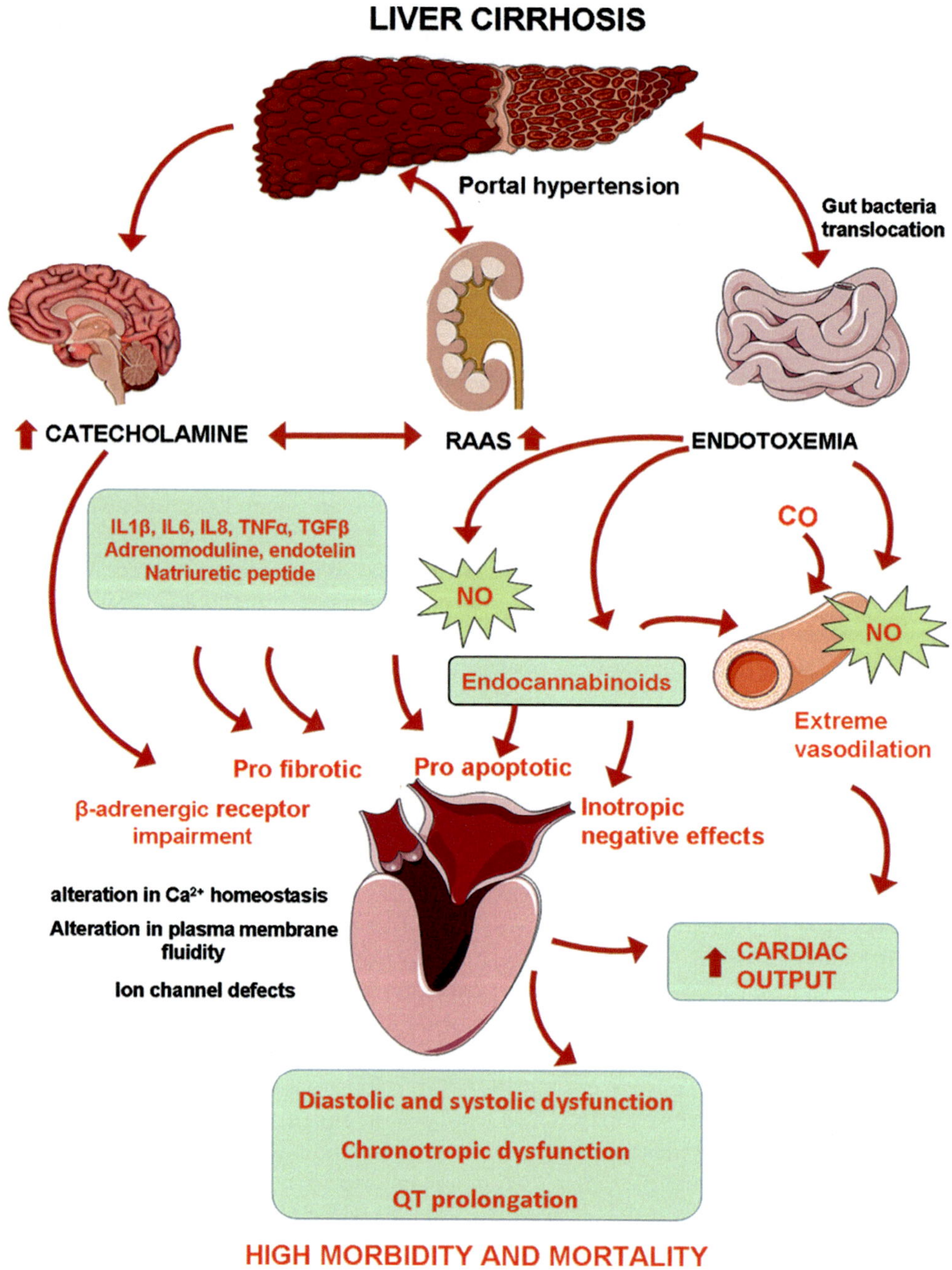

Fig. 29.2 Pathophysiological mechanisms of cirrhotic cardiomyopathy. RAAS = renin-angiotensin-aldosterone system; CO = carbon monoxide; IL1β = interleukin-1β; IL-6 = interleukin-6; IL-8 = interleukin-8; TNF-α = tumor necrosis factor-α; TGF-β = transforming growth factor β; NO = nitric oxide

All patient with LC must undergo clinical, biological, electrocardiographic and imaging evaluation for early diagnosis of CCM [13, 16]. However, CCM is generally latent, and is not so evident on routine examination. With the progression of liver disease, when the patients are subjected to stress, the cardiac dysfunction becomes manifest [11, 16]. In early stages, diastolic precede systolic dysfunction, both being concomitant with the progression of the disease ([16] Torregrosa et al. 2005).

Different complementary imaging techniques were developed within the field of cardiology in the last years. However, in LC patients, **echocardiography** is by far the most useful method for the diagnosis of cardiac dysfunction. There is limited experience with other imaging modalities such as **cardiac magnetic resonance** (CMR) and **myocardial scintigraphy**. Chest X-Ray evaluation is usually normal, or may reveal in advanced stages left atrial or ventricular enlargement, and cardiomegaly with pleural effusion.

29.5.1 Echocardiography

The actual definition of CCM includes impaired contractile responsiveness to stress and/or altered diastolic function associated with electrophysiological abnormalities. However, this definition is too vague, because there are many echocardiographic parameters available for the estimation of diastolic and systolic function. Moreover, diastolic dysfunction evaluation changes a lot in the last years, and a new and more complete algorithm is now available [17, 18]. In this light, a new consensus regarding CCM definition is still lacking, and important unanswered questions should be discussed: the optimal echocardiographic parameters, the role of new TDI and STE methods, the minimum number of criteria required for the CCM diagnosis, utility of stress echocardiography to unmask myocardial dysfunction, and the feasibility of this investigation in cirrhotic patients. A specific algorithm for the diagnosis of CCM has not yet been validated.

29.5.2 Systolic Dysfunction

Systolic dysfunction is mostly latent in LC patients. Although left ventricular systolic function (LVEF) at rest is normal in cirrhotic patients, there are subtle alterations that could be detected in stressful conditions or by using new echocardiographic techniques at rest, such TDI and STE (Mor-Avi et al. 2011). LVEF by 2D echocardiography is the most widely used parameter of global LV systolic function assessment. Most studies have found that LVEF is increased in LC patient in the resting state. The disk summation method in two orthogonal planes (modified Simpson's rule) is still the method of choice. Although three-dimensional echocardiography (3DE) is becoming more available in clinical practice, this imaging technique is highly dependent on image quality, breath hold making it more prone to artifacts. These issues may limit its applicability in decompensated cirrhotic patients with tachycardia and unable to hold their breath. Moreover, volumes obtained with 3DE are larger than 2DE derived volumes and should not be used interchangeably in serial measurements [19]. To the best of our knowledge, there are no studies comparing 3DE, 2DE and CMR in liver cirrhosis. Hence, its validity in this specific setting remains unproven (Sampaio et al. 2016).

According to the current consensus, an LVEF of less than 52% in men and 54% in women, using 2DE, suggests systolic dysfunction. Higher cut-off values should be considered for 3DE and CMR [20]. However, since LVEF is highly dependent on loading conditions, a higher cut-off value may need to be considered in patients with LC due to the decreased afterload. This probably explains the finding of normal resting LVEF in the majority of the studies in cirrhosis (Sampaio et al. 2016). Although the LVEF is normal at rest, contractile response to stress is impaired, which becomes evident when challenged. Similar result was proved in a study by Sampaio and Pimenta [20] examining the LVEF response, as measured by magnetic resonance myocardial stress testing with low-dose dobutamine.

LC patients have blunted responsiveness to volume and postural challenge, exercise or pharmacological stimulation. The altered response to active tilt also suggests an impaired myocardial contractility. During 5 min of standing, cirrhotic patients experienced a decrease in the LV end-systolic volume, SVR and CO despite marked increments in heart rate and in the activity of neuro-humoral systems (Sampaio et al. 2016). On the other hand, in LC patients there is an abnormal LV response during exercise manifested by an increase in CO and LVEF less than expected, by comparison to normal subjects, emphasizing the theory of impaired contractile response in cirrhotic patients (Sampaio et al. 2016). Several studies have demonstrated blunted cardiac responsiveness to vasoactive drugs. The infusion of angiotensin or terlipressin produced a normalization of SVR, and an increase in pulmonary wedge capillary pressure (PCWP), but not an increase in CO (Krag et al. 2010). These findings suggest that the normalization of the afterload may unmask LV dysfunction at rest. Stimulation by β-adrenergic agonists reduces the inotropic and chronotropic responses of the heart in LC patients. Furthermore, administration of dobutamine, a β1-adrenergic receptor agonist, causes only a slight increase in stroke volume, and the dose of isoproterenol needed to increase the heart rate is higher in cirrhotic patients than in normal subjects, which indicate chronotropic incompetence in cirrhotic patients ([20] Krag et al. 2010).

Myocardial strain imaging by STE has been validated for the assessment of regional myocardial function (Mor-Avi et al. 2011). Furthermore, a new parameter of systolic dysfunction, global longitudinal systolic strain (GLS), has been proposed for the assessment of early cardiac dysfunction in LC patients. 2D-STE, which objectively measures intrinsic deformation of myocardial fibre, is less likely to be preload or afterload dependent when compared with standard echocardiographic measures, and now we have cut-off value of −20% for healthy subjects. This makes STE very useful in LC patients, more sensitive and accurate to detect subtle systolic dysfunction ([18] Sampaio et al. 2016).

Recently, Sampaio et al. (2016) and Altekin et al.[21] found that patients with cirrhosis had reduced longitudinal systolic function, despite still having normal LVEF. Conversely, circumferential shortening, is augmented as a compensatory [7, 21]. Moreover, Nazar et al. [6] and Rimbas et al. [18] using 2D-STE, found no differences in GLS in LC patients with different grades of LV diastolic dysfunction. The prognosis value of GLS in LC patients is still controversial ([18] Krag et al. 2010; Sampaio et al. 2016).

Changes in systolic function post liver transplant have also been evaluated in six studies. Three of them showed statistically significant decline in LVEF post-LT, but the decline was clinically insignificant [22]. The systolic response to stress showed significant improvement 9 months after transplant in one study [16]. More recently, studies analysing

GLS showed that although strain values remained within normal range, there was an improvement at 18 months after LT in the LV deformation (−18.5% to −21%, $p < 0.01$) [23].

Recently, it has become possible to perform real-time 3DE. This method allows quantification of LV, RV, and LA volumes closely correlated to those measured by CMR. However, this imaging technique was not incorporated in the diagnostic work-up of CCM yet. There is no single study designed to use 3DE for the assessment of LVEF in LC patients and to define prognostic role of this parameter.

29.5.3 Diastolic Dysfunction

Diastolic dysfunction is the prominent feature of cirrhotic cardiomyopathy ([5, 8] Mota et al. 2013). The prevalence of DD in cirrhotic patients is about 46%. It is considered to be a sensitive marker for the development of hepato-renal syndrome and a predictor of mortality (Ruiz-del-Arbol et al. 2016). Moreover, 75% of patients with cirrhosis and DD have LV hypertrophy (Torregrosa et al. 2005).

All key biological mediators involved in CCM pathogenesis affect mainly diastolic proprieties of the LV, with decreased compliance, relaxation, and abnormal filling pattern. The pathophysiological background of DD is an increased stiffness of the myocardial wall, resulting from a combination of mild myocardial hypertrophy, fibrosis, myocytes apoptosis, and sub endothelial oedema [14].

DD can be determined both by invasive (measuring PCWP and end diastolic pressure) and non-invasive (echocardiography, CMR) methods. Reduced SVR and central hypovolemia explain increased cardiopulmonary pressure with normal mean left atrial pressure [24]. Nowadays, CCM should be understood as a specific type of heart failure with preserved ejection fraction (HFpEF), in which DD is the prominent feature, in the context of central hypovolemia. Similar to other type of HFpEF, transthoracic echocardiography plays the key role for the detection of DD.

Echocardiographic changes in CCM includes left atrial (LA) dilatation with increased left atrial volume indexed (LAVi), increased LV diameter, LV mass, and thickness of the LV walls, without an increase in LV volume. In the present definition of CCM, DD is expressed as decreased peak E velocity (early rapid filling phase), prolonged deceleration time (TDE) and isovolumetric relaxation time (IVRT), and an increased atrial contribution to the late ventricular filling (A wave) with a decreased E/A ratio [12]. Older studies used only mitral inflow profile to define CCM (E/A ratio, IVRT). All recent studies use TDI and STE methods, currently not included in the definition criteria. Moreover, in the current definition, DD refers only to impaired relaxation pattern, completely excluding all other types of DD [18]. However, DD assessed using the present definition of CCM was reported as a predictor of mortality in LT patients [25]. Since E/A ratio is significantly dependent of loading conditions and LC is characterize by important variability of preload and afterload, additional parameters for the evaluation of DD should be used. Patients with ascites have lower E/A ratio than LC patients without ascites. After paracentesis, by reducing the A-wave velocity, E/A ratio increases [11]. Paracentesis reduces the preload by lowering increased plasma renin activity, aldosterone, norepinephrine, and epinephrine. However, systolic function is not affected by paracentesis [11].

TDI is a well validated imaging technique. By TDI we can measure diastolic tissue velocity of mitral annulus (E′) at the basal and septal level. E′ is considered a more accurate marker for the evaluation of DD than E and E/A ratio, due to the partial independency of loading conditions. At present, the *E*/*E*′ ratio is used to estimate LV filling pressure (LVFP), and recommended by the guidelines for the evaluation of DD [17] However, these parameters (E′ and E/E′ ratio) are not included in the present definition of CCM. Different studies suggested that DD is related to mortality assessed by using new guidelines indication, and *E*/*E*′ ratio was found as an independent predictor of mortality ([26] Cazzaniga et al. 2007). However, these data are presently discordant and are not confirmed by other studies ([6, 8, 18] Alexopoulou et al. 2012). All these studies did not find an association between any of the echocardiographic parameters (new and old) and short or long-term mortality. Indeed, different methods used to assess LV diastolic function in LC might explain different results from studies. Therefore larger, multicentric, adequately powered studies using new definition criteria for quantification of DD are required to confirm or exclude an effect of DD on survival in patients with LC.

Moreover, LAVi is a mandatory measurement for the assessment of DD in the last guidelines for the assessment of LV function [17]. An increase in LAVi has been reported in cirrhosis, and was interpreted as a marker of DD in these patients [4]. Other studies have found that LA enlargement is related to loading conditions and should not be used as a single marker of DD. LA longitudinal deformation seems to correlate better with LVFP than LAVi or E/E′ ratio [21, 27].

Severity of DD is usually classified from mild grade 1 to severe grade 3. Majority of cirrhotic patients have DD grade 1 or moderate grade 2. Only a minority of them have a restrictive pattern (grade 3) [18]. DD correlates with severity of liver disease and high MELD score [9, 26]. The present algorithm for DD diagnosis in patients with preserved LVEF, includes TDI mitral annulus velocities (septal E′, lateral E′), PW Doppler mitral inflow (E wave, E/A ratio), E/E′ ratio, tricuspid velocity (TV) and LAVi. Guidelines recommend four variables for identifying DD, and their specific cut-off values: annular E′ velocity: septal E′ < 7 cm/s or lateral E′

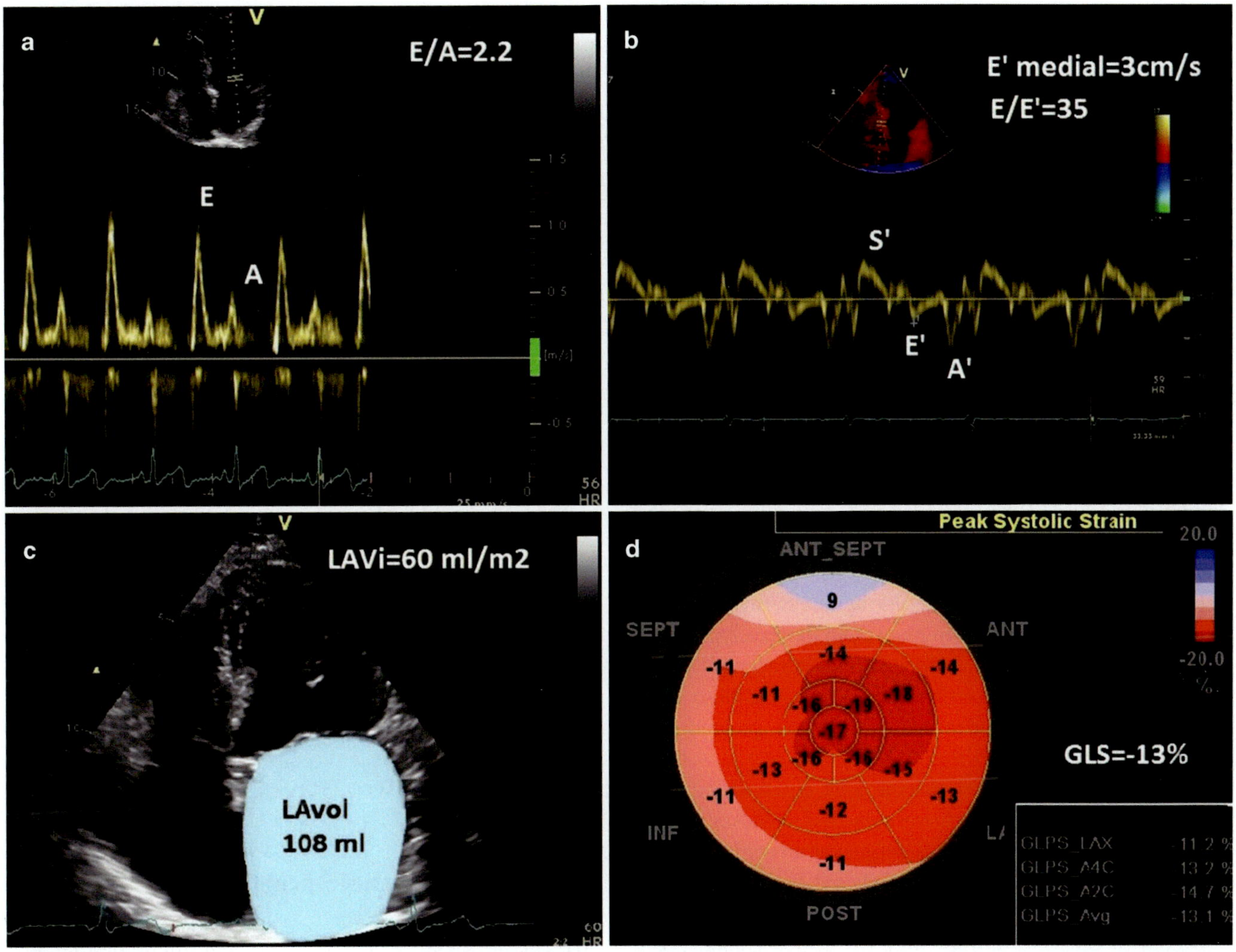

Fig. 29.3 Echocardiographic evaluation of cirrhotic cardiomyopathy. An example of a liver cirrhotic patient with Child-Pugh C, and severe diastolic dysfunction grade 3. Panel A. Pulsed wave Doppler at the level of mitral inflow: E = peak velocity blood flow in early diastole; A = peak velocity blood flow in late diastole; E/A ratio = the ratio between peak velocity blood flow in early diastole to peak velocity blood flow in late diastole; E/A = 2.2 suggesting a restrictive pattern (grade 3) of diastolic dysfunction. Panel B: TDI evaluation of myocardial velocities at the level of mitral annulus: S′ = systolic velocity; E′ = early diastolic velocity; A' = late diastolic velocity; E′ medial = early diastolic velocity at septal site; E/E′ = 35 suggesting high left ventricular filling pressure. Panel C: LAvol = left atrial volume; LAVi = left atrial indexed volume (LAvol/BSA); LAVi = 60 ml/m2 suggesting an important LA dilatation. Panel D: GLS = global longitudinal strain of the left ventricle. GLS = -13% suggesting a significantly decreased longitudinal systolic dysfunction

<10 cm/s, average E/E′ ratio >14, and LAVi >34 mL/m^2 and elevated pulmonary artery pressure predicted by TV > 2.8 m/s [17]. If ≥3 variables are abnormal, DD is present, and E-wave and E/A ratio determines its severity or grading. None of these criteria were included in the actual definition of CCM. We recommend the use of this algorithm for an accurate DD diagnosis in LC patients (Fig. 29.3).

Although it is often believed that CCM reverses after LT, the data are limited and do not support entirely this idea. In fact, the data suggest that diastolic function may not improve after transplant and may actually worsen. The only criterion of CCM that has been shown to improve after liver transplant is QTc prolongation. More importantly, the presence of the DD may be associated with adverse outcomes and mortality after transplant [22]. In this light, it is obvious why is so important to reach a reference standard definition for the assessment of myocardial dysfunction, and to define its contribution to mortality in LC patients.

Since many of the clinical features are unmasked by different stressful conditions (LT, infection, bleeding, other surgical procedure), it seems reasonable that by simulating the effect of these stressful stimuli on cardiovascular system we could reveal cardiac dysfunction. In patients with DD and normal LVFP despite delayed myocardial relaxation, diastolic stress test may uncover increased LVFP in response to exercise [28]. Exercise echocardiography might be useful to assess diastolic as well as systolic response in LC patients. Till now, there are conflicting data regarding the utility of the stress echocardiography in CCM diagnosis. Stress echocardiography was found to be inconclusive because of the inability to achieve the predicted target heart rate in LC patients, as a result of chronotropic incompetence [3]. Dahl et al. [29] found that patients with early LC had a normal chronotropic and inotropic response to pharmacological stress. Krag et al. [30] used CMR to assess LV volumes and CO at rest and during maximal heart rate induced by increasing dosages of dobutamine and atropine. They confirmed that in early stages of LC, the chronotropic and inotropic response to stress is normal [30]. When comparing LC patients with controls, the normal increase in CO and LVEF in response to graded exercise testing is significantly suppressed, with the most pronounced inability to increase cardiac performance seen in decompensated patients (Wong et al. 2001). Recently, Barbosa et al. [31] suggested dobutamine stress echocardiography (DSE) as a reliable tool for the diagnosis of CCM. They measured E/E′ ratio at rest and after stress. They suggested that stress echocardiography could unmask patients with DD not recognized at rest, but with impaired myocardial relaxation during stress (average E/E′ ratio increase). This finding might explain the development of acute pulmonary edema after trans-jugular intrahepatic porto-systemic shunt (TIPS) insertion and LT, because these interventions generate a sudden increase in the preload and, consequently, a rise in LVFP [31].

DSE is widely used for detection of chronotropic dysfunction, as part of the cardiovascular risk assessment pre-LT. Chronotropic dysfunction is defined as an achieved heart rate less than 85% of maximal predicted heart rate. It is a strong independent predictor of major cardiovascular events. It occurs in 26–37% of end stage LC patients undergoing DSE ([32] Williams et al. 2000). However, the predictive value in detection of CCM in patients with cirrhosis is not well established ([31] Rudzinski et al. 2012).

Taking in consider all new data about diagnostic potential and limitations of the old and new echocardiographic parameters, we suggest that the definition of CCM should be updated, according to new guidelines for the diagnosis of DD. TDI-derived parameters and global longitudinal strain by STE should be included in the definition criteria of CCM. Since each parameter alone has some potential limitation, the diagnosis of DD should not rely on a single measurement but rather a multi-parameter approach should be used, in order to better classify the severity of DD and, importantly, to estimate LVFP in the context of high preload conditions. Stress echocardiography should be used in selected cases to unmask DD.

29.5.4 Cardiac Scintigraphy

There is limited data available on myocardial scintigraphy in the evaluation algorithm of CCM. A lower increase in LVEF after physiological stress can be revealed by scintigraphy in cirrhotic patients when compared to non-cirrhotic patients, revealing a blunted contractile response to stress in cirrhotic patients. However data regarding the diagnosis and prognosis utility of this imaging technique is lacking [24].

29.5.5 Cardiac Magnetic Resonance

Cardiac magnetic resonance is considered as a gold standard for accurate assessment of the LVEF, volumes of cardiac chambers, myocardial fibrosis, and oedema prior to the onset of LV dysfunction. Studies using CMR in cirrhotic patients have shown a hyperdynamic LV with increased LA volume, LV thickness, and raised LV end diastolic volume [33]. One study has investigated structural changes in CCM with contrast-enhanced CMR and found that myocardial changes were similar to the findings in patients with myocarditis, showing a patchy distribution (Lossnitzer et al. 2010). CMR has been used for evaluation of tissue characterization, and identification of specific cardiac lesions in cirrhotic patients proposed for LT. The presence of late-gadolinium enhancement (LGE) seems to be a promising tool to identify patients with CCM. LGE can be detected regardless of the cause of liver disease, even if it is more pronounced in patients with alcoholic liver cirrhosis ([33] Lossnitzer et al. 2010).

29.5.6 Electrophysiological Changes

LC generate electromechanical uncoupling, prolongation of QT interval, and chronotropic dysfunction. One of the supportive diagnostic criteria for CCM according to current definition is **QT prolongation** on electrocardiogram (Fig. 29.1). This is one of the most common electrophysiological changes in cirrhosis, with a prevalence of 37–84% (Bernardi et al. 2010). However, it is inadequate, alone, to diagnose CCM. ECG abnormalities in CCM include prolonged QT interval as the earliest and the most prevalent alteration, atrial and ventricular premature contractions, bundle branch block and ST segment depression in more advanced stages. Twenty-four-hour Holter monitoring has better sensitivity to identify bradyarrhythmia and tachyarrhythmia, and can aid in the diagnosis of subclinical disease [34, 35].

Loss of K^+ channels on plasma membrane and their dysfunction, sympathetic over-activity, exposure of different cytokines through porto-systemic shunts are responsible for QT prolongation. It is worth noting that patients undergoing LT are found to have prolonged QTc interval $\geq$500 ms. Moreover, QTc > 440 ms correlated with 1-year mortality, but only in patients with DD ([18] Trevisani et al. 2012). All studies showed significant improvement in QTc after LT, and some of them found improvement or normalization in >80% of the patients [22].

Electromechanical dyssynchrony: LC patients have a dyssynchronous contractile response of systole to electrical signals, due to decreased concentration of L-type calcium channels (Bernardi et al. 1991). Electromechanical dyssynchrony has two components, pre-ejection phase (time interval between ventricular depolarization and ventricular ejection) and LV ejection phase. Pre-ejection time delay and electromechanical delay have been reported among LC patients both at rest and after exercise, suggesting electromechanical dyssynchrony. Moreover, cirrhotic patients with prolonged QT interval have more chances of electromechanical uncoupling (Henriksen et al. 2002).

Chronotropic incompetence: Chronotropic incompetence is defined as inability of heart to proportionally increase its rate in response to metabolic challenges. It is characterized as an achieved HR less than 85% of maximal predicted HR. In early stages (Child A and B) chronotropic response to dobutamine remains normal. Chronotropic incompetence is observed in advance cirrhosis in response to exercise, pharmacologic stimuli, paracentesis and infections. Reduced sensitivity of activation in sympathetic nervous system (SNS) due to down regulation and desensitization to beta adrenergic receptors in sino-atrial node is the proposed mechanism for chronotropic incompetence [29].

29.5.7 Cardiac Biomarkers

Biomarkers, especially troponin I, BNP, and NT-proBNP are elevated in cirrhosis, and they seem to be useful in clinical practice for early detection of cirrhotic cardiomyopathy [12].

Troponin I elevation has been associated to a decrease in CO and increased LV mass, but without any correlation to the severity of cirrhosis [5]. Troponin C level was recently found well correlated with severity of LC and mortality [12, 33].

BNP and NT-proBNP are biomarkers recommended to rule out heart failure, but not to establish the diagnostic. They have very high to high negative predictive values, but the positive predictive values are lower. In patient with cirrhosis, BNP and NT-proBNP levels are elevated. They indicate a myocardial origin because of the stretching of cardiomyocytes from LV overload, which increases the expression of the gene responsible for BNP transcription (Wong 2009). Increased levels of BNP and NT-proBNP are associated to the severity of cirrhosis and to cardiac dysfunction, but not to hyperdynamic circulation [14]. These peptides can be used as a screening test in an asymptomatic cirrhotic patient, in order to detect CCM. They could be also biomarkers of successful therapeutic intervention in cirrhosis (Wong et al. 2001). One study identified those patients who have plasma levels of NT-proBNP >290 pg/ml are at increased risk and should be referred for further cardiac investigations (Ziada et al. 2011).

BNP and NT-proBNP have shown good correlations with PCWP and E/E′ ratios in LC patients, even with normal LV function [26]. Moreover, they were found to correlate with LV septal thickness, LV end-diastolic diameter, and QT interval. However, the highest correlation is seen with end diastolic pressures, suggesting that the diastolic stretch is one of the major determinants of BNP increasing [26]. NT-proBNP was recently indicated to be a better indicator for early cardiac dysfunction than BNP because of its stability and longer biological half-life (Campbell et al. 2000). Elevated levels of **Atrial Natriuretic Peptide (ANP)** and **BNP** as biomarkers of cardiac dysfunction have been found as an indicator of compromised myocardial contractility and impaired diastole among cirrhotics. ANP is predominantly synthesized at the atrial level as a result of direct wall stress. Plasma levels of ANP are increased in patients with cirrhosis and ascites, but only in some pre-ascitic LC patients [12, 22]. Different studies indicated that proANP is a superior predictor for outcome than ANP, probably because proANP undergoes less enzymatic degradation and has a lower affinity to receptors, having higher and more stable circulating plasma levels [12, 33].

New biomarkers of cardiac injury: Galectin and copeptin are newly investigated cardiac biomarker for myocardial injury. Galectin-3 level is found to be high in LC patients, and is linked to myocardial fibrosis [36]. The prognostic role and the cut-off values for all these biomarkers in LC patients are not well established yet.

In summary, all established and potential diagnostic methods for CCM and their role are summarized in Table 29.2.

29.6 Prognosis and Correlation with Liver Disease Severity

It has been already demonstrated that CCM is a latent but frequent complication in patients with LC, and the mechanisms of cardiac involvement are complex and multifactorial. Thus, CCM remains a challenge in clinical practice. The data regarding a correlation between the severity of LC and the stage of cardiomyopathy is still controversial, although most of the studies suggested that diastolic and systolic dysfunction are directly related to the severity of liver dysfunction and portal hypertension. Despite this, it is known that cardiac dysfunction can negatively interfere in the prognostic of cirrhotic patients, reducing survival and induce complications [5–9].

All components of cardiac impairment (systolic, diastolic and electrocardiographic changes) are present concomitant to the progression of the hepatic disease (Ripoll et al. 2011). DD usually precedes systolic dysfunction, the last being unmasked when the patient is subjected to hemodynamic stress (Mota et al. 2013). Acute exacerbation of heart failure is rare because of the peripheral vasodilatation with reduced afterload (Wong 2009). Despite this, situations of increased demand for CO such as LT, infection, and TIPS can induce overt heart failure (Henriksen et al. 2003). Indeed, heart failure secondary to CCM has been reported as the most common cause of death in patients who undergo LT [8, 9].

CCM may also contribute to the pathogenesis of hepatorenal syndrome by an inadequate contractile response to the stress of infection in the face of marked peripheral vasodilatation. Moreover, CCM is associated in the pathogenesis of post-paracentesis circulatory dysfunction secondary to inadequate albumin intake and quick removal of large ascitic volume (Zardi et al. 2010). It seems that the mechanism lays in the chronotropic dysfunction of cirrhotic patient, the inability to increment the heart rate despite arterial hypotension, and intense activation of SNS [6].

One of the diagnostic criteria for CCM according to expert consensus committee in 2005 is QT prolongation on electrocardiogram. It has been demonstrated that the prevalence of QT prolongation increases simultaneous with the severity of the hepatic disease, defined by the Child-Pugh score and the hepatic venous pressure gradient [9]. QT prolongation can cause serious rhythm disturbances including torsades des pointes and sudden cardiac death. Contrary, sudden cardiac death is reported to be rare in cirrhotic patients (Zambruni et al. 2008). Currently, it has been demonstrated that gastrointestinal haemorrhage lengthens QT interval, and increase mortality in this setting (Trevisani et al. 2012). Moreover, patients with QT prolongation undergoing LT have a worse outcome (Zambruni et al. 2008). Generally, CCM worsens with the progression of the underlying liver disease, with a major impact on prognosis of cirrhotic patients.

29.7 Management Options

At present, there are no well-established guidelines regarding the treatment of CCM. Because most patients remain asymptomatic in resting conditions, treatment is usually initiated when symptoms appear. Management of CCM should follow the same recommendations as for non-cirrhotic HFpEF, with sodium restriction, diuretics, and β-blockers. Special care should be taken with the use of ACE-inhibitors and aldosterone antagonist, which have not demonstrated long-term efficacy [37]. Moreover, ACE-inhibitors may aggravate systemic vasodilatation and precipitate hypotension [11]. ACE-inhibitors improve diastolic function in cirrhotic patients by decreasing ventricular thickness and dilatation, and can only be used in early cirrhosis (Child A). Major concerns with these drugs are hypotension. Currently, there is no definite data available about use of ACE-inhibitors in CCM (Pozzi et al. 2005). Aldosterone antagonists have also shown reduction in ventricular wall thickness and end diastolic volume in early cirrhosis (Pozzi et al. 2005).

Loop diuretics are used to relieve symptoms by decreasing volume overload, which is a challenge in cirrhotic patients, who already have baseline arterial hypotension [38]. β-blockers reduce prolonged QT interval to normal values and prevent variceal bleeding by lowering portal pressure. However, administration of β-blockers correlates with poor long term survival in patients with cirrhosis and refractory ascites (Sersté et al. 2011). Moreover, a recent prospective randomized clinical trial in patients with LC regarding β-blockers efficacy in reduction of CCM (abnormal cardiac output response under DSE) did not find any positive impact [39]. The uses of cardiac glycosides, such as digitalis, are not effective in increasing cardiac contraction in cirrhotic patients [37]. Currently, if medical treatment has any benefits on mortality needs to be further elucidated.

In summary, CCM is a complication of cirrhosis with no specific treatment. Because of the central role of the cirrhosis itself in the development of circulatory abnormalities, focus should be put on treating underlying cirrhotic disease [11]. Liver transplantation seems to be the only established effective treatment [11, 22]. The time course of potential cardiac recovery is consider to be between 6 and 12 months post-transplantation, although the factors that induce reversibility are not completely understood [11]. Although cardiac function potentially recovers after LT, the presence of CCM is a risk factor for post-operative complications [38]. High PCWP has the risk of post-reperfusion hemodynamic instability, a major cause of immediate death after LT (Fouad et al. 2009). Some studies demonstrated a complete regression in DD, ventricular wall thickness, and a recovery in systolic function and exercise capacity after transplantation [11]. Moreover, there is a diminished CO, lower heart rate, decreased pulmonary artery pressure, an increase in SVR and blood pressure following LT [38].

Changes in systolic function post-transplant have been evaluated in six studies [22]. Although three of them showed statistically significant decline in LVEF post-transplant, the decline was clinically insignificant [22]. The systolic response to stress before and after LT showed significant improvement 9 months after transplant (Torregrosa et al. 2005). More recently, global longitudinal strain showed that although strain values remained within normal range, there was improvement 18 months after transplant in the left ventricle (−18.5 to −21%, $P < 0.01$) and in right ventricle (−21 to −23%, $P < 0.01$) (Chen et al. 2015).

Diastolic function worsened in three studies and improved in one study post-transplant ([22, 40] Acosta et al. 1999; Therapondos et al. 2002). Therapondos et al. (2002) showed that IVRT was increased, before and after transplant with further increase 3 months after transplant. E/E′ ratio, a surrogate to best measure LVFP was assessed in two studies. While Dowsley et al. (2012) showed increase in E/E′ ratio at 3 months post liver transplant, Chen et al. [23] did not reveal significant change in E/E′ ratio 18 months post-transplant. Changes in LA enlargement in relation to transplant were investigated in three studies. Two studies showed no significant changes after transplant on short and long term, respectively ([40] Dowsley et al. 2012). All studies showed significant improvement in QTc after liver transplant. The median time to improvement in QTc prolongation was 6 months. Although the QTc decreased after LT, it remained significantly longer than in the age/gender matched healthy individuals [22].

CCM is consider the main factor for survival in cirrhotic patients undergoing procedures as TIPS that dramatically increase the preload due to a shift of a large volume of blood from the splanchnic to the central circulation (Lee and Liu 2007). Heart failure and acute pulmonary oedema are the most reported complications after TIPS. DD and pre-TIPS state of central blood volume influence the outcome of TIPS (Lee and Liu 2007). Patients with hypovolemia have a considerable improvement of diastolic function while a pre-TIPS DD is associated with a reduced ascites mobilization. Patients with persistence DD 28 days after TIPS have an increased mortality during follow-up [38].

In summary, there are limited evidences demonstrating the complete reversibility of CCM after LT. Because of the current limited therapeutic options, general knowledge regarding the treatment options of heart failure should be adapted to patients with CCM. However, a critical need for more effective imagistic criteria for the diagnosis of CCM, and for newer agents capable to treat this condition still remains [38].

29.8 Conclusions

Cirrhotic cardiomyopathy represent a new clinical phenotype, characterized mainly by subtle systolic and diastolic dysfunction at rest, associated with electrophysiological abnormalities, chronotropic dysfunction, and electromechanical dyssynchrony. Myocardial dysfunction is frequently underdiagnosed in cirrhotic patients, due to low peripheral vascular resistance. However, CCM contributes to the high cardiovascular morbidity and mortality related to TIPS insertion and LT. To date, there is no clear consensus on how to efficiently diagnose cirrhotic cardiomyopathy. With the remarkable developments in cardiac imaging, and especially in echocardiography, a critical revision of the current definition criteria is highly required, probably including TDI and STE parameters, and in specific situation stress test echocardiography, in order to unmasked myocardial dysfunction. Future studies are needed to establish which echocardiographic parameters serves better to characterize and monitor the cardiac changes in cirrhotic patients. Detailed prospective assessment of this entity will help identify patients at risk for worse outcomes after liver transplant. Treatment of cirrhotic cardiomyopathy is nonspecific, and the only effective treatment seems to be liver transplantation. Moreover, there is also a need for studies with the objective of identifying potential treatment that can change the natural history of cardiac dysfunction in cirrhotic patients, especially in the asymptomatic phase.

Self Study

Questions

1. **Cirrhotic cardiomyopathy is an entity described in patients with liver cirrhosis. It consists of:**
   (a) Prolonged QT interval
   (b) Subtle diastolic and systolic dysfunction
   (c) Inotropic and chronotropic incompetence
   (d) All the above
2. **The commonest electrophysiological abnormalities found in cirrhotic cardiomyopathy is:**
   (a) Atrial fibrillation
   (b) Prolonged QT interval
   (c) Frequent atrial and ventricular ectopic beats
   (d) Torsades des point
3. **Cardiac dysfunction from cirrhotic cardiomyopathy is related to several pathophysiological changes. Which one of the following is correct?**
   (a) Various gases such as nitric oxide and carbon monoxide causing direct suppressive action on the cardiomyocytes
   (b) Inflammatory cytokines stimulated form intestinal endotoxemia in liver cirrhosis exerting a pro-fibrotic and pro-inflammatory action on the cardiomyocytes
   (c) There is altered cardiomyocyte plasma membrane fluidity
   (d) All the above

Answers

1. **Cirrhotic cardiomyopathy is an entity described in patients with liver cirrhosis. It consists of:**
   Answer: (d).
2. **The commonest electrophysiological abnormalities found in cirrhotic cardiomyopathy is:**
   Answer: (b).
3. **Cardiac dysfunction from cirrhotic cardiomyopathy is related to several pathophysiological changes. Which one of the following is correct?**
   Answer: (d).

References

1. Martin P, DiMartini A, Feng S, Brown R Jr, Fallon M. Evaluation for liver transplantation in adults: 2013 practice guideline by the American Association for the Study of Liver Diseases and the American Society of Transplantation. Hepatology. 2014;59:1144–65.
2. Mocarzel LOC, Rossi MM, Miliosse B de M, Lanzieri PG, Gismondi RA. Cirrhotic cardiomyopathy: a new clinical phenotype. Arq Bras Cardiol. 2017;108:564–8.
3. Zaky A, Bendjelid K. Appraising cardiac dysfunction in liver transplantation: an ongoing challenge. Liver Int. 2015;35:12–29.
4. Møller S, Hove JD, Dixen U, Bendtsen F. New insights into cirrhotic cardiomyopathy. Int J Cardiol. 2013;167:1101–8.
5. Merli M, Calicchia A, Ruffa A, Pellicori P, Riggio O, Giusto M, et al. Cardiac dysfunction in cirrhosis is not associated with the severity of liver disease. Eur J Intern Med. 2013;24:172–6.
6. Nazar A, Guevara M, Sitges M, Terra C, Solà E, Guigou C, Arroyo V, Ginès P. Left ventricular function assessed by echocardiography in cirrhosis: relationship to systemic hemodynamic and renal dysfunction. J Hepatol. 2013;58:51–7.
7. Sampaio F, Pimenta J, Bettencourt N, Fontes-Carvalho R, Silva AP, Valente J, et al. Systolic and diastolic dysfunction in cirrhosis: a tissue-Doppler and speckle tracking echocardiography study. Liver Int. 2013;33:1158–65.
8. Sampaio F, Pimenta J, Bettencourt N, Fontes-Carvalho R, Silva AP, Valente J, et al. Systolic dysfunction and diastolic dysfunction do not influence medium-term prognosis in patients with cirrhosis. Eur J Intern Med. 2014;25:241–6.
9. Naqvi IH, Mahmood K, Naeem M, Vashwani AS, Ziaullah S. The heart matters when the liver shatters! Cirrhotic cardiomyopathy: frequency, comparison, and correlation with severity of disease. Gastroenterol Rev. 2016;11:247–56.
10. Enache I, Oswald-Mammosser M, Woehl-Jaegle M-L, Habersetzer F, Di MP, Charloux A, Doutreleau S. Cirrhotic cardiomyopathy and hepatopulmonary syndrome: Prevalence and prognosis in a series of patients. Respir Med. 2013;107:1030–6.
11. Gassanov N, Caglayan E, Semmo N, Massenkeil G, Er F. Cirrhotic cardiomyopathy: a cardiologist's perspective. World J Gastroenterol. 2014;20:15492–8.
12. Wiese S, Hove JD, Bendtsen F, Møller S. Cirrhotic cardiomyopathy: pathogenesis and clinical relevance. Nat Rev Gastroenterol Hepatol. 2014;11:177–86.
13. Horvatits T, Drolz A, Rutter K, Roedl K, Kluge S, Fuhrmann V. Hepato-cardiac disorders. World J Hepatol. 2014;6:41–54.
14. Møller S, Bernardi M. Interactions of the heart and the liver. Eur Heart J. 2013;34:2804–11.
15. Mota VG, Markman Filho B. Echocardiography in chronic liver disease: systematic review. Arq Bras Cardiol. 2013;100:376–85.
16. Liu H, Jayakumar S, Traboulsi M, Lee SS. Cirrhotic cardiomyopathy: implications for liver transplantation. Liver Transpl. 2017;23:826–35.
17. Nagueh SF, Smiseth OA, Appleton CP, Benjamin F, Dokainish H, Edvardsen T, et al. Recommendations for the evaluation of left ventricular diastolic function by echocardiography: an update from the American Society of Echocardiography and the European Association of Cardiovascular Imaging. J Am Soc Echocardiogr. 2016;29:277–314.
18. Rimbaş RC, Baldea SM, Guerra RDGA, Visoiu SI, Rimbaş M, Pop CS, Vinereanu D. New definition criteria of myocardial dysfunction in patients with liver cirrhosis: a speckle tracking and tissue Doppler imaging study. Ultrasound Med Biol. 2018;44:562–74.
19. Lang RM, Badano LP, Mor-Avi V, Afilalo J, Armstrong A, Ernande L, et al. Recommendations for cardiac chamber quantification by echocardiography in adults: an update from the American Society of Echocardiography and the European Association of Cardiovascular Imaging. J Am Soc Echocardiogr. 2015;28:1–39.
20. Sampaio F, Lamata P, Bettencourt N, Alt SC, Ferreira N, Kowallick JT, et al. Assessment of cardiovascular physiology using dobutamine stress cardiovascular magnetic resonance reveals impaired contractile reserve in patients with cirrhotic cardiomyopathy. J Cardiovasc Magn Reson. 2015;17:61.
21. Altekin RE, Caglar B, Karakas MS, Ozel D, Deger N, Demir I. Evaluation of subclinical left ventricular systolic dysfunction using two-dimensional speckle-tracking echocardiography in patients with non-alcoholic cirrhosis. Hell J Cardiol. 2014;55:402–10.
22. Izzy M, Oh J, Watt KD. Cirrhotic cardiomyopathy after transplantation: neither the transient nor innocent bystander. Hepatology. 2018; https://doi.org/10.1002/hep.30040.
23. Chen Y, Chan AC, Chan SC, Chok SH, Sharr W, Fung J, Liu JH, et al. A detailed evaluation of cardiac function in cirrhotic patients and its alteration with or without liver transplantation. J Cardiol. 2016;67:140–6.
24. Naqvi IH, Mahmood K, Talib A, Rizvi NZ. Looking beyond liver! cirrhotic cardiomyopathy: pathophysiology, clinical presentation and management strategies. J Gastroenterol Liv Pancr Dis. 2017;2:1009.
25. Carvalheiro F, Rodrigues C, Adrego T, Viana J, Vieira H, Seco C, et al. Diastolic dysfunction in liver cirrhosis: prognostic predictor in liver transplantation? Transplant Proc. 2016;48:128–31.
26. Ruiz-Del-Arbol L, Achecar L, Serradilla R, Rodriguez-Gandia MA, Rivero M, Garrido E, Natcher JJ. Diastolic dysfunction is a predictor of poor outcomes in patients with cirrhosis, portal hypertension and a normal creatinine. Hepatology. 2013;58:1732–41.
27. Sampaio F, Pimenta J. Left ventricular function assessment in cirrhosis: current methods and future directions. World J Gastroenterol. 2016;22:112–25.
28. Oh JK, Kane GC. Diastolic stress echocardiography: the time has come for its integration into clinical practice. J Am Soc Echocardiogr. 2014;27:1060–3.
29. Dahl EK, Møller S, Kjær A, Petersen CL, Bendtsen F, Krag A. Diastolic and autonomic dysfunction in early cirrhosis: a dobutamine stress study. Scand J Gastroenterol. 2014;49:362–72.
30. Krag A, Bendtsen F, Dahl EK, Kjær A, Petersen CL, Møller S. Cardiac function in patients with early cirrhosis during maximal beta-adrenergic drive: a dobutamine stress study. PLoS One. 2014;9:e109179.
31. Barbosa M, Guardado J, Marinho C, Rosa B, Quelhas I, Lourenço A, et al. Cirrhotic cardiomyopathy: isn't stress evaluation always required for the diagnosis? World J Hepatol. 2016;8:200–6.
32. Umphrey LG, Hurst RT, Eleid MF, Lee KS, Reuss CS, Hentz JG, et al. Preoperative dobutamine stress echocardiographic findings and subsequent short-term adverse cardiac events after orthotopic liver transplantation. Liver Transpl. 2008;14:886–92.
33. Wiese S, Hove JD, Møller S. Cardiac imaging in patients with chronic liver disease. Clin Physiol Funct Imaging. 2017;37:347–56.
34. Mozos I. Arrhythmia risk in liver cirrhosis. World J Hepatol. 2015;7:662–72.
35. Pall A, Czifra A, Vitális Z, Papp M, Paragh G, Szabó Z. Pathophysiological and clinical approach to cirrhotic cardiomyopathy. J Gastrointestin Liver Dis. 2014;23:301–10.
36. Kimer N, Goetze JP, Bendtsen F, Moller S. New vasoactive peptides in cirrhosis: organ extraction and relation to the vasodilatory state. Eur J Clin Investig. 2014;44:441–52.
37. Chayanupatkul M, Liangpunsakul S. Cirrhotic cardiomyopathy: review of pathophysiology and treatment. Hepatol Int. 2014;8:308–15.
38. Ruiz-del-Árbol L, Serradilla R. Cirrhotic cardiomyopathy and circulatory function. World J Gastroenterol. 2015;21:11502–21.

39. Silvestre OM, Farias AQ, Ramos DS, Furtado MS, Rodrigues AC, Ximenes RO, et al. β-Blocker therapy for cirrhotic cardiomyopathy: a randomized-controlled trial. Eur J Gastroenterol Hepatol. 2018;30:930–7.
40. Sonny A, Ibrahim A, Schuster A, Jaber WA, Cywinski JB. Impact and persistence of cirrhotic cardiomyopathy after liver transplantation. Clin Transpl. 2016;30:986–93.

Further Reading

Acosta F, De La Morena G, Villegas M, Sansano T, Reche M, Beltran R, Roques V, et al. Evaluation of cardiac function before and after liver transplantation. Transplant Proc. 1999;31:2369–70.

Alexopoulou A, Papatheodoridis G, Pouriki S, Chrysohoou C, Raftopoulos L, Stefanadis C, Pectasides D. Diastolic myocardial dysfunction does not affect survival in patients with cirrhosis. Transpl Int. 2012;25:1174–81.

Baik SK, Fouad TR, Lee SS. Cirrhotic cardiomyopathy. Orphanet J Rare Dis. 2007;2:15–27.

Bolognesi M, Sacerdoti D, Piva A, Di Pascoli M, Zampieri F, Quarta S, Baik SK, Fouad TR, Lee SS. Carbon monoxide-mediated activation of large conductance calcium-activated potassium channels contributes to mesenteric vasodilatation in cirrhotic rats. J Pharmacol Exp Ther. 2007;321:187–94.

Bernardi M, Rubboli A, Trevisani F, Cancellieri C, Ligabue A, Baraldini M, et al. Reduced cardiovascular responsiveness to exercise-induced sympatho-adrenergic stimulation in patients with cirrhosis. J Hepatol. 1991;12:207–16.

Bernardi M, Calandra S, Colantoni A, Trevisani F, Raimondo ML, Sica G, Schepis F, Mandini M, Simoni P, Contin M, et al. Q-T interval prolongation in cirrhosis: prevalence, relationship with severity, and etiology of the disease and possible pathogenetic factors. Hepatology. 1998;27:28–34.

Bonz A, Laser M, Kullmer S, Kniesch S, Babin-Ebell J, Popp V, Ertl G, Wagner JA. Cannabinoids acting on CB1 receptors decrease contractile performance in human atrial muscle. J Cardiovasc Pharmacol. 2003;41:657–64.

Cameli M, Lisi M, Mondillo S, Padeletti M, Ballo P, Tsioulpas C, Bernazzali S, Maccherini M. Left atrial longitudinal strain by speckle tracking echocardiography correlates well with left ventricular filling pressures in patients with heart failure. Cardiovasc Ultrasound. 2010;8:14.

Campbell DJ, Mitchelhill KI, Schlicht SM, Booth RJ. Plasma amino-terminal pro-brain natriuretic peptide: a novel approach to the diagnosis of cardiac dysfunction. J Card Fail. 2000;6:130–9.

Cazzaniga M, Salerno F, Pagnozzi G, Dionigi E, Visentin S, Cirello I, Meregaglia D, Nicolini A. Diastolic dysfunction is associated with poor survival in patients with cirrhosis with transjugular intrahepatic portosystemic shunt. Gut. 2007;56:869–75.

Dowsley TF, Bayne DB, Langnas AN, Dumitru I, Windle JR, Porter TR, Raichlin E. Diastolic dysfunction in patients with end-stage liver disease is associated with development of heart failure early after liver transplantation. Transplantation. 2012;94(6):646–51.

Fouad TR, Abdel-Razek WM, Burak KW, Bain VG, Lee SS. Prediction of cardiac complications after liver transplantation. Transplantation. 2009;87:763–70.

Garcia-Estan J, Ortiz MC, Lee SS. Nitric oxide and renal and cardiac dysfunction in cirrhosis. Clin Sci. 2002;102:213–22.

Henriksen JH, Fuglsang S, Bendtsen F, Christensen E, Møller S. Dyssynchronous electrical and mechanical systole in patients with cirrhosis. J Hepatol. 2002;36:513–20.

Henriksen JH, Gotze JP, Fuglsang S, Christensen E, Bendtsen F, Moller S. Increased circulating pro-brain natriuretic peptide (proBNP) and brain natriuretic peptide (BNP) in patients with cirrhosis: relation to cardiovascular dysfunction and severity of disease. Gut. 2003;52:1511–7.

Hoyert D, Xu J. Deaths: preliminary data for 2011. Natl Vital Stat Rep. 2012;61:1–51.

Kazankov K, Holland-Fischer P, Andersen NH, Torp P, Sloth E, Aagaard NK, Vilstrup H. Resting myocardial dysfunction in cirrhosis quantified by tissue Doppler imaging. Liver Int. 2011;31:534–40.

Kowalski HJ, Abelmann WH. The cardiac output at rest in Laennec's cirrhosis. J Clin Invest. 1953;32:1025–33.

Krag A, Bendtsen F, Mortensen C, Henriksen JH, Møller S. Effects of a single terlipressin administration on cardiac function and perfusion in cirrhosis. Eur J Gastroenterol Hepatol. 2010;22:1085–92.

Lee SS, Liu H. Cardiovascular determinants of survival in cirrhosis. Gut. 2007;56:746–8.

Liu H, Gaskari SA, Lee SS. Cardiac and vascular changes in cirrhosis: pathogenic mechanisms. World J Gastroenterol. 2006;12:837–42.

Lossnitzer D, Steen H, Zahn A, Lehrke S, Weiss C, Weiss KH, et al. Myocardial late gadolinium enhancement cardiovascular magnetic resonance in patients with cirrhosis. J Cardiovasc Magn Reson. 2010;12:47.

Ma Z, Miyamoto A, Lee SS. Role of altered beta-adrenoceptor signal transduction in the pathogenesis of cirrhotic cardiomyopathy in rats. Gastroenterology. 1996;110:1191–8.

Madhwal S, Atreja A, Albeldawi M, Lopez R, Post A, Costa MA. Is liver transplantation a risk factor for cardiovascular disease? A meta-analysis of observational studies. Liver Transpl. 2012;18:1140–6.

McCaughan GW. Trekking new ground: overcoming medical and social impediments for extended criteria liver transplant recipients. Liver Transpl. 2012;18(Suppl 2):S39–46.

Møller S, Henriksen JH. Cirrhotic cardiomyopathy. J Hepatol. 2010;53:179–90.

Mor-Avi V, Lang RM, Badano LP, Belohlavek M, Cardim NM, Derumeaux G, et al. Current and evolving echocardiographic techniques for the quantitative evaluation of cardiac mechanics: ASE/EAE consensus statement on methodology and indications endorsed by the Japanese Society of Echocardiography. Eur J Echocardiogr. 2011;12:167–205.

Murray JF, Dawson AM, Sherlock S. Circulatory changes in chronic liver disease. Am J Med. 1958;24:358–67.

Pozzi M, Grassi G, Ratti L, Favini G, Dell'Oro R, Redaelli E, et al. Cardiac, neuroadrenergic, and portal hemodynamic effects of prolonged aldosterone blockade in postviral child A cirrhosis. Am J Gastroenterol. 2005;100:1110–6.

Rudzinski W, Waller AH, Prasad A, Sood S, Gerula C, Samanta A, Koneru B, Klapholz M. New index for assessing the chronotropic response in patients with end-stage liver disease who are undergoing dobutamine stress echocardiography. Liver Transpl. 2012;18:355–60.

Ripoll C, Yotti R, Bermejo J, Bañares R. The heart in liver transplantation. J Hepatol. 2011;54:810–22.

Ruiz-del-Arbol L, Monescillo A, Arocena C, Valer P, Gines P, Moreira V, et al. Circulatory function and hepatorenal syndrome in cirrhosis. Hepatology. 2005;42:439–47.

Sersté T, Francoz C, Durand F, Rautou PE, Melot C, Valla D, Moreau R, Lebrec D. Beta-blockers cause paracentesis-induced circulatory dysfunction in patients with cirrhosis and refractory ascites: a cross-over study. J Hepatol. 2011;55:794–9.

Therapondos G, Flapan AD, Dollinger MM, Garden OJ, Plevris JN, Hayes PC. Cardiac function after orthotopic liver transplantation and the effects of immunosuppression: a prospective randomized trial comparing cyclosporin (Neoral) and tacrolimus. Liver Transpl. 2002;8:690–700.

Torregrosa M, Aguadé S, Dos L, Segura R, Gónzalez A, Evangelista A, et al. Cardiac alterations in cirrhosis: reversibility after liver transplantation. J Hepatol. 2005;42:68–74.

Trevisani F, Di Micoli A, Zambruni A, Biselli M, Santi V, Erroi V, et al. QT interval prolongation by acute gastrointestinal bleeding in patients with cirrhosis. Liver Int. 2012;32:1510–5.
Williams K, Lewis JF, Davis G, Geiser EA. Dobutamine stress echocardiography in patients undergoing liver transplantation evaluation. Transplantation. 2000;69:2354–6.
Wong F, Girgrah N, Graba J, Allidina Y, Liu P, Blendis L. The cardiac response to exercise in cirrhosis. Gut. 2001;49:268–75.
Wong F, Siu S, Liu P, Blendis LM. Brain natriuretic peptide: is it a predictor of cardiomyopathy in cirrhosis? Clin Sci. 2001;101:621–8.
Wong F. Cirrhotic cardiomyopathy. Hepatol Int. 2009;3:294–304.
Yang YY, Lin HC. The heart: pathophysiology and clinical implications of cirrhotic cardiomyopathy. J Chin Med Assoc. 2012;75:619–23.
Zardi EM, Abbate A, Zardi DM, Dobrina A, Margiotta D, Van Tassell BW, et al. Cirrhotic Cardiomyopathy. J Am Coll Cardiol. 2010;56:539–49.
Ziada D, Gaber R, Kotb N, Ghazy M, Nagy H. Predictive value of N-terminal pro B-type natriuretic peptide in tissue Doppler-diagnosed cirrhotic cardiomyopathy. Heart Mirror J. 2011;5:264–70.
Zambruni A, Trevisani F, Di Micoli A, Savelli F, Berzigotti A, Bracci E. Effect of chronic beta-blockade on QT interval in patients with liver cirrhosis. J Hepatol. 2008;48:415–21.

30 Benign Liver Tumours

Emilio De Raffele

30.1 Introduction

Benign liver tumours are a heterogeneous group of solid or cystic focal liver lesions (FLL) deriving from different cell types [1, 2].

Solid benign liver tumours may have hepatocellular, biliary, vascular and mesenchymal origin, respectively [2]. A descriptive classification of the lesions of hepatocellular origin has been proposed in 1994 by an international panel of experts sponsored by the World Congress of Gastroenterology [3], and includes: regenerative lesions, comprising regenerative nodules, nodular regenerative hyperplasia (NRH) and focal nodular hyperplasia (FNH); and dysplastic and neoplastic lesions, comprising hepatocellular adenoma (HA), dysplastic nodules and hepatocellular carcinoma (HCC). Benign biliary lesions are quite unfrequent and include the bile duct adenoma, the biliary hamartoma, and the biliary cystadenoma. Vascular lesions include the hepatic hemangioma (HH), which is the most common benign hepatic tumour, and other unfrequent tumours. Mesenchymal lesions include a heterogeneous group of rare tumours.

Cystic lesions of the liver (CLL) represent a miscellaneous group of disorders, with heterogeneous etiology, prevalence, and clinical manifestations. The most common cystic lesions of the liver include: simple (solitary) hepatic cysts (SHC); polycystic liver disease (PLD); parasitic cysts, comprising hydatid cysts; primary neoplastic cysts, comprising biliary cystadenoma (BCA) and cystadenocarcinoma (BCAC); and duct related cysts, comprising Caroli's disease and bile duct duplication [4].

FLLs are increasingly being discovered, in otherwise asymptomatic patients in most cases, because of the extensive use of medical imaging in clinical practice [1, 5–8], including ultrasonography (US), computed tomography (CT), and magnetic resonance imaging (MRI). An accurate evaluation of FLL is of paramount importance to identify primary liver malignancies, especially HCC and cholangiocarcinoma (CCA), and liver metastases at an early, potentially curable stage.

An appropriate diagnostic approach to FLLs requires a detailed clinical history and consideration of risk factors [1, 8], physical examination, laboratory test findings, different imaging modalities, and histopathology in selected cases [1, 5]. Radiological evaluation is the most important aspect in the characterization of FLLs. Even though US is usually the first imaging test obtained because is safe and cost-effective, contrast-enhanced imaging techniques are needed in most cases to reach a diagnosis [1, 8], including contrast-enhanced triphasic CT scan or gadolinium-enhanced MRI; the use of gadolinium-containing contrast agents with both extracellular blood pool and hepatocyte-specific properties has further improved liver MR imaging [6]; hepatobiliary (HPB)-specific MR contrast agents include gadobenate dimeglumine (Gd-BOPTA) and gadoxetic acid (Gd-EOB-DTPA). In the context of HCC and liver transplantation, a recent consensus conference has underlined the importance of standardizing the technical specifications for CT and MRI in the diagnosis of HCC [9]; the same technical specifications for CT or MRI should be applied to the evaluation of FLLs [5]. Contrast-enhanced US (CEUS) is an emerging technique that can add further information in selected cases. An appropriate contrast-enhanced imaging technique should include a late arterial phase, a portal venous phase, and a delayed venous phase [5, 6]. 18-Fluoro-deoxyglucose positron emission tomography (FDG-PET), eventually associated with a CT scan (FDG-PET/TC), is rarely indicated. If the diagnosis remains uncertain after extensive radiographic imaging, a liver biopsy or even a surgical resection for histopathological examination should be performed [1]. A well-sampled core biopsy should be preferred to fine-needle aspiration biopsy (FNAB), since it consents the assessment of both architectural and cytological features and provides tissue for additional testing, including immunohistochemistry (IHC) [5, 10].

E. De Raffele (✉)
Unità Operativa di Chirurgia Generale, Dipartimento dell'Apparato Digerente, Azienda Ospedaliero-Universitaria di Bologna, Policlinico S. Orsola-Malpighi, Bologna, Italy
e-mail: e.deraffele@aosp.bo.it

F. Radu-Ionita et al. (eds.), *Liver Diseases*, https://doi.org/10.1007/978-3-030-24432-3_30

Key Concepts
- Benign liver tumours are a heterogeneous group of solid or cystic focal liver lesions deriving from different cell types. Solid benign liver tumours may have hepatocellular, biliary, vascular and mesenchymal origin, respectively. Cystic liver lesions represent a miscellaneous group of disorders, including simple cysts, polycystic disease, parasitic cysts, neoplastic cysts, and duct related cysts.
- An accurate evaluation of FLL is essential to identify primary liver malignancies at an early, potentially curable stage. Radiological evaluation is the most important issue, and includes US, CEUS, CT and MRI.

30.2 Focal Nodular Hyperplasia

30.2.1 Introduction and Epidemiology

Focal nodular hyperplasia, also known as benign hepatoma, focal or lobar cirrhosis, hepatic hamartoma, hamartomatous cholangiohepatoma, hepatic pseudotumor, solitary hyperplastic nodule, is a benign, usually polyclonal, epithelial liver tumour characterized by nodular hyperplasia of liver parenchyma in a fibrous meshwork around a central scar containing an aberrant artery. It usually develops in otherwise normal liver parenchyma, and is considered as a proliferative cell response to arterial malformation [1, 3, 6–8].

It is the second most common benign lesion of the liver, after hemangioma, with a prevalence of 0.3–3.0% in autopsy series and of 0.2–1.6% at imaging series [5, 6]. FNH is seen predominantly in women, with a male:female ratio of 1:8 or 1:9, between 20 and 50 years of age [1, 7, 8]; however it has been observed throughout the age spectrum, including children [6]. FNHs are usually solitary, multiple in 20–30% of cases, and measure less than 5 cm, but may be larger. They are often associated with liver haemangiomas, less frequently with hepatic adenomas [1, 3, 6].

FNH may be responsive to estrogens [8, 11]. The higher prevalence in women and the evidence that FNH is usually larger, more vascular, and develop earlier in females suggested that female sex hormones and the use of oral contraceptives (OCPs) might influence tumour evolution; recent studies however did not confirm the role of modern OCPs and of pregnancy in the development or progression of FNH [1, 5–7]. Since this issue remains somewhat controversial, women bearing FNH who wish to continue OCPs treatment should undergo US evaluation every 6–12 months for 2–3 years to monitor any size changes of their tumours [6].

30.2.2 Pathogenesis

FNH is presently considered a regenerative response to hyperperfusion by the anomalous arteries typically found in the center of these lesions (International Working Party 2006 [6, 8]). The hypothesis that FNH derives from congenital vascular anomalies is further supported by its frequent association with other vascular malformations, including cavernous HHs, hereditary hemorrhagic telangiectasia (Osler-Weber-Rendu disease), hemihypertrophy and vascular malformations (Klippel-Trénaunay-Weber syndrome). FNHs with similar features at CT and MR imaging have been reported in identical twins, supporting a potential pathogenetic role of congenital vascular anomalies and also a possible genetic predisposition to these lesions [12].

30.2.3 Pathology

The gross appearance of a typical FNH is that of a firm, well-demarcated but not encapsulated lesion. Well-developed and sizable nodules have a lobulated appearance with a central or eccentric stellate fibrous scar. Fibrous bands extend outward from this scar and surround parenchymal nodules [1, 6, 13]. The central scar contains an aberrant large artery with multiple branches radiating through the fibrous septa to the periphery and draining into adjacent hepatic veins; this radiating pattern of the arterial branches determines the "spoke-wheel" appearance typically seen on angiography and on contrast-enhanced imaging techniques [6].

Histologically, FNH is composed of normal appearing hepatocytes arranged into multiple small nodules or cords usually partially delineated by the fibrous septa originating from the central scar. Fibrous septa contain large dystrophic vessels with eccentrically thickened walls. Various degrees of ductular proliferation and inflammatory cells are frequently present at the interface between fibrous septa and parenchymal nodules [1, 8, 13]. The minimal microscopic key features for the diagnosis of classical FNH are nodular architecture, abnormal vessels, and proliferation of bile ductules [14]. Sinusoids and Kupffer cells are typically present, and help to distinguish FNH from HCAs, which generally do not have bile ducts and Kupffer cells [14].

Atypical forms of FNH are frequent and include FNH without a central scar, which is usually absent in lesions smaller than 3 cm; FNH with significant steatosis, focal or diffuse; with cytologic atypia resembling dysplasia of large cell type; with areas of sinusoidal dilatation; subtle FNH, that defines lesions at an early stage of development that may lack some key features [1, 13, 14]. Telangiectatic FNH has been shown to be a variant of the inflammatory HCA. Multiple FNHs are generally observed in patients with underlying vascular liver diseases, including Budd-Chiari syndrome, obliterative portal venopathy and congenital disorders, such as hereditary haemorrhagic telangiectasia and portal vein agenesis [1].

The diagnosis of FNH is usually made on a hematoxylin and eosin (H&E) stain, in resected specimen or in a liver biopsy, when the key features are present. IHC staining for glutamine synthetase (GS) is distinctive of FNH and permits a definite differentiation from other hepatocellular nodules [6, 15]; large hepatocytic areas expressing GS are usually sited around hepatic veins, whereas hepatocytes close to fibrous septa containing vessels, inflammatory cells, and ductules, do not express GS; thus, areas over-expressing GS are in the periphery of the nodules and have a characteristic "map-like" pattern, that is found in all types of FNH, whether classical or atypical [15]. IHC staining for keratin 7 or 19 may be useful to demonstrate the associated ductular reaction [13]. IHC staining for β-catenin is normal, since it remains normally expressed on the hepatocyte membranes.

30.2.4 Clinical Features

FNHs are usually asymptomatic and discovered incidentally, but about 20–40% may present with symptoms [1, 5–7]. Larger tumours may present as an abdominal mass, sometimes symptomatic (epigastric and abdominal pain), and may rarely compress vessels, the biliary tree, or adjacent organs, such as the stomach. FNHs have no risk of malignant transformation, and hemorrhage, necrosis, or infarction are exceptional [6, 7]. Liver tests are most often normal, but mild elevation of gamma-glutamyl transferase (GGT) and alkaline phosphatise (ALP) levels might be observed if large FNH causes extrinsic compression of intrahepatic biliary ducts [7]. Serum levels of alpha-fetoprotein (AFP) are normal.

30.2.5 Diagnosis

A confident diagnosis can usually be achieved through a combination of imaging techniques that evidence the typical features of FNH [1, 5–8], and usually permit the differential diagnosis with other solid benign tumours, including HCA, large regenerative nodules, sometimes hemangioma, and malignant tumours, including HCC, fibrolamellar carcinoma, and hypervascular metastases. FNH is usually slightly hypo or isoechoic, rarely hyperechoic at US; sometimes only the presence of a pseudocapsule, due to compression of the surrounding hepatic tissue or vessels, may suggest the presence of the tumour; the central scar is visualized in a minority of cases; on Power Doppler ultrasound central arteries may have the typical "spoke-wheel" pattern. CEUS has significantly improved characterization of FNH [6], and usually shows a lesion with strong and homogeneous enhancement on arterial phase, with a central vascular supply, which becomes similar to adjacent liver parenchyma on portal and delayed phases [1, 6, 16].

At CT scan, FNH may be hypo or isodense on non-contrast imaging, with an evident central scar in a minority of patients, shows a strong and homogeneous enhancement on arterial phase, resulting hyperdense compared to the surrounding parenchyma, and becomes generally isodense during the portal venous and delayed phases, although the central scar may become hyperdense as contrast diffuses into the scar [1, 7, 16].

At MR imaging, FNH is typically isointense or slightly hypointense on T1w images and slightly hyperintense or isointense on T2w images; the central scar is typically hypointense on T1w images and hyperintense on T2w images, due to vessels or edema; at gadolinium-enhanced imaging, the tumour shows intense homogeneous enhancement during the arterial phase, except for the central scar, and becomes isointense or occasionally slightly hyperintense to the surrounding liver parenchyma during the portal venous and delayed phases, while the central scar enhances on delayed phase because of the slower diffusion of the contrast medium through the fibrous tissue. MRI has the highest sensitivity among imaging techniques and a specificity of almost 100% for the diagnosis of FNH [1, 7]; its sensitivity is lower for smaller tumours without the central scar; in these cases, combination of CEUS and MRI provides the highest diagnostic accuracy [1, 7, 16]. The use of the HPB-specific MR contrast agents Gd-BOPTA and Gd-EOB-DTPA has further improved MR imaging of the liver [6]; FNH is composed of functional hepatocytes with abnormal bile ductules, and is expected to accumulate HPB-specific contrast agents, while HCA does not contain bile ductules and is supposed not to accumulate such contrast agents [17]. At MRI with HPB-specific contrast agents, FNH shows early arterial enhancement, which persists during delayed phases to a greater degree than in the surrounding normal liver because of the presence of normal hepatocytes and abnormal bile ductules; most FNHs are iso or hyperintense during the delayed hepatobiliary phase; on the contrary, HCAs are classically hypointense relative to liver during the hepatobiliary phase [7, 18, 19]. The sensitivity of MRI with HPB-specific contrast agents approaches 90%, and the sensitivity and specificity to differentiate FNH from HCA ranges from 92 to 97% and from 91 to 100%, respectively [1, 17–19]. FNH can have unusual features at MRI in presence of steatosis, focal or diffuse, so mimicking HCA, or if there is an atypical scar [7].

30.2.6 Treatment

FNHs are usually asymptomatic and stable over time [6], without malignant transformation and with rare complications [1, 8]. Asymptomatic patients where the diagnosis of FNH is reasonably definite should be managed conservatively [1, 7]. Monitoring the tumour every 3–6 months after the initial diagnosis is usually sufficient to confirm that the tumour is stable. Enlargement of FNH is exceptional, usually in patients that use OCPs and during pregnancy. OCPs can be maintained with appropriate follow-up imaging studies [7]. Only large FNHs may represent a risk for pregnancy and should be considered for liver resection.

If the diagnosis remains unclear, a liver resection should be considered [1, 5, 6, 8]. A liver resection should be also selectively considered for symptomatic tumours, in case of enlargement, and for exophytic or pedunculated tumours [6–8]. Non-surgical therapies, including trans-arterial embolization (TAE) and radiofrequency thermal ablation (RFTA), should be considered in patients unfit for surgery [1, 5–7].

Key Concepts

- FNH is a benign epithelial liver tumour which usually develops in otherwise normal liver parenchyma. It is predominant in women, mostly between 20 and 50 years of age. The role of female sex hormones and of OCPs is uncertain.
- Histologically, FNHs are composed of normal appearing hepatocytes arranged into nodular architecture, with abnormal vessels, and proliferation of bile ductules; sinusoids and Kupffer cells are typically present. Atypical forms of FNH are frequent. Multiple FNHs are generally observed in patients with underlying vascular liver diseases.
- FNHs are usually asymptomatic and discovered incidentally; 20–40% of patients may present with symptoms. FNHs have no risk of malignant transformation, and complications are exceptional.
- A confident diagnosis can mostly be achieved through a combination of imaging techniques, including CEUS, CT and MRI. Contrast-enhanced MRI has the highest sensitivity and specificity among imaging techniques.
- FNHs are usually asymptomatic and stable over time and should be managed conservatively. A liver resection should be considered if the diagnosis remains unclear, in case of enlargement, symptomatic tumours, and exophytic or pedunculated tumours.

30.3 Hepatocellular Adenoma

30.3.1 Introduction and Epidemiology

Hepatocellular adenoma, also known as liver cell adenoma, liver adenoma and benign hepatoma, is a benign monoclonal epithelial liver tumour that develops in otherwise normal liver parenchyma, usually related to metabolic or hormonal abnormalities [5, 6]. HCA is rare, with an estimated prevalence between 0.001% and 0.004%, predominantly found in women of child bearing age, with a reported female:male ratio of 10:1, solitary in most cases but sometimes multifocal, and usually asymptomatic [1, 5–7]. Liver adenomatosis is defined by the presence of more than ten HCAs in the liver [20], based on the number of tumours identified at imaging studies. Since larger adenomas have a significant risk of spontaneous rupture and haemorrhage, and also of malignant transformation, differentiation from other nodular lesions of the liver is essential [5].

30.3.2 Etiology and Incidence

HCAs are associated with the use of OCPs, anabolic androgens, less frequently with pregnancy. The incidence of HCAs raised in the last decades in young women coinciding with the introduction of OCPs [6, 7]. HCAs are larger, more numerous, and at higher risk of rupture and bleeding in patients who take OCPs [21], their development correlates with the dose and duration of hormonal treatment [7], may regress after discontinuation of OCPs and also recur during readministration or pregnancy [6].

The use of anabolic steroids, typically in young men, has been associated with the development of HCAs [1, 6, 7], which frequently disappear after treatment discontinuation [22]; as for OCPs, androgens seem to predispose to multiple tumours [22]. Individuals with high levels of endogenous estrogens and androgens are also at risk of developing HCA [1, 6, 7].

The increased prevalence in men has been associated with the rising prevalence of obesity and metabolic syndrome [1, 5, 23]. Obesity and clinical features of the metabolic syndrome, including diabetes, insulin resistance, dyslipidemia and hypertension, have been recently recognized as significant risk factors for the development of HCAs [24, 25], and seem to promote either the development or the progression of HCAs [24]. Obesity and metabolic syndrome in association with OCPs use determine an increased risk for the development of HCAs in women [24, 25]. Nonetheless, the prevalence of malignant transformation of HCAs is ten times more likely in males, especially in patients bearing a metabolic syndrome [26]. Obesity and the metabolic syndrome are becoming the dominant risk factors for HCA [7].

Patients with type I, III and IV glycogen storage diseases (GSD) have a significant lifelong risk of developing HCA [1, 5, 6, 23], with a 2:1 male:female ratio and a substantial increase of the incidence in patients >25 years of age [5, 6]; HCAs in GSD patients are usually of the inflammatory subtype, and may regress following adequate dietary regimens and metabolic control [1, 5, 6].

Less frequent are the association with maturity onset diabetes type 3 (MODY3), iron overload due to β-thalassemia or hemochromatosis, and some rare hepatic vascular abnormalities [1, 5, 7, 23]. Regardless of these multiple risk factors, otherwise healthy patients—both male and female—with no history of use of OCPs or anabolic androgenic steroids, without obesity and metabolic syndrome and without other underlying metabolic conditions may develop HCAs [6].

30.3.3 Pathology

HCAs are solitary in 70–80% of the cases, with size varying from few millimeters to several centimeters. They are soft and well demarcated, but without a fibrous capsule. The tumours may appear lighter or darker than the surrounding liver tissue [1, 27]. Large blood vessels are often present on the surface and within the tumour, frequently with areas of hemorrhage and necrosis [1, 23]. Since they have no capsule, hemorrhagic foci within the tumour can easily extend into the surrounding normal liver.

Microscopically, HCAs are composed of large plates of benign hepatocytes, of normal size or larger than normal hepatocytes [1, 13]. Their cytoplasm can be either normal or contain glycogen and lipids. The nuclei are small and regular, and mitoses are very uncommon. Nuclear atypia, mitoses and acinar growth patterns are remarkably rare; if present, the differential diagnosis with very well-differentiated HCC may be very difficult [23]. The normal hepatic architecture is absent, with the adenomatous cells arranged in normal or thickened trabeculae supplied by thin-walled arteries and sinusoids without satellite bile ductules. Regular septa and portal tracts are absent. Kupffer cells may be present, but are rare and nonfunctional, so that most adenomas cannot take up technetium Tc-99m sulfur colloid.

30.3.4 Genotype and Phenotype Classification

Based on the underlying gene mutations, the molecular classification of HCAs has evolved with time [13, 23, 28], and has been recently updated in six subgroups [20, 29]: (1) hepatocyte nuclear factor 1α (HNF1 α)-inactivated HCA (H-HCA) (30–35%); (2) inflammatory HCA (IHCA), with multiple mutated genes, mainly IL6 (30–35%); (3) β-catenin-activated HCA mutated in exon 3 (β-catenin HCA exon 3) (7%); (4) β-catenin-activated HCA mutated in exon 7–8 (β-catenin HCA exon 7–8) (3%); (5) sonic hedgehog HCA (shHCA) (4%); (6) unclassified (not otherwise specified) HCAs (UHCAs) (7%). About 50% of β-catenin-mutated HCAs (either in exon 3 or in exon 7–8) are also inflammatory. Risk factors, histology, imaging and clinical features related to the different subgroups have been recently reviewed [20, 23, 29]. HCAs, especially β-catenin-mutated HCAs, have malignant potential and can evolve into HCC [23], while shHCA are associated with bleeding [20, 29]. In clinical practice, H&E stain combined with IHC usually allows appropriate classification [13, 20, 29], while molecular biology analysis is reserved to cases where interpretation is uncertain [28].

H-HCAs. Are associated with inactivation of HNF-1α, a transcription factor implied in hepatocyte differentiation and metabolism control [1]; HNF-1α mutations are usually of somatic origin and in a minority of cases of germline origin; patients with germline mutations of HNF1A are younger, frequently have a family history of liver adenomatosis and sometimes have clinical diabetes, usually the MODY3. H-HCAs have a yellowish gross appearance. At histology are characterized by the presence of diffuse steatosis without cytologic abnormalities or inflammatory infiltrates; at IHC adenomatous cells do not express the liver fatty acid binding protein (LFABP), which is normally expressed by the surrounding normal hepatocytes; in case of adenomatosis, multiple nodules of H-HCA of different size coexist with numerous steatotic micronodules.

I-HCAs. Represent a heterogeneous subgroup of HCA with respect to the variety of gene mutations, all resulting in the activation of the JAK/STAT pathway [30]. I-HCA are usually observed in patients with obesity, metabolic syndrome, high alcohol consumption. Systemic inflammatory syndrome, evidenced by increased levels of serum C-reactive protein (CRP) and fibrinogen, can regress after the removal of the tumour [1]. Histology shows inflammatory infiltrates, with dystrophic arteries and sinusoidal dilatation; the inflammatory infiltrates are focally distributed within the tumour and contain mainly mononuclear cells, lymphocytes and histiocytes, with few polymorphonuclear cells and plasma cells; at IHC adenomatous cells express acute phase inflammatory proteins such as serum amyloid protein A (SAA) and CRP. This subgroup includes the telangiectatic HCA (THCA), previously classified as telangiectatic FNH [6]; the development of THCA has been associated with OCPs use, hormonal treatments and obesity [5, 6]; similarly to HCAs, THCAs are likely to be symptomatic, may contain focal necrosis and are predisposed to rupture and bleeding; their potential of malignant transformation is unknown; as a consequence, these adenomas should be routinely considered for surgical resection [5, 6].

β-catenin-mutated HCAs. Are characterized by β-catenin activation within the tumour cells due to mutations of the β-catenin gene (CTNNB1). β-HCA are more frequent in males and have an increased potential for malignant transformation in HCC [1]. At histology show frequent cytologic abnormalities, pseudo-glandular formation, and sometimes cholestasis; because of the cytologic and architectural abnormalities, the differential diagnosis with well-differentiated HCC may be difficult in some cases; moreover, these tumours are more frequently associated with unequivocal HCC; at IHC adenomatous cells have various degrees of cytoplasmic expression of GS and of aberrant nuclear and cytoplasmic positivity of β-catenin.

shHCAs. At histology often contain haemorrhagic foci; for this subgroup no specific IHC markers are presently available.

Unclassified HCAs. Account for 5–10% of HCA. These tumours do not have any of the gene mutations previously described and do not show peculiar morphological features [1]; this group includes tumours with such an extensive necrosis and/or hemorrhage to prevent a correct characterization.

The available combinations of antibodies for immunostaining (LFABP, GS, β-catenin, SAA/CRP) can subtype the majority of HCA, however at present routine molecular subtyping of HCAs is not recommended [1].

30.3.5 Clinical Features

Most of HCA are diagnosed in young women with a history of prolonged OCPs use. The clinical presentation of HCA is extremely variable. These tumours are often symptomatic [5, 6], but are usually incidentally discovered during abdominal imaging for unrelated causes, inflammatory syndrome, or liver function test abnormalities [7]. Symptomatic tumours typically cause abdominal pain localized to the epigastrium or right upper quadrant, which may reflect an enlarged liver, intratumoral bleeding or necrosis. Less commonly an abdominal mass is found on clinical examination. About one-third of patients with I-HCA have an inflammatory syndrome with fever [7]. Spontaneous rupture and intraperitoneal bleeding present as a sudden, severe pain associated with hypotension, and is fatal in up to 20% if not diagnosed and appropriately treated [21]. HCAs have been associated with an increased risk of bleeding in the presence of abdominal pain, a history of long duration of OCPs use, tumour size larger than 35–50 mm, visualization of lesional arteries, exophytic tumour and subcapsular location [1, 7, 31]. Jaundice has been sometimes reported. Liver function test abnormalities are rare and usually associated with large tumours [7]. Serum AFP is normal in the absence of malignant transformation. During its natural evolution, HCA may increase in size, remain stable, or even regress; regression is more frequent in adenomas related to androgenic-anabolic steroids after hormone withdrawal, and in glycogenosis after an appropriate dietary regimen.

Risk of malignant transformation. Malignant transformation of HCAs to HCC is well known, but is considered quite rare [1, 7]. It has been more frequently associated with tumour diameter >5 cm, independent of the subtype, and with male sex, androgenic-anabolic steroid exposure, glycogenosis type I and familial adenomatous polyposis; all these conditions are usually associated with β-catenin-mutated HCAs. This subtype determines a higher risk of developing HCC in men. Prevalence of HCC within HCA is 10 times more frequent in men than in women, and the metabolic syndrome seem to predispose to malignant transformation of HCA in men [1, 26]. HCA harboring CTNNB1 mutations have an increased potential for malignant transformation; however CTNNB1 mutations are important events in clonal benign hepatocellular tumorigenesis, but not *per se* sufficient to determine malignant transformation of HCAs; on the contrary, somatic mutations of the telomerase reverse transcriptase (*TERT*) promoter are not required for clonal benign hepatocellular tumorigenesis, but are critical for malignant transformation of HCA in association with CTNNB1 mutations; it has been suggested that TERT promoter mutations and activation of the Wnt/b-catenin pathway could cooperate to promote malignant hepatocellular transformation [32]. A progressive increase of the tumour size on sequential imaging studies or rising levels of serum AFP suggest malignant transformation. HCCs within adenoma are typically well-differentiated, without vascular invasion or satellite nodules, with normal serum α-fetoprotein levels, and are associated with a favorable prognosis after liver resection [7].

Adenomatosis. Hepatocellular adenomatosis (HCadenomatosis) is defined by the presence of more than ten HCAs in the liver, and was classified as a distinct pathological entity at its first description in 1985 [20]. In the last decade however this distinction has become arbitrary, since numerous studies have demonstrated that all subtypes of HCA can be solitary, multiple <10 or multiple >10, including adenomas associated with administration of androgenic-anabolic steroids and with GSD [5, 6]. Also the management of HCadenomatosis may not differ from solitary or multiple HCAs, even though embolization and liver transplantation are more often indicated because other conventional therapies usually considered for HCAs may be inappropriate or too risky.

The natural history of HCadenomatosis is uncertain because of the limited number of cases reported. Hemorrhage seems to be common, especially for tumours >4 cm with subcapsular location. Also malignant transformation has been well documented. Nonetheless, in patients with multiple HCAs, only tumours >5 cm should be resected [6, 7]. In female patients where the tumours are all <5 cm, pathological confirmation is not required, surgery is usually not indicated and a regular follow-up is an appropriate strategy [7].

30.3.6 Diagnosis

The diagnosis is often difficult and is based upon the clinical setting, imaging studies, and/or surgical resection. When a HCA is suspected, percutaneous liver biopsy or FNAB should be avoided because of the significant risk of bleeding following biopsy [5, 6], and also because the tissue obtained is not rarely insufficient to accomplish a definite diagnosis. Common diagnostic dilemmas are FNH and HCC [16]. Multiple imaging procedures may be required to achieve a definite diagnosis, including US, CT and MRI, which is the modality of choice to characterize the different subtypes of HCA [33, 34]. The presence of intratumoral necrosis and/or hemorrhage may help characterization. When the diagnosis remains uncertain, surgical resection may be selectively indicated, and is at the same time the most appropriate therapeutic option.

HCAs are usually first detected by US. However, sonographic features are usually non-specific and may mimic other benign or malignant liver tumours. HCAs may appear as a well demarcated and hyperechoic lesion due to the high intralesional fat content, but can also be heterogeneous because of intratumoral necrosis and/or hemorrhage. CEUS may help refine the diagnosis in selected cases; HCA usually shows homogeneous contrast enhancement in the arterial phase, usually with rapid complete centripetal enhancement; in the early portal venous phase, the tumour usually becomes isoechoic but may remain slightly hyperechoic [16, 34].

At CT scan, HCAs often have intralesional areas of necrosis, hemorrhage, or fibrosis, giving them a heterogeneous appearance. H-HCAs are typically well demarcated hypodense lesions on non-enhanced CT; on contrast-enhanced CT scans they show variable grade of enhancement during the arterial phase and rapid washout during the portal venous and the late dynamic phases [16]. I-HCAs are heterogeneously hypodense on non-enhanced CT, sometimes with hyperdense areas due to recent intralesional bleeding; on contrast-enhanced CT scans typically show intense arterial enhancement with persistent enhancement in the delayed phase [16]. β-catenin-mutated HCAs have less specific characteristics, and are heterogeneously hypo or isodense on non-enhanced CT; on contrast-enhanced CT scans show arterial enhancement and portal venous or delayed washout, with sometimes heterogeneous content [16].

MR imaging is currently the procedure of choice to characterize HCAs and the respective subtypes [16, 33, 34]. The specific MR imaging features vary on the basis of histopathology, and are related to intralesional fat distribution, sinusoidal dilatation and the eventually associated complications. The two most common complications of HCAs are the intratumoral bleeding, sometimes associated with rupture and intraperitoneal bleeding, and the malignant transformation into HCC; as mentioned above, different subtypes of adenoma have variable complication rates [16, 33]. H-HCAs appear homogeneous on MRI; are predominantly hyper or isointense on T1w images; the diffuse and homogeneous signal drop-off on chemical shift T1w sequences is peculiar of this subtype because of the presence of intralesional steatosis; have a variable signal on T2w sequences, usually slightly hyperintense on non-fat suppressed sequence and iso or hypointense on fat suppressed T2w sequences; on gadolinium-enhanced T1w images show intense enhancement during the arterial phase, that persists in the portal venous and delayed phases [16, 33]; using the diffuse and homogeneous signal drop-off on chemical shift T1w sequences, the sensitivity and specificity of MRI to diagnose H-HCA range from 87% to 91% and from 89% to 100%, respectively [1, 7]. I-HCAs are isointense or mildly hyperintense on T1w images, with minimal or no signal drop-off with chemical shift sequence, and diffusely hyperintense on T2w images, with higher signal intensity at the periphery of the tumour due to dilated sinusoids; on gadolinium-enhanced T1w images usually show intense enhancement during the arterial phase, that persists in the portal venous and delayed phases [16, 33]; in the presence of diffuse hyperintensity on T2w images and persistent contrast enhancement on delayed phase determine, the sensitivity and specificity of MRI to diagnose I-HCA range from 85% to 88% and from 88% to 100%, respectively [1, 7]. β-catenin-mutated HCAs have less specific MR imaging patterns and may show hypointense signal on T1w sequences and homogeneous or heterogeneous hyperintense signal on T2w sequences, depending on the presence of intralesional necrosis and/or hemorrhage; on gadolinium-enhanced T1w images usually show intense enhancement during the arterial phase, that may or may not persist on the portal venous and delayed phases [1, 16, 33]; these subtype of adenoma may mimic HCC at imaging. MRI with HPB-specific MR contrast agents can help differentiate between HCAs and FNH [6, 17].

Nuclear imaging with Technetium Tc-99m sulfur colloid may be helpful in the differential diagnosis with FNH. As mentioned above, HCAs may contain Kupffer cells, but usually in small numbers and generally nonfunctional [35]. As a consequence, most adenomas do not take up technetium Tc-99m sulfur colloid and the scintigram shows a "cold" spot within the liver; however some adenomas take up the technetium Tc-99m sulfur colloid and are indistinguishable from FNH at nuclear imaging.

30.3.7 Treatment

The natural history and prognosis of HCAs varies according to the different subtypes and to the clinical context. Treatment strategies are related to the certainty of the diagnosis, the presence of symptoms, the size, number and location of the tumour(s), and to the risk of complications, including hemorrhage and malignant transformation. Actually, the treatment of HCAs may require more aggressive therapeutic strategies than for most other benign hepatic tumours [5, 6]. Asymptomatic HCAs <5 cm can be managed conservatively since the risk of rupture or malignant transformation is very low [5, 6, 23]. However, HCAs diagnosed in men have a significantly higher risk of malignant transformation and should be resected irrespective of size [26]. In women, HCAs <5 cm have a very low risk of rupture or malignant transformation; thus discontinuation of OCPs and control of body weight, along with monitoring the tumour(s) with MRI, may represent an appropriate strategy [6, 7].

Patients with symptoms referable to the adenoma should receive surgical resection. Also asymptomatic patients with tumours persistently >5 cm or growing in size at reassessments after baseline imaging should be considered for resection [1, 7]. Spontaneous rupture with hemorrhage has been reported in 11–29% of HCAs cases, usually (but not exclusively) in lesions >5 cm [5, 6, 36]. In case of rupture with active bleeding, a temporaneous conservative management to achieve hemodynamic stability and avoid emergent liver resection is suggested, since emergent surgery has higher perioperative risks [5, 6]. The appropriate control of the haemorrhage can be obtained with an emergent TAE of the hepatic artery or with surgery, including liver packing, emergent liver resection, or even liver transplantation [5, 6]. TAE is usually effective to control active bleeding and to prevent emergent resection; at follow-up CT scan, TAE may also result in partial or complete regression of the tumour, so that a conservative non-operative approach with MRI surveillance can be considered; in case of persistent HCA tissue in a large-sized lesion, a surgical resection is indicated [6, 7]. Malignant transformation of HCAs into HCCs is relatively rare, with a reported overall frequency of about 4%; it usually occurs in tumours >5 cm, but has been reported also in smaller adenomas [37]. β-catenin-mutated HCAs have the higher risk of malignant transformation and should be routinely considered for surgical resection [5, 23]. TAE is used to manage bleeding HCA and occasionally to reduce tumour size before liver resection; it may represent an alternative to surgery in high risk patients or for tumours in difficult anatomical locations [1, 7, 38, 39]; after TAE complete tumour disappearance has been observed in 10% of patients, and partial regression in 75% [38]. RFTA has been proposed as an alternative to liver resection in selected cases [39], usually for tumours <4 cm [7]. Also liver transplantation may be exceptionally indicated, usually for GSD or multiple adenomas [7].

Discontinuation of OCPs or androgenic-anabolic steroids with close observation of the adenoma(s) with repeated imaging is usually followed by regression of the tumour(s) [6]. Nevertheless, some HCAs may increase in size despite steroid withdrawal, and malignant transformation has been reported despite regression in size [5, 6]. As a consequence, HCAs should be monitored with imaging techniques every 6 months for at least 2 years to define any growth patterns and ascertain malignant transformation, and subsequently with annual imaging in case of tumour stability or regression [5, 6]. Female patients with HCAs should be aware of the potential risks of pregnancy, and should be discouraged from pregnancy in selected cases, since the behavior of adenomas during pregnancy is unpredictable [40], but the risk of tumour growth is substantial [7]. Even though pregnancy is usually not discouraged when lesions are <5 cm [1, 5], tumour resection or ablation prior to pregnancy may represent the best option in selected cases [40]. If an adenoma is incidentally found during pregnancy, a close follow-up is necessary with US every 6–12 weeks to monitor size; growing tumours are associated with an increased risk of rupture; surgical resection should be considered for large or growing symptomatic tumours; surgery performed during the second trimester have limited operative risks for both the mother and the foetus [41].

The clinical presentation, the risk of bleeding and of malignant transformation in patients with adenomatosis are similar to those in patients with a single HCA, and is related to the size of the largest lesion(s), rather than the number of nodules [42]. Regression of tumour burden has been reported, even though in a minority of patients, after significant lifestyle changes, including withdrawal of OCPs or appropriate dietary restrictions with weight loss [42]. The management of patients with multiple HCAs should be based on the size of the largest tumour(s) [1].

Key Concepts

- HCA is a benign monoclonal epithelial liver tumour that develop in otherwise normal liver parenchyma, usually related to metabolic or hormonal abnormalities. HCA is rare, predominantly found in women of child bearing age, solitary in most cases. Liver adenomatosis is defined by the presence of >10 HCAs. Larger adenomas have a significant risk of spontaneous rupture, hemorrhage, and of malignant transformation.
- HCAs are associated with the use of OCPs, anabolic androgens, sometimes with pregnancy. HCAs in men are associated with the rising prevalence of obesity and metabolic syndrome, with higher risk of malignant transformation. HCAs occur also in patients with GSD, MODY3, iron overload, some rare hepatic vascular abnormalities, but also without evident risk factors.
- Histologically, HCAs are composed of large plates of benign hepatocytes without the normal hepatic

architecture. Based on the underlying gene mutations, the molecular classification of HCAs has evolved with time, and has been recently updated in six subgroups.

- HCAs are usually incidentally discovered during abdominal imaging, although these tumours are often symptomatic. Spontaneous rupture and intraperitoneal bleeding may occur and may be fatal if unrecognized. The risk of malignant transformation is quite rare, mostly associated with β-catenin-mutation, tumour diameter of >5 cm, male sex, androgenic-anabolic steroid exposure.
- The diagnosis is often difficult. Multiple imaging procedures may be required. MRI is the modality of choice to characterize the different subtypes of HCA. When a HCA is suspected, percutaneous liver biopsy or FNAB should be avoided because of the significant risk of bleeding.
- Asymptomatic HCAs <5 cm in women can be managed conservatively and monitored with imaging techniques. Liver resection should be routinely considered in male patients, for tumours >5 cm, in symptomatic patients, and in case of tumour enlargement. Spontaneous rupture with hemorrhage should be treated conservatively whenever possible, with emergent TAE, to achieve hemodynamic stability and avoid emergent liver resection. Elective TAE and RFTA should be considered in patients unfit for surgery.
- Female patients with HCAs should be aware of the potential risks of pregnancy, since the risk of tumour growth is substantial. Tumour resection or ablation prior to pregnancy may represent the best option in selected cases.

30.4 Hepatic Hemangioma

30.4.1 Introduction and Epidemiology

Hepatic hemangiomas, also known as cavernous hemangiomas, are the most common benign mesenchymal liver tumours, with an estimated prevalence ranging from 0.4% to 20% [1, 5, 7, 8, 43]; the highest estimates have been derived from autopsy series; HHs are increasingly recognized in asymptomatic patients undergoing radiologic imaging evaluation of the abdomen for aspecific abdominal complaints; US studies have placed the frequency at 0.7–1.5% [6]. They can be diagnosed at any age, in most cases in patients between 30 and 50 years. In adults, the female:male ratio ranges from 1.2:1 to 6:1 [1, 5, 43]. HHs are often solitary, but multiple lesions are not unfrequent. They are small, less than 4–5 cm, in most cases, but may also reach 20 cm in diameter [1, 7, 43]. HHs >4 cm have been termed giant hemangiomas. An accurate differential diagnosis is often required in patients at risk of primary or metastatic malignant liver tumours, including cirrhotics and patients with primary tumours potentially metastasizing to the liver.

30.4.2 Pathogenesis

The etiology of HHs is incompletely understood. They are regarded as congenital vascular malformations or hamartomas, possibly with hormonal dependence [1]. Hormonal influence over tumour behavior is suggested by its growth during pregnancy and estrogen and progesterone based therapies, with possible regression after withdrawal [6]; nonetheless, tumour growth has been reported also in the absence of hormonal therapy and in postmenopausal women [5, 6].

30.4.3 Pathology

HHs are single or multiple tumours, with a variable size from a few millimeters to over 20 cm, well demarcated and often surrounded by a thin capsule. They are located either deeply or in the periphery of liver, and may infrequently be pedunculated. On gross examination, hemangiomas are well delineated; the cut surface is red-brown and spongy, with cystic or honeycomb patterns; areas of thrombosis, hemorrhage, scarring, and, occasionally, calcifications, may be present, especially in larger tumours, suggesting regressive changes; sometimes the entire lesion may be sclerosed (sclerosed hemangioma) [1, 44].

Microscopically, cavernous HHs are composed of cavernous vascular spaces of varied sizes, lined by a single layer of flattened endothelium, separated by thin fibrous septae [7, 44]. Larger tumours may contain collagenous scars or fibrous nodules, and rarely also focal stromal calcifications. Fresh and organizing fibrin thrombi may also be evident. Smaller cavernous HHs are in most cases well delineated from the surrounding liver parenchyma with a distinct fibrous interface; however, Zimmermann and Baer in giant hemangiomas (defined as >4 cm) described four different interface patterns: fibrous, interdigitating, compression, and irregular/spongy [45]; in larger lesions, lesional dilated vascular spaces filled with blood, termed hemangioma-like vessels, may extend into the adjacent parenchyma 0.1–2.0 cm beyond the margins of the main tumour [46].

30.4.4 Clinical Features

HHs are typically discovered incidentally during an imaging test performed for unrelated conditions [5–7]. Symptoms occur in 11–14% of cases [6], mostly in larger tumours, usually abdominal pain and discomfort or fullness at the right upper quadrant; some patients refer nausea, vomiting, anorexia, dyspepsia, and early satiety, usually related to large hemangiomas compressing adjacent organs [5, 6]. Acute thrombosis or bleeding within the tumour may cause acute abdominal pain; moreover, giant HHs have a low but relevant risk of rupture and intraperitoneal bleeding, particularly when peripherally located and exophytic [47]. Physical examination is usually unremarkable, but occasionally show a palpable mass [6, 7]. Liver function tests are usually normal [6, 7]. Alpha-fetoprotein is normal.

In children giant HHs have been associated with high-output cardiac failure [48]. Cutaneous hemangiomas in children may be a marker for hepatic hemangiomas [49]. The Kasabach-Merritt syndrome (KMS) is an infrequent but potentially fatal complication of giant HHs in children, characterized by thrombocytopenia and consumption coagulopathy [1, 5–7]. It may exceptionally occur also in adults [1, 7]. Symptoms disappear after tumour removal [7]. KMS may complicate haemangiomas of any site, especially those larger than 5 cm, particularly the tufted angioma and the kaposiform hemangioendothelioma [1].

The natural history of HHs is incompletely understood. Progression rates in different series range from 18% to 39% over 1–10 years of follow-up [43, 50]. The risk of spontaneous rupture is low but relevant, up to 3%, particularly when peripherally located and exophytic [47]. Traumatic rupture following blunt abdominal trauma is also rare. Iatrogenic rupture or intratumoral bleeding have been reported following liver biopsy or FNAB; thus liver biopsy is rarely considered for diagnostic confirmation.

30.4.5 Diagnosis

HHs have specific features that can suggest the diagnosis on US, CT or MRI [1, 5–7]. In a minority of cases the tumour(s) are atypical and may require multiple imaging tests to define diagnosis. MRI is considered the best imaging technique, with sensitivity and specificity of 84% and 100%, respectively [16]. At US examination, HHs typically appear as a well delineated, homogeneous, hyperechoic mass [8], but may be hypoechoic in patients with liver steatosis, due to the bright signal from the surrounding liver tissue. Color Doppler identifies blood flow within the tumour in a minority of cases, and thus has limited diagnostic value. US findings are also related to the size of HHs: tumours >5 cm usually show mixed echogenicity because of intratumoral thrombosis and fibrosis [1, 8, 43]. In case of incidental lesions with US features atypical of HHs, further evaluation is recommended, with confirmatory contrast-enhanced CT or MRI. If US diagnoses a HH with typical appearance, recommendations regarding the appropriate follow-up are somewhat conflicting, ranging from confirmatory contrast-enhanced CT or MRI to repeat US after a time interval. Since the US appearances of HHs may coincide, at least in part, with those of HCC and liver metastases, the appropriate strategy of follow-up should depend upon the single patient risk of primary or metastatic liver malignancy. We suggest that all patients with a history of liver disease (i.e. chronic hepatitis, liver cirrhosis, etc.) or known or suspected extrahepatic malignancy should receive a validating contrast-enhanced CT or MRI. Patients without evidence of liver disease or extrahepatic malignancy and typical US appearances, may alternatively repeat US examination at 3–6 months, to exclude changes in size and morphology. At CEUS examination, HHs typically have a peripheral globular contrast enhancement in the early phase, that becomes larger in later phases; this typical pattern has been described in 74% of cases [51].

At unenhanced CT scan HHs appear as a well delineated hypodense lesion; larger lesions may contain calcifications; in patients with hepatic steatosis the tumour may appear as hyperdense relative to the surrounding liver parenchyma. The administration of contrast typically determines a peripheral nodular or globular enhancement in the arterial phase, with a centripetal progression or "filling in" in the portal venous and delayed phases [16]; this pattern is observed in up to 94% of HHs >4 cm; an enhancement pattern isodense to the aorta and blood vessels is observed in 67% of the cases and is useful to distinguish HHs from liver metastases. HHs typically opacify after a delay of three or more minutes and remain isodense or hyperdense on delayed scans [8]. Larger tumours, usually giant HHs >4–5 cm, may show a residual central hypodense portion, due to the presence of cystic areas or scar tissue.

MR imaging is at present the most accurate technique for diagnostic confirmation of suspected HH [1, 16], especially for tumours <3 cm [6]. The typical MRI appearance is a homogeneous mass with smooth, well-defined margins, hypointense on T1w images and markedly hyperintense on T2w images [7, 16]; areas of intratumoral fibrosis result hypointense on T2w images. Administration of extracellular contrast agents, as the gadolinium diethylenetriaminepentaacetic acid (Gd-DTPA), determines early peripheral discontinuous nodular or globular enhancement of the tumour in the arterial phase, with progressive centripetal enhancement or "filling in" in the portal venous and delayed phases; this pattern of contrast enhancement is typical of HHs >2 cm. Smaller high-flow hemangiomas usually show a hypervascular pattern, with uniform enhancement in the early arterial phase images, which may persist in the portal venous and delayed phases [52]; small hemangiomas with rapid and uniform enhancement may be difficult to distinguish from HCC or hypervascular metastases [16].

Diffusion-weighted (DW) MRI evaluates the attenuation of T2w signal based on how easily water molecules are able to diffuse in the liver tumour and surrounding parenchima, and is considered useful to characterize focal liver lesions, especially cystic tumours and HHs, if they show high signal intensity on both T2w and b 0 s/mm^2, with a progressive and strong decrease with increasing b-values; as a consequence, the apparent diffusion co-efficient (ADC) value is high [1, 7, 16].

Planar scintigraphy and Single-photon emission CT (SPECT) with Technetium-99m pertechnetate-labeled red blood cell (99mTc-RBC) typically show hypoperfusion during the early arterial phase, followed by gradual radioactivity "fill in" that peaks at 30–50 min from injection; radioactivity usually remains within the tumour in the delayed phases [53]; sensitivity and specificity for lesions >2 cm reach 92% and almost 100%, respectively; SPECT with 99mTc-RBC further increases sensitivity and accuracy for lesions >1 cm [53].

The role of percutaneous needle biopsy or FNAB when the diagnosis is still uncertain after complete imaging, is still being debated, due to the risk of bleeding [5, 6], especially for larger tumours with subcapsular location; nevertheless, if the tumour is surrounded by a cuff of normal hepatic parenchyma, needle biopsy is not contraindicated and may allow a definite diagnosis in most cases [1, 7].

30.4.6 Treatment

HHs are most often small tumours discovered incidentally; they are usually asymptomatic, and do not grow or develop complications, even though may change in size over time [43, 50]. Asymptomatic patients with a first diagnosis of typical hemangioma at US <5 cm and at low risk (i.e. without chronic liver disease or primary tumours potentially metastasizing to the liver), should repeat imaging within 3–6 months, to confirm diagnosis and size stability. Patients with larger lesions may experience progressive tumour growth, sometimes rapid, and should receive periodic re-evaluation, every 6–12 months, with appropriate imaging techniques, TC or MRI. Asymptomatic patients with HHs surrounded by normal liver parenchyma and without changes in size should receive a conservative treatment [5–7]. The impact of OCPs use or pregnancy in uncertain, since the role of estrogens on the development or growth of on HHSs is poorly understood [5, 6]. As a consequence, pregnancy and the use of OCPs usually are not contraindicated in case of stable asymptomatic tumours [1, 7]. HHs have mostly an indolent course and complications are rare in tumours <10 cm; even though enlargement is not unusual, spontaneous intratumoral or intraperitoneal bleeding are rare [47]. Patients who complain of pain or symptoms suggestive of compression of adjacent organs should be considered for surgical resection [5]. However, other possible causes of pain should be excluded prior to surgery [6]. Liver resection is rarely indicated, usually in patients with uncertain diagnosis, with large lesions determining severe symptoms (including KMS), with tumours enlarging, exophytic, pedunculated or extensively exposed on liver surface, or exceptionally with rupture and intraperitoneal bleeding [1, 5]. HHs can be resected safely by either enucleation or anatomic resection [7]; enucleation however can preserve normal liver parenchyma and has been associated with lower incidence of perioperative complications [6]. TAE has been used to manage symptomatic tumours, as an emergent procedure to treat acute bleeding, or electively either prior to surgical resection to shrink giant HHs and limit the perioperative bleeding, or as an alternative to surgery in selected patients [1]. Also orthotopic liver transplantation has been successfully performed to treat symptomatic patients with unresectable giant HHs, including those associated with KMS [1, 6, 7].

Key Concepts

- HHs are the most common benign mesenchymal liver tumours, increasingly recognized in asymptomatic patients undergoing radiologic imaging evaluation. HHs can be diagnosed at any age, mostly in patients of 30–50 years, prevalently of female sex. HHs are usually small, but may also reach 20 cm in diameter; tumours >4 cm have been termed giant HHs.
- Histologically, cavernous HHs are composed of cavernous vascular spaces of varied sizes, lined by a single layer of flattened endothelium, separated by thin fibrous septae.
- HHs are typically discovered incidentally during abdominal imaging. Symptoms are usually related to larger tumours; acute thrombosis or bleeding within the tumour may cause acute abdominal pain; giant HH have a low but relevant risk of rupture and intraperitoneal bleeding. In children giant HH may determine high-output cardiac failure, or the Kasabach-Merritt syndrome, characterized by thrombocytopenia and consumption coagulopathy.
- HHs have usually specific features that can suggest the diagnosis on US, CT, or MRI. Sometimes are atypical and more difficult to diagnose. MRI is considered the best imaging technique, with sensitivity and specificity proximal to 100%. A history of liver disease or known or suspected extrahepatic malignancy should suggest confirmation of US diagnosis

with a validating contrast-enhanced CT or MRI. Percutaneous needle biopsy should be avoided, due to the risk of bleeding.

- Asymptomatic patients with stable HHs surrounded by normal liver parenchyma should receive a conservative treatment. Liver resection should be considered in patients with uncertain diagnosis, large symptomatic lesions, tumours enlarging, exophytic, pedunculated or extensively exposed on liver surface. HHs can be resected safely by either enucleation or anatomic resection.

30.5 Cystic Liver Lesions

30.5.1 Introduction

Cystic lesions of the liver represent a miscellaneous group of disorders that occur in about 5–10% of the population [54], with heterogeneous etiology, prevalence, clinical course and prognosis. CLL are mostly found incidentally on imaging studies and in asymptomatic patients, even though larger cysts may sometimes cause symptoms and occasionally severe complications, including spontaneous intracystic infection or bleeding, bile duct compression, spontaneous intraperitoneal or intrabiliary rupture [5, 6]. Biliary cystadenomas may evolve into malignant tumours [5, 6]. Some of these complications may sometimes require elective or urgent surgery.

Key Concepts

- CLLs represent a miscellaneous group of disorders that occur in about 5–10% of the population, with heterogeneous etiology, prevalence, clinical course and prognosis. CLL are mostly found incidentally on imaging studies and in asymptomatic patients, even though larger cysts may sometimes cause symptoms and occasionally severe complications that may require elective or urgent surgery.

30.6 Simple Hepatic Cysts

30.6.1 Epidemiology and Pathogenesis

Simple hepatic cysts (SHC) are cystic lesions containing clear fluid, without communication with the intrahepatic biliary tree. They are thought to derive during embryogenesis from congenital exclusions of hyperplastic bile duct rests disconnected from biliary ducts [6]. The reported prevalence in the general population ranged between 2.5% and 10.5% in ultrasound series, and reached 15–18% in CT series [5, 6]; however only a minority of SHC becomes clinically relevant. Their size ranges from a few millimeters up to 30 cm [4], containing several liters of fluid. The prevalence of SHC increases with age and is higher in women, with a female:male ratio of approximately 1.5:1 for asymptomatic simple cysts, which rises considerably for symptomatic or complicated simple cysts; larger symptomatic cysts are prevalently found in women over 50 [4, 6, 55]. However, no clear correlation with OCPs use or pregnancy has been documented [5, 6].

30.6.2 Pathology

SHC are composed of an outer layer of fibrous tissue lined by a cuboid or columnar epithelium identical to biliary epithelium, that produces cystic fluid [6].

30.6.3 Clinical Features

SHC are usually asymptomatic; symptoms occur in less than 4% of cases, usually associated with cysts >5 cm, and include right upper quadrant or epigastric pain, abdominal distension or discomfort, epigastric fullness, early satiety, nausea, vomiting, dyspnea, fatigue, fever; physical examination may reveal an abdominal mass or hepatomegaly; jaundice and/or portal hypertension may be present [4–6, 56]. Larger cysts may determine atrophy of the adjacent liver tissue, or even the complete atrophy of a hepatic lobe with compensatory hyperplasia of the other lobe. Larger cysts may complicate with spontaneous intracystic hemorrhage, bacterial infection, rupture in the peritoneum, torsion of pedunculated cyst, or biliary obstruction [4–6, 55]. Intracystic hemorrhage is rare and usually presents with severe abdominal pain [4, 56]. Although the natural history of SHC is not completely elucidated, they are not believed to be premalignant precursors of BCAs or BCACs.

30.6.4 Diagnosis

The differential diagnosis with mucinous cystic neoplasms, hydatid cysts, and other rare primary or metastatic tumours can be sometimes difficult, but is extremely important, since parasitic and neoplastic cystic lesions have different clinical significance and therapeutic implications. The presence of multiple cysts, cysts >4–5 cm, irregular walls, calcifications, intracystic heterogeneity, septations, loculations, daughter cysts, enhancing internal components, or the occurrence of symptoms at presentation, are not characteristic of SHC and should motivate further diagnostic evaluation [5, 16, 56]. US is probably the most appropriate initial test and can be also used for the follow-up studies, since is highly sensitive and specific, non-invasive and cost-effective [4, 6]. SHCs appear as anechoic, fluid filled lesions without internal septations, spherical or oval shaped with sharp smooth borders, and accentuation of posterior wall echoes [4, 16]. Also CEUS can be used to differentiate between SHC and other cystic lesions [56]. On CT scan SHCs appear as well-demarcated water density lesions without contrast enhancement [4, 16, 56]. On MR imaging SHCs appear as well-defined water density lesions, with very low signal intensity on T1w sequences, isointense to fluid, and very high signal intensity on T2w sequences, without enhancement after administration of intravenous Gadolinium. Intracystic hemorrhage may alter the typical aspect and lead to confusion with other cystic lesions, especially MCNs, with or without invasive carcinoma; US can show a hyperechoic pattern combined with internal echoes mimicking septations or solid lesions; at CT scan intracystic haemorrhage appears hyperdense; on MR imaging it is hyperintense on both T1w and T2w images [55, 56]. Aspiration is rarely indicated for diagnosing cysts with a typical appearance at imaging. When it is performed, the intracystic fluid may vary from a clear straw color to brown, is usually sterile, with negative testing for cytology and normal carbohydrate antigen 19-9 levels (CA 19-9); high levels of carcinoembryonic antigen (CEA) in the cystic fluid have been reported in MCNs evolving to invasive carcinoma.

30.6.5 Treatment

Asymptomatic SHCs do not usually require any treatment. Since their natural history is uncertain and they have no malignant potential, asymptomatic cysts do not usually require serial imaging [5, 16]. The presence of symptoms related to intracystic hemorrhage, infection, rupture, biliary obstruction, or increasing size, should raise concern about the diagnosis, since SHCs tend to remain stable in size and complications are rare. Also the causal relationship between symptoms and a simple cyst should be adequately evaluated to exclude other possible etiologies, including cholelithiasis, gastroesophageal reflux disease, peptic ulcer disease, and other causes of dyspepsia. Therapeutic approaches described for symptomatic, large SHCs, include needle aspiration with or without injection of alcohol or other sclerosing agents, also known as sclerotherapy, wide surgical fenestration, also known as deroofing or marsupialization, and rarely liver resection. Simple percutaneous needle aspiration and percutaneous needle aspiration with sclerotherapy are generally safe, effective, and relatively noninvasive [57]. Sclerotherapy determines the destruction of the intracystic epithelial lining to limit intracystic fluid secretion; drainage of the intracystic fluid is followed by injection of water-soluble contrast to exclude communication with adjacent bile duct or peritoneal cavity; the solution containing sclerosing agents is then injected in the cyst and aspirated before the catheter is removed [55]. An intracystic drainage can be left for some time in selected cases. Sclerotherapy is contraindicated in case of intracystic bleeding and fistula between the cyst and biliary tree or peritoneum [55]. Due to high recurrence rates, however, percutaneous aspiration eventually followed by sclerotherapy should be reserved for patients unfit for surgery and general anesthesia [4–6, 16, 55].

Wide surgical fenestration or resection of SHCs have been reported to be successful in up to 90% of the cases with a relatively low incidence of perioperative complications and of recurrence [4–6, 16, 55]. Laparoscopic fenestration is at present the standard surgical approach compared with open procedures, because of similar success rates along with reduced perioperative morbidity and length of hospital stay [5]. Laparoscopic fenestration may be technically difficult in case of superior or posterior location of the cyst, with higher recurrence rates. No associated mortality has been reported, and morbidity ranges from 0% to 15% [55]. The decision to pursue surgical intervention is often derived by the uncertainty of the diagnosis of SHCs, and the inability to exclude premalignant or malignant neoplasms, mainly BCAs and BCACs, without histological evaluation. In the absence of adequate comparative studies between percutaneous aspiration with or without sclerotherapy, surgical fenestration, and laparoscopic versus open surgical approaches, the therapeutic strategy should be established according to the local availability of radiologic and surgical expertise and to patient preference, on an individual basis [5].

Key Concepts

- SHCs of the liver are cystic lesions containing clear fluid, without communication with the intrahepatic biliary tree. Their prevalence ranges between 2.5% and 18%, increases with age and is higher in women.
- Histologically, SHCs are composed of an outer layer of fibrous tissue lined by a cuboid or columnar epithelium identical to biliary epithelium, that produces cystic fluid.
- SHCs are usually asymptomatic. Symptoms occur in less than 4% of cases. Larger cysts may complicate with spontaneous intracystic hemorrhage, bacterial infection, rupture in the peritoneum, or biliary

obstruction. SHCs are not believed to be premalignant precursors of BCAs or BCACs.

- The differential diagnosis with MCN, hydatid cysts, and other rare primary or metastatic tumours can be difficult, but is essential, since parasitic and neoplastic cysts have different clinical significance and therapeutic implications. US is the most appropriate initial test. CEUS and contrast-enhanced CT and MRI can be used to confirm the diagnosis. Aspiration is rarely indicated.
- Asymptomatic SHCs do not require any treatment. The therapeutic approaches described for symptomatic, large SHCs, include needle aspiration with or without sclerotherapy, followed by recurrence in most cases; wide surgical fenestration, and rarely liver resection, either with open or with laparoscopic approach.

30.7 Polycystic Liver Disease

30.7.1 Epidemiology and Pathogenesis

Polycystic liver disease is characterized by the presence of multiple liver cysts. Current literature defines PLD as >20 liver cysts [58]; however the International PLD Registry steering committee has recently come to a consensus to consider PLD as >10 cysts [59]. PLD occurs in the context of two distinct hereditary disorders, either as a primary presentation of autosomal dominant polycystic liver disease (ADPLD), or in association with polycystic kidneys in autosomal dominant polycystic kidney disease (ADPKD). PLD results from germline mutations in *PKD1* or *PKD2* in ADPKD, or *PRKCSH*, *SEC63*, *LRP5* in ADPLD [59]. These different diseases have different clinical course and prognosis. Patients with ADPKD develop in most cases hypertension, a progressive decline of renal function up to renal failure, multiple renal complications, and require the accurate monitoring of renal function; at the same time, the liver function usually remains substantially intact until very late in the course of disease, even when the liver architecture is seriously affected by PLD; most patients with PLD are asymptomatic, while about 20% of them complain of compressive symptoms including abdominal pain and distension, back pain, early satiety and gastroesophageal reflux [60]. The severity of the liver disease in PLD is extremely variable, and the phenotype of patients bearing the same genetic mutation may range from normal liver with only few cysts to disabling disease with massive hepatomegaly. The prevalence and size of liver cysts, and of the related symptoms, increase with age, with a female predilection, probably because the disease progresses much faster in females; these differences may be related to the hormonal status of women, to previous pregnancy and also to the use of OCPs [5, 59]; even if this point is still controversial, some authors suggest to stop taking OCPs containing oestrogen [59].

30.7.2 Clinical Features

Most patients with PLD remain asymptomatic through the years, until the number and volume of cysts do not determine significant hepatomegaly. The occurrence of abdominal symptoms motivates imaging studies and reveals hepatomegaly. Patients with moderate to severe hepatomegaly usually refer a sudden abdominal distension associated with symptoms related to PLD, including abdominal pain, loss of appetite, early satiety, nausea, dyspepsia. PLD-related symptoms can be evaluated in specific questionnaires to score the burden of disease and to assess the efficacy of the available treatments [59]. The severity of disease can be further classified through imaging studies, based on the number, size, and location of liver cysts and the amount of remaining liver parenchyma [61]. Also the liver volume has a prognostic role, affecting either symptom burden or quality of life, and can be used to evaluate the effects of the available treatments; based on the liver volume, PLD can be classified in mild, moderate and severe disease [62]. Patients with mild PLD are usually asymptomatic and cysts are incidentally found on abdominal imaging studies; sometimes patients complain of pain located to the back and flank [62], eventually related to a large dominant cyst stretching the liver capsule. Surveillance of asymptomatic patients is not recommended. Patients with moderate disease have symptoms related to hepatomegaly, including pain in the abdomen, flank or back, nausea, early satiety, gastroesophageal reflux, and dyspnea, that significantly diminish the quality of life; the liver is palpable below the costal margin [59]. Patients with severe PLD are typically females aged between 30 and 50 years; compression of the stomach may lower food intake and determine weight loss and sarcopenia; a massive hepatomegaly is evident, with the right liver lobe extending into the pelvis; liver function remains preserved in most cases, even though compression of hepatic veins and of inferior vena cava causes hepatic venous outflow obstruction, sometimes associated with liver fibrosis, that can determine ascites formation and liver failure after liver resection [59].

Intracystic complications. Intracystic haemorrhage predominantly occurs in larger cysts and may happen asymptomatically or determine acute pain in the upper abdomen or flank; intracystic hemorrhage with mild symptoms can be treated conservatively, while the presence of severe symptoms may require fenestration or enucleation [63]. Intracystic infection, probably related to translocation of bacteria across the intestinal barrier, mostly *Escherichia coli* and *Klebsiella* species, determines pain in the right upper quadrant, malaise and fever [58]; FDG-PET has been proven useful to confirm the diagnosis and to differentiate between hepatic or renal cyst infection [64], although the identification of inflammatory cells and bacteria from intracystic fluid is the most reliable diagnostic procedure; therapy with one or more antibiotics is usually effective; in case of antibiotic failure, percutaneous drainage of the infected cyst is resolutive. Rupture of a cyst is extremely rare, probably due to a significant cyst enlargement, either spontaneous or related to haemorrhage or trauma; rupture determines severe abdominal pain and sometimes haemodynamic instability; radiological imaging demonstrates free fluid around the liver and usually the residual hepatic cyst; monitoring and percutaneous drainage of ascites and of the hepatic cyst is the proper strategy in most cases; the occurrence of acute abdominal pain and haemodynamic instability usually require an emergent surgical intervention [59].

Liver volume-related complications. These rare complications result from severe compression on adjacent organs, either by a single cyst or by the enlarged liver volume, and include obstructive jaundice, portal hypertension with varices, portal vein occlusion, Budd-Chiari syndrome, compression of the inferior vena cava determining peripheral oedema and ascites [59]. Treatment strategies are usually individualized according to the severity of the liver disease and to clinical features of the single patient [59].

30.7.3 Diagnosis

Radiological findings of PLD are similar to those of simple hepatic cysts; cysts are multiple, bilobar, with variable size and numerous microcysts; signs of intracystic haemorrhage are more frequent; MR imaging is more sensitive for the detection of intracystic complications [16].

30.7.4 Treatment

Patients with symptomatic PLD and hepatomegaly usually require treatment, at least to relief symptoms and improve the quality of life. Treatment choice depends on therapeutic goals, features of the cystic disease, including size, location, hepatomegaly, and overall patient conditions. Somatostatin analogues (SAs) substantially modify the natural course of PLD by decreasing the liver volume and ultimately improving quality of life [58]. Somatostatin and analogues (long-acting lanreotide and octreotide) inhibit the production of cAMP in cystic cholangiocytes and reduce fluid secretion and proliferation [59]. If symptoms are related to one or more dominant cysts, multiple treatment strategies can be considered. Patients with symptoms caused by one dominant cyst are eligible for needle aspiration and sclerotherapy, to reduce the cyst volume and related symptoms; sclerotherapy is safe and usually effective to reduce symptoms [57], despite high recurrence rates. In patients with symptoms determined by multiple larger cysts, fenestration may represent an appropriate solution, combining aspiration and surgical deroofing of multiple cysts in a single session; recurrence is less frequent; the laparoscopic approach is preferred whenever possible, since determines better perioperative results than the open approach; complications include perioperative ascites, pleural effusion, and bleeding [65].

Liver resection, with or without fenestration, is indicated in selected patients where sclerotherapy or fenestration are not possible, because of the number and/or distribution of the cysts, especially in symptomatic and severe hepatomegaly; liver resection can be performed with acceptable morbidity and mortality rates, prompt and durable relief of symptoms, and maintenance of liver function [66], even though major surgery may complicate future liver transplantation because of multiple adhesions. Liver transplantation is the only curative treatment option, but is indicated in a minority of patients with PLD, including those with massive hepatomegaly and severe malnutrition, sarcopenia, low serum albumin, or severe complications such as recurrent intracystic infections, portal hypertension, ascites [59]; patient and graft survival rates after liver transplantation for PLD were 92.3% and 87.5%, respectively, in the European Liver Transplantation Registry [67]. Combined liver-kidney transplantation in patients with ADPKD and renal failure is selectively indicated, and is associated with more favourable results than liver transplantation alone [68].

Key Concepts

- PLD is characterized by the presence of multiple (>10) liver cysts. PLD occurs in the context of two distinct hereditary disorders, either as a primary presentation of autosomal dominant polycystic liver disease (ADPLD), or in association with polycystic kidneys in autosomal dominant polycystic kidney disease (ADPKD). These different diseases have different clinical course and prognosis. Patients with ADPKD develop in most cases hypertension, a progressive decline of renal function up to renal failure, multiple renal complications, while the liver function usually remains substantially intact for a long time.
- The severity of the liver disease in PLD is extremely variable, ranging from normal liver with only few cysts to disabling disease with massive hepatomeg-

aly. The prevalence and size of liver cysts, and of the related symptoms, increase with age, with a female predilection.

- Most patients with PLD remain asymptomatic through the years, until the development of significant hepatomegaly, with the related symptoms. The severity of disease can be classified according to symptoms, to the number, size, location of liver cysts and the amount of remaining liver parenchyma, and to the liver volume. Intracystic complications include haemorrhage, infection, and exceptionally the rupture of a cyst.
- Radiological findings of PLD are similar to those of simple hepatic cysts; cysts are multiple, bilobar, with variable size and numerous microcysts; signs of intracystic haemorrhage are more frequent.
- Patients with symptomatic PLD and hepatomegaly should be treated, at least to relief symptoms and improve the quality of life. Somatostatin analogues (SAs) decrease liver volume and ultimately improve quality of life. Symptoms caused by one dominant cyst can be resolved with needle aspiration and sclerotherapy. Symptoms determined by multiple larger cysts may require surgical fenestration, either with open or with laparoscopic approach. Liver resection, with or without fenestration, is selectively indicated for more advanced disease. Liver transplantation or combined liver-kidney transplantation are indicated in selected cases.

30.8 Benign Biliary Cystic Tumours (Cystadenoma)

30.8.1 Epidemiology and Pathogenesis

Biliary cystic tumors, that include BCA and BCAC, are rare neoplasms that occur within the liver parenchyma, or less frequently in the extrahepatic biliary system, including the gallbladder [6, 69]. BCTs represent less than 5% of all liver cysts, with a diameter ranging from 1.5 to 35 cm [5, 6, 16, 54, 56]. However, BCAs are the most frequent primary cystic tumours of the liver, comprising up to 10% of all cysts >4 cm [6, 8]. BCAs occur predominantly in females (90%), with a mean age of 45–50 years at presentation [6, 54, 69–71]. BCAs with ovarian-type stroma express estrogen and progesterone receptors [72], which might explain the high incidence among females, the frequent occurrence reported in patients on hormonal therapy, and the size increase during pregnancy [54]. It has been hypothesized that BCTs derive from ectopic rests of embryonic bile ducts [73], or from intrahepatic peribiliary glands [69].

30.8.2 Pathology

On gross pathology, BCTs are generally solitary, multilocular cystic neoplasms with mucinous or serous fluid contents [5, 69]; papillary projections that form thick, compact septa are sometimes evident [5]. Multifocal BCTs are rare. BCTs frequently contain blood or chocolate-colored material. The left hepatic lobe is the more frequent site [70], although this point is controversial [56]. BCTs are occasionally centered on extrahepatic bile ducts [6, 70]. BCAs present biliary immunophenotype [6], with an outer layer of fibrous connective tissue lined by a cuboidal to columnar epithelium [54]. Typically, BCAs have been characterized by ovarian-type mesenchymal stroma that expresses estrogen and progesterone receptors [6, 72]. Wheeler and Edmondson defined BCA according to the presence of mesenchymal stroma [73]; cystadenoma with mesenchymal stroma showed an outer layer of cellular stroma composed of spindle cells; the stromal element appeared similar to primitive mesenchyme with variable differentiation toward fibroblasts, smooth muscle, adipose tissue and capillaries; this histotype occurred only in young and middle-aged women; in contrast, cystadenoma without mesenchymal stroma occurred at a mean age of 53.4 years, without female predominance. Multiple studies have reported BCAs either with or without the presence of ovarian-like mesenchymal stroma between the inner epithelial lining and the outer fibrous capsule [6, 73–75]. In 2010 however, the World Health Organization (WHO) defined BCAs of the liver as mucinous cystic neoplasms (MCN) with ovarian stroma [70, 76]: the criteria established for the classification of cystic neoplasms of the pancreas have been applied also to the hepatobiliary tract, and the nonspecific diagnosis of "hepatobiliary cystadenoma/cystadenocarcinoma" has been eliminated and replaced by more specific entities, including MCN defined by the presence of ovarian stroma; moreover, it has been assessed that not all biliary-lined cysts are MCNs [70].

According to the new classification, MCNs are composed of an outer layer containing variable amounts of ovarian stroma, containing progesterone receptors, estrogen receptors and inhibin at IHC staining, and a lining epithelium classified as either mucinous or biliary nonmucinous [70]; ovarian stroma can be focal or hypo/atrophic [70]; the degree of cytoarchitectural dysplasia can be defined according either to the 3-tiered grading system (low, intermediate, and high-grade intraepithelial neoplasia) [76], or to the recently modified 2-tiered grading system (low and high-grade intraepithelial neoplasia), as has been adopted for intraepithelial neoplasia in the pancreas [77]; complex epithelial proliferations may form intracystic papillary/polypoid nodules, with various grades of cytoarchitectural dysplasia, but mural nodules may also be formed by polypoid projections of the ovarian stroma, sometimes with hemorrhage, necrosis, stromal inflammation, fibrosis, and other degenerative changes [70]. Epithelial cells of BCT are characterized by mucin production and are immunoreactive to cytokeratins (CAM5.2, AE1, AE3), CEA, CA 19-9, and epithelial membrane antigen [54, 69, 72].

BCAs have malignant potential [4, 5, 54, 73]. Areas of benign BCA epithelium have been detected in a large number of BCACs [6, 69]. It has been suggested that the nonmucinous biliary epithelium might constitute the initial phase of MCNs, with the mucinous epithelium representing the next step in tumorigenic progression [70, 71]; papillary proliferation of the epithelium and the formation of nodules with high-grade intraepithelial neoplasia might represent the most advanced state of this carcinogenetic pathway [70, 71, 73]. Stromal invasion is the next crucial event in the carcinogenetic sequence, and can be followed by the development of metastases [73]. The entire process of malignant epithelial transformation of MCN might require many years in most cases, since the mean age of patients with malignant MCNs is significantly higher than those with benign MCNs [6, 71, 73]. Not all BCAC originate from pre-existing MCNs; BCAC without mesenchymal stroma might arise either directly from bile ducts or from malignant transformation of cystic liver lesions other than MCNs [69, 70, 73]. The overall rate of malignant transformation ranges from 2% to 30% [6, 56, 70, 74]. Male sex has been associated with an increased risk of BCAC [74]. The presence of ovarian stroma has been reported to have significant prognostic implications. BCAC without ovarian stroma occurs in both men and women, while those with ovarian stroma develop almost exclusively in females [54, 69, 70, 73]. BCACs without ovarian stroma progress to malignancy more frequently, develop more rapidly and are associated with worse prognosis [69, 71], even though these data are still controversial [74]. BCAs with ovarian stroma develop carcinomatous changes in about 5% of the cases [70]. BCA ovarian stroma can regress during carcinomatous transformation [69].

30.8.3 Clinical Features

Clinical presentation of BCAs is extremely variable. Most lesions are discovered incidentally on imaging studies for different indications and in asymptomatic patients [4–6, 54, 70]. Symptoms are very ambiguous and usually nonspecific, often related to enlarging lesions, and include indeterminate abdominal pain and distension in up to 90% of the patients, right upper quadrant mass or discomfort, nausea, early satiety, anorexia, diaphragmatic compression with breathing difficulties [5, 8, 54, 70, 74]. Laboratory values are normal in most cases [4], although approximately 20% of patients exhibit abnormal liver function tests, including increased bilirubin levels. Obstructive jaundice and cholangitis occur rarely, usually with extrahepatic BCAs, while intracystic hemorrhage, infection with fever, and cyst rupture are exceptional [6, 54, 71, 74].

30.8.4 Diagnosis

The differential diagnosis of patients with complex cystic lesions of the liver includes BCT with invasive carcinoma, hydatid cyst, post-traumatic cyst, liver abscess, simple hepatic cyst, including those with intracystic hemorrhage, and other rare primary or metastatic tumours. Differential diagnosis also includes biliary intraductal papillary mucinous neoplasm (IPMN), a recently recognized neoplasm characterized by mucin production, prominent intraductal papillary proliferation, and biliary tree communication [54, 72], with clinicopathologic features different from BCA [54, 72]. While cross-sectional imaging with US, CT and MRI is effective in characterizing simple hepatic cystic lesions, its accuracy in defining and characterizing different types of complex cystic lesions is considerably lower [6, 16, 56, 70, 75]. Single hepatic cyst, located in the left hepatic lobe, with biliary duct dilation, can be predictive of BCT [54, 74]. Larger BCTs are at higher risk of containing areas of malignant transformation [54, 70].

At ultrasonography, BCTs are anechoic or hypoechoic, with thickened irregular walls and hyperechoic internal septations [4, 5, 16, 78]; thickened septa, papillary projections and mural and/or septal nodules are typical of BCTs [4, 8, 16]; calcifications are frequent [4–6]. CEUS may add significant information; simple liver cysts typically have no enhancement on CEUS, while BCTs show enhancement of the cystic wall and septa, and eventually of mural nodes, during the arterial phase, and hypoenhancement during the portal and late phases [16, 56, 71]. On CT scan, BCTs appear as single, well-demarcated water density lesions with thick fibrous capsule [16], without intralesional contrast enhancement; internal septations, irregular papillary growths, and nodular areas sometimes enhance with intravenous contrast [4, 5, 16, 56, 78]; CT allows better visualization of any calcifications [56]. On MR imaging, BCTs are multilocular water density lesions with thickened irregular walls and internal septations [16, 78], with low signal intensity on T1w sequences, isointense to fluid, and high signal intensity on T2w sequences; signal intensity on T1w and T2w images depends on cystic fluid protein content [5, 16]; intra-cystic septations determine linear low signal intensity within high-intensity cysts on T2w images. The addition of DW-MRI to conventional MRI sequences has been reported to be useful in characterization of cystic hepatic lesions and detection of malignancy [4]. MR cholangiopancreatography identifies internal septations, and can demonstrate the relationship or the presence of cyst communication with the biliary tree [54]. Cross-sectional imaging with contrast-enhanced CT an MR delineates anatomic relationships within the liver and is essential for surgical planning in candidates to liver resection.

BCA and BCAC cannot be reliably distinguished with preoperative imaging [4, 71]; both tumours appear as solitary, multilocular cystic lesions; larger lesions with irregular thickness of the cystic wall and of the intracystic septations, contrast enhancement of cyst wall and intracystic septations, hypervascularity, the presence of mural nodules, solid component, papillary projection, calcification, intracystic hemorrhage, and biliary ductal dilatation, might suggest a higher risk of malignant transformation; however these features are not pathognomonic for malignancy [4, 16, 56, 70, 71, 74]. Tumor location in the right hemiliver has been associated with higher risk of BCAC [74]. FNAB and core-needle biopsy of suspected BCTs should be avoided because of the limited sensitivity, the low likelihood of identifying malignant cells, and of the risk of pleural and peritoneal dissemination [4, 5, 8, 78]; CEA e CA 19-9 levels in the cystic fluid have been reported to be useful to differentiate BCTs from other benign cystic lesions, but their role is controversial, especially in distinguishing BCAs from BCACs [6, 54].

30.8.5 Treatment

If BCT is suspected on imaging, complete surgical excision is recommended, because of its attitude to recur if incompletely excised, the malignant potential, the difficulty of preoperative identification of BCAC [4–6, 70, 71, 74]; inappropriate treatment of these lesions, including partial excision, is invariably associated with recurrence and with worse prognosis compared with complete resection [71, 74]. Simple percutaneous needle aspiration, percutaneous needle aspiration with sclerotherapy, internal drainage, marsupialization, surgical fenestration or partial resection are inappropriate whenever a diagnosis of BCT is plausible. When a presumed simple cyst recurs rapidly after percutaneous aspiration, a BCT should be suspected. BCTs should be surgically resected with negative margins whenever possible [54, 70]. The appropriate surgical treatment, either formal liver resection or enucleation, depends on the anatomic site of the tumour and its relationships with intrahepatic vessels and bile ducts [71, 78]; patients with peripheral BCT or tumours located in a hemiliver can receive a formal liver resection, in case of appropriate surgical risk, while centrally located tumours adjoining central vascular or biliary structures can require enucleation, which is usually technically feasible because of the presence of a thick pseudocapsule [5, 71]. Extrahepatic BCTs require liver resection with resection of the involved bile duct. Surgical resection can be achieved either with open conventional or with laparoscopic approach, with similar results [5, 79]. Intraoperative frozen-section analysis should not be used to define the surgical strategy, since small areas of malignant transformation are usually missed with partial sampling and the intraoperative diagnosis of BCAC is unachievable in most cases [78]. After complete surgical excision, an extensive sampling of the tumour is essential to exclude focal malignant transformation [70]. In a recent multicentric series of 248 patients who underwent surgical resection of BCT [74], overall 1, 3, and 5 year recurrence-free survival was 89.1%, 72.6%, and 61.4%, respectively; recurrences were significantly higher after uncomplete tumour resection, occurring in 48.6% of the patients who underwent tumour unroofing/fenestration; 1, 3, and 5 year overall survival was 95.0%, 86.8%, and 84.2%, respectively, significantly lower in patients with BCAC than in those with BCA. Patients with BCAC invading the liver parenchyma or neighboring organs have a poor prognosis [71]. Orthotopic liver transplantation has been proposed in highly selected patients with symptomatic, unresectable BCT [54].

Key Concepts

- BCTs, that include BCA and BCAC, are rare neoplasms that occur within the liver parenchyma, or less frequently in the extrahepatic biliary system. BCTs represent less than 5% of all liver cysts, and occur predominantly in females (90%), with a mean age of 45–50 years at presentation. BCAs with ovarian-type stroma express estrogen and progesterone receptors, which might explain the high incidence among females and in patients on hormonal therapy, and the size increase during pregnancy.
- Histologically, BCAs present biliary immunophenotype, with an outer layer of fibrous connective tissue lined by a cuboidal to columnar epithelium. Typically, BCAs have been characterized by ovarian-type mesenchymal stroma; however, multiple studies have also reported BCAs without mesenchymal stroma; the WHO has recently defined BCAs of the liver as mucinous cystic neoplasms (MCN) with ovarian stroma, applying the criteria established for the classification of cystic neoplasms of the pancreas.
- The degree of cytoarchitectural dysplasia of the lining epithelium can be defined according either to the 3-tiered grading system (low, intermediate, and high-grade intraepithelial neoplasia), or to the

recently modified 2-tiered grading system (low and high-grade intraepithelial neoplasia). BCAs have malignant potential. Malignant epithelial transformation of MCNs probably requires many years in most cases. The overall rate of malignant transformation ranges from 2% to 30%.

- Most BCAs are discovered incidentally in asymptomatic patients. Symptoms are very ambiguous and usually nonspecific, often related to enlarging lesions. Complications are rare; obstructive jaundice and cholangitis may occur in extrahepatic BCAs, while intracystic hemorrhage, infection, and cyst rupture are exceptional.
- The differential diagnosis of patients with complex cystic lesions of the liver is usually difficult and usually requires a combination of US, CEUS, CT and MRI. Thickened septa, papillary projections, mural and/or septal nodules, calcifications, are typical of BCTs. BCA and BCAC cannot be reliably distinguished with preoperative imaging. Percutaneous needle biopsy or FNAB should be avoided because of the limited accuracy, and of the risk of dissemination.
- If a BCT is suspected on imaging, complete surgical excision is recommended, because of its attitude to recur if incompletely excised, the malignant potential, the difficulty of preoperative identification of BCAC. Formal liver resection or complete enucleation can be achieved with either open or laparoscopic approach. After complete surgical excision, an extensive sampling of the tumour is essential to exclude focal malignant transformation.

30.9 Conclusions

Benign liver tumours are a heterogeneous group of solid or cystic focal liver lesions deriving from different cell types, that are increasingly being discovered, usually in otherwise asymptomatic patients, because of the extensive use of medical imaging in clinical practice. An appropriate diagnostic approach is essential to differentiate benign lesions from primary and metastatic liver malignancies, and should include a detailed clinical history and evaluation of risk factors, physical examination, laboratory test findings, different imaging modalities, and eventually histopathology. New genetic and biomolecular criteria have been developed and can be selectively useful to define more precise diagnostic and therapeutic strategies. Radiological evaluation is the most important aspect and includes conventional and contrast-enhanced US, CT, MRI, and FDG-PET/TC in selected cases. Standardization of the technical specifications for CT and MRI should be systematically applied to the evaluation of FLLs; an appropriate contrast-enhanced imaging technique should include a late arterial phase, a portal venous phase, and a delayed venous phase. MRI is highly accurate for the detection and characterization of liver masses because of its multiparametric potentialities. When the diagnosis remains uncertain after extensive radiographic imaging, a liver biopsy or even a surgical resection for histopathological examination should be performed. However, percutaneous liver biopsy should be considered with caution, either for the risk of bleeding in some vascularized lesions, or for the low probability of detecting areas of malignancy in heterogeneous lesions. The management of benign hepatic tumors ranges from conservative to aggressive, depending on the nature of the lesions. Asymptomatic benign tumours usually do not require any specific treatment. Larger lesions however may sometimes determine significant symptoms or have a high risk of complications, including rupture and bleeding, and should be considered for surgery, or alternatively for ablation or TAE in selected cases. Some tumours have a well known risk of malignant transformation and should undergo radical resection. Further improvements in the knowledge of the natural history and in cross-sectional imaging of benign tumours, and also the development of new genetic and biomolecular markers, may favour the development of more tailored diagnostic and therapeutic approaches, according to the nature of the tumour and to the features of the single patient.

References

1. European Association for the Study of the Liver. EASL clinical practice guidelines on the management of benign liver tumours. J Hepatol. 2016;65:386–98. https://doi.org/10.1016/j.jhep.2016.04.001.
2. Colombo M, Sangiovanni A, Lencioni R. Benign liver tumors. In: Sanyal AJ, Boyer TD, Terrault N, Lindor KD, editors. Zakim and Boyer's hepatology: a textbook of liver disease. 7th ed. Philadelphia: Elsevier; 2018. p. 720–35.
3. International Working Party. Terminology of nodular hepatocellular lesions. Hepatology. 1995;22:983–93.
4. Lantinga MA, Gevers TJ, Drenth JP. Evaluation of hepatic cystic lesions. World J Gastroenterol. 2013;19:3543–54. https://doi.org/10.3748/wjg.v19.i23.3543.
5. Marrero JA, Ahn J, Rajender Reddy K, American College of Gastroenterology. ACG clinical guideline: the diagnosis and management of focal liver lesions. Am J Gastroenterol. 2014;109:1328–47. https://doi.org/10.1038/ajg.2014.213.
6. Shaked O, Siegelman ES, Olthoff K, Reddy KR. Biologic and clinical features of benign solid and cystic lesions of the liver. Clin Gastroenterol Hepatol. 2011;9:547–62. https://doi.org/10.1016/j.cgh.2011.03.007.
7. Belghiti J, Cauchy F, Paradis V, Vilgrain V. Diagnosis and management of solid benign liver lesions. Nat Rev Gastroenterol Hepatol. 2014;11:737–49. https://doi.org/10.1038/nrgastro.2014.151.

8. Bonder A, Afdhal N. Evaluation of liver lesions. Clin Liver Dis. 2012;16:271–83. https://doi.org/10.1016/j.cld.2012.03.001.
9. Pomfret EA, Washburn K, Wald C, Nalesnik MA, Douglas D, Russo M, Roberts J, Reich DJ, Schwartz ME, Mieles L, Lee FT, Florman S, Yao F, Harper A, Edwards E, Freeman R, Lake J. Report of a national conference on liver allocation in patients with hepatocellular carcinoma in the United States. Liver Transpl. 2010;16:262–78. https://doi.org/10.1002/lt.21999.
10. International Consensus Group for Hepatocellular Neoplasia. Pathologic diagnosis of early hepatocellular carcinoma: a report of the international consensus group for hepatocellular neoplasia. Hepatology. 2009;49:658–64. https://doi.org/10.1002/hep.22709.
11. Nakanuma Y. Non-neoplastic nodular lesions in the liver. Pathol Int. 1995;45:703–14.
12. Mindikoglu AL, Regev A, Levi JU, Casillas J, Schiff ER. Focal nodular hyperplasia in identical twins. Am J Gastroenterol. 2005;100:1616–9. https://doi.org/10.1111/j.1572-0241.2005.41898.x.
13. Bioulac-Sage P, Frulio N, Balabaud CP. Benign hepatocellular tumors. In: Saxena R, editor. Practical hepatic pathology: a diagnostic approach. 2nd ed. Philadelphia: Elsevier; 2018. p. 507–26.
14. Nguyen BN, Fléjou JF, Terris B, Belghiti J, Degott C. Focal nodular hyperplasia of the liver: a comprehensive pathologic study of 305 lesions and recognition of new histologic forms. Am J Surg Pathol. 1999;23:1441–54.
15. Bioulac-Sage P, Laumonier H, Rullier A, Cubel G, Laurent C, Zucman-Rossi J, Balabaud C. Over-expression of glutamine synthetase in focal nodular hyperplasia: a novel easy diagnostic tool in surgical pathology. Liver Int. 2009;29:459–65. https://doi.org/10.1111/j.1478-3231.2008.01849.x.
16. Grazioli L, Ambrosini R, Frittoli B, Grazioli M, Morone M. Primary benign liver lesions. Eur J Radiol. 2017;95:378–98. https://doi.org/10.1016/j.ejrad.2017.08.028.
17. McInnes MD, Hibbert RM, Inácio JR, Schieda N. Focal nodular hyperplasia and hepatocellular adenoma: accuracy of gadoxetic acid-enhanced MR imaging. A systematic review. Radiology. 2015;277:413–23. https://doi.org/10.1148/radiol.2015142986.
18. Seale MK, Catalano OA, Saini S, Hahn PF, Sahani DV. Hepatobiliary-specific MR contrast agents: role in imaging the liver and biliary tree. Radiographics. 2009;29:1725–48. https://doi.org/10.1148/rg.296095515.
19. Cogley JR, Miller FH. MR imaging of benign focal liver lesions. Radiol Clin N Am. 2014;52:657–82. https://doi.org/10.1016/j.rcl.2014.02.005.
20. Nault JC, Paradis V, Cherqui D, Vilgrain V, Zucman-Rossi J. Molecular classification of hepatocellular adenoma in clinical practice. J Hepatol. 2017;67:1074–83. https://doi.org/10.1016/j.jhep.2017.07.009.
21. Klatskin G. Hepatic tumors: possible relationship to use of oral contraceptives. Gastroenterology. 1977;73:386–94.
22. Carrasco D, Prieto M, Pallardó L, Moll JL, Cruz JM, Muñoz C, Berenguer J. Multiple hepatic adenomas after long-term therapy with testosterone enanthate. Review of the literature. J Hepatol. 1985;1:573–8.
23. Bioulac-Sage P, Sempoux C, Balabaud C. Hepatocellular adenoma: classification, variants and clinical relevance. Semin Diagn Pathol. 2017;34:112–25. https://doi.org/10.1053/j.semdp.2016.12.007.
24. Bunchorntavakul C, Bahirwani R, Drazek D, Soulen MC, Siegelman ES, Furth EE, Olthoff K, Shaked A, Reddy KR. Clinical features and natural history of hepatocellular adenomas: the impact of obesity. Aliment Pharmacol Ther. 2011;34:664–74. https://doi.org/10.1111/j.1365-2036.2011.04772.x.
25. Bioulac-Sage P, Taouji S, Possenti L, Balabaud C. Hepatocellular adenoma subtypes: the impact of overweight and obesity. Liver Int. 2012;32:1217–21. https://doi.org/10.1111/j.1478-3231.2012.02786.x.
26. Farges O, Ferreira N, Dokmak S, Belghiti J, Bedossa P, Paradis V. Changing trends in malignant transformation of hepatocellular adenoma. Gut. 2011;60:85–9. https://doi.org/10.1136/gut.2010.222109.
27. Sempoux C, Balabaud C, Bioulac-Sage P. Pictures of focal nodular hyperplasia and hepatocellular adenomas. World J Hepatol. 2014;6:580–95. https://doi.org/10.4254/wjh.v6.i8.580.
28. Bioulac-Sage P, Sempoux C, Balabaud C. Hepatocellular adenomas: morphology and genomics. Gastroenterol Clin N Am. 2017;46:253–72. https://doi.org/10.1016/j.gtc.2017.01.003.
29. Védie AL, Sutter O, Ziol M, Nault JC. Molecular classification of hepatocellular adenomas: impact on clinical practice. Hepatol Oncol. 2018;5:HEP04. https://doi.org/10.2217/hep-2017-0023.
30. Nault JC, Bioulac-Sage P, Zucman-Rossi J. Hepatocellular benign tumors-from molecular classification to personalized clinical care. Gastroenterology. 2013;144:888–902. https://doi.org/10.1053/j.gastro.2013.02.032.
31. Bieze M, Phoa SS, Verheij J, van Lienden KP, van Gulik TM. Risk factors for bleeding in hepatocellular adenoma. Br J Surg. 2014;101:847–55. https://doi.org/10.1002/bjs.9493.
32. Nault JC, Mallet M, Pilati C, Calderaro J, Bioulac-Sage P, Laurent C, Laurent A, Cherqui D, Balabaud C, Zucman-Rossi J. High frequency of telomerase reverse-transcriptase promoter somatic mutations in hepatocellular carcinoma and preneoplastic lesions. Nat Commun. 2013;4:2218. https://doi.org/10.1038/ncomms3218.
33. Katabathina VS, Menias CO, Shanbhogue AK, Jagirdar J, Paspulati RM, Prasad SR. Genetics and imaging of hepatocellular adenomas: 2011 update. Radiographics. 2011;31:1529–43. https://doi.org/10.1148/rg.316115527.
34. Laumonier H, Cailliez H, Balabaud C, Possenti L, Zucman-Rossi J, Bioulac-Sage P, Trillaud H. Role of contrast-enhanced sonography in differentiation of subtypes of hepatocellular adenoma: correlation with MRI findings. AJR Am J Roentgenol. 2012;199:341–8. https://doi.org/10.2214/AJR.11.7046.
35. Lubbers PR, Ros PR, Goodman ZD, Ishak KG. Accumulation of technetium-99m sulfur colloid by hepatocellular adenoma: scintigraphic-pathologic correlation. AJR Am J Roentgenol. 1987;148:1105–8. https://doi.org/10.2214/ajr.148.6.1105.
36. van Aalten SM, de Man RA, IJzermans JN, Terkivatan T. Systematic review of haemorrhage and rupture of hepatocellular adenomas. Br J Surg. 2012;99:911–6. https://doi.org/10.1002/bjs.8762.
37. Stoot JH, Coelen RJ, De Jong MC, Dejong CH. Malignant transformation of hepatocellular adenomas into hepatocellular carcinomas: a systematic review including more than 1600 adenoma cases. HPB (Oxford). 2010;12:509–22. https://doi.org/10.1111/j.1477-2574.2010.00222.x.
38. van Rosmalen BV, Coelen RJS, Bieze M, van Delden OM, Verheij J, Dejong CHC, van Gulik TM. Systematic review of transarterial embolization for hepatocellular adenomas. Br J Surg. 2017;104:823–35. https://doi.org/10.1002/bjs.10547.
39. Silva JP, Klooster B, Tsai S, Christians KK, Clarke CN, Mogal H, Clark GT. Elective regional therapy treatment for hepatic adenoma. Ann Surg Oncol. 2018; https://doi.org/10.1245/s10434-018-6802-1.
40. Noels JE, van Aalten SM, van der Windt DJ, Kok NF, de Man RA, Terkivatan T, Ijzermans JN. Management of hepatocellular adenoma during pregnancy. J Hepatol. 2011;54:553–8. https://doi.org/10.1016/j.jhep.2010.07.022.
41. Terkivatan T, de Wilt JH, de Man RA, Ijzermans JN. Management of hepatocellular adenoma during pregnancy. Liver. 2000;20:186–7.
42. Bioulac-Sage P, Laumonier H, Couchy G, Le Bail B, Sa Cunha A, Rullier A, Laurent C, Blanc JF, Cubel G, Trillaud H, Zucman-Rossi J, Balabaud C, Saric J. Hepatocellular adenoma management and phenotypic classification: the Bordeaux experience. Hepatology. 2009;50:481–9. https://doi.org/10.1002/hep.22995.

43. Gandolfi L, Leo P, Solmi L, Vitelli E, Verros G, Colecchia A. Natural history of hepatic haemangiomas: clinical and ultrasound study. Gut. 1991;32:677–80.
44. Suriawinata AA. Miscellaneous liver tumors and tumor-like lesions. In: Saxena R, editor. Practical hepatic pathology: a diagnostic approach. 2nd ed. Philadelphia: Elsevier; 2018. p. 583–99.
45. Zimmermann A, Baer HU. Fibrous tumor-liver interface in large hepatic neoplasms: its significance for tumor resection and enucleation. Liver Transpl Surg. 1996;2:192–9.
46. Kim GE, Thung SN, Tsui WM, Ferrell LD. Hepatic cavernous hemangioma: underrecognized associated histologic features. Liver Int. 2006;26:334–8.
47. Mocchegiani F, Vincenzi P, Coletta M, Agostini A, Marzioni M, Baroni GS, Giovagnoni A, Guerrieri M, Marmorale C, Risaliti A, Vivarelli M. Prevalence and clinical outcome of hepatic haemangioma with specific reference to the risk of rupture: a large retrospective cross-sectional study. Dig Liver Dis. 2016;48:309–14. https://doi.org/10.1016/j.dld.2015.09.016.
48. Luks FI, Yazbeck S, Brandt ML, Bensoussan AL, Brochu P, Blanchard H. Benign liver tumors in children: a 25-year experience. J Pediatr Surg. 1991;26:1326–30.
49. Canty KM, Horii KA, Ahmad H, Lowe LH, Nopper AJ. Multiple cutaneous and hepatic hemangiomas in infants. South Med J. 2014;107:159–64. https://doi.org/10.1097/SMJ.0000000000000070.
50. Hasan HY, Hinshaw JL, Borman EJ, Gegios A, Leverson G, Winslow ER. Assessing normal growth of hepatic hemangiomas during long-term follow-up. JAMA Surg. 2014;149:1266–71. https://doi.org/10.1001/jamasurg.2014.477.
51. Dietrich CF, Mertens JC, Braden B, Schuessler G, Ott M, Ignee A. Contrast-enhanced ultrasound of histologically proven liver hemangiomas. Hepatology. 2007;45:1139–45.
52. Lencioni R, Cioni D, Crocetti L, Della Pina C, Bartolozzi C. Magnetic resonance imaging of liver tumors. J Hepatol. 2004;40:162–71.
53. el-Desouki M, Mohamadiyeh M, al-Rashed R, Othman S, al-Mofleh I. Features of hepatic cavernous hemangioma on planar and SPECT Tc-99m-labeled red blood cell scintigraphy. Clin Nucl Med. 1999;24:583–9.
54. Soares KC, Arnaoutakis DJ, Kamel I, Anders R, Adams RB, Bauer TW, Pawlik TM. Cystic neoplasms of the liver: biliary cystadenoma and cystadenocarcinoma. J Am Coll Surg. 2014;218:119–28. https://doi.org/10.1016/j.jamcollsurg.2013.08.014.
55. Machedo FI. Current management of noninfectious hepatic cystic lesions: a review of the literature. World J Hepatol. 2013;5:462–9. https://doi.org/10.4254/wjh.v5.i9.462.
56. Mavilia MG, Pakala T, Molina M, Wu GY. Differentiating cystic liver lesions: a review of imaging modalities, diagnosis and management. J Clin Transl Hepatol. 2018;6:208–16. https://doi.org/10.14218/JCTH.2017.00069.
57. Wijnands TF, Görtjes AP, Gevers TJ, Jenniskens SF, Kool LJ, Potthoff A, Ronot M, Drenth JP. Efficacy and safety of aspiration sclerotherapy of simple hepatic cysts: a systematic review. Am J Roentgenol. 2017;208:201–7. https://doi.org/10.2214/AJR.16.16130.
58. Gevers TJ, Drenth JP. Diagnosis and management of polycystic liver disease. Nat Rev Gastroenterol Hepatol. 2013;10:101–8. https://doi.org/10.1038/nrgastro.2012.254.
59. van Aerts RMM, van de Laarschot LFM, Banales JM, Drenth JPH. Clinical management of polycystic liver disease. J Hepatol. 2018;68:827-37. https://doi.org/10.1016/j.jhep.2017.11.024.
60. Chapman AB, Devuyst O, Eckardt KU, Gansevoort RT, Harris T, Horie S, Kasiske BL, Odland D, Pei Y, Perrone RD, Pirson Y, Schrier RW, Torra R, Torres VE, Watnick T, Wheeler DC, Conference Participants. Autosomal-dominant polycystic kidney disease (ADPKD): executive summary from a Kidney Disease: Improving Global Outcomes (KDIGO) controversies conference. Kidney Int. 2015;88:17–27. https://doi.org/10.1038/ki.2015.59.
61. Gigot JF, Jadoul P, Que F, Van Beers BE, Etienne J, Horsmans Y, Collard A, Geubel A, Pringot J, Kestens PJ. Adult polycystic liver disease: is fenestration the most adequate operation for long-term management? Ann Surg. 1997;225:286–94.
62. Kim H, Park HC, Ryu H, Kim K, Kim HS, Oh KH, Yu SJ, Chung JW, Cho JY, Kim SH, Cheong HI, Lee K, Park JH, Pei Y, Hwang YH, Ahn C. Clinical correlates of mass effect in autosomal dominant polycystic kidney disease. PLoS One. 2015;10:e0144526. https://doi.org/10.1371/journal.pone.0144526.
63. Fong ZV, Wolf AM, Doria C, Berger AC, Rosato EL, Palazzo F. Hemorrhagic hepatic cyst: report of a case and review of the literature with emphasis on clinical approach and management. J Gastrointest Surg. 2012;16:1782–9. https://doi.org/10.1007/s11605-012-1922-6.
64. Lantinga MA, de Sévaux RG, Drenth JP. 18F-FDG PET/CT during diagnosis and follow-up of recurrent hepatic cyst infection in autosomal dominant polycystic kidney disease. Clin Nephrol. 2015;84:61–4. https://doi.org/10.5414/CN108495.
65. Drenth JP, Chrispijn M, Nagorney DM, Kamath PS, Torres VE. Medical and surgical treatment options for polycystic liver disease. Hepatology. 2010;52:2223–30. https://doi.org/10.1002/hep.24036.
66. Schnelldorfer T, Torres VE, Zakaria S, Rosen CB, Nagorney DM. Polycystic liver disease: a critical appraisal of hepatic resection, cyst fenestration, and liver transplantation. Ann Surg. 2009;250:112–8. https://doi.org/10.1097/SLA.0b013e3181ad83dc.
67. van Keimpema L, Nevens F, Adam R, Porte RJ, Fikatas P, Becker T, Kirkegaard P, Metselaar HJ, Drenth JP, European Liver and Intestine Transplant Association. Excellent survival after liver transplantation for isolated polycystic liver disease: an European Liver Transplant Registry study. Transpl Int. 2011;24:1239–45. https://doi.org/10.1111/j.1432-2277.2011.01360.x.
68. Coquillard C, Berger J, Daily M, Shah M, Mei X, Marti F, Gedaly R. Combined liver-kidney transplantation for polycystic liver and kidney disease: analysis from the United Network for Organ Sharing dataset. Liver Int. 2016;36:1018–25. https://doi.org/10.1111/liv.13041.
69. Devaney K, Goodman ZD, Ishak KG. Hepatobiliary cystadenoma and cystadenocarcinoma. A light microscopic and immunohistochemical study of 70 patients. Am J Surg Pathol. 1994;18:1078–91.
70. Quigley B, Reid MD, Pehlivanoglu B, Squires MH 3rd, Maithel S, Xue Y, Hyejeong C, Akkas G, Muraki T, Kooby DA, Sarmiento JM, Cardona K, Sekhar A, Krasinskas A, Adsay V. Hepatobiliary mucinous cystic neoplasms with ovarian type stroma (so-called "hepatobiliary cystadenoma/cystadenocarcinoma"): clinicopathologic analysis of 36 cases illustrates rarity of carcinomatous change. Am J Surg Pathol. 2018;42:95–102. https://doi.org/10.1097/PAS.0000000000000963.
71. Bakoyiannis A, Delis S, Triantopoulou C, Dervenis C. Rare cystic liver lesions: a diagnostic and managing challenge. World J Gastroenterol. 2013;19:7603–19. https://doi.org/10.3748/wjg.v19.i43.7603.
72. Zen Y, Pedica F, Patcha VR, Capelli P, Zamboni G, Casaril A, Quaglia A, Nakanuma Y, Heaton N, Portmann B. Mucinous cystic neoplasms of the liver: a clinicopathological study and comparison with intraductal papillary neoplasms of the bile duct. Mod Pathol. 2011;24:1079–89. https://doi.org/10.1038/modpathol.2011.71.
73. Wheeler DA, Edmondson HA. Cystadenoma with mesenchymal stroma (CMS) in the liver and bile ducts. A clinicopathologic study of 17 cases, 4 with malignant change. Cancer. 1985;56:1434–45.
74. Arnaoutakis DJ, Kim Y, Pulitano C, Zaydfudim V, Squires MH, Kooby D, Groeschl R, Alexandrescu S, Bauer TW, Bloomston M, Soares K, Marques H, Gamblin TC, Popescu I, Adams R, Nagorney D, Barroso E, Maithel SK, Crawford M, Sandroussi C, Marsh

W, Pawlik TM. Management of biliary cystic tumors: a multi-institutional analysis of a rare liver tumor. Ann Surg. 2015;261:361–7. https://doi.org/10.1097/SLA.0000000000000543.
75. Kishida N, Shinoda M, Masugi Y, Itano O, Fujii-Nishimura Y, Ueno A, Kitago M, Hibi T, Abe Y, Yagi H, Tanimoto A, Tanabe M, Sakamaoto M, Kitagawa Y. Cystic tumor of the liver without ovarian-like stroma or bile duct communication: two case reports and a review of the literature. World J Surg Oncol. 2014;12:229. https://doi.org/10.1186/1477-7819-12-229.
76. Bosman FT, World Health Organization, International Agency for Research on Cancer. WHO classification of tumours of the digestive system. 4th ed. Lyon: International Agency for Research on Cancer; 2010.
77. Adsay V, Mino-Kenudson M, Furukawa T, Basturk O, Zamboni G, Marchegiani G, Bassi C, Salvia R, Malleo G, Paiella S, Wolfgang CL, Matthaei H, Offerhaus GJ, Adham M, Bruno MJ, Reid MD, Krasinskas A, Klöppel G, Ohike N, Tajiri T, Jang KT, Roa JC, Allen P, Fernández-del Castillo C, Jang JY, Klimstra DS, Hruban RH, Members of Verona Consensus Meeting, 2013. Pathologic evaluation and reporting of intraductal papillary mucinous neoplasms of the pancreas and other tumoral intraepithelial neoplasms of pancreatobiliary tract: recommendations of verona consensus meeting. Ann Surg. 2016;263:162–77. https://doi.org/10.1097/SLA.0000000000001173.
78. Sang X, Sun Y, Mao Y, Yang Z, Lu X, Yang H, Xu H, Zhong S, Huang J. Hepatobiliary cystadenomas and cystadenocarcinomas: a report of 33 cases. Liver Int. 2011;31:1337–44. https://doi.org/10.1111/j.1478-3231.2011.02560.x.
79. Koffron A, Rao S, Ferrario M, Abecassis M. Intrahepatic biliary cystadenoma: role of cyst fluid analysis and surgical management in the laparoscopic era. Surgery. 2004;136:926–36. https://doi.org/10.1016/j.surg.2004.06.031.

Liver Cancer

31

Emilio De Raffele

31.1 Introduction

Hepatocellular carcinoma (HCC) and intrahepatic cholangiocarcinoma (iCCA) are the most frequent primary liver malignancies, with increasing incidence rates worldwide. These cancers have significantly higher prevalence in patients with chronic liver or biliary disease, related to persistent inflammation and hepatocellular and/or biliary damage. The risk for liver cancer is influenced by the etiology and the stage of underlying liver disease. Screening of patients at risk of malignant primary tumours is essential to diagnose premalignant or malignant lesions at an early stage, when the available treatments are most effective. In most cases however liver cancer is still diagnosed at an intermediate or advanced stage, with less favourable prognosis despite the availability of multiple therapeutic strategies. We review the biological and clinical features of the most common malignant liver neoplasms, HCC and iCCA, that are implicated in their prevention, surveillance, diagnosis and management strategies.

31.2 Hepatocellular Carcinoma

Hepatocellular carcinoma is the most frequent primary liver cancer, with an increasing incidence worldwide. Liver cirrhosis, infection from primary hepatotropic viruses, non-alcoholic fatty liver disease (NAFLD), are well-known risk factors and need different surveillance protocols. Early detection is essential because tumours at an early stage are potentially curable. In the past decade, however, treatment of HCC has substantially evolved and effective therapeutic strategies are available also for more advanced tumours.

E. De Raffele (✉)
Unità Operativa di Chirurgia Generale, Dipartimento dell'Apparato Digerente, Azienda Ospedaliero-Universitaria di Bologna, Policlinico S. Orsola-Malpighi, Bologna, Italy
e-mail: e.deraffele@aosp.bo.it

31.2.1 Epidemiology and Risk Factors

Liver cancer is the fifth most common cancer in the world, and the second most frequent cause of cancer mortality [1, 2], with increasing incidence rates in Europe and worldwide. HCC represents more than 90% of primary liver cancer [3, 4] and is the most common cause of death among cirrhotic patients [5–7]. The incidence of HCC increases with age; a progressive ageing of HCC patients has been reported in recent years in most Western countries, with the peak incidence in septuagenarians [8], and in Japan, where the incidence is higher in men aged 70–79 years [9]; in Chinese and black African populations the peak incidence occurs at an earlier age [4]. The male to female ratio ranges between is 2:1 and 4:1 [3, 4]. The global distribution of HCC varies according to geographic location, in parallel with different etiologies, being mostly related to the distribution of infections from hepatitis B (HBV) and hepatitis C (HCV) viruses, with the highest incidence rates in East Asia, where China has the greatest burden, and Sub-Saharan Africa [3–5]; in some of these areas however, the progressive diffusion of vaccination programs against HBV has recently determined a substantial decline in viral hepatitis and a concurrent decrease of HCC incidence [4, 5, 7]. HCC incidence is lower in Europe, except for Southern Europe [10]; Mediterranean countries, including Italy, Spain, and Greece, have intermediate incidence rates of 10–20 per 100,000 individuals [11]; recently, a notable decrease of HCC incidence has occurred also in France and Italy [5, 7]. However, the global incidence of HCC is growing, with an increase in most developed Western countries, including USA, Canada, Australia, New Zealand and most European countries [3–5]. It has been estimated that in 2030 liver cancer will become the third leading cause of cancer mortality in the USA [12]. However, the diffusion of vaccination programs and effective therapies against HBV infection and the development and diffusion of new antiviral agents against HCV will probably determine its gradual decline in the next decades [4, 7, 8].

F. Radu-Ionita et al. (eds.), *Liver Diseases*, https://doi.org/10.1007/978-3-030-24432-3_31

The single most relevant risk factor for development of HCC is liver cirrhosis of any aetiology, which is present in 70–90% of liver cancer patients [13], and about 30–35% of all cirrhotic patients will develop HCC over time [14]. The annual risk of developing HCC has been estimated between 1% and 8% in cirrhotics [8], and the 5-year cumulative risk for the development of HCC in cirrhotics ranges between 5% and 30%, according to the aetiology (with the highest risk among those infected with HCV), region or ethnic group, and stage of liver disease [6]. The risk of developing HCC has been reported to increase progressively in male patients, with advanced age, and progressive, worsening liver disease [8]. HBV is the leading risk factor for HCC, globally accounting for at least 50% of all cases of HCC [5, 15]. In Asia and Africa HBV infection is endemic, and 60% of HCC is associated with HBV, 20% with HCV, and the remaining with other risk factors; the risk of developing HCC among chronic HBV carriers is 10- to 100-fold greater compared with that of uninfected people [3]. HCV infection is the most important factor in North America, Europe and Japan [6, 11], being detected in 80–90% of HCC cases in Japan, 44–66% in Italy, and 30–50% in the United States [5, 6]. NAFLD is at present the leading cause of chronic liver disease in the United States and is increasingly diffusing in most developed and developing countries [5, 8, 11, 16]; features of the metabolic syndrome (MS), defined by the presence of central obesity, dyslipidemia, hypertension and impaired glucose metabolism, are present in virtually all cases of NAFLD; the MS has been recently associated with an increased risk of developing HCC [5, 16, 17]. Other well known risk factors are alcohol abuse, obesity, type 2 diabetes mellitus (DM), the ingestion of food contaminated with aflatoxins, tobacco smoking, while other factors are relatively less frequent [5, 6, 8, 11]. Some patients may have multiple risk factors, including HBV/HCV, alcohol abuse plus viral infection, etc.

HBV infection. HBV is a well known cause of HCC also in the absence of cirrhosis, even though most HBV-related HCCs develop in cirrhotic livers [6]. Chronic HBV infection determines a lifetime risk of HCC of 10–25% [3]. The risk of HCC among HBV carriers is related to multiple factors: male sex; age; the viral load, expressed by serum HBV-DNA levels [5, 18], serum hepatitis B surface antigen (HBsAg) and hepatitis B envelope antigen (HBeAg) levels [19, 20]; genotype C and some common variants in the precore and basal core promoter regions of the viral genome [21, 22]; perinatal transmission of HBV and maternal virus load [23]. Baseline liver stiffness values have been reported to predict HCC development in chronic HBV carriers [24]. Vaccination drastically reduces the incidence of chronic HBV infection and the related risk of HCC [3]; also antiviral therapy significantly reduces the risk of HCC in chronic HBV carriers with or without cirrhosis, especially among patients with sustained virological response (SVR) [3].

HCV infection. The relative risk of developing HCC among HCV carriers is estimated to be 17-fold [11]. HCV appears to increase the risk of HCC either inducing hepatic inflammation and fibrosis, or directly promoting malignant transformation of infected hepatocytes. The risk progressively increases in patients with advanced fibrosis and cirrhosis, respectively [3]. Other significant risk factors in chronic HCV carriers are male sex, older age, HCV genotype 1b, coinfection with HBV or HIV, alcohol abuse, obesity and presence of DM [3]. Patients with HBV/HCV coinfection have an increased risk of HCC [3, 5].

Metabolic diseases. NAFLD and nonalcoholic steatohepatitis (NASH) determine a significant risk of developing liver cancer, which is higher in the presence of advanced liver fibrosis and cirrhosis. Recent data seem to indicate that NAFLD can progress to NASH even in the absence of hepatocellular injury and inflammation [25]. The estimated overall prevalence of NASH ranges between 2% and 3% [26], with a significant proportion of NASH evolving towards advanced liver fibrosis and cirrhosis over time [27]. The incidence of HCC in patients with NASH cirrhosis has been reported to be 2.3–4.0% per year [3]. Some reports however indicate that HCC may occur in NAFLD patients even in the absence of cirrhosis, even though the exact incidence rates and the related pathophysiological mechanisms are still under investigation [3, 8, 11, 16, 28]. NAFLD, with or without NASH, is the hepatic manifestation of MS. Metabolic syndrome and its features, including overweight and obesity, have been recently associated with a substantial risk of HCC [3, 5]. DM determines a 2.0–2.5 relative risk of developing HCC and is considered to be independent of other risk factors [3, 5]; diabetes of long duration and treatment with insulin or sulfonylureas have a higher risk, while metformin treatment has been associated with a lower risk of HCC [29]. NAFLD has become the most common liver disorder in some developed countries and is at present a noticeable risk factor for the development of HCC; moreover, the role of NAFLD, NASH and MS in liver cancer has been estimated to increase in the near future [3, 5, 28]. Also the number of candidates to liver transplantation for HCC due to NASH is rapidly growing [30].

Alcohol consumption and tobacco smoking. Alcohol abuse significantly increases the risk of liver cancer and the increased risk is dose-related [3, 5]; cessation of alcohol consumption determines a progressive decrease of the liver cancer risk [31]. Alcohol has a synergistic effect with other causative agents of chronic liver disease, including HBV and HCV infection, fatty liver disease and NAFLD, obesity, diabetes, and smoking, to further increase the risk of HCC [3]. Tobacco smoking has been recently associated with an increased risk of liver cancer [3, 5].

Aflatoxin. Aflatoxin B1 is an aflatoxin produced by *Aspergillus flavus* and *Aspergillus parasiticus*; it is a major hepatocarcinogen that contaminates a variety of foods, and is more common in areas where HBV is endemic, including sub-Saharan Africa, Southeast Asia, and China; in these regions, higher levels of Aflatoxin B1 are found among chronic HBV carriers [32]; Aflatoxin B1 has a synergistic effect in increasing the risk of HCC with HBV infection [33], alcohol intake, and also HCV infection [3].

Other causes. Also liver cirrhosis of less frequent aetiology has an increased risk of HCC, including genetic hemochromatosis, primary biliary cholangitis (PBC), autoimmune hepatitis, and Wilson disease [3]. Host genetics may favour progression to HCC, including some variants of tumour necrosis factor (TNF) and null genotypes of glutathione S-transferase (GST) genes [3].

Key Concepts

- Liver cancer is amongst the most frequent causes of cancer mortality in the world, with increasing incidence rates worldwide.
- The most relevant risk factors for development of HCC include liver cirrhosis of any aetiology, HBV infection, HCV infection, NAFLD, metabolic syndrome, alcohol abuse, obesity, diabetes mellitus, ingestion of food contaminated with aflatoxins, tobacco smoking; other factors are relatively less frequent; some patients may have multiple risk factors.

31.2.2 Prevention

The most common risk factor for HCC is chronic HBV infection, so that strategies to prevent liver cancer related to HVB include vaccination to reduce new infections, antiviral therapies to suppress viral replication and limit liver disease progression, and adequate surveillance of patients at risk, with the aim of detecting HCC at an earlier, potentially curable stage [3–5]. The extensive vaccination programs to prevent new HBV infections in endemic areas resulted in a substantial decline in HBV infections and incidence of HCC [13]. The national vaccination program against HBV started between 1984 and 1990 in Taiwan significantly reduced the incidence of acute and chronic hepatitis B, of liver cirrhosis, and specifically of HCC by more than 80% [5]. Similar results have been achieved in endemic regions of China [3]. Persistent HBV replication with high and also moderate levels of serum HBV-DNA results in substantial risk of developing HCC [34]. As a consequence, antiviral treatment that reduce serum viral loads can reduce the incidence of cancer. Lamivudine monotherapy has been demonstrated to significantly decrease the risk of HCC in chronic HBV carriers with advanced fibrosis and cirrhosis [35]. Similar results have been obtained with other available antiviral agents, including standard or pegylated interferon-alpha (IFNa), and oral nucleos(t)ide analogues [36]. The risk of HCC is significantly lower in patients with sustained viral response (SVR) and favourable clinical outcome [3–5]. However suppression of viral replication in chronic HBV carriers by antiviral treatment significantly reduce but do not eliminate the risk of HCC, especially in the presence of cirrhosis [37], so that also responders to antiviral agents should undergo regular surveillance [3].

Also among chronic HCV carriers, the risk of HCC is significantly reduced in patients with SVR after interferon or interferon plus ribavirin treatment [38]. However, as for chronic HBV carriers, the risk of HCC in HCV patients with SVR, though remarkably reduced, remains relatively high, especially in older patients and in the presence of cirrhosis, and requires surveillance [3, 5, 39]. The recent availability of direct-acting antiviral (DAA) therapies has substantially increased the percentage of chronic HCV carriers with SVR [3]; however there is no evidence at present that successful DAA therapies will decrease the incidence of liver cancer in HCV cirrhotics [3, 5].

As previously discussed, NAFLD and NASH have been associated with a significant risk of developing liver cancer, which is higher in the presence of advanced liver fibrosis and cirrhosis, although may occur even in the absence of cirrhosis [3, 28]. NAFLD and NASH are the hepatic manifestation of MS. Also MS and its features, including overweight, obesity and diabetes, have been recently associated with a substantial risk of HCC, and their role in liver cancer has been estimated to increase in the near future [3, 28], both in developed and developing countries; as a consequence, major efforts should be devoted to reduce the load of factors determining NAFLD and NASH, explaining and supporting the role of healthier dietary habits, lifestyle modifications, including regular walking, exercise, and weight loss, to the general population, and especially to patients at risk or affected by metabolic derangements [3, 5]. Moreover, patients with established NAFLD and NASH should be considered for periodic HCC screening [40]. Coffee consumption has been definitely associated with a decreased risk of developing HCC [5, 41]. Some observational studies suggest a reduction of HCC risk in patients assuming statins, but these effects need to be further confirmed [5, 41].

Key Concepts

- HBV vaccination reduces the risk of HCC and is recommended for all infants and high-risk groups, and should be implemented worldwide.
- Treatment of chronic liver disease may prevent progression of liver disease; antiviral therapies against HBV and HCV that achieve SVR have been demonstrated to prevent progression to cirrhosis and HCC development.
- In patients with established cirrhosis, antiviral therapies are beneficial in preventing cirrhosis progression, decompensation, and cancer development, although SVR reduces but does not eliminate the risk of HCC occurrence.
- Major efforts should be devoted by governmental health agencies to prevent viral transmission and chronic alcohol abuse, and to reduce the load of factors determining NAFLD, metabolic syndrome and obesity, by encouraging healthier dietary habits, lifestyle modifications, and weight loss.
- Coffee consumption has been demonstrated to decrease the risk of HCC in patients with chronic liver disease.

31.2.3 Pathogenesis

Development of HCC is a complex multistep process related to a persistent inflammation determined by hepatocyte necrosis and regeneration, associated with progressive fibrosis. Evolution to cirrhosis substantially increases the risk of HCC. Multiple somatic genomic alterations and epigenetic modifications determine the vast molecular heterogeneity of HCC [42]. Multiple pathways have been advocated to be involved in the hepatocarcinogenesis of HCC, and some of the molecules associated with these pathways represent the target of the systemic therapies selectively used for advanced tumours. [41]. The mitogen-activated protein kinase (MAPK) cascade consists of serine/threonine kinases, which convert extracellular molecules (growth factors, hormones, tumor-promoting substances, differentiation factors, etc.) into intracellular signals for regulating cell growth and differentiation; there are four core protein kinases, Ras, Raf, MEK and ERK, in the Ras/Raf/MEK/ERK signaling pathway; this is a common downstream pathway for multiple tyrosine kinase receptors, including epidermal growth factor receptor (EGFR), vascular endothelial growth factor receptor (VEGFR), platelet-derived growth factor receptor (PDGFR), and type I insulin-like growth factor receptor (IGF-1R); the activation of this pathway has been reported in HCC; Sorafenib is a multikinase inhibitor of Raf serine/threonine kinase, of VEGFR, PDGFR, and of other receptors involved in this pathway [43]. Other pathways have been found to be activated in HCC tissue samples, including the PI3K-AKT–mammalian target of rapamycin (mTOR) pathway, which plays a key role in cell growth and regulation; the Wnt-β-catenin pathway; the proangiogenic pathways, where multiple factors, such as VEGF, PDGF, fibroblast growth factor (FGF), and hepatocyte growth factor (HGF) induce signaling via the Ras-Raf-mTOR-Wnt pathways, activate angiogenesis and play a substantial role in the vascularization, invasiveness, and metastatic potential of the HCC; the EGFR pathway, that may activate angiogenesis, cell proliferation and adhesion, and inhibition of apoptosis [41].

Key Concepts

- Development of HCC is a complex multistep process related to a persistent inflammation, determined by hepatocyte necrosis and regeneration, associated with progressive fibrosis. Evolution to cirrhosis increases the risk of HCC.
- Multiple pathways have been advocated to be involved in the hepatocarcinogenesis of HCC, and some of the molecules associated with these pathways represent the target of the systemic therapies selectively used for advanced cancer stages.

31.2.4 Diagnosis

Ultrasonography. Ultrasonography (US) is the most widely used imaging modality for screening and surveillance of liver cancer [44–46], because is noninvasive, well tolerated, widely available and cost-effective, with a reported sensitivity of 40–81% and specificity of 80–100% for HCC [3]. HCC does not have a characteristic appearance on US; nodules larger than 1 cm are typically hypoechoic, but may be isoechoic, hyperechoic with or without a hypoechoic rim, or mixed [44]. Although the overall sensitivity of US is 94% for detection of HCC at any stage, significantly lower rates of detection have been reported in cirrhotics and in obese patients [44]. Because of significantly lower sensitivity and positive predictive value than other imaging techniques, B-mode US is not indicated for diagnostic confirmation [47]. Contrast-enhanced ultrasonography (CEUS) using microbubble contrast agents has been demonstrated to be effective for characterizing liver tumours [48], sharing most of the enhancement features of dynamic computed tomography (CT) and magnetic resonance imaging (MRI), although a discordant enhancement pattern has been observed for intrahepatic cholangiocarcinoma (iCCA) [3, 5]; recent studies have shown that a wash-out time >55–60 s accurately identifies HCCs, while a wash-out time <55–60 s correctly identifies most non-HCC malignancies [3, 44]. CEUS has been used for lesion characterization and diagnosis of HCC with a specificity of 93–100% [49, 50], and has been reported to have comparable accuracy than dynamic CT and MRI also for small HCCs [47]. At present CEUS is considered a cost-effective second-line imaging modality to characterize focal liver lesions identified at conventional US examination, while dynamic multidetector CT (MDCT) and MRI remain the most appropriate modalities to characterize solid lesions suspicious for HCC in cirrhotic patients [2–4].

Dynamic computed tomography and magnetic resonance imaging. At contrast enhanced imaging, HCC typically appears as a well-defined nodule with hepatic arterial pathologic neovascularization [51]. When a typical enhancement pattern is evident with dynamic MDCT and MRI, a confident diagnosis of HCC can be usually obtained without biopsy confirmation, since MDCT/MR imaging specificity approaches 100% [3, 5, 44, 52, 53]. The most reliable imaging modalities for HCC diagnosis are quadruple-phase dynamic MDCT and dynamic MRI, that include precontrast phase, late hepatic arterial phase, about 30 s after rapid-bolus intravenous contrast injection, portal venous phase, 60–70 s after injection, and delayed phase imaging, 3–5 min after contrast injection [3, 54]. HCCs with typical pattern of enhancement at MDCT show avid contrast enhancement in the late arterial phase, as their blood supply mainly derive from intrahepatic arterial vessels; during the portal venous phase the tumour typically shows a rapid washout and becomes hypodense relative to the surrounding liver parenchyma, as the blood supply to the liver comes predominantly from the portal vein, while HCC lacks a portal venous supply; sometimes the washout is evident only in the delayed phase [3, 44, 54]. During the portal venous or delayed phases, a thin ring of enhancement is often evident, due to the presence of a true fibrous capsule or of a pseudocapsule made of compressed vessels and liver parenchyma, which is a relevant imaging feature of HCC [3, 54]. Vascular invasion, mainly the presence of a portal tumour thrombus, but also in the hepatic veins and in the vena cava, is typical of advanced HCCs [55].

MRI examination of the liver generally consists of T1-weighted (T1w) sequences, T2-weighted (T2w) sequences, and diffusion-weighted imaging (DWI) with apparent diffusion coefficient (ADC) map [54]. HCCs are usually hypointense on T1w imaging and hyperintense on T2w sequences. Contrast-enhanced T1w sequences with extracellular gadolinium-based contrast medium are similar to MDCT, with hyperenhancement at hepatic arterial phase, washout in the portal venous and delayed phases, and eventually the presence of a capsule/pseudocapsule in the portal venous and delayed phases [54]. Increased signal on DWI with corresponding low intensity on the generated ADC map indicates hypercellularity and may be useful to diagnose malignant lesions [54]. The typical pattern of arterial enhancement followed by washout in the later phases has sensitivity and specificity of 90% and >95%, respectively, with a positive predictive value approximating 100% in cirrhotics [3, 52–54]. According to recent studies comparing the diagnostic accuracy of US, CT, and MRI, the overall per-lesion sensitivity for nodular HCC is 77–100% and 68–91% for MRI and CT, respectively, with MRI showing equivalent or higher per-lesion sensitivity compared with CT [47, 56]; the per-lesion sensitivity stratified by size, was 100% for both modalities for HCCs >2 cm, 44–47% and 40–44% for MRI and CT, respectively, for HCCs measuring 1–2 cm, and 29–43% and 10–33% for MRI and CT, respectively, for HCCs <1 cm [3].

Recently, MRI performed with liver specific intracellular contrast agents other than nonspecific extracellular gadolinium-based agents have shown to be highly sensitive for detection of HCC, including smaller tumours [3, 54]. Hepatobiliary (HPB)-specific contrast media gadoxetate disodium (Gd-EOB-DTPA) and gadobenate dimeglumine (Gd-BOPTA), are progressively transported into hepatocytes and excreted through bile ducts; the scan phases can be divided into the distribution phase, where the HPB-Gd agents act as an extracellular contrast agent, consisting of the hepatic arterial phase (about 20–30 s after injection) and the portal venous phase (about 60 s after injection); and the hepatobiliary (HBP) phase, where the HPB-Gd agents are transported into hepatocytes; HBP phase starts about 60 s after the injection of HPB-Gd agents, and hepatic enhancement is complete about 20 min after injection; the transitional phase represents the transitional time between the distribution and the HBP phase, 2–5 min after injection, where the signal is a mixture of the distribution and the HBP phases [57]. MRI with HPB-Gd agents have shown higher overall sensitivity than dynamic CT or MRI using nonspecific extracellular gadolinium-based agents [3, 52, 54, 56]. Gd-EOB-DTPA-enhanced MRI has been included as a first-line diagnostic method for HCC in the guidelines of the Japan Society of Hepatology (JSH) and the Liver Cancer Study Group of Japan (LCSGJ) [58], and in the HCC guidelines of the Asian Pacific Association for the Study of the Liver (APASL) [3], but not in the guidelines of the European Association for the Study of the Liver (EASL) [4]. Gd-EOB-DTPA-enhanced MRI and/or CEUS using Sonazoid are considered useful to distinguish HCC from benign hypervascular lesions, iCCA or combined HCC-CCA in case of hypervascular tumours; and to identify early carcinogenetic processes in case of iso or hypovascular tumours, including precancerous dysplastic nodules, early HCC, and nodule-in-nodule liver cancer [3];

the HBP phase of Gd-EOB-DTPA-enhanced MRI is believed to detect the earliest carcinogenetic changes suggestive of HCC [3].

Hypovascular nodules associated with liver cirrhosis include low-grade dysplastic nodules (LGDN), high-grade dysplastic nodules (HGDN), early HCCs, and well-differentiated HCCs [55, 59]. The sensitivity of dynamic MDCT and/or MRI in detection of these borderline lesions is quite low [59]. Early HCCs may be more frequently visible on the HBP images of Gd-EOB-DTPA-enhanced MRI as hypointense nodules [58, 60], and hypointensity at HBP images is considered a strong predictor of premalignancy or malignancy, favouring a diagnosis of HGDN or early HCC rather than LGDN or simple cirrhotic nodule [58, 60, 61]. At present however it is quite difficult to distinguish early HCC from preneoplastic nodular lesions based on MRI evaluation. The recent updates of the guidelines of the JSH and of the APASL suggest that hypointense nodules in the HBP images of Gd-EOB-DTPA-enhanced MRI should undergo CEUS with Sonazoid, which can correctly diagnose HCCs if hypervascularity and/or a decreased uptake in the Kupffer phase of the exams are observed [3, 58, 60].

To standardize the performance, interpretation, reporting and data collection of the available contrast-enhanced imaging modalities, including CT, MRI, and most recently CEUS, the American College of Radiology (ACR) supported the development of the Liver Imaging Reporting and Data System (LI-RADS) [44, 46, 62], to be applied to patients at high risk of HCC. LI-RADS includes five major categories, where LR-5 indicates a definite HCC, LR-1 a definite benign lesion, and LR-4, LR-3, and LR-2 indicate decreasing likelihood of HCC; tumour evaluation is based on the presence of major and minor criteria. Major criteria include arterial phase enhancement, where only lesions with unequivocal arterial phase hyperenhancement (APHE) are categorized as LR-5, particularly in the late arterial phase, when the portal vein is at least partially enhanced, as some HCCs demonstrate contrast enhancement during the late hepatic arterial phase only [46]; observation size (diameter), where tumours with APHE are categorized as LR-5 only if the diameter size is >10 mm; washout appearance during the portal venous phase or also the delayed phase, defined by the ACR as "nonperipheral visually assessed temporal reduction in enhancement relative to liver from an earlier to a later phase resulting in hypoenhancement in the extracellular phase" [44]; an enhancing "capsule", defined by the ACR as a "smooth, uniform, sharp border around most or all of the observation, unequivocally thicker or more conspicuous than fibrotic tissue around background nodules, and visible as an enhancing rim on portal venous phase, delayed phase, or transitional phase" [44]; and threshold growth, defined as an observation with a diameter increase of a minimum of 5 mm and either >50% growth in ≤6 months or with ≥100% growth after 6 months, or a new observation ≥10 mm. A series of minor criteria or ancillary features can be used to upgrade or downgrade an observation; these may suggest a different liver cancer, or a HCC with atypical behavior, when the diagnosis of malignancy is not definitive according to the major criteria; ancillary features suggesting malignancy include the presence of a nonenhancing capsule, hypointensity on HBP and transitional phases at MRI with HPB-Gd agents, mild to moderate hyperintensity on T2w imaged, restricted diffusion, lesional fat or iron sparing, intralesional hemorrhage, size increase less than the threshold growth, and other features suggestive of malignancy [44, 46, 62]. The LR-5 category in the 2017 LI-RADS version maintains a specificity approaching 100% [44], although a small percentage of HCCs are hypovascular and thus difficult to characterize [63]. A diagnostic algorithm has been recently approved by the ACR also for the use of CEUS in patients at high risk of HCC, which shares many features with the conventional 2017 LI-RADS version [50].

Positron-emission tomography. 18F-Fluorodeoxyglucose (FDG)-positron emission tomography (PET) and PET-TC have a limited value in diagnostic evaluation, since HCCs are not very avid for FDG; well differentiated tumours are usually FDG-PET negative; on the contrary, more advanced tumours may show FDG uptake, usually associated with increased serum alpha-fetoprotein (AFP), vascular invasion and overall poor prognosis [4]. Because of its potential prognostic value, FDG-PET may facilitate the selection of candidates to liver resection or transplantation [64, 65].

Tumour markers. Tumour markers for HCC are useful for diagnosis, even in surveillance programs, in treatment evaluation and during the follow-up after treatment. Serum AFP has been used as a diagnostic test for HCC since the 1970s, but its usefulness is limited because higher levels of AFP are usually found in advanced HCC, while smaller tumours may have normal or slightly altered AFP levels. At present the suggested cut-off values of AFP in surveillance programs is set at 200 ng/mL instead of 20 ng/mL when used with US [66]. Moreover, AFP has lower specificity in patient at high risk of HCC, since its levels increase with necroinflammation and regeneration in patients with active hepatitis or cirrhosis and without HCC, while decrease in chronic HBV and HCV carriers responsive to antiviral therapies [3]. Other tumour markers include the des-gamma-carboxyprothrombin (DCP), an abnormal prothrombin protein also known as prothrombin induced by vitamin K absence-II (PIVKA-II), and the *Lens culinaris* agglutinin-reactive fraction of AFP (AFP-L3), a variant of AFP that can differentiate an increase in AFP levels related to HCC rather than to benign liver diseases [66].

Key Concepts

- Diagnosis of HCC in cirrhotic patients should be based on non-invasive criteria whenever possible, limiting liver biopsy to uncertain lesions.
- US is a screening test and should not be used for diagnostic confirmation. CEUS is useful for characterization of liver nodules found at US, and is currently considered as sensitive as dynamic CT or MRI in the diagnosis of HCC.
- Dynamic MDCT, dynamic MRI, or MRI with HPB-specific contrast media represent the first-line diagnostic techniques for HCC. Diagnosis is based on the presence of the typical hallmarks of HCC: APHE with washout in the portal venous or delayed phases on MDCT and MRI using extracellular contrast agents, APHE with washout in the portal venous phase on MRI using Gd-EOB-DTPA.
- To standardize the interpretation and reporting of the available dynamic imaging modalities, including MDCT, MRI, and more recently CEUS, the ACR has supported the development of the LI-RADS categorization, to be applied to patients at high risk of HCC; LI-RADS includes five major categories, where LR-5 indicates a definite HCC, LR-1 a definite benign lesion, and LR-4, LR-3, and LR-2 indicate decreasing likelihood of HCC; categorization is based on the presence of major and minor criteria.
- FDG-PET is not effective to diagnose early HCC, but can have prognostic value in candidates to surgery.
- Serum AFP levels have limited value in early HCC stages, either in surveillance or as a confirmatory test.

31.2.5 Surveillance

The progressive diffusion of surveillance programs in patients at risk of developing HCC have the aim to reduce cancer-related mortality, and may allow earlier diagnosis, when the stage of the tumour is still susceptible to potentially curative therapies with expected 5-year survival rates beyond 50–70%, such as surgical resection, ablation and liver transplantation [5, 8, 67]. Surveillance has been found to be cost-effective, and should be undertaken in groups of patients with a significant risk of HCC development, mainly cirrhotics with HBV or HCV infection, NASH, primary biliary cirrhosis, selected groups of adult Asian and African chronic HBV carriers even in the absence of cirrhosis, patients with chronic hepatitis C and bridging fibrosis, patients with NAFLD without underlying cirrhosis [3, 5, 41]. Suppression of viral replication in chronic HBV and HCV carriers by antiviral treatment does not eliminate the risk of HCC, especially in the presence of cirrhosis, so that surveillance should be maintained [3, 5]. Multiple scoring systems to stratify the risk of HCC have been proposed to identify the optimal population for HCC surveillance [3, 41]. Cost-effectiveness of surveillance is related to the potential of receiving curative treatments in case of HCC occurrence; thus patients with severe liver disease or comorbidities ineligible for treatments are not appropriate candidates to HCC surveillance [3, 5]. Several Eastern and Western non-randomized studies have demonstrated that patients at risk of developing HCC enrolled into surveillance programs were diagnosed at an earlier stage, more frequently underwent potentially curative treatments, and had better survival rates [45, 67]. These results have been confirmed by an extensive randomized study from China, where HBV infected patients screened with US and AFP test every 6 months had a HCC mortality reduced by 37% than unscreened controls; in the screened group the HCC was subclinical in 60.5% of patients, small in 45.3% and the resection was achieved in 46.5% [68]. In 1967 a nationwide HCC surveillance program was established in Japan through the LCSGJ, with the institution of a prospective registry of all patients with HCC diagnosed throughout Japan; patients with chronic HBV and/or HCV infection and/or liver cirrhosis are considered at high risk of developing HCC and undergo US and serum concentration of tumour markers every 3–6 months [69, 70]; the updated results of the LCSGJ surveillance program have shown a dramatic improvement of the long term survival of patients with HCC observed over about 30 years [69].

US is the most diffuse imaging procedure for surveillance of HCC, because it is noninvasive, well tolerated and has relatively moderate costs [3, 5]. Although US efficacy is related to the tumour size, with a sensitivity of about 63% for early-stage HCC, the overall sensitivity approaches 95% [71]. The efficacy of the surveillance strategies are substantially related to the quality of the equipment and the expertise of the ultrasonographers [3, 5]. US-based surveillance performed biannually by experienced ultrasonographers is considered effective for early detection of HCC <3 cm [72]. At present there is no evidence to support the use of dynamic CT or MRI in routine surveillance strategies for HCC. Conflicting results have been obtained combining imaging modalities with serum biomarkers, usually AFP levels [3, 5]; however, some guidelines suggest to perform biannually a combination of US and measurement of serum AFP levels for surveillance in patients at risk of HCC [3]. On the basis of the available data, patients at risk of HCC should be screened every 6 months, a time interval considered more effective to achieve early detection and survival than longer intervals [3, 5].

Key Concepts

- Implementation of screening programs in patients at high risk of HCC has been demonstrated to reduce cancer-related mortality because of earlier diagnosis, when tumours are still susceptible to potentially curative therapies, and to be cost-effective in selected patients.
- Patients at high risk of HCC should be entered into surveillance programs, including those with compensated liver cirrhosis and chronic HBV or HCV infection; the role of surveillance for patients with NAFLD without cirrhosis is still unclear.
- Surveillance should be performed by experienced personnel with appropriate equipment in high-risk populations, using abdominal US and eventually AFP every 6 months.

31.2.6 Staging

Several staging systems have been proposed to stratify the tumour burden, and in most cases the liver function, and to determine the most appropriate treatment strategy for the different stages [5, 41, 73]. The tumor-node-metastasis (TNM) classification has been developed by the American Joint Committee on Cancer (AJCC) and International Union for Cancer Control (UICC) and has been regularly updated since the first edition of 1977; it is based on the size of the tumour, the extent of regional lymph node involvement, and the presence of distant metastases; the seventh edition of the TNM staging system is currently available [73]. Neoplastic lymphovascular invasion plays a major role in the T classification of the TNM system, where the presence of microscopic vascular invasion differentiates pT1 from pT2, and also clinical stage I from clinical stage II [74]; microvascular invasion is the most important independent prognostic factor of overall survival after LR and LT, and is found in up to 50% of resected HCCs [75, 76]. Microvascular invasion correlates with tumour size and multiple tumours [76]. The most important limitation of the TNM classification for HCC is that it does not consider the liver function and/or the performance status of the patients, which are determinant prognostic factors. The Okuda classification system was developed in 1985 and was the first classification to consider both the tumor size and the liver function, as measured by the serum albumin level, bilirubin level, and presence of ascites [77]. The Cancer of the Liver Italian Program (CLIP) score was proposed in 1998 and incorporates four covariates, Child-Pugh grade, tumor morphology, serum AFP level and portal vein thrombosis [78]. The Japan Integrated Staging (JIS) score was developed in 2003 and is based on the combination of the Child-Pugh grade and of the TNM stage, based on the criteria of the LCSGJ [79]. The Barcelona Clinic Liver Cancer (BCLC) staging system was first proposed in 1999 and subsequently updated [5], and is the staging system endorsed by the AASLD and the EASL [4, 80]; this model includes four elements: the tumour burden, that incorporates the number of tumours, tumour size, and presence of portal vein invasion or extrahepatic metastasis; the liver functional reserve; the physical status according to the ECOG performance status (PS); and cancer-related symptoms; patients are subsequently assigned to five categories (0, A, B, C and D) based on these parameters. BCLC stage of 0 (very early stage disease) comprises patients diagnosed with one asymptomatic nodule measuring <2 cm, without vascular invasion or satellites and preserved liver function; BCLC stage of A (early-stage disease) includes patients diagnosed with one nodule of any size or a maximum of three nodules measuring <3 cm and preserved liver function; BCLC stage of B (intermediate-stage disease) comprises patients diagnosed with multiple nodules without vascular invasion or extrahepatic metastasis and preserved liver function; BCLC stage of C (advanced-stage disease) includes patients with vascular invasion or extrahepatic metastasis, preserved liver function, and cancer-related symptoms (PS 1–2); finally, BCLC stage of D (terminal stage disease) comprises patients with end-stage liver function, in any tumour stage and cancer-related symptoms (PS > 2). Based on the stage of the disease, a treatment strategy is recommended. The BCLC staging system has been validated in various studies, although it has some substantial limitations [3, 73, 81]. The Hong Kong Liver Cancer (HKLC) classification has been developed in 2014 [82], and is based on four prognostic factors including ECOG PS, Child-Pugh grade, liver tumour status, and presence of extrahepatic vascular invasion or metastasis; based on these prognostic factors, patients are assigned to five main stages and nine substages; substantial differences with the BCLC classification in terms of treatment recommendations include that patients with preserved liver function and multifocal tumours or presence of intrahepatic vascular invasion may be considered for LR, and that intrahepatic vascular invasion is not considered a contraindication for intra-arterial treatments; this classification seems to exhibit better prognostic value than the BCLC classification, but also to better reflect clinical practices [3, 41, 73]; however more extensive validation is required to confirm these important issues [5].

Key Concepts

- Several staging systems have been proposed to determine the most appropriate treatment strategy for the different stages of HCC; patients are usually stratified according to the tumour burden and the liver function.
- The TNM classification developed by AJCC-UICC is regularly updated, and is based on the size of the tumour, the extent of regional lymph node involvement, and the presence of distant metastases; this classification however does not consider the liver function and/or the performance status of the patients, limiting its clinical usefulness.
- The BCLC staging system, proposed in 1999 and currently endorsed by the EASL and the AASLD, has been extensively validated and is the present the most diffuse classification; this model is based on tumour burden, liver functional reserve, physical status, and cancer-related symptoms; patients are assigned to five categories (0, A, B, C and D) from very early stage disease to terminal stage disease. Based on the stage of the disease, a treatment strategy is recommended.
- Staging systems from Asian counties are also based on a combination of liver tumour status and liver functional reserve. Contrary to BCLC classification, however, in these staging systems LR is considered also in patients with preserved liver function and more advanced liver tumours, and intrahepatic vascular invasion is not considered a contraindication for intra-arterial treatments.

31.2.7 Pathology

Premalignant hepatocellular lesions. HCC develops in most cases in the background of chronic liver disease following a multistep sequence, through a series of intermediate lesions considered premalignant. The current nomenclature for these lesions has been proposed in 1995 and further updated in 2008 [83, 88]. Premalignant lesions include dysplastic foci (DF) and dysplastic nodules (DN), while small cancerous lesions, up to 2 cm, can be either early HCC (eHCC) or progressed HCC (pHCC) [41, 84]. DFs are uniform cluster of hepatocytes, <1 mm in size, with cellular atypia, but no evidence of malignancy; DF are typically found within the liver parenchyma in chronic liver disease, particularly in cirrhotic livers, are considered to be premalignant lesions, and may contain dysplastic hepatocytes with small cell changes (previously called small cell dysplasia), with increased nuclear/cytoplasmic ratio, or dysplastic hepatocytes with large cell changes (previously called large cell dysplasia), with enlarged nucleus and cytoplasm, and preserved nuclear/cytoplasmic ratio; DF have a definite precancerous role [41, 84]. DNs are lesions >1 mm and up to 2 cm, that typically arise in cirrhotic livers. According to the degree of cytologic and architectural atypia, dysplastic nodules can be classified into low-grade DN (LGDN) and high-grade DN (HGDN) [41, 84]. LGDNs are lesions with features suggestive of a regenerative growth, without major architectural alterations, and with an overall non-malignant morphology; since LGDNs share a number of features with non-neoplastic regenerative nodules, differentiation between these two lesions can be difficult; LGDNs are composed of hepatocytes with normal to slightly increased nuclear/cytoplasmic ratio, minimal cellular atypia and no mitotic figures; the liver architecture is well preserved, with normal hepatocyte plates and portal tracts, and a reticulin network; nodules have rounded borders and do not compress adjacent hepatic tissue. HGDNs are lesions with some degree of cytologic and architectural atypia, but insufficient to define a malignant morphology; HGDNs are composed of hepatocytes with an increased nuclear/cytoplasmic ratio, sometimes basophilic cytoplasm and peripheral nuclei, and occasional mitotic figures; the architecture of the nodules is irregular with thicker hepatocyte plates, sometimes with pseudogland formation, and abnormal arterial supply. DNs are premalignant lesions, and sometimes contain early malignant foci, defined "nodule-in-nodule lesion" [85]; patients with DNs, especially those with HGDNs, have a significant risk of progression to HCC [86]; HGDNs are sometimes difficult to differentiate from early HCC nodules; immunohistochemical staining for keratins CK7 and CK19 and CD34 can be useful in differentiation [41]. Immunohistochemical panels including glypican 3, glutamine synthetase, clathrin heavy chain, and heat shock protein 70, have also been suggested for detection of HCC [5, 41].

Gross pathology. The gross appearance of HCC is widely variable. Tumour size ranges from less than 1 to over 30 cm in diameter; the average size at diagnosis is usually smaller for tumours occurring in cirrhotic livers. HCC smaller than 2 cm are defined as "small HCC" [87], further differentiated into "vaguely nodular HCC", biologically at an earlier stage with a better prognosis, and "distinctly nodular HCC" [88]. At gross examination, HCC may have a nodular, infiltrative, or diffuse pattern [84]. The nodular or expanding pattern is the most common, typically found in cirrhotic livers; nodules are soft masses of variable colour, from gray to light brown to yellow-green, and may contain areas of hemorrhage or necrosis; nodules may be solitary or multiple, which may represent intrahepatic metastases or even multifocal independent tumours; small nodules adjacent to the main tumour are considered to be satellite nodules; nodular HCC is usually well-delineated and may be surrounded by a fibrous capsule, either complete or incomplete. The infiltrative or massive pattern is usually found in noncirrhotic livers; it usually appears as a large mass of variable size, with ill-defined, invasive borders. Advanced HCC, either nodular or infiltrative, may diffuse into large veins, mostly the portal vein, although hepatic veins, the inferior vena cava, and even the right atrium may be invaded; the invasion of large bile ducts is less frequent, and may determine biliary obstruction and hemobilia. The diffuse pattern is the least common and is characterized by a widespread infiltration by numerous small nodules that replace wide areas of the liver.

Microscopic pathology. At histology, the architecture is irregular, with atypical arteries and distorted portal tracts; neoplastic hepatocytes may have increased nuclear/cytoplasmic ratio and irregular nuclei, with a growth pattern ranging from well-differentiated thin sheets to trabecular or pseudoglandular patterns; steatosis, steatohepatitis, hyaline globules, and Mallory bodies are commonly found [41]. Regarding tumour cells, the Edmondson and Steiner's classification system is still considered the gold standard for classifying HCC into grades [89]: grade I or well-differentiated HCC, characterized by small neoplastic cells with abundant eosinophilic cytoplasm and slightly enlarged nuclei, arranged in thin trabeculae; these cells are almost identical to normal hepatocytes; grade II or moderately differentiated HCC, where neoplastic cells are larger, with increased nuclear/cytoplasmic ratio and abnormal nuclei; pseudoglandular structures may be evident; grade III or poorly differentiated HCC, where neoplastic cells show larger hyperchromatic, clearly irregular nuclei with very prominent nucleoli; and grade IV HCC, characterized by neoplastic cells with very high nuclear/cytoplasmic ratio, presence of anaplastic giant cells, and loss of trabecular pattern.

Different architectural growth patterns may be observed [84]. In the trabecular growth pattern, neoplastic hepatocytes are arranged in plates of 2 to more than 20 cells in thickness, resembling the trabecular architecture of the normal liver; neoplastic hepatocytes are arranged along simplified sinusoids with few or no Kupffer cells; the reticulin framework is mostly sparse or absent. In the compact or solid pattern the trabeculae are very close and the sinusoids compressed or non visible. The acinar or pseudoglandular pattern derives either from the dilatation of the bile canaliculi between neoplastic hepatocytes, where the lumina may contain bile, or from central degeneration of trabeculae, where the lumina contain degenerative material with fibrin; stroma is typically sparse. The scirrhous pattern is rare; neoplastic hepatocytes have cytologic and phenotypic features of typical HCC, but are surrounded by an abundant fibrous stroma. At the interface with surrounding liver parenchyma, HCCs may have an expansive growth, where the tumour expands compressing the adjacent nontumorous tissue, eventually delimitated by a complete or incomplete fibrous capsule; or an infiltrative growth, where the tumour merges into the adjacent nontumorous tissue, replacing the normal hepatocyte plates.

Immunohistochemistry. HCCs express many immunoreactive substances, but only few are useful for differential diagnosis with cholangiocarcinoma and metastatic adenocarcinoma [84, 90]. The most commonly used antibodies for the diagnosis of HCC include hepatocyte paraffin 1 (HepPar-1), a monoclonal antibody reacting with an epitope of liver mitochondria, that produces positive staining in approximately 90% of cases of HCC; arginase-1, an enzyme expressed by normal hepatocytes, that has shown higher sensitivity and specificity in differentiating HCC from metastatic tumours; polyclonal antiserum to carcinoembryonic antigen (CEA), that stains bile canaliculi of both normal liver and HCC, where a canalicular staining pattern indicates the presence of biliary glycoprotein I specific for HCCs in 60–90% of cases; immunostaining with other substances, including AFP and aberrant keratins CK7, CK20 and CK19, is less useful and have selective indications.

Key Concepts

- HCC develops in most cases in the background of chronic liver disease following a multistep sequence, through a series of intermediate lesions considered premalignant, that include dysplastic foci, <1 mm in size, and dysplastic nodules (DN), >1 mm and up to 2 cm. DN can be further classified into low-grade DN (LGDN) and high-grade DN (HGDN), and sometimes contain early malignant foci, defined "nodule-in-nodule lesion". Small HCC, up to 2 cm, can be either early HCC or progressed HCC. HGDNs are sometimes difficult to differentiate from early HCC nodules.
- The gross appearance of HCC is widely variable; neoplastic nodules may be solitary or multiple. HCC smaller than 2 cm are defined as "small HCC". At gross examination, HCC may have a nodular, infiltrative, or diffuse pattern; the nodular or expanding pattern is the most common, typically found in cirrhotic livers, is usually well-delineated and may be surrounded by a fibrous capsule. Advanced HCC may diffuse into large veins, mostly the portal vein, or into large bile ducts.
- At histology the architecture of HCC is irregular, with atypical arteries and distorted portal tracts. Regarding tumour cells, the Edmondson and Steiner's classification system is still considered the

gold standard for classifying HCC into grades, from grade I or well-differentiated HCC, to grade IV or poorly differentiated HCC. Architectural growth pattern may be trabecular, acinar or pseudoglandular, and scirrhous. At the interface with surrounding liver parenchyma, HCCs may have an expansive or an infiltrative growth.
- HCCs express many immunoreactive substances, but only few are useful for differential diagnosis with cholangiocarcinoma and metastatic adenocarcinoma. The most commonly used antibodies include HepPar-1, arginase-1, polyclonal antiserum to CEA, AFP, and aberrant keratins CK7, CK20 and CK19.

31.2.8 Clinical Features

Early HCCs in cirrhotics are usually asymptomatic. Clinical manifestations include abdominal pain or discomfort, palpable abdominal mass, hepatomegaly, or nonspecific symptoms such as weight loss, anorexia, dyspepsia and malaise, splenomegaly, ascites; these symptoms may also be related, at least in part, to the underlying chronic liver disease. Routine liver function tests may be substantially normal or even variably abnormal, mostly reflecting the underlying chronic liver disease. Serum AFP is usually raised in advanced, symptomatic HCC, while early HCCs show slightly elevated or even normal AFP levels. HCCs arising in noncirrhotic patients usually present with evidence of malignancy; symptoms may be related to the intrahepatic diffusion of the tumour, with jaundice, the occurrence of distant metastases, or severe complications, including portal vein thrombosis or biliary obstruction.

Key Concepts

- Early HCCs in cirrhotics are usually asymptomatic. Clinical manifestations are variable and may also be related, at least in part, to the underlying chronic liver disease. HCCs arising in noncirrhotic patients usually present with symptoms related to intrahepatic diffusion, distant metastases, or severe complications.

31.2.9 Treatment

Multiple treatments are available for HCC and the choice is based on the burden of the tumour and the liver function, especially in cirrhotic patients; moreover different options are suggested by major guidelines worldwide; on this basis, patients diagnosed with HCC should be referred to multidisciplinary teams involving surgeons, hepatologists, interventional radiologists, pathologists, and oncologists [3, 5].

31.2.9.1 Liver Surgery

The optimal surgical strategy for HCC is still somewhat controversial, with substantial differences among major guidelines worldwide [91]. Liver resection is the first approach in many instances, but liver transplantation theoretically represents the best treatment strategy, at least in patients with chronic liver disease or established cirrhosis, because may cure both the diseased liver and the liver cancer. LR, either open or laparoscopic, represents one of the most valuable curative options for HCC, based on the extent of the liver resection to achieve a radical procedure, and on the accurate evaluation of the volume and of the functional reserve of the future liver remnant (FLR), especially in case of advanced liver fibrosis or cirrhosis. LT provides the best treatment of HCC from an oncologic point of view, because removes both the tumour and the diseased liver, which represents *per se* a preneoplastic condition and exposes to the risk of recurrence; LT however has a limited role, because of the scarcity of organ donations, especially in Asian countries, high costs, and the progressive ageing of HCC patients [5, 6, 8, 92].

The role of LR is still widely debated regarding the tumour burden and the hepatic functional reserve suitable for surgery with adequate survival. In the current most relevant Western guidelines, including those of the EASL and the AASLD, LR is recommended only for patients with very early and early stage tumours based on the BCLC classification [4, 5, 93], specifically with a single nodule and preserved liver function without evidence of portal hypertension. Most Western surgeons evaluate serum bilirubin levels and portal pressure to select appropriate candidates to LR [5]. The 5-year survival rates of patients with normal bilirubin levels and without significant portal hypertension may reach 70%, while decrease to 50% in patients with both adverse factors [94]. Moreover, the presence of significant portal hypertension may increase the risk of adverse results both in the postoperative period and in the long term [95]. In current clinical practice however, many tertiary referral centers worldwide routinely consider LR also for patients with more advanced HCC according to the BCLC classification, with acceptable perioperative and long-term outcomes [81, 94]. Similarly, guidelines from Asian countries contemplate LR also for more advanced HCC in patients with more diseased liver; most of these guidelines consider LR also for tumours of any size, if curatively resectable, with multiple nodules, and/or with macrovascular invasion [3]. The 2017 revision of the APASL HCC guidelines does not include strictly defined criteria for LR, that can be considered for resectable tumours of any size and number, also with macrovascular invasion, in Child–Pugh class A and B patients; it is suggested that the decision about resectability should be discussed by a multidisciplinary team, including surgeons and hepatologists [3]. Laparoscopic LR is less invasive than conventional surgery, and has been recently reported to achieve better perioperative results with comparable long-term oncological outcomes [96, 97]. Hepatic recurrence, due to intrahepatic dissemination or de novo HCC, and distant metastases occur in 64–77% of patients after LR or local ablation [98]. At present there is no clear evidence that the proposed neoadjuvant or adjuvant strategies can significantly reduce the risk of either intrahepatic or distant recurrences [5]. Some beneficial effects have been suggested for postoperative infusion therapies via the hepatic artery of chemotherapeutic agents or of I-131 lipiodol [99] and for adjuvant immunotherapy with autologous cytokine-induced killer cells [5].

Although LT represents the only chance of cure for both liver cancer and the underlying liver disease, the shortage of organs and the possibility of tumor recurrence favoured by immunosuppression are determinant limiting factors. In terms of tumour burden, the Milan criteria are at present the most widely used to minimize HCC recurrence: LT is restricted to patients with solitary HCC <5 cm in diameter or within three nodules <3 cm in diameter, without radiological evidence of vascular invasion or distant metastasis [100]; patients within the Milan criteria have recurrence rates lower than 15% and 5-year survival rates higher than 70% after LT for HCC [5, 100]. In recent years however multiple criteria have been suggested to expand the Milan criteria without compromising oncological results. The University of California, San Francisco (UCSF) expanded criteria are the most diffuse: LT is restricted to patients with solitary HCC ≤65 mm in diameter, or 2–3 tumours, each with diameter ≤45 mm and total tumour diameter ≤80 mm, without radiological evidence of vascular invasion or distant metastasis [101]. In general, although the Milan criteria are probably too strict and could be expanded to some extent without significantly compromising the oncological and clinical outcomes, substantial expansion of the criteria regarding tumour size and/or number may worsen the overall posttransplant results [5, 102]. Although the Milan criteria are currently used also in Asian countries to select HCC patients for LT, the relevant diffusion of living-donor liver transplantation (LDLT) determines considerably less restrictions, with significant differences among countries and institutions. Criteria for LDLT are usually expanded; in some countries the UCSF criteria are basically adopted, while in others each transplant center has developed institutional expansion criteria; also the National Insurance coverage varies among different Asiatic countries [3]. The expansion of the criteria for LT in patients with HCC and the use of organs from living donors may expose to increased recurrence rates and worsen overall outcomes, although the impact of LDLT compared to deceased-donor LT for HCC is still controversial [103]. Substantial differences also exist between Western and Asian countries, regarding the liver functional reserve to consider the indication to LT for HCC; in Western countries LT is deliberated according to the model for end-stage liver disease (MELD) score with additional points [102], thus LT can be offered also to Child–Pugh class A patients that fulfil the Milan criteria [104]; in contrast, in Asian countries, where liver grafts from deceased-donors are extremely scarce, LT is recommended for patients with HCC and decompensated liver cirrhosis (Child-Pugh class B and C) [3].

Key Concepts

- Liver resection is a first-line curative treatment for HCC in patients with compensated cirrhosis when resectability is confirmed by appropriate multidisciplinary evaluation of liver function, extent of LR, expected volume of the FLR, performance status and co-morbidities of the single patient.
- The indication to LR is still controversial, since Western guidelines recommend LR for HCC at early stages, while Eastern guidelines support LR also for resectable tumours at more advanced stages, including tumours of any size, with multiple nodules, and/or with macrovascular invasion. Laparoscopic LR is less invasive than conventional surgery, with better perioperative results and comparable long-term oncological outcomes.
- Liver transplantation represents the best curative treatment option for HCC from an oncologic point of view, because removes both the tumour and the diseased liver, which represents *per se* a preneoplastic condition and exposes to the risk of recurrence. LT should be selectively considered as a first-line treatment for HCC, especially among Child-Pugh class B and C patients, but scarcity of organ donations, high costs, and progressive ageing of HCC patients represent substantial limitations to its use.
- Selection of candidates to LT is usually made according to the Milan criteria, where LT is restricted to patients with solitary HCC <5 cm in diameter or within three nodules <3 cm in diameter, without radiological evidence of vascular invasion or distant metastasis. Cautious expansion of the Milan criteria has been proposed in recent years. However, substantial expansion of the criteria regarding tumour size and/or number may worsen the overall oncological outcomes.
- The relevant diffusion of living-donor liver transplantation has determined considerably less restrictions in the selection of candidates to LT, with significant differences among countries and institutions.

31.2.9.2 Local Ablation

Image-guided percutaneous ablation therapies include radiofrequency ablation (RFA), ethanol injection (PEI), and microwave ablation (MWA). These minimally invasive techniques are increasingly used [70, 105], especially in case of small HCC [5, 106], because are considered potentially curative, can be easily repeated in case of recurrence, and in selected patients are more cost-effective than surgery with potentially similar results. Child-Pugh class A or B patients with a limited tumour burden, usually ≤3 nodules of ≤3 cm in diameter, are considered the most appropriate candidates to percutaneous local ablation [3]. RFA is at present the most diffused ablation technique for liver tumours [70, 105]; perioperative morbidity and mortality rates are 0.9–7.9% and 0–1.5%, respectively, with local tumour progression rates of 2.4–27.0%, and 5-year overall survival rates of 39.9–68.5% [3]; combination of RFA with TACE or PEI may increase the volume of tumoral necrosis and ameliorate the clinical outcome [105]. PEI has long been the standard technique for percutaneous ablation of HCC [107], with perioperative morbidity and mortality rates of 0–3.2% and 0–0.4%, respectively, local tumour progression rates of 6–31% according to the tumour size, and 5-year overall survival rates of 38–60% [3]; at present it is reserved to selected patients where RFA is contraindicated, usually with HCC adjacent or adherent to the gastrointestinal tract [3, 5]. Other techniques of local ablation are available, including percutaneous MWA and irreversible electroporation, but the available data about their efficacy and the overall clinical and oncological outcome are limited. Comparative studies have demonstrated that percutaneous RFA achieved better treatment response, lower recurrence rates and better overall survival rates than PEI [3, 5, 70, 105].

Key Concepts

- Image-guided percutaneous ablation therapies, including RFA, PEI, and MWA, are increasingly used, especially in case of small HCC, because are considered potentially curative, can be easily repeated in case of recurrence, and in selected patients are more cost-effective than surgery with potentially similar results.
- Child-Pugh class A or B patients with a limited tumour burden, usually ≤3 nodules of ≤3 cm in diameter, are considered the most appropriate candidates to percutaneous local ablation.
- RFA is at present the most diffused ablation technique for liver tumours, and is recommended as the first-line percutaneous ablation technique. Combination of RFA with TACE or PEI may increase the volume of tumoral necrosis and ameliorate the clinical outcome. PEI at present is reserved to selected patients where RFA is contraindicated, usually with HCC adjacent or adherent to the gastrointestinal tract.

31.2.9.3 Liver Resection vs Local Ablation

Multiple studies have compared LR with local ablative therapies, with controversial results [5, 105, 106]. Four randomized controlled trials (RCT) have compared LR and RFA [3]; in three of them overall and disease-free survival rates were similar between groups, while in the remaining study LR achieved significantly better overall and disease-free survival rates than RFA; perioperative results, including complications and length of hospital stay, were worse after LR than RFA. Interesting data came from the 19th nationwide follow-up survey of primary liver cancer in Japan made by the LCSGJ [70]; in patients treated with LR cumulative survival rates at 1, 5 and 10 years were 90.2%, 56.8% and 32.0%, respectively; were 91.5%, 61.4% and 37.3%, respectively, in class A patients according to the liver damage classification by LCSGJ; and were 93.7%, 67.0% and 39.0%, respectively, in patients with a single tumour; cumulative survival rates at 1, 5 and 10 years according to tumour size were 97.1%, 73.9% and 40.2%, respectively, for tumours measuring <2 cm, 93.6%, 63.1% and 35.1, respectively, for tumours measuring 2–3 cm, 91.5%, 59.7% and 36.5%, respectively, for tumours measuring 3–5 cm, 85.9%, 52.4% and 31.0%, respectively, for tumours measuring 5–10 cm, and 77.8%, 45.4% and 31.0% at 1, 5 and 8 years, respectively, for tumours measuring >10 cm; in comparison, in patients treated in the same period with local ablative therapies, cumulative survival rates at 1, 5 and 10 years were 93.9%, 47.0% and 17.0%, respectively; were 96.3%, 55.7% and 21.3%, respectively, in class A patients according to the liver damage classification by LCSGJ; and were 95.2%, 52.9% and 20.8%, respectively in patients with a single tumour; cumulative survival rates at 1, 5 and 10 years according to tumour size were 95.9%, 53.7% and 18.9%, respectively, for tumours measuring 1–2 cm, 94.0%, 41.3% and 15.3%, respectively, for tumours measuring 2–3 cm, 89.4%, 34.2% and 10.8%, respectively, for tumours measuring 3–5 cm, and 77.2%, 24.6% and 13.1%, respectively, for tumours measuring >5 cm; the overall results of LR were superior when compared to those reported for local ablative therapies, even though statistical evaluations were not available. Further evaluation of a subgroup of patients of the same registry, including those with liver function classified as liver damage A or B defined by the LCSGJ, with ≤3 tumours and a maximum tumour diameter ≤3 cm, suggested that LR may offer significant advantage over RFA and PEI in terms of both overall survival and time to recurrence in patients with less advanced HCC [98]. Moreover, data collected from 1978 in the same registry demonstrated marked improvements, over almost 30 years, in overall survival rates of HCC patients treated either with LR or with ablation; the 5-year overall survival of patients treated between 2001 and 2005 was 58.4% and 47.6% after LR and ablation, respectively, and the median overall survival was 74 and 59 months, respectively [70]. A recent overview of meta-analyses comparing the results of the management of HCC has shown that LR is superior to RFA because of higher overall survival rates [105]. Similar conclusions have been drawn for small HCC, with LR being superior to nonsurgical ablative therapies, and with RFA being the most effective single nonsurgical ablative treatment [106]. The advent of laparoscopic LR also for HCC will probably further reduce perioperative morbidity rates and postoperative hospital stay without adverse impact on overall and recurrence-free survivals [96]. However most studies suggest that RFA may represent an appropriate alternative to LR in selected patients with HCC smaller than 2–3 cm, because is minimally invasive and achieves better perioperative results and similar long-term outcome [3, 5].

Key Concepts

- Multiple studies have compared LR with local ablative therapies, with controversial results. LRs seem to achieve better oncological results than local ablative therapies, also in patients with small HCC.
- However RFA may represent an appropriate alternative to LR in selected patients with HCC smaller than 2–3 cm, because is minimally invasive and achieves better perioperative results and similar long-term outcome.

31.2.9.4 Transarterial Chemoembolization

TACE is based on the selective administration of chemotherapeutic agents, mixed with Lipiodol, followed by embolization of the arteries feeding the tumour with different types of particles, while sparing the surrounding liver parenchyma [108]; alternatively, chemotherapeutic agents can be delivered by drug-eluting beads (DEB-TACE) [109]. As a consequence, selective or superselective TACE are usually effective in inducing tumour necrosis with a limited impact on the surrounding liver parenchyma also in patients with advanced liver fibrosis or cirrhosis, with perioperative severe complications and mortality rates lower than 5% [3, 5]. TACE can achieve objective response rates of 58–86%, with complete response rates of 20–41% [3]. Several studies have shown that TACE determines a significant survival advantage in selected patients with unresectable HCC and preserved liver function [110, 111]; median survival rates of 30–40 months have been reported in case of adequate patient selection and optimal treatment delivery [5]. Several scoring systems have been proposed to predict the clinical and oncological outcome of TACE, and to select patients suitable for multiple TACE sessions [3]; patients with bulky tumours and compromised liver function are reported to achieve worse overall results [112]. At present TACE is considered as a first-line noncurative treatment for unresectable, large/multifocal HCCs without vascular invasion or extrahepatic spread in the guidelines published by the EASL and AASLD [4, 5, 93]. TACE can also be considered in patients with HCC at an early stage where LR or RFA are not indicated because of difficult locations and/or medical conditions [113], and for downstaging tumours exceeding the criteria for LT. DEB-TACE has shown similar objective response rates compared to conventional TACE, but with improved tolerability due to lower rates of liver toxicity and systemic adverse effects [114]. After initial tumour response with TACE, HCC may recur and can be retreated with further TACE sessions; however retreatment is considered not indicated when significant necrosis is not achieved after two sessions, in case of major progression, including vascular invasion, extensive intrahepatic involvement, distant metastases, or even in case of deteriorating liver function [4, 5].

Transarterial radioembolization is based on the injection of implantable radioactive microspheres into arteries feeding the tumour, while sparing the surrounding liver parenchyma. TARE using yttrium-90 has been proposed as a complement or as an alternative to TACE [4], with tumour response rates of 40–80% [5]. Further evidence confirming the clinical and oncological benefits of TARE compared with conventional TACE is required.

Key Concepts

- At present TACE is considered as a first-line noncurative treatment for unresectable, large/multifocal HCCs without vascular invasion or extrahepatic spread.
- Selective or superselective TACE should be attempted to achieve appropriate effects, preserve nontumorous liver parenchyma, and minimize complications.
- Selective TACE can also be considered in patients with HCC at an early stage, where LR or RFA are not indicated because of difficult locations and/or medical comorbidities.
- TARE with yttrium-90-loaded resin/glass beads has been proposed as a complement or as an alternative to TACE.

31.2.9.5 Radiation Therapy

HCC is considered to be radiosensitive, but also the liver is a radiosensitive organ. The development of technologies for targeting HCC precisely with RT, including stereotactic body radiotherapy (SBRT), can improve the oncological and clinical benefits with reduced risks on the surrounding liver parenchyma. At present however, only small series have evaluated the possible role of RT in the treatment of HCC, with promising results [3].

31.2.9.6 Systemic Therapy

Systemic therapy has been approved for the treatment of patients with advanced-stage HCC, including macrovascular invasion and/or extrahepatic metastases, who are not suitable for locoregional treatments, and have an adequate liver functional reserve [3, 4]. Sorafenib is a multikinase inhibitor of RAF, VEGFR, PDGFR, c-KIT, FLT3, and RET [43], with antiangiogenic and antiproliferative effects, and is at present recommended for the first-line treatment of patients with advanced-stage HCC, including macrovascular invasion and/or extrahepatic metastases, who are not suitable for locoregional treatments, and with preserved liver function [3, 4]. Regorafenib is a novel multikinase inhibitor with more potent inhibitory activities against multiple angiogenic pathways (VEGFR, PDGFR, TIE2, and FGF receptor) and oncogenic pathways (RET, KIT, c-RAF/RAF-1, and BRAF) than Sorafenib [115], and has been proposed as a second-line treatment in HCC patients with preserved liver function who had progression on Sorafenib [5].

Key Concepts

- Systemic therapy with Sorafenib is the first-line treatment of patients with advanced-stage HCC, including macrovascular invasion and/or extrahepatic metastases, who are not suitable for locoregional treatments, and have an adequate liver functional reserve. Regorafenib is a novel multikinase inhibitor proposed as a second-line treatment in HCC patients who had progression on Sorafenib.

31.3 Intrahepatic Cholangiocellular Carcinoma

Cholangiocarcinoma (CCA) includes a heterogeneous group of cancers originating from the biliary system, and is the second most common tumor of the liver, accounting for 10–20% of all hepatobiliary neoplasms [116, 117]. Based on the anatomical origin, CCA are classified as intrahepatic (iCCA), arising above the second-order bile ducts, perihilar, or distal CCA; there is at present enough evidence to consider these tumours as three distinct entities, considering the differences in epidemiology, pathobiology, clinical presentations, and management [116–119]. Intrahepatic CCA may develop in a normal or in a diseased liver, and is pathologically classified as an adenocarcinoma; combined hepatocellular-cholangiocarcinomas (cHCC-CCA) account for 1–5% of liver neoplasms and are more frequent in chronic liver disease [116, 117, 120].

31.3.1 Epidemiology and Risk Factors

The incidence of iCCA is high in the Far East and much lower in Western countries, but is rapidly increasing worldwide, with a concomitant increase in mortality rates [116, 121–123]. The overall incidence is similar in both sex, with a slight male predominance (male to female ratio 1.2–1.5:1). Intra and extrahepatic CCAs likely develop through a multistep, multifactorial carcinogenic process in a context of different risk factors associated with genetic, ethnic, cultural and environmental predispositions [116, 124]. Well-known risk factors for CCA include primary sclerosing cholangitis, mainly associated with perihilar and distal CCA; infections by hepatobiliary flukes *Opisthorchis viverrini* and *Clonorchis sinensis*, that colonize the biliary tree determining persistent inflammation [125], and have been associated either with perihilar and distal CCA or with iCCA; hepatolithiasis, mostly diffused in some Asiatic regions, with or without concomitant parasitic infection, that has been associated with a substantial risk of developing iCCA [126]; choledochal cysts diseases, including the Caroli's disease, uncommon inherited abnormalities of the biliary ducts resulting in persistent reflux of pancreatic enzymes, cholestasis, biliary lithiasis and chronic inflammation, mostly encountered in Asian than Western countries, that have an impressive overall lifetime risk of CCA of 5–30%, including iCCA [126, 127]; exposure to Thorotrast, a contrast medium containing radioactive thorium dioxide, and used as a contrast agent until the 1950s. All these factors are associated with chronic inflammation and increased cellular turnover of the bile ducts, predisposing to carcinogenesis [116, 124]. In recent years however, chronic liver disease has been recognized as a significant risk factor for iCCA, as for HCC, suggesting that chronic inflammation may represent the common pathogenic pathway for CCA. Cirrhosis of any aetiology has been reported to represent an independent risk factor for iCCA with an estimated risk of 5–14 [116, 126–128]. A strong association has been also reported between iCCA and HBV and HCV related chronic hepatitis, either in Eastern or in Western countries [116, 126–128]; in a recent meta-analysis, HBV and HCV infection were significantly associated with iCCA, with an OR of 5.5 and 4.8, respectively [128]. Metabolic syndrome and obesity have been recently suggested to represent independent risk factors for the development of iCCA [116, 128], while the association of diabetes to iCCA has been suggested by some studies [127, 128], but is still controversial. The role of alcohol consumption and tobacco smoking as risk factors of iCCA is uncertain [116, 128]. It has been suggested that also host genetic polymorphism may have a role in CCA predisposition [116, 124].

Key Concepts
- The incidence of iCCA is high in the Far East and is rapidly increasing worldwide, with a concomitant increase in mortality rates.
- Intra and extrahepatic CCAs likely develop through a multistep, multifactorial carcinogenic process in a context of different risk factors associated with genetic, ethnic, cultural and environmental predispositions.
- Well-known risk factors include primary sclerosing cholangitis, infections by hepatobiliary flukes, hepatolithiasis, choledochal cysts diseases, exposure to Thorotrast. Recently also chronic liver disease has been recognized as a significant risk factor for iCCA, including cirrhosis of any aetiology, HBV and HCV related chronic hepatitis, metabolic syndrome and obesity.

31.3.2 Molecular Pathogenesis

Molecular pathogenesis of CCA is a complex topic, although in recent years there has been considerable progress in understanding the mechanisms of cholangiocarcinogenesis and progression of CCA. Malignant transformation of biliary epithelium is believed to occur in a context of chronic inflammation of the bile ducts and persistent cholestasis, determining increased production of cytokines and reactive oxygen species, iterative damage of cholangiocytes, and finally their malignant transformation. However, recent evidence suggests that iCCA has multiple cellular origins, including intrahepatic biliary epithelial cells/cholangiocytes, differentiated hepatocytes, pluripotent stem cells, either hepatic stem/progenitor cells or biliary tree stem/progenitor cells, and peribiliary gland [129]; the contribution of multiple cell subtypes, including differentiated hepatocytes, to cholangiocarcinogenesis might explain the role of chronic viral hepatitis, advanced fibrosis and cirrhosis as independent risk factors for iCCA [117]. Many different factors have been hypothesized to be involved in cholangiocarcinogenesis, such as stem cells, differentiated liver cell subtypes, genetic and epigenetic changes, cancer microenvironment and exposure to carcinogenic agents, all of which may lead to the heterogeneity observed between patients, but also within the same cancer; these complex and interrelated mechanisms of cholangiocarcinogenesis and progression of CCA have been summarized in several noteworthy reviews [116–119, 128, 129], and are beyond the scope of this chapter.

Key Concepts
- Malignant transformation of biliary epithelium is believed to occur in a context of chronic inflammation of the bile ducts and persistent cholestasis, determining iterative damage of cholangiocytes, and finally their malignant transformation.
- Recent evidence, however, suggests that iCCA has multiple cellular origins, including intrahepatic biliary epithelial cells/cholangiocytes, differentiated hepatocytes, pluripotent stem cells, either hepatic stem/progenitor cells or biliary tree stem/progenitor cells, and peribiliary gland, which might explain the role of chronic liver disease and cirrhosis as independent risk factors for iCCA.

31.3.3 Pathology and Classification

At pathological examination, CCAs are usually tubular adenocarcinomas or mucinous carcinomas, with varying degrees of desmoplasia that surrounds the carcinomatous cells. Based on the anatomic site, CCAs are classified into intrahepatic, perihilar, and distal, that approximately account for the 25%, 50% and 25% of the cases, respectively [117]. At gross pathology, iCCAs may present as single or multiple gray-white to tan tumours, with or without satellite nodules. Microscopically, iCCA may mimic metastatic adenocarcinoma of the pancreas or other adenocarcinomas from any site. The malignant cells are epithelial cells usually with eosinophilic and granular cytoplasm. Various degrees of intracytoplasmic or extracellular mucin can be usually demonstrated. Typically, the carcinomatous cells form glands, but also solid nests, cords, or papillary structures [123], with different degrees of differentiation, from well to moderate to poor [120], with some rare variants [117, 123]. iCCA has been classified into mass-forming (60–80%), periductal-infiltrating (15–35%), intraductal (8–29%), undefined and mixed subtypes, with different prognostic implications [120, 130, 131].

Intrahepatic CCAs derive from the hepatic stem/progenitor cells, which are located either in the peribiliary glands, contained in the large bile ducts, or in the small bile ducts and ductules of Hering, which might explain the heterogeneity of iCCAs arising from different anatomical sites [131]. On this basis, iCCA can be divided into two main classes, large duct or bile duct type, and small duct or peripheral type [74, 120, 131, 132]; glandular morphology has been suggested to coincide with distinct molecular defects, and different therapeutic implications [74]. Large duct type (also known as "bile duct" type) iCCAs are characterized by large, dilated glands with mucin formation and desmoplastic stromal fibrosis; are usually more centrally located, and resemble the epithelium of larger bile ducts and/or the mucinous epithelium of the peribiliary glands; this subtype is associated with chronic biliary disease; precursor biliary lesions are represented by biliary intraepithelial neoplasia (BilIN) and intraductal papillary neoplasm of bile duct (IPNB); large duct type iCCAs express S100P and trefoil factor 1 (TFF1). Small duct type (also known as cholangiolar, cholangiolocellular, or cholangiocellular type) iCCAs are characterized by cuboidal cells with uniform round nuclei, forming small tubular or trabecular structures, typically surrounded by a dense collagenous stroma; this subtype is associated with chronic liver disease and cirrhosis; small duct type iCCAs characteristically express CD56 (neural cell adhesion molecule/NCAM), N-cadherin, and C-reactive protein (CRP) [74]. In addition to the main subtypes, rare variants of iCCA have been described, that may represent examples of the morphologic variability of the large or small duct type, but also truly different tumours with distinct unique molecular features; the most frequent include lymphoepithelioma-like iCCA, sarcomatoid iCCA, and undifferentiated carcinoma. [74]. Three most relevant precursor lesions of iCCA are the biliary intraepithelial neoplasia (BilIN), the intraductal papillary neoplasm of bile duct (IPNB), and the mucinous cystic neoplasm (MCN) [74]. BilIN is a flat dysplasia that can occur anywhere in the biliary tract, but more frequently in the larger intrahepatic bile ducts and the extrahepatic biliary tree; BilIN usually arises in the setting of chronic inflammation; based on the degree of cytologic and architectural atypia, BilIN can be distinguished into three grades, with progressively worsening atypia. IPNB (also known as papillary carcinoma in situ and intraductal growth type CCA, if there is no invasion through the basement membrane of the bile duct) is histologically similar to intraductal papillary mucinous neoplasm of the pancreas; based on cytologic and architectural changes, IPNB can be differentiated into low, intermediate, and high grade dysplasia. MCN of the biliary tract is a cystic tumour without communication with the biliary ducts, composed by an inner epithelial lining surrounded by ovarian type stroma; epithelial proliferation within the cyst can be distinguished into low, intermediate, and high grade dysplasia.

Key Concepts

- At pathological examination, CCAs are tubular adenocarcinomas or mucinous carcinomas, with varying degrees of desmoplasia. Based on the anatomic site, CCAs are classified into intrahepatic, perihilar, and distal.
- At gross pathology, iCCAs may present as single or multiple tumours, with or without satellite nodules.
- Microscopically, iCCA may mimic metastatic adenocarcinoma from any site. Typically, the carcinomatous cells form glands, with different degrees of differentiation, from well to moderate to poor, with some rare variants.
- iCCAs derive from the hepatic stem/progenitor cells, located either in the peribiliary glands, contained in the large bile ducts, or in the small bile ducts and ductules of Hering. On this basis, iCCA has been divided into large duct or bile duct type, and small duct or peripheral type; glandular morphology has been suggested to coincide with distinct molecular defects, and different therapeutic implications.

31.3.4 Clinical Features

Intracellular CCA presents with nonspecific symptoms. At earlier stages the tumour is usually asymptomatic, while at more advanced stages patients complain of abdominal pain or discomfort, anorexia, malaise, weight loss, hepatomegaly or a palpable abdominal mass, sometimes jaundice; biliary tract obstruction occurs infrequently; night sweats are referred in advanced disease. iCCA should be suspected in patients with known hepatolithiasis or choledochal cysts diseases and worsening clinical conditions.

Key Concepts

- At earlier stages iCCA is usually asymptomatic, while at more advanced stages patients complain of abdominal pain or discomfort, hepatomegaly or a palpable mass. iCCA should be suspected in patients with known hepatolithiasis or choledochal cysts diseases and worsening clinical conditions.

31.3.5 Diagnosis

Asymptomatic iCCAs may be incidentally discovered by cross-sectional imaging performed for other reasons, often during routine imaging surveillance for HCC in cirrhotic patients [119]. In more advanced stages, iCCAs are usually large mass-forming lesions, single or often multifocal, with satellite nodules. Segmental dilatation of intrahepatic bile ducts associated with the tumour is typical and may help characterization [54]. On US, iCCAs appear as a hypoechoic mass, eventually associated with dilatation of bile ducts close to the tumour. CEUS usually demonstrates an arterial contrast enhancement, but its role in characterizing iCCA is still controversial [3, 44]. On dynamic MDCT, iCCAs typically appear as a hypodense hepatic mass with irregular margins in the precontrast phase, peripheral rim enhancement in the arterial phase, and progressive centripetal enhancement during the venous and delayed phases [54, 116, 119]; regional atrophy with retraction of the liver capsule, the presence of segmental dilatation of bile ducts close to the tumour, the encasement of intrahepatic vessels without grossly visible tumour thrombus, the absence of a capsule or pseudocapsule, are typical features of iCCA that can help in differential diagnosis [54]. Dynamic MDCT is useful in most cases to differentiate iCCA from HCC: the progressive centripetal contrast enhancement over several minutes, from the arterial phase to the venous and especially the delayed phase, is related to the fibrotic tissue within the cancer [54], and is observed in up to 81% of iCCA, while HCC typically shows rapid enhancement during the late arterial phase, with evident washout in the venous or delayed phases [116]. Smaller iCCAs, however, may sometimes have arterial enhancement, resembling HCC [116]. On MRI, iCCAs tend to appear hypointense on T1w images and hyperintense on T2w images [54, 116]; augmented signal on DWI with consequent low ADC map value can be observed [54]. T2w images may also show central hypointensity, which correspond to areas of severe fibrosis, necrosis, or mucin [54, 116]. As for dynamic MDCT, dynamic T1w images show peripheral rim enhancement in the arterial phase, followed by progressive centripetal enhancement during the venous and delayed phases; the prolonged enhancement in the delayed phase is indicative of intralesional fibrous stroma and suggest an iCCA [54, 116, 119]. MDCT and MRI have equivalent efficacy in the detection of primary and satellite iCCA lesions [119]. MRI with cholangiopancreatography (MRCP) is useful to depict the dilated intrahepatic bile ducts and the intrahepatic vessels, and consequently to determine the tumour extent [54, 116] and to plan liver surgery. FDG-PET scan can detect mass-forming iCCA as small as 1 cm, with a reported sensitivity of 85–95%, but is less useful for infiltrating tumours [116]; moreover, FDG-PET may be helpful in diagnosis of metastatic disease [117].

However, a confident diagnosis of iCCA can be obtained according to dynamic imaging criteria only in the absence of cirrhosis or extrahepatic primary malignancies [116]. As a consequence, although the diagnosis of iCCA can be achieved referring to clinical presentation, laboratory findings and radiologic evaluation, liver biopsy is often required for definitive diagnosis, especially in patients with cirrhosis, or with other primary malignancies, or even with small solid hepatic lesions without specific radiologic features [116, 117, 119, 123]. Core biopsies are preferable. The risk of tumour seeding is uncertain. At histology, iCCA is similar to adenocarcinomas arising in extrahepatic sites that can give metastases to the liver, including pancreas, esophagus, stomach, and lung [133]. The expression of keratins CK7 and CK20 may be helpful to ascertain a biliary origin [134]. Differentiation with mixed HCC tumours may require the use of specific immunohistochemical markers including Hep-Par-1, GPC3, HSP70, glutamine synthetase [5, 41].

Serum levels of tumour biomarkers, including Carbohydrate Antigen (CA) 19-9 and CEA, may have some diagnostic value, although their low sensitivity for iCCA at earlier stages limit their diagnostic efficacy. The sensitivity and specificity of CA 19-9 for iCCA is only 62% and 63%, respectively [116]. However, CA 19-9 levels are significantly higher in patients with more advanced, often unresectable tumours, and CA 19-9 levels >1,000 U/ml have been related with the presence of metastatic CCA [119].

Key Concepts

- On US, iCCAs appear as a hypoechoic mass; CEUS usually demonstrates an arterial contrast enhancement.
- On dynamic MDCT, iCCAs typically appear as hypodense hepatic lesions with irregular margins in the precontrast phase, peripheral rim enhancement in the arterial phase, and progressive centripetal enhancement during the venous and delayed phases; other typical features include regional atrophy with retraction of the liver capsule, segmental dilatation of bile ducts close to the tumour, encasement of intrahepatic vessels without grossly visible tumour thrombus, absence of a capsule or pseudocapsule.
- The typical behaviour of iCCA at dynamic MDCT, with the progressive centripetal contrast enhancement over several minutes, from the arterial phase to the venous and especially the delayed phase, differs from that observed in HCC, which typically shows rapid enhancement during the late arterial phase and rapid washout in the venous or delayed phases.
- On MRI, iCCAs tend to appear hypointense on T1w images and hyperintense on T2w images, with augmented signal on DWI and low ADC map value;

T2w images may also show central hypointensity. Dynamic T1w images show peripheral rim enhancement in the arterial phase, with progressive prolonged centripetal enhancement during the venous and delayed phases. MRCP is useful to depict the dilated intrahepatic bile ducts and the intrahepatic vessels.
- FDG-PET scan can detect mass-forming iCCA as small as 1 cm, and may be helpful in diagnosis of metastatic disease.
- A confident diagnosis of iCCA, however, can be obtained according to dynamic imaging criteria only in the absence of cirrhosis or extrahepatic primary malignancies. Otherwise, liver biopsy may be required for definitive diagnosis. Core biopsies are preferable.
- Serum levels of tumour biomarkers, including CA 19-9 and CEA, may have some diagnostic value, but have low sensitivity for iCCA at earlier stages.

31.3.6 Staging

The TNM classification of CCA is different for iCCA, perihilar and distal CCA, respectively, and is based on surgical specimen. The TNM classification is defined by AJCC, UICC and LCSGJ, and is regularly updated in new editions [41, 135]. In the TNM classification of iCCA, the lymphovascular invasion and the multifocal disease (including multiple separate tumours, satellitosis, and intrahepatic metastasis) are included in the T component; microvascular invasion and multifocal disease have been demonstrated to represent adverse prognostic factors of survival [74, 136]. More recent classification systems, specifically developed for iCCA, are based on preoperative clinical and radiological features, including number of tumours, vascular invasion, lymph node status, and presence of metastatic disease [137], but require further evaluation.

Key Concepts
- The TNM classification of CCA is different for iCCA, perihilar and distal CCA, respectively, and is based on surgical specimen.
- More recent classification systems, specifically developed for iCCA, are based on preoperative clinical and radiological features, including number of tumours, vascular invasion, lymph node status, and presence of metastatic disease.

31.3.7 Treatment

31.3.7.1 Liver Resection and Liver Transplantation

LR remains the mainstay for potentially curative treatment of iCCA, although surgical outcomes are still poor, since in most cases iCCA are in an advanced stage at the time of diagnosis and may require major LR [116, 117, 119]. After curative resection however the median overall survival may approach 80 months [138]. Following radical resection of iCCA, the 1-year and 5-year survival rates have been 72.4% and 30.4%, respectively, in one series [139], although the actuarial overall survival may significantly decrease over time, up to 16% at 8 years [140]. The reported median disease-free survival rates are 12–36 months [119]. Predictors of unfavourable oncological outcome include large tumour size, multiple intrahepatic lesions, and regional lymph-node involvement [136, 141]; also liver cirrhosis seems to represent an independent factor of worse survival rates after LR [142].

Although iCCA has been traditionally considered a contraindication to LT due to high recurrence rates and the poor overall oncological outcome, a recent multi-institutional series reported a 5-year survival of 65% in patients with very early iCCA, defined as a single tumour ≤2 cm in diameter, and of 45% in those with advanced iCCA, defined as a single tumour >2 cm or multifocal disease [143]. In another multi-institutional series, a small number of patients undergoing LT for very early iCCA in cirrhosis achieved a 5-year actuarial survival of 73% [144]. These results suggest that LT might represent a potentially curative treatment option in very selected patients with early iCCA [117, 119].

Key Concepts
- LR remains the mainstay for potentially curative treatment of iCCA, although oncological outcomes are often unsatisfying. Predictors of unfavourable outcome include large tumour size, multiple intrahepatic lesions, regional lymph-node involvement and also liver cirrhosis.
- Although iCCA has been traditionally considered a contraindication to LT due to high recurrence rates and poor overall oncological outcome, some recent studies suggest that LT might represent a potentially curative treatment option in very selected patients with early iCCA.

31.3.7.2 Locoregional Therapies

Locoregional therapies are an appropriate treatment strategy for advanced, unresectable iCCA. In patients with unresectable iCCA limited to the liver, TACE may represent a safe option [116, 117] and has been associated with median overall survival of 12–15 months [119]. DEB-TACE might achieve better oncological results than conventional TACE [145]. Also TARE with yttrium-90 microspheres has shown to be safe and achieved reasonable oncological efficacy [146], even for iCCA refractory to conventional chemotherapy [147]. Ongoing technological advances have improved the safety and effectiveness of RT for CCA [119]; advanced EBRT techniques, including 3D conformal radiotherapy (3D–CRT) and intensity-modulated radiotherapy (IMRT), are used to deliver conformal radiation to the tumour tissue while sparing surrounding unaffected liver; alternatively, stereotactic body radiotherapy (SBRT) can improve the oncological and clinical benefits minimizing the risk on the surrounding liver parenchyma; these techniques have been proposed to treat CCA, and for local ablation of unresectable iCCA [64, 65]. To date, the different locoregional treatments for local ablation of unresectable iCCA have not been compared, and appropriate clinical trials are expected.

Key Concepts

- Locoregional therapies are an appropriate treatment strategy for advanced, unresectable iCCA. Conventional TACE, DEB-TACE and TARE with yttrium-90 microspheres may be proposed to patients with unresectable iCCA limited to the liver.
- Radiotherapeutic technologies for targeting CCA precisely with reduced risks on the surrounding liver parenchyma, including SBRT, have been also proposed for local ablation of unresectable iCCA.

31.3.7.3 Systemic Therapy

The combination of gemcitabine and cisplatin is the current first-line chemotherapy for patients with unresectable, advanced-stage CCA not eligible to locoregional treatments, irrespective of anatomical subtype, although the oncological results are modest [148]. Capecitabine has shown to be effective as an adjuvant treatment in patients who received R0 or R1 surgical resection for CCA [119]; in another study however adjuvant chemotherapy with gemcitabine and oxaliplatin (GEMOX) after R0 or R1 surgical resection of CCA did not improve the recurrence-free survival rates [119]; these conflicting data demonstrate the need of further evaluation regarding the role of adjuvant chemotherapy after LR [119].

A growing number of clinical trials are evaluating the efficacy of targeted therapies for CCA, alone or in combination with traditional chemotherapy, including erlotinib, panitumumab, cetuximab, sorafenib, and bevacizumab; the rationale and results of these trials, the molecular targets and the evaluated targeted therapies have been extensively reviewed [116, 117, 119, 120, 129].

Key Concepts

- The combination of gemcitabine and cisplatin is the current first-line chemotherapy for patients with unresectable, advanced-stage CCA not eligible to locoregional treatments, irrespective of anatomical subtype; the oncological results are modest.
- The role of adjuvant chemotherapy after surgical resection of CCA is still controversial.
- A growing number of clinical trials are evaluating the efficacy of targeted therapies for CCA, alone or in combination with traditional chemotherapy, including erlotinib, panitumumab, cetuximab, sorafenib, and bevacizumab.

31.4 Combined Hepatocellular-Cholangiocarcinoma

Combined hepatocellular-cholangiocarcinoma (cHCC-CCA), also known as combined or mixed or biphenotypic hepatobiliary carcinoma, or hepatocholangiocarcinoma, is a biphenotypic primary liver cancer with both typical HCC and typical iCCA, in adjacent but spatially distinct areas, with a morphologic transition from one phenotype to the other [74, 149–151]. These tumours have been suggested to derive from stem/progenitor cells [151]. cHCC-CCAs account for approximately 2–5% of primary liver cancers [151], although increasingly recognized, and are usually difficult to diagnose.

Microscopic pathology. According to the World Health Organization (WHO) classification of digestive tumors, histologic diagnosis of cHCC-CCA requires unequivocal presence of both hepatocellular and cholangiocellular elements within the same tumour [74, 149, 152]. The hepatocellular component may be well, moderately or poorly differentiated; hepatocellular differentiation is confirmed by specific immunoreaction with HepPar1, glypican-3, arginase-1 [149–151]. The cholangiocellular component corresponds to an adenocarcinoma variably arranged, associated with dense fibrous stroma, and sometimes containing mucins; cholangiocellular differentiation usually shows immunoreaction with keratins CK7 and CK19, but markers of hepatocellular differentiation are absent [149, 150]. Moreover, cHCC-CCAs often show areas of intermediate morphology, composed of cells with features between those of hepatocytes and cholangiocytes, and associated with a desmoplastic stroma; at immunohistochemistry these areas demonstrate mixed hepatocytic and cholangiocytic phenotypes, and also stem/progenitor cell phenotypes [74, 149]. Stem/progenitor cell features or phenotypes consist of small cells with scant cytoplasm, high nuclear/cytoplasmic ratio, and hyperchromatic nuclei, typically found at the interface of the tumour and its surrounding stroma; mitotic activity is uncommon; immunohistochemical markers include keratin CK19, CD56/NCAM, CD117/KIT, EpCAM/MOC-31, and others [74, 151]. cHCC-CCAs can develop either in a background of cirrhosis or in noncirrhotic livers.

Dynamic MDCT and MRI. Few publications report the radiological appearances of cHCC-CCA. On dynamic MDCT and MRI, these tumours show some form of APHE, most commonly peripheral or rim-like [153–155]. Washout is common and mostly peripheral. Delayed central enhancement is frequent. Most commonly these imaging features coincide partially with those of iCCA [154]; however, cHCC-CCAs may sometimes show the classical behavior of HCC, with diffuse APHE and diffuse or patchy washout appearance, or features of both typical HCC and iCCA [153]. Dynamic imaging features are related to the predominant histopathological component of HCC and iCCA, respectively [151]. Using the LI-RADS analysis, most cHCC-CCAs were categorized in a single series as unknown liver malignant tumours (LR-M; probably malignant, not specific for HCC) [155]; however, LI-RADS has been formulated for the diagnosis of HCC in populations at risk, while cHCC-CCA may occur in patients without cirrhosis or other known risk factors for HCC. In case of undetermined tumours with atypical imaging features and without established clinical risk factors, a core liver biopsy is suggested [74, 151].

Clinical features and treatment. Although little is known about the clinical and oncological behaviour of these cancers, the available data suggest that they may be aggressive, and likely represent a unique subset of primary liver cancers, with distinctive features [151]. Serum CA 19-9 and AFP levels may be increased, with the elevated CA19-9 levels reflecting the iCCA component and AFP the HCC component [150]. Regional lymph node metastases at presentation are more frequent than in conventional HCC [156], so that hilar lymph node dissection during LR should be achieved when a diagnosis of cHCC-CCA is suspected before surgery. The overall prognosis falls in between that of iCCA and HCC [157, 158], and is driven by the cholangiocarcinoma component [159]. Combined tumors are staged in the TNM system using the CCA protocol because the CCA components tend to drive prognosis; nonetheless, cHCC-CCA should be considered sufficiently distinct from CCAs and probably require a unique staging system [150]. At present it is virtually impossible to predict the outcome of cHCC-CCA after liver resection and transplantation; how these cancers respond to locoregional therapies, including conventional and DEB-TACE, TARE, RT; how these tumours react to systemic therapies currently administered for HCC or iCCA, including the available targeted agents. In a very limited series of cHCC-CCA who underwent LR, recurrent or metastatic deposits replicated the heterogeneity of the primary cHCC-CCA, while HCC and iCCA components demonstrated different tropism in distant organs, indicating that the behaviour of recurrent/metastatic cHCC-CCA is unpredictable [160]. These very limited data suggest that more accurate elucidation of the biologic and clinical behaviour of cHCC-CCA is needed.

Key Concepts

- Combined hepatocellular-cholangiocarcinoma (cHCC-CCA) is a biphenotypic primary liver cancer with both typical HCC and typical iCCA, in adjacent but spatially distinct areas, with a morphologic transition from one phenotype to the other. cHCC-CCA has been suggested to derive from stem/progenitor cells.
- According to the WHO classification of digestive tumours, a histologic diagnosis of cHCC-CCA requires unequivocal presence of both hepatocellular and cholangiocellular elements within the same tumour. Moreover, cHCC-CCAs often show areas of intermediate morphology, composed of cells with features between those of hepatocytes and cholangiocytes, and also of stem/progenitor cell phenotypes. cHCC-CCAs can develop either in a background of cirrhosis or in noncirrhotic livers.
- The radiological appearance of cHCC-CCA is variable. On dynamic MDCT and MRI, these tumours usually show features similar to those of iCCA, sometimes of HCC, or of both typical HCC and iCCA. Dynamic imaging features are related to the predominant histopathological component of HCC and iCCA, respectively.
- In case of tumours with atypical imaging features and without established clinical risk factors, a core liver biopsy is suggested.

Little is known about the clinical and oncological behaviour of these cancers, which likely represent a unique subset of primary liver cancers, with distinctive features. At present it is virtually impossible to predict the outcome of cHCC-CCA in case of LR, transplantation, locoregional therapies, including conventional and DEB-TACE, TARE, RT, and systemic therapies currently administered for HCC or iCCA, including the available targeted agents. More accurate elucidation of the biologic and clinical behaviour of cHCC-CCA is needed.

Self Study

Questions

1. **Which groups of patients at risk of HCC should undergo surveillance?**
   (a) Cirrhotic patients with:
   - HBV infection.
   - HCV infection.
   - NASH.
   - Primary biliary cirrhosis.

   (b) Noncirrhotic patients with:
   - Chronic HBV hepatitis, in Asian and African countries where HBV infection is endemic.
   - Chronic HCV hepatitis and bridging fibrosis.
   - NAFLD.

   (c) Patients treated for chronic viral hepatitis:
   - With sustained HBV-DNA suppression or HBeAg seroconversion in chronic hepatitis B.
   - With sustained viral response in chronic hepatitis C with advanced fibrosis or cirrhosis.

   (d) All these groups.
2. **Which is the typical behaviour of intrahepatic cholangiocellular carcinoma at dynamic CT?**
   (a) Arterial phase hyperenhancement (APHE) with washout in the portal venous or delayed phases.
   (b) Peripheral rim enhancement in the arterial phase, and progressive centripetal enhancement during the venous and delayed phases, commonly lasting several minutes.
   (c) Peripheral nodular or globular enhancement in the arterial phase, with a centripetal progression or "filling in" in the portal venous and delayed phases; the tumour opacifies after a delay of three or more minutes and remains isodense or hyperdense on delayed scans.

Answers

1. **Which groups of patients at risk of HCC should undergo surveillance?**
   (a) Cost-effectiveness studies suggest that an incidence of HCC of ≥1.5% per year would require implementing surveillance strategies of HCC in cirrhotic patients, irrespective of its aetiology; HBV and HCV infection, NASH and primary biliary cirrhosis are related to high risk of HCC occurrence.
   (b) HCC can occur even in the absence of cirrhosis in patients with chronic HBV hepatitis, in Asian and African countries where HBV infection is endemic; with chronic HCV hepatitis and bridging fibrosis; and with NAFLD.
   (c) Successful antiviral treatments determining sustained HBV-DNA suppression or HBeAg seroconversion in chronic hepatitis B, and sustained virological response in chronic hepatitis C, reduce, but do not eliminate the risk of developing HCC. As a consequence, treated patients with chronic hepatitis B who remain at risk of HCC occurrence because of baseline factors, and those with HCV-related advanced fibrosis or cirrhosis, should undergo surveillance even after achieving sustained viral response.
   (d) **CORRECT**. All these groups are at risk of developing HCC and should receive appropriate surveillance.
2. **Which is the typical behaviour of intrahepatic cholangiocellular carcinoma at dynamic CT?**
   (a) Hepatocellular carcinoma typically shows arterial phase hyperenhancement (APHE) with washout in the portal venous or delayed phases on CT and MRI using extracellular contrast agents, and APHE with washout in the portal venous phase on MRI using Gd-EOB-DTPA.
   (b) **CORRECT**. Intrahepatic cholangiocellular carcinoma typically appears as a hypodense hepatic mass with irregular margins in the precontrast phase on CT, with peripheral rim enhancement in the arterial phase, and progressive centripetal enhancement during the venous and delayed phases, over several minutes, related to the fibrotic tissue within the cancer.
   (c) Hepatic hemangioma typically appears as a well delineated hypodense lesion in the precontrast phase on CT, with peripheral nodular or globular enhancement in the arterial phase, with a centripetal progression or "filling in" in the portal venous and delayed phases; the tumour typically opacifies after a delay of three or more minutes and remain isodense or hyperdense on delayed scans; this pattern is observed in up to 94% of hemangiomas larger than 4 cm.

References

1. Global Burden of Disease Liver Cancer Collaboration, Akinyemiju T, Abera S, Ahmed M, Alam N, Alemayohu MA, Allen C, et al. The burden of primary liver cancer and underlying etiologies from 1990 to 2015 at the global, regional, and national level. JAMA Oncol. 2017;3:1683–91. https://doi.org/10.1001/jamaoncol.2017.3055.
2. Marrero JA, Kulik LM, Sirlin CB, Zhu AX, Finn RS, Abecassis MM, Roberts LR, Heimbach JK. Diagnosis, staging, and management of hepatocellular carcinoma: 2018 practice guidance by the American Association for the Study of Liver Diseases. Hepatology. 2018;68:723–50. https://doi.org/10.1002/hep.29913.
3. Omata M, Cheng AL, Kokudo N, Kudo M, Lee JM, Jia J, Tateishi R, Han KH, Chawla YK, Shiina S, Jafri W, Payawal DA, Ohki T, Ogasawara S, Chen PJ, Lesmana CRA, Lesmana LA, Gani RA, Obi S, Dokmeci AK, Sarin SK. Asia-Pacific clinical practice guidelines on the management of hepatocellular carcinoma: a 2017

update. Hepatol Int. 2017;11:317–70. https://doi.org/10.1007/s12072-017-9799-9.
4. European Association for the Study of the Liver. EASL clinical practice guidelines: management of hepatocellular carcinoma. J Hepatol. 2018;69:182–236. https://doi.org/10.1016/j.jhep.2018.03.019.
5. Forner A, Reig M, Bruix J. Hepatocellular carcinoma. Lancet. 2018;391:1301–14. https://doi.org/10.1016/S0140-6736(18)30010-2.
6. El-Serag HB. Hepatocellular carcinoma. N Engl J Med. 2011;365:1118–27. https://doi.org/10.1056/NEJMra1001683.
7. Petrick JL, Braunlin M, Laversanne M, Valery PC, Bray F, McGlynn KA. International trends in liver cancer incidence, overall and by histologic subtype, 1978-2007. Int J Cancer. 2016;139:1534–45. https://doi.org/10.1002/ijc.30211.
8. Pascual S, Herrera I, Irurzun J. New advances in hepatocellular carcinoma. World J Hepatol. 2016;8:421–38. https://doi.org/10.4254/wjh.v8.i9.421.
9. Qiu D, Katanoda K, Marugame T, Sobue T. A Joinpoint regression analysis of long-term trends in cancer mortality in Japan (1958–2004). Int J Cancer. 2009;124:443–8. https://doi.org/10.1002/ijc.23911.
10. Bosetti C, Levi F, Boffetta P, Lucchini F, Negri E, La Vecchia C. Trends in mortality from hepatocellular carcinoma in Europe, 1980–2004. Hepatology. 2008;48:137–45. https://doi.org/10.1002/hep.22312.
11. Mittal S, El-Serag HB. Epidemiology of hepatocellular carcinoma: consider the population. J Clin Gastroenterol. 2013;47:S2–6. https://doi.org/10.1097/MCG.0b013e3182872f29.
12. El-Serag HB, Kanwal F. Epidemiology of hepatocellular carcinoma in the United States: where are we? Where do we go? Hepatology. 2014;60:1767–75. https://doi.org/10.1002/hep.27222.
13. El-Serag HB. Epidemiology of viral hepatitis and hepatocellular carcinoma. Gastroenterology. 2012;142:1264–73. https://doi.org/10.1053/j.gastro.2011.12.061.
14. Sangiovanni A, Prati GM, Fasani P, Ronchi G, Romeo R, Manini M, Del Ninno E, Morabito A, Colombo M. The natural history of compensated cirrhosis due to hepatitis C virus: a 17-year cohort study of 214 patients. Hepatology. 2006;43:1303–10. https://doi.org/10.1002/hep.21176.
15. de Martel C, Maucort-Boulch D, Plummer M, Franceschi S. World-wide relative contribution of hepatitis B and C viruses in hepatocellular carcinoma. Hepatology. 2015;62:1190–200. https://doi.org/10.1002/hep.27969.
16. Wong CR, Nguyen MH, Lim JK. Hepatocellular carcinoma in patients with non-alcoholic fatty liver disease. World J Gastroenterol. 2016;22:8294–303. https://doi.org/10.3748/wjg.v22.i37.8294.
17. Welzel TM, Graubard BI, Zeuzem S, El-Serag HB, Davila JA, McGlynn KA. Metabolic syndrome increases the risk of primary liver cancer in the United States: a study in the SEER-Medicare database. Hepatology. 2011;54:463–71. https://doi.org/10.1002/hep.24397.
18. Chen CJ, Iloeje UH, Yang HI. Long-term outcomes in hepatitis B: the REVEAL-HBV study. Clin Liver Dis. 2007;11:797–816. https://doi.org/10.1016/j.cld.2007.08.005.
19. Tseng TC, Liu CJ, Yang HC, Su TH, Wang CC, Chen CL, Hsu CA, Kuo SF, Liu CH, Chen PJ, Chen DS, Kao JH. Serum hepatitis B surface antigen levels help predict disease progression in patients with low hepatitis B virus loads. Hepatology. 2013;57:441–50. https://doi.org/10.1002/hep.26041.
20. Liaw YF. HBeAg seroconversion as an important end point in the treatment of chronic hepatitis B. Hepatol Int. 2009;3:425–33. https://doi.org/10.1007/s12072-009-9140-3.
21. Liu CJ, Kao JH. Global perspective on the natural history of chronic hepatitis B: role of hepatitis B virus genotypes A to J. Semin Liver Dis. 2013;33:97–102. https://doi.org/10.1055/s-0033-1345716.
22. Yang HI, Yeh SH, Chen PJ, Iloeje UH, Jen CL, Su J, Wang LY, Lu SN, You SL, Chen DS, Liaw YF, Chen CJ, REVEAL-HBV Study Group. Associations between hepatitis B virus genotype and mutants and the risk of hepatocellular carcinoma. J Natl Cancer Inst. 2008;100:1134–43. https://doi.org/10.1093/jnci/djn243.
23. Chen CH, Chen YY, Chen GH, Yang SS, Tang HS, Lin HH, Lin DY, Lo SK, Du JM, Chang TT, Chen SC, Liao LY, Kuo CH, Lin KC, Tai DI, Changchien CS, Chang WY, Sheu JC, Chen DS, Liaw YF, Sung JL. Hepatitis B virus transmission and hepatocarcinogenesis: a 9 year retrospective cohort of 13676 relatives with hepatocellular carcinoma. J Hepatol. 2004;40:653–9. https://doi.org/10.1016/j.jhep.2003.12.002.
24. Jung KS, Kim SU, Ahn SH, Park YN, Kim DY, Park JY, Chon CY, Choi EH, Han KH. Risk assessment of hepatitis B virus-related hepatocellular carcinoma development using liver stiffness measurement (FibroScan). Hepatology. 2011;53:885–94. https://doi.org/10.1002/hep.24121.
25. McPherson S, Hardy T, Henderson E, Burt AD, Day CP, Anstee QM. Evidence of NAFLD progression from steatosis to fibrosing-steatohepatitis using paired biopsies: implications for prognosis and clinical management. J Hepatol. 2015;62:1148–55. https://doi.org/10.1016/j.jhep.2014.11.034.
26. Bellentani S, Scaglioni F, Marino M, Bedogni G. Epidemiology of non-alcoholic fatty liver disease. Dig Dis. 2010;28:155–61. https://doi.org/10.1159/000282080.
27. Matteoni CA, Younossi ZM, Gramlich T, Boparai N, Liu YC, McCullough AJ. Nonalcoholic fatty liver disease: a spectrum of clinical and pathological severity. Gastroenterology. 1999;116:1413–9.
28. Desai A, Sandhu S, Lai JP, Sandhu DS. Hepatocellular carcinoma in non-cirrhotic liver: a comprehensive review. World J Hepatol. 2019;11:1–18. https://doi.org/10.4254/wjh.v11.i1.1.
29. Wang P, Kang D, Cao W, Wang Y, Liu Z. Diabetes mellitus and risk of hepatocellular carcinoma: a systematic review and meta-analysis. Diabetes Metab Res Rev. 2012;28:109–22. https://doi.org/10.1002/dmrr.1291.
30. Wong RJ, Cheung R, Ahmed A. Nonalcoholic steatohepatitis is the most rapidly growing indication for liver transplantation in patients with hepatocellular carcinoma in the U.S. Hepatology. 2014;59:2188–95. https://doi.org/10.1002/hep.26986.
31. Heckley GA, Jarl J, Asamoah BO, G-Gerdtham U. How the risk of liver cancer changes after alcohol cessation: a review and meta-analysis of the current literature. BMC Cancer. 2011;11:446. https://doi.org/10.1186/1471-2407-11-446.
32. Sun CA, Wu DM, Wang LY, Chen CJ, You SL, Santella RM. Determinants of formation of aflatoxin-albumin adducts: a seven-township study in Taiwan. Br J Cancer. 2002;87:966–70. https://doi.org/10.1038/sj.bjc.6600584.
33. Ross RK, Yuan JM, Yu MC, Wogan GN, Qian GS, Tu JT, Groopman JD, Gao YT, Henderson BE. Urinary aflatoxin biomarkers and risk of hepatocellular carcinoma. Lancet. 1992;339:943–6.
34. Chen JD, Yang HI, Iloeje UH, You SL, Lu SN, Wang LY, Su J, Sun CA, Liaw YF, Chen CJ, Risk Evaluation of Viral Load Elevation and Associated Liver Disease/Cancer in HBV (REVEAL-HBV) Study Group. Carriers of inactive hepatitis B virus are still at risk for hepatocellular carcinoma and liver-related death. Gastroenterology. 2010;138:1747–54. https://doi.org/10.1053/j.gastro.2010.01.042.
35. Liaw YF, Sung JJ, Chow WC, Farrell G, Lee CZ, Yuen H, Tanwandee T, Tao QM, Shue K, Keene ON, Dixon JS, Gray DF, Sabbat J, Cirrhosis Asian Lamivudine Multicentre Study Group. Lamivudine for patients with chronic hepatitis B and advanced liver disease. N Engl J Med. 2004;351:1521–31. https://doi.org/10.1056/NEJMoa033364.
36. Papatheodoridis GV, Lampertico P, Manolakopoulos S, Lok A. Incidence of hepatocellular carcinoma in chronic hepatitis B patients receiving nucleos(t)ide therapy: a systematic review. J Hepatol. 2010;53:348–56. https://doi.org/10.1016/j.jhep.2010.02.035.

37. Cho JY, Paik YH, Sohn W, Cho HC, Gwak GY, Choi MS, Lee JH, Koh KC, Paik SW, Yoo BC. Patients with chronic hepatitis B treated with oral antiviral therapy retain a higher risk for HCC compared with patients with inactive stage disease. Gut. 2014;63:1943–50. https://doi.org/10.1136/gutjnl-2013-306409.
38. Yu ML, Lin SM, Chuang WL, Dai CY, Wang JH, Lu SN, Sheen IS, Chang WY, Lee CM, Liaw YF. A sustained virological response to interferon or interferon/ribavirin reduces hepatocellular carcinoma and improves survival in chronic hepatitis C: a nationwide, multicentre study in Taiwan. Antivir Ther. 2006;11:985–94.
39. El-Serag HB, Kanwal F, Richardson P, Kramer J. Risk of hepatocellular carcinoma after sustained virological response in veterans with hepatitis C virus infection. Hepatology. 2016;64:130–7. https://doi.org/10.1002/hep.28535.
40. Chalasani N, Younossi Z, Lavine JE, Diehl AM, Brunt EM, Cusi K, Charlton M, Sanyal AJ. The diagnosis and management of nonalcoholic fatty liver disease: practice Guideline by the American Association for the Study of Liver Diseases, American College of Gastroenterology, and the American Gastroenterological Association. Hepatology. 2012;55:2005–23. https://doi.org/10.1002/hep.25762.
41. Prenner S, Kulik L. Hepatocellular carcinoma. In: Sanyal AJ, Boyer TD, Lindor KD, Terrault NA, editors. Zakim and Boyer's hepatology: a textbook of liver disease. 7th ed. Philadelphia, PA: Elsevier; 2018. p. 668–92.
42. Schulze K, Nault JC, Villanueva A. Genetic profiling of hepatocellular carcinoma using next-generation sequencing. J Hepatol. 2016;65:1031–42. https://doi.org/10.1016/j.jhep.2016.05.035.
43. Wilhelm S, Carter C, Lynch M, Lowinger T, Dumas J, Smith RA, Schwartz B, Simantov R, Kelley S. Discovery and development of sorafenib: a multikinase inhibitor for treating cancer. Nat Rev Drug Discov. 2006;5:835–44. https://doi.org/10.1038/nrd2130.
44. Gupta M, Gabriel H, Miller FH. Role of imaging in surveillance and diagnosis of hepatocellular carcinoma. Gastroenterol Clin North Am. 2018;47:585–602. https://doi.org/10.1016/j.gtc.2018.04.013.
45. Bolondi L, Sofia S, Siringo S, Gaiani S, Casali A, Zironi G, Piscaglia F, Gramantieri L, Zanetti M, Sherman M. Surveillance programme of cirrhotic patients for early diagnosis and treatment of hepatocellular carcinoma: a cost effectiveness analysis. Gut. 2001;48:251–9.
46. Elsayes KM, Hooker JC, Agrons MM, Kielar AZ, Tang A, Fowler KJ, Chernyak V, Bashir MR, Kono Y, Do RK, Mitchell DG, Kamaya A, Hecht EM, Sirlin CB. 2017 version of LI-RADS for CT and MR imaging: an update. Radiographics. 2017;37:1994–2017. https://doi.org/10.1148/rg.2017170098.
47. Hanna RF, Miloushev VZ, Tang A, Finklestone LA, Brejt SZ, Sandhu RS, Santillan CS, Wolfson T, Gamst A, Sirlin CB. Comparative 13-year meta-analysis of the sensitivity and positive predictive value of ultrasound, CT, and MRI for detecting hepatocellular carcinoma. Abdom Radiol (NY). 2016;41:71–90. https://doi.org/10.1007/s00261-015-0592-8.
48. D'Onofrio M, Crosara S, De Robertis R, Canestrini S, Mucelli RP. Contrast-enhanced ultrasound of focal liver lesions. AJR Am J Roentgenol. 2015;205:W56–66. https://doi.org/10.2214/AJR.14.14203.
49. Roberts LR, Sirlin CB, Zaiem F, Almasri J, Prokop LJ, Heimbach JK, Murad MH, Mohammed K. Imaging for the diagnosis of hepatocellular carcinoma: a systematic review and meta-analysis. Hepatology. 2018;67:401–21. https://doi.org/10.1002/hep.29487.
50. Lyshchik A, Kono Y, Dietrich CF, Jang HJ, Kim TK, Piscaglia F, Vezeridis A, Willmann JK, Wilson SR. Contrast-enhanced ultrasound of the liver: technical and lexicon recommendations from the ACR CEUS LI-RADS working group. Abdom Radiol (NY). 2018;43:861–79. https://doi.org/10.1007/s00261-017-1392-0.
51. Tajima T, Honda H, Taguchi K, Asayama Y, Kuroiwa T, Yoshimitsu K, Irie H, Aibe H, Shimada M, Masuda K. Sequential hemodynamic change in hepatocellular carcinoma and dysplastic nodules: CT angiography and pathologic correlation. AJR Am J Roentgenol. 2002;178:885–97. https://doi.org/10.2214/ajr.178.4.1780885.
52. Choi JY, Lee JM, Sirlin CB. CT and MR imaging diagnosis and staging of hepatocellular carcinoma: part II. Extracellular agents, hepatobiliary agents, and ancillary imaging features. Radiology. 2014;273:30–50. https://doi.org/10.1148/radiol.14132362.
53. Neri E, Bali MA, Ba-Ssalamah A, Boraschi P, Brancatelli G, Alves FC, Grazioli L, Helmberger T, Lee JM, Manfredi R, Martì-Bonmatì L, Matos C, Merkle EM, Op De Beeck B, Schima W, Skehan S, Vilgrain V, Zech C, Bartolozzi C. ESGAR consensus statement on liver MR imaging and clinical use of liver-specific contrast agents. Eur Radiol. 2016;26:921–31. https://doi.org/10.1007/s00330-015-3900-3.
54. Lo EC, Rucker A, Federle MP. Hepatocellular carcinoma and intrahepatic cholangiocarcinoma: imaging for diagnosis, tumor response to treatment and liver response to radiation. Semin Radiat Oncol. 2018;28:267–76. https://doi.org/10.1016/j.semradonc.2018.06.010.
55. Choi JY, Lee JM, Sirlin CB. CT and MR imaging diagnosis and staging of hepatocellular carcinoma: part I. Development, growth, and spread: key pathologic and imaging aspects. Radiology. 2014;272:635–54. https://doi.org/10.1148/radiol.14132361.
56. Lee YJ, Lee JM, Lee JS, Lee HY, Park BH, Kim YH, Han JK, Choi BI. Hepatocellular carcinoma: diagnostic performance of multidetector CT and MR imaging-a systematic review and meta-analysis. Radiology. 2015;275:97–109. https://doi.org/10.1148/radiol.14140690.
57. Nakamura Y, Toyota N, Date S, Oda S, Namimoto T, Yamashita Y, Beppu T, Awai K. Clinical significance of the transitional phase at gadoxetate disodium-enhanced hepatic MRI for the diagnosis of hepatocellular carcinoma: preliminary results. J Comput Assist Tomogr. 2011;35:723–7. https://doi.org/10.1097/RCT.0b013e3182372c40.
58. Kudo M, Matsui O, Izumi N, Iijima H, Kadoya M, Imai Y, Okusaka T, Miyayama S, Tsuchiya K, Ueshima K, Hiraoka A, Ikeda M, Ogasawara S, Yamashita T, Minami T, Yamakado K, Liver Cancer Study Group of Japan. JSH consensus-based clinical practice guidelines for the management of hepatocellular carcinoma: 2014 update by the Liver Cancer Study Group of Japan. Liver Cancer. 2014;3:458–68. https://doi.org/10.1159/000343875.
59. Choi BI, Lee JM, Kim TK, Dioguardi Burgio M, Vilgrain V. Diagnosing borderline hepatic nodules in hepatocarcinogenesis: imaging performance. AJR Am J Roentgenol. 2015;205:10–21. https://doi.org/10.2214/AJR.14.12655.
60. Kudo M. Early hepatocellular carcinoma: definition and diagnosis. Liver Cancer. 2013;2:69–72. https://doi.org/10.1159/000343842.
61. Golfieri R, Grazioli L, Orlando E, Dormi A, Lucidi V, Corcioni B, Dettori E, Romanini L, Renzulli M. Which is the best MRI marker of malignancy for atypical cirrhotic nodules: hypointensity in hepatobiliary phase alone or combined with other features? Classification after Gd-EOB-DTPA administration. J Magn Reson Imaging. 2012;36:648–57. https://doi.org/10.1002/jmri.23685.
62. Mitchell DG, Bruix J, Sherman M, Sirlin CB. LI-RADS (liver imaging reporting and data system): summary, discussion, and consensus of the LI-RADS Management Working Group and future directions. Hepatology. 2015;61:1056–65. https://doi.org/10.1002/hep.27304.
63. Bolondi L, Gaiani S, Celli N, Golfieri R, Grigioni WF, Leoni S, Venturi AM, Piscaglia F. Characterization of small nodules in cirrhosis by assessment of vascularity: the problem of hypovascular hepatocellular carcinoma. Hepatology. 2005;42:27–34. https://doi.org/10.1002/hep.20728.
64. Hong G, Suh KS, Suh SW, Yoo T, Kim H, Park MS, Choi Y, Paeng JC, Yi NJ, Lee KW. Alpha-fetoprotein and (18)F-FDG positron emission tomography predict tumor recurrence better than Milan criteria in living donor liver transplantation. J Hepatol. 2016;64:852–9. https://doi.org/10.1016/j.jhep.2015.11.033.

65. Hong TS, Wo JY, Yeap BY, Ben-Josef E, McDonnell EI, Blaszkowsky LS, Kwak EL, Allen JN, Clark JW, Goyal L, Murphy JE, Javle MM, Wolfgang JA, Drapek LC, Arellano RS, Mamon HJ, Mullen JT, Yoon SS, Tanabe KK, Ferrone CR, Ryan DP, TF DL, Crane CH, Zhu AX. Multi-institutional phase II study of high-dose hypofractionated proton beam therapy in patients with localized, unresectable hepatocellular carcinoma and intrahepatic cholangiocarcinoma. J Clin Oncol. 2016;34:460–8. https://doi.org/10.1200/JCO.2015.64.2710.
66. Tateishi R, Yoshida H, Matsuyama Y, Mine N, Kondo Y, Omata M. Diagnostic accuracy of tumor markers for hepatocellular carcinoma: a systematic review. Hepatol Int. 2008;2:17–30. https://doi.org/10.1007/s12072-007-9038-x.
67. Díaz-González Á, Forner A. Surveillance for hepatocellular carcinoma. Best Pract Res Clin Gastroenterol. 2016;30:1001–10. https://doi.org/10.1016/j.bpg.2016.10.006.
68. Zhang BH, Yang BH, Tang ZY. Randomized controlled trial of screening for hepatocellular carcinoma. J Cancer Res Clin Oncol. 2004;130:417–22. https://doi.org/10.1007/s00432-004-0552-0.
69. Kudo M, Izumi N, Sakamoto M, Matsuyama Y, Ichida T, Nakashima O, Matsui O, Ku Y, Kokudo N, Makuuchi M, Liver Cancer Study Group of Japan. Survival analysis over 28 years of 173,378 patients with hepatocellular carcinoma in Japan. Liver Cancer. 2016;5:190–7. https://doi.org/10.1159/000367775.
70. Kudo M, Izumi N, Ichida T, Ku Y, Kokudo N, Sakamoto M, Takayama T, Nakashima O, Matsui O, Matsuyama Y. Report of the 19th follow-up survey of primary liver cancer in Japan. Hepatol Res. 2016;46:372–90. https://doi.org/10.1111/hepr.12697.
71. Singal A, Volk ML, Waljee A, Salgia R, Higgins P, Rogers MA, Marrero JA. Meta-analysis: surveillance with ultrasound for early-stage hepatocellular carcinoma in patients with cirrhosis. Aliment Pharmacol Ther. 2009;30:37–47. https://doi.org/10.1111/j.1365-2036.2009.04014.x.
72. Sato T, Tateishi R, Yoshida H, Ohki T, Masuzaki R, Imamura J, Goto T, Kanai F, Obi S, Kato N, Shiina S, Kawabe T, Omata M. Ultrasound surveillance for early detection of hepatocellular carcinoma among patients with chronic hepatitis C. Hepatol Int. 2009;3:544–50. https://doi.org/10.1007/s12072-009-9145-y.
73. Kinoshita A, Onoda H, Fushiya N, Koike K, Nishino H, Tajiri H. Staging systems for hepatocellular carcinoma: current status and future perspectives. World J Hepatol. 2015;7:406–24. https://doi.org/10.4254/wjh.v7.i3.406.
74. Matsukuma KE, Yeh MM. Update on the pathology of liver neoplasms. Ann Diagn Pathol. 2019;38:126–37. https://doi.org/10.1016/j.anndiagpath.2018.10.005.
75. Lauwers GY, Terris B, Balis UJ, Batts KP, Regimbeau JM, Chang Y, Graeme-Cook F, Yamabe H, Ikai I, Cleary KR, Fujita S, Flejou JF, Zukerberg LR, Nagorney DM, Belghiti J, Yamaoka Y, Vauthey JN, International Cooperative Study Group on Hepatocellular Carcinoma. Prognostic histologic indicators of curatively resected hepatocellular carcinomas: a multi-institutional analysis of 425 patients with definition of a histologic prognostic index. Am J Surg Pathol. 2002;26:25–34.
76. Pawlik TM, Delman KA, Vauthey JN, Nagorney DM, Ng IO, Ikai I, Yamaoka Y, Belghiti J, Lauwers GY, Poon RT, Abdalla EK. Tumor size predicts vascular invasion and histologic grade: implications for selection of surgical treatment for hepatocellular carcinoma. Liver Transpl. 2005;11:1086–92. https://doi.org/10.1002/lt.20472.
77. Okuda K, Ohtsuki T, Obata H, Tomimatsu M, Okazaki N, Hasegawa H, Nakajima Y, Ohnishi K. Natural history of hepatocellular carcinoma and prognosis in relation to treatment. Study of 850 patients. Cancer. 1985;56:918–28.
78. CLIP Investigators. A new prognostic system for hepatocellular carcinoma: a retrospective study of 435 patients: the Cancer of the Liver Italian Program (CLIP) investigators. Hepatology. 1998;28:751–5. https://doi.org/10.1002/hep.510280322.
79. Kudo M, Chung H, Osaki Y. Prognostic staging system for hepatocellular carcinoma (CLIP score): its value and limitations, and a proposal for a new staging system, the Japan Integrated Staging Score (JIS score). J Gastroenterol. 2003;38:207–15. https://doi.org/10.1007/s005350300038.
80. Heimbach JK, Kulik LM, Finn RS, Sirlin CB, Abecassis MM, Roberts LR, Zhu AX, Murad MH, Marrero JA. AASLD guidelines for the treatment of hepatocellular carcinoma. Hepatology. 2018;67:358–80. https://doi.org/10.1002/hep.29086.
81. Torzilli G, Belghiti J, Kokudo N, Takayama T, Capussotti L, Nuzzo G, Vauthey JN, Choti MA, De Santibanes E, Donadon M, Morenghi E, Makuuchi M. A snapshot of the effective indications and results of surgery for hepatocellular carcinoma in tertiary referral centers: is it adherent to the EASL/AASLD recommendations? An observational study of the HCC East-West Study Group. Ann Surg. 2013;257:929–37. https://doi.org/10.1097/SLA.0b013e31828329b8.
82. Yau T, Tang VY, Yao TJ, Fan ST, Lo CM, Poon RT. Development of Hong Kong liver cancer staging system with treatment stratification for patients with hepatocellular carcinoma. Gastroenterology. 2014;146:1691–1700.e3. https://doi.org/10.1053/j.gastro.2014.02.032.
83. International Working Party. Terminology of nodular hepatocellular lesions. Hepatology. 1995;22:983–93.
84. Roncalli M, Park YN, Borzio M, Sangiovanni A, Sciarra A, Di Tommaso L. Premalignant and early malignant hepatocellular lesions in chronic hepatitis/cirrhosis. In: Saxena R, editor. Practical hepatic pathology: a diagnostic approach. 2nd ed. Philadelphia, PA: Elsevier; 2018. p. 487–505.
85. Arakawa M, Kage M, Sugihara S, Nakashima T, Suenaga M, Okuda K. Emergence of malignant lesions within an adenomatous hyperplastic nodule in a cirrhotic liver. Observations in five cases. Gastroenterology. 1986;91:198–208.
86. Borzio M, Fargion S, Borzio F, Fracanzani AL, Croce AM, Stroffolini T, Oldani S, Cotichini R, Roncalli M. Impact of large regenerative, low grade and high grade dysplastic nodules in hepatocellular carcinoma development. J Hepatol. 2003;39:208–14.
87. Hytiroglou P, Park YN, Krinsky G, Theise ND. Hepatic precancerous lesions and small hepatocellular carcinoma. Gastroenterol Clin North Am. 2007;36:867–87. https://doi.org/10.1016/j.gtc.2007.08.010.
88. International Consensus Group for Hepatocellular Neoplasia. The International Consensus Group for Hepatocellular Neoplasia. Pathologic diagnosis of early hepatocellular carcinoma: a report of the international consensus group for hepatocellular neoplasia. Hepatology. 2009;49:658–64. https://doi.org/10.1002/hep.22709.
89. Edmondson HA, Steiner PE. Primary carcinoma of the liver: a study of 100 cases among 48,900 necropsies. Cancer. 1954;7:462–503.
90. Kakar S, Gown AM, Goodman ZD, Ferrell LD. Best practices in diagnostic immunohistochemistry: hepatocellular carcinoma versus metastatic neoplasms. Arch Pathol Lab Med. 2007;131:1648–54. https://doi.org/10.1043/1543-2165(2007)131[1648:BPIDIH]2.0.CO;2.
91. Song P, Tobe RG, Inagaki Y, Kokudo N, Hasegawa K, Sugawara Y, Tang W. The management of hepatocellular carcinoma around the world: a comparison of guidelines from 2001 to 2011. Liver Int. 2012;32:1053–63. https://doi.org/10.1111/j.1478-3231.2012.02792.x.
92. Wong TC, Lo CM. Resection strategies for hepatocellular carcinoma. Semin Liver Dis. 2013;33:273–81. https://doi.org/10.1055/s-0033-1351782.
93. Bruix J, Reig M, Sherman M. Evidence-based diagnosis, staging, and treatment of patients with hepatocellular carcinoma. Gastroenterology. 2016;150:835–53. https://doi.org/10.1053/j.gastro.2015.12.041.
94. Ishizawa T, Hasegawa K, Aoki T, Takahashi M, Inoue Y, Sano K, Imamura H, Sugawara Y, Kokudo N, Makuuchi M. Neither multiple tumors nor portal hypertension are surgical contraindications

for hepatocellular carcinoma. Gastroenterology. 2008;134:1908–16. https://doi.org/10.1053/j.gastro.2008.02.091.
95. Berzigotti A, Reig M, Abraldes JG, Bosch J, Bruix J. Portal hypertension and the outcome of surgery for hepatocellular carcinoma in compensated cirrhosis: a systematic review and meta-analysis. Hepatology. 2015;61:526–36. https://doi.org/10.1002/hep.27431.
96. Perini MV, Starkey G, Fink MA, Bhandari R, Muralidharan V, Jones R, Christophi C. From minimal to maximal surgery in the treatment of hepatocarcinoma: a review. World J Hepatol. 2015;7:93–100. https://doi.org/10.4254/wjh.v7.i1.93.
97. Wakabayashi G, Cherqui D, Geller DA, Buell JF, Kaneko H, Han HS, Asbun H, O'Rourke N, Tanabe M, Koffron AJ, Tsung A, Soubrane O, Machado MA, Gayet B, Troisi RI, Pessaux P, Van Dam RM, Scatton O, Abu Hilal M, Belli G, Kwon CH, Edwin B, Choi GH, Aldrighetti LA, Cai X, Cleary S, Chen KH, Schön MR, Sugioka A, Tang CN, Herman P, Pekolj J, Chen XP, Dagher I, Jarnagin W, Yamamoto M, Strong R, Jagannath P, Lo CM, Clavien PA, Kokudo N, Barkun J, Strasberg SM. Recommendations for laparoscopic liver resection: a report from the second international consensus conference held in Morioka. Ann Surg. 2015;261:619–29. https://doi.org/10.1097/SLA.0000000000001184.
98. Hasegawa K, Kokudo N, Makuuchi M, Izumi N, Ichida T, Kudo M, Ku Y, Sakamoto M, Nakashima O, Matsui O, Matsuyama Y. Comparison of resection and ablation for hepatocellular carcinoma: a cohort study based on a Japanese nationwide survey. J Hepatol. 2013;58:724–9. https://doi.org/10.1016/j.jhep.2012.11.009.
99. Moran A, Ramos LF, Picado O, Pendola F, Sleeman D, Dudeja V, Merchant N, Yakoub D. Hepatocellular carcinoma: resection with adjuvant hepatic artery infusion therapy vs resection alone. A systematic review and meta-analysis. J Surg Oncol. 2019;119:455–63. https://doi.org/10.1002/jso.25338.
100. Mazzaferro V, Regalia E, Doci R, Andreola S, Pulvirenti A, Bozzetti F, Montalto F, Ammatuna M, Morabito A, Gennari L. Liver transplantation for the treatment of small hepatocellular carcinomas in patients with cirrhosis. N Engl J Med. 1996;334:693–9. https://doi.org/10.1056/NEJM199603143341104.
101. Yao FY, Ferrell L, Bass NM, Watson JJ, Bacchetti P, Venook A, Ascher NL, Roberts JP. Liver transplantation for hepatocellular carcinoma: expansion of the tumor size limits does not adversely impact survival. Hepatology. 2001;33:1394–403. https://doi.org/10.1053/jhep.2001.24563.
102. Toso C, Mazzaferro V, Bruix J, Freeman R, Mentha G, Majno P. Toward a better liver graft allocation that accounts for candidates with and without hepatocellular carcinoma. Am J Transplant. 2014;14:2221–7. https://doi.org/10.1111/ajt.12923.
103. Liang W, Wu L, Ling X, Schroder PM, Ju W, Wang D, Shang Y, Kong Y, Guo Z, He X. Living donor liver transplantation versus deceased donor liver transplantation for hepatocellular carcinoma: a meta-analysis. Liver Transpl. 2012;18:1226–36. https://doi.org/10.1002/lt.23490.
104. Vitale A, Morales RR, Zanus G, Farinati F, Burra P, Angeli P, Frigo AC, Del Poggio P, Rapaccini G, Di Nolfo MA, Benvegnù L, Zoli M, Borzio F, Giannini EG, Caturelli E, Chiaramonte M, Trevisani F, Cillo U, Italian Liver Cancer Group. Barcelona clinic liver cancer staging and transplant survival benefit for patients with hepatocellular carcinoma: a multicentre, cohort study. Lancet Oncol. 2011;12:654–62. https://doi.org/10.1016/S1470-2045(11)70144-9.
105. Qi X, Zhao Y, Li H, Guo X, Han G. Management of hepatocellular carcinoma: an overview of major findings from meta-analyses. Oncotarget. 2016;7:34703–51. https://doi.org/10.18632/oncotarget.9157.
106. Dong W, Zhang T, Wang ZG, Liu H. Clinical outcome of small hepatocellular carcinoma after different treatments: a meta-analysis. World J Gastroenterol. 2014;20:10174–82. https://doi.org/10.3748/wjg.v20.i29.10174.
107. Shiina S, Yasuda H, Muto H, Tagawa K, Unuma T, Ibukuro K, Inoue Y, Takanashi R. Percutaneous ethanol injection in the treatment of liver neoplasms. AJR Am J Roentgenol. 1987;149:949–52. https://doi.org/10.2214/ajr.149.5.949.
108. Yamada R, Sato M, Kawabata M, Nakatsuka H, Nakamura K, Takashima S. Hepatic artery embolization in 120 patients with unresectable hepatoma. Radiology. 1983;148:397–401. https://doi.org/10.1148/radiology.148.2.6306721.
109. Nouri YM, Kim JH, Yoon HK, Ko HK, Shin JH, Gwon DI. Update on transarterial chemoembolization with drug-eluting microspheres for hepatocellular carcinoma. Korean J Radiol. 2019;20:34–49. https://doi.org/10.3348/kjr.2018.0088.
110. Llovet JM, Bruix J. Systematic review of randomized trials for unresectable hepatocellular carcinoma: chemoembolization improves survival. Hepatology. 2003;37:429–42. https://doi.org/10.1053/jhep.2003.50047.
111. Llovet JM, Bruix J. Novel advancements in the management of hepatocellular carcinoma in 2008. J Hepatol. 2008;48(Suppl 1):S20–37. https://doi.org/10.1016/j.jhep.2008.01.022.
112. Lee S, Kim BK, Song K, Park JY, Ahn SH, Kim SU, Han KH, Kim DY, Korea Central Cancer Registry. Subclassification of Barcelona clinic liver cancer B and C hepatocellular carcinoma: a cohort study of the multicenter registry database. J Gastroenterol Hepatol. 2016;31:842–7. https://doi.org/10.1111/jgh.13218.
113. El-Serag HB, Marrero JA, Rudolph L, Reddy KR. Diagnosis and treatment of hepatocellular carcinoma. Gastroenterology. 2008;134:1752–63. https://doi.org/10.1053/j.gastro.2008.02.090.
114. Lammer J, Malagari K, Vogl T, Pilleul F, Denys A, Watkinson A, Pitton M, Sergent G, Pfammatter T, Terraz S, Benhamou Y, Avajon Y, Gruenberger T, Pomoni M, Langenberger H, Schuchmann M, Dumortier J, Mueller C, Chevallier P, Lencioni R, PRECISION V Investigators. Prospective randomized study of doxorubicin-eluting-bead embolization in the treatment of hepatocellular carcinoma: results of the PRECISION V study. Cardiovasc Intervent Radiol. 2010;33:41–52. https://doi.org/10.1007/s00270-009-9711-7.
115. Wilhelm SM, Dumas J, Adnane L, Lynch M, Carter CA, Schütz G, Thierauch KH, Zopf D. Regorafenib (BAY 73-4506): a new oral multikinase inhibitor of angiogenic, stromal and oncogenic receptor tyrosine kinases with potent preclinical antitumor activity. Int J Cancer. 2011;129:245–55. https://doi.org/10.1002/ijc.25864.
116. Bridgewater J, Galle PR, Khan SA, Llovet JM, Park JW, Patel T, Pawlik TM, Gores GJ. Guidelines for the diagnosis and management of intrahepatic cholangiocarcinoma. J Hepatol. 2014;60:1268–89. https://doi.org/10.1016/j.jhep.2014.01.021.
117. Razumilava N, Lazaridis KN, Gores GJ. Cholangiocarcinoma. In: Sanyal AJ, Boyer TD, Lindor KD, Terrault NA, editors. Zakim and Boyer's hepatology: a textbook of liver disease. 7th ed. Philadelphia, PA: Elsevier; 2018. p. 693–707.
118. Blechacz B, Komuta M, Roskams T, Gores GJ. Clinical diagnosis and staging of cholangiocarcinoma. Nat Rev Gastroenterol Hepatol. 2011;8:512–22. https://doi.org/10.1038/nrgastro.2011.131.
119. Rizvi S, Khan SA, Hallemeier CL, Kelley RK, Gores GJ. Cholangiocarcinoma – evolving concepts and therapeutic strategies. Nat Rev Clin Oncol. 2018;15:95–111. https://doi.org/10.1038/nrclinonc.2017.157.
120. Lendvai G, Szekerczés T, Illyés I, Dóra R, Kontsek E, Gógl A, Kiss A, Werling K, Kovalszky I, Schaff Z, Borka K. Cholangiocarcinoma: classification, histopathology and molecular carcinogenesis. Pathol Oncol Res. 2018; https://doi.org/10.1007/s12253-018-0491-8.
121. Patel T. Worldwide trends in mortality from biliary tract malignancies. BMC Cancer. 2002;2:10.
122. Khan SA, Toledano MB, Taylor-Robinson SD. Epidemiology, risk factors, and pathogenesis of cholangiocarcinoma. HPB (Oxford). 2008;10:77–82. https://doi.org/10.1080/13651820801992641.

123. Yeh MM. Benign and malignant tumors of bile ducts. In: Saxena R, editor. Practical hepatic pathology: a diagnostic approach. 2nd ed. Philadelphia: Elsevier; 2018. p. 545–54.
124. Khan SA, Thomas HC, Davidson BR, Taylor-Robinson SD. Cholangiocarcinoma. Lancet. 2005;366:1303–14. https://doi.org/10.1016/S0140-6736(05)67530-7.
125. Shin HR, Lee CU, Park HJ, Seol SY, Chung JM, Choi HC, Ahn YO, Shigemastu T. Hepatitis B and C virus, clonorchis sinensis for the risk of liver cancer: a case-control study in Pusan. Korea Int J Epidemiol. 1996;25:933–40.
126. Lee TY, Lee SS, Jung SW, Jeon SH, Yun SC, Oh HC, Kwon S, Lee SK, Seo DW, Kim MH, Suh DJ. Hepatitis B virus infection and intrahepatic cholangiocarcinoma in Korea: a case-control study. Am J Gastroenterol. 2008;103:1716–20. https://doi.org/10.1111/j.1572-0241.2008.01796.x.
127. Welzel TM, Mellemkjaer L, Gloria G, Sakoda LC, Hsing AW, El Ghormli L, Olsen JH, McGlynn KA. Risk factors for intrahepatic cholangiocarcinoma in a low-risk population: a nationwide case-control study. Int J Cancer. 2007;120:638–41.
128. Palmer WC, Patel T. Are common factors involved in the pathogenesis of primary liver cancers? A meta-analysis of risk factors for intrahepatic cholangiocarcinoma. J Hepatol. 2012;57:69–76. https://doi.org/10.1016/j.jhep.2012.02.022.
129. Wei M, Lü L, Lin P, Chen Z, Quan Z, Tang Z. Multiple cellular origins and molecular evolution of intrahepatic cholangiocarcinoma. Cancer Lett. 2016;379:253–61. https://doi.org/10.1016/j.canlet.2016.02.038.
130. Razumilava N, Gores GJ. Cholangiocarcinoma. Lancet. 2014;383:2168–79. https://doi.org/10.1016/S0140-6736(13)61903-0.
131. Nakanuma Y, Tsutsui A, Ren XS, Harada K, Sato Y, Sasaki M. What are the precursor and early lesions of peripheral intrahepatic cholangiocarcinoma? Int J Hepatol. 2014;2014:805973. https://doi.org/10.1155/2014/805973.
132. Aishima S, Oda Y. Pathogenesis and classification of intrahepatic cholangiocarcinoma: different characters of perihilar large duct type versus peripheral small duct type. J Hepatobiliary Pancreat Sci. 2015;22:94–100. https://doi.org/10.1002/jhbp.154.
133. Goodman ZD. Neoplasms of the liver. Mod Pathol. 2007;20(Suppl 1):S49–60. https://doi.org/10.1038/modpathol.3800682.
134. Rullier A, Le Bail B, Fawaz R, Blanc JF, Saric J, Bioulac-Sage P. Cytokeratin 7 and 20 expression in cholangiocarcinomas varies along the biliary tract but still differs from that in colorectal carcinoma metastasis. Am J Surg Pathol. 2000;24:870–6.
135. Dodson RM, Weiss MJ, Cosgrove D, Herman JM, Kamel I, Anders R, Geschwind JF, Pawlik TM. Intrahepatic cholangiocarcinoma: management options and emerging therapies. J Am Coll Surg. 2013;217:736–750.e4. https://doi.org/10.1016/j.jamcollsurg.2013.05.021.
136. Mavros MN, Economopoulos KP, Alexiou VG, Pawlik TM. Treatment and prognosis for patients with intrahepatic cholangiocarcinoma: systematic review and meta-analysis. JAMA Surg. 2014;149:565–74. https://doi.org/10.1001/jamasurg.2013.5137.
137. Nathan H, Aloia TA, Vauthey JN, Abdalla EK, Zhu AX, Schulick RD, Choti MA, Pawlik TM. A proposed staging system for intrahepatic cholangiocarcinoma. Ann Surg Oncol. 2009;16:14–22. https://doi.org/10.1245/s10434-008-0180-z.
138. DeOliveira ML, Cunningham SC, Cameron JL, Kamangar F, Winter JM, Lillemoe KD, Choti MA, Yeo CJ, Schulick RD. Cholangiocarcinoma: thirty-one-year experience with 564 patients at a single institution. Ann Surg. 2007;245:755–62. https://doi.org/10.1097/01.sla.0000251366.62632.d3.
139. Jonas S, Thelen A, Benckert C, Biskup W, Neumann U, Rudolph B, Lopez-Häänninen E, Neuhaus P. Extended liver resection for intrahepatic cholangiocarcinoma: a comparison of the prognostic accuracy of the fifth and sixth editions of the TNM classification. Ann Surg. 2009;249:303–9. https://doi.org/10.1097/SLA.0b013e318195e164.
140. Spolverato G, Kim Y, Ejaz A, Alexandrescu S, Marques H, Aldrighetti L, Gamblin TC, Pulitano C, Bauer TW, Shen F, Sandroussi C, Poultsides G, Maithel SK, Pawlik TM. Conditional probability of long-term survival after liver resection for intrahepatic cholangiocarcinoma: a multi-institutional analysis of 535 patients. JAMA Surg. 2015;150:538–45. https://doi.org/10.1001/jamasurg.2015.0219.
141. Endo I, Gonen M, Yopp AC, Dalal KM, Zhou Q, Klimstra D, D'Angelica M, DeMatteo RP, Fong Y, Schwartz L, Kemeny N, O'Reilly E, Abou-Alfa GK, Shimada H, Blumgart LH, Jarnagin WR. Intrahepatic cholangiocarcinoma: rising frequency, improved survival, and determinants of outcome after resection. Ann Surg. 2008;248:84–96. https://doi.org/10.1097/SLA.0b013e318176c4d3.
142. Li YY, Li H, Lv P, Liu G, Li XR, Tian BN, Chen DJ. Prognostic value of cirrhosis for intrahepatic cholangiocarcinoma after surgical treatment. J Gastrointest Surg. 2011;15:608–13. https://doi.org/10.1007/s11605-011-1419-8.
143. Sapisochin G, Facciuto M, Rubbia-Brandt L, Marti J, Mehta N, Yao FY, Vibert E, Cherqui D, Grant DR, Hernandez-Alejandro R, Dale CH, Cucchetti A, Pinna A, Hwang S, Lee SG, Agopian VG, Busuttil RW, Rizvi S, Heimbach JK, Montenovo M, Reyes J, Cesaretti M, Soubrane O, Reichman T, Seal J, Kim PT, Klintmalm G, Sposito C, Mazzaferro V, Dutkowski P, Clavien PA, Toso C, Majno P, Kneteman N, Saunders C, Bruix J, iCCA International Consortium. Liver transplantation for "very early" intrahepatic cholangiocarcinoma: international retrospective study supporting a prospective assessment. Hepatology. 2016;64:1178–88. https://doi.org/10.1002/hep.28744.
144. Sapisochin G, Rodríguez de Lope C, Gastaca M, Ortiz de Urbina J, Suarez MA, Santoyo J, Castroagudín JF, Varo E, López-Andujar R, Palacios F, Sanchez Antolín G, Perez B, Guiberteau A, Blanco G, González-Diéguez ML, Rodriguez M, Varona MA, Barrera MA, Fundora Y, Ferron JA, Ramos E, Fabregat J, Ciria R, Rufian S, Otero A, Vazquez MA, Pons JA, Parrilla P, Zozaya G, Herrero JI, Charco R, Bruix J. "Very early" intrahepatic cholangiocarcinoma in cirrhotic patients: should liver transplantation be reconsidered in these patients? Am J Transplant. 2014;14:660–7. https://doi.org/10.1111/ajt.12591.
145. Kuhlmann JB, Euringer W, Spangenberg HC, Breidert M, Blum HE, Harder J, Fischer R. Treatment of unresectable cholangiocarcinoma: conventional transarterial chemoembolization compared with drug eluting bead-transarterial chemoembolization and systemic chemotherapy. Eur J Gastroenterol Hepatol. 2012;24:437–43. https://doi.org/10.1097/MEG.0b013e3283502241.
146. Hoffmann RT, Paprottka PM, Schön A, Bamberg F, Haug A, Dürr EM, Rauch B, Trumm CT, Jakobs TF, Helmberger TK, Reiser MF, Kolligs FT. Transarterial hepatic yttrium-90 radioembolization in patients with unresectable intrahepatic cholangiocarcinoma: factors associated with prolonged survival. Cardiovasc Intervent Radiol. 2012;35:105–16. https://doi.org/10.1007/s00270-011-0142-x.
147. Rafi S, Piduru SM, El-Rayes B, Kauh JS, Kooby DA, Sarmiento JM, Kim HS. Yttrium-90 radioembolization for unresectable standard-chemorefractory intrahepatic cholangiocarcinoma: survival, efficacy, and safety study. Cardiovasc Intervent Radiol. 2013;36:440–8. https://doi.org/10.1007/s00270-012-0463-4.
148. Valle J, Wasan H, Palmer DH, Cunningham D, Anthoney A, Maraveyas A, Madhusudan S, Iveson T, Hughes S, Pereira SP, Roughton M, Bridgewater J, ABC-02 Trial Investigators. Cisplatin plus gemcitabine versus gemcitabine for biliary tract cancer. N Engl J Med. 2010;362:1273–81. https://doi.org/10.1056/NEJMoa0908721.
149. Paradis V, Bedossa P. Biphenotypic primary liver carcinoma. In: Saxena R, editor. Practical hepatic pathology: a diagnostic approach. 2nd ed. Philadelphia, PA: Elsevier; 2018. p. 665–8.

150. Torbenson MS. Morphologic subtypes of hepatocellular carcinoma. Gastroenterol Clin North Am. 2017;46:365–91. https://doi.org/10.1016/j.gtc.2017.01.009.
151. Brunt E, Aishima S, Clavien PA, Fowler K, Goodman Z, Gores G, Gouw A, Kagen A, Klimstra D, Komuta M, Kondo F, Miksad R, Nakano M, Nakanuma Y, Ng I, Paradis V, Nyun Park Y, Quaglia A, Roncalli M, Roskams T, Sakamoto M, Saxena R, Sempoux C, Sirlin C, Stueck A, Thung S, WMS T, Wang XW, Wee A, Yano H, Yeh M, Zen Y, Zucman-Rossi J, Theise N. cHCC-CCA: consensus terminology for primary liver carcinomas with both hepatocytic and cholangiocytic differentiation. Hepatology. 2018;68:113–26. https://doi.org/10.1002/hep.29789.
152. Theise ND, Nakashima O, Park YN, Nakanuma Y. Combined hepatocellular-cholangiocarcinoma. In: Bosman FT, Carneiro F, Hruban R, Theise ND, editors. WHO classification of tumours of the digestive system volume 3. 4th ed. Lyon: International Agency for Research on Cancer; 2010. p. 225–7.
153. Wells ML, Venkatesh SK, Chandan VS, Fidler JL, Fletcher JG, Johnson GB, Hough DM, Roberts LR. Biphenotypic hepatic tumors: imaging findings and review of literature. Abdom Imaging. 2015;40:2293–305. https://doi.org/10.1007/s00261-015-0433-9.
154. Fowler KJ, Sheybani A, Parker RA, Doherty S, Brunt EM, Chapman WC, Menias CO. Combined hepatocellular and cholangiocarcinoma (biphenotypic) tumors: imaging features and diagnostic accuracy of contrast-enhanced CT and MRI. Am J Roentgenol. 2013;201:332–9. https://doi.org/10.2214/AJR.12.9488.
155. Potretzke TA, Tan BR, Doyle MB, Brunt EM, Heiken JP, Fowler KJ. Imaging features of biphenotypic primary liver carcinoma (hepatocholangiocarcinoma) and the potential to mimic hepatocellular carcinoma: LI-RADS analysis of CT and MRI features in 61 cases. Am J Roentgenol. 2016;207:25–31. https://doi.org/10.2214/AJR.15.14997.
156. Yin X, Zhang BH, Qiu SJ, Ren ZG, Zhou J, Chen XH, Zhou Y, Fan J. Combined hepatocellular carcinoma and cholangiocarcinoma: clinical features, treatment modalities, and prognosis. Ann Surg Oncol. 2012;19:2869–76. https://doi.org/10.1245/s10434-012-2328-0.
157. Yeh MM. Pathology of combined hepatocellular-cholangiocarcinoma. J Gastroenterol Hepatol. 2010;25:1485–92. https://doi.org/10.1111/j.1440-1746.2010.06430.x.
158. Lee JH, Chung GE, Yu SJ, Hwang SY, Kim JS, Kim HY, Yoon JH, Lee HS, Yi NJ, Suh KS, Lee KU, Jang JJ, Kim YJ. Long-term prognosis of combined hepatocellular and cholangiocarcinoma after curative resection. Comparison with hepatocellular carcinoma and cholangiocarcinoma. J Clin Gastroenterol. 2011;45:69–75. https://doi.org/10.1097/MCG.0b013e3181ce5dfa.
159. Cao J, Huang L, Liu C, Li J, Zhang X, Shen J, Li J, Lu L, Xu F, Yan J, Wu M, Lau WY, Yan Y. Double primary hepatic cancer (hepatocellular carcinoma and intrahepatic cholangiocarcinoma) in a single patient: a clinicopathologic study of 35 resected cases. J Gastroenterol Hepatol. 2013;28:1025–31. https://doi.org/10.1111/jgh.12143.
160. De Vito C, Sarker D, Ross P, Heaton N, Quaglia A. Histological heterogeneity in primary and metastatic classic combined hepatocellular-cholangiocarcinoma: a case series. Virchows Arch. 2017;471:619–29. https://doi.org/10.1007/s00428-017-2196-x.

Acute Liver Failure

32

Diana Toma, Ovidiu Lazar, and Ecaterina Bontas

Key Concepts

- Acute liver failure is defined by the deterioration of liver function tests, hepatic encephalopathy, and potentially associated dysfunction of other organs (such as acute respiratory distress syndrome, acute kidney injury, gastrointestinal bleeding, pancreatitis, sepsis) in a patient without underlying chronic liver disease.
- Untreated, the prognosis of acute liver failure is very poor, with a high mortality.
- Early recognition of acute liver failure, establishment of the etiology and relocation to a liver transplantation center, or tertiary intensive care specialized in acute liver failure are primordial measures in treating acute liver failure patients.

32.1 Introduction

Acute liver failure (ALF) is defined as the acute episode of hepatocellular severe dysfunction characterized by the deterioration of liver function tests, hepatic encephalopathy (HE), and potentially associated dysfunction of other organs [such as acute respiratory distress syndrome, acute kidney injury (AKI), gastrointestinal bleeding, pancreatitis, sepsis] in a patient without underlying chronic liver disease [1]. Untreated, the prognosis of ALF is very poor, with a high mortality. The patients with ALF should be managed in Intensive Care Unit (ICU) where therapy should be applied based on the specific etiology of ALF and should be started as early as possible. Broadly, the medical management of ALF is supportive until recovery of the native liver or until the liver transplantation is an option. Accordingly, liver transplantation is the only proven treatment option for patients who do not recover spontaneously.

D. Toma · O. Lazar
Life Memorial Hospital—Medlife, Bucharest, Romania

E. Bontas (✉)
"Prof. C.C. Iliescu" Emergency Institute for Cardiovascular Diseases, Bucharest, Romania

32.2 Definition

ALF is the clinical entity defined by the presence of encephalopathy and coagulopathy (impaired synthetic function with INR $\geq$1.5) within <26 weeks of the onset of symptoms, in a patient without cirrhosis or underlying chronic liver disease [1, 2]. When patients develop coagulopathy without any alteration of their consciousness level is defined as ***acute liver injury*** (ALI) [1]. A severe form of ALI can precede the installation of ALF. Other used terms for ALF are "fulminant hepatic failure", "acute hepatic necrosis", "fulminate hepatic necrosis" or "fulminant hepatitis".

In 1999 the International Association for the Study of the Liver (IASL) defined the subcategories of ALF based on the duration of disease from the beginning until the occurrence of hepatic encephalopathy (HE): ***hyperacute ALF*** as less than 10 days, ***fulminant ALF*** as 10–30 days and ***subacute hepatic failure*** as 5–24 weeks [3]. The fulminant type of ALF requires the presence of HE, severe coagulopathy, markedly increases serum transaminases, and jaundice; whereas the subacute type of ALF does not necessarily have HE and is mainly characterized by severe jaundice and ascites, mild/moderate coagulopathy and serum transaminases level [1].

Acute deterioration of liver function in case of patients with chronic liver disease known also as acute-on-chronic liver failure; or after extensive liver resection or liver trauma; liver injury secondary to systemic diseases; and secondary to alcohol abuse (alcoholic hepatitis) may fulfill clinical features of ALF, but they are not considered ALF. However, exceptions are considered in case of de

F. Radu-Ionita et al. (eds.), *Liver Diseases*, https://doi.org/10.1007/978-3-030-24432-3_32

novo presentation of patients with Wilson disease, vertically acquired hepatitis B, Budd-Chiari syndrome, or autoimmune hepatitis, which may be considered ALF despite of cirrhosis, if their disease has been manifested for less than 26 weeks [1, 2].

32.3 Etiology

Through the last decades, the etiology of ALF changed, with the declining incidence of hepatitis A and B, and elevation of paracetamol (acetaminophen) overdose, especially in Western Europe and United States [1, 2]. Moreover, there are also differences in etiology between developing and developed countries such as Europe and United States characterized by high incidence of paracetamol toxicity along with drug-induced liver injury (DILI) due to prescription agents. By contrast, South Asia and Hong Kong have a higher incidence of viral hepatitis.

Etiologies of ALF are the best indicators of prognosis, and require specific management options, such as an emergency liver transplantation (LT). The clinical course of different ALF etiologies is presented in Table 32.1 [1].

Lastly, European Association for the Study of the Liver recommends the classification of ALF based on their etiologies. Therefore, the etiologies of ALF are further divided in etiologies **with** possible indication for emergency LT, and etiologies **with no** indication for emergency LT [1].

Table 32.1 The clinical course of different ALF aetiologies with permission [1]

Precipitant	Examples	Presentation
Viral	Hepatitis A, E, B (less frequent CMV, HSV, VZV, Dengue)	Acute/fulminant
Drugs/ toxins	Paracetamol (acetaminophen), phosphorous, *Amanita phalloides* Anti-tuberculous, chemotherapy, statins, NSAI, phenytoin, carbamazepine, ecstasy, flucloxacillin	Acute/fulminant and subacute/ subfulminant Acute/fulminant
Vascular	Budd Chiari Hypoxic hepatitis	Acute/fulminant and subacute/ subfulminant Acute/fulminant
Pregnancy	Pre-eclamptic liver rupture, HELLP, fatty liver of pregnancy	Acute/fulminant
Other	Wilson disease, autoimmune, lymphoma, malignancy, HLH	Acute/fulminant and subacute/ subfulminant

CMV cytomegalovirus, *HSV* Herpes simplex, *NSAI* non-steroidal anti-inflammatory, *HELLP* haemolysis, elevated liver enzymes, low platelets, *HLH* haemophagocytic lymphohistiocytosis

32.3.1 Etiologies with Possible Indication for Emergency LT

The main causes of ALF with possible indication of LT are drug related hepatotoxicity (paracetamol, idiosyncratic drug reaction), toxin-related hepatotoxicity, viral hepatitis, autoimmune hepatitis, Wilson disease, Budd-Chiari syndrome, and pregnancy related liver failure) [1].

32.3.1.1 Drug-Related Hepatotoxicity

Many drugs could be the cause of drug-induced liver injury (DILI) which is a leading cause for emergency LT [4], especially in developed countries.

32.3.1.2 Acetaminophen (Paracetamol) Toxicity

Even if paracetamol—a widely used drug to ameliorate pain—rarely determines hepatotoxicity at therapeutic dose (<4 g/day in adults), this may occur after ingestion of large doses for suicidal purposes or nonintentional (ingestion of excessive amounts of paracetamol containing compounds such as opioid-paracetamol compounds). Hepatotoxicity can even occur at therapeutic dose, if other factors exist, like decreased glutathione reserves (in alcohol ingestion, fasting, malnutrition) or with medication known to induce cytochrome P450 system (anticonvulsants).

In the very early stages of paracetamol ingestion, the clinical syndrome is mainly characterized by severe metabolic acidosis, high lactate level, mild elevation of transaminases, minimal or any coagulopathy; being the consequence of the drug effect with liver functional mitochondrial standstill [1]. Subsequently, paracetamol hepatotoxicity is characterized by extreme high level of serum aminotransferase >10,000 IU/L, normal bilirubin level, hypoglycemia, and acute kidney injury (AKI). The progression of paracetamol induced hepatotoxicity is often rapidly to HE with coma and multiple organ failure [1].

32.3.1.3 Idiosyncratic Drug Reaction

ALF due to idiosyncratic drug reactions known as drug induced liver injury (DILI) may occur after any type of medication. It is a finding of older patients >60 years [1]. The most common implicated drugs are ***antibiotics*** (ampicillin-clavulanate, tetracyclines, macrolides, ciprofloxacin, nitrofurantoin), ***antituberculosis drugs*** (isoniazid, pyrazinamide), ***anticonvulsants*** (phenytoin, valproate), ***antidepressants*** (amitriptyline, nortriptyline), ***non-steroidal anti-inflammatory*** (NSAIDs), ***immunosuppressive agents*** (cyclophosphamide, methotrexate), and ***halothane***.

Shortly, mechanisms involved in hepatic injury are (1) the disruption of intracellular calcium homeostasis; (2) injury of the canalicular transport pumps, such as multidrug resistance–associated protein 3; (3) T cells mediated immunologic injury; (4) triggering of apoptotic pathways by tumor necrosis factor-α; and (5) the inhibition of mitochondrial beta oxidation [5].

Herbal supplements, alternative medicine, weight loss agents and other nutritional supplements have been also associated with idiosyncratic hypersensitivity reactions, such as Ginseng, Kawakawa and St. John's Wort.

Some illicit drugs (ecstasy, cocaine and phencyclidine) have been associated with idiosyncratic hypersensitivity reactions. For instance, ecstasy induced liver injury presents as an "heat shock related liver injury" with severe hyperthermia, multiple organ dysfunction, profound coagulopathy, and severe rhabdomyolysis [1, 6].

Even rarely, consider ***DRESS syndrome*** or **D**rug **R**eaction with **E**osinophilia and **S**ystemic **S**ymptom **S**yndrome, in case of clinical picture with (1) fever; (2) severe cutaneous rash; (3) lymphadenopathy and (4) eosinophilia [1]. DRESS syndrome is a hypersensitivity drug reaction and is most frequently associated with antiepileptic or anticonvulsivants, some antibiotics/antivirals, sulphur containing compounds, and NSAIDs [1]. Broadly, DRESS syndrome is characterized by skin rash, fever, pharyngitis, lymphadenopathy, and visceral organ involvement, typically presenting within eight weeks of therapy. Liver is one of the most common organs involved in DRESS Syndrome and liver failure is the most common cause of death in these patients. Liver abnormalities manifest with hepatomegaly, increased level of serum aminotransferases, hepatitis or even liver failure. Recent studies have suggested a close relationship between Herpes Viruses and DRESS syndrome. Management of this syndrome include withdrawal of the causative drug, supportive therapy in ICU, and systemic steroids.

32.3.1.4 Toxin-Related Hepatotoxicity

Different toxins are associated with dose-related toxicity:

- *Amanita phalloides* mushroom toxin—this mushrooms poisoning is more common in Europe compared with United States, and it is manifested in the first phases by muscarinic effects (sweating, salivation, vomiting, diarrhea, and so on). Later, after 4–8 days is associated with ALF.
- Organic solvents (e.g., carbon tetrachloride)
- Yellow phosphorus
- Aflatoxins—are defined as a family of toxins produced by certain fungi—*Aspergillus flavus* and *Aspergillus parasiticus*, that are found in agricultural crops such as maize (corn), peanuts, cottonseed, and tree nuts.

32.3.1.5 Viral Hepatitis

Although viral hepatitis has become a relatively infrequent cause of ALF in Europe or United States, it remains the commonest cause of ALF in Asia and Africa, with hepatitis virus type A, B and E involvement. Importantly, if HBV is the main cause of ALF in Far East countries, hepatitis E virus (HEV) is more common in India [7], and hepatitis A virus in United States.

32.3.1.6 Hepatitis B Virus (HBV)

Hepatitis caused by virus type B can evolve to ALI or ALF. HBV infection is classified de novo (acute primary infection), reactivation of HBV infection (occurred during or after treatment-induced immunosuppression after solid organ or for hematological malignancies transplantation), or superinfection with hepatitis D virus (HDV). In the last situation, the identification of patients at risk and the administration of antiviral prophylactic treatment before the initiation of immunosuppressive therapy are mandatory with benefits [8].

32.3.1.7 Hepatitis A Virus (HAV)

Hepatitis A virus is mainly transmitted by food or drinking water polluted with infected feces being common in India [9, 10]. ALF occurs in less than 1% of cases of acute hepatitis A but could be a form of HAV evolution in older adulthood, or in patients with preexisting chronic liver disease [1]. Vaccination, as a form of prevention, is recommended for adults traveling in endemic area or for high-risk group.

32.3.1.8 Hepatitis E Virus (HEV)

Infection caused by HEV is rare in USA or Western Europe, but it is a significant cause of liver failure in endemic areas such as Russia, Pakistan, Mexico, and India. ALF due to hepatitis E has a worse outcome in elderly, pregnant women, and patients with underlying chronic liver disease [11].

32.3.1.9 Hepatitis D Virus (HDV)

ALF occurs in 2.5–6% of HDV infections. The coinfection of HBV and HDV, or superinfection of a chronic HBV patient with HDV, can both lead to ALF, but with a higher risk in those with coinfection.

32.3.1.10 Hepatitis C Virus (HCV)

Acute hepatitis C rarely causes ALF.

32.3.1.11 Other Viral Infection

Some viruses are implied in the etiology of ALF including herpes simplex virus 1 and 2 (HSV 1, 2), varicella-zoster virus, cytomegalovirus, Epstein-Barr virus, yellow fever virus, adenovirus, and parvovirus B19 especially in immunosuppress patients. Moreover, virus infection may be a cofactor for DILI development.

To date, ALF is a rare complication of HSV or varicella-zoster infection, which may appear especially in immunocompromised patients (such transplanted recipients or HIV infected patients), pregnant women (usually in the third trimester), those with cancer or myelodysplastic syndromes, and rarely in immunocompetent patients. In 50% of patients with ALF caused by HSV, the skin lesion may be missing and in this case liver biopsy could be helpful for making the diagnosis. Treatment should be initiated with acyclovir (5–10 mg/kg every 8 h for at least 7 days) for suspected or documented cases [12]. As a side note, Epstein-Barr virus and CMV infection are rare causes of ALF, but blood screening for these two viruses should be done for all patients with unclear etiology of ALF.

32.3.1.12 Autoimmune Hepatitis

Patients with autoimmune hepatitis (AIH), same to Wilson disease, may have unrecognized preexisting chronic liver disease. However, if they develop hepatic failure, they should be considered as having ALF, if their disease has been manifested for less than 26 weeks. AIH should be suspected in patients with other autoimmune disorders presented with ALF. The diagnostic can be established by laboratory tests (fraction of globulin elevated, positive autoantibodies) or by liver biopsy [1].

AIH patients that develop ALF represent the most severe form of the disease; and they have the generally recommendation to receive corticosteroid therapy in early stages, if possible. Nonetheless, steroid treatment may be effective, sometimes the lack of improvement requires emergency LT.

32.3.1.13 Wilson Disease

Patients with Wilson disease represent 6–12% from ALF cases. These patients are generally young women <20 years old which present hemolytic anemia (Coombs negative), very high serum bilirubin and low alkaline phosphatase, and very increased serum and urinary cooper [13]. Accordingly, ALF in patients with Wilson disease may be precipitated by a viral infection. Common diagnostic testing for Wilson's disease includes serum ceruloplasmin, and assessment of serum and urinary cooper. Only that, the tests have high false-positive and false-negative rates, but this is unlikely to alter the management of ALF caused by Wilson's disease where LT is the ultimate choice.

32.3.1.14 Budd-Chiari Syndrome

Budd-Chiari syndrome is an uncommon condition induced by thrombotic or non-thrombotic obstruction of the hepatic venous outflow. It is characterized by hepatomegaly, ascites, and abdominal pain, and rarely presents as ALF. Early recognition and prompt treatment with anticoagulant therapy, thrombolytic therapy, and interventional radiology may result in good recovery.

32.3.1.15 Pregnancy: Acute Fatty Liver of Pregnancy and HELLP Syndrome

Acute fatty liver of pregnancy (AFLP) is a rare and severe complication of the third trimester of the pregnancy (30–38 week of gestation), caused by the free fatty acids accumulation in maternal blood and hepatocytes with the infiltration of the liver, which may cause ALF. The initial symptoms in patients with AFLP are usually nonspecific (nausea, vomiting, abdominal pain, malaise, headache), but often associate hypertension, with or without proteinuria, possibly due to preeclampsia. Signs and symptoms of ALF, including jaundice, ascites, encephalopathy, disseminated intravascular coagulopathy, and hypoglycemia can rapidly progress. Most patients develop acute kidney injury, and often progress to multiorgan failure [14]. Laboratory findings are elevated serum aspartate aminotransferase/alanine aminotransferase (AST/ALT), hypoglycemia, elevated levels of bilirubin and blood ammonia, low platelet count, and low fibrinogen. If it is not diagnosed and treated promptly, AFLP can result in high maternal and neonatal morbidity and mortality. Management of AFLP includes prompt delivery of the fetus, maternal stabilization and support, with the goals to recover damaged liver. Liver transplantation for fulminant hepatic failure caused by AFLP has been reported, but transplantation is unlikely to be needed with early diagnosis and prompt delivery of the fetus [15, 16].

HELLP syndrome defined by haemolysis, elevated liver enzyme levels, and low platelet levels, is a life-threatening condition through the third trimester of the pregnancy. Presently, the etiology of HELLP is not clear, but same to preeclampsia is due to an inadequate placental perfusion that results in placenta hypoxia and secondary in activation of coagulation cascade, thrombocytopenia, microvascular organs damage, with hepatic damage.

Same to AFLP, its presentation has nonspecific symptoms such as general altered state, nausea, vomiting, epigastric or right upper quadrant pain, and edema. The laboratory tests reveal thrombocytopenia, anemia and increase bilirubin level (secondary to hemolysis), elevated serum aspartate aminotransferase/alanine aminotransferase (AST/ALT) and lactate dehydrogenase (LDH) levels (secondary to liver dysfunction), low fibrinogen level and increased D-dimers due to fibrinolysis/DIC. Accordingly, the most common liver histological lesions are periportal necrosis and microvascular thrombosis which can evolve into subcapsular hematomas and even to hepatic rupture. Management of HELLP syndrome consists in early recognition, stabilization of the mother, seizure prophylaxis (intravenous magnesium sulfate), treatment of hypertension, corticosteroid therapy and delivery.

32.3.2 Etiologies with No Indication of LT

32.3.2.1 Malignancies

Briefly, malignancies associated with hepatic failure can be divided into primary liver tumor (hepatocarcinoma and cholangiocarcinoma), and secondary liver tumor such as metastatic infiltration of the liver with adenocarcinoma (e.g.

breast, lung, colon, and gastric cancer), lymphoma, and leukemia. Laboratory blood tests usually highlight elevated alkaline phosphatase and gamma-glutamyl transferase level, or in case of lymphoma, high serum level of lactate dehydrogenase.

32.3.2.2 Vascular Causes

Acute ischemic injury of the liver. Hypoxic hepatitis (HH) is usually a consequence of another severe illness such as cardiac, circulatory or respiratory failure, being more common in ICU settings with an incidence 2.5–10%. Pathophysiological mechanism of HH is represented by the reduction of the hepatic blood flow, hypoxemia, and hepatocyte lesions ischemic or through reperfusion. Laboratory tests reveal massive and rapid raise of serum aminotransferases caused by reduced oxygen delivery to the liver. The main treatment of the HH is the correction of the underlying disease state. Using of N-acetylcysteine, other antioxidants or molecular adsorbent recirculating system (MARS) for the management of liver dysfunction is known, but published evidence does not support their effectiveness or regular use [17]. Unfortunately, the poor prognosis with hospitalization mortality rate >50% represents the most frequent cause of death due to the predisposing condition and not to the liver injury itself [18]. Liver transplantation is rarely indicated for the treatment of HH [19].

32.3.2.3 Portal Vein Thrombosis (PVT)

As already known, portal vein results by the confluence of mesenteric superior and splenic veins, and could be occluded in patients with cirrhosis, prothrombotic disorders like neoplasms (21–24%), myeloproliferative disorders and hypercoagulable disorders (10–12%), abdominal trauma, surgery, inflammatory bowel disease, or idiopathic causes (8–15%). Patients with acute PVT present pain with sudden onset in the right hypochondrium, nausea, fever, followed by acute portal hypertension, and intestinal ischemia. The diagnosis can be established by ultrasonography, endoscopic ultrasonography (EUS), MRI and magnetic resonance angiography (MRA), and CT scan. The principles of treatment are the anticoagulant treatment or thrombolysis, the treatment of underlying disease, and the treatment of complications caused by acute portal hypertension (variceal bleeding, ascites, and encephalopathy)

32.4 Epidemiology

The commonest worldwide cause of ALF remains viral hepatitis (hepatitis A, E and B). The incidence of viral etiology of ALF has declined in Europe and USA, but in case of developing countries from Asia and Africa remains the main cause of ALF. On the other side, South Asia and Hong Kong still have higher incidence of hepatitis viruses (hepatitis E in Pakistan and hepatitis B in Hong Kong).

In Europe, the commonest cause of ALF is DILI (drug induced liver injury). In developed countries from Europe and USA, drug induced liver injury (DILI) and especially paracetamol or acetaminophen induced ALF represent nowadays the most frequent etiology. In USA, nearly half of all cases of ALF over a period of 17 years (US ALFSG Adult Registry 1998–2014) were represented by paracetamol induced ALF, and in United Kingdom paracetamol remains the predominant etiology of ALF, but an exponential rise in severe poisoning was effectively controlled by the restriction imposed on drug sales in 1998 [20].

32.5 Pathophysiology

ALF is a severe organ damage having the onset with nonspecific symptoms such as malaise, nausea, vomiting, abdominal pains and dehydration, followed by the appearance of jaundice, hepatic encephalopathy, coma, coagulopathy, metabolic abnormalities, and afterwards with progression to multiorgan failure (cardiovascular, hemodynamic, respiratory, and renal systems). Therefore, the severity of clinical signs and illness depends upon the adverse metabolic consequences of liver dysfunction, the side effects of toxins released by the necrotic liver, and the degree of liver regeneration [21].

In a simplified manner, ALF is defined by a significant liver necrosis with (1) coagulopathy; and (2) HE; in a patient without underling liver disorder. It has to be noted, that liver necrosis is missing in acute fatty liver of pregnancy. It follows that a necrotic liver release neurotoxic (ammonia) and inflammatory mediators (TNF, IL-1, IL-6). As a consequence, there is a continual alteration of blood-brain barrier with its dysfunction. Glutamine accumulation due to ammonia, crosses blood-brain barrier with further alteration and increasing of oxidative stress. Inflammatory mediators cause microglial activation. Finally, dysfunction of blood-brain barrier is associating astrocyte swelling and cerebral edema.

Encephalopathy. In ALF, the encephalopathy develops in the early stages of liver failure, sometimes suddenly; it may precede the jaundice, and it manifests through drowsiness, agitation, delirium, convulsions with rapid progression to decerebrate rigidity and deep coma. As a note, HE usually develops after 7 days of jaundice [1]. Also, patients with noted jaundice who develop HE between 8 and 28 days of jaundice, develop further ALF [1]. On the other side, patients with jaundice over 3 weeks and without HE are diagnosed with chronic liver disease [1].

One well known classification of HE is based on the underlying disease [22]. ***Type A*** is associated with acute liver failure resulting from severe inflammatory and/or necrotic

Table 32.2 West Haven Criteria and Clinical Description. From [22] with **permission**

West Haven criteria including minimal HE	ISHEN	Description	Suggested operative criteria	Comment
Unimpaired		No encephalopathy at all, no history of HE	Tested and proved to be normal	
Minimal	Covert	Psychometric or neuropsychological alterations of tests exploring psychomotor speed/executive functions or neurophysiological alterations without clinical evidence of mental change	Abnormal results of established psychometric or neuropsychological tests without clinical manifestations	No universal criteria for diagnosis Local standards and expertise required
Grade I		• Trivial lack of awareness • Euphoria or anxiety • Shortened attention span • Impairment of addition or subtraction • Altered sleep rhythm	Despite oriented in time and space (see below), the patient appears to have some cognitive/behavioral decay with respect to his or her standard on clinical examination or to the caregivers	Clinical findings usually not reproducible
Grade II	Overt	• Lethargy or apathy • Disorientation for time • Obvious personality change • Inappropriate behavior • Dyspraxia • Asterixis	Disoriented for time (at least three of the followings are wrong: day of the month, day of the week, month, season, or year) ± the other mentioned symptoms	Clinical findings variable, but reproducible to some extent
Grade III		• Somnolence to semistupor • Responsive to stimuli • Confused • Gross disorientation • Bizarre behavior	Disoriented also for space (at least three of the following wrongly reported: country, state [or region], city, or place) ± the other mentioned symptoms	Clinical findings reproducible to some extent
Grade IV		Coma	Does not respond even to painful stimuli	Comatose state usually reproducible

All conditions are required to be related to liver insufficiency and/or PSS (portosystemic shunting). Where **ISHEN**—International Society for Hepatic Encephalopathy and Nitrogen Metabolism

rapid onset liver disease, is associated with increased intracranial pressure (ICP) due to cerebral edema that progresses rapidly and may lead to brain herniation and death; ***type B*** is associated with portosystemic bypass without parenchymal liver disorders; ***type C*** accompanies chronic liver disease (cirrhosis) and portal hypertension with portosystemic shunts (with three subcategories: episodic, persistent and minimal); and ***type D*** associated with disorders of the urea cycle [22]. It has to be underlined, that types B and C have similar clinical manifestations [22].

Another useful classification of HE known as The West Haven Criteria is based on the severity of manifestations. The West Haven Criteria are described in Table 32.2 [22].

32.6 Diagnosis

The typical scenario of ALF is the association of **liver damage** (a 2–3 times elevation of serum transaminases) with **altered hepatic function** (jaundice and coagulopathy) in a patient without chronic liver disease [1].

The diagnostic of acute liver failure must be considered in patients with recent onset <26 weeks of mental status changes, jaundice, but also of nonspecific symptoms such as nausea, vomiting, malaise, right upper quadrant pain [1, 2].

Based on the definition of ALF, the diagnosis work up must encompass all three criteria:

- Elevated aminotransferases level
- Hepatic encephalopathy (HE)
- Coagulopathy (prolonged INR $\geq$ 1.5 or increased PT (prothrombin time)).

Besides, the establishing of ALF diagnosis has to go through careful medical history, physical examination, laboratory evaluation, imaging studies, and liver biopsy if is necessary.

Notably, it is the early identification of the ALF etiology, because prognosis and specific treatment of ALF are dependent of its etiology, and also for the early identification of those patients who may benefit from urgent liver transplantation. When the main pathogenetic mechanism is cell necrosis or liver necrosis, patients have extremely increased serum transaminases (aminotransferases) [23]. If the liver injury is steady, patients have lower serum hepatic transaminases but severe hyperbilirubinemia [23].

Without a doubt, **medical history** can bring essential information from patient and/or from patient's family (if severe encephalopathy is present) regarding the etiology of ALF, such as medication use (including herbal and dietary supplements, illicit drugs), alcohol abuse, risks factor for acute viral hepatitis (travel in endemic areas, transfusions, unprotected sexual contacts, occupation, body piercing), toxin exposure (mushrooms, organic solvents, phosphorus), suicidal intentions or depression, pregnancy, hepatic ischemia, malignancy, and family history of liver disease.

Physical examination of a patient with ALF must be complete and aims to identify the possible cause of ALF, and further the complications of ALF and/or the impact of ALF on other organs or systems (cerebral edema, renal failure, ARDS, and infections). It appears that the jaundice, a common sign in patients with ALF, is not always seen at presentation in paracetamol toxicity or in herpes simplex virus infection. Right upper quadrant palpation and percussion can identify hepatomegaly (in viral hepatitis, in malignant infiltration, congestive heart failure, or acute Budd-Chiari syndrome). Conversely, small liver indicates a significant loss of volume due to hepatic necrosis. The presence of ascites, especially if it develops rapidly and is accompanied by pain, suggests the possibility of hepatic vein thrombosis (Budd-Chiari syndrome).

A very important part of the physical examination is the neurologic examination in order to identify and estimate the severity of HE, and also for early identification of intracranial hypertension (ICH) or cerebral edema signs. If in patients with grade I or II HE cerebral edema is uncommon, it is present in 25–35% in those with grade III HE, and in 75% with grade IV HE [24].

Clinical signs and symptoms suggestive for intracranial hypertension caused by brain edema are reactivity of pupils, systolic hypertension, bradycardia, respiratory depression/apnea, seizure, increased muscles tension or tonus (opisthotonus or opisthotonos, decerebrate posturing). However, intracranial hypertension may increase rapidly before the onset of any clinical sign and may further result in brain death before any treatment can be initiated [24].

32.6.1 Laboratory Evaluation

Obligatory tests for ALF patients:

- Prothrombin time or INR > 1.5 is part of the ALF definition. Coagulation parameters should be monitoring 3–4 times/day but is not helpful to estimate the patient's risk for bleeding.
- Liver blood tests
  - AST and/or ALT—usual markedly elevated (very high levels >3500 IU/L in acetaminophen overdose, ischemic liver injury; high levels 1000–2000 IU/L in hepatitis B, Herpes simplex virus hepatitis, and Wilson disease). These parameters should be monitored daily.
  - Bilirubin conjugated/unconjugated level should be monitored daily—usually it is elevated. The decrease of prothrombin time/INR and bilirubin levels is seen in recovering patients, but they are raising in patients with poor prognosis.
  - Alkaline phosphatase
  - GGT
- Complete blood cell (CBC)—monitored 3–4 times/day
  - Thrombocytopenia <150,000 per mmc
  - Anemia
  - Leukocytosis or leukopenia (in Herpes simplex virus hepatitis)
- Serum chemistries—metabolic panels should be monitored more than once/day
  - Glucose—possible very low
  - Creatinine, blood urea nitrogen—possible elevated
  - Ammonia (arterial)—probably elevated
  - Serum electrolytes—sodium, potassium, chloride, bicarbonate, calcium, magnesium, phosphate
  - LDH—elevated
  - Albumin
  - Amylase, lipase
- Toxicology screening—Acetaminophen level in blood, or urine toxicology
- Viral hepatitis serology—anti-HAVA IgM, anti-HBV IgM, hepatitis B surface antigen, anti-HCV virus antibodies, anti-herpes simplex/varicella zoster virus antibodies IgM, anti-HEV IgM, serologic testing for HIV
- Autoimmune markers
- Arterial blood gas analysis—metabolic acidosis, high lactate level
- For pregnant women—AST and/or ALT (<1000 UI/L), bilirubin level, low platelet count, urinalysis (proteinuria)
- For Wilson disease—AST/ALT (>2), Alkaline phosphatase/total bilirubin (<4), ceruloplasmin level (low <5 mg/dL), serum cooper (elevated >200 μg/dL), test Coombs (negative), anemia
- Infections surveillance—cultures for respiratory tract, blood, urine

32.6.2 Imaging Study

- Abdominal CT scan—for liver dimensions, density, spleen dimensions, evidence of hepatocellular carcinoma or intrahepatic metastases, hepatic vein occlusion
- Abdominal ultrasound—same information as CT scan but it is more available, no risk, noninvasive, and cheaper; with Doppler—establish the presence of flow in the hepatic veins, hepatic artery, and the portal vein.
- Cerebral CT scan/MRI—cerebral edema, hemorrhage

Liver biopsy is indicated when medical past history, laboratory evaluation or imaging studies failed to identify the etiology of ALF, or patient needs liver transplantation. If coagulopathy is present, percutaneous biopsy is contraindicated, although transjugular liver biopsy is a choice. Nonetheless, the results of liver biopsy can bring useful information in malignant infiltration, autoimmune hepatitis, lymphoma, herpes simplex hepatitis (viral inclusions), and Wilson disease [1].

32.7 Treatment

32.7.1 General Principles and Organ Specific Management

ALF is a highly unpredictable disease, which can evolve to a life-threatening situation within few hours. The main part of ALF patients should be managed in ICU, and moreover, or in centers specialized on liver transplantation. If a patient with ALF is admitted in a hospital without liver transplantation, this patient must to be transferred in a liver transplantation center as soon as possible [1], before the progression of coagulopathy or HE, and the onset of increased intracranial pressure. Briefly, it is recommended to take in consideration the transfer of the patient to a liver transplantation center or tertiary intensive care unit in case of evolution into grade II HE, INR > 1.5 and the onset of hypoglycemia.

Cardiovascular management. Hemodynamic disturbances in ALF patients are caused by low systemic vascular resistance and intravascular volume depletion by extravasation of fluid in extravascular space. So that, there is positive response to appropriate volume loading. Hypotensive ALF patients should be initially resuscitated with crystalloids, or sometimes normal saline fluids [1]. A keynote factor it is to avoid hyperchloraemia because of its severe side effects [1]. Later, volume loading may be done by the association of crystalloid fluids with Ringers lactate or balanced solution. Dextrose solution should be added in patients with hypoglycemia. Albumin is not indicated, because its role in ALF has not been investigated [1]. When fluids are administrated it is important to avoid excessive volume loading because it may worsen cerebral edema [24] and prognosis.

When fluid resuscitation is not efficient, vasopressor support is required in order to maintain the mean arterial pressure of 60–75 mmHg and the cerebral perfusion pressure of 50–60 mmHg. The first drug of choice is norepinephrine with a dose starting of 0.05 μg/kg/min IV. Vasopressin in low dose of 1–2 U/h, is the second choice, for patients who do not respond adequately to norepinephrine, but it has been suggested to be detrimental with cerebral complications [25].

Respiratory management. In case of encephalopathy progression, hypoxia or respiratory failure, the patients with ALF may require invasive or noninvasive ventilatory support. Ventilation settings and parameters should be protective such as low tidal volume 6–8 mL/kg (ideal body weight) and PEEP to maintain an open lung with low tidal volume [26]. The main outcome is to avoid hypo- or hypercapnia. Obviously, adequate airway care, physiotherapy and periodic infections surveillance assure good prognosis.

Metabolic and nutritional management. Nutritional support is essential for the treatment of ALF patients, because they have increased resting energy expenditure. Oral or enteral nutrition is preferred whenever is possible, in order to counteract the loss of muscle mass, gastrointestinal hemorrhage and gut microbiome translocation, together with the monitoring of serum ammonia. If enteral nutrition is not possible or enough, parenteral nutrition is an option. Proton pump inhibitors should be used only for the period of parenteral nutrition, taking into account the possible risk of ventilator associated pneumonia and *Clostridium difficile* infection.

Hypoglycemia is a particular risk for ALF patients, especially when ALF is caused by paracetamol (acetaminophen) overdose, and it is associated with increased mortality. Nevertheless, the symptoms of hypoglycemia may be confused or overlapped with those of HE. Consequently, frequent monitoring of blood glucose level (at 2 h) is mandatory. Correction of hypoglycemia with concentrated glucose/dextrose bolus therapy or boluses may sometimes be necessary but can cause hyperglycemia that exacerbates an elevated intracranial pressure.

Renal management. Acute kidney injury (AKI) is a complication of ALF in 30–50% of cases, and it is associated with increased hospitalization and mortality. Risk factors for developing AKI in ALF patients are paracetamol induced ALF, prolonged hypotension, preexisting kidney disease, increased age, systemic inflammatory response syndrome (SIRS) and infection [27]. Measures to avoid the appearance of AKI are prompt treatment of hypotension, infections, and avoiding nephrotoxic drugs (including radiological contrast agents). If acute renal failure develops, renal replacement therapy must be set up early preferably by using venovenous hemofiltration technique. In ALF patients with AKI, the main indications for renal replacement therapy are hyperammonemia, acidosis, hyponatremia and others metabolic disturbances, fluid balance and temperature control [28].

Infection surveillance and management. Patients with ALF are at high risk for developing infections (viral, bacterial or fungal), sepsis and septic shock. The main sites of infections are respiratory tract (pneumonia), urinary tract and blood stream. The most frequently involved microorganisms are Gram-negative enteric bacilli, Gram-positive cocci, fungal organisms and sometimes reactivation of a preexisting infection with CMV. Clinical diagnosis is difficult because the signs and symptoms of infections may be absent, and the only indirect sign is worsening of HE or renal dysfunction. Routine and frequent microbiological surveillance (sputum, urine, blood) is the safest way to detect and treat on time ALF associated with infections. Prophylactic antibiotics can reduce the incidence of infections, but studies have shown no benefit on survival [29]. Antibiotics should be given only in case of infection signs, positive culture results, clinical deterioration of HE, or for patients waiting emergency liver transplantation [1].

32.7.2 Treatment for Specific Etiology of ALF

It has to be noted that advanced liver injury or damage with ALF may not benefit from specific therapies [23].

Acetaminophen overdose. Paracetamol or acetaminophen overdose has characteristically at presentation AST > 10,000 IU/L and at least twice the value of ALT, and normal bilirubin [1]. N-acetylcysteine (NAC) is the specific antidote for acetaminophen or paracetamol overdose. However, NAC should be prescribed for ALF of unknown etiology, because it has benefits regarding cerebral edema, hemodynamic, oxygen delivery, consumption, and prognosis. If NAC is given during first 8 h after acetaminophen overdose, it decreases dramatically the hepatotoxicity and death. The dose of NAC for ALF patients is 150 mg/kg/1 h, followed by 12.5 mg/kg/h for 4 h and 6.25 mg/kg/h for the next 67 h. However, it is advisable to exclude NAC in case of "advanced coma" [23].

Viral hepatitis. In case of ALF secondary to hepatitis virus B infection, antiviral therapy with nucleoside/nucleotide analogues such as LAM, adefovir (ADV), entecavir may be useful. They also need to be administered in patient with indication for liver transplantation in order to prevent post-transplantation recurrence.

Patients with herpes simplex virus infections and hepatitis should receive Acyclovir (5–10 mg/kg every 8 h) for at least 7 days.

Mushroom poisoning. ALF secondary to *Amanita phalloides* poisoning benefits from early administration of activated charcoal that binds the amatoxin. It is highly recommended.

Autoimmune hepatitis. Also, autoimmune hepatitis may benefit from corticosteroids. They reduce the need for liver transplantation.

Budd-Chiari syndrome. Patients can benefit from anticoagulant therapy, thrombolytic therapy, interventional radiology (TIPS—transjugular intrahepatic portosystemic shunt placement), and surgical decompression, all in order to restore hepatic venous drainage.

Wilson disease. These patients benefit from plasma exchange for copper removal until liver transplantation is an available option.

Acute fatty liver of pregnancy. The main treatment is emergency delivery, after mother stabilization.

32.7.3 Specific Treatment of ALF

Management of ALF patients is primarily tackling the main manifestations that defines ALF such as coagulopathy, HE, and cerebral edema.

Treatment of coagulopathy. Severe coagulopathy in ALF is caused by the inadequate liver production of coagulation factors—II, V, VII, IX and X, often doubled by the fall of platelet number less than 100,000 per mmc. Prophylactic administration of fresh frozen plasma is not recommended, because published data has not shown to decrease mortality, and further can interfere with the tests for liver assessment function and may lead to fluid overloading. Exception is made in case of a planned invasive procedure or in the presence of profound coagulopathy (INR > 7). Platelet administration is recommended when platelet count is below 10,000 per mmc, or before an invasive procedure when platelet count is <50,000 per mmc.

Hepatic encephalopathy. The treatment of HE is focused on the decreasing ammonia production by gut microbiota and the avoiding of aggravating factors of HE such as infections, gastrointestinal bleeding, constipation, and sedatives. One option treatment is Lactulose (nonabsorbable disaccharide) but it has controversial efficacy in ALF, and it is associated with bowel distention, dehydration secondary to diarrhea, and hypernatremia. Usually it is oral administered, and a better option is lactulose enema. Other alternatives are Metronidazole—but may be neurotoxic in ALF, Neomycin—should be avoided because is nephrotoxic, Rifaximin—used often for HE in patients with chronic liver disease.

Cerebral edema. It is a finding of 25–35% patients with grade III HE, and of 75% of patients with grade IV HE. Cerebral edema followed by elevated ICP, brain ischemia and finally by brainstem herniation is the most common cause of death in patients with ALF. Liver transplantation is the only choice treatment for cerebral edema, and the rest of measures reduces cerebral edema and elevated ICP being only supportive until transplantation. An ICP > 30 mmHg and an arterial ammonia >200 μg/dL are predictive for brain herniation and death.

Intracranial pressure monitoring. It is an indication for patient with grade III/IV HE—in order to diagnose elevated ICP and guiding the treatment. Even if the monitoring of ICP can be done using epidural, subdural, parenchymal or intraventricular catheters, in the case of patients with ALF are preferred the use of epidural/subdural catheters because they are less invasive, with lower risk for hemorrhagic complications and infections. Prior to catheter placement, a CT scan of brain should be done, and coagulopathy must be corrected. ICP should be maintained <20 mmHg.

Transcranial Doppler ultrasound is a noninvasive investigation that can be used to estimate the ICP, as an alternative to invasive monitoring.

32.7.3.1 Measures to Prevent ICP Elevation

- Treatment of elevated ICP aims to maintain the ICP less than 20–25 mmHg, and the cerebral perfusion pressure above 50–60 mmHg.
- Minimizing patient agitation or stimulation—placing patient in quiet rooms, reduction of sensorial stimulation, nasogastric tube placement only in intubated and sedated patient with gentle and rare endotracheal suctions.
- Patient head elevation at 30° improves jugular venous outflow.
- Avoid volume overloading.
- Administration of hypertonic saline to induce hypernatremia with maintaining of serum sodium level between 145 and 155 mEq/L will decrease water influx into brain and reduce cerebral edema.
- Hyperosmotic agents can reduce brain edema, but only temporary. A bolus of Mannitol 0.5–1 g/kgc administrated IV, repeated once or twice can correct episodes of ICP elevation and improves survival [24], with the condition to maintain serum osmolality less than 320 mOsm/L.
- Hyperventilation is a method to reduce elevated ICP, but with limited efficacy over time (after 48 h). Every mmHg reduction of $PaCO_2$, reduces the cerebral blood flow by 2–3% and restore autoregulation. Moderate hyperventilation, with a $PaCO_2$ between 25 and 30 mmHg is indicated in patients with severe elevated ICP and at risk of brain herniation.
- Induced coma with barbiturates (pentobarbital, thiopental) or propofol, in order to reduce cerebral metabolic rate and cerebral blood flow in refractory patients.
- Glucocorticoids are not indicated and should not be used, because studies have not shown to be beneficial in ALF patients.

32.7.4 Experimental Therapies

- Induction of moderate hypothermia with core temperature 34–35 °C by cooling blankets, has been shown to reduce ICP and improves cerebral perfusion pressure but with the risk of cardiac depression or arrhythmias, shivering, infection, and bleeding.
- Indometacin (indomethacin) in bolus of 0.5 mg/kg can be considered in patients with elevated ICP refractory to standard treatment [30].

32.7.5 Artificial Liver Support Devices

The aim of **extracorporeal systems** use is to be a "bridging therapy" until liver transplantation.

- Extracorporeal albumin dialysis. Extracorporeal systems that uses albumin as a scavenging molecule are MARS (Molecular Adsorbent Recirculation System) and SPAD (Single-Pass Albumin Dialysis) [31]. Prometheus (Fractionated Plasma Separation and Adsorption) is another form of albumin dialysis [31]. Bleeding is a significant problem for MARS [31]. Even if, MARS is the most studied albumin dialysis technology in ALF, further randomized studies are needed [31]. Overall, extracorporeal liver support systems seem to increase survival in ALF [32] but further studies are a requisite.
- **BAL (Bioartificial liver) system** is a bioreactor with liver cells which temporarily replaces the hepatic functions. BAL systems are a temporary option in therapy of ALF or the treatment of acute-on-chronic liver failure [33, 34]. They also can assure for short term the endogenous regeneration of the native liver [33].
- **Plasma exchange** has been shown to improve survival in patients with ALF, and to modulate immune dysfunction, if used on timely (first 3 days after ICU admission) [1].

32.7.6 Liver Transplantation

Orthotopic liver transplantation is the only therapeutic choice in end-stage liver disorders such as cirrhosis, chronic hepatitis, ALF, chronic hepatic failure or metabolic diseases [35]. Contraindications for liver transplantation are malignancy, irreversible brain damage, uncontrolled infection, and severe pancreatitis [1].

32.8 Prognosis

One important step in the management of ALF patients is the early selection of patients who recover spontaneously, or of those who benefit from liver transplantation, and of those who do not benefit from liver transplantation [1]. For this reason, several criteria for emergency liver transplantation have been developed. Newly, it seems that the combination of hypoglycemia, coagulopathy, and lactic acidosis predicts better death or liver transplant in comparison with the King's College criteria [36].

King's College Criteria for transplant is the most widely model used for ALF selection that benefit from liver transplantation Table 32.3 [1, 2].

Model for End-stage liver disease (MELD) score is a scoring system also used to predict survival among ALF patients based on the laboratory values of serum bilirubin, creatinine and the INR. MELD score >32 are predictive for high mortality.

Table 32.3 King's College Criteria adapted from [2] with permission

Acetaminophen overdose	Nonacetaminophen overdose
Arterial pH < 7.30 *or* **all of the following**:	Prothrombin time > 100 s (INR > 6.5) *or* **any three of the following**:
• Prothrombin time > 100 s (INR > 6.5)	• Non-A, non-B hepatitis; idiosyncratic drug reaction; halothane etiology
• Creatinine level >3.4 mg/dL (>300 μmol/L)	• Time from jaundice to encephalopathy >7 days
• Grade 3/4 encephalopathy	• Age <10 years or >40 years
	• Prothrombin time >50 s (INR > 3.5)
	• Serum bilirubin level >17.4 mg/dL (300 μmol/L)

32.9 Conclusions

ALF is a life-threatening illness, with multiorgan damaging associated with numerous complications, and very poor prognosis, being caused by various etiologies. Despite the numerous advances on pathophysiology, intensive care treatment, and transplantation techniques from the last decades, is still characterized by increased mortality.

Early recognition of ALF, establishment of the etiology and relocation to a liver transplantation center, or tertiary intensive care specialized in ALF are primordial measures in treating ALF patients.

Equally important is the identification of patients with great probability of spontaneous recovery but also of patients who may benefit from emergency liver transplantation.

Liver transplantation is the only one proven liver replacement therapy that reduces mortality. One year survival rates following emergency liver transplantation are >80% [1].

Self Study

Questions

1. **Which statement is true?**
   (a) Cirrhosis with Budd-Chiari syndrome is considered ALF when diagnosed within 26 weeks
   (b) Paracetamol hepatotoxicity is characterized by extreme high level of serum aminotransferase (AST/ALT) > 10,000 IU/L.
   (c) Ecstasy induced liver injury presents with no hyperthermia
   (d) Drug-induced liver injury (DILI) is a leading cause for emergency liver transplantation
2. **Which statement/statements is/are true?**
   (a) Drug induced liver injury may occur after any type of medication
   (b) HELLP syndrome defined by haemolysis, elevated liver enzyme levels
   (c) N-acetylcysteine (NAC) is the specific antidote for acetaminophen or paracetamol overdose
   (d) Extracorporeal systems that uses albumin as a scavenging molecule are MARS (Molecular Adsorbent Recirculation System) and SPAD (Single-Pass Albumin Dialysis)

Answers

1. **Which statement is true?**
   (a) Correct.
   (b) Correct.
   (c) Ecstasy induced liver injury presents as an "heat shock related liver injury" with severe hyperthermia, multiple organ dysfunction, profound coagulopathy, and severe rhabdomyolysis.
   (d) Correct.
2. **Which statement/statements is/are true?**
   (a) Correct
   (b) Correct
   (c) Correct
   (d) Correct

References

1. European Association for the Study of the Liver. EASL clinical practical guidelines on the management of acute (fulminant) liver failure. J Hepatol. 2017;66(5):1047–81. https://doi.org/10.1016/j.jhep.2016.12.003.
2. Fix OK. Acute liver failure: peritransplant management and outcomes. Clin Liver Dis. 2013;2:165–8. https://doi.org/10.1002/cld.219.
3. Tandon BN, Bernauau J, O'Grady J, Gupta SD, Krisch RE, Liaw YF, Okuda K, Acharya SK. Recommendations of the International Association for the Study of the Liver Subcommittee on nomenclature of acute and subacute liver failure. J Gastroenterol Hepatol. 1999;14(5):403–4.
4. Alempijevic T, Zec S, Milosavljevic T. Drug-induced liver injury: do we know everything? World J Hepatol. 2017;9(10):491–502. https://doi.org/10.4254/wjh.v9.i10.491.
5. Chalasani N, Fontana RJ, Bonkovsky HL, Watkins PB, Davern T, Serrano J, Yang H, Rochon J, Drug Induced Liver Injury Network (DILIN). Causes, clinical features, and outcomes from a prospective study of drug-induced liver injury in the United States. Gastroenterology. 2008;135(6):1924–34., 1934.e1–4. https://doi.org/10.1053/j.gastro.2008.09.011.
6. Lange-Brock N, Berg T, Müller AR, Fliege H, Neuhaus P, Wiedenmann B, Klapp BF, Mönnikes H. Acute liver failure fol-

lowing the use of ecstasy (MDMA). Z Gastroenterol. 2002;40(8):581–6. [Article in German]
7. Kumar S, Ratho RK, Chawla YK, Chakraborti A. The incidence of sporadic viral hepatitis in North India: a preliminary study. Hepatobiliary Pancreat Dis Int. 2007;6(6):596–9.
8. Torres HA, Davila M. Reactivation of hepatitis B virus and hepatitis C virus in patients with cancer. Nat Rev Clin Oncol. 2012;9(3):156–66. https://doi.org/10.1038/nrclinonc.2012.1.
9. Khuroo MS, Kamili S. Aetiology and prognostic factors in acute liver failure in India. J Viral Hepat. 2003;10(3):224–31.
10. Acharya SK, Dasarathy S, Kumer TL, et al. Fulminant hepatitis in a tropical population: clinical course, cause, and early predictors of outcome. Hepatology. 1996;23(6):1448–55.
11. Dalton HR, Bendall R, Ijaz S, Banks M. Hepatitis E: an emerging infection in developed countries. Lancet Infect Dis. 2008;8(11):698–709. https://doi.org/10.1016/S1473-3099(08)70255-X.
12. Peters DJ, Greene WH, Ruggiero F, McGarrity TJ. Herpes simplex-induced fulminant hepatitis in adults: a call for empiric therapy. Dig Dis Sci. 2000;45(12):2399–404.
13. Korman JD, Volenberg I, Balko J, Webster J, Schiodt FV, Squires RH Jr, Fontana RJ, Lee WM, Schilsky ML, Pediatric and Adult Acute Liver Failure Study Groups. Screening for Wilson disease in acute liver failure: a comparison of currently available diagnostic tests. Hepatology. 2008;48(4):1167–74. https://doi.org/10.1002/hep.22446.
14. Nelson DB, Yost NP, Cunningham FG. Acute fatty liver of pregnancy: clinical outcomes and expected duration of recovery. Am J Obstet Gynecol. 2013;209(5):456.e1–7. https://doi.org/10.1016/j.ajog.2013.07.006.
15. Westbrook RH, Dusheiko G, Williamson C. Pregnancy and liver disease. J Hepatol. 2016;64(4):933–45. https://doi.org/10.1016/j.jhep.2015.11.030.
16. Remiszewski P, Pawlak J, Skwarek A, et al. Orthotopic liver transplantation for acute liver failure resulting from “acute fatty liver of pregnancy”. Ann Transplant. 2003;8(3):8–11.
17. Fuhrmann V, Jäger B, Zubkova A, Drolz A. Hypoxic hepatitis – epidemiology, pathophysiology and clinical management. Wien Klin Wochenschr. 2010;122(5-6):129–39. https://doi.org/10.1007/s00508-010-1357-6.
18. Waseem N, Chen PH. Hypoxic hepatitis: a review and clinical update. J Clin Transl Hepatol. 2016;4(3):263–8. https://doi.org/10.14218/JCTH.2016.00022.
19. Polson J, Lee WM, American Association for the Study of Liver Disease. AASLD position paper: the management of acute liver failure. Hepatology. 2005;41(5):1179–97. https://doi.org/10.1002/hep.20703.
20. Hawton K, Bergen H, Simkin S, Dodd S, Pocock P, Bernal W, Gunnell D, Kapur N. Long term effect of reduced pack sizes of paracetamol on poisoning deaths and liver transplant activity in England and Wales: interrupted time series analyses. BMJ. 2013;346:f403. https://doi.org/10.1136/bmj.f403.
21. Pyleris E, Giannikopoulos G, Dabos K. Pathophysiology and management of acute liver failure. Ann Gastroenterol. 2010;23(4):257–65.
22. Vilstrup H, Amodio P, Bajaj J, Cordoba J, Ferenci P, Mullen KD, Weissenborn K, Wong P. Hepatic encephalopathy in chronic liver disease: 2014 practice guideline by the American Association for the Study of Liver Diseases and the European Association for the Study of the Liver. Hepatology. 2014;60(2):715–35. https://doi.org/10.1002/hep.27210.
23. Bernal W, Lee WM, Wendon J, Larsen FS, Williams R. Acute liver failure: a curable disease by 2024? J Hepatol. 2015;62(1 Suppl):S112–20. https://doi.org/10.1016/j.jhep.2014.12.016.
24. Eric G, Chopra S. Acute liver failure in adults: management and prognosis uptodate. Waltham, MA: UpToDate Inc. http://www.uptodate.com. Accessed 2 Aug 2018.
25. Shawcross DL, Davies NA, Mookerjee RP, Hayes PC, Williams R, Lee A, Jalan R. Worsening of cerebral hyperemia by the administration of terlipressin in acute liver failure with severe encephalopathy. Hepatology. 2004;39(2):471–5.
26. Futier E, Constantin JM, Paugam-Burtz C, Pascal J, Eurin M, Neuschwander A, Marret E, Beaussier M, Gutton C, Lefrant JY, Allaouchiche B, Verzilli D, Leone M, De Jong A, Bazin JE, Pereira B, Jaber S, IMPROVE Study Group. A trial of intraoperative low-tidal-volume ventilation in abdominal surgery. N Engl J Med. 2013;369(5):428–37. https://doi.org/10.1056/NEJMoa1301082.
27. Leithead JA, Ferguson JW, Bates CM, Davidson JS, Lee A, Bathgate AJ, Hayes PC, Simpson KJ. The systemic inflammatory response syndrome is predictive of renal dysfunction in patients with non-paracetamol-induced acute liver failure. Gut. 2009;58(3):443–9. https://doi.org/10.1136/gut.2008.154120.
28. Slack AJ, Auzinger G, Willars C, Dew T, Musto R, Corsilli D, Sherwood R, Wendon JA, Bernal W. Ammonia clearance with haemofiltration in adults with liver disease. Liver Int. 2014;34(1):42–8. https://doi.org/10.1111/liv.12221.
29. Karvellas CJ, Cavazos J, Battenhouse H, Durkalski V, Balko J, Sanders C, Lee WM, US Acute Liver Failure Study Group. Effects of antimicrobial prophylaxis and blood stream infections in patients with acute liver failure: a retrospective cohort study. Clin Gastroenterol Hepatol. 2014;12(11):1942–9.1e. https://doi.org/10.1016/j.cgh.2014.03.011.
30. Tofteng F, Larsen FS. The effect of indomethacin on intracranial pressure, cerebral perfusion and extracellular lactate and glutamate concentrations in patients with fulminant hepatic failure. J Cereb Blood Flow Metab. 2004;24(7):798–804.
31. Karvellas CJ, Gibney N, Kutsogiannis D, Wendon J, Bain VG. Bench-to-bedside review: current evidence for extracorporeal albumin dialysis systems in liver failure. Crit Care. 2007;11(3):215.
32. Stutchfield BM, Simpson K, Wigmore SJ. Systematic review and meta-analysis of survival following extracorporeal liver support. Br J Surg. 2011;98(5):623–31. https://doi.org/10.1002/bjs.7418.
33. Nicolas CT, Hickey RD, Chen HS, Mao SA, Lopera Higuita M, Wang Y, Nyberg SL. Concise review: liver regenerative medicine: from hepatocyte transplantation to bioartificial livers and bioengineered grafts. Stem Cells. 2017;35(1):42–50. https://doi.org/10.1002/stem.2500.
34. Lee CW, Chen YF, Wu HH, Lee OK. Historical perspectives and advances in mesenchymal stem cell research for the treatment of liver diseases. Gastroenterology. 2018;154(1):46–56. https://doi.org/10.1053/j.gastro.2017.09.049.
35. Hansel MC, Davila JC, Vosough M, Gramignoli R, Skvorak KJ, Dorko K, Marongiu F, Blake W, Strom SC. The use of induced pluripotent stem cells for the study and treatment of liver diseases. Curr Protoc Toxicol. 2016;67:14.13.1–14.13.27. https://doi.org/10.1002/0471140856.tx1413s67.
36. Levine M, Stellpflug SJ, Pizon AF, Peak DA, Villano J, Wiegand T, Dib C, Thomas SH. Hypoglycemia and lactic acidosis outperform King’s College criteria for predicting death or transplant in acetaminophen toxic patients. Clin Toxicol (Phila). 2018;56(7):622–5. https://doi.org/10.1080/15563650.2017.1420193.

Chronic Liver Failure and Acute-on-Chronic Liver Failure

33

Rita Garcia-Martinez, Raquel Diaz-Ruiz, Jesus Millan, and Rafael Bañares

Abbreviations

ACLF	Acute-on-chronic liver failure
AKI	Acute kidney injury
BCLC	Barcelona clinic liver cancer
BT	Bacterial translocation
cACLD	Compensated advanced chronic liver disease
CLF	Chronic liver failure
CRP	C-reactive protein
Crs	Serum creatinine
DAMP	Damage-associated molecular pattern
DM	Diabetes mellitus
GA	Glutaminase
GS	Glutamine synthetase
HCC	Hepatocellular carcinoma
HE	Hepatic encephalopathy
HPS	Hepatopulmonary syndrome
HRS	Hepatorenal syndrome
LT	Liver transplantation
LVP	Large volume paracentesis
MELD	Model for end-stage liver disease
NAFLD	Non-alcoholic fatty liver disease
NSAIDs	Nonsteroidal anti-inflammatory drugs
NSBB	Non-selective beta blockers
PAMP	Pathogen-associated molecular pattern
PH	Portal hypertension
PPHT	Portopulmonary hypertension
PSS	Portosystemic shunts
SBP	Spontaneous bacterial peritonitis
TIPS	Transjugular intrahepatic portosystemic shunt

Key Concepts

- Cirrhosis and CLF are the consequences of chronic and progressive liver injury. Etiological treatment may halt and reduce liver damage, particularly in early stages of the disease, so cirrhosis is considered potentially reversible.
- Clinical stages of cirrhosis are based on different outcomes and have prognostic value. The progression of the disease parallels liver damage, inflammatory features and hemodynamic alterations, although this progression is not predictable.
- Progressive chronic liver failure driven by hemodynamic and inflammatory alterations may impact on

R. Garcia-Martinez (✉)
Servicio de Medicina Interna, Hospital General Universitario Gregorio Marañón, Madrid, Spain

Instituto de Investigación Sanitaria Gregorio Marañón, Madrid, Spain

Centro de Investigación Biomédica en Red de Enfermedades Hepáticas y Digestivas (CIBERehd), Madrid, Spain

Facultad de Medicina, Universidad San Pablo CEU, Madrid, Spain

R. Diaz-Ruiz
Servicio de Aparato Digestivo, Hospital General Universitario Gregorio Marañón, Madrid, Spain

Facultad de Medicina, Universidad Complutense Madrid, Madrid, Spain

J. Millan
Servicio de Medicina Interna, Hospital General Universitario Gregorio Marañón, Madrid, Spain

Facultad de Medicina, Universidad Complutense Madrid, Madrid, Spain
e-mail: jesus.millan@salud.madrid.org

R. Bañares
Instituto de Investigación Sanitaria Gregorio Marañón, Madrid, Spain

Centro de Investigación Biomédica en Red de Enfermedades Hepáticas y Digestivas (CIBERehd), Madrid, Spain

Servicio de Aparato Digestivo, Hospital General Universitario Gregorio Marañón, Madrid, Spain

Facultad de Medicina, Universidad Complutense Madrid, Madrid, Spain

F. Radu-Ionita et al. (eds.), *Liver Diseases*, https://doi.org/10.1007/978-3-030-24432-3_33

the performance of different organs, leading to clinical decompensation and dysfunction of multiple organs and systems. So, chronic liver failure is considered a multisystem disease.

- Management of chronic liver failure aims to treat primary liver disease, screening, prevent and controlling complications, and consider LT in patients with advanced stages.
- ACLF is an acute decompensation characterized by organ failure and high short-term mortality. It is a very dynamic syndrome, which may improve/resolve in up to 50% of cases. So, prognosis is highly dependent on the early clinical course during hospitalization among other factors.

33.1 Introduction

Chronic liver failure is the result of chronic liver inflammation of any cause including viral hepatitis, alcoholic liver disease, autoimmune liver disease, non-alcoholic fatty liver disease (NAFLD) or genetic conditions, leading to parenchymal necrosis, fibrogenesis, angiogenesis and profound vascular changes. Regardless of the aetiology, chronic liver failure is characterized by the progressive reduction in liver functions such as, synthesis of essential serum proteins (albumin, coagulation factors, hormonal and growth factors, …), metabolism of many endogen and exogenous compounds (bilirubin, ammonia, drugs, …), and leading to intrahepatic vascular resistance (secondary to both mechanical obstacle and vasoconstriction) [1, 2].

Liver cirrhosis is defined histopathologically as an advanced state of liver fibrosis with prominent architectural distortion and formation of regenerative nodules. Cirrhosis evolves from a compensated (no or minor symptoms) to a decompensated state characterized by the development of typical complications such as gastrointestinal bleeding secondary to portal hypertension (PH), ascites, hepatic encephalopathy (HE), jaundice, bacterial infections and multiorgan failure [1, 2]. Severe fibrosis and cirrhosis are often not possible to be distinguished in asymptomatic patients in the era of non-invasive methods to assess liver fibrosis and they are considered as a continuum, so the term "compensated advanced chronic liver disease" (cACLD) has been proposed to better reflect this transition [3]. Since cirrhosis is associated with a large and increasing number of organ and system dysfunctions is, therefore, considered a multisystem disease [4–6]. Cirrhosis is also currently considered potentially reversible since it may return from decompensated to compensated or even precirrhotic phase if the cause of the disease is removed [7–10].

Mechanisms involved in progression and decompensation of cirrhosis include increasing portal pressure, hyperdynamic circulation, dysbiosis of microbiota, bacterial translocation and systemic inflammation.

Clinical manifestations, quality of life and prognosis vary according to the progression of the disease, thus relevant clinical stages have been proposed (Fig. 33.1) [3, 11]. These clinical stages are based on the outcome and have prognostic value, but they do not follow a predictable pathway. Acute-on-chronic liver failure is a recently described syndrome occurring frequently in patients with cirrhosis characterized by acute decompensation, development of organ failure and high short-term mortality [12, 13]. ACLF is among the most common causes of death in patients with cirrhosis together with infections, hepatocellular carcinoma (HCC), renal failure and PH related bleeding.

Herein, pathogenesis and manifestations of CLF and ACLF are reviewed focusing in the multisystem dimension and potential reversibility of the disease.

33.2 Pathogenesis of Chronic Liver Failure

Regardless of the aetiology, several mechanisms are associated with the progression of CLF and risk of decompensation, compromising the outcome of patients with cirrhosis.

33.2.1 Portal Hypertension and Hyperdynamic Circulation

PH is a common and serious complication of CLF considered clinically significant when hepatic venous pressure gradient increases above 10 mmHg. Both, the architectural distortion secondary to liver fibrosis and dysfunction of sinusoidal endothelial cells contribute to the development of PH. Also, hepatic stellate cells contraction has been proposed to be implicated in the syndrome. Other factors such as mesenteric hypervolemia secondary to splanchnic vasodilatation further contributes and aggravates PH.

This scenario results in a series of hemodynamic alterations and clinical complications. In patients with cirrhosis PH is associated with splanchnic vasodilatation, consequently leading to high cardiac output, increased heart rate, and a reduced peripheral vascular resistance culminating in a reduction in mean arterial pressure which in turn, activates compensatory mechanisms associated with arteriolar vasoconstriction of several territories (kidney, muscle, brain, skin, …) [14]. This particular cardiovascular scenario, known as *circulatory dysfunction*, deteriorates with the advance of liver failure leading to a progressive decrease in cardiac output, a reduction in the effective arterial blood volume and a progressive reduction

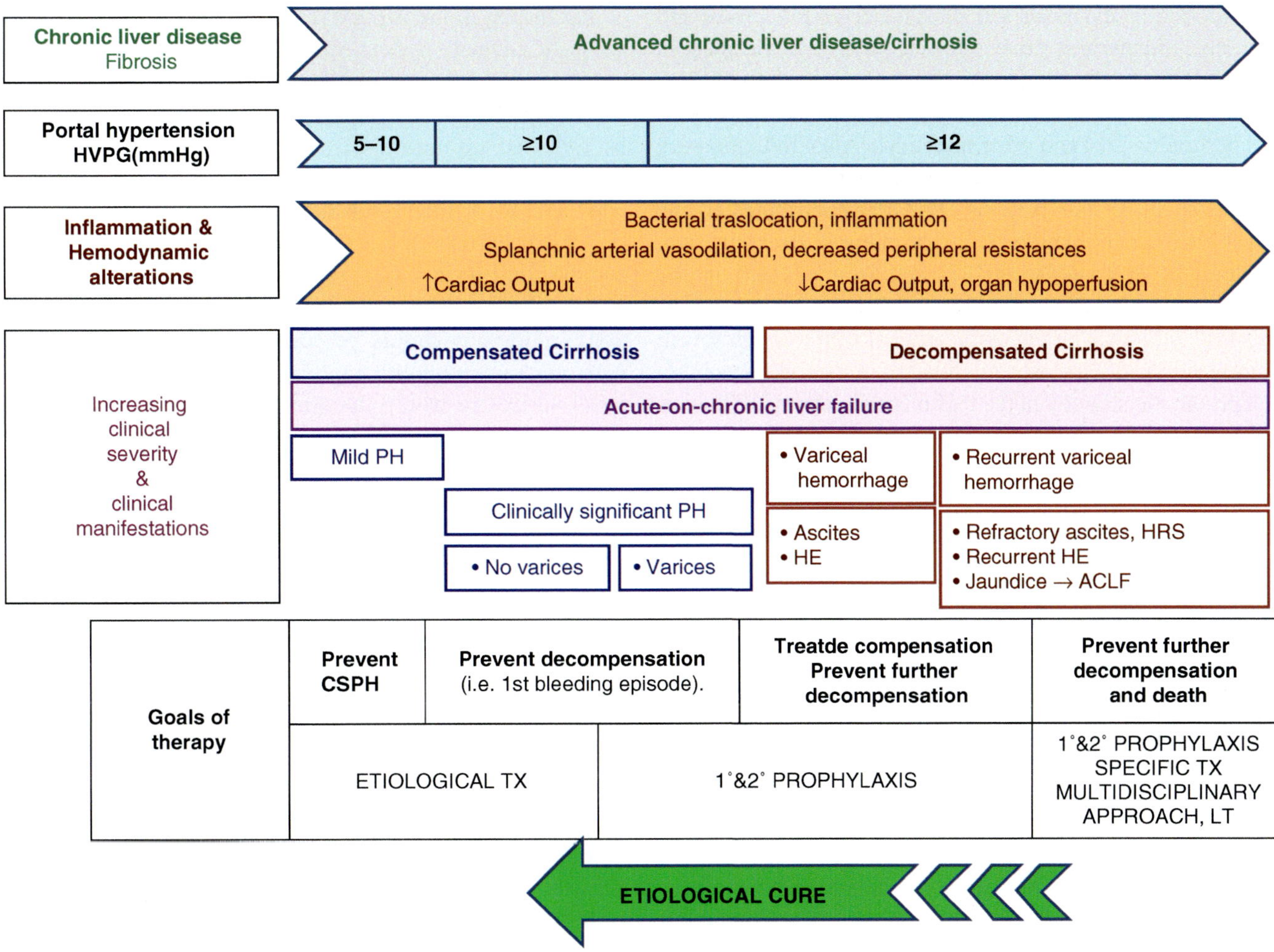

Fig. 33.1 Physiopathology, progressive clinical manifestations and therapeutic goals in cirrhosis (Adapted from D'Amico G with permission [11])

in individual organ perfusion [2, 15]. In fact, liver failure causes high morbidity and its mortality remains disturbingly elevated without LT [16].

33.2.2 Dysbiosis, Bacterial Translocation and Systemic Inflammation

Gut microbiota comprises trillions of microorganisms that reside in our gastrointestinal tract. The latest deep sequencing techniques allowed a better understanding of microbiome (genome of microorganisms of flora) in health and disease.

In CLF, several changes in composition and function of gut microbiota have been described, known as dysbiosis (alteration of the normal equilibrium in gut flora) [17, 18]. So, a shift towards a greater abundance of potentially pathogenic bacteria (*Enterobacteriaceae*, *Bacteroidaceae and Enterococcaceae*) and a decrease in autochthonous bacteria has been observed (i.e. *Lachnospiraceae/ Ruminococcus and Clostridiales*) [19, 20] which correlates with the severity of liver disease.

In fact, cirrhotic patients exhibit several features that increase the risk of dysbiosis including decreased intestinal motility, higher gastric pH, reduced bile acid concentration in colon and alterations in local and systemic immune response. These alterations may favour intestinal bacterial overgrowth [21]. Other factors that may contribute to dysbiosis are diet modifications, use of antibiotics and the exposition to health care system [17]. Indeed, small intestinal bacterial overgrowth in cirrhosis was demonstrated [21, 22].

The passage of viable bacteria but also microbial products (endotoxins, bacterial DNA, …) across the intestinal barrier from the gut lumen to the mesenteric lymph nodes and other extraintestinal organs and sites is known to happen in cirrhosis. Mechanisms involved in this phenomenon, named bacterial translocation (BT), are not well-known; although dysbiosis, increased intestinal permeability and alterations in local host immune system are involved [17, 21].

Importantly, dysbiosis and BT have deleterious local and systemic effects and drive relevant clinical consequences [23]. In fact, dysbiosis and BT are associated with clinical decompensation precipitating HE [24], spontaneous bacterial peritonitis [25] and other infections. Also, inflammatory response secondary to circulating bacterial or pathogen-associated molecular patterns (PAMPs) contributes to the hyperdynamic circulation [26], worsening in liver function, impairment in coagulation [27] and is implicated in the pathogenesis of ACLF, multiorgan failure and death in cirrhosis [13, 28]. Given the implication of dysbiosis on severe complications of cirrhosis, modulation of the gut microbiota is a promising strategy in the treatment of patients with liver diseases [29].

33.3 Clinical Manifestations

Recent advances in the knowledge of the hepatic and extrahepatic alterations observed in CLF led to an increased number of organs and systems affected has and to a better understanding of the organ dysfunctions [5, 13]. Among the reasons for a multisystem involvement of CLF are the multifunctional qualities of the liver: (a) liver is a key organ in the synthesis of essential proteins including coagulation factors, hormonal and growth factors, …; (b) liver has a major role in several metabolic routes (glucose, fatty acids, …) and the metabolism and removal of many endogen and exogenous compounds (bilirubin, ammonia, drugs, …); (c) liver has also a high blood flow supplied from portal vein and hepatic artery which is softly accommodated in healthy conditions; (d) liver has a reticulo-endothelial cell network and plays an important role in the host defence against invading microorganisms [30].

33.3.1 Gastrointestinal Bleeding Secondary to PH

The development of oesophageal varices because of clinically significant PH can be complicated with one of the most feared complications in cirrhosis: variceal bleeding. Varices are present in up to 40% of patients with compensated cirrhosis at the first evaluation and in up to 60% of those with decompensation [31]. If untreated, bleeding occurs in 10–30% within 2 years and it is associated with a 6-weeks mortality of 12–20%. If no effective treatment is provided, bleeding will recur in 2/3 of patients within 2 years. Before effective treatment was routinely available the prognosis was much worst, with a mortality over 40% within the first month [32]. So, screening strategies, primary and secondary prophylaxis and effective haemostatic therapies are fundamental in patients with cirrhosis.

According to the experts' recommendations [3], patients with cACLD with liver stiffness measured by transient elastography <20 kPa and platelets >150,000 have a very low risk of varices and can safely avoid screening endoscopy and be followed up yearly. In any other circumstances, these patients should be screened with esophagogastroduodenoscopy. Follow-up afterwards depends on the presence of varices, the occurrence of active liver disease/etiological cure and the clinical situation. For patients with small varices and ongoing liver injury (active drinker, active hepatitis C infection), endoscopy should be conducted every year. Patients with no varices but with ongoing liver injury and those with small varices in whom the etiological factor was removed and without comorbidities, surveillance endoscopy should be repeated at 2-year intervals. Patients with no varices and etiological factor removed, surveillance endoscopy should be repeated at 3 years.

Importantly, patients with small varices with red wale marks or Child-Pugh C class should be treated with non-selective beta blockers (NSBB). In patients with medium-large varices, either NSBB or endoscopic band ligation (depending on local resources, expertise, comorbidities, …) are recommended.

Etiological therapy may be particularly effective in patients with cACLD without clinically significant PH since the aim of treatment is to prevent the PH to become clinically significant. In patients with significant PH it also has a pivotal role since it may reduce PH and prevent complications [7–10].

In the advent of variceal bleeding, clinical management requires airway maintenance and hemodynamic stabilization with fluids resuscitation plus vasoactive drugs (somatostatin, terlipressin) and further control with endoscopic techniques. Red blood cells transfusion should be done conservatively [33] and antibiotic prophylaxis should be started as soon as possible. Early TIPS (transjugular intrahepatic portosystemic shunt) with polytetrafluoroethylene (PTFE)-covered stent within 72 h must be considered in patients at high risk of treatment failure [34, 35]. PTFE-covered TIPS should also be considered for persistent or severe early rebleeding. Prevention of recurrent variceal bleeding should be based on the combination of NSBB plus endoscopic variceal ligation. Caution should be taken in patients with advanced decompensated cirrhosis (refractory ascites) receiving NSBB since recently has been suggested that NSBB may have deleterious effects on these patients [36, 37]. An individualized use of these drugs is recommended until randomized trials clarify its risk/benefit at this advanced stage of the disease [3, 38].

Acute or chronic gastrointestinal bleeding may also occur as a consequence of hypertensive gastropathy, hypertensive enteropathy, portal colopathy or anorectal varices. NSBB should be the treatment option and TIPS could be considered with uncontrolled bleeding, transfusion dependent [39] after excluding other aetiologies.

33.3.2 Ascites

Ascites, the accumulation of ascitic fluid in the peritoneal cavity is the most common complication of cirrhosis. Up to 60% of compensated patients will develop ascites during the course of the disease and mortality rises up to 50% at 2 years [37, 40, 41]. Clinical evaluation at the presentation should include clinical and physical exam, liver and kidney laboratory test, ultrasound and a diagnostic paracentesis. Ascitic fluid analysis is important in order to exclude other potential aetiologies (heart or renal failure, pancreatic or infectious disease, neoplastic origin) and will also be helpful in the identification of complications such us spontaneous bacterial peritonitis (SBP). So, diagnostic paracentesis is recommended for all patients with new onset ascites, patients with clinical deterioration and those hospitalized for any complication of cirrhosis [42].

Current management of ascites includes moderate sodium intake restriction and diuretics titrated according to the degree of ascites and diuretic response [42]. Anti-mineralocorticoids are the diuretics of choice. Furosemide can be associated in case of low response or limited use of anti-mineralocorticoids because of secondary effects. Diuretics should be adjusted to the lowest effective dose. In the case of refractory ascites (either diuretic-resistant or diuretic intractable because of serious side effects) large volume paracentesis (LVP) plus albumin administration is the first line of treatment [43, 44]. However, LVP doesn't prevent re-accumulation of ascites, and refractory ascites is linked to poor prognosis [45], so these patients should be evaluated for LT. First studies comparing uncovered TIPS with repeated LVP, showed that the former was better than LVP to prevent ascites recurrence but with a higher incidence of hepatic encephalopathy post-TIPS. A meta-analyses using individual patient data of the same studies, showed a significant improvement of transplant-free survival in patients treated with TIPS, which was strongly influenced by three prognostic variables (age, bilirubin and sodium) revealing the importance of careful patient selection [46]. A recent randomized controlled trial showed that PTFE-covered TIPS improves control of ascites and survival compare to large volume paracentesis in recurrent ascites. So it may be a very good option for these patients [47]. However, TIPS requires a careful selection of patients in order to maximise beneficial effects and avoid complications since it may have detrimental effects in the most advanced stages of cirrhosis. For patients not candidates to TIPS, they can be evaluated for Alfapump® insertion in experienced centers since it helps to control ascites [48, 49]. Since this system is linked to a high risk of adverse events (infections, renal dysfunction, …) and technical troubles patients should follow close monitoring.

33.3.3 Renal Impairment

Renal failure was traditionally defined as a creatinine increase >50% above 1.5 mg/dL in cirrhosis. Given the limitations of serum creatinine (Crs) in cirrhotic patients, and the new diagnostic criteria for acute renal failure (now acute kidney injury—AKI) in general population, the definition of AKI in cirrhosis was recently revised [50]. So, AKI is defined as an increase of Crs > 0.3 mg/dL in 48 h or 50% from baseline value within 7 days. According to its severity AKI can be stratified into three stages (Table 33.1).

Table 33.1 New definition, stages of acute kidney injury and diagnostic criteria of hepatorenal syndrome in patients with cirrhosis proposed by the International Club of Ascites [50]

Definition of AKI	Increase of Crs ≥ 0.3 mg/dL in 48 h Increase Crs ≥ 50% with respect to its baseline value in 7 days	
Stages of AKI	Stage 1[a]: increase Crs > 0.3 mg/dL; or increase of Crs > 1.5 to twofold from baseline	
	Stage 2: increase of Crs > two- to threefold from baseline	
	Stage 3: increase of Crs > threefold from baseline; or increase Crs ≥ 4 mg/dL with acute increase Crs ≥ 0.3 mg/dL; or renal replacement therapy	
Clinical forms of AKI	Prerenal AKI: in relation to hypovolemia and renal hypoperfusion because of diuretics, diarrhea, digestive hemorrhage, …	
	Intrinsic AKI: mainly represented by acute tubular necrosis in relation to shock, nephrotoxicity, …	
	Post-renal AKI	
	HRS-AKI (previously type 1 HRS): new diagnostic criteria	• Diagnosis of cirrhosis and ascites • Diagnosis of AKI according to the classification of the International Club of ascites • Absence of response after 2 days to the withdrawal of diuretics and expansion with albumin (1 g/kg of weight) • Absence of shock • No current/recent use of nephrotoxic drugs (NSAIDs, aminoglycosides, iodinated contrasts, …) • Absence of macroscopic signs of structural kidney damage: – Absence of proteinuria (>500 mg/day) – Absence of microhematuria (>50 erythrocytes per high power field) – Absence of morphological alterations in ultrasound

[a]It has been suggested that patients in stage 1 may have different outcomes according to value of Crs supporting an sub-classification in Stage 1A Crs ≤ 1.5 mg/dL and stage 1B Crs > 1.5 mg/dL [91]

Once AKI is identified, it is important to differentiate among the clinical forms of AKI, since all of them can occur in cirrhosis but they have prognostic and therapeutic implications. Prerenal AKI is the most common form accounting for up to 70% of cases in hospitalized cirrhotic patients. Post-renal AKI is very infrequent. Intrinsic AKI is mainly represented by acute tubular necrosis. Given that most prerenal forms resolve with volume expansion, this form constitutes the main differential diagnosis with HRS-AKI. The new diagnostic criteria of HRS-AKI include the elimination of the cut-off point of Crs > 2.5 mg/dL (Table 33.1). This has relevant implications in the management of patients favouring that patients can be treated with lower creatinine levels.

AKI should be suspected in patients with cirrhosis and oliguria or nonspecific symptoms. The cause of AKI should be investigated and managed as soon as possible. So, risk factors should be sought and corrected including: withdrawal of nephrotoxic drugs (NSAIDs, vasodilators, diuretics, beta blockers), seek and treatment of infections (SBP, urine, pneumonia, …) and correction of hypovolemia. In the AKI stage >1A and no clear origin, volume expansion with albumin (1 g/kg of weight) is also recommended for 2 days [50].

As specific measures, patients who meet SHR-AKI criteria should be treated with vasoconstrictors plus albumin that requires close monitoring. The drug of choice is terlipressin. It can be used intravenously at the initial dose of 1 mg every 4–6 h or by continuous infusion at the initial dose of 2 mg/day. If there is no decrease of Crs > 25% by the third day it can be increased up to a maximum of 12 mg/day [42]. Terlipressin plus albumin is also effective in the formerly known type II HRS, now HRS-non-AKI. However, since the impact of treatment on long-term outcome is controversial it is not recommended in this setting.

LT is the best therapeutic option for patients suffering HRS. TIPS could be evaluated in patients with HRS-non-AKI [51], whereas there is no enough data to promote TIPS in HRS-AKI [52].

33.3.4 Immune Dysfunction

Cirrhosis associated immune dysfunction involves a state of immunodeficiency, and in parallel a state of persistent activation of the immune system cells [53].

Immunodeficiency affects both the innate and the adaptive immune response with numerous defects. Excluding monocytes, cirrhosis leads to reduced numbers of circulating immune system cells, which is particularly profound for neutrophils. In addition, mononuclear phagocytic cells and neutrophils show reduced phagocytic capacity, T and B cells show hypo-proliferative response and NK cells display low cytotoxic activity. Furthermore, cirrhosis results in reticuloendothelial dysfunction, due to reduced number of liver reticuloendothelial mononuclear cells and porto-systemic shunting. This lowers the liver ability to clear bacteria and decreases hepatic synthesis of molecules of the innate immune response, such as complement components and secreted-pattern recognition receptors.

These defects coexist with systemic inflammation in form of induced expression of activation molecules on the surface of immune cells and the increased synthesis of pro-inflammatory cytokines.

The pathogenesis of this immune dysfunction is multifactorial, including persistent immune system cells stimulation by pathogen- and damage-associated molecular patterns (PAMPs, DAMPs), decreased hepatic synthesis of trophic factors, hypersplenism, and the etiological factors of cirrhosis such as alcohol. Furthermore, the continuous stimulation of the immune system may lead to exhaustion of the immune response that might further increase the susceptibility to bacterial infections.

33.3.5 Infections

Spontaneous bacterial peritonitis (infection of ascitic fluid unrelated to surgically treatable infection) is a characteristic bacterial infection in decompensated cirrhotic patients. Its mortality decreased from 90% to 20% with early diagnosis and treatment. Diagnosis is based on ascitic fluid analysis. Since some patients can be asymptomatic, or have minor/unspecific symptoms, diagnostic paracentesis is required in all cirrhotic patients with ascites admitted to hospital or presenting any clinical deterioration.

Early diagnosis and treatment are crucial and associated to better outcomes [54]. Empiric antibiotic should be selected according to the characteristics of the infection (site of acquisition, clinical severity), local bacterial epidemiology and avoiding nephrotoxic drugs. Clinical monitoring and second paracentesis 48 hours after empiric therapy should be done. Failure to empiric treatment must be suspected if no improvement in control paracentesis or clinical deterioration is noticed. De-escalation according to bacterial susceptibility is recommended and treatment duration should be at least 5–7 days, followed by antibiotic prophylaxis [42]. Albumin, a multifunctional protein [44, 55], reduces the incidence of HRS-AKI and mortality in patients with SBP [56]. So, its concomitant administration is recommended although it may not be needed in low risk patients [57].

Non-SBP infections are a heterogeneous group of infections which often occur in cirrhotic patients and are associated with up to 60% 1-year mortality [58]. Endocarditis, secondary peritonitis, pneumonia and bacteraemia have the worse prognosis. Early diagnosis and treatment are also crucial and often require high clinical suspicion. Like in SBP, empiric antibiotic should be chosen according characteristics of the infection with special attention to the site of acquisition and local bacterial epidemiology and clinical severity [42].

33.3.6 Neurological Manifestations

Hepatic encephalopathy is a brain dysfunction caused by liver failure and/or the presence of portosystemic shunts (PSS) involving a wide range of clinical manifestations [59]. Overt HE will occur in 30–40% of cirrhotic patients at some point of their disease and there is a risk of recurrence in those who survive [60].

The physiopathology of HE is not well understood. CLF and the presence PSS favour brain exposure to substances that under normal conditions would have been efficiently metabolized and excreted by the liver. Ammonia has traditionally been considered one of the most important factors in the development of HE. Other factors may facilitate brain dysfunction such as inflammation, hyponatremia, nutritional deficits and comorbidities [61] (Fig. 33.2).

- Ammonia. Under physiological conditions, ammonia enters the portal circulation from the gut where it derives from colonic bacteria and the deamidation of glutamine in the small bowel (action catalyzed by the enzyme glutaminase—GA). Through the portal vein it reaches the liver where 90% is metabolized in urea (through the urea cycle) and excreted in the urine. In liver failure or PSS, the liver clearance decreases, and ammonia reaches the systemic circulation and cerebral parenchyma causing its toxic effects [61]. Apart from liver and intestine, muscle and kidney have a relevant role in ammonia homeostasis. So, muscle can eliminate ammonia by synthesizing glutamine (through the action of glutamine synthetase—GS). Kidneys generate ammonia from the deamination of glutamine, a reaction involved in the regulation of plasma and urinary PH. So, ammonia excretion may be affected by dehydration or hypokalemia and increases in conditions of hyperammonemia [62].
- Manganese. Brain magnetic resonance studies documented an increase in signal in the basal ganglia that has been attributed to a manganese accumulation. It could be linked to the extrapyramidal alterations of patients with persistent HE [61].
- Inflammation. Inflammatory response has been associated to the development of HE [63]. This proinflammatory component may be particularly relevant in patients with HE and acute-on-chronic liver failure, where the inflammatory response is marked [64].

Clinical manifestations of HE involve a broad spectrum of neuropsyquiatric alterations and can occur in patients with very diverse liver disorders. Thus, HE should be classified according to various criteria [59] (Table 33.2): underlying

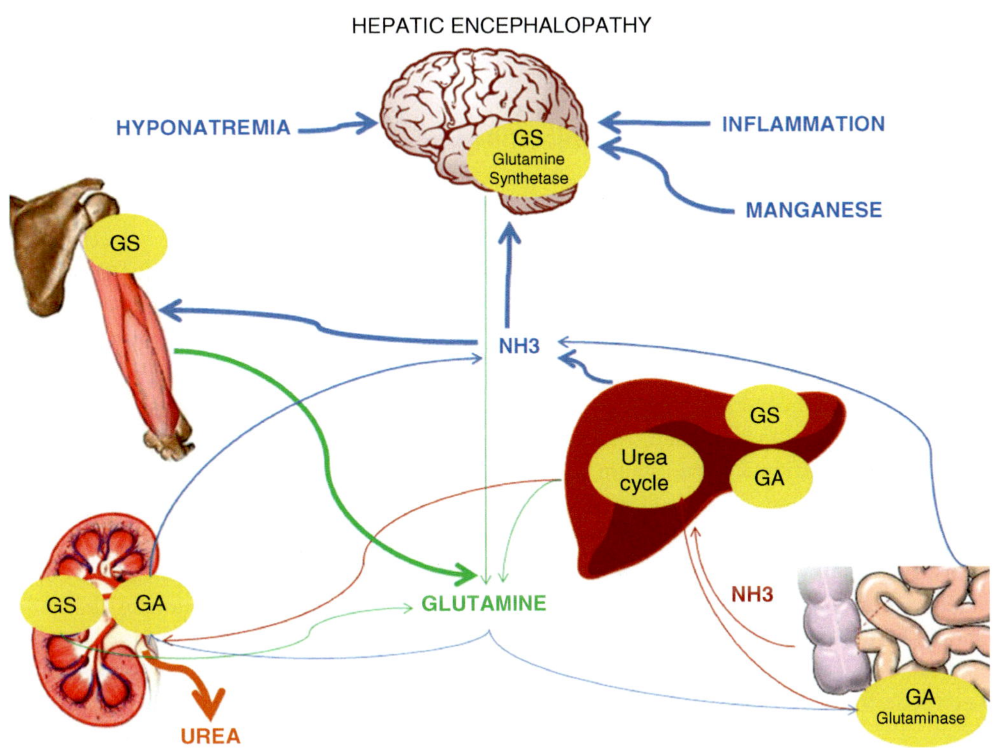

Fig. 33.2 Physiopathology of hepatic encephalopathy

Table 33.2 Classification of hepatic encephalopathy according to different criteria

Type	Clinical severity		Time course	Precipitating factors
A (acute liver failure)	Minimal HE	(COVERT)	Episodic	Nonprecipitated
	Grade 1			
B (PSS)	Grade 2	(OVERT)	Recurrent (>2 episodes in 6 months)	Precipitated (infections, diuretic overdose, constipation, …)
C (CLD)	Grade 3		Persistent (cognitive alterations always present)	
	Grade 4			

liver disease; severity of clinical manifestations; time course and the existence of precipitating factors. West Haven classification has been used widely to assess the severity of HE. However, it has been questioned for its lack of specificity and inter-observer variations. Given that HE is a continuum, it has been proposed to reclassify the HE in two sub-categories: Covert HE, (includes minimal and grade I HE) and Overt HE (HE $\geq$ grade II). Precipitating factors (infections, diuretic overdose, constipation, …) should be systematically sought and treated.

The diagnosis of HE is based on the presence of compatible clinical symptoms, the existence of an underlying disease that justifies it, and the exclusion of other causes of brain dysfunction. Since there is no laboratory data or additional explorations specific to the disease, HE diagnosis remains to be a diagnosis of exclusion of other potential causes [65].

The management of patients with HE includes general and specific measures which will be deeply discussed separately in this book.

Other neurological disorders, such as hepatic myelopathy or polyneuropathy, have been associated to CLF or to the aetiology of the liver disease. These entities in many cases share symptoms with HE [66] and may coexist. Adequate diagnosis would allow optimal management of these patients.

33.3.7 Cardiopulmonary Complications

Cirrhotic cardiomyopathy is a cardiac dysfunction characterized by an impaired systolic response to stress and altered diastolic function, often concomitant with electrophysiological abnormalities (i.e. prolonged QTc interval) in the absence of known cardiovascular disease [67]. Heart failure may become obvious during certain procedures (TIPS insertion, large volume paracentesis, liver transplantation) in patients previously asymptomatic. Diagnosis requires dynamic stress echocardiography since hyperdynamic circulation may mask systolic dysfunction at rest. Decreased cardiac output is associated with the development of HRS-AKI after infections, providing its prognostic significance. Prolonged QTc interval may also indicate poor outcome in cirrhosis and should be evaluated [42]. Normalization of cardiac function and improvement of electrophysiological abnormalities has been seen following LT [68]

Hepatopulmonary syndrome (HPS) is a pulmonary disorder characterized by gas exchange abnormalities caused by intrapulmonary vasodilatation or pleuro-pulmonary arteriovenous communications in the setting of portal hypertension [69]. It is more frequently associated to cirrhosis (11–32%), although it may occur in pre-hepatic PH, Budd-Chiari (28%) and even in acute or chronic hepatitis (10%). Pathophysiology is complex in relation to a vasodilators predominance and angiogenesis, resulting in an altered ventilation/perfusion mismatch and hypoxemia. Diagnosis requires demonstration of gas exchange abnormalities ($pO_2 < 80$ mmHg; alveolar-arterial oxygen gradient $\geq$15 mmHg or >20 mmHg in older than 65 years) and intrapulmonary vasodilatation (contrast-enhanced echocardiography or Technetium-99-labeled macro-aggregated albumin scanning) in patients with PH. For patients with severe hypoxemia ($paO_2 < 60$ mmHg) long-term oxygen is recommended despite the lack of data on long-term effectiveness. Medical therapy or TIPS are not recommended based on available data. LT is associated with resolution of HPS in >80% patients, so patients with severe hypoxemia should be evaluated for LT. Since very severe hypoxemia ($paO_2 <$ 45–50 mmHg) is linked to increased post-LT mortality, caution and close follow-up should be carried out order to facilitate prioritisation on waiting list [42].

Portopulmonary hypertension (PPHT) refers to the pulmonary arterial hypertension in the absence of other causes in a patient with PH. It occurs in up to 10% of patients with cirrhosis and is associated higher mortality rate than predicted by MELD (Model for End-stage Liver Disease) score. Pathophysiology is largely unknown, probably related to the effect of vasoactive substances that reach the pulmonary circulation in the presence of PSS/CLF. Transthoracic Doppler echocardiography is the main screening tool and right heart catheterisation provides diagnostic confirmation. Medical management includes different drugs such as prostacyclin analogues and PDP5 inhibitors. NSBB should be stopped in this particular group of patients and varices managed by endoscopic therapy. LT has been associated with treatment discontinuation in the follow-up in up to 64% of patients with moderate to severe PPHT, however, this patients should be treated before aggressively to lower mPAP and improve right ventricular function [42].

33.3.8 Nutrition and Muscle Mass

Malnutrition and sarcopenia are common and progressive complications in cirrhosis associated with the progression of CLF. Aetiology is multifactorial including decreased oral intake, malabsorption and impaired capacity of the liver to metabolize and save nutrients. Both sarcopenia and malnutrition are associated with development of complications of cirrhosis, and worsen quality of life and survival [70–72]. Therefore, strategies addressed to assess and improve nutritional status and muscle mass showed to be of benefit and should be considered [73]. Those include repeated snacks, including late-evening snacks [73, 74], protein/branched chain amino acid supplementation if needed [73, 75] or moderate aerobic exercise [73, 76].

33.3.9 Bone Disease

Bone disease (osteopenia, osteoporosis) has been reported in up to 55% of patients with cirrhosis, and it is associated with a higher risk of fracture (5–20%). Prevalence is higher in patients with cholestatic liver disease. It has a negative impact on quality of life and is crucial to identify and treat it before LT because bone disease worsens during the first year after transplantation [77]. Prevention and treatment of bone disease in patients with CLF include screening for all of them, elimination of modifiable risk factors (alcohol, smoking), and consideration of calcium and vitamin D supplementation together with other specific therapies (biphosphonates, hormonal therapy, raloxifene, calcitonin) [73, 78]. However, the lack of conclusive studies on safety and efficacy in cirrhosis for the majority of specific therapies preclude formal recommendations, and those should be evaluated on individual basis.

33.3.10 Endocrinopathies

Relative adrenal insufficiency has been described in cirrhotic patients either critically ill (69%) or non-critically ill (42%). Its presence is associated with higher probability of sepsis, HRS-AKI and higher short-term mortality. Diagnosis should be based on the recommendations of the American College of Critical Care Medicine. The effect of corticosteroid supplementation is still controversial in critically ill cirrhotic patients and cannot be currently recommended [42].

Disorders of glucose metabolism are very frequent in CLF ranging from 20% to 70%. Prevalence of diabetes mellitus (DM) is higher in advanced stages of CLF and in some aetiologies (i.e. alcohol, NAFLD or hepatitis C virus). DM is associated with higher rate of complications and worse prognosis. Treating diabetes may be challenging in cirrhotic patients because of the liver' metabolic impairments and because the most appropriate pharmacologic treatment is not well-defined [79].

Liver disease may interfere with thyroid hormone metabolism and conversely, thyroid dysfunction may also alter liver function [80, 81].

Sexual dysfunction is often observed in patients with CLD in relation to hormonal disturbances inducing feminization in men and infertility and amenorrhoea in women [80].

33.3.11 Haematological Alterations

A myriad of hematologic manifestations have been observed in patients with CLF, including alterations on cellular and soluble components of blood. Cellular abnormalities, particularly cytopenias are very common and of multifactorial origin [82]. On the other hand, liver synthesizes most of coagulation factors (both procoagulants and anticoagulants), So, in CLF there is a decrease in plasma levels of the liver derived coagulation factors, leading to a fragile rebalance of homeostasis. This rebalance may shift toward hypercoagulable or bleeding complications in the course of the disease [83].

33.3.12 Skin Manifestations

Palmar erythema, spider angioma, caput medusa, pigmentary skin alterations or hair and nail changes are among the numerous cutaneous alterations related to CLF. They are easily recognized and can be the first sign allowing early diagnosis and adequate management [84].

33.3.13 Hepatocellular Carcinoma

The incidence of HCC is increasing worldwide. It occurs in 2–8% cirrhotic patients per year, and the risk is higher in older or male patients, those with clinically significant PH, higher body mass index, platelet <100,000 cells/μL, esophageal varices and decompensated cirrhosis. Median survival after detection is 9 months in untreated patients and 2 years in treated patients, ranging from >10 years in Barcelona Clinic Liver Cancer (BCLC) stage 0 to <6 months in stage D. HCC requires a multidisciplinary approach in order to shape personalized treatment options [85].

33.3.14 Acute-on-Chronic Liver Failure

In the routine clinical practice, it is noticed that a proportion of patients with acute decompensation of cirrhosis also develop failure of different organs which is associated with poor short-term prognosis. This concept, traditionally called *acute-on-chronic liver failure*, generated several definitions proposed by different societies. However, none of them has been universally accepted, partially justified by disagreements regarding the underlying liver disease, precipitating factors, prognostic criteria and management [86]. Among the most widely used are the definitions proposed by the Asian Pacific Association for the Study of the Liver (APASL), World North American Consortium for the Study of End-Stage Liver Disease (NACSELD) and The European Association for the Study of the Liver-Chronic Liver Failure (EASL-CLIF) Consortium of whom, the last two are based on prospective studies. The NACSELD included only patients with cirrhosis and bacterial infections whereas the CANONIC study, conducted by the EASL-CLIF Consortium is the most comprehensive registry to understand outcomes on hospitalized cirrhotic patients since it included 1343 subjects admitted for any cirrhosis-related complication.

The CANONIC study aimed to determine which patients with acute decompensation of cirrhosis (variceal bleeding, ascites, bacterial infection, HE) were at high risk of short-term mortality, set at 28-day mortality ≥15%. Organ failure seems a key component of the syndrome and it was evaluated using an adapted version of the *Sequential Organ Failure Assessment—SOFA-score* to patients with cirrhosis, later simplified into the CLIF-C-OF score (Table 33.3). Thus, ACLF was identified according to the type and number of organ failure, and it was classified in three stages according to its severity (Table 33.4) [12]. Prevalence of ACLF in the CANONIC study was 30% (20% at admission and 10% during hospitalization). Patients with ACLF were younger and main cirrhosis causes were alcohol in 60% and hepatitis C in 13%. Kidney was the most common organ failure (56%). Patients with no history of acute decompensation (23% of them) developed a more severe ACLF. The most frequent precipitating events were bacterial infections and active alcoholism. Interestingly, in 40% of cases no precipitating event could be identified. In addition, markers of systemic inflammation, such as white cell count and plasma C-reactive protein (CRP), were higher in ACLF patients [12]. In concordance, other markers of systemic inflammation, such as proinflammatory cytokines and chemokines, were found higher in patients with ACLF and correlated with the progression and prognosis of the disease [28]. These findings lead to the currently widely accepted hypothesis that systemic inflammation has a relevant role of in the pathogenesis of ACLF [13].

Although the initial ACLF stage is linked to prognosis (Table 33.4), ACLF is a dynamic and potentially reversible syndrome which may resolve or improve (49% of patients), remain stable or fluctuating (30%) or worsen (20%) during the hospitalization. Indeed, the clinical course during hospitalization was the most important determinant of short-term mortality, independently of the initial grade [87]. More than 80% of patients achieved the final ACLF grade within the first week. Therefore, ACLF-grade at days 3–7 predicts significantly better 28- and 90-day mortality rates than ACLF grade at diagnosis.

Patients with severe early course (final ACLF-2 or -3) were younger, presented a more intense systemic inflammatory reaction (higher white cell count), higher prevalence of cerebral, circulatory, coagulation, and liver failure; without history of prior decompensation. Mortality was independent of the presence and type of precipitating events.

Table 33.4 Diagnostic criteria for ACLF

	28-days mortality (%)	Grade
No organ failure	39/879 (4.4%)	→ No ACLF
1 Single organ failure (no kidney) with creatinine < 1.5 mg/dL and no EH	8/128 (6.3%)	
Single kidney failure	16/86 (18.6%)	→ ACLF-1
1 Single organ failure + creatinine 1.5–1.9 mg/dL year old HE grade I–II	15/54 (27.7%)	
2 Organ failures	31/97 (32.0%)	→ ACLF-2
3 Organ failures	17/25 (68.0%)	→ ACLF-3
4–6 Organ failures	12/18 (88.9%)	

Table 33.3 CLIF-C-OF-score

Organ system	Parameter	Score = 1	Score = 2	Score = 3
Liver	Bilirubin (mg/dL)	< 6	6–12	**≥12**
Kidney	Creatinine (mg/dL)	<2	**2–3.5**	**≥3.5 old RRT**
Brain	Hepatic encephalopathy (West-Haven)	0	1–2	**3–4**
Clotting	INR	<2.0	2.0–2.5	**≥2.5**
Circulation	MAP (mmHg)	>70	<70	**Vasopressors**
Respiratory	PaO_2/FiO_2	>300	≤300 year > 200	**≤200**
	$SatO_2/FiO_2$	>357	>214 year ≤ 357	**≤214**

Organ failure is defined by the indicated value of parameter in bold font
The index is obtained by adding together the score for each of the different organs or systems (minimum 6, maximum 18 points)
FiO_2 fraction of inspired oxygen, *INR* international normalised ratio, *MAP* mean arterial pressure, *PaO_2* partial pressure of oxygen in arterial blood, *SpO_2* oxygen saturation, *RRT* renal replacement therapy

In the view of the mortality-related factors, a new prognostic score with greater prognostic capability than Child-Pugh, MELD or CLIF-C-OF was developed: CLIF-C-ACLF score. This score incorporated CLIF-C-OF and also age and inflammatory markers. Its sequential application during hospitalization could help to make decisions such as treatment continuation, potential consideration for LT, or discontinuation due to futility [87].

The general management of ACLF includes a rapid identification and treatment of potential triggers, measures that prevent progression of the syndrome and the support of failed organs. So, these patients should ideally be treated in intermediate/intensive care units and potential candidates for liver transplantation should be transferred to a transplant centre. Since LT is the definitive treatment in liver failure, if no absolute contraindication, patients should be evaluated for liver transplant. However, it is complex and controversial, particularly in those subjects with worse ACLF stages because of their high short-term mortality, presence of contraindications, narrow window for the LT and potential futility. Data on the prognosis of patients with ACLF after LT is still scarce, and coming from retrospective studies [87–89]. In the CANONIC study, patients who received a LT were highly selected (only 9%) and no patients with respiratory failure were included. Almost all ACLF-3 patients presented complications after LT, especially pulmonary, respiratory or infectious; therefore, a special management is needed in this subgroup of patients. However, results are optimistic considering that 28-day survival in patients with severe ACLF raised from less than 20% to 80%. Nevertheless, evidence of the impact of ACLF in the outcome post-LT is very limited and more data are needed in order to establish objective recommendations on selection, inclusion and prioritisation or list withdrawal of these patients [90]. Other treatments with pathophysiological effects such as immunomodulatory and regenerative therapies are currently under investigation.

33.4 Conclusions/Summary

CLF is a multisystem disease secondary to chronic and persistent liver damage. It progresses from a compensated to a decompensated phase driven by hemodynamic disturbances associated with PH and systemic inflammation. Etiological cure may prevent the progression of the disease and even induce reversibility to a compensated or precirrhotic phase.

ACLF is an acute decompensation characterized by the development of organ failure and high short-term mortality. Systemic inflammatory response seems to be a key factor in the pathogenesis and prognosis. Despite a high short-term mortality, ACLF is highly dynamic and may improve/resolve so it is potentially reversible. There is no specific treatment and currently clinical management includes early detection and treatment of triggers, support of the failed organs and potentially LT.

Acknowledgement *Conflict of interest*: None.

Self Study

Questions

1. Regarding AKI in Cirrhosis Which Is FALSE
   (a) Clinical manifestations are prominent and drive the diagnosis.
   (b) Once diagnosis is made, risk factors should be sought and corrected
   (c) Diagnostic criteria for AKI and HRS-AKI has been updated leading to the elimination of the Crs cut-off point of 2.5 mg/dL
   (d) The subtype HRS-AKI requires close monitoring and specific treatment based on vasoconstrictors and albumin infusion

2. With Regard to the Physiopathology of HE Which Is TRUE
   (a) Ammonia is the only element involved and its serum level is diagnostic.
   (b) The amount of ammonia that enters portal vein is the result of catabolism of proteins by gut bacteria and deamination of glutamine in the gut.
   (c) Systemic inflammation is not important in the pathogenesis of HE.
   (d) Kidney eliminates ammonia in urea form and is not implicated in the ammoniagenesis.

Answers

1. Regarding AKI in Cirrhosis Which Is FALSE
   Right answer: a.
   AKI doesn't have prominent manifestations, it has to be suspected in patients with oliguria and unspecific symptoms. All the others are correct.

2. With Regard to the Physiopathology of HE Which Is TRUE
   Right answer: b.
   Ammonia is an important factor in the physiopathology *of HE together with others. Inflammation is also important, especially in clinical situations where the inflammatory response is marked as ACLF. The determination of plasma ammonia levels may suggest HE but there are no cut-off points to confirm or exclude HE. Ammonia that enters portal vein* from the gastrointestinal tract derives

from colonic bacteria and the deamidation of glutamine in the small bowel *Muscle and kidney are important organs in ammonia homeostasis. Kidney can either eliminate or generate ammonia (through glutamine metabolism).*

References

1. Tsochatzis EA, Bosch J, Burroughs AK. Liver cirrhosis. Lancet. 2014;383(9930):1749–61.
2. Sanyal AJ, Bosch J, Blei A, Arroyo V. Portal hypertension and its complications. Gastroenterology. 2008;134(6):1715–28.
3. de Franchis R. Expanding consensus in portal hypertension: report of the Baveno VI consensus workshop: stratifying risk and individualizing care for portal hypertension. J Hepatol. 2015;63(3):743–52.
4. Golding PL, Smith M, Williams R. Multisystem involvement in chronic liver disease. Studies on the incidence and pathogenesis. Am J Med. 1973;55(6):772–82.
5. Minemura M, Tajiri K, Shimizu Y. Systemic abnormalities in liver disease. World J Gastroenterol. 2009;15(24):2960–74.
6. Thomson MJ, Tapper EB, Lok ASF. Dos and don'ts in the management of cirrhosis: a view from the 21st century. Am J Gastroenterol. 2018;113(7):927–31.
7. Lens S, Alvarado-Tapias E, Marino Z, et al. Effects of all-oral antiviral therapy on HVPG and systemic hemodynamics in patients with hepatitis C virus-associated cirrhosis. Gastroenterology. 2017;153(5):1273–83.
8. Muntaner L, Altamirano JT, Augustin S, et al. High doses of beta-blockers and alcohol abstinence improve long-term rebleeding and mortality in cirrhotic patients after an acute variceal bleeding. Liver Int. 2010;30(8):1123–30.
9. Di M, Calvaruso V, Ferraro D, et al. Effects of eradicating hepatitis C virus infection in patients with cirrhosis differ with stage of portal hypertension. Gastroenterology. 2016;151(1):130–9.
10. Luca A, Garcia-Pagan JC, Bosch J, et al. Effects of ethanol consumption on hepatic hemodynamics in patients with alcoholic cirrhosis. Gastroenterology. 1997;112(4):1284–9.
11. D'Amico G, Morabito A, D'Amico M, et al. Clinical states of cirrhosis and competing risks. J Hepatol. 2018;68(3):563–76.
12. Moreau R, Jalan R, Gines P, et al. Acute-on-chronic liver failure is a distinct syndrome that develops in patients with acute decompensation of cirrhosis. Gastroenterology. 2013;144(7):1426, 1437.
13. Arroyo V, Moreau R, Kamath PS, et al. Acute-on-chronic liver failure in cirrhosis. Nat Rev Dis Primers. 2016;2:16041.
14. Bosch J, Arroyo V, Betriu A, et al. Hepatic hemodynamics and the renin-angiotensin-aldosterone system in cirrhosis. Gastroenterology. 1980;78(1):92–9.
15. Bosch J, Pizcueta P, Feu F, Fernandez M, Garcia-Pagan JC. Pathophysiology of portal hypertension. Gastroenterol Clin N Am. 1992;21(1):1–14.
16. Pimpin L, Cortez-Pinto H, Negro F, et al. Burden of liver disease in Europe: epidemiology and analysis of risk factors to identify prevention policies. J Hepatol. 2018;69(3):718–35.
17. Giannelli V, Di G, Iebba V, et al. Microbiota and the gut-liver axis: bacterial translocation, inflammation and infection in cirrhosis. World J Gastroenterol. 2014;20(45):16795–810.
18. Acharya C, Sahingur SE, Bajaj JS. Microbiota, cirrhosis, and the emerging oral-gut-liver axis. JCI Insight. 2017;2(19):pii: 94416.
19. Chen Y, Yang F, Lu H, et al. Characterization of fecal microbial communities in patients with liver cirrhosis. Hepatology. 2011;54(2):562–72.
20. Bajaj JS, Heuman DM, Hylemon PB, et al. Altered profile of human gut microbiome is associated with cirrhosis and its complications. J Hepatol. 2014;60(5):940–7.
21. Wiest R, Lawson M, Geuking M. Pathological bacterial translocation in liver cirrhosis. J Hepatol. 2014;60(1):197–209.
22. Bauer TM, Steinbruckner B, Brinkmann FE, et al. Small intestinal bacterial overgrowth in patients with cirrhosis: prevalence and relation with spontaneous bacterial peritonitis. Am J Gastroenterol. 2001;96(10):2962–7.
23. Ponziani FR, Zocco MA, Cerrito L, Gasbarrini A, Pompili M. Bacterial translocation in patients with liver cirrhosis: physiology, clinical consequences, and practical implications. Expert Rev Gastroenterol Hepatol. 2018;12(7):641–56.
24. Bajaj JS, Ridlon JM, Hylemon PB, et al. Linkage of gut microbiome with cognition in hepatic encephalopathy. Am J Physiol Gastrointest Liver Physiol. 2012;302(1):G168–75.
25. Runyon BA, Squier S, Borzio M. Translocation of gut bacteria in rats with cirrhosis to mesenteric lymph nodes partially explains the pathogenesis of spontaneous bacterial peritonitis. J Hepatol. 1994;21(5):792–6.
26. Bellot P, Garcia-Pagan JC, Frances R, et al. Bacterial DNA translocation is associated with systemic circulatory abnormalities and intrahepatic endothelial dysfunction in patients with cirrhosis. Hepatology. 2010;52(6):2044–52.
27. Thalheimer U, Triantos CK, Samonakis DN, Patch D, Burroughs AK. Infection, coagulation, and variceal bleeding in cirrhosis. Gut. 2005;54(4):556–63.
28. Claria J, Stauber RE, Coenraad MJ, et al. Systemic inflammation in decompensated cirrhosis: characterization and role in acute-on-chronic liver failure. Hepatology. 2016;64(4):1249–64.
29. Wiest R, Albillos A, Trauner M, Bajaj JS, Jalan R. Targeting the gut-liver axis in liver disease. J Hepatol. 2017;67(5):1084–103.
30. Ishibashi H, Nakamura M, Komori A, Migita K, Shimoda S. Liver architecture, cell function, and disease. Semin Immunopathol. 2009;31(3):399–409.
31. Berzigotti A, Seijo S, Reverter E, Bosch J. Assessing portal hypertension in liver diseases. Expert Rev Gastroenterol Hepatol. 2013;7(2):141–55.
32. Graham DY, Smith JL. The course of patients after variceal hemorrhage. Gastroenterology. 1981;80(4):800–9.
33. Villanueva C, Colomo A, Bosch A, et al. Transfusion strategies for acute upper gastrointestinal bleeding. N Engl J Med. 2013;368(1):11–21.
34. Garcia-Pagan JC, Caca K, Bureau C, et al. Early use of TIPS in patients with cirrhosis and variceal bleeding. N Engl J Med. 2010;362(25):2370–9.
35. Procopet B, Giraldez A, Amitrano L, et al. Preemptive-TIPS improves outcome in high-risk variceal bleeding: an observational study. Hepatology. 2019;69(1):282–93.
36. Serste T, Melot C, Francoz C, et al. Deleterious effects of beta-blockers on survival in patients with cirrhosis and refractory ascites. Hepatology. 2010;52(3):1017–22.
37. Mandorfer M, Bota S, Schwabl P, et al. Nonselective beta blockers increase risk for hepatorenal syndrome and death in patients with cirrhosis and spontaneous bacterial peritonitis. Gastroenterology. 2014;146(7):1680–90.
38. Reiberger T, Mandorfer M. Beta adrenergic blockade and decompensated cirrhosis. J Hepatol. 2017;66(4):849–59.
39. Urrunaga NH, Rockey DC. Portal hypertensive gastropathy and colopathy. Clin Liver Dis. 2014;18(2):389–406.
40. Madonia S, D'Amico G, Traina M, et al. Prognostic indicators of successful endoscopic sclerotherapy for prevention of rebleeding from oesophageal varices in cirrhosis: a long-term cohort study. Dig Liver Dis. 2000;32(9):782–91.

41. Ripoll C, Groszmann R, Garcia-Tsao G, et al. Hepatic venous pressure gradient predicts clinical decompensation in patients with compensated cirrhosis. Gastroenterology. 2007;133(2):481–8.
42. EASL. EASL clinical practice guidelines for the management of patients with decompensated cirrhosis. J Hepatol. 2018;69(2):406–60.
43. Bernardi M, Caraceni P, Navickis RJ, Wilkes MM. Albumin infusion in patients undergoing large-volume paracentesis: a meta-analysis of randomized trials. Hepatology. 2012;55(4):1172–81.
44. Garcia-Martinez R, Caraceni P, Bernardi M, Gines P, Arroyo V, Jalan R. Albumin: pathophysiologic basis of its role in the treatment of cirrhosis and its complications. Hepatology. 2013;58(5):1836–46.
45. Salerno F, Borroni G, Moser P, et al. Survival and prognostic factors of cirrhotic patients with ascites: a study of 134 outpatients. Am J Gastroenterol. 1993;88(4):514–9.
46. Salerno F, Camma C, Enea M, Rossle M, Wong F. Transjugular intrahepatic portosystemic shunt for refractory ascites: a meta-analysis of individual patient data. Gastroenterology. 2007;133(3):825–34.
47. Bureau C, Thabut D, Oberti F, et al. Transjugular intrahepatic portosystemic shunts with covered stents increase transplant-free survival of patients with cirrhosis and recurrent ascites. Gastroenterology. 2017;152(1):157–63.
48. Bellot P, Welker MW, Soriano G, et al. Automated low flow pump system for the treatment of refractory ascites: a multi-center safety and efficacy study. J Hepatol. 2013;58(5):922–7.
49. Bureau C, Adebayo D, de RM C, et al. Alfapump(R) system vs. large volume paracentesis for refractory ascites: a multicenter randomized controlled study. J Hepatol. 2017;67(5):940–9.
50. Angeli P, Gines P, Wong F, et al. Diagnosis and management of acute kidney injury in patients with cirrhosis: revised consensus recommendations of the International Club of Ascites. J Hepatol. 2015;62(4):968–74.
51. Testino G, Ferro C, Sumberaz A, et al. Type-2 hepatorenal syndrome and refractory ascites: role of transjugular intrahepatic portosystemic stent-shunt in eighteen patients with advanced cirrhosis awaiting orthotopic liver transplantation. Hepato-Gastroenterology. 2003;50(54):1753–5.
52. Guevara M, Gines P, Bandi JC, et al. Transjugular intrahepatic portosystemic shunt in hepatorenal syndrome: effects on renal function and vasoactive systems. Hepatology. 1998;28(2):416–22.
53. Albillos A, Lario M, Alvarez-Mon M. Cirrhosis-associated immune dysfunction: distinctive features and clinical relevance. J Hepatol. 2014;61(6):1385–96.
54. Kim JJ, Tsukamoto MM, Mathur AK, et al. Delayed paracentesis is associated with increased in-hospital mortality in patients with spontaneous bacterial peritonitis. Am J Gastroenterol. 2014;109(9):1436–42.
55. Garcia-Martinez R, Andreola F, Mehta G, et al. Immunomodulatory and antioxidant function of albumin stabilises the endothelium and improves survival in a rodent model of chronic liver failure. J Hepatol. 2015;62(4):799–806.
56. Sort P, Navasa M, Arroyo V, et al. Effect of intravenous albumin on renal impairment and mortality in patients with cirrhosis and spontaneous bacterial peritonitis. N Engl J Med. 1999;341(6):403–9.
57. Poca M, Concepcion M, Casas M, et al. Role of albumin treatment in patients with spontaneous bacterial peritonitis. Clin Gastroenterol Hepatol. 2012;10(3):309–15.
58. Arvaniti V, D'Amico G, Fede G, et al. Infections in patients with cirrhosis increase mortality four-fold and should be used in determining prognosis. Gastroenterology. 2010;139(4):1246, 1256.
59. Vilstrup H, Amodio P, Bajaj J, et al. Hepatic encephalopathy in chronic liver disease: 2014 practice guideline by the American Association for the Study of Liver Diseases and the European Association for the Study of the Liver. Hepatology. 2014;60(2):715–35.
60. Amodio P, Del PF, Petteno E, et al. Prevalence and prognostic value of quantified electroencephalogram (EEG) alterations in cirrhotic patients. J Hepatol. 2001;35(1):37–45.
61. Cordoba J, Minguez B. Hepatic encephalopathy. Semin Liver Dis. 2008;28(1):70–80.
62. Olde Damink SW, Jalan R, Deutz NE, et al. The kidney plays a major role in the hyperammonemia seen after simulated or actual GI bleeding in patients with cirrhosis. Hepatology. 2003;37(6):1277–85.
63. Shawcross DL, Davies NA, Williams R, Jalan R. Systemic inflammatory response exacerbates the neuropsychological effects of induced hyperammonemia in cirrhosis. J Hepatol. 2004;40(2):247–54.
64. Cordoba J, Ventura-Cots M, Simon-Talero M, et al. Characteristics, risk factors, and mortality of cirrhotic patients hospitalized for hepatic encephalopathy with and without acute-on-chronic liver failure (ACLF). J Hepatol. 2014;60(2):275–81.
65. Vilstrup H, Schousboe A. Hepatic encephalopathy: an enigma from patient to enzyme and back. Metab Brain Dis. 2013;28(2):117.
66. Feltracco P, Cagnin A, Carollo C, Barbieri S, Ori C. Neurological disorders in liver transplant candidates: Pathophysiology and clinical assessment. Transplant Rev (Orlando). 2017;31(3):193–206.
67. Zardi EM, Abbate A, Zardi DM, et al. Cirrhotic cardiomyopathy. J Am Coll Cardiol. 2010;56(7):539–49.
68. Torregrosa M, Aguade S, Dos L, et al. Cardiac alterations in cirrhosis: reversibility after liver transplantation. J Hepatol. 2005;42(1):68–74.
69. Machicao VI, Balakrishnan M, Fallon MB. Pulmonary complications in chronic liver disease. Hepatology. 2014;59(4):1627–37.
70. Montano-Loza AJ, Meza-Junco J, Prado CM, et al. Muscle wasting is associated with mortality in patients with cirrhosis. Clin Gastroenterol Hepatol. 2012;10(2):166–73, 173.
71. Lucidi C, Lattanzi B, Di G. V et al. A low muscle mass increases mortality in compensated cirrhotic patients with sepsis. Liver Int. 2018;38(5):851–7.
72. Ebadi M, Tandon P, Moctezuma-Velazquez C, et al. Low subcutaneous adiposity associates with higher mortality in female patients with cirrhosis. J Hepatol. 2018;69(3):608–16.
73. EASL. Clinical practice guidelines on nutrition in chronic liver disease. J Hepatol. 2019;70(1):172–93.
74. Amodio P, Bemeur C, Butterworth R, et al. The nutritional management of hepatic encephalopathy in patients with cirrhosis: International Society for Hepatic Encephalopathy and Nitrogen Metabolism Consensus. Hepatology. 2013;58(1):325–36.
75. Les I, Doval E, Garcia-Martinez R, et al. Effects of branched-chain amino acids supplementation in patients with cirrhosis and a previous episode of hepatic encephalopathy: a randomized study. Am J Gastroenterol. 2011;106(6):1081–8.
76. Roman E, Garcia-Galceran C, Torrades T, et al. Effects of an exercise programme on functional capacity, body composition and risk of falls in patients with cirrhosis: a randomized clinical trial. PLoS One. 2016;11(3):e0151652.
77. Patel N, Muoz SJ. Bone disease in cirrhosis. Clin Liver Dis. 2015;6(4):96–9.
78. Handzlik-Orlik G, Holecki M, Wilczynski K, Dulawa J. Osteoporosis in liver disease: pathogenesis and management. Ther Adv Endocrinol Metab. 2016;7(3):128–35.
79. Elkrief L, Rautou PE, Sarin S, Valla D, Paradis V, Moreau R. Diabetes mellitus in patients with cirrhosis: clinical implications and management. Liver Int. 2016;36(7):936–48.
80. Burra P. Liver abnormalities and endocrine diseases. Best Pract Res Clin Gastroenterol. 2013;27(4):553–63.
81. Diaz-Fontenla F, Castillo-Pradillo M, Diaz-Gomez A, et al. Refractory hepatic encephalopathy in a patient with hypothyroidism: Another element in ammonia metabolism. World J Gastroenterol. 2017;23(28):5246–52.

82. Marks PW. Hematologic manifestations of liver disease. Semin Hematol. 2013;50(3):216–21.
83. Tripodi A, Primignani M, Mannucci PM, Caldwell SH. Changing concepts of cirrhotic coagulopathy. Am J Gastroenterol. 2016;112:274.
84. Ghosn SH, Kibbi AG. Cutaneous manifestations of liver diseases. Clin Dermatol. 2008;26(3):274–82.
85. EASL. EASL clinical practice guidelines: management of hepatocellular carcinoma. J Hepatol. 2018;69(1):182–236.
86. Bajaj JS, Moreau R, Kamath PS, et al. Acute-on-chronic liver failure: getting ready for prime-time. Hepatology. 2018;68(4):1621–32.
87. Gustot T, Fernandez J, Garcia E, et al. Clinical course of acute-on-chronic liver failure syndrome and effects on prognosis. Hepatology. 2015;62(1):243–52.
88. Artru F, Louvet A, Ruiz I, et al. Liver transplantation in the most severely ill cirrhotic patients: a multicenter study in acute-on-chronic liver failure grade 3. J Hepatol. 2017;67(4):708–15.
89. Levesque E, Winter A, Noorah Z, et al. Impact of acute-on-chronic liver failure on 90-day mortality following a first liver transplantation. Liver Int. 2017;37(5):684–93.
90. Putignano A, Gustot T. New concepts in acute-on-chronic liver failure: implications for liver transplantation. Liver Transpl. 2017;23(2):234–43.
91. Fagundes C, Barreto R, Guevara M, et al. A modified acute kidney injury classification for diagnosis and risk stratification of impairment of kidney function in cirrhosis. J Hepatol. 2013;59(3):474–81.

Further Reading and Related Links

http://www.efclif.com/

https://www.gastrojournal.org/article/S0016-5085(13)00291-6/pdf

https://www.journal-of-hepatology.eu/article/S0168-8278(18)31966-4/pdf

https://www.journal-of-hepatology.eu/article/S0168-8278(15)00349-9/pdf

https://www.journal-of-hepatology.eu/article/S0168-8278(14)00390-0/pdf

https://www.ncbi.nlm.nih.gov/pubmed/27277335

Part II

Diagnostic Methods

History and Physical Examination

34

Ana-Maria Vintilă, Mihaela Horumbă, and Vlad Damian Vintilă

Abbreviations

BMI	Body mass index
HCC	Hepatocellular carcinoma
HCV	Hepatitis C virus
VEGF	Vascular endothelial growth factor

Key Concepts

- A thorough history should be obtained, including information about alcohol and drug abuse, exposure to blood products and family history of liver disease.
- Fever is a sign of either acute hepatic necrosis or bacterial involvement in a coexisting liver condition (cholecystitis or cholangitis).
- The combination of spider nevi, Dupuytren contracture and ascites is common in patients with alcoholic cirrhosis.
- The color of urine and stool may help orient the diagnosis in a patient with jaundice.

A.-M. Vintilă (✉)
Carol Davila University of Medicine and Pharmacy, Bucharest, Romania

Department of Internal Medicine and Cardiology, Colțea Clinical Hospital, Bucharest, Romania

M. Horumbă
Department of Internal Medicine and Cardiology, Colțea Clinical Hospital, Bucharest, Romania

V. D. Vintilă
Carol Davila University of Medicine and Pharmacy, Bucharest, Romania

Department of Cardiology, Emergency University Hospital, Bucharest, Romania

34.1 Introduction

Chronic liver disease and cirrhosis were listed, in 2015 as the fifth leading cause of death in the United States in people aged 25–44 and the fourth in 45–65 year-olds [1], rendering this condition one of particular importance in terms of early diagnosis and treatment. Cirrhosis is the result of long-standing liver injury caused by alcohol consumption, chronic hepatitis or non-alcoholic fatty liver disease. Other, less common causes of chronic liver failure are Wilson's disease, hemochromatosis and primary biliary cirrhosis etc.

Cirrhosis is often asymptomatic for many years; symptoms only occur once 80–90% of the liver parenchyma has been destroyed [2].

History taking should include questions regarding risk factors such as alcohol consumption, preexisting autoimmune disorders, workplace or sexual exposure to viral infections, tattoos, piercings, travel history to endemic areas, intravenous drug use, previous transfusions or dental work and last, but not least, family history of liver disease. Further information should be obtained about ongoing medication, including herbal remedies and over the counter drugs. In cases where alcohol abuse is suspected, focused questioning should collect data on the quantity, frequency, pattern of drinking, changes in behavior, feelings of guilt and difficulty in maintaining relationships or adequate work performance.

34.2 Symptoms of Liver Disease

Early signs of liver disease include loss of appetite (anorexia), weakness (asthenia) and fatigue, while patients with end-stage liver disease may show signs of portal hypertension (ascites, variceal bleeding etc.) or patent hepatocellular failure (ecchymoses, jaundice, encephalopathy etc.).

Abdominal pain associated with liver disease may have a variety of different causes.

The liver parenchyma lacks nerve fibers thus is unable to elicit pain; however, the acute distention of the liver capsule

F. Radu-Ionita et al. (eds.), *Liver Diseases*, https://doi.org/10.1007/978-3-030-24432-3_34

produces dull pain in the epigastrium or right upper quadrant accentuated by palpation or percussion. Capsular distention occurs in acute hepatitis, neoplasia and acute congestion (in Budd-Chiari syndrome due to hepatic vein occlusion or right-sided heart failure).

Chronic liver disorders like non-alcoholic fatty liver disease and chronic hepatitis may produce vague discomfort in the epigastric region and right upper quadrant without any specific aggravating or alleviating factors.

Episodic, steady epigastric or right upper quadrant pain, radiating to the back or chest, with an abrupt onset and lasting for at least 30 min, after a fatty meal, with or without nausea and vomiting, may be a sign of gallbladder dysfunction. In a patient running a fever and a painful episode lasting longer than six hours, acute cholecystitis may be suspected. Sharp pain irradiating along the entire upper abdomen in a patient previously known with gallstones may indicate acute pancreatitis. Moreover, gallbladder dyskinesia or chronic acalculous gallbladder dysfunction may produce a similar type of pain in patients without ultrasound evidence of lithiasis and normal liver and pancreatic tests [3].

Fatigue, appetite loss (anorexia) and **malaise** are non-specific symptoms common in patients with liver disease, but may also occur in patients with unrelated disorders such a neoplasia or tuberculosis. **Weight gain** may be encountered in patients with ascites due to an increase in the amount of intraabdominal fluid and not fatty deposits. Moreover, patients with cirrhosis exhibit wasting of fat and muscle mass, leading to cachexia through a combination of reduced food intake (anorexia) and malabsorption, both due to frequent episodes of endotoxinemia [4].

Nausea and **vomiting** may occur in acute inflammation of intraabdominal organs (acute hepatitis, cholecystitis, pancreatitis), and do not necessarily alleviate the abdominal discomfort they accompany. Therefore, nausea and vomiting with an abrupt onset, following a large meal, hint to gallbladder dysfunction. Moreover, patients with portal hypertension and ruptured esophageal varices may vomit blood (**hematemesis**).

Fever (pyrexia) may be a sign of acute hepatic necrosis (hepatitis), be it of viral, alcoholic or drug induced etiology or bacterial infection as is the case in cholecystitis, cholangitis and spontaneous bacterial peritonitis. Moreover, prolonged fever could be associated with liver abscess or neoplasia.

Encephalopathy is a neuropsychiatric complication of liver failure. Ammonia buildup has been linked to encephalopathy and may be caused by a high protein diet, infection, gastrointestinal bleeding or constipation. Patients with low grade encephalopathy present with a disturbance in sleep patterns characterised by nocturnal insomnia and daytime drowsiness. According to the time elapsed between the onset of liver failure and the development of encephalopathy, liver failure may be classified into: hyperacute (less than 7 days), acute (8–28 days) and subacute (more than 28 days) [5]. Fulminant liver failure may be induced by viral hepatitis (hepatitis A and E in endemic regions through a fecal-oral route or hepatitis B and C via contact with infected bodily fluids), toxic agents like acetaminophen (either through accidental overdose or after attempted suicide), ischemic hepatitis, autoimmune hepatitis, Wilson disease, Budd-Chiari syndrome, neoplasia or sepsis. Pregnancy-related acute liver failure is due to acute fatty liver, HELLP syndrome (hemolysis, elevated liver enzymes, and low platelets) or eclampsia.

34.3 Clinical Examination in Liver Disease

A complete physical examination should be performed in the patient with suspected liver disease, including inspection, palpation, percussion and auscultation (Fig. 34.1).

> The room in which the clinical examination is to take place must be well lit (preferably by natural light), and the room temperature should be adequate so as not to make the patient uncomfortable. The patient should lie supine with arms outstretched, completely relaxed. The examiner may ask the patient to bend their knees so as to further relax the abdominal muscles. Avoid allowing the patient to observe the clinical maneuvers as neck flexing may hinder relaxation of the abdomen. The examiner will stand to the patient's right side, introduce themselves and ask for permission to perform the clinical exam.

34.3.1 Auscultation

The auscultation of the abdomen provides little information but should be performed before other maneuvers as palpation and percussion may shift intraabdominal gas.

An accentuation of **intestinal sounds** may be present in diarrheic syndromes associated with acute hepatitis.

A **peritoneal rub** is a scratchy sound produced by fibrin buildup (similar to pericardial or pleural rubs) audible after liver infarcts, in acute inflammation or cancer; the sound is more evident with the patient's breathing as the intraabdominal organs shift with the movement of the diaphragm.

A **hepatic arterial bruit** is a systolic murmur audible over the projection of the liver due to an increase in arterial blood flow. Primary and metastatic tumors produce arterial bruits as a consequence of neovasculature, while cirrhosis and liver cancer may hinder arterial flow through the presence of regeneration or neoplastic nodules.

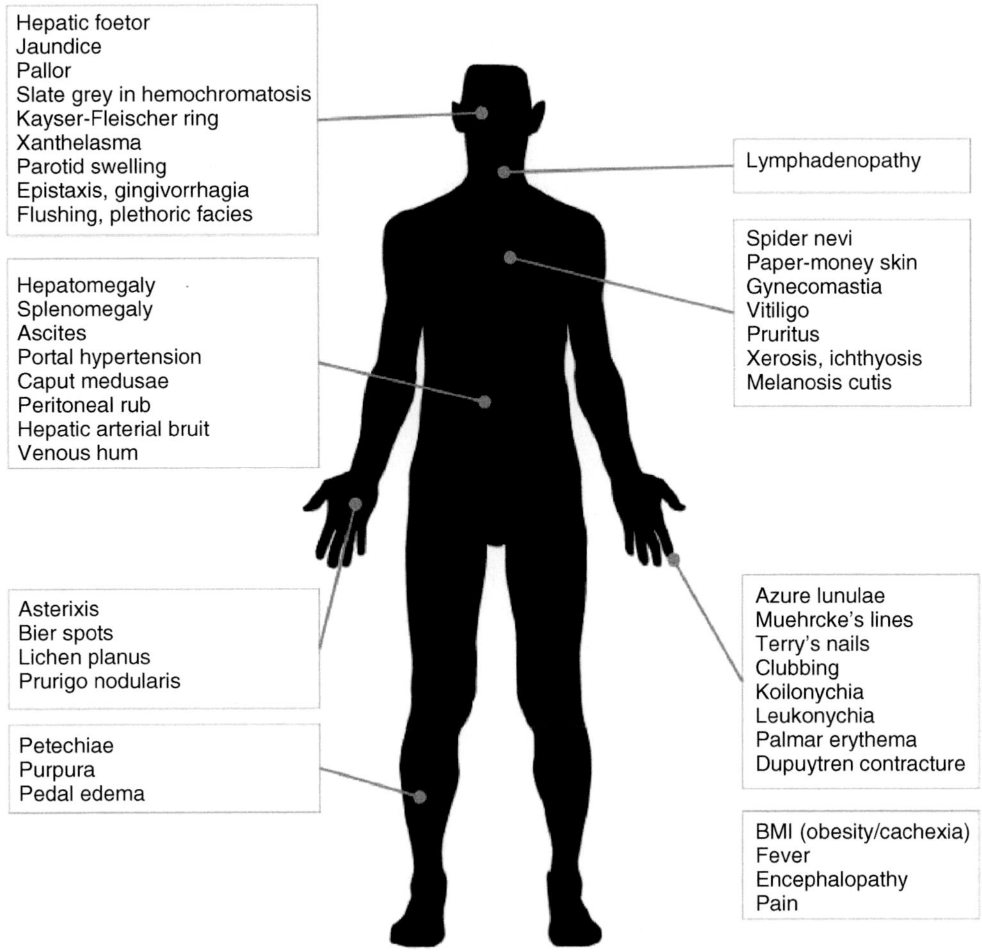

Fig. 34.1 Clinical examination in a patient with liver disease

A **venous hum** is a low frequency, continuous hum heard over the epigastrium or right upper quadrant due to a well-developed collateral circulation in portal hypertension. **Cruveilhier-Baumgarten disease** is the association of a congenitally atrophic liver with a patent umbilical vein that produce portal hypertension and an abdominal venous hum. If, however, portal hypertension and the abdominal venous hum result from other causes of liver disease, the term used is **Cruveilhier-Baumgartner syndrome** [6].

In order to examine the mucosae, ask the patient to sit in natural lighting and look upward; retract the lower lid in order to expose the conjunctiva and the sclera. Furthermore, ask the patient to extend their tongue and examine the hard palate, then ask the patient to touch the tip of their tongue to the roof of the mouth in order to examine de sublingual mucosa.

34.3.2 Inspection

Note must be made of the general aspect of the patient, cutaneous and mucosal lesions, shape of the abdomen, scars and stretch marks (rapid accumulation of fluid), respiratory movement, presence of peristalsis and aspect of the umbilicus. Care must be taken in order to identify both direct and indirect signs of liver disease. Occasionally, gross hepatomegaly or splenomegaly may be observed through inspection of the abdomen as a bulge in the upper right or left quadrant, respectively.

Hepatic foetor is a form of halitosis specific to patients with liver disease, generally associated with a higher concentration of mercaptan produced in the bowel which the liver cannot fully process; it may be encountered in patients with liver necrosis and/or significant portal hypertension.

Asterixis (**flapping tremor**) is a jerky rhythmical tremor perceived due to periodic brief pauses in striated muscle activity. Asterixis may also be encountered in hyponatremia, hypoglycemia and non-ketonic hyperglycemia [7], however, when associated with liver disease it is a sign of hepatic **encephalopathy** (Table 34.1).

Ask the patient to sit, extend their arms, dorsiflex the hands and close their eyes.

Table 34.1 Grading of encephalopathy according to mental status and presence of asterixis [8]

Grade	Description
0	Normal mental status. Asterixis absent
1	Mild confusion. Asterixis can be detected
2	Lethargy with inappropriate behaviors. Obvious asterixis
3	Somnolent with incomprehensible speech and marked confusion
4	Coma

Jaundice (icterus) is the yellowish discoloration of the skin and mucosae due to accumulation of bilirubin over the threshold of 2.5–3 mg/dl (Fig. 34.2 - panel A). According to the type of bilirubin—direct, indirect or both, jaundice may be classified into:

- prehepatic jaundice is due to erythrocyte destruction: extravascular hemolysis takes place in the reticuloendothelial cells of the spleen, liver or bone marrow; it is a process through which senescent or damaged cells undergo apoptosis. Hemolytic anemia is caused by destruction of abnormal red blood cells and leads to a pale yellow discoloration of the skin and mucosae due to a combination of hyperbilirubinemia and anemia.
- hepatocellular jaundice is due to chronic liver disease where the rate of bilirubin formation surpasses the rate of conjugation, leading to the accumulation of both direct and indirect bilirubin. In cirrhosis, portosystemic shunts lead to decreased blood flow to the hepatocytes and a lower conjugation rate. In congenital conjugation defects such as Gilbert and Crigler-Najjar syndromes, hyperbilirubinemia is due solely to unconjugated bilirubin [9]. Rotor and Dubin-Johnson syndromes are characterized by conjugated non-hemolytic hyperbilirubinemia due to defects in biliary transport and hepatic storage of conjugated bilirubin respectively [10].
- posthepatic jaundice is a result of cholestasis and, due to the accumulation of bile salts in the skin, has a slightly greenish tint; moreover, the high levels of urobilin determine alterations in the color of urine and stool (see below). A rare, intriguing condition consisting of hemolytic anemia, cholestatic jaundice and transient hyperlipidemia occurring after alcohol abuse is named **Zieve's syndrome** [11].
- **Urine semiology**—the color of urine may be influenced by the presence of bilirubin or urobilin; hence, in patients with hemolytic anemia, due to the high urobilin content, urine appears reddish while in patients with cholestasis urine is dark, due to the high bilirubin content, and frothy due to bile salts.
- **Stool semiology**—depending on the presence of stercobilin (after intestinal reduction of colorless urobilin), stool may be helpful in diagnosing liver pathology. Thus, a darker stool due to stercobilin excess may be encountered in patients with hemolytic anemia; in cases of cholestasis the stool appears discolored, whitish. Moreover, in patients with variceal bleeding due to portal hypertension, the stool may be black (**melena**).

As a case in point, a patient presenting with jaundice, pale mucosae, who also exhibits reddish urine and dark stools may have hemolytic anemia, while a patient with cholestasis may exhibit a darker, greenish form of jaundice accompanied by dark, frothy urine and discolored stools.

Pallor is a sign of anemia. Liver disease may produce anemia through a variety of mechanisms: variceal bleeding, portal gastropathy, gingivorrhagia, epistaxis, hematuria, hypersplenism and hepatic malignancy. Variceal bleeding is often of abrupt onset and may manifest in patients with significant portal hypertension. Tachycardia and orthostatic hypotension hint to a large amount of blood lost, usually through either hematemesis or melena.

In a well lit room, ask the patient to look up over their head and carefully draw their lower eyelid so as to expose the conjunctiva; ask the patient to extend their arms and supinate the wrists so as to examine the palms; ask the patient to touch the tip of their tongue to the roof of their mouth.

Hemorrhage under the skin may be due to thrombocytopenia (hypersplenism, reduction in hepatic synthesis of thrombopoietin, bone marrow micromedium disturbance by hepatitis C virus) or defects in the synthesis/consumption of clotting factors (coagulopathy or disseminated intravascular coagulopathy). Skin lesions vary from **petechiae** (small—<3 mm, round, non-confluent, reddish spots disseminated on the limbs or abdomen) to **purpura** (3–10 mm in size, resulted from petechial confluence) and **ecchymoses** (patches of varying sizes, usually over 1 cm, with colors ranging from red to purple to green to yellow according to the degree of red blood cell destruction in the local macrophages and bilirubin formation [9]—thus acting like time stamps for previous trauma). None of the above mentioned lesions blanches on pressure (as opposed to spider angiomata).

Ascites is due to intraabdominal accumulation of fluid with subsequent bilateral flank bulging. Large ascites may hinder the movement of the patient and tense ascites may push out the umbilicus, resulting in an umbilical hernia. For clinical signs of ascites to be present, a minimum quantity of 1500 ml of liquid must accumulate [2].

Spider nevi (*sg. **nevus***) also known as **spider angiomata** (*sg. **angioma***) are dilated, superficial arterioles that appear as reddish spots with fine branching vessels radiating outward (Fig. 34.2 - panel C); these telangiectasias are found on the upper half of the body—trunk, arms and face—the distribution territory of the superior vena cava. The preferential disposition is based on regional differences in peripheral circulation, a consequence of variation in sympathetic nervous system reactivity in patients with liver cirrhosis [12, 13]. Though mucosal distribution is uncommon, case reports of massive bleeding from lesions of the colon or pleura have been cited. Furthermore, a higher prevalence of spider angiomata has been described in relation to young age and elevated VEGF (vascular endothelial growth factor) and to alcoholic etiology of liver disease due to the angiogenic properties of alcohol [12]. Their appearance is due to the increase in estradiol to testosterone ratio, secondary to impaired catabolism of androstenedione with consequent shunting of estrogen production and buildup of estradiol. Since estradiol buildup is the cause, spider nevi may also be encountered in young women taking oral contraceptives and during pregnancy in the absence of liver disease. They may also appear in patients with thyrotoxicosis and rheumatoid arthritis.

> Apply pressure onto the suspected lesion until it disappears; as the pressure stops, the spider nevus refills with blood from the central arteriole toward the periphery.

Paper-money skin is a condition associated with alcoholic cirrhosis and consists of numerous, fine superficial capillaries randomly dispersed over the torso. The name comes from the resemblance of the needle-like capillaries to the fine silk thread in dollar bills [12, 14, 15].

Bier spots are small, irregularly shaped areas of hypopigmentation found on the arms and legs, associated with small vessel damage and venous stasis in the skin.

> Apply pressure to Bier spots and, much like spider nevi, they disappear. Moreover, raising the limb causes the spots to disappear as opposed to true hypopigmentation.

Portal hypertension—Varicose veins become engorged due to portal hypertension and may be visible along the flanks (cavo-caval collateral circulation - Fig. 34.2, panel B, yellow arrows) or around the umbilicus (porto-caval collateral circulation - Fig. 34.2, panel B, red arrows). **Caput medusae** is a sign of severe portal hypertension, where varicose veins radiating from the umbilicus become engorged; the name originates from the Greek legend of Medusa whose hair had been turned into snakes (Fig. 34.2).

Flushing and plethoric facies are due to vasodilation occurring in the vessels of the face and are more common in alcoholic cirrhosis. Moreover, patients with a history of alcohol abuse tend to also exhibit sialadenosis—asymptomatic bilateral parotid gland enlargement that does not affect the function of the salivary gland. Historically, this condition has been attributed to a vitamin deficit due to its association with alcoholism, malnutrition, anorexia or bulimia nervosa [16].

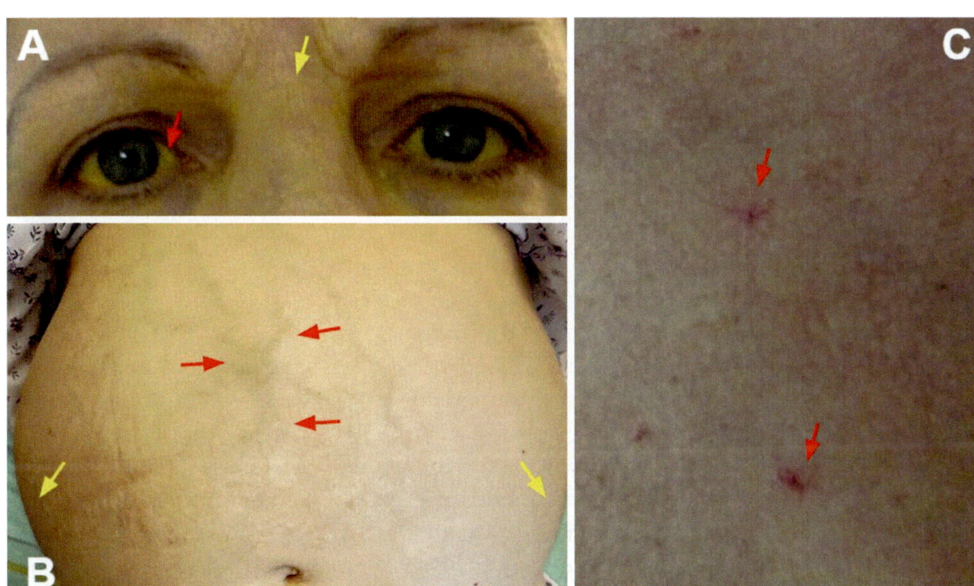

Fig. 34.2 (**a**) Jaundice as seen in the sclera (red arrow) and skin (yellow arrow); (**b**) porto-caval collateral circulation (red arrows) in a patient with voluminous ascites and flank bulging (yellow arrows); (**c**) spider angiomata. Source: personal collection of author

Palmar erythema is a symmetrical, non-pruritic, non-painful, non-scaling, slightly warmer, reddish discoloration of the hypothenar/thenar eminence, palmar aspect of the phalanges or the dorsal surface of the proximal nail folds. It is due to a combination of local vasodilation, high cardiac output (hyperdynamic circulation) and estradiol buildup. This finding is also associated, though to a lower extent, with rheumatoid arthritis, thyrotoxicosis and diabetes mellitus, drug induced liver damage due to amiodarone or gemfibrozil. It may also occur in the absence of pathology as primary palmar erythema due to heredity, pregnancy or use of salbutamol [17].

Ask the patient to extend their arms, palm side up and observe the reddish discoloration of the thenar or hypothenar eminences, palmar aspect of the phalanges or proximal aspect of the dorsal phalanges.

Dupuytren contracture is the progressive fibrosis of the tendons in the palmar fascia with subsequent retraction of fingers and phalangeal ankylosis and is common in alcoholic liver disease. Other risk factors for Dupuytren's contracture include: age (>50 years), gender (higher incidence in men), ancestry (familial aggregation, more common in North European), tobacco use and diabetes (probably due to microangiopathy). Fasciectomy may be curative in these patients [14].

Have the patient extend their fingers, palm side up; if one or more fingers cannot be extended and the tendon is visible as a firm, non-painful structure under the skin, the patient has Dupuytren contracture. The differential diagnosis must include stenosing tenosynovitis (pain and overuse), trigger finger (pain upon flexion), a ganglion cyst (small, mobile, tender nodule) or a soft tissue mass.

Gynecomastia is the enlargement of the male breast secondary to hyperestrogenism—glandular tissue may be palpated around the areola and it must be differentiated from lipomastia, where the breast becomes enlarged due to disposition of subcutaneous fat tissue in patients with obesity. Furthermore, spironolactone, a drug commonly used in cirrhosis and a known inhibitor of testosterone synthesis may give rise to gynecomastia and mastodynia. Additional signs of hyperestrogenism are testicular atrophy, loss of axillary and pubic hair and female distribution of hair.

Xanthelasma are non-pruritic, yellowish, soft plaques due to cholesterol deposits in the histiocytes of the eyelids [15]. **Xantomata** (sg. **xantoma**) have a similar appearance, though may be larger in side and are cholesterol deposits commonly located on the extensor surface of upper or lower limbs. Both lesions are indicative of hypercholesterolemia and may be associated with primary biliary cirrhosis [14, 15].

Vitiligo is an autoimmune condition where patches of hypopigmentation appear on the skin and may be associated with other autoimmune phenomena such as hepatitis or primary biliary cirrhosis. Interferon-induced vitiligo is associated with hepatitis C infection treated with interferon and the lesions resolve with treatment interruption.

Pruritus manifests through itchiness of the palms, soles or back. Though a definite etiology has yet to be established, the current theory is that pruritus may be a result of bile salts buildup in the skin and consequent activation of opioid receptors. Henceforth, the current treatments include bile salts sequestrants such as cholestyramine and serotonin reuptake inhibitors or opioid antagonists [18].

- **Prurigo nodularis** are pruritic nodules associated with hepatitis C or HIV infection, bacterial infection or kidney failure. Treatment consists of topic steroids and antihistamines; low doses of thalidomide have been proven to be safe and effective [14].
- **Lichen planus** is a lesion associated with HCV infection, described by the "5 P's": pruritic, planar, polygonal, purple papules [14]; it often affects the wrists or ankles and may resolve by itself within 6 months or become chronic and lead to scaling and atrophy of the skin, especially if found on the scalp—lichen planopilaris.

Ask the patient about an itching sensation; useful instruments are the Visual Analog Scale (VAS) and the 5-D itch scale (Duration, Degree, Direction, Distribution, Disability) in order to determine the extents of symptoms and their impact on quality of life [19]. Furthermore, examine the skin for scratch marks (excoriations).

Cutaneous xerosis is one of the most common findings in chronic liver disease with a cited prevalence of up to 72% [18]. Xerosis or dry skin is due to the disruption of the stratum corneum, dehydration and altered differentiation of keratinocytes and may also be encountered in various dermatoses or otherwise healthy patients.

Melanosis cutis is due to excessive melanin secretion from giant melanosomes [12] which leads to hyperpigmentation of palmar creases and accentuation of perioral, periorbital and areolar hyperpigmentation; these pigmentary lesions are more evident in primary biliary cirrhosis and alcoholic liver disease.

Hemochromatosis used to be known as "bronze diabetes" due to accumulation of iron in the skin causing "slate grey" [20] or brown-bronze hyperpigmentation in areas exposed to sunlight. The iron deposits in the skin induce excess melanin production in response to UV light. Treatment of iron overload may alleviate organ function (as excess iron is also stored in other organs) but cutaneous manifestations are less responsive [14].

Ichthyosis is another finding related to hemochromatosis and leads to dry, scale-like skin [14].

Porphyria cutanea tarda leads to blistering of the skin after exposure to sun light and eventually increase of local hair growth [20]; there is a defect in heme synthesis due to the liver's inability to produce uroporphyrin-decarboxylase and, though it is associated with liver disease in general, there seems to be a higher prevalence among patients with chronic hepatitis C infection [14].

Disseminated superficial porokeratosis—white, scaly papules that coalesce into plaques and are due to a keratinization defect of monoclonal origin that may evolve into squamous cell carcinoma; it is associated with alcoholic liver disease; once liver function is restored the skin lesions also improve [14].

Necrolytic acral erythema presents as erythematous plaques with or without scales and a burning sensation, affecting mainly the dorsal aspect of the feet, particularly the halluces and is characteristic of hepatitis C infection.

Kayser-Fleischer ring is the brown-green discoloration surrounding the pupil in patients with Wilson's disease and is due to copper accumulation.

Azure lunulae represent the bluish discoloration of the lunulae occurring in Wilson's disease [21].

Muehrcke's nails are paired horizontal white bands separated by normal color [2] caused by hypoalbuminemia (<2.2 g/dl) [12]; they are also common in nephrotic syndrome, glomerulonephritis and malnutrition.

Terry's nails—ground-glass opacity of the nail plate with no visible lunula and a narrow strip of sparred nail at the distal end (due to hyperplasia of the nail bed connective tissue [2, 12, 14]. Though classically associated with chronic liver disease, they may also be seen in chronic heart failure, thyrotoxicosis, renal failure, adult-onset diabetes mellitus and with advanced age [12]. The differential diagnosis includes half-and-half nails (opacification of half the nail plate) and true **leukonychia** (abnormality of the nail plate rather than the nail bed) [22].

34.3.3 Palpation

Palpation is the most important maneuver used in the clinical examination of the abdomen. In describing intraabdominal organs, note must be made of the dimensions, consistency, characters of the lower edge and presence of tenderness.

> Palpation of the abdomen is done with the palm extended, moving in small circles in order to detect any change in size or shape.

The patient must be asked beforehand about the existence of spontaneous abdominal pain and examination must start from the opposite side, leaving the painful area toward the end of the examination. Touch must be gentle in order to avoid unnecessary discomfort and the patient's face must be carefully observed for any sign of pain; all the while the examiner must ask questions in order to deter attention from the examination and differentiate real from simulated pain.

> Palpation of the liver is done with both hands pointing upward toward the rib cage, starting from the flank and slowly moving cranially. Only in the case that the liver cannot be felt using this maneuver, the examiner may stand facing the patient's feet and, using flexed hands as a hook may try to sense the inferior margin as it lowers during inspiration. Obese patients may be examined using a left lateral decubitus that helps to shift the abdominal fat toward away from the viscera.

Palpation allows for the assessment of the inferior edge of the liver along the right coastal margin toward the epigastric region. In patients without an underlying hepatic pathology, due to its soft consistency, the liver is difficult to palpate and is non-tender.

Dimension assessment includes the diameters measured along the midclavicular line (between the superior—generally in the fifth intercostal space—and inferior liver edges, normally spanning 7–12 cm) and the midsternal line (between the cardiohepatic angle obtained through percussion and the inferior liver edge, spanning 6–8 cm). A size greater than normal exposes **hepatomegaly** (acute hepatitis, non-alcoholic fatty liver disease and liver malignancy), while a smaller than normal liver may reveal **hepatic atrophy** (some forms of cirrhosis).

The inferior liver edge may vary in **shape** and **consistency**: a round inferior edge may be encountered in acute (soft consistency) or chronic hepatitis (firm consistency), while in patients with cirrhosis the edge may become sharp.

The **surface** may provide additional information: thus, a smooth surface is encountered in chronic hepatitis and non-alcoholic fatty liver disease, while a nodular surface may be present in patients with cirrhosis or HCC (hepatocellular carcinoma).

Tenderness on palpation is indicative of capsule dilation and should orient the diagnosis toward either acute hepatitis or tumors with capsular involvement.

The gallbladder is not normally accessible to palpation. However, in specific cases, a round structure may be felt along the inferior margin of the liver—highly painful in acute cholecystitis, mildly tender in gallbladder hydrops (accumulation of sterile and colorless mucin through chronic cystic duct obstruction) and non-tender in pancreatic cancer (Courvoisier-Terrier sign) or a highly calcific gallbladder.

Since the normal spleen lies behind the rib cage, a spleen accessible on palpation automatically diagnoses **splenomegaly**.

The patient lies in a right lateral decubitus with the left arm outstretched over their head; the examiner may palpate the spleen from the patient's right side or try to hook it from the left. One must keep in mind that the anterior margin of the spleen is irregular and moves anteriorly and caudally with inspiration.

Lymphadenopathy in a patient presenting with jaundice may raise the clinical suspicion of epidemic hepatitis or a viral infection such as infectious mononucleosis. **Generalized lymphadenopathy** is more commonly associated with malignant processes that may also affect the liver such as lymphoma.

Use the pads of all four fingers in a circular fashion along the anterior and posterior regions of the neck and jaw, axillae, elbows, inguinal region and knees.

Pedal edema is due to the accumulation of free fluid in the interstitium; in liver disease, pedal edema is associated with a decrease in oncotic pressure (the pressure that normally maintains fluid inside the blood vessels) due to faulty production of albumin.

Ask the patient to lie in bed with legs outstretched; press your thumb against the tibial surface so as to force the fluid out of the interstitium. In a patient with pedal edema pitting will be elicited.

34.3.4 Percussion

Percussion of the abdomen is a useful tool in determining approximate organ size and the presence of intraabdominal fluid.

Percussion is done in a radial fashion starting from the umbilicus, radiating outward to every segment of the abdomen. If dullness is detected, percussion will be repeated from the epigastrium in a radial fashion toward the mesogastrium and flanks so as to delineate the upper limit of the intraabdominal fluid.

The distance between the upper limit of the free intraperitoneal fluid and a horizontal line drawn through the umbilicus is used to measure the amount of fluid.

Flank dullness—percuss the patient in a supine position; tympany is noted periumbilically, while the flanks remain dull.

Shifting dullness—the patient is asked to roll into lateral decubitus first onto the right side, then onto the left; while in a lateral decubitus position, percussion will find that tympany has moved upward, while dullness has shifted to the flank according to the repositioning of the intraabdominal fluid.

The **wave sign** is elicited by asking a partner to push their hands down the midline of the abdomen, while the examiner taps one side of the abdomen all the while palpating the opposite side of the abdomen; a wave of ascites is perceived by the examiner's hand as the impulse is transmitted through the fluid.

The puddle sign—ask the patient to assume the genupectoral position (on elbows and knees) and percuss periumbilically—dullness is noted due to the shifting of the ascites; this position is particularly useful in patients with a small quantity of ascites.

Percussion of the liver helps establish the upper and lower limits of the liver.

> The upper margin may be found by percussing along the right midclavicular line from the second intercostal space caudally—generally located in the fifth intercostal space. By continuing toward the flank, the examiner will encounter the inferior liver margin at the interface of dullness and tympany.

The lower hepatic edge is generally situated within 1 cm of the rib cage. A lower edge beyond the 1 cm limit may reveal either **hepatomegaly** or **liver ptosis** (the upper limit is also shifted caudally in case of ptosis). Percussion of the lower edge is of particular importance in cases where the liver is not readily accessible by palpation. In Chilaiditi syndrome, the colon is interposed between the skin and the hepatic parenchyma, rendering percussion ineffective.

Percussion of the spleen helps identify splenomegaly, either a consequence of portal hypertension or a sign of hematologic malignancy.

> **Castell's method**. With the patient supine, percussion will be performed along the left anterior axillary line in the lowest intercostal space, after full inspiration followed by full expiration—shifting from tympany to dullness is called Castell's sign and signals **splenomegaly**.
>
> **Traube's (semilunar) space** is defined by the sixth rib (sup.), left midaxillary line (lateral) and left costal margin (inferior). With the patient supine and left arm abducted, percuss Traube's space from its medial to its lateral aspect—dullness during normal breathing will signal **splenomegaly**.
>
> **Nixon's method**: Ask the patient to sit in a right lateral decubitus with the left arm in an abducted position. Percuss along the posterior axillary line for the lowest level of pulmonary resonance. Proceed diagonally toward the left costal margin. The normal spleen produces an area of dullness 6–8 cm above the left costal margin, a greater size reveals **splenomegaly**.

34.4 Conclusions/Summary

Due to its high prevalence and mortality, liver disease is of particular importance nowadays. Thus, physicians must maintain a high index of suspicion, actively enquire about risk factors and perform a thorough clinical examination so as to diagnose liver disease from its earliest signs. The most common disorders of the liver—acute hepatitis, cirrhosis and HCC—vary in terms of clinical presentation and faster diagnosis and treatment may be instated after careful examination of the patient.

Self Study

Questions

1. Which of the following statements is true?
   (a) An abdominal venous hum may be encountered in patients with acute hepatitis
   (b) Infection with HCV may be present with a plethora of cutaneous manifestations like lichen planus, porphyria cutanea tarda and necrolytic acral erythema
   (c) Posthepatic jaundice is due to the accumulation of unconjugated bilirubin, made evident by a reddish discoloration of urine and clay-colored stools
   (d) A patient presenting with fever and ascites is more likely to have acute cholecystitis than spontaneous bacterial peritonitis
2. Which of the following statements is true?
   (a) The spleen will be examined with the patient in an erect position as this brings the inferior pole closer to the examiner
   (b) The genupectoral position is most commonly used for assessment of ascites, especially in patients with tense ascites
   (c) In examining the liver note must be taken of the dimensions, consistency, surface, character of the inferior edge and tenderness
   (d) The presence of asterixis is assessed by gently pulling down the patient's eyelid so as to be able to observe both the conjunctiva and the sclera

Answers

1. Which of the following statements is true?
   (a) An abdominal venous hum may be encountered in patients with portal hypertension as a consequence of a well-developed collateral circulation
   (b) Infection with HCV may be present with a plethora of cutaneous manifestations like lichen planus, porphyria cutanea tarda and necrolytic acral erythema—CORRECT
   (c) Posthepatic jaundice is due to extrahepatic obstruction of the bile ducts, thus leading to a rise in conjugated bilirubin with dark, frothy urine and clay-colored stools

(d) A patient presenting with fever and ascites is more likely to have spontaneous bacterial peritonitis; in patients with decompensated cirrhosis, ascites is likely to get infected leading to abdominal pain, fever and signs of peritoneal irritation

2. Which of the following statements is true?
   (a) The spleen will be examined with the patient in a recumbent position, in a left lateral decubitus, so as to shift the intraabdominal fat and fluid and allow for a correct assessment of the spleen
   (b) The genupectoral position is sometimes used to certify the existence of a small quantity of intraabdominal fluid
   (c) In examining the liver note must be taken of the dimensions, consistency, surface, character of the inferior edge and tenderness—CORRECT
   (d) The presence of asterixis is assessed by asking the patient to hold their arms outstretched, wrists extended and fingers apart so as to reveal a fluttering of the phalanges associated with encephalopathy. The color of the sclera and the conjunctiva will be evaluated in order to diagnose jaundice and anemia.

References

1. National Center for Health Statistics (US). Health, United States, 2016: with chartbook on long-term trends in health. Hyattsville, MD: National Center for Health Statistics (US); 2017.
2. Heidelbaugh JJ, Bruderly M. Cirrhosis and chronic liver failure: part I. Diagnosis and evaluation. Am Fam Physician. 2006;74(5):756–62.
3. Hansel SL, DiBaise JK. Functional gallbladder disorder: gallbladder dyskinesia. Gastroenterol Clin N Am. 2010;39(2):369–79.
4. Plauth M, Schütz E-T. Cachexia in liver cirrhosis. Int J Cardiol. 2002;85(1):83–7.
5. Ostapowicz G, Fontana RJ, Schiødt FV, Larson A, Davern TJ, Han SH, et al. Results of a prospective study of acute liver failure at 17 tertiary care centers in the United States. Ann Intern Med. 2002;137(12):947–54.
6. Hardison JE. Auscultation of the liver. In: Walker HK, Hall WD, Hurst JW, editors. Clinical methods: the history, physical, and laboratory examinations. 3rd ed. Boston, MA: Butterworths; 1990.
7. Karnath B. Stigmata of chronic liver disease. MedGen. 2003;39(7):14–20.
8. Blei AT, Córdoba J, Gastroenterology PPCotACo. Hepatic encephalopathy. Am J Gastroenterol. 2001;96(7):1968–76.
9. Roy-Chowdhury N, Roy-Chowdhury J. Classification and causes of jaundice or asymptomatic hyperbilirubinemia. UpToDate. 2011;2011:1–11.
10. Strassburg CP. Hyperbilirubinemia syndromes (Gilbert-Meulengracht, Crigler-Najjar, Dubin-Johnson, and Rotor syndrome). Best Pract Res Clin Gastroenterol. 2010;24(5):555–71.
11. Liu M-X, Wen X-Y, Leung Y-K, Zheng Y-J, Jin M-S, Jin Q-L, et al. Hemolytic anemia in alcoholic liver disease: Zieve syndrome: a case report and literature review. Medicine (Baltimore). 2017;96(47):e8742.
12. Ghosn SH, Kibbi A-G. Cutaneous manifestations of liver diseases. Clin Dermatol. 2008;26(3):274–82.
13. Okumura H, Aramaki T, Katsuta Y, Terada H, Satomura K, Akaike M, et al. Regional differences in peripheral circulation between upper and lower extremity in patients with cirrhosis. Scand J Gastroenterol. 1990;25(9):883–9.
14. Hazin R, Abu-Rajab TT, Abuzetun JY, Zein NN. Recognizing and treating cutaneous signs of liver disease. Cleve Clin J Med. 2009;76(10):599–606.
15. Godara SK, Thappa DM, Pottakkatt B, Hamide A, Barath J, Munisamy M, et al. Cutaneous manifestations in disorders of hepatobiliary system. Indian Dermatol Online J. 2017;8(1):9.
16. Guggenheimer J, Close JM, Eghtesad B. Sialadenosis in patients with advanced liver disease. Head Neck Pathol. 2009;3(2):100–5.
17. Serrao R, Zirwas M, English JC. Palmar erythema. Am J Clin Dermatol. 2007;8(6):347–56.
18. Maia NC, Araújo FC, Pires CAA, Conde SRSS, Nunes HM, Soares MCP. Manifestações dermatológicas em uma casuística de doença hepática crônica de um hospital de referência em Belém, Estado do Pará, Brasil. Rev Pan-Amazônica Saúde. 2014;5(2):43–51.
19. Elman S, Hynan L, Gabriel V, Mayo M. The 5-D itch scale: a new measure of pruritus. Br J Dermatol. 2010;162(3):587–93.
20. Koulaouzidis A, Bhat S, Moschos J. Skin manifestations of liver diseases. J Clin Exp Hepatol. 2007;6(3):181–4.
21. Dogra S, Jindal R. Cutaneous manifestations of common liver diseases. J Clin Exp Hepatol. 2011;1(3):177–84.
22. Witkowska AB, Jasterzbski TJ, Schwartz RA. Terry's nails: a sign of systemic disease. Indian J Dermatol. 2017;62(3):309.

Further Reading

Bacon BR. Harrison's principles of internal medicine 19e. Williamston, NC: AccessMedicine; 2015.

Bates B, Hoekelman RA. A guide to physical examination. Philadelphia, PA: Lippincott Williams & Wilkins; 1983.

Goldman L, Ausiello DA, editors. Cecil medicine. Philadelphia, PA: Saunders Elsevier; 2008.

Macleod J. Macleod's clinical examination. Philadelphia, PA Elsevier Health Sciences; 2009.

35 Assessment of Liver Function

Zain Moosvi, Felix H. Lui, and Douglas Nguyen

Key Concepts

- As many of the coagulation factors are produced in the liver, prothrombin time (PT) and international normalized ratio (INR) can be used to assess liver synthetic function.
- Albumin is a protein that is manufactured by the liver and can be used to assess liver synthetic function.
- Elevated serum bilirubin levels cause jaundice, and severity is loosely proportional to the bilirubin level.
- Abnormal liver chemistries can be characterized by a hepatocellular pattern (elevated AST and ALT) or cholestatic pattern (elevated ALP).
- Alanine transaminase (ALT) and aspartate transaminase (AST) are markers for hepatocellular injury. AST to ALT ratio greater than 2 is consistent with alcoholic liver disease. A AST to ALT ratio of less than 2 is indicative of a myriad of conditions, including NASH and hepatitis C cirrhosis

35.1 Introduction: Standard Liver Panel

35.1.1 Total Bilirubin

Bilirubin is involved in the catabolism of heme. It is excreted in bile and ultimately feces as stercobilin, and in urine as urobilin and urobilinogen [1]. Bilirubin exists in two forms: Conjugated bilirubin and unconjugated bilirubin. Elevated bilirubin levels, referred to as hyperbilirubinemia, can cause jaundice, which is yellow discoloration of the skin and eyes. Serum bilirubin reflects the balance between bilirubin production and clearance. Accordingly, hyperbilirubinemia is caused by overproduction of bilirubin, impaired uptake, conjugation, or excretion, or leakage from damaged hepatocytes or bile ducts [2]. Serum bilirubin levels usually correlate with severity of jaundice, though this can be affected by compounds such as sulfonamides, salicylates, and albumin [3].

Unconjugated hyperbilirubinemia is typically a product of overproduction or reduced uptake or conjugation of bilirubin. Other etiologies include hemolysis, extravasation of blood, and dyserythropoiesis [4]. Conjugated hyperbilirubinemia, on the other hand, is usually caused by reduced excretion or leakage from hepatocytes or the biliary system, and is thus a more accurate indicator of hepatobiliary dysfunction or pathology. Conjugated hyperbilirubinemia can also result in bilirubin in the urine. On the contrary, unconjugated bilirubin is bound to albumin, and as such is not filtered by the glomerulus into the urine [3].

35.1.2 Transaminases

Alanine transaminase (ALT) is a transaminase enzyme that is found in a variety of body tissues, but is most commonly present in the liver. It is involved in the Cahill cycle, but is used clinically as a biomarker for liver function and health [5]. Elevations in ALT suggest hepatocellular injury, though etiologies vary from primary liver disorders to infections, malignancy, and heart failure [6].

Similar to ALT, aspartate transaminase (AST) is another transaminase enzyme used as a biomarker for liver health. It differs from ALT in that AST is more widely present in tissues outside of the liver, making it a less specific biomarker for hepatocellular injury [6].

35.1.3 AST/ALT Ratio

The ratio of AST to ALT can sometimes be used to determine the etiology of liver disease. Classically, AST to ALT ratio greater than 2 is consistent with alcoholic liver disease, par-

Z. Moosvi (✉) · F. H. Lui · D. Nguyen
Department of Medicine, UC Irvine Health, Orange, CA, USA
e-mail: zmoosvi@uci.edu; luif@uci.edu; douglaln@uci.edu

F. Radu-Ionita et al. (eds.), *Liver Diseases*, https://doi.org/10.1007/978-3-030-24432-3_35

ticularly in the setting of an elevated gamma glutamyl transpeptidase [7]. Several other pathologies confer an elevated AST to ALT ratio that is usually less than 2, including nonalcoholic steatohepatitis (NASH), cirrhosis from hepatitis C, and Wilson's disease [8]. Of note, elevated AST to ALT ratio is not considered diagnostic of liver disease, as it may also be elevated in myopathy as well, such as dermatomyositis.

35.1.4 Alkaline Phosphatase

Alkaline phosphatase (ALP) is an enzyme involved in dephosphorylating compounds and is most commonly found in liver, bone, and placenta [9]. As such, elevations in ALP can be secondary to processes involving any of the aforementioned organs. In contrast to ALP elevations from bone and placenta, ALP elevation from liver disease is characterized by concomitant elevation in gamma glutamyl transpeptidase and 5′-nucleotidase [9].

35.1.5 Gamma Glutamyl Transpeptidase

Gamma glutamyl transpeptidase (GGT) is found in hepatocytes, biliary epithelial cells, and pancreas cells, in addition to a variety of organs outside of the gastrointestinal system [10]. Elevations in GGT reflect abnormalities in any of the aforementioned organ systems. The primary utility of GGT in medicine is in determining the etiology of ALP elevation. Elevations in both ALP and GGT strongly suggest a hepatobiliary pathology [11].

35.1.6 Albumin

Albumin refers to a family of water soluble globular proteins that are found in blood plasma. It is the most abundant blood plasma protein, and accounts for approximately 50% of all plasma protein [12]. The primary function of serum albumin is to regulate oncotic pressure of the blood. Additionally, albumin also binds water, cations, fatty acids, hormones, thyroxine, bilirubin, and a multitude of pharmaceutical compounds [12].

As serum albumin is produced in the liver, it can be used as a surrogate marker for liver synthetic function. Hypoalbuminemia is more common in chronic liver disease rather than acute pathologies [13].The Child-Turcotte-Pugh, for instance, uses serum albumin level in addition to other liver chemistries to determine the severity of cirrhosis. However, low serum albumin is not specific to liver disease, as it can also be a product of extrahepatic etiologies including nephrotic syndrome and malnutrition [13].

35.1.7 Other Tests

35.1.7.1 5′-Nucleotidase

5′-Nucleotidase is a membrane-bound enzyme that facilitates the conversion of nucleotides to nucleosides. It is found in the liver, intestines, endocrine pancreas and blood vessels. Despite this, it is only released into the serum by the hepatobiliary system [14]. Therefore, similar to GGT, 5′-nucleotidase is used as a biomarker to differentiate ALP elevation from hepatobiliary disease from nonhepatic etiologies [15].

35.1.7.2 Ceruloplasmin

Ceruloplasmin is a ferroxidase enzyme and is the major copper-carrying protein in blood. As it is synthesized in the liver, ceruloplasmin levels may be reduced in liver disease [16]. The most common use of ceruloplasmin is in the diagnosis of Wilson disease, a genetic disorder due to a mutation in a copper transporter protein. However, low ceruloplasmin levels can be seen in patients without Wilson disease, and normal or elevated levels can be seen in patients with Wilson disease [17].

35.1.7.3 Alpha-Fetoprotein

Alpha-fetoprotein (AFP) is a glycoprotein normally produced during gestation by the fetal liver and yolk sac. It is the most commonly used as a tumor marker for hepatocellular carcinoma (HCC) [18]. Serum AFP levels correlate with the progression of the malignancy, as early HCC may be accompanied by lower serum AFP levels compared to advanced disease [19]. Higher levels are more specific but less sensitive. A serum AFP level greater than 400 ng/mL in a high risk patient is considered diagnostic of HCC [20]. Elevated serum AFP levels may also be seen in acute or chronic viral hepatitis, germ cell and non-germ cell tumors, and gastric cancer [18].

35.1.7.4 Coagulation Studies

The majority of the coagulation factors are synthesized in the liver. These include factor I, factor II, factor V, factor VII, factor IX, factor X, factor XII, and factor XIII. As such, deficiencies in these coagulation factors occur frequently in chronic liver disease, and is reflected in the prothrombin time (PT) or international normalized ratio (INR) [21]. Thus, similar to serum albumin, PT or INR can be used as a marker for liver synthetic function, where an elevated PT or INR indicates compromised synthetic function.

35.1.7.5 Serum Glucose

Glucose is a simple sugar and the most abundant monosaccharide, a subtype of carbohydrate. The primary role of glucose in the body is to produce energy in the form of adenosine triphosphate via cellular respiration. The liver functions to maintain normal levels of serum glucose through a variety of mechanisms, including glycogenesis, glycogenolysis, gluconeogenesis, and glycolysis. The association between liver disease and carbohydrate metabolism has been well-studied. Glycogenolysis is reduced in cirrhosis, owing to low glycogen stores and reduced levels of the catabolizing enzyme, glucose-6-phosphatase. Gluconeogenesis is also reduced [22]. Impaired glucose tolerance and fasting hyperglycemia are present in at least 50% of patients with cirrhosis. This is thought to be caused by insulin resistance as opposed to insulin deficiency [23]. Contrastingly, hypoglycemia is usually seen in acute liver failure, though it can also be present in cirrhosis due to decreased hepatic glycogen stores, decreased response to glucagon, and reduced glycogen synthesis capacity [22].

35.1.8 Lactate Dehydrogenase

Lactate dehydrogenase (LDH) is a cytoplasmic enzyme present in a variety of body tissues. Because it is released during tissue damage, it can be used as a marker for cellular injury. However, it has a poor sensitivity and specificity, and is now primarily used as a marker for hemolysis and to distinguish ischemic hepatitis from viral hepatitis [24].

35.1.8.1 Elevated Transaminases

Abnormal liver chemistries can be characterized by a hepatocellular pattern, when the predominant elevated chemistries are ALT and AST, or cholestatic pattern, when the predominant elevated chemistry is ALP. The magnitude of transaminase elevation depends on the etiology of hepatocellular injury, and can be characterized by their relation to the upper limit of normal (ULN) range for the liver chemistry (Table 35.1).

Table 35.1 Common liver diseases with their associated abnormal liver chemistry studies

Disease	AST	ALT	ALP	Bilirubin	Other features
Acute viral hepatitis	↑↑↑ (>25× ULN)	↑↑↑ (>25× ULN)	Normal to ↑	Normal to ↑↑↑	Exposure history, fatigue, nausea/vomiting, RUQ pain
Chronic viral hepatitis	↑ (<2× ULN)	↑↑ (< 2× ULN)	Normal to ↑	↑ if advanced	History of exposure to infected blood or body fluids
Nonalcoholic steatohepatitis	↑ (<4× ULN)	↑ (<4× ULN)	Normal to ↑	Normal	History of metabolic syndrome
Alcoholic hepatitis	↑↑ (<8× ULN)	Normal or ↑ (<5× ULN)	↑	Normal to ↑↑↑	History of alcohol abuse
Acute autoimmune hepatitis	↑↑↑	↑↑↑	Normal to ↑	Normal to ↑↑	Type I: Antinuclear antibodies (ANA) and anti-smooth muscle antibodies (ASMA) Type II: anti-liver-kidney microsome-1 antibodies (ALKM-1) and anti-liver cytosol antibody-1 (ALC-1)
Chronic autoimmune hepatitis	↑	↑↑	Normal to ↑	Normal	Type I: Antinuclear antibodies (ANA) and anti-smooth muscle antibodies (ASMA) Type II: anti-liver-kidney microsome-1 antibodies (ALKM-1) and anti-liver cytosol antibody-1 (ALC-1)
Wilson disease	↑	↑	Low	↑ (Unconjugated)	Low serum ceruloplasmin. Neurologic symptoms
Alpha 1 antitrypsin deficiency	↑	↑	Normal	↑ If advanced	Early onset COPD in absence of smoking history
Hemochromatosis	Normal	Normal	Normal	Normal	Bronze skin, diabetes, CHF, family history
Primary biliary cirrhosis	↑	↑	↑↑↑	↑ If advanced	Middle-aged female, antimitochondrial antibody
Primary sclerosing cholangitis	↑	↑	↑↑↑	↑ If advanced/ severe structuring	Highly associated with ulcerative colitis
Duct obstruction	↑	↑	↑↑	↑↑	Dilated ducts on imaging
Hepatic ischemia	↑↑↑ (>50× ULN)	↑↑↑ (>50× ULN)	Normal	Normal	AST > 5000 U/L, recent episode of hypotension
Celiac disease	Normal or ↑	Normal or ↑	Normal or ↑	Normal	Iron deficiency anemia, dermatitis herpetiformis
Infiltrative liver disease	↑	↑	↑↑↑	Normal	Malignancy, sarcoidosis, amyloidosis, mycobacterial/fungal infection

Adapted from [25] [American College of Physicians. Gastroenterology and Hepatology. MKSAP: Medical Knowledge Self-Assessment 18. Philadelphia, PA: American College of Physicians. ISBN 978-1-938245-50-319881989. Page 50]

Initial workup of abnormal liver tests should include imaging. Ultrasound (US) is considered first-line as it does not require intravenous access and is relatively cost-effective. Additionally, it does not require the administration of contrast, which may be a relative contraindication in patients with kidney disease. However, ultrasound can potentially be limited by patient body habitus and user error. It also carries a lower sensitivity for liver masses compared to computed tomography (CT) or magnetic resonance imaging (MRI). MRI has numerous advantages over CT. Namely, it does not expose the patient to radiation and requires visualization of the biliary tree with magnetic resonance cholangiopancreatography (MRCP) [26].

Other diagnostic tests include histologic assessment via liver biopsy, however this has been largely replaced by serologic markers and imaging (US or MRI elastography) (Fig. 35.1).

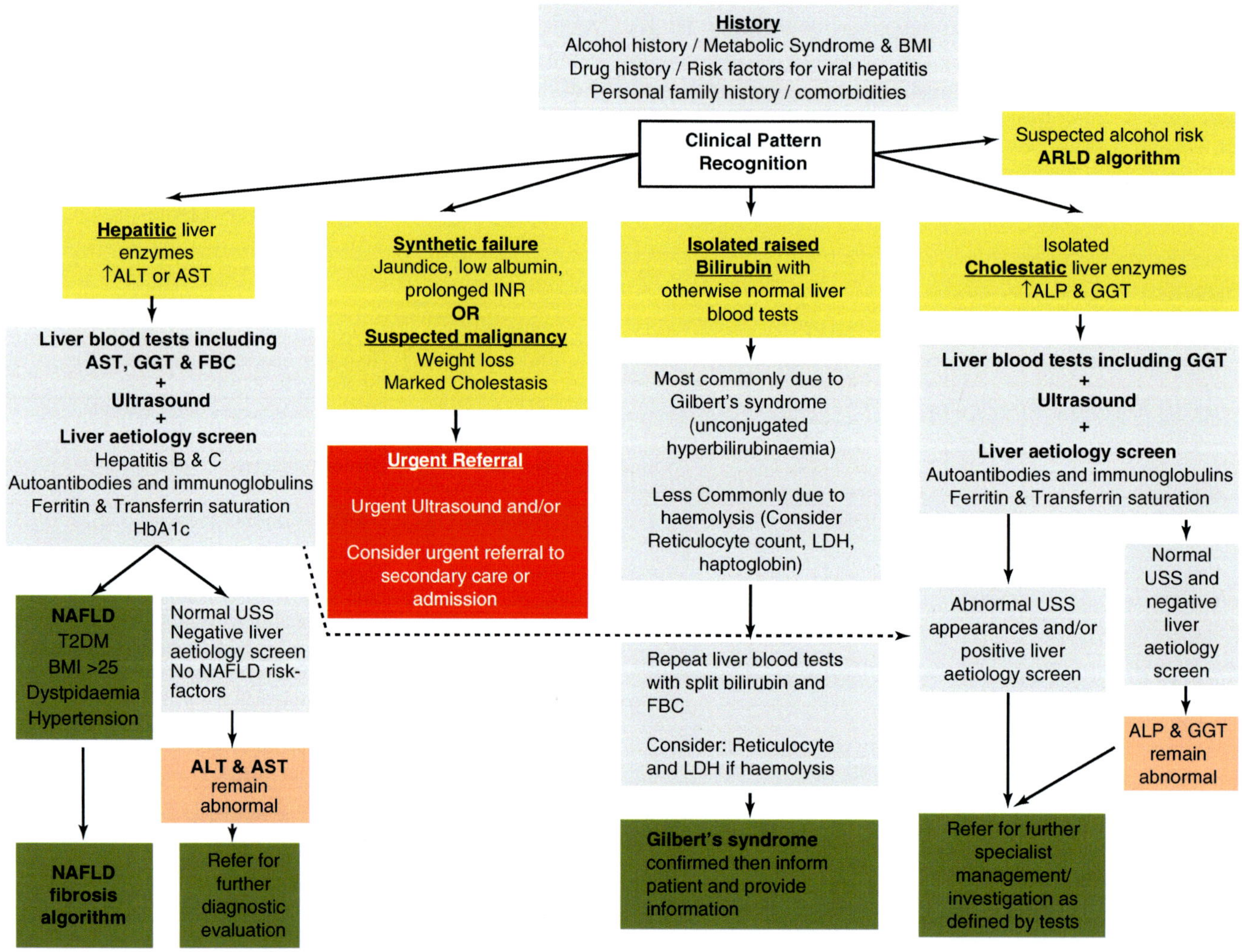

Fig. 35.1 Response to abnormal liver blood tests. This figure details the initial response to abnormal liver blood tests. Boxes in yellow indicate the initial evaluation of the clinical presentation. Patients with marked derangement of liver blood tests, synthetic failure and/or suspicious clinical symptoms/signs should be considered for urgent referral to secondary care (red box). For the remainder, a clinical history alongside evaluation of the pattern of liver blood test derangement will determine choice of pathway and is shown in the grey boxes. A grey box indicates all the tests that should be requested at that stage rather than a hierarchy within it. The presence of metabolic syndrome criteria should be sought to support a diagnosis of NAFLD. For children, the text should be consulted for modification of recommendation. Areas of diagnostic uncertainty are indicated in orange boxes and the decision for repeat testing or referral to secondary care will be influenced by the magnitude of enzyme elevation and clinical context. Green boxes indicate final/definitive outcomes for users of the pathway. (Asterisk) Abnormal USS may well include extrahepatic biliary obstruction due to malignancy, which should result in urgent referral. *ALP* alkaline phosphatase, *ALT* alanine aminotransferase, *ARLD* alcohol-related liver disease, *AST* aspartate aminotransferase, *BMI* body mass index, *FBC* full blood count, *GGT* γ-glutamyltransferase, *INR* international normalised ratio, *LDH* lactate dehydrogenase, *NAFLD* non-alcoholic fatty liver disease, *T2DM* type 2 diabetes mellitus, *USS* ultrasound scan. From [27] [Newsome PN, et al. Guidelines on the management of abnormal liver blood tests. **Gut. 2018** Jan;67(1):6–19. doi: https://doi.org/10.1136/gutjnl-2017-314,924.]. **It is open access article** [*This is an Open Access article distributed in accordance with the terms of the Creative Commons Attribution (CC BY 4.0) license, which permits others to distribute, remix, adapt and build upon this work, for commercial use, provided the original work is properly cited. See: http://creativecommons.org/licenses/by/4.0/*]

35.2 Viral Hepatitis

35.2.1 Hepatitis A

Hepatitis A is caused by the hepatitis A virus (HAV). HAV is a member of the genus *Hepatovirus* in the family Picornaviridae [28]. Infection and vaccination confer lifelong immunity.

HAV is usually a self-limited illness that does not become chronic. Presentation is usually relatively mild, with acute liver failure occurring in less than 1% of cases. Typical symptoms of acute HAV include jaundice, fatigue, fever, diarrhea, and mild RUQ abdominal pain. Symptoms and lab abnormalities typically resolve within 3 months [29].

The incubation period of HAV is 2–6 weeks. Transmission occurs via fecal-oral route. For this reason, the prevalence of HAV infection is highest in countries of lower socioeconomic status and poorly developed sanitation systems, including Central America, South Asia, and the majority of Africa [28]. IgG antibodies to HAV indicate previous exposure or vaccination.

HAV vaccination or immune globulin is indicated in individuals who have been exposed to the virus within the past 2 weeks and have not been previously vaccinated/infected. Furthermore, immune globulin is indicated for adults over the age of 40 years of age, individuals with chronic liver disease, and individuals who are immunocompromised [29]. There is no definitive treatment for hepatitis A, and therapy is usually supportive care.

35.2.2 Hepatitis B

Hepatitis B virus (HBV) is a DNA virus belonging to the family hepadnaviruses. HBV infection is a global public health problem, as it is the most prevalent of all the viral hepatitides worldwide, with about 350 million individuals infected as of 2015. Approximately 600,000 individuals die each year from HBV-related disease [31] (Tables 35.2 and 35.3). In contrast to HAV infection, HBV infection can be both acute and chronic. Transmission occurs via parenteral contact, vertically, or sexually. Extrahepatic manifestations of HBV infection include serum sickness-like syndrome, polyarthritis, polyarteritis nodosa, cryoglobulinemia, and glomerulonephritis [30] (Fig. 35.2).

The immune tolerant phase is most commonly seen in patients who acquire HBV infection at birth (vertical transmission). This phase usually manifests as a normal ALT level in the setting of positive hepatitis B e antigen (HBeAg). Histology usually will only demonstrate mild hepatocyte injury during this phase.

The immune clearance and reactivation phases, which together comprise the immune active phase, are characterized by positive HBeAg, elevated ALT, and HBV DNA greater than 10,000 IU/mL. The inactive carrier or control phase can be identified by normal ALT levels and HBV DNA less than 10,000 IU/mL [30].

Treatment of HBV is indicated for patients who present with acute liver failure, chronic HBV infection with elevated ALT and HBV DNA less than 10,000 IU/mL, or who are

Table 35.2 Hepatitis B serologies and their respective clinical scenarios

Clinical scenario	HBsAg	Anti-HBs	IgM anti-Hbc	IgG anti-Hbc	HBeAg	Anti-HBe	HBV DNA (IU/mL)
Acute hepatitis B; rarely reactivation of chronic hepatitis B	+	–	+	–	+	–	>20,000
Resolved previous infection	–	+	–	+	–	+/–	Undetected
Immunity from vaccination	–	+	–	–	–	–	Undetected
False positive anti-HBc or resolved previous infection	–	–	–	+	–	–	Undetected
Immune control (chronic hepatitis B, inactive)	+	–	–	+	–	+	<10,000
Immune tolerant (perinatally acquired)	+	–	–	+	+	–	>1 million
Immune active	+	–	–	+	+	–	>10,000
Reactivation	+	–	–	+	–	+	>10,000

Adapted from [25] [American College of Physicians. Gastroenterology and Hepatology. MKSAP: Medical Knowledge Self-Assessment 18. Philadelphia, PA: American College of Physicians. ISBN 978-1-938245-50-319881989. Page 50]

Table 35.3 Chronic HBV infection divided into phases of disease [30]

Phase	HBeAg/anti-HBe status	HBV DNA	ALT level	Liver biopsy	Treatment candidate
Immune tolerant	HBeAg+	>20,000 IU/mL	Normal	Normal or minimal activity	No
Immune clearance/ reactivation	HBeAg+ or anti-HBe+	>2000 IU/mL	Elevated	Active inflammation	Yes
Inactive carrier	HBeAg negative/anti-HBe+	<2000 IU/mL	Normal	Normal or minimal activity	No

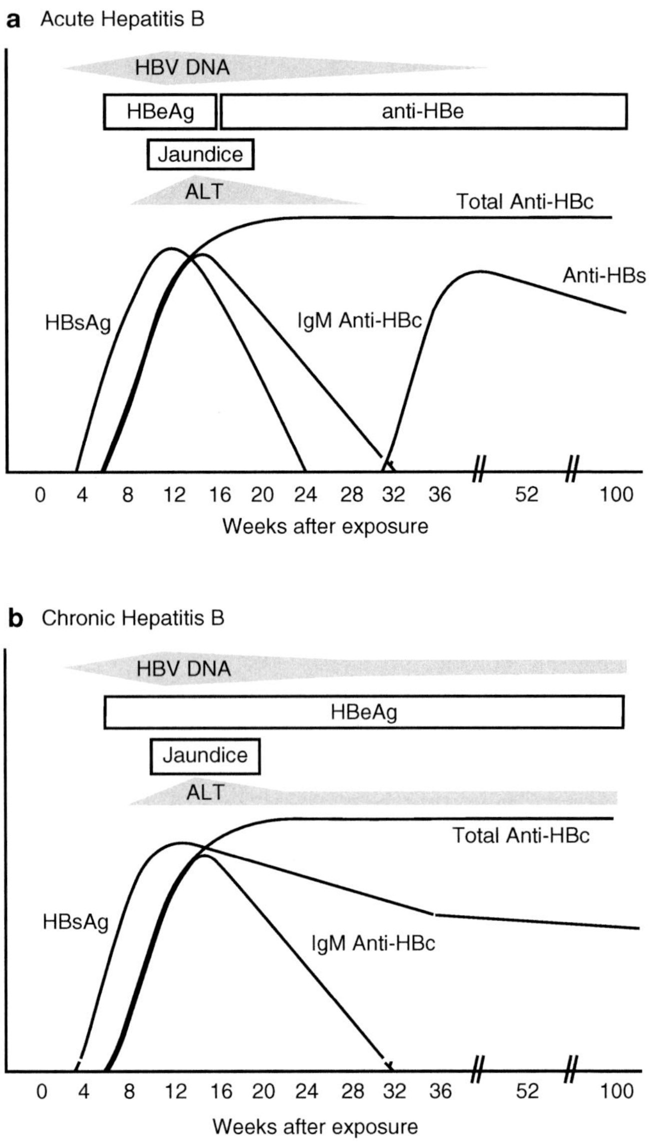

Fig. 35.2 The clinical course and serologic profiles of (**a**) acute and (**b**) chronic hepatitis B. From [30] [Liang TJ. Hepatitis B: the virus and disease. Hepatology. 2009 May;49(5 Suppl):S13–21. doi: https://doi.org/10.1002/hep.22881] with permission

receiving immunosuppressive therapy. Antivirals such as tenofovir and entecavir are first-line treatment, with pegylated interferon reserved for patients without cirrhosis who have high ALT levels and low HBV DNA levels. Treatment is aimed at normalizing ALT and reducing HBV DNA to less than 50 IU/mL [32].

Complications of chronic untreated HBV include hepatocellular carcinoma (HCC) and cirrhosis. Successful treatment reduces the risk of developing the aforementioned complications [30]. Certain populations carry an increased risk of progression to HCC, and for these patients ultrasound surveillance every 6 months is indicated. These groups include patients with cirrhosis, Asian men older than 40 years, Asian women older than 50 years, African patients older than 20 years, patients with persistent inflammatory activity (elevated ALT and HBV greater than 10,000 IU/mL for multiple years), and patients with family history of HCC [33].

35.2.3 Hepatitis C

Hepatitis C is caused by the hepatitis C virus (HCV). It is the most common bloodborne disease in the United States, with approximately four million individuals infected [34]. The virus is contracted primarily through exposure to blood, for this reason intravenous drug users are at the highest risk for HCV. The virus can also be transmitted sexually, though the risk is 0.07% per year, as well as vertically. Men who have sex with men are at an elevated risk for transmission [34]. Current guidelines by the U.S. Preventive Services Task Forces recommend screening for individuals born between 1945 and 1965 [33].

HCV rarely presents as an acute infection. Chronic HCV infection will often be asymptomatic, with fatigue and right upper quadrant pain the most common symptoms. Extrahepatic manifestations of HCV include cryoglobulinemia, porphyria cutanea tarda, and membranoproliferative glomerulonephritis [34].

HCV is diagnosed via anti IgG antibodies and HCV RNA PCR. Once diagnosis is confirmed, individuals should also be tested for human immunodeficiency virus (HIV), and HBV given the common modes of transmission and rapid progression of liver disease with coinfection. Lab tests in hepatitis C will be nonspecific, ranging from normal ALT/AST to mild elevation [35]. If therapy is planned, quantitative HCV RNA should be ordered as well. Liver biopsy, which demonstrates lymphocytic portal inflammation and variable levels of fibrosis, has become less popular with the less invasive ways to assess for cirrhosis, including MRE [26].

HCV treatment is aimed at achieving sustained virologic response (SVR), which is defined as undetectable HCV RNA 6 months after completion of treatment. SVR is associated with a decrease in all-cause mortality, liver-related mortality, and need for liver transplantation. It is less likely to achieve in the setting of cirrhosis [3]. Treatment regimens vary depending on the viral genotype. HCV genotype 1, which is most prevalent in the United States, is treated with the antivirals sofosbuvir and ledipasvir, which lead to SVR in 95% of patients. Other less common treatment regimens for this genotype include the combination of ombitasvir and paritaprevir, and ritonavir and dasabuvir. Ribavirin may be added to either of the aforementioned regimens [35].

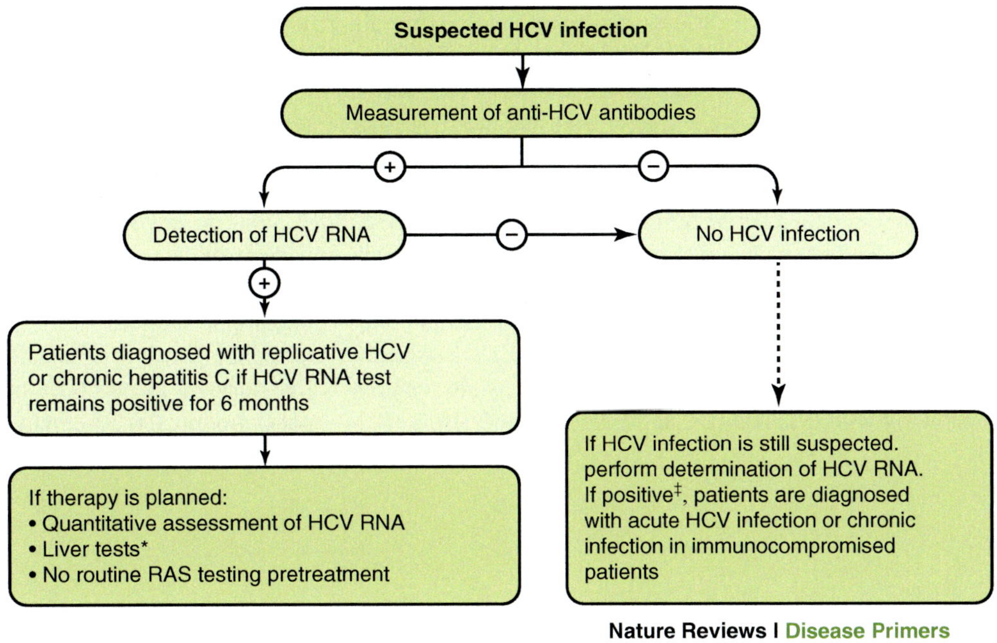

Fig. 35.3 Diagnostic algorithm for HCV infection. From [34] [Manns MP et al. Hepatitis C virus infection. Nat. Rev. Dis. Primers Nature Reviews Disease Primers, volume 3, Article number: 17006 (2017). doi: https://doi.org/10.1038/nrdp.2017.6] with permission

Surveillance imaging with abdominal ultrasound every 6 months is indicated for patients with cirrhosis to monitor for HCC, even in the setting of SVR. Individuals with cirrhosis should also receive upper endoscopy screening for esophageal varices [33].Transplantation is indicated in patients with decompensated disease or localized HCC that meets Milan criteria [36].

Variability in the HCV envelope protein has greatly hindered the development of a vaccine. Individuals infected with HCV who are not immune to HAV or HBV should be vaccinated against these viruses [35] (Fig. 35.3).

35.2.4 Hepatitis D

Hepatitis D (HDV) is a defective RNA virus that requires the presence of HBV for infection. HDV infection can occur in three scenarios: acute HBV/HDV coinfection, acute HDV superinfection of chronic HBV carrier, or chronic HDV infection [35]. Coinfection and superinfection increase the likelihood of severe complications including acute liver failure with rapid progression to cirrhosis, and HCC in chronic infections. HDV coinfection and superinfections carry a mortality rate of 20%, the highest of all hepatitis infections [36]. HBsAg is necessary for the diagnosis of HDV infection. Furthermore, IgM antibody to HBc is necessary for the diagnosis of acute HBV/HDV coinfection. Treatment is with pegylated interferon, however the efficacy rate is approximately 20%. For this reason, treatment is typically reserved with patients with worsening liver disease despite HBV treatment [37].

35.2.5 Hepatitis E

Hepatitis E virus (HEV) is an RNA virus that is most similar to HAV with regards to geographic distribution and clinical presentation [35]. Similar to HAV, it diagnosed by IgM antibody and is usually a self-limited infection. In pregnant women, however, the risk of acute liver failure is elevated. Women in the third trimester of pregnancy are at a particularly high risk, as the infection carries a mortality rate of approximately 20% in this demographic [36].

35.2.6 Alcohol-Induced Liver Disease

Excessive alcohol consumption is associated with a variety of liver diseases, ranging from alcoholic fatty liver disease to hepatitis to cirrhosis. Individuals who consume greater than two alcoholic drinks per day are at an increased risk of cirrhosis, though the vast majority of individuals will not develop cirrhosis [36].

Alcohol abuse is very common worldwide. In the United States, alcohol abuse has an estimated lifetime prevalence of 18% among adults [38].

Complications from alcohol abuse include steatosis, steatohepatitis, cirrhosis, and HCC. Hepatic steatosis, or fatty liver, is the first stage of liver disease, and occurs on the macrovesicular level. It affects approximately 90% of heavy drinkers, and can be caused both by binge drinking or chronic alcohol abuse. Individuals with steatosis are usually asymptomatic. Steatosis can resolve within 4–6 weeks with abstinence [38].

Steatohepatitis is the next stage of alcohol-induced liver disease, and can be characterized by hepatic steatosis with inflammation. It carries a much higher risk of cirrhosis than simple steatosis. Most patients are asymptomatic, and may be associated with mild elevations in aminotransferase levels [39].

Alcoholic hepatitis (AH) can be distinguished from steatosis and steatohepatitis by clinical presentation and lab findings. Patients with AH typically present with anorexia, jaundice, and hepatomegaly [38]. Aminotransferase levels are frequently elevated, but usually below 300–400 U/L. Additionally, the ratio of AST to ALT is classically greater than 2. A direct hyperbilirubinemia may also be present, along with leukocytosis, and coagulopathy [39].

The severity of AH is assessed using the Maddrey discriminant function (MDF) score. Patients with MDF less than 32 are considered to have mild disease, and are treated with supportive measures. On the other hand, a MDF greater than 32 is associated with a high mortality rate, and treatment is indicated. Prednisone is first-line therapy for AH with MDF greater than 32, with pentoxifylline being reserved for patients presenting with infection, variceal hemorrhage, or acute kidney injury [39].

Decompensation of alcoholic cirrhosis, defined as complications such as ascites, variceal bleeding, or hepatic encephalopathy, dramatically reduces the 5-year transplant-free survival rate to 60% in individuals who cease alcohol consumption and 30% in those who do not [39] (Fig. 35.4).

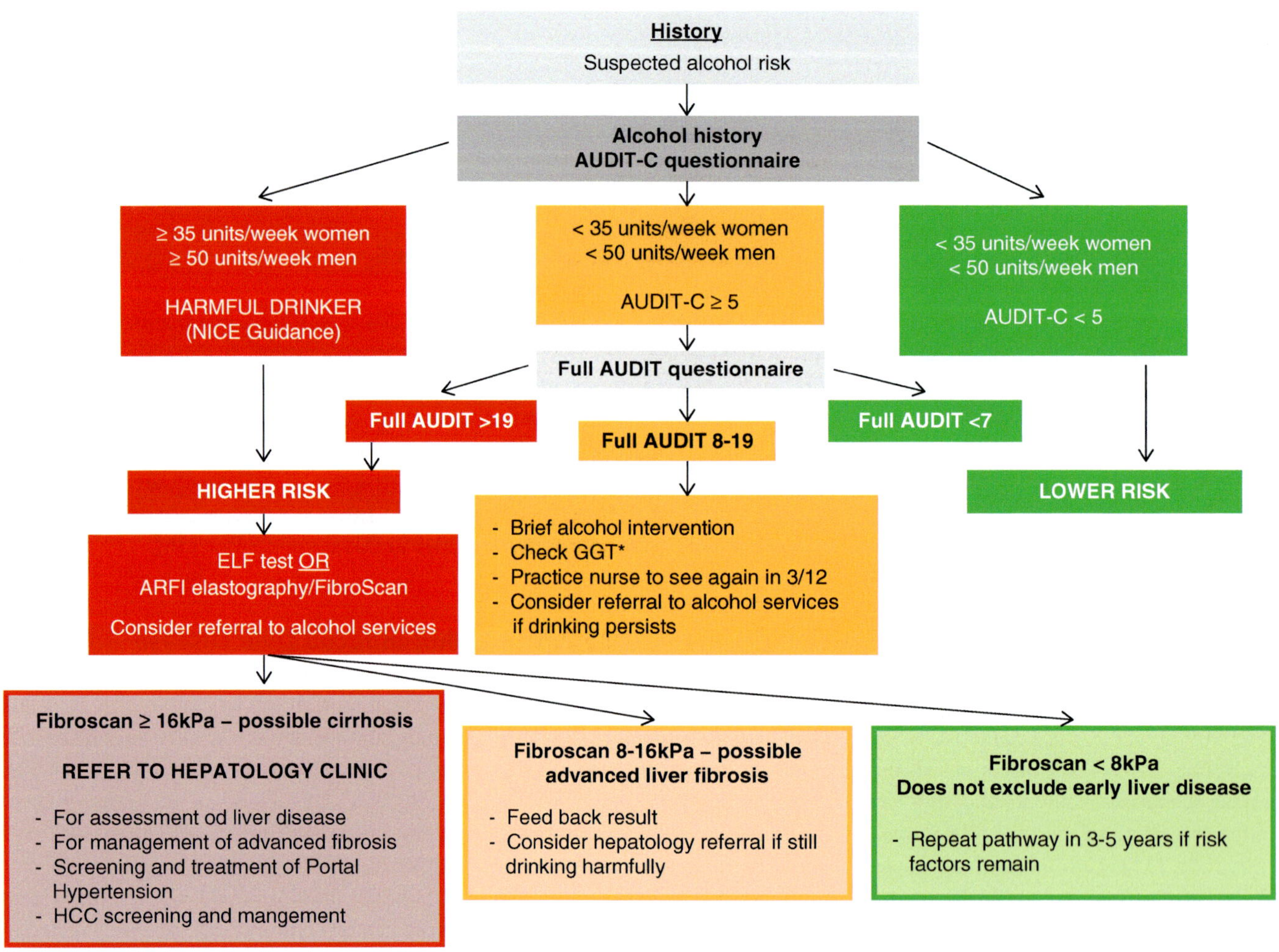

Fig. 35.4 Alcohol-related liver disease algorithm. In patients in whom alcohol is suspected to be the main injurious factor, the extent of consumption influences early decision-making. For those drinking at harmful levels, ≥35 U/week women and ≥50 U/week men, an assessment of liver fibrosis is the critical next step. For other patients, administration of the AUDIT C questionnaire alongside brief intervention is recommended initially. For patients who continue to drink at hazardous levels consideration should be given to assessment as for the higher-risk category according to liver fibrosis evaluation. This is particularly important for those with a GGT of >100 U/L. Cut-off points for ARFI vary according to manufacturer and thus should be tailored to the device used. ARFI, acoustic radiation force impulse; ELF, enhanced liver fibrosis; GGT, γ-glutamyltransferase; HCC, hepatocellular carcinoma. From [27] [Newsome PN, et al. Guidelines on the management of abnormal liver blood tests. **Gut. 2018** Jan;67(1):6–19. doi: https://doi.org/10.1136/gutjnl-2017-314,924.] **It is open access article** [*This is an* ***Open Access*** *article distributed in accordance with the terms of the Creative Commons Attribution (CC BY 4.0) license, which permits others to distribute, remix, adapt and build upon this work, for commercial use, provided the original work is properly cited. See: http://creativecommons.org/licenses/by/4.0/*]

35.2.7 Drug-Induced Liver Injury

Drug-induced liver injury (DILI) can be caused by a variety of prescription and over-the-counter medications, in addition to herbs and supplements. There are over 900 drugs that are known to cause DILI [40]. Clinical presentations are also varied, ranging from mild elevations in liver chemistries to acute liver failure. It is responsible for approximately 50% of all acute liver failures. The most common offending agents are antimicrobials, antiepileptics (phenytoin, valproate), and antituberculosis drugs (isoniazid, rifampin) [40].

The diagnosis of DILI requires a history of exposure to a drug, a hepatotoxicity pattern that fits the profile of the drug suspected, improvement after the drug is removed, and absence of any preexisting hepatobiliary disease [25]. A hepatocellular pattern (elevated aminotransferases) are seen in DILI caused by allopurinol, isoniazid, phenytoin, and valproate. A cholestatic pattern (elevated ALP) is seen in DILI from amoxicillin-clavulanate, carbamazepine, erythromycin, and sulfonamides. A mixed pattern can be seen in DILI caused by azathioprine and ibuprofen [40].

The most common cause of DILI and acute liver failure worldwide is acetaminophen overdose. Initial workup for suspected DILI from acetaminophen should include acetaminophen serum concentrations. Treatment with N-acetylcysteine (NAC) is indicated for patients with levels above 150 μg/mL at 4 h after ingestion, or 18.8 μg/mL at 16 h after ingestion [40]. NAC works by capturing the toxic metabolite of acetaminophen, N-acetyl-p-benzoquinone imine (NAPQI) [36].

35.2.8 Ischemic Hepatitis

Ischemic hepatitis, also known as shock liver, is a cause of acute liver injury and can often be severe enough to cause acute liver failure. It arises from insufficient blood flow to the liver, which is usually due to shock of some variety.

Patients will usually present with fatigue, low urine output, and mental confusion. Hepatic encephalopathy may be present in the setting of acute liver failure [41]. Less commonly, patients will have symptoms of acute viral hepatitis, including nausea/vomiting and right upper quadrant pain.

Liver chemistries will demonstrate an early rapid rise in lactate dehydrogenase (LDH) levels, in addition to markedly elevated aminotransferases, with both AST and ALT often exceeding 10,000 U/L. Hepatic synthetic function typically remains unaffected, and though bilirubin and ALP can also be elevated in ischemic hepatitis, these lab findings are relatively uncommon and less prominent [42]. Other etiologies of acute liver failure should be ruled out as well.

Ischemic hepatitis can be differentiated from other causes of acute liver injury by several key lab findings. Firstly, a rapid rise in LDH is unusual in viral hepatitis, and a serum alanine aminotransferase to LDH ratio of less than 1.5 is suggestive of ischemic hepatitis. Additionally, a rapid fall of serum aminotransferases after the initial rise is consistent with ischemic injury. Lastly, as the etiology of ischemic hepatitis is due to hypoperfusion, other findings of hypoperfusion are usually present, including acute kidney injury from acute tubular necrosis [41]. Therapy is directed towards treatment of the underlying cause of shock to restore and maintain adequate blood pressure.

35.2.9 Acute Liver Failure

Acute liver failure (ALF) is defined by hepatic encephalopathy and INR greater than or equal to 1.5 in the absence of prior liver disease. The most common causes of ALF in the United States are acetaminophen overdose, followed by idiopathic causes and HBV [43]. Patients diagnosed with ALF should be considered for transfer to liver transplant center as early as possible. Complications of ALF include hypoglycemia, hypophosphatemia, acute kidney injury, and worsening hepatic encephalopathy, for which close monitoring is required. Hepatic encephalopathy by itself may require ICU admission as the risk of cerebral edema and intracranial hypertension increases with worsening of the disease [43]. Signs of worsening intracranial pressure include cranial nerve palsies, papilledema, and Cushing's triad.

ALF from acetaminophen toxicity is characterized by aminotransferase levels in the thousands preceded by ingestion of usually greater than 10 g of acetaminophen in the past 24 h. Activated charcoal is indicated for patients who present within 3–4 h of acetaminophen ingestion. NAC should be administered as early as possible, as mortality rates increase dramatically with longer time intervals between acetaminophen ingestion and NAC administration [43].

35.2.10 Autoimmune Hepatitis

Autoimmune hepatitis is a chronic inflammatory liver disease frequently associated with other autoimmune conditions, most commonly ulcerative colitis, autoimmune thyroiditis, and type 1 diabetes. It is usually seen in women with a female to male ratio of 3.6–1, and can occur at any age, but most commonly is seen in patients in their fifth and sixth decade of life [44].

Clinical presentations drastically vary, and include asymptomatic patients as well as those with ALF. Lab findings associated with autoimmune hepatitis included elevated serum IgG and aminotransferase levels, which can be elevated in the thousands in the case of ALF. Elevated anti-smooth muscle or antinuclear antibodies titers are also suggestive of type 1 autoimmune hepatitis, while type 2 autoimmune hepatitis is characterized by the presence of antibodies to liver/kidney microsomes (ALKM-1) and/or to liver cytosol antigen (ALC-1) [44].

Liver biopsy is usually needed to confirm the diagnosis. According to the Association for the Study of Liver Diseases guidelines, treatment is indicated in patients with severe disease and consists of prednisone and/or azathioprine [44].

35.3 Metabolic Liver Disease

35.3.1 Nonalcoholic Fatty Liver Disease

NAFLD is the most common cause of liver disease in the United States, with approximately 30% of Americans affected. Risk factors for NAFLD include metabolic syndrome. Approximately 20% of patients with NAFLD have nonalcoholic steatohepatitis (NASH), characterized by steatosis and chronic inflammation and fibrosis. Of this 20%, 10% will progress to advanced fibrosis. Risk factors for disease progression include age greater than 50 years old, diabetes mellitus, and BMI greater than or equal to 28 kg/m^2 [45]. Liver chemistries are similar to those in other etiologies of chronic liver disease.

Treatment consists of controlling risk factors for insulin resistance. Weight loss in particular, achieved via diet, exercise, or bariatric surgery, confers a large risk reduction of disease progression. There is some evidence that vitamin E therapy can result in delayed disease progression and even reversal, however follow-up studies have been inconclusive [45].

35.3.2 Hereditary Hemochromatosis

Hereditary hemochromatosis is a hereditary condition characterized by abnormally high iron stores due to increased intestinal absorption. It is inherited in an autosomal recessive pattern, and is caused by a mutation in the *HFE* gene, which regulates interactions with transferrin and its receptor [46]. It is most commonly seen in people of Eastern European descent. Men usually present in their fifth and sixth decade of life, while women may present decades later due to iron loss from menstruation [47]. Patients are often diagnosed after incidental findings on liver chemistries and iron panels.

Hereditary hemochromatosis classically presents as the triad of cirrhosis, bronze skin, and diabetes, but patients also commonly have arthropathy and fatigue. Less common manifestations include congestive heart failure, erectile dysfunction, and deafness [46]. Initial workup includes iron studies. In particular, fasting transferrin saturation has been found to be the most useful lab test in initial screening for hemochromatosis. Transferrin saturation values greater than 45% in men and 35% in premenopausal women warrant additional evaluation, while values greater than 62% are strongly suggestive of homozygosity for HFE mutation [46]. Serum ferritin is typically elevated, though it can be normal in early disease. Ferritin greater than 1000 ng/mL is strongly suggestive of hemochromatosis. Phlebotomy is first-line treatment, and is indicated in patients whose serum ferritin is greater than 500 ng/mL. Alternative therapy is with desferrioxamine, an iron-chelating compound [47].

35.3.3 Alpha-1 Antitrypsin Deficiency

Alpha-1 antitrypsin (A1AT) deficiency is a hereditary condition that causes lung and liver disease. Inherited in an autosomal-codominant pattern, it is caused by a mutation in the *SERPINA1* gene and results in reduced levels of alpha-1 antitrypsin [48]. This allows for unregulated activity of neutrophil elastase and buildup of abnormal A1AT in the liver. It is most common in individuals of European ancestry. The most significant risk factor for lung disease is smoking. Patients with lung involvement may present between 20 and 50 years of age. Life expectancy for patients who smoke is around 50 years, while those who do not have a normal life expectancy [48]. Complications include COPD from increased neutrophil elastase activity and cirrhosis from abnormal A1AT buildup [36].

A1AT deficiency remains undiagnosed in many patients, as patients are often times diagnosed with only COPD. Patients typically present with respiratory symptoms, include dyspnea and wheezing. Early onset emphysema in the absence of smoking, usually between 30 and 50 years of age, should raise suspicion for A1AT deficiency. Testing should be performed in all patients who are diagnosed with COPD, as approximately 1% of these patients have A1AT deficiency as well. Initial testing consists of a serum A1AT level. A low A1AT level is considered diagnostic of A1AT deficiency diagnostic, and should be followed up by A1AT genotyping and phenotyping [28].

Treatment of lung disease is identical to COPD and includes bronchodilators and inhaled steroids. Severe cases may require lung transplantation. Liver transplantation is the definitive treatment for liver disease.

35.3.4 Wilson Disease

Wilson disease is a hereditary disorder caused by abnormal buildup of copper in the body, resulting in liver and neurologic disease. It is inherited in an autosomal recessive pattern, and is caused by a mutation in the *ATP7B* gene, which regulates copper excretion into bile and plasma [36]. It affects 1 in 30,000 live births. Approximately 5% of patients will present with ALF, while about 50% of patients will present with neuropsychiatric symptoms [49].

Patients usually present between ages of 5 and 35 years depending on organ involvement. Patients with liver problems present during childhood and teenage years, often with ALF. Patients with neuropsychiatric symptoms usually present in their 20s and 30s [49].

Diagnosis is achieved via exam and lab tests. The hallmark of Wilson disease is Kayser-Fleischer rings, brownish or green rings in the cornea observable on slit-lamp exam that arise from copper sulfate deposition. They are seen in 50–60% of patients with hepatic involvement and over 90% of patients with neurologic disease. Liver chemistries will demonstrate a low ALP and mildly elevated aminotransferases. Serum ceruloplasmin cannot be used by itself to establish diagnosis, as it can be elevated or normal in Wilson disease, and low in a plethora of other hepatic pathologies. Copper levels will also be abnormally low, in addition to elevated urine copper [36]. Liver biopsy is usually not needed but can be used to confirm diagnosis if laboratory findings are equivocal.

Treatment is with the copper-chelating agent penicillamine. Trientine hydrochloride is considered second-line therapy and is indicated in patients who suffer from side effects from penicillamine, including drug-induced lupus, myasthenia, or worsening of neuropsychiatric symptoms. Liver transplant is reserved for patients with acute liver failure who do not respond to medical therapy and those with advanced chronic liver disease. Liver transplant has not been shown to be of benefit in patients with only neuropsychiatric manifestations and is thus not indicated in this subset of patients [49].

35.4 Cholestatic Liver Diseases

35.4.1 Primary Biliary Cholangitis

Primary biliary cholangitis (PBC), formerly known as primary biliary cirrhosis, is an autoimmune disease of the liver resulting from progressive destruction of intrahepatic bile ducts. PBC is much more common in women, with a female to male ratio of at least 9:1 [50]. Similar to other autoimmune conditions, patients with PBC also suffer from a variety of other autoimmune diseases, including Sjogren's syndrome, systemic sclerosis, rheumatoid arthritis, and systemic lupus erythematosus [51].

Patients typically present with fatigue, jaundice, and pruritus, with the latter two symptoms arising from hyperbilirubinemia. Xanthelasma, xanthomas, and hyperpigmentation may be present on exam. As disease progresses to cirrhosis, this may be reflected in exam findings.

Initial workup of PBC includes serum antimitochondrial antibodies, which are present in 90–95% of patients with PBC, and liver chemistries, which will demonstrate a cholestatic pattern [50]. Bilirubin will be elevated in advanced disease. Other autoantibodies that may be present include antinuclear antibody, which are not specific to PBC, anti-glycoprotein-210 antibodies, and anti-centromere antibodies. The latter two correlate with end-stage liver disease and portal hypertension, respectively [51]. US, MRCP, or CT may be used to rule out bile duct obstruction from other etiologies, including gallstones. Liver biopsy is not needed to confirm the diagnosis but is used to determine the stage of the disease.

First-line therapy is ursodeoxycholic acid, though its efficacy remains controversial. Although a Cochrane review in 2012 demonstrated improvement in liver chemistries and histopathologic staging, ursodeoxycholic acid did not show any benefits in mortality, liver transplantation, or symptoms [52]. Other adjuvant therapies include cholestyramine, a bile acid sequestrant used to treat pruritus from hyperbilirubinemia, and the lipid-dependent vitamins A, D, E, and K [50]. In advanced disease, liver transplantation may be indicated. Liver transplantation has been shown to be effective, with disease recurrence rate of approximately 20% [51].

35.4.2 Primary Sclerosing Cholangitis

Primary sclerosing cholangitis (PSC) is a fibroinflammatory disorder of the intrahepatic and extrahepatic bile ducts. In contrast to PBC, PSC can affect large ducts in addition to small ducts. The exact cause and pathogenesis of PSC are unknown. Eighty percentage of patients with PSC have IBD, usually ulcerative colitis. However, only 3–7.5% of patients with ulcerative colitis have PSC [53]. There is a higher prevalence of PSC in men compared to women, with a male to female ratio of 2–3 to 1. Most patients are diagnosed in their fourth and fifth decades of life [54]. Patients are often asymptomatic, with diagnostic workup pursued after routine liver chemistries demonstrate a cholestatic pattern.

The diagnosis of PSC requires two of the following three criteria: serum ALP greater than 1.5 times the upper limit of normal for more than 6 months, cholangiography demonstrating biliary strictures/irregularities, and liver biopsy that demonstrates PSC [53].

Malignancy is the most serious complication of PSC. Cholangiocarcinoma is the most common form of cancer in PSC patients, occurring in approximately 10–15% of patients with PSC. The risk of cholangiocarcinoma is 400-fold greater in patients with PSC compared to the general population. For this reason, some experts recommend surveillance for cholangiocarcinoma with annual liver chemistries, CA 19-9, and imaging [54]. The risk of colorectal

Table 35.4 Liver etiology table for patients with non-acute abnormal liver blood tests

	Standard liver aetiology panel	Extended liver aetiology panel
Viral hepatitis	Hepatitis B surface antigen AND hepatitis C antibody (with follow-on PCR if positive)	Anti-HBc and anti-HBs hepatitis B DNA quantification of hepatitis delta in high-prevalence areas
Iron overload	Ferritin AND transferrin saturation	Haemochromatosis gene testing
Autoimmune liver disease (excluding PSC)	Anti-mitochondrial antibody, anti-smooth muscle antibody, antinuclear antibody, serum immunoglobulins	Anti-LKM antibody and coeliac antibodies (consider ANCA in the presence of cholestatic liver blood tests)
Metabolic liver disease		Alpha-1-antitrypsin level; thyroid function tests; ceruloplasmin (age >3 and <40 years) ± urinary copper collection

From [27] [Newsome PN, et al. Guidelines on the management of abnormal liver blood tests. **Gut. 2018** Jan;67(1):6–19. doi: https://doi.org/10.1136/gutjnl-2017-314,924]. **It is open access article** [*This is an Open Access article distributed in accordance with the terms of the Creative Commons Attribution (CC BY 4.0) license, which permits others to distribute, remix, adapt and build upon this work, for commercial use, provided the original work is properly cited. See: http://creativecommons.org/licenses/by/4.0/*]
ANCA antineutrophil cytoplasmic antibodies, *LKM* liver kidney microsome, *PCR* polymerase chain reaction, *PSC* primary sclerosing cholangitis

cancer is also elevated in the setting of PSC, approximately tenfold greater than the general population. Accordingly, colonoscopy at the time of diagnosis is recommended [53].

There is no effective medical therapy for PSC. Liver transplantation is the most effective albeit not definitive treatment, as the recurrence rate of disease post-transplantation is between 12% and 20% [53] (Table 35.4).

35.5 Complications of Chronic Liver Disease

35.5.1 Cirrhosis

Cirrhosis affected 2.89 million individuals In the United States in 2015, and accounted for 1.3 million deaths during that time. NAFLD, HCV, and alcoholic liver disease are the most common causes of cirrhosis in the United States. Together they account for approximately 80% of individuals on the liver transplantation waitlist [55]. Other etiologies of cirrhosis include HBV, autoimmune hepatitis, primary sclerosing cholangitis, and primary biliary cholangitis.

Individuals who develop cirrhosis may present with nonspecific symptoms, including anorexia, weight loss, lethargy in addition to peripheral manifestations of liver disease. These include findings in the head and neck, abdomen, skin, extremities, in addition to features from hormonal changes and hemodynamic changes.

Cirrhosis may result in several changes in the skin. The most common is jaundice, which is yellowing of the skin and mucous membranes due to hyperbilirubinemia. Jaundice is usually not present until the serum bilirubin is greater than 2 or 3 mg/dL, and can be accompanied by pruritus [55]. Spider angiomata are vascular lesions consisting of a central arteriole surrounded by several smaller vessels. They are usually found on the trunk and upper limbs. They are believed to be a result of sex hormone metabolism, and the number and size of spider angiomata correlates with severity of underlying cirrhosis [56].

Head and neck findings in cirrhosis include parotid gland enlargement and fetor hepaticus. The former is typically seen in cirrhosis from alcohol abuse, and is due to fatty infiltration, fibrosis, and edema. Fetor hepaticus is characterized by a sweet smell to the breath caused by increasing dimethyl sulfide levels from portal-systemic shunting [55].

Hormonal changes are also relatively common in cirrhosis. Women with cirrhosis may develop amenorrhea or oligomenorrhea from chronic anovulation, while men may develop impotence, infertility, and testicular atrophy from hypogonadism. Men may also develop gynecomastia. While not completely understood, the mechanism of gynecomastia is thought to be increased production of androstenedione from the adrenal glands, enhanced aromatization of androstenedione to estrone, and increased conversion of estrone to estradiol [56]. Other features of feminization in men include loss of chest and axillary hair and inversion of normal male pubic hair pattern [55].

As may be expected, there are various abdominal findings in cirrhosis. The cirrhotic liver may be enlarged, normal sized, or small. Splenomegaly results from red pulp congestion from portal hypertension, though the differential diagnosis of this exam finding includes many extrahepatic etiologies as well. Caput medusae refer to the engorged superficial epigastric veins that occur as a result of portal hypertension. The veins of the lower abdominal wall normal drain inferiorly into the iliofemoral system, while those of the upper abdominal wall drain superiorly into the thoracic wall and axilla. Portal hypertension causes the umbilical vein to reopen. This results in a shunt from the portal venous system through the periumbilical veins into the umbilical vein and superficial epigastric veins, causing them to become distended and engorged [5]. The Cruveilhier-Baumgarten murmur occurs in the setting of portal hypertension due to collateral connections between the portal system and the remnant umbilical vein. The murmur is increased with maneuvers that increase intraabdominal pressure, such as Valsalva, and reduced by applying pressure on the skin superior to the umbilicus [56].

Changes in extremities in cirrhotic individuals include palmar erythema, clubbing, hypertrophic osteoarthropathy, Dupuytren's contracture. Palmar erythema, frequently found on the thenar and hypothenar eminences, is believed to be caused by changes in sex hormone metabolism [55]. Clubbing refers to the angle between the nail bed and proximal nail fold being greater than 180°. Hypertrophic osteoarthropathy is a painful chronic periostitis of the long bone. Neither clubbing nor hypertrophic osteopathy are specific for liver disease. Asterixis, or flapping of the hands, is suggestive of hepatic encephalopathy.

Hemodynamics are also affected by cirrhosis. Cirrhosis is the most common cause of portal hypertension, which is defined as a hepatic venous pressure gradient (HVPG). It is the measurement of pressure between the wedged hepatic venous pressure (WHVP) and free hepatic venous pressure [55]. Hence, it can be used as a measurement of the pressure gradient between the portal vein and inferior vena cava. HVPG is a measurement of the pressure. An HVPG greater than or equal to 5 mmHg is diagnostic of portal hypertension. HVPG greater than 12 mmHg drastically increases the risk for variceal hemorrhage [57]. As cirrhosis progresses, individuals typically have a reduction in mean arterial pressure. This is thought to be due to nitric oxide release from splanchnic vasculature as a response to portal hypertension. It is this mechanism that is also believed to be the etiology of hepatorenal syndrome (HRS) [55].

Portal hypertension causes the majority of complications that arise from cirrhosis. Decompensated cirrhosis is defined as cirrhosis in the setting of any of the following: HE, variceal hemorrhage, ascites, spontaneous bacterial peritonitis, hepatorenal syndrome, jaundice, or HCC [56].

Liver enzymes are usually moderately elevated in individuals with cirrhosis, with AST being more often elevated than ALT. ALP is also usually elevated in the setting of cirrhosis at a value less than 2–3 times the ULN [55]. Values higher than this are typically seen in cholestatic liver disease, such as choledocholithiasis, primary sclerosing cholangitis, and primary biliary cholangitis. Gamma-glutamyl transpeptidase (GGT) is an enzyme specific to the liver. As ALP elevations can be derived from liver or bone etiology, GGT can serve to ascertain the specific source of pathology. Bilirubin is typically normal in the early stages of cirrhosis, with a gradual rise correlating with the progression of the liver disease [56].

Albumin and INR serve as surrogate markers for liver synthetic function. Albumin and coagulation factors are exclusively synthesized in the liver. Accordingly, albumin levels fall and INR rises as synthetic function declines over time due to worsening cirrhosis. Hyponatremia is another common lab finding in cirrhosis, and is related to elevated levels of antidiuretic hormone (ADH) [55]. Thrombocytopenia which is also frequently seen in cirrhosis, is caused by primarily by portal hypertension resulting in splenic sequestration. Reduced thrombopoietin levels also contribute to thrombocytopenia, albeit to a lesser degree. Anemia can be caused by a variety of mechanisms in the setting of cirrhosis: Acute on chronic gastrointestinal blood loss, folate deficiency, alcohol toxicity, hypersplenism, bone marrow suppression, anemia of chronic disease, and hemolysis. Leukopenia and neutropenia may also be present, both as a result of hypersplenism [56].

Imaging studies used in the diagnosis of cirrhosis include US, CT, and MRI. Findings consistent with cirrhosis include shrunk liver, irregular contour, and nodular. US is considered the imaging modality of choice to evaluate liver parenchyma and to detect extrahepatic manifestations of cirrhosis [57]. Liver biopsy is generally not needed if cirrhosis is strongly suggested by clinical, laboratory, and radiologic data [55]. It is important to determine the underlying cause of cirrhosis, as it may help predict prognosis and further treatment.

35.6 Complications of Cirrhosis

35.6.1 Portal Hypertension

Portal hypertension is characterized in hypertension in the hepatic portal system. Etiologies can be classified as prehepatic, intrahepatic, and posthepatic. The most common cause of portal hypertension is cirrhosis, which is an intrahepatic cause [57]. Prehepatic causes include portal or splenic vein thrombosis, while post-hepatic causes include Budd-Chiari syndrome and inferior vena cava obstruction.

The treatment of portal hypertension classically has consisted of portosystemic shunts such as splenorenal or H-shunts. More recently, transjugular intrahepatic portosystemic shunting (TIPS) has become the treatment of choice in managing portal hypertension. It has the benefit of being a technically less challenging procedure and less disruptive to the hepatic vasculature, with worsening of hepatic encephalopathy being the most common adverse effect [58].

35.6.2 Esophageal Varices

Esophageal varices are extremely dilated superficial veins of the distal third of the esophagus that arise from portal hypertension. Eighty-five percentage of patients with CTP class C have esophageal varices, while only 40% of patients with CTP class A have them [59]. Variceal hemorrhage carries a high mortality rate, as 15–20% of patients die within 6 weeks of initial hemorrhage [60].

In acute variceal hemorrhage, treatment is directed towards achieving hemostasis and maintaining adequate blood pressure. Two large-bore intravenous lines should be placed for fluid resuscitation, and blood should be transfused to achieve a goal hemoglobin of greater than 7 g/dL [61]. Higher hemoglobin goals have been associated with increased portal pressure and bleeding. Continuous octreotide infusion for 3–5 days should also be initiated to help reduce portal pressure and hemorrhage [59]. Intravenous proton-pump inhibitor therapy is indicated for the same reason. Prophylactic antibiotics should be administered to prevent spontaneous bacterial peritonitis and other infections, as up to 50% of patients with cirrhosis and acute gastrointestinal bleed develop infections within 1 week [60]. Treatment with oral norfloxacin or intravenous ciprofloxacin for 7 days is recommended. Ceftriaxone is preferred in patients with CTP class B and C cirrhosis, patients on fluoroquinolone prophylaxis, or in geographic areas with high rates of fluoroquinolone resistance [59]. Therapeutic endoscopy with variceal ligation with banding or sclerotherapy is considered the mainstay of acute treatment. In instances where this may not be readily available, balloon tamponade with a Sengstaken-Blakemore tube is indicated to serve as a bridge until endoscopy can be performed. Nonselective β-blocker (e.g. propranolol or nadolol) should be administered after patient is stabilized following therapeutic endoscopy. Surveillance endoscopy is indicated every 2–4 weeks, and may be spaced out to every 6–12 months if findings are stable [60]. TIPS may be indicated in patients with early rebleeding or uncontrolled bleeding.

Patients with known varices should receive treatment to reduce the risk of bleeding. Non-selective β-blockers are considered first-line therapy. If β-blocker therapy is contraindicated, as in patients with severe uncontrolled reactive airway disease, prophylactic endoscopic variceal ligation is indicated [60].

35.6.3 Gastric Varices and Portal Hypertensive Gastropathy

Gastric varices are a relatively common complication of cirrhosis, with a prevalence of 20% [59]. Unlike in the management of esophageal varices, primary prophylaxis is not indicated for gastric varices. Management of acute gastric variceal hemorrhage is similar to that of esophageal variceal hemorrhage, involving hemodynamic resuscitation with IV fluids and blood, prophylactic antibiotics, and portal pressure reduction with octreotide. Gastric varices that are extensions of esophageal varices can be treated successfully with band ligation. Cyanoacrylate (glue) injection is recommended for treatment of all other gastric variceal bleeds, though band ligation can be used if glue is not available. TIPS can be considered for uncontrolled bleeding or rebleeding [59].

Portal hypertensive gastropathy (PHG) is a congestive gastropathy that is results from portal hypertension. Contrary to varices, PHG commonly causes chronic mild bleeding. Treatment includes non-selective β-blockers and iron supplementation [58].

35.6.4 Hepatic Encephalopathy

Hepatic encephalopathy (HE) is a neuropsychiatric syndrome that develops in patients with cirrhosis. Severity of HE is graded from 0 to IV. Diagnosis is made via history and physical exam. Ammonia levels may be of use but trending ammonia levels is not recommended. HE grade II or greater usually warrants hospitalization [62]. The vast majority of patients with HE will have a precipitating factor, most commonly infection or gastrointestinal bleeding [55]. Inappropriate lactulose dosing or noncompliance, TIPS, or hypoglycemia can also cause HE. First-line treatment is lactulose, and should be dosed to achieve a goal of three bowel movements per day [62]. Rifaximin or neomycin can be added as adjunctive therapy, as studies have shown addition of rifaximin hastens the resolution of HE compared to lactulose alone [63].

35.6.5 Hepatopulmonary Syndrome

Hepatopulmonary syndrome (HPS) is a sequela of chronic liver disease that causes platypnea (worsening dyspnea when upright) and orthodeoxia (worsening arterial oxygen saturation when upright). The mechanism involves intrapulmonary arteriovenous dilatation due to increased concentrations of vasodilators, including nitric oxide [55]. This causes overperfusion and subsequent ventilation-perfusion mismatch and hypoxemia, defined as an arterial oxygen tension of less than 80 mmHg on room air. An arterial blood gas will demonstrate an alveolar-arterial oxygen gradient greater than 15 mmHg and echocardiography will show evidence of intrapulmonary shunting. The only definitive treatment for hepatopulmonary syndrome is liver transplantation [64].

35.6.6 Portopulmonary Hypertension

Portopulmonary hypertension (PPH) is pulmonary hypertension in the presence of portal hypertension from cirrhosis. Similar to hepatopulmonary syndrome, it stems from increased vasodilators such as nitric oxide [56]. However in contrast to HPS, PPH results from a compensatory increase in intrapulmonary vasoconstrictors, most notably endothelin-1 [64]. Patients will usually present with dyspnea, usually at exertion, in the setting of cirrhosis. Diagnostic testing involves echocardiography and subsequent right heart catheterization if right ventricular systolic pressures are found to be markedly elevated. Medical therapy mirror that of isolated pulmonary hypertension and consists of prostacyclin analogues, endothelin antagonists, and phosphodiesterase inhibitors [64].

35.6.7 Ascites

Ascites is characterized by abnormal buildup of fluid in the abdomen. It is the most common complication of cirrhosis. Approximately half of all patients with cirrhosis will develop ascites within 10 years of diagnosis [55]. Diagnosis can be achieved with physical exam, which may demonstrate a fluid wave and shifting dullness, or by ultrasound. Treatment involves low sodium diet (less than 2 g daily), diuretics, therapeutic paracentesis, and TIPS [58]. If paracentesis is performed, ascitic fluid should be analyzed for albumin and total protein to calculate serum-ascites albumin gradient (SAAG), in addition to cell count, gram stain, and bacterial culture if infection is suspected. SAAG can be used to assess etiology of ascites. A SAAG greater than or equal to 1.1 g/dL with an ascitic total protein of less than 2.5 g/dL is consistent with cirrhosis [55].

35.6.8 Spontaneous Bacterial Peritonitis

Spontaneous bacterial peritonitis (SBP) is a bacterial infection in the peritoneum that causes peritonitis. E.coli and klebsiella are the common causative bacteria, with gram positive bacteria accounting for less than 25% of all cases [65]. Patients typically present with abdominal pain, fever, or HE. Diagnostic workup consists of a diagnostic paracentesis, and ascitic fluid should be analyzed for cell count, gram stain, and bacterial culture. Diagnosis is confirmed with greater than 250 neutrophils/μL [55]. Treatment consists of antibiotics, usually a third-generation cephalosporin such as cefotaxime or ceftriaxone. Patients with serum creatinine greater than 1 mg/dL, total bilirubin greater than 4 mg/dL, or blood urea nitrogen greater than 30 mg/dL should be treated with albumin, with 1.5 g/kg given on the day of diagnosis followed by 1 g/kg given 2 days later [66]. Prophylaxis with norfloxacin or ciprofloxacin are indicated for primary prevention in patients who are considered to be high risk. This includes patients with ascitic fluid protein less than 1.5 g/dL and any of the following: CTP class B or C, serum sodium less than or equal to 130 mEq/L, serum creatinine greater than or equal to 1.2 mg/dL, blood urea nitrogen greater than or equal to 25 mg/dL, or serum bilirubin greater than or equal to 3 mg/dL [65]. All patients with SBP should receive prophylaxis for secondary prevention [58].

35.6.9 Hepatorenal Syndrome

Hepatorenal syndrome (HRS) is characterized by rapidly declining renal function in the setting of cirrhosis or ALF [55]. It is defined as an increase in serum creatinine to greater than 1.5 mg/dL, lack of response to albumin challenge of 1 g/kg/day for 2 days in the absence of any other causes of acute kidney injury. Type 1 HRS is more severe, and is defined by doubling of serum creatinine to a level greater than 2.5 mg/dL in less than 2 weeks. Type 2 HRS has a more gradual progression, with the hallmark of ascites not responsive to diuretics [67]. Type 1 HRS is treated with midodrine, octreotide, and albumin on the medicine ward, or with albumin and norepinephrine in the ICU [58]. Patients with type 1 HRS who do not respond to medical therapy should receive liver transplantation with or without kidney transplantation. Without transplantation, the life expectancy of patients with type 1 HRS is on the order of weeks [67].

35.6.10 Hepatocellular Carcinoma

Hepatocellular carcinoma (HCC) is the most common type of primary liver cancer, and is the most common cause of death of patients with cirrhosis. Although cirrhosis of any etiology is the greatest risk factor for HCC, cirrhosis from viral hepatitis accounts for approximately 80% of HCC cases worldwide. HCC is most prevalent in Asia and sub-Saharan Africa, which correlates with the prevalence of HBV [68]. In the US, HCC is caused from cirrhosis due to HCV, NASH, and alcohol abuse [69].

Patients may present with worsening symptoms of chronic liver disease, in addition to anorexia, unintentional weight loss, and fatigue.

HCC screening plays an integral role in the management of chronic liver disease. In the US, the American Association for the Study of Liver Diseases (AASLD) recommends screening patients with cirrhosis with ultrasound every 6 months, with or without measurement of the serum tumor marker alpha-fetoprotein [33].

Diagnosis is based on imaging and lab findings. AFP has been shown to reflect tumor size and volume, as more poorly differentiated tumors tend to produce higher levels of AFP [70]. Prognosis drastically worsens with serum AFP levels greater than 1000 ng/ml [71]. Imaging is an integral part of diagnostic workup and includes multiphasic contrast CT or MRI. US was previously used but has been replaced due to low sensitivity and positive predictive value in setting of cirrhosis. Extrahepatic spread is evaluated by contrast CT or PET. Liver biopsy has traditionally been considered the gold standard for the diagnosis of HCC, owing to its sensitivity and specificity of 96% and 95% respectively. However, current guidelines hold that biopsy is not necessary if clinical, laboratory, and radiographic findings are strongly suggestive of HCC [20].

Treatment of HCC depends on the stage of the disease as well as the patient's surgical candidacy. Surgical resection of tumor is usually not attempted as it is associated with high morbidity and mortality in addition to a recurrence rate of 50–60% [72]. Liver transplantation has become increasingly popular due to improving surgical techniques and the adoption of the Milan criteria, which has been used to assess if patients are appropriate candidates for transplant. It is largely responsible for marked improvement in survival rates compared to when liver transplantation was initially used [69]. Other treatment modalities include ablation, including radiofrequency ablation (RFA), cryoablation, and percutaneous ethanol injection (PEI) [72].

Additionally, transcatheter arterial chemoembolization (TACE) can be performed for unresectable tumors or as temporary treatment in anticipation of liver transplantation. It involves the injection of a chemotherapeutic agent, usually cisplatin, in addition to an embolic agent into the right or left hepatic artery. By restricting the tumor's vascular supply, TACE has been shown to improve survival rates and downstage HCC to allow patients to meet Milan criteria for liver transplantation [72].

Systemic chemotherapy may be considered in patients with metastatic disease. Sorafenib, an oral multikinase inhibitor, is the only systemic agent and first-line treatment for advanced HCC. It has been shown to have mild improvement in survival rates [20].

35.7 Determining Prognosis

35.7.1 MELD

The Model for End-Stage Liver Disease, or MELD, is a scoring system used to assess the severity of chronic liver disease and predict short-term mortality. It was originally developed based on survival data from patients who underwent TIPS procedure [73]. It has more recently been adopted by the United Network for Organ Sharing (UNOS) to prioritize allocation of deceased donor organs for liver transplantation [74]. Variables that are included in the MELD calculation include total bilirubin, serum sodium, INR, and serum creatinine [75]. The higher the MELD score, the lower the 3-month survival. The MELD score has fewer limitations than the CTP score as it only includes objective data and can discriminate more accurately between abnormal laboratory values [76].

35.7.2 Child-Turcotte-Pugh

Child-Turcotte-Pugh (CTP) is another scoring system used to categorize chronic liver disease and predict mortality. It was initially developed in 1964 to risk-stratify patients undergoing shunt surgery for portal decompression [77]. Variables include total bilirubin, serum albumin, INR, ascites, and hepatic encephalopathy, and are used to stratify patients into Classes A, B, and C [78]. Class A are associated with the highest 1 and 2 year survival rates, while Class C are associated with the lowest. The CTP score has several drawbacks. Firstly, it has limited capacity to discriminate patients based on abnormal lab results. For instance, a patient with a serum bilirubin of 20 mg/dL would be assigned the same score as a patient with a serum bilirubin of 3.5 mg/dL. Additionally, equal weight is given to all parameters. Moreover, two of the five parameters (ascites and encephalopathy) must be determined subjectively. Lastly, several key prognostic factors, including serum creatinine and variceal hemorrhage, are not accounted for in the CTP score [76].

35.8 Future Directions

The field of hepatology has recently seen a surge in the area of translational research. Serum biomarkers have in particular been at the center of a large effort to develop noninvasive methods to more accurately diagnose and monitor hepatobiliary diseases. In the following section, we discuss some of the most prominent and well-studied molecular structures with an emphasis on their potential to serve as novel biomarkers for various liver diseases.

35.8.1 Cytokeratin 18

Cytokeratin 18 (CK18) is a type I cytokeratin that is expressed in single layer epithelial tissues of the body. It serves to provide a flexible intracellular scaffolding to structure cytoplasm, resist external stress applied to the cell, and maintain mitochondrial structures [79]. Mutations in this gene have been linked to cryptogenic cirrhosis. Studies have demonstrated that plasma CK18 fragment levels correlate with the magnitude of hepatocyte apoptosis and may be used as an independent predictor of NASH [80, 81]. Thus, CK18 may have utility in the future as a noninvasive biomarker for NASH.

35.8.2 MicroRNA

MicroRNAs (miRNAs) are small RNAs that regulate gene expression by inhibiting turnover of mRNAs. Recent studies have shown that miRNAs are released into the peripheral circulation, and that circulating miRNAs may serve as optimal biomarkers for various disease processes, owing to their simple chemical structure, stability, and lack of post-processing modifications [82]. Circulating miRNAs can be bound to serum proteins and lipoproteins or carried in extracellular vesicles such as exosomes and microvesicles [83]. Because exosomes are released by various hepatic cells and transferred to other hepatic cells to regulate gene expression, they were thought to play an integral role in cell-cell communication, particularly with regards to liver disease pathophysiology [84].

Indeed, miRNAs have been implicated in playing a role in various liver diseases, with the potential to serve as biomarkers for ALF, liver fibrosis, NAFLD, cirrhosis, AIH, PSC, PBC, and HCC [84]. In studies on acetaminophen (APAP)-induced ALF in mice, liver specific miR-122 and miR-192 were found to be elevated in sera [82]. Specifically, serum miR-122 levels were detectable in a large cohort of APAP-induced ALF soon after initial liver intoxication, at which point serum ALT levels were still normal [82]. Another study demonstrated that miR-138 had a sensitivity and specificity of 89.3% and 71.43% respectively for prediction of early stage fibrosis and of 89.3% and 93.02% respectively for prediction of late stage fibrosis [83]. Even more promisingly, recent meta-analysis on miR-21 showed a pooled sensitivity and specificity of 81.2% and 84.8% for the diagnosis of HCC [85]. This in particular is a very encouraging finding, as diagnosis of chronic liver disease can be challenging and early diagnosis can improve survival rates. Additionally, miR-122, one of the most well-studied miRNA in liver diseases, has been strongly linked to HCC. Specifically, decreased exosomal miR-122 expression has been seen in HCC. Moreover, miR-122 also has the potential to be a target for cancer therapy, as knockdown of miR-122 has been shown to improve HCC cell viability by inhibiting apoptosis [86].

Still, despite its promise as a potential diagnostic and prognostic tool, several issues may prevent the routine clinical use of miRNA. Difficulty with data normalization due to a lack of an RNA housekeeping gene and inter-platform differences in miRNA quantification that reduce comparability between studies. Additionally, most studies thus far have been performed at a single center with a small amount of patients.

35.8.3 Extracellular Vesicles

Extracellular vesicles (EVs) are vesicles secreted by virtually all cells. They contain a variety of material, including proteins, lipids, miRNAs, and mRNAs to regulate target cell function. EVs are grouped by size into three categories: exosomes (40–100 nm), microvesicles (MVs) (0.1–1 μm), and apoptotic bodies (1–4 μm) [87]. As described above, there has been great interest in identifying exosomes and their cargo miRNA to serve as biomarkers of various liver diseases. However, recent findings have also demonstrated the use of exosomes as therapeutic tools in liver diseases. Injection of exosomes isolated from human mesenchymal stem cells (MSCs) into mouse liver have been shown to improve carbon tetrachloride-induced liver fibrosis by suppressing collagen and pro-inflammatory cytokines such as TGF-β1 [88]. Similarly, intrasplenic injection of MSCs can enhance protein expression ultimately aiding in liver recovery from carbon tetrachloride-induced liver damage in mice [89]. MVs have also shown potential as novel therapeutic agents. MVs from liver stem cells have been shown to inhibit HCC cell growth, hypothesized to be facilitated by their various cargo miRNAs.

Self Study

Questions

1. Which statement is true?
   (a) Bilirubin is exclusively synthesized in the liver.
   (b) Unconjugated hyperbilirubinemia will result in bilirubin in the urine.
   (c) Hyperbilirubinemia is caused by overproduction of bilirubin, impaired uptake, conjugation, or excretion, or leakage from hepatocytes or bile ducts.
   (d) Hyperbilirubinemia is always accompanied by elevated transaminases.
2. Which statement is true?
   (a) An AST/ALT ratio of less than 2 is consistent with alcoholic liver disease.
   (b) ALP elevation in the setting of normal GGT level is suggestive of liver disease.
   (c) An elevated INR is suggestive of increased liver synthetic function.
   (d) While elevated serum AFP levels are suggestive of HCC, they can also be elevated in other malignancies as well as hepatitis.
3. Which statement is true?
   (a) Hepatitis A is treated with antiviral therapy.
   (b) Hepatitis C is the most prevalent of all viral hepatitides worldwide.
   (c) All patients with chronic hepatitis B should receive antiviral therapy.
   (d) Sustained virologic response (SVR) is defined as undetectable hepatitis C virus RNA 6 months after the completion of antiviral therapy.
4. Which statement is true?
   (a) Pentoxifylline is first-line treatment of alcoholic hepatitis.
   (b) Hepatic steatosis is reversible with cessation of alcohol consumption.
   (c) Five-year transplant-free survival rate is not affected by the cessation of alcohol consumption.
   (d) Patients with alcoholic hepatitis are usually asymptomatic.

5. Which statement is true?
   (a) Drug-induced liver injury is most commonly caused by antibiotics.
   (b) A serum ALT to LDH ratio of greater than 1.5 is suggestive of ischemic hepatitis.
   (c) Serum transferrin levels are elevated in hereditary hemochromatosis.
   (d) Antibodies to liver/kidney microsomes are suggestive of primary sclerosing cholangitis.
6. Which statement is true?
   (a) The presence of antimitochondrial antibodies are suggestive of primary biliary cholangitis.
   (b) Wilson's disease is characterized by low ceruloplasmin levels.
   (c) Primary biliary cholangitis is strongly associated with inflammatory bowel disease.
   (d) The malignancy that is most strongly associated with primary sclerosing cholangitis is hepatocellular carcinoma.

Answers

1. Which statement is true?
   (a) Bilirubin is made both in the bone marrow and in the liver. It is exclusively conjugated in the liver.
   (b) Conjugated hyperbilirubinemia will result in bilirubin in the urine. Unconjugated bilirubin is bound to albumin, and is not filtered by the glomerulus into the urine.
   (c) **Correct**: Hyperbilirubinemia can be caused by a variety of pathologies but all are related to overproduction, reduced excretion, impaired conjugation, or leakage.
   (d) Hyperbilirubinemia can be caused by a multitude of etiologies. Only liver disease such as cirrhosis will cause elevated transaminases as well.
2. Which statement is true?
   (a) An AST to ALT ratio greater than 2 is consistent with alcoholic liver disease. An AST to ALT ratio less than 2 is suggestive of NASH and Wilson's disease.
   (b) GGT is found in hepatocytes, in addition to a myriad of other cells. ALP is found in liver, bone, and placenta. Therefore, an elevated ALP in the setting of an elevated, not normal GGT, is suggestive of liver disease.
   (c) INR is a marker for coagulation function. It is affected by coagulation factors, which are made in the liver. Therefore, reduced, not elevated synthetic function, would cause an elevated INR.
   (d) **Correct**: AFP is not specific to HCC. It can also be elevated in gastric cancer, germ-cell tumors, and non-germ cell tumors.
3. Which statement is true?
   (a) Hepatitis A is a self-remitting illness and therefore should be treated with supportive care only.
   (b) Hepatitis B, not hepatitis C, is the most common of the viral hepatitides worldwide.
   (c) Patients with chronic hepatitis B should only receive antiviral treatment if serum ALT is elevated and HBV DNA is less than 10,000 IU/mL.
   (d) **Correct**: Sustained virologic response is a term used to define successful antiviral treatment of hepatitis C and is based on HCV viral load.
4. Which statement is true?
   (a) Prednisone, not pentoxifylline, is first-line treatment for alcoholic hepatitis. Pentoxifylline should be used in the setting of infection, variceal hemorrhage, or acute kidney injury.
   (b) **Correct**: Hepatic steatosis, the first stage of alcohol-induced liver disease, is reversible with cessation of alcohol consumption, as no fibrosis has occurred at this point.
   (c) Five-year transplant-free survival rate is doubled from 30% to 60% if patients cease alcohol consumption.
   (d) Patients with alcoholic hepatitis usually present with anorexia, jaundice, hepatomegaly, and abdominal pain. Patients with hepatic steatosis are usually asymptomatic.
5. Which statement is true?
   (a) Drug-induced liver injury is most commonly caused by acetaminophen, not antibiotics.
   (b) A serum ALT to LDH ratio of less than, not greater than 1.5 is suggestive of ischemic hepatitis.
   (c) **Correct**: Serum transferrin levels are the best initial screening test for hereditary hemochromatosis. Transferrin saturation values greater than 45% in men and 35% in premenopausal women necessitate further workup.
   (d) Antibodies to liver/kidney microsomes are suggestive of primary biliary cirrhosis, not primary sclerosing cholangitis.
6. Which statement is true?
   (a) **Correct**: Antimitochondrial antibodies are present in between 90% and 95% of patients with PBC.
   (b) Serum ceruloplasmin can be elevated or normal in Wilson's disease. Serum copper levels will be low.
   (c) Primary sclerosing cholangitis, not primary biliary cholangitis, is strongly associated with inflammatory bowel disease.
   (d) The malignancy that is most strongly associated with primary sclerosing cholangitis is cholangiocarcinoma, not hepatocellular carcinoma.

References

1. Sticova E, Jirsa M. New insights in bilirubin metabolism and their clinical implications. World J Gastroenterol. 2013;19:6398.
2. Raymond GD, Galambos JT. Hepatic storage and excretion of bilirubin in man. Am J Gastroenterol. 1971;55:135.
3. Schmid R, Diamond I, Hammaker L, Gundersen CB. Interaction of bilirubin with albumin. Nature. 1965;206:1041.
4. VanWagner LB, Green RM. Evaluating elevated bilirubin levels in asymptomatic adults. JAMA. 2015;313:516–7.
5. Karmen A, Wroblewski F, Ladue JS. Transaminase activity in human blood. J Clin Invest. 1955;34(1):126–31.
6. Kwo PY, Cohen SM, Lim JK. ACG clinical guideline: evaluation of abnormal liver chemistries. Am J Gastroenterol. 2017;112:18.
7. Moussavian SN, Becker RC, Piepmeyer JL, et al. Serum gamma-glutamyl transpeptidase and chronic alcoholism. Influence of alcohol ingestion and liver disease. Dig Dis Sci. 1985;30:211.
8. Cohen JA, Kaplan MM. The SGOT/SGPT ratio-an indicator of alcoholic liver disease. Dig Dis Sci. 1979;24:835.
9. Sharma U, Pal D, Prasad R. Alkaline phosphatase: an overview. Indian J Clin Biochem. 2014;29(3):269–78.
10. Goldberg DM. Structural, functional, and clinical aspects of gamma-glutamyltransferase. CRC Crit Rev Clin Lab Sci. 1980;12:1.
11. Lum G, Gambino SR. Serum gamma-glutamyl transpeptidase activity as an indicator of disease of liver, pancreas, or bone. Clin Chem. 1972;18:358.
12. Rothschild MA, Oratz M, Schreiber SS. Serum albumin. Hepatology. 1988;8:385.
13. Farrugia A. Albumin usage in clinical medicine: tradition or therapeutic? Transfus Med Rev. 2010;24(1):53–63.
14. Eschar J, Rudzki C, Zimmerman HJ. Serum levels of 5′-nucleotidase in disease. Am J Clin Pathol. 1967;47:598.
15. Hill PG, Sammons HG. An assessment of 5′-nucleotidase as a liver-function test. Q J Med. 1967;36:457.
16. Brewer GJ, Yuzbasiyan-Gurkan V. Wilson disease. Medicine (Baltimore). 1992;71:139.
17. Gibbs K, Walshe JM. A study of the caeruloplasmin concentrations found in 75 patients with Wilson's disease, their kinships and various control groups. Q J Med. 1979;48:447.
18. Marrero JA, Feng Z, Wang Y, et al. Alpha-fetoprotein, des-gamma carboxyprothrombin, and lectin-bound alpha-fetoprotein in early hepatocellular carcinoma. Gastroenterology. 2009;137:110.
19. Lok AS, Sterling RK, Everhart JE, et al. Des-gamma-carboxy prothrombin and alpha-fetoprotein as biomarkers for the early detection of hepatocellular carcinoma. Gastroenterology. 2010;138:493.
20. Bialecki ES, Di Bisceglie AM. Diagnosis of hepatocellular carcinoma. HPB (Oxford). 2005;7:26.
21. Marks PW. Hematologic manifestations of liver disease. Semin Hematol. 2013;50:216.
22. Johnston DG, Alberti KGMM, Binder C, Faber OK, Wright R, Orskov H. Hormonal and metabolic changes in hepatic cirrhosis. Horm Metab Res. 1982;14:34–9.
23. Megyesi C, Samols E, Marks V. Glucose tolerance and diabetes in chronic liver disease. Lancet. 1967;2:1051–6.
24. Ellis G, Goldberg DM, Spooner RJ, Ward AM. Serum enzyme tests in diseases of the liver and biliary tree. Am J Clin Pathol. 1978;70:248.
25. American College of Physicians. Gastroenterology and Hepatology. MKSAP: Medical Knowledge Self-Assessment 18. Philadelphia, PA: American College of Physicians. p. 50. isbn:978-1-938245-50-3 19881989.
26. Sahani DV, Sanjeeva PK. Imaging the liver. Oncologist. 2004;9:385–97.
27. Newsome PN, et al. Guidelines on the management of abnormal liver blood tests. Gut. 2018 Jan;67(1):6–19. https://doi.org/10.1136/gutjnl-2017-314924.
28. Matheny SC, Kingery JE. Hepatitis A. Am Fam Physician. 2012;86(11):1027–34. quiz 1010–1012
29. Dienstag JL. Acute viral hepatitis. In: Kasper D, Fauci A, Hauser S, Longo D, Jameson J, Loscalzo J, editors. Harrison's principles of internal medicine. 19th ed. New York, NY: McGraw-Hill; 2015. isbn:978-0-07-180215-4.
30. Liang TJ. Hepatitis B: the virus and disease. Hepatology (Baltimore, MD). 2009;49(5 Suppl):S13–21.
31. Vos T, Allen C, Arora M, et al. Global, regional, and national incidence, prevalence, and years lived with disability for 310 diseases and injuries, 1990–2015: a systematic analysis for the Global Burden of Disease Study 2015. Lancet. 2016;388:1545–602.
32. Lok A, McMahon B, Brown R, Wong JB, Ahmed HT, Wigdan F, et al. Antiviral therapy for chronic hepatitis B virus infection in adults: a systematic review and meta-analysis. Hepatology. 2015;63:284–06.
33. CDC (2009) Guidelines for viral hepatitis surveillance and case management. http://www.cdc.gov/hepatitis/Statistics/Surveillance Guidelines.htm. Accessed 26 Nov 2011
34. Manns MP, Buti M, Gane E, Pawlotsky JM, Razavi H, Terrault N, et al. Hepatitis C virus infection. Nat Rev Dis Primers. 2017;3:17006.
35. Rutherford A, Dienstag JL. Viral hepatitis. In: Greenberger NJ, Blumberg RS, Burakoff R, editors. Current diagnosis & treatment: gastroenterology, hepatology, & endoscopy. 3rd ed. New York, NY: McGraw-Hill; 2016. isbn:978-0-07-183772-9.
36. Khalili M, Burman B. Liver disease. In: Hammer GD, McPhee SJ, editors. Pathophysiology of disease: an introduction to clinical medicine. 7th ed. New York, NY: McGraw-Hill; 2013.
37. Hsieh TH, Liu CJ, Chen DS, Chen PJ. Natural course and treatment of hepatitis D virus infection. J Formos Med Assoc. 2006;105:869–81.
38. Menon KV, Gores GJ, Shah VH. Pathogenesis, diagnosis, and treatment of alcoholic liver disease. Mayo Clin Proc. 2001;76(10):1021–9.
39. Osna NA, Donohue TM Jr, Kharbanda KK. Alcoholic liver disease: pathogenesis and current management. Alcohol Res. 2017;38(2):147–61.
40. Fontana R, Hayashi P. Clinical features, diagnosis, and natural history of drug-induced liver injury. Seminars in liver disease. 2014;34(2):134–44.
41. Bynum TE, Boitnott JK, Maddrey WC. Ischemic hepatitis. Dig Dis Sci. 1979;24:129–35.
42. Fuchs S, Bogomolski-Yahalom V, Paltiel O, Ackerman Z. Ischemic hepatitis: clinical and laboratory observations of 34 patients. J Clin Gastroenterol. 1998;26:183–6.
43. Bernal W, Wendon J. Acute liver failure. N Engl J Med. 2013;369:2525–34.
44. Czaja AJ. Diagnosis and management of autoimmune hepatitis: current status and future directions. Gut Liver. 2016;10:177–203.
45. Benedict M, Zhang X. Non-alcoholic fatty liver disease: an expanded review. World J Hepatol. 2017;9:715–32.
46. Bacon BR, Adams PC, Kowdley KV, Powell LW, Tavill AS. Diagnosis and management of hemochromatosis: 2011 practice guideline by the American Association for the Study of Liver Diseases. Hepatology. 2011;54(1):328–43.
47. Crownover BK, Covey CJ. Hereditary hemochromatosis. Am Fam Physician. 2013;87:183–90.
48. Stoller JK, Aboussouan LS. A review of alpha1-antitrypsin deficiency. Am J Respir Crit Care Med. 2012;185:246–59.
49. Roberts EA, Schilsky ML. A practice guideline on Wilson disease. Hepatology. 2003;37:1475–92.
50. Lindor KD, Gershwin ME, Poupon R, Kaplan M, Bergasa NV, Heathcote EJ. Primary biliary cirrhosis. Hepatology. 2009;50:291–308.
51. Kaplan MM, Gershwin ME. Primary biliary cirrhosis. N Engl J Med. 2005;353:1261–73.

52. Rudic JS, Poropat G, Krstic MN, Bjelakovic G, Gluud C. Ursodeoxycholic acid for primary biliary cirrhosis. Cochrane Database Syst Rev. 2012;12:CD000551.
53. Lazaridis KN, LaRusso NF. Primary sclerosing cholangitis. N Engl J Med. 2016;375:1161–70.
54. Karlsen TH, Folseraas T, Thorburn D, Vesterhus M. Primary sclerosing cholangitis—a comprehensive review. J Hepatol. 2017;67(6):1298–323.
55. Tsochatzis EA, Bosch J, Burroughs AK. Liver cirrhosis. Lancet. 2014;383:1749–61.
56. Schuppan D, Afdhal NH. Liver cirrhosis. Lancet. 2008;371:838–51.
57. Procopet B, Berzigotti A. Diagnosis of cirrhosis and portal hypertension: imaging, non-invasive markers of fibrosis and liver biopsy. Gastroenterol Rep. 2017;5(2):79–89.
58. Ge PS, Runyon BA. Treatment of patients with cirrhosis. N Engl J Med. 2016;375:767–77.
59. Garcia-Tsao G, Bosch J. Management of varices and variceal hemorrhage in cirrhosis. N Engl J Med. 2010;362(9):823–32.
60. Haq I, Tripathi D. Recent advances in the management of variceal bleeding. Gastroenterol Rep. 2017;5:113–26.
61. Villanueva C, et al. Transfusion strategies for acute upper gastrointestinal bleeding. N Engl J Med. 2013;368(1):11–21.
62. Ferenci P. Hepatic encephalopathy. Gastroenterol Rep. 2017;5(2):138–47.
63. Sharma BC, et al. A randomized, double-blind, controlled trial comparing rifaximin plus lactulose with lactulose alone in treatment of overt hepatic encephalopathy. Am J Gastroenterol. 2013;108(9):1458–63.
64. Porres-Aguilar M, Altamirano JT, Torre-Delgadillo A, Charlton MR, Duarte-Rojo A. Portopulmonary hypertension and hepatopulmonary syndrome: a clinician-oriented overview. Eur Respir Rev. 2012;21:223–33.
65. Dever JB, Sheikh MY. Review article: spontaneous bacterial peritonitis—bacteriology, diagnosis, treatment, risk factors and prevention. Aliment Pharmacol Ther. 2015;41:1116–31.
66. Sort P, et al. Effect of intravenous albumin on renal impairment and mortality in patients with cirrhosis and spontaneous bacterial peritonitis. N Engl J Med. 1999;341(6):403–9.
67. Ng CKF, Chan MHM, Tai MHL, Lam CWK. Hepatorenal syndrome. Clin Biochem Rev. 2007;28:11–7.
68. Ferenci P, et al. Hepatocellular carcinoma (HCC): a global perspective. J Clin Gastroenterol. 2010;44:239–45.
69. Forner A, Llovet JM, Bruix J. Hepatocellular carcinoma. Lancet. 2012;379:1245–55.
70. Tangkijvanich P, Anukulkarnkusol N, Suwangool P, et al. Clinical characteristics and prognosis of hepatocellular carcinoma. Analysis based in serum αfetoprotein levels. J Clin Gastroenterol. 2000;31(4):302–8.
71. Hanazaki K, Kajikawa S, Koide N, Adachi W, Amano J. Prognostic factors after hepatic resection for hepatocellular carcinoma with hepatitis C viral infection: univariate and multivariate analysis. Am J Gastroenterol. 2001 Apr;96(4):1243–50.
72. Heimbach J, Kulik LM, Finn R, et al. AASLD guidelines for the treatment of hepatocellular carcinoma. Hepatology. 2018;67(1):358–80.
73. Malinchoc M, Kamath PS, Gordon FD, Peine CJ, Rank J, ter Borg PC. A model to predict poor survival in patients undergoing transjugular intrahepatic portosystemic shunts. Hepatology. 2000;31:864–71.
74. Wiesner R, Edwards E, Freeman R, et al. Model for end-stage liver disease (MELD) and allocation of donor livers. Gastroenterology. 2003;124:91–6.
75. Cholongitas E, Marelli L, Shusang V, Senzolo M, Rolles K, Patch D, et al. A systematic review of the performance of the model for end-stage liver disease (MELD) in the setting of liver transplantation. Liver Transpl. 2006;12:1049–61.
76. Cholongitas E, Papatheodoridis GV, Vangeli M, Terreni N, Patch D, Burroughs AK. Systematic review: the model for end-stage liver disease–should it replace Child-Pugh's classification for assessing prognosis in cirrhosis? Aliment Pharmacol Ther. 2005;22(11–12):1079–89.
77. Child CG, Turcotte JG. Surgery and portal hypertension. Major Probl Clin Surg. 1964;1:1–85.
78. Durand F, Valla D. Assessment of prognosis of cirrhosis. Semin Liver Dis. 2008;28:110–22.
79. Weng Y, Cui Y, Fang J. Biological functions of cytokeratin 18 in cancer. Mol Cancer Res. 2012;10:485–93.
80. Maher MM, Ibrahim WA, Saleh SA, Shash L, Abou Gabal H, Tarif M, et al. Cytokeratin 18 as a non invasive marker in diagnosis of NASH and its usefulness in correlation with disease severity in Egyptian patients. Egypt J Med Hum Genet. 2015;16(1):41–6. https://doi.org/10.1016/j.ejmhg.2014.11.003.
81. Feldstein AE, Wieckowska A, Lopez AR, Liu YC, Zein NN, McCullough AJ. Cytokeratin-18 fragment levels as noninvasive biomarker for nonalcoholic steatohepatitis: A multicenter validation study. Hepatology. 2009;50:1072–8.
82. Wang K, Zhang S, Marzolf B, Troisch P, Brightman A, Hu Z, Hood LE, Galas DJ. Circulating microRNAs, potential biomarkers for drug-induced liver injury. Proc Natl Acad Sci U S A. 2009 Mar 17;106(11):4402–7.
83. Cortez MA, Bueso-Ramos C, Ferdin J, Lopez-Berestein G, Sood AK, Calin GA. MicroRNAs in body fluids—the mix of hormones and biomarkers. Nat Rev Clin Oncol. 2011;8(8):467–77.
84. Loosen SH, Schueller F, Trautwein C, et al. Role of circulating microRNAs in liver diseases. World J Hepatol. 2017;9:586–94.
85. El-Ahwany E, Nagy F, Zoheiry M, Shemis M, Nosseir M, Taleb HA, El Ghannam M, Atta R, Zada S. Circulating miRNAs as predictor markers for activation of hepatic stellate cells and progression of HCV-induced liver fibrosis. Electr Phys. 2016;8(1):1804–10.
86. Wu X, Wu S, Tong L, Luan T, Lin L, Lu S, et al. MiR-122 affects the viability and apoptosis of hepatocellular carcinoma cells. Sci J Gastroenterol. 2009;44:1332–9.
87. Sato K, Meng F, Glaser S, Alpini G. Exosomes in liver pathology. J Hepatol. 2016;65:213–21.
88. Li T, Yan Y, Wang B, Qian H, Zhang X, Shen L, et al. Exosomes derived from human umbilical cord mesenchymal stem cells alleviate liver fibrosis. Stem Cells Dev. 2013;22:845–54.
89. Tan CY, Lai RC, Wong W, Dan YY, Lim SK, Ho HK. Mesenchymal stem cell-derived exosomes promote hepatic regeneration in drug-induced liver injury models. Stem Cell Res Ther. 2014;5:76.

Noninvasive Biomarkers for Liver Fibrosis

36

Gamal Shiha and Nasser Mousa

Key Concepts

- The liver fibrosis is a pathological state caused by different etiology and is associated with significant morbidity and mortality.
- Noninvasive diagnosis of liver fibrosis is one of the fields that has growth more quickly in current days.
- For the diagnosis of significant fibrosis, a combination of noninvasive biomarkers tests with concordance may provide the peak diagnostic accuracy.
- Newly discovered biomarkers may have vital role preceding the therapy by non-specialists to build sure that patients with severe fibrosis/cirrhosis are referred for proper definite specialist assessment.
- Noninvasive evaluation with any serum biomarkers can be used to check improvement in liver fibrosis throughout antiviral treatment.
- Successful diagnosis of liver fibrosis needs more reliable biomarkers which are specific to the liver.

36.1 Introduction

Five different types of cells occupy about 80% of the liver volume. The residual 20% include the extracellular spaces and components of the extracellular matrix [1]. Liver fibrosis is a reversible wound-healing response to cellular injury reflects an equilibrium between liver repair and scar formation. Throughout acute damage, the changes in liver architecture are temporary and reversible, while in chronic damage, there is progressive replacement of the liver parenchyma by scar tissue [2]. So that, liver fibrosis is the terminal result of an imbalance between the deposition-removal of extracellular matrix (ECM), which disrupts the standard architecture of the liver. The description of the basic mechanisms of liver fibrogenesis has pointed that, fibrosis is a dynamic course involving the increased synthesis of matrix components and a non success of physiological mechanisms of matrix turnover [3–6]. The maestro of hepatic fibrosis is the hepatic stellate cell (HSC), that orchestrating the deposition of ECM in healthy and fibrotic liver. HSCs are resident perisinusoidal cells within the subendothelial space between hepatocytes and sinusoidal endothelial cells (Fig. 36.1). They're well placed to closely interact with hepatocytes, endothelial cells, and nerve endings through their several processes extending across the space of Disse [7, 8].

In injured liver, the activated phenotype of HSCs is a myofibroblast, that secrete extracellular matrix components and expressing α-smooth muscle actin and linked to the establishment of the fibrotic state. By distinction, clearance of fibrotic scar tissue is related to HSC apoptosis or de-differentiation of HSCs [9].

In the space of Disse' of the normal liver, an organized group of proteins known as the extracellular matrix (ECM) can be observed in direct contact with the basal lamina (low-density material similar to the "basal membrane" that is formed by type IV collagen together with laminin and entactin along the sinusoidal wall. This ECM is the support for the parenchymatous cells and reinforcing the organ's architecture [10, 11].

In the advanced stage of fibrotic liver (cirrhosis), the elements of the ECM are large in amount. These large amounts are firstly placed within the portal tract and/or central vein, resulting in the event of fibrous networks between the vascular structures followed by capillarization of sinusoidal endothelium and loss of microvilli of the hepatocytes. This leads to interruption of the normal vascularization of the hepatic lobe, shunting of the portal and arterial blood directly into

G. Shiha (✉)
Department of Internal Medicine and Hepatology, Mansoura University, Mansoura, Egypt

Egyptian Liver Research Institute and Hospital (ELRIH), Sherbin, El-Mansoura, Mansoura, Egypt

N. Mousa
Departments of Tropical Medicine, Mansoura University, Mansoura, Egypt

F. Radu-Ionita et al. (eds.), *Liver Diseases*, https://doi.org/10.1007/978-3-030-24432-3_36

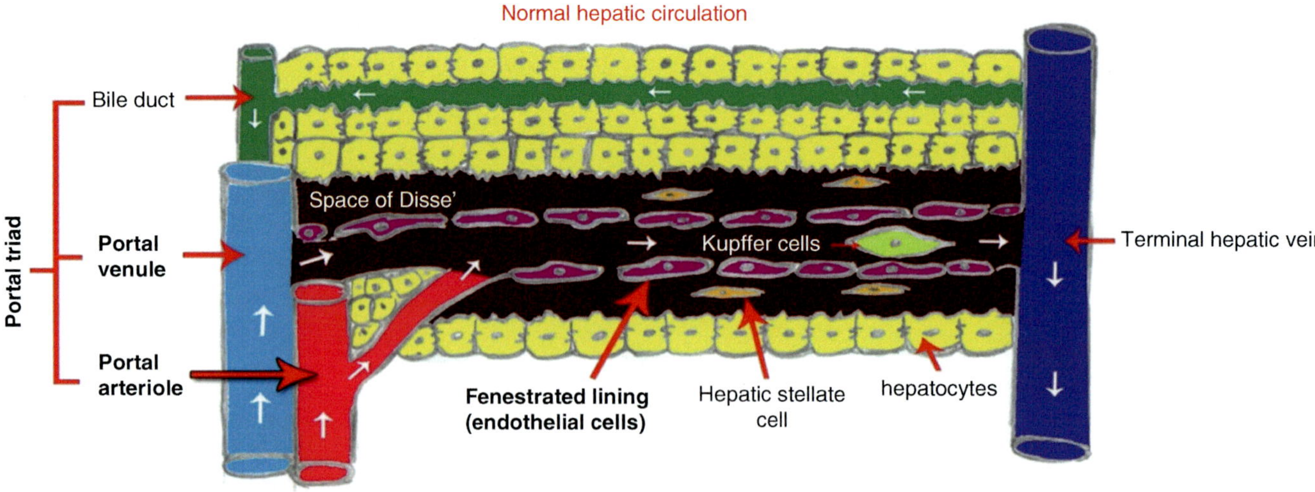

Fig. 36.1 Normal hepatic circulation. In healthy liver, the blood runs comes from the mesenteric circulation to the liver through terminal portal vein and terminal hepatic artery in portal tracts. The blood goes through the hepatic sinusoids then through the fenestrated sinusoidal endothelium which lie on space of Disse (consists of loose connective tissue) where the metabolic exchange between blood and hepatocytes occurs. After metabolic exchange, the sinusoidal blood is collected and drained by central hepatic into hepatic veins and lastly the caval vein

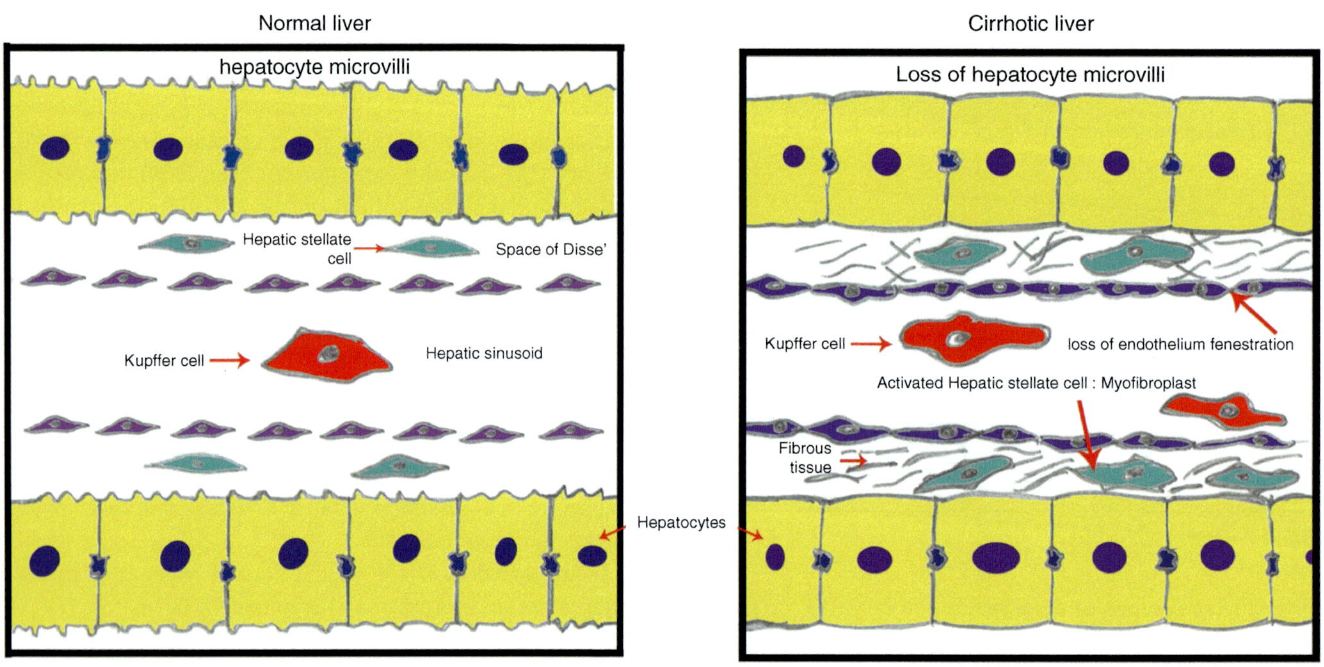

Fig. 36.2 In cirrhotic liver there are, transdifferentiation of activated hepatic stellate to matrix-synthesizing myofibroblasts that produce excess extracellular matrix (ECM), loss of hepatocyte microvilli, disappearance of endothelial fenestrations with capillarization of the sinusoids, fibrous portal tract expansion, fibrosis of the central vein, congestion of the space of Disse' with ECM, and departure of perisinusoidal hepatocyte from sinusoidal blood flow by collagenous septa. Lastly, the blood is directly forced from terminal portal veins and arteries to central veins, with resultant portal hypertension

the hepatic outflow (central veins), impaired interchange between hepatic sinusoids and the hepatocytes and deterioration of the liver function (Fig. 36.2) [12, 13]. Cirrhosis and its related vascular distortion are traditionally considered to be irreversible however recent knowledge suggested that, cirrhosis maybe reversal [14, 15].

36.2 Extracellular Matrix (ECM) from Normal to Fibrotic Liver

In normal liver, an organized cluster of proteins known as extracellular matrix (ECM) is found in space of Disse in direct contact with low-density basal lamina (similar to the basal membrane, that's comprised mainly of collagens IV and VI) with glycoproteins, proteoglycans and glycosaminoglycan's (hyaluronic acid) [10].

Liver fibrosis is associated with major alterations in each amount and composition of ECM. In advanced stage, fibrotic liver contains 3–10 times additional ECM than normal liver which comprising the fibril forming interstitial collagens (I, III and basement membrane collagen type IV), fibronectin, elastin, laminin, hyaluronic acid (HA) and proteoglycans [16]. The chief hepatic ECM manufacturing cells are myofibroblasts that either originate from activated hepatic stellate cells (HSC) or perivascular fibroblasts [12, 17]. The homeostasis of ECM during hepatic injury is incredibly vital. This homeostasis depends on, the well balance between matrix metalloproteinases (MMPs) and their inhibitors (tissue inhibitors of matrix metalloproteinases) (TIMPs) [18].

Degradation of ECM of liver is due to action of MMP. Three MMPs are present in humans, MMP-1 (collagenases), MMP-2 (gelatinase A) and MMP-9 (gelatinase B) [19]. These enzymes are manufactured intra-cellular and secreted as zymogens and inhibited by tissue inhibitors of metalloproteinases (TIMPs) [20]. In liver fibrosis, there'll be inverse correlation between levels of MMP-1 and histological severity [21]. MMP-2 secreted from hepatic stellate cells. It has been found that, a 2.4-fold increase in the levels of MMP-2 was in fibrotic patients compared with controls [22]. MMP-9 from Kupffer cells has negative correlation with histological severity [23]. ECM degradation by MMPs is inhibited by TIMPs. TIMP-1 will interact with nearly all the 3MMPs whereas TIMP-2 precisely interacts with MMP-2. Through advance of liver disease, serum levels of TIMPs will increase. MMP-1/TIMP-1 ratio is beneficial for the diagnosis of hepatic fibrosis and correlates with degree of portal inflammation [24]. Additionally, in hepatic fibrosis, there was, an accumulation of other matrix proteins, including elastin, hyaluronan, proteoglycans and fibronectin. This type of matrix has the capacity to activate quiescent HSCs, producing disappearance of endothelial fenestrations and hepatocyte microvilli (Fig. 36.2) [25].

The alteration of ECM proteins influences cellular behavior and resulting in vanishing of endothelial fenestrations impairs the transport of solutes from the sinusoid to the hepatocytes, So that encourage hepatocyte dysfunction [26].

36.3 Liver Biopsy

At present and since 50 years the sole accepted gold standard method for the diagnosis of the fibrotic stages of chronic liver disease is a liver biopsy. Also to permit histological grading of inflammation and the staging of fibrosis. The added benefits of liver biopsy are to be confirmed the etiology of liver disease, assessing potential disease co-factors such as hepatic steatosis, iron overload. However, the biopsy is clearly invasive with risks of pain, bleeding or perforation and rarely death. Additionally, liver biopsy is expensive and [27, 28]. Also many restrictions of the liver biopsy include, inefficiently reflection of the fibrotic changes occurring in the entire liver because an optimally sized biopsy contains 5–11 complete portal tracts and [29]. Moreover the process of hepatic fibrosis is not linear, and biopsies from different areas have shown different stages of fibrosis [30]. Also a number of papers have shown that, cirrhosis may be lost in 10–30% of patients [31]. Lastly disagreements between pathologists occur according to the experience of the pathologist [32]. This disadvantage of liver biopsy greatly restrict the frequency of utilization and therefore prevents accurate fibrosis assessment within the majority of patients with chronic liver disease.

36.4 Noninvasive Biomarkers of Liver Fibrosis

More recently, there has been growing attention in recognizing and describing hepatic fibrosis via the utilization of noninvasive biomarkers for the diagnosis of liver fibrosis. Initially developed in chronic viral hepatitis and now, dilated to incorporate all causes of CLD. Actuality these markers are noninvasive with nearly no problems, few sampling mistakes, measurements can be done frequently, thus allowing supervising the disease progression or regression [33]. These markers can be divided into (Table 36.1).

Table 36.1 Biomarkers of liver fibrosis

Indirect markers	Direct markers
Simple liver function tests: • Aminotransferases (ALT, AST) • Platelets (thrombocytes) • Bilirubin • Albumin • Prothrombin time • Glutamyltransferase (GGT), • α 2-macroglobulin • Cholesterol • Apolipoprotein A-I • Haptoglobin • Alkaline phosphatase • Pseudo-cholinesterase (PCHE)	1. Collagens – PICP – PIIINP – Type IV collagen 2. Collagenases and their inhibitors – MMPs – TIMPs 3. Glycoproteins and polysaccharides – Hyaluronic acid – Laminin – YKL-40 4. Cytokines – TGF-β1 – PDGF 5. Cytokeratin-18 fragments – Microfibril associated protein-4 6. Proteomic markers. – Phosphoproteomics – N-glycosylation of total serum protein 7. Genetic markers – SNP of AZIN1, TLR4, TRPM5, AQP2, STXBP5L

MMP matrix metalloproteinase, *PICP* procollagen I carboxy peptide, *PIIINP* procollagen III amino peptide, *TIMP* tissue inhibitors of metalloproteinase, *SNP* single nucleotide polymorphisms

(a) **Indirect "simple" markers**: This indirect markers measure component not directly intricate in the fibrosis course but reflect the changes in liver functions and are molecules released into the blood due to liver inflammation, but they do not correlate with ECM turnover [5, 34]. They have the advantage of being fairly cheap and easy to perform, but, they lack the diagnostic accuracy for the detection of hepatic fibrosis [35].
(b) **Direct "complex" markers**: Are direct markers of fibrosis and reflect the molecular pathogenesis and turnover of liver ECM. They are pathophysiologically markers derived from ECM turnover and/or from changes of the fibrogenic cell types in liver through the fibrosis process [34, 36]. Despite the fact that, there's no standard fibrosis marker, various molecules or algorithms are known as helpful indicators, once they are managed together [37]. Ultimately, both types of serum biomarkers are complementary.

36.5 Characteristics of Ideal Marker

- Great sensitivity and specificity to recognize different stages of fibrosis.
- Be ready available, safe, inexpensive, and can be repeated.
- Lack of false positive results for example, in individuals with inflammation related to other diseases.
- Be valid to the checking of the hepatic disease progression or regression.
- In this review, we try to understand the diagnostic accuracy, advantages and limitations of noninvasive Biomarkers of Liver Fibrosis (Table 36.2).

Table 36.2 Advantages and limitation of non-invasive biomarkers of fibrosis

Limitation	Advantages
Absence of organ specific, affected by unrelated sites of inflammation	Less invasive
Numerous of these markers are not regularly presented in many laboratories	Little hazard of sampling mistake
No one of the biomarkers have a high degree of accuracy	May be performed repeatedly over time
Influenced by impaired biliary and urinary excretion	Allowing for ongoing monitoring of fibrosis
Certain biomarkers lack standardization due to variable values and the different upper used by different laboratories	Relative low cost
All studies that evaluated the accuracy of NIBMs used the liver biopsy as the gold standard reference	Not associated with morbidity or mortality
Incapable to distinguish between intermediate stages of fibrosis	Can be performed in the out patient clinic
	Validated biomarkers with scores may be useful for monitoring therapy

36.5.1 Indirect Markers

36.5.1.1 Aspartate Aminotransferase (AST) and Alanine Aminotransferase (ALT) Ratio (AAR)

Serum alanine aminotransferase (ALT) is a vital indicator used to assess liver disease [12]. It has shown that, serum ALT level (2.25-fold) greater than the normal levels predicts liver histology [38]. However, serum ALT levels are affected from different aspects such as, sex, body mass index, and the use of hepatotoxic drugs [39, 40]. The AAR index is a simple index that used for evaluation of liver fibrosis and can be calculated by dividing the levels of the two enzyme (AST and ALT). It has been validated in different forms of liver disease [41, 42] and a ratio of >1 is predictive of cirrhosis [43, 44]. However, Shiha et al. found that, AAR is not a reliable predictor to differentiate significant fibrosis or advanced fibrosis in patients with chronic hepatitis B infection [45]. In certain acute and chronic hepatitis and/or steatosis this ratio is ≤1, but ratio >2 suggests alcoholic hepatitis [43, 46].

36.5.1.2 APRI

APRI is the index is dependent to two routine tests (aspartate aminotransferase and platelet count) and simply calculated by this formula:

$$\frac{(\text{AST / upper limit of the normal range})\times 100}{\text{PLT}\left(10^{9}\ \text{L}^{-1}\right)}$$

APRI was developed in 2003. The APRI of greater than 1.5 showed an area under the receiver operating curve of (0.8, and a 0.89) for advanced fibrosis F3–F4 and cirrhosis respectively [47]. Several studies had revealed that (APRI) is of great value and has great accuracy in predicting advanced fibrosis in dissimilar types of hepatic disease [45, 48, 49]. Conversely, when using the APRI alone, the stage of fibrosis is wrongly classified in 40–65% of cases [50]. The diagnostic accuracy of APRI was enhanced by Lok et al. by the combination of ALT and the international normalized ratio (INR) [51]. Additionally, the APRI was also found to be of great diagnostic accuracy in evaluating the advance of fibrosis in post liver transplant patients [52].

36.6 Immune Fibrosis Index (IFI) Score

Immune fibrosis index (IFI) is a novel noninvasive test, can be used easily for the prediction of liver fibrosis stage in CHC patients. IFI score utilize five biochemical markers and the score produced areas under curve of 0.949, 0.947, and 0.806 for differentiation of significant fibrosis (F2–F4), advanced fibrosis (F3–F4), and cirrhosis (F4) respectively.

The score is calculated as = 3.07 + 3.06 × CD4/CD8 + 0.02 × α-fetoprotein (U/L) − 0.07 × alanine aminotransferase ratio − 0.005 × platelet count (10/L) − 1.4 × albumin (g/dL) [53].

36.6.1 Prothrombin Time

Prothrombin time (PT) is marker that reveals the hepatic synthetic function and consequently is one of the early pointers of cirrhosis. In severe hepatocellular damage, PT remains raised for a longer time [20]. Additional studies confirmed that, PTs were correlated with the histologic fibrosis score [54], and with the occurrence and size of the esophageal varices [55].

36.6.2 The FIB-4 Score

The FIB-4 index is calculated using the formula: FIB-4 = Age (years) × AST (U/L)/[PLT (10^9 L^{-1}) × ALT1/2 (U/L)] [56]. Yang et al. reported that FIB-4 index had a significant power for differentiation between patients with mild and significant fibrosis in nonalcoholic fatty liver disease (0.24 ± 0.12 vs. 0.31 ± 0.21, P = 0.010) and the AUROC of FIB4 was 0.810. They reported that FIB4 might be useful as a noninvasive hepatic fibrosis scores for predicting hepatic fibrosis in patients with NAFLD [57]. This score was first developed to evaluate fibrosis in HIV/HCV co-infected, and was later valid for detection of fibrosis with AUCs of 0.85 and 0.81 for severe fibrosis, for isolated HCV and HBV infection, respectively [58]. In patients with chronic HBV infection, FIB-4 could reliably distinguish significant fibrosis, advanced fibrosis and cirrhosis [45].

$$\text{FIB}-4 = \frac{\text{Age}(\text{years}) \times \text{AST}(\text{U}/\text{L})}{\text{Platelet count}\left(10^9\ \text{L}^{-1}\right)} \times \sqrt{\text{ALT}(\text{U}/\text{L})}$$

36.7 Fibrofast; FIB-5

A simple non-invasive score (Fibrofast, FIB-5) was settled using five regular laboratory tests (ALT, AST, alkaline phosphatase, albumin and platelets count) for the discovery of significant hepatic fibrosis in patients with chronic hepatitis C. The performance characteristics of FIB-5 at ≥7.5 and FIB-4 at ≤1.45 for the distinction between non-significant fibrosis and significant fibrosis were: specificity 94.4%, PPV 85.7%, and specificity 54.9%, PPV 55.7% respectively [59].

36.7.1 The NAFLD Fibrosis Score

Components of this score include, six usually measured objects (age, hyperglycemia, BMI, platelet count, albumin and AST/ALT ratio) [60]. Shah et al. studied diagnostic accuracy of this scoring model in 541 adults with NAFLD for estimation of liver fibrosis and found an AUROC (95% confidence interval [CI] of 0.768; 0.720–0.816) for this model [61].

$$\begin{aligned}\textbf{NAFLD fibrosis score} &= -1.675 + 0.037 \times \text{age}(\text{years}) \\ &+ 0.094 \times \text{BMI}\left(\text{kg}/\text{m}^2\right) \\ &+ 1.13 \times \text{IFG}/\text{diabetes}(\text{yes} = 1, \text{no} = 0) \\ &+ 0.99 \times \text{AST}/\text{ALT ratio} - 0.013 \\ &\times \text{platelets}\left(10^9\ \text{L}^{-1}\right) - 0.66 \times \text{albumin}(\text{g}/\text{dL})\end{aligned}$$

36.7.2 Fibro Index

This index was settled by Koda et al. The score developed from platelet count, AST and γGT to assess fibrosis [62]. A cut-off of 2.25, was correlated with F2–F3 fibrosis and has 90% NPV. but, further validation showed this score has fewer diagnostic accuracy [63].

$$\begin{aligned}\text{Fibro index} &= 1.738 - 0.064 \times \text{platelet count}\left(10^4\ \text{mm}^{-3}\right) \\ &+ 0.005 \times \text{AST}(\text{IU}/\text{L}) + 0.463 \text{gamma globulin}(\text{g}/\text{dL})\end{aligned}$$

36.7.3 FibroTest (FibroSURE in USA)

Fibrotest is comprising panel of five biomarkers that suggested for assessment of liver fibrosis stage. Constituents of this index are, the age, gender, plus five serum biochemical parameters including, serum haptoglobin, α2-macroglobulin, apolipoprotein A1, γ-glutamyltransferase, and bilirubin which was developed by Poynard and colleagues [64]. FT is the best studied test and various studies suggested this test has significant ability for discrimination of liver fibrosis without noteworthy discrepancy among liver diseases. For example its ability on hepatitis C, hepatitis B, alcoholic and nonalcoholic fatty liver disease was shown [65]. The advantages of FT comprise great applicability (>95%), prevalent availability, and inter-laboratory reproducibility [66]; yet, there are also several disadvantages such as price, unsuccessful external validation, absence of specificity for liver disease (can be markedly impaired by comorbidities, i.e., Gilbert' s syndrome or hemolysis) [67], and difficulty in differentiating intermediate stages of fibrosis [68]. For practice deriving, Salkic et al. propose that, FibroTest is of brilliant value for excluding cirrhosis in patients with CHB, but has suboptimal performance in discovery of significant fibrosis and cirrhosis and in exclusion of significant fibrosis [69].

36.8 Fibro Test Is Calculated as Below

$$\begin{aligned} z = {} & 4.467 \times \log_{10}\left[\text{alpha2macroglobulin}(g/L)\right] - 1.357 \\ & \times \log_{10}\left[\text{haptoglobin}(g/L)\right] \\ & + 1.017 \times \log_{10}\left[\gamma GT(\text{IU}/L)\right] + 0.0281 \\ & \times \left[\text{age}(\text{years})\right] + 1.737 \times \log_{10}\left[\text{bilirubin}(\mu\text{mol}/L)\right] \\ & - 1.184 \times \left[\text{apolipoprotein A1}(g/L)\right] \\ & + 0.301 \times \text{sex}(\text{female} = 0, \text{male} = 1) \end{aligned}$$

36.8.1 FibroMax

Three blood tests were combined to produce FibroMax. These tests offer assessment of fibrosis (Fibro Test), steatosis (SteatoTest), and nonalcoholic steatohepatitis (NASH Test). The outcomes of these three tests are present collectively on one page provides doctors with a data for assessment of the hepatic lesion associated with nonalcoholic fatty liver disease. The tests include, the patient's age, sex, height and weight, α2-macroglobulin, haptoglobin, apolipoprotein A1, γ-glutamyltransferase, total bilirubin, ALT, AST, total cholesterol, triglycerides, and glucose (fasting) [70].

36.9 Serum Leptin and Homeostasis Model Assessment-IR Model

As a novel predictor of fibrosis among patients with chronic Hepatitis B virus infection, Mousa et al, demonstrated that, serum leptin and HOMA-IR in non diabetic HBV-infected patients may be used as a non-invasive marker of early liver fibrosis liver with ROC/AUC analysis for serum leptin levels cut off of >11.5 ng/mL with 93.2 sensitivity and 73.6 specificity. PPV of 90.3 and NPV of 80.3 for differentiation between non fibrosis and early fibrosis (F1-F2) [71].

36.9.1 Neutrophil to Lymphocyte Ratio

Recently, Neutrophil to lymphocyte ratio (NLR) was validated in combination with HOMA-IR as novel noninvasive marker for predication of liver fibrosis in patients with chronic HCV infection, and it was found that, patients with advanced fibrosis (F3–4) had an elevated N/L ratio [2.4 ± 0.99] compared with patients with fibrosis stage 1–2 [1.86 ± 0.66], *(P* < 0.001) [72].

36.9.2 The PGA Index

The PGA index was proposed by Poynard et al. as a marker to assess alcoholic liver disease. **it's** calculated by the sum of, prothrombin index, GGT and apolipoprotein A [73]. The accuracy of this index has been **augmented** from 65% to 70% by addition of α2 macroglobulin (PGAA) [74] studies informed that this score has highest accuracy for detecting cirrhosis in patients with alcoholic liver disease [75].

PGAA index is the sum of the below

- PT (% of control): ≥80 = 0; 70–79 = 1; 60–69 = 2; 50–59 = 3; <50 = 4
- γGT (IU/L): <20 = 0; 20–49 = 1; 50–99 = 2; 100–199 = 3; ≥200 = 4
- Apolipoprotein A1 (mg/dL): ≥200 = 0; 175–199 = 1; 150–174 = 2; 125–149 = 3; <125 = 4
- α2 macroglobulin (g/L): <1.25 = 0; 1.25–1.74 = 1; 1.75–2.24 = 2; 2.25–2.74 = 3; ≥2.75 = 4

36.9.3 The Forns Index

This index was described by Forns et al., in 2002 for fibrosis predication and replace endoscopy in detecting esophageal varices. The score is calculated depending on, age, platelet count, gamma GT, and total cholesterol. Some studies suggest that, the score can distinguish mild fibrosis from advanced fibrosis at a cut-off value of 6.9 [76, 83].

36.10 Forns Index

$$\begin{aligned} \text{Forns Index} = {} & 7.811 - 3.131 \times \ln\left(\text{platelet count}\left[10^9\ L^{-1}\right]\right) \\ & + 0.781 \times \ln\left(\gamma GT[\text{IU}/L]\right) \\ & + 3.467 \times \ln(\text{age}) - 0.014 \times \text{cholestrol}(\text{mg}/\text{dL}) \end{aligned}$$

36.10.1 HepaScore

It was developed by Australian investigators to predict the severity of liver fibrosis in patients with chronic hepatitis C. It Combines, alpha2-macroglobulin, hyaluronic acid, bilirubin and gamma-glutamyltranspeptidase, as well as age and gender [77]. The study of Huang et al. established that, Hepascore is a good score to assess the severity of liver fibrosis and high diagnostic performance to exclude cirrhosis in patients with chronic liver disease [78].

36.10.2 Platelet Volume and Neutrophil to Lymphocyte Ratio

In patients with NAFLD, a model that join in, the mean platelet volume (MPV), neutrophil–lymphocyte (N/L) ratio, ALT, and platelets was created via logistic regression. MPV and the N/L ratio were higher in NASH patients versus non-NASH persons, and in patients with marked fibrosis (F3–4) in comparison to initial fibrosis (F1–2). They can be utilize as noninvasive markers to expect progression of the disease.

The equation of this model was.

$$\left[-12.7531 + 0.4321 \times \text{MPV}(\text{fL}) + 0.7645 \times \text{N / L ratio-} + 0.0762 \times \text{ALT}(\text{IU / L}) + 0.0129 \times \text{platelets}\left(\times 10^{3}\ \text{mm}^{-3}\right)\right].$$

The area under the ROC curve for the prediction of NASH was 0.913 (95% CI: 0.854–0.963). A cut-off value of 0.398, with a specificity of 88.5% and a sensitivity of 91%, has a NPV of 86% and a PPV of 88% [79].

36.10.3 FibroMeter

Is a combination of the platelet count, prothrombin index, AST, α2 macroglobulin, hyaluronate, blood urea nitrogen and age. The results of FibroMeter has two major diagnostic values; first, is staging of fibrosis and second, is fibrosis quantification in each of the three major causes of chronic liver diseases (chronic viral hepatitis, ALD and NAFLD) [80].

Several Fibrometers are now commercially available at BioLiveScale (Angers, France) for assessment of fibrosis in different chronic liver diseases.

36.10.4 SteatoTest

This test is used in patients with NAFLD, SteatoTest, ActiTest and are non-invasive tests that offer a contrasting option to biopsy, and they correlate with the simple grading/staging of the SAF scoring system across the three rudimentary highlights of NAFLD: steatosis, inflammatory activity and fibrosis [81]. It fuses the five components of the Fibro test (*α*2 macroglobulin, haptoglobin, apolipoprotein A1, GGT, and total bilirubin) and the Acti Test (ALT as well, body mass index, serum cholesterol, triglycerides, and glucose, adjusted for age and gender) [82]. Also, in patients with morbid obesity, Lassailly et al. confirmed that, the diagnostic performances of the FibroTest, SteatoTest, and ActiTest were statistically significant, so perhaps decreasing the requirement for biopsy in this patients [83].

36.10.5 The Proteomics Based Tests

These tests evaluate patterns of protein or glycoprotein via mass spectroscopy by means of serum samples. Callewaert et al. [84] established tests built on the changed N-glycosylation of total serum protein (GlycoCirrhoTest and GlycoFibroTest). The developed Phosphoproteomics tests serve the aim of improving and understanding the pathogenesis of liver fibrosis to more than improving of clinical diagnostics. An example is phosphoproteomics based tests predict the fibrosis of the liver have been used to profile the phosphorylated (i.e. activated) forms of the major signaling proteins in visceral adipose samples of patients with NAFLD [85].

36.11 Direct Noninvasive Biomarkers (NIBMs) for Assessing Liver Fibrosis

36.11.1 Direct Markers Related to Matrix Deposition

36.11.1.1 Procollagen I Carboxy Peptide and Procollagen III Amino Peptide

The comments two types of procollagen (collagen precursor) in normal liver are, Procollagen type I (carboxy-terminal peptide) and procollagen type III (amino-terminal peptide) [86]. Procollagen undergoes enzymatic cleavage by procollagen C-peptidase and procollagen N-peptidase at its carboxy-terminal (type 1 (PC1CP)) and amino-terminal (type III (PCIIINP)), leading to the production of collagen [6]. through the separation of type III collagen, the N-terminal propeptide of procollagen type III (PIIINP) is removed from procollagen type III, and released into the serum. Thus, the measure of propeptide of procollagen type III can be a direct indicator of collagen synthesis and its estimations can be used to measure matrix deposition [87]. But, the low sensitivity and specificity (78% and 81%) of these marker have restricted their clinical utilize. Although, PIIINP levels correlate with the aminotransferase levels and reflecting the grade of fibrosis, it is not accurate to hepatic fibrosis as it can be establish in other conditions, such as acromegaly, chronic pancreatitis, and rheumatic diseases [6, 84]. A number of studies establish that, the serum levels of PCIIINP represent the stage of hepatic fibrosis [88]. No correlation between procollagen I carboxy peptide and PIIINP serum levels and grading of liver fibrosis. Therefore, these are not reliable to found fibrosis grading [87].

36.11.1.2 Type IV Collagen

It is the principal element of all basement membrane proteins. Type IV collagen is capable of forming networks with itself and is thus also called network forming collagen; this property differentiates type IV collagen from other collagen types [89]. Type IV collagen is one of the important components of the extracellular matrix. It does not undergo proteolysis and is deposited unbroken in the matrix, and so, its serum estimation is indicative of matrix degradation. Type IV collagen is positively correlated with the stage of hepatic fibrosis. Patients with advanced hepatic fibrosis have elevated type IV collagen concentrations [90, 91].

36.11.1.3 Laminin

It is the main basement membrane glycoprotein produced by the HSC. in the course of fibrosis, laminin increases around the vessels, in the perisinusoidal spaces and portal triad [91]. Laminin levels have been estimated for diagnosis of fibrosis in a study of 87 patients with chronic HBV, it provided 71.9% sensitivity and 80.0% specificity for significant fibrosis [92]. Studies demonstrated that, grouping of laminin plus Hyaluronic acid (HA) showed positive correlation with the stages of liver fibrosis [91, 93–97].

36.11.1.4 Hyaluronic Acid (HA)

HA is a polysaccharide present in ECM and raised in serum in patients with hepatic fibrosis [98]. In healthy liver, the uptake and degradation of HA is mediated via sinusoidal endothelial cells. Increased HA levels attributed either to decreased removal or increased manufacture. Great levels have been found in liver fibrosis with varied etiology specially, with cirrhosis [36]. HA has been studied in CHC, NAFLD, alcoholic liver disease, and CHB and has been found of great value in detecting advanced fibrosis [99–101]. Several studies established that the major utility of this marker is to exclude the advanced fibrosis and cirrhosis [84].

36.11.1.5 YKL-40 (Chondrex)

YKL-40 is intensely expressed in the liver and play a role in remodeling or degradation of the extracellular matrix [102]. Serum levels of YKL-40 are strongly linked to the grade of fibrosis [103]. It can be used as a marker to assess liver fibrosis and helps distinguish between mild stage and extensive stage of liver fibrosis [104].

36.11.2 Direct Markers Linked to Matrix Degradation [Metalloproteinases (MMPs) and Tissue Inhibitors of Matrix Metalloproteinases (TIMPs)]

The ECM are degraded by matrix metalloproteinases. The three most commonly studied MMPs in human are, (1) MMP-1 (collagenases), (2) MMP-2 (gelatinase A) and (3) MMP-9 (gelatinase B). These enzymes are synthesized intracellular and is secreted by activated HSCs [105]. MMPs are activated by membrane-type MMP and inhibited by tissue inhibitors of metalloproteinases (TIMPs) [20]. In hepatic fibrosis, there will be inverse correlation between levels of MMP-1 and histological severity [21]. MMP-2 is synthetized by activated HSCs; increased levels of MMP-2 have been detected in several liver diseases [106]. Throughout hepatic fibrogenesis, the expression of MMP-2 is markedly increased. The possibility of MMP-2 for expecting liver fibrosis still vague as some conflicting knowledge's have been reported by many studies [21, 107] . MMP-9 in one study has negative correlation with histological severity [23]. Tissue inhibitors of matrix metalloproteinases are proteins that interact with MMPs and control their activation and working. TIMP-1 controls activity of most MMPs, but TIMP-2 precisely inhibits MMP-2. TIMPs-dependent inhibition of ECM degradation may encourage liver fibrosis; raising of TIMPs' levels has been detected in chronic liver disease. It was established that, chronic hepatitis C produced increase of both TIMP-1 and TIMP-2 in corollary with fibrosis advancement [107]. ECM degradation by MMPs is inhibited by TIMPs, which affect MMPs function. TIMP-1 will interact with almost all the 3MMPs whereas TIMP-2 specifically interacts with MMP-2. With progression of liver disease, serum levels of TIMPs will increase. MMP-1/TIMP-1 ratio is useful for the diagnosis of hepatic fibrosis and correlates with degree of portal inflammation [24].

36.11.3 Cytokines

36.11.3.1 Transforming Growth Factor (TGF)-β1 and TGFα

During liver fibrosis, TGF-α enhances proliferation of HSCs and correlates well with progression of the disease [108, 109]. TGF-β1 share in ECM production by HSCs and prevents hepatocyte growth and proliferation in liver fibrosis [110]. High levels of TGF-β1 correlate with progression of hepatic fibrosis, and correlation between TGF-β**1** levels and the rate of fibrosis advancement is generally accepted, but certain limitations of levels of TGF-β1 is due to contamination of sample by platelet TGF-β [111, 112].

36.11.3.2 Connective Tissue Growth Factor (CTGF)

It is manufactured by activated HSC as well as hepatocytes via stimulation of TGF-β. Yet, serum CTGF levels decline within the end-stage cirrhosis [113].

36.11.3.3 Platelet-Derived Growth Factor-Beta

PDGF-B is expressed by platelets, fibroblasts, endothelial cells, mast cells and macrophages [36]. It is the chief drive for proliferation of HSC and its migration. Serum levels of PDGF-BB have correlation with severity of hepatic fibrosis. Although, early studies demonstrated that, PDGF-BB mRNA expression was found to be markedly elevated in chronic liver disease [114, 115], some studies showed decreased serum levels of PDGF-BB in liver fibrosis [116, 117].

36.11.3.4 Microfibrillar-Associated Protein 4

It is a ligand for integrins present in ECM including elastin and collagen [118]. Quantitative investigation of MFAP-4 serum levels indicated a good diagnostic accuracy for the prediction of non-diseased liver in comparison to cirrhosis (AUROC = 0.97) also, stage 0 against stage 4 fibrosis (AUROC = 0.84), and stages 0–3 versus stage 4 fibrosis (AUROC = 0.76) [119]. MPAF4 is n perfect serum marker among liver-specific proteins [120].

36.11.3.5 Cytokeratin-18 Fragments

The major intermediate filament present in hepatocyte are cytokeratin-18 fragments (CK18). Caspase-induced apoptosis takes place by cleavage of CK18 in different positions and results in the formation of CK18 fragments [121]. The levels of M30 antigen (a neoepitope in CK18) and M65 (cytosolic pool of CK18) can distinguish between mild and advanced fibrosis [122, 123]. Moreover, CK18 could be a hopeful non-invasive biomarker for NASH in **youngsters** with fatty liver disease [124].

36.11.4 Genetic Markers for Liver Fibrosis

Genetics of progression in liver fibrosis is multifactorial and result from interaction between genes and environment insults (e.g. viruses), and the host response. Genome studies have permitted the discovery of single nucleotide polymorphisms (SNPs) in specific genes which are linked with liver fibrosis [125, 126]. There are ethnic-dependent factors prompting the degree and outcome of hepatic fibrogenesis [125]. Numerous gene variations and polymorphisms recognized that surge the risk of hepatic fibrosis, e.g., in the Asian origin, the alcohol addiction, is one of the main damaging of the liver, was revealed to be directly exaggerated by variations in the genes encoding alcohol dehydrogenase and aldehyde dehydrogenase [127]. Huang and colleagues observed nearly 25,000 SNPs in 1020CHC patients and establish seven gene polymorphisms related with cirrhosis [128]. Two novel markers, located in the gene encoding DEAD box polypeptide 5 (DDX5) and carnitine palmitoyltransferase 1A (CPT1A) were significantly linked with marked hepatic fibrosis [129]. Although the precise influence of gene polymorphisms sited within the coding region of the TGFB1 gene continues to be controversially discussed [130–134]. Hall et al. identified seven genomic loci on chromosomes 4, 5, 7, 12 and 17 which influences fibrosis phenotypes based on quantitative trait locus analysis [135]. Also, seven single nucleotide polymorphisms located in (IL-28B) genes were identified by Lopez-Rodriguez et al. in severe necroinflammatory activity grade of chronic hepatitis C patients [136]. Small, noncoding micro RNAs (miRNAs) control gene expression by binding to mRNA and control diverse biological functions viz., apoptosis, cell proliferation and differentiation [137, 138]. Alterations of intracellular miRNAs have a vital role in pathophysiology of chronic liver disease. Normal liver homoeostasis requires miR-122 which controls genes that are involved in hepatic cholesterol and lipid metabolism [139]. After chronic liver injury, HSCs' proliferation and differentiation into myofibroblast-like cells are regulated by mi-R221. miR-9, miR-21 and miR-188 regulate activation of myofibroblast, synthesis of extracellular proteins and collagen deposition. The broad variety of miRNAs which are involved in liver fibrosis and enters into systemic circulation can serve as potential biomarkers [140]. A number of studies have revealed that, increased levels of iron that promote iron deposition and chronic inflammation are independent risk factors for liver fibrosis-and cirrhosis. The C282Y mutation of the haemochromatosis gene (HFE), for example, is connected with disease progressive in chronic HCV, suggesting a role of HFE mutations as main risk factors for disease progression [141–143].

36.12 Combined Direct and Indirect Markers

The combination of different biomarkers can really increase the sensitivity and specificity of these markers.

36.12.1 The Fibrometer Test

Was described by Cal'es et al. In 2005. The test has been validated in viral hepatitis and ALD and demonstrates AUCs of 0.883 and 0.962, respectively, for the detection of marked fibrosis (F2–F4) [80]. The Fibrometer has also been validated in NAFLD, with a reported AUC of 0.943 [144]. When compared to other indirect tests the Fibrometer showed an AUC of 0.892 for detecting stage F2–F4 fibrosis in CHC and CHB. This value was higher than those obtained for the Fibro test, Forns index, and APRI, which were 0.808, 0.82, and 0.794, respectively [145].

36.12.2 Enhanced Liver Fibrosis Test (ELF)

The combination of the hyaluronic acid, PIIINP, and TIMP-1 has been proposed for the detection of moderate-fibrosis. Results were entered into the established algorithm and expressed as ELF scores. The ELF test shows good performance and considerable diagnostic value for the prediction of histological fibrosis stage [146].

36.12.3 TGF-ß1, HA, PIIINP and TIMP-1 Panel

A pro-fibrogenic cytokine (TGF-ß1) and special matrix deposition markers [hyaluronic acid, PIIINP and TIMP-1] associated with liver injury during CHC. Their combination could offer a possible valuable tool to assess liver fibrosis in adults [147].

36.12.4 Combination of sFas with TGF-ß1, HA, PIIINP

The addition of apoptosis markers (particularly sFas) joint with TGF-ß1, hyaluronic acid, PIIINP in adult patients have found to have a high degree of estimation of liver fibrosis severity. The diagnostic accuracy evaluation demonstrated a good performance for sFas to assess advanced fibrosis in adults (AUROC: 0.8) [148].

36.12.5 Fibrospect II Test

This test contains three markers; hyaluronic acid, TIMP-1, and $\alpha 2$ macroglobulin. In a study that carried out on 696 HCV patients via the creative research team of this scoring system they reported that, an AUROC of 0.830 for the diagnosis of significant fibrosis [149].

36.12.6 SHASTA Index

Consists of serum hyaluronic acid, AST, and albumin. Was evaluated in a cohort of 95 patients with HIV/HCV co-infection. This index first time presented by Kelleher et al. it is valuable for differentiation of mild from advanced fibrosis [150].

This index can be calculated by the following formula.

$$\begin{aligned}\text{Risk score} = &-3.84 + 1.70(1 \text{ if HA } 41-85\text{ng/mL}, 0 \text{ otherwise})\\ &+3.28(1 \text{ if HA} > 85\text{ng/mL}, 0 \text{ otherwise})\\ &+1.58(\text{albumin} < 3.5\text{g/dL}, 0 \text{ otherwise})\\ &+1.78(1 \text{ if AST} > 60 \text{ IU/L}, 0 \text{ otherwise}).\end{aligned}$$

36.12.7 European Liver Fibrosis Panel (ELF) Test

This test is a model of a panel of markers (which focus on matrix turnover). It includes, age, tissue inhibitor of matrix metalloproteinase 1 (TIMP 1), hyaluronic acid, and amino-terminal peptide of pro-collagen III (P3NP) [151]. One study validated the performance of the ELF panel and has revealed that, it has the capacity to distinguish different degrees of fibrosis in an independent cohort of patients with NAFLD. The study proposed that, the modification of the formula by removing age simplifies the panel while not losing any diagnostic accuracy [152].

36.12.8 Hyaluronic Acid Vascular Score

Hyaluronic acid vascular score (HAV score) is a grouping of direct markers [hyaluronic acid (HA) and vascular endothelial growth factor (VEGF)] and indirect markers [aspartate aminotransferase (AST)/alanine aminotransferase (ALT) ratio (AAR)]. By the HAV score we can differentiated between significant and advanced fibrosis where is, the areas under curve of 0.979 and 0.994 for significant (F2–F4) and advanced fibrosis (F3–F4) and the cut off = 0.583 and 6.3, respectively [153].

36.13 Consensus Guidelines on Non-invasive Assessment of Hepatic Fibrosis

The Asian-Pacific Association for the Study of the Liver (APASL) provided the medical field a consensus guidelines for non-invasive markers of hepatic fibrosis, they recommended that, circulating serum biomarkers of hepatic fibrosis universally can give reasonable recognition of both significant fibrosis-cirrhosis or exclude both. These biomarkers could be used either stepwise or in combination with other non-invasive tests such as imaging or elastography to get better the accuracy of hepatic fibrosis. Also they recommended that, Fibrotest and APRI are the preferred noninvasive tests to evaluate liver cirrhosis, and APRI is favored in resource-limited conditions [154].

The European Association for the Study of the Liver and Asociaciòn Latinoamericana para el Estudio del Hígado guidelines recommended that, non-invasive tests should always be interpreted by hepatologist, according to the clinical background, considering the results of other tests (biochemical, radiological and endoscopic). Serum biomarkers can be used in clinical practice due to their high applicability (>95%) and good inter laboratory reproducibility [155].

36.14 Conclusions/Summary

Successful management of chronic liver disease depends on the accurate staging of liver fibrosis.

- Although the liver biopsy an invasive maneuver, it is still considered as a gold standard diagnostic tool for liver fibrosis.

- In fact, the noninvasive biomarkers for diagnosis of hepatic fibrosis, including the extracellular matrix have diagnostic importance, but they are not organ specific and may also correlate with inflammation in other sites.
- It is essential to point out that the majority of non-invasive tests are not able to exactly differentiate the early stages of fibrosis.

36.15 Future Perspectives for Liver Fibrosis Markers

- Considering the limitations of noninvasive markers, successful management of liver fibrosis needs more specific and vital liver biomarkers.
- Continued research in area of noninvasive diagnosis of liver fibrosis will give us the opportunity to offer our patients more accurately and noninvasive diagnostic tools.
- Many and Many studies on serum fibrosis markers and more validation efforts on large cohorts of patients with chronic liver diseases are needed.

Self Study

Questions

1. **Which statement is true?**
   (a) Hepatic stellate cells are the key cell of liver fibrosis
   (b) Hepatic stellate cells resident in portal tract
   (c) Hepatic stellate cells transdifferentiate into Kupffer cells
   (d) Hepatic stellate cells synthetized albumin
2. **Which statement/statements is/are true?**
   (a) After chronic liver injury, necrotic cells will be replaced by regenerated parenchymal cells
   (b) In chronic hepatitis, hepatocytes synthesize laminin
   (c) Activated hepatic stellate cells transdifferentiate into myofibroblast-like cells
   (d) Liver fibrosis is not linked with changes in composition of ECM
3. **Which statement/statements is/are true as regard biomarkers of liver fibrosis?**
   (a) Associated with morbidity or mortality
   (b) Biomarkers are more expensive
   (c) Direct markers are not organ specific, influenced by unrelated sites of inflammation
   (d) Not sensitive enough to discriminate intermediate stages of fibrosis
   (e) All of these markers are routinely available in all laboratories
4. **Which statement/statements is/are true?**
   (a) ECM homeostasis based on, the well equilibrium between matrix metalloproteinases and inhibitors tissue inhibitors of matrix metalloproteinases
   (b) The constituents of the ECM are similar in both normal and fibrotic liver
   (c) Normal liver includes collagens (I, III and IV)
   (d) The progressive fibrosis are correlated with the marked decrease of tissue inhibitors of matrix metalloproteinases (TIMP1 and 2)

Answers

1. **Which statement is true?**
   a
2. **Which statement/statements is/are true?**
   a and c
3. **Which statement/statements is/are true as regard biomarkers of liver fibrosis?**
   c and d
4. **Which statement/statements is/are true?**
   a

References

1. Rojkind M, Greenwel P. The extracellular matrix and the liver. In: Arias IM, Boyer JL, Fausto N, et al., editors. The liver: biology and pathology. 3rd ed. New York, NY: Raven Press; 1994. p. 843–68.
2. Lee UE, Friedman SL. Mechanisms of hepatic fibrogenesis. Best Pract Res Clin Gastroenterol. 2011;25(2):195–206.
3. Iredale JP. Models of liver fibrosis: exploring the dynamic nature of inflammation and repair in a solid organ. J Clin Invest. 2007;117:539–48.
4. Hernandez-Gea V, Friedman SL. Pathogenesis of liver fibrosis. Annu Rev Pathol. 2011;6:425–56.
5. Baranova A, Lal P, Birerdinc A, Younossi M. Noninvasive markers for hepatic fibrosis. BMC Gastroenterol. 2011;11:article 91.
6. Bataller R, Brenner DA. Liver fibrosis. J Clin Invest. 2005;115:209–18.
7. Wake K. Structure of the sinusoidal wall in the liver. In: Wisse E, Knook DL, Wake K, editors. Cells of the hepatic sinusoid. Leiden: The Kupffer Cell Foundation; 1995. p. 241–6.
8. Bioulac-Sage P, Lafon ME, Saric J, et al. Nerves and perisinusoidal cells in human liver. J Hepatol. 1990;10:105–12.
9. Kisseleva T, Brenner DA. Role of hepatic stellate cells in fibrogenesis and the reversal of fibrosis. J Gastroenterol Hepatol. 2007;22(Suppl):S73–8.
10. Schuppan D, Afdhal N. Liver cirrhosis. Lancet. 2008;371(9615):838–51.
11. Bedossa P, Paradis V. Liver extracellular matrix in health and disease. J Pathol. 2003;200:504–15.
12. Friedman SL. Molecular regulation of hepatic fibrosis, an integrated cellular response to tissue injury. J Biol Chem. 2000;275:2247–50.
13. Schaffner H, Popper H. Capillarization of the sinusoids. Gastroenterology. 1963;44:339–42.
14. Desmet VJ, Roskams T. Cirrhosis reversal: a duel between dogma and myth. J Hepatol. 2004;40:860–7.

15. Wanless IR, Nakashima E, Sherman M. Regression of human cirrhosis. Morphologic features and the genesis of incomplete septal cirrhosis. Arch Pathol Lab Med. 2000;124:1599–607.
16. Scott LF. Hepatic fibrosis. In: Schiff ER, Sorrell MF, Maddrey WC, editors. Schiff 's diseases of the liver. 11th ed. Singapore: Wiley-Blackwell; 2012. p. 297–305.
17. Schuppan D, Krebs A, Bauer M, Hahn EG. Hepatitis C and liver fibrosis. Cell Death Differ. 2003;10(Suppl 1):S59–67.
18. Guo J, Friedman SL. Hepatic fibrogenesis. Semin Liver Dis. 2007;27:413–26.
19. Sun J. Matrix metalloproteinases and tissue inhibitor of metalloproteinases are essential for the inflammatory response in cancer cells. J Signal Transduct. 2010;2010:985132.
20. Grigorescu M. Noninvasive biochemical markers of liver fibrosis. J Gastrointestin Liver Dis. 2006;15:149–59.
21. Murawaki Y, Ikuta Y, Idobe Y, Kawasaki H. Serum matrix metalloproteinase − 1 in patients with chronic viral hepatitis. J Gastroenterol Hepatol. 1999;14(2):138–45.
22. Boeker KHW, Haberkorn CI, Michels D, Flemming P, Manns MP, Lichtinghagen R. Diagnostic potential of circulating TIMP-1 and MMP-2 as markers of liver fibrosis in patients with chronic hepatitis. Clin Chim Acta. 2002;316(1–2):71–81.
23. Badra G, Lotfy M, El Refaie A, et al. Significance of serum matrix metalloproteinase-9 and tissue inhibitor of metalloproteinase-1 in chronic hepatitis patients. Acta Microbiol Immunol Hung. 2010;57(1):29–42.
24. Zhang BB, Min C, Weng HL, et al. Diagnostic value of platelet derived growth factor-BB, transforming growth factor α1, matrix metalloproteinase − 1 in serum and peripheral blood mononuclear cells for hepatic fibrosis. World J Gastroenterol. 2003;9(11):2490–6.
25. Schuppan D, Ruehl M, Somasundaram R, Hahn EG. Matrix as a modulator of hepatic fibrogenesis. Semin Liver Dis. 2001;21:351–72.
26. McGuire RF, Bissell DM, Boyles J, Roll FJ. Role of extracellular matrix in regulating fenestrations of sinusoidal endothelial cells isolated from normal rat liver. Hepatology. 1992;15:989–97.
27. Sebastiani G, Alberti A. Non invasive fibrosis biomarkers reduce but not substitute the need for liver biopsy. World J Gastroenterol. 2006;12:3682–94.
28. Piccinino F, Sagnelli E, Pasquale G, Giusti G. Complications following percutaneous liver biopsy. A multicentre retrospective study on 68 276 biopsies. J Hepatol. 1986;2:165–73.
29. Lavanchy D. The global burden of hepatitis C. Liver Int. 2009;29(Suppl 1):74–81.
30. Moorman A, Gordon S, Rupp L, et al. Base line characteristics and mortality among people in care for chronic hepatitis: the chronic hepatitis cohort study. Clin Infect Dis. 2012;56(1):40–50.
31. Cainelli F. Liver diseases in developing countries. World J Hepatol. 2012;4(3):66–7.
32. Bravo A, Sheth G, Chopra S. Liver biopsy. N Engl J Med. 2001;344(7):495–500.
33. Zhou K, Lu LG. Assessment of fibrosis in chronic liver diseases. Dig Dis. 2009;10:7–14.
34. Pinzani M, Rombouts K, Colagrande S. Fibrosis in chronic liver diseases: diagnosis and management. J Hepatol. 2005;42(Suppl 1):S22–36.
35. Morling J, Guha I. Biomarkers of liver fibrosis. Clin Liver Dis. 2016;7(6):139–42.
36. Grigorescu M. Noninvasive biochemical markers of liver fibrosis. J Gastrointestinal Liver Dis. 2006;15:149–59.
37. Baranova A, Lal P, Birerdinc A, et al. Non-invasive markers for hepatic fibrosis. BMC Gastroenterol. 2011;11:91.
38. Pradat P, Alberti A, Poynard T, et al. Predictive value of ALT levels for histologic findings in chronic hepatitis C: a European collaborative study. Hepatology. 2002;36(4):973–7.
39. Prat D, Taioli E, Zanella A, et al. Updated definitions of healthy ranges for serum alanine aminotransferase levels. Ann Intern Med. 2002;137(1):1–9.
40. Akbar Hand Fallatah H. Serum ALT levels in a cohort of healthy blood donors and volunteers from Saudi Arabia: the influence of sex and body mass index. Ann Gastroenterol Hepatol. 2010;1:13–9.
41. Haukeland J, Schreiner L, Lorgen I, Oskar Frigstad S, Bang C, Raknerud N. ASAT/ALAT ratio provides prognostic information independently of Child-Pugh class, gender and age in non-alcoholic cirrhosis. Scand J Gastroenterol. 2008;43(10):1241–8.
42. McPherson S, Stewart F, Henderson E, Burt A, Day C. Simple non-invasive fibrosis scoring systems can reliably exclude advanced fibrosis in patients with non-alcoholic fatty liver disease. Gut. 2010;59(9):1265–9.
43. Giannini E, Risso D, Botta F, et al. Validity and clinical utility of the aspartate aminotransferase-alanine aminotransferase ratio in assessing disease severity and prognosis in patients with hepatitis C virus-related chronic liver disease. Arch Intern Med. 2003;163(2):218–24.
44. Sebastiani G, Vario A, Guido M, Alberti A. Sequential algorithms combining non-invasive markers and biopsy for the assessment of liver fibrosis in chronic hepatitis B. World J Gastroenterol. 2007;13(4):525–31.
45. Shiha G, Mousa N, Salah M, Soliman R, Abed S, Elbasiony M, et al. Noninvasive markers for staging fibrosis in chronic hepatitis B patients. Med J Viral Hepat. 2018;2(2):17–23.
46. Green R, Flamm S. AGA technical review on the evaluation of liver chemistry tests. Gastroenterology. 2002;123:1367–84.
47. Wai C, Greenson J, Fontana R, et al. A simple noninvasive index can predict both significant fibrosis and cirrhosis in patients with chronic hepatitis C. Hepatology. 2003;38(2):518–26.
48. da Silva JR, Fakhouri R, Do-Nascimento T, Santos I, Barbosa L. Aspartate aminotransferase to-platelet ratio index for fibrosis and cirrhosis prediction in chronic hepatitis C patients. Braz J Infect Dis. 2008;12(1):15–9.
49. Loaeza-del-Castillo A, Paz-Pineda F, Oviedo-C'ardenas E, S'anchez-Avila F, Vargas-Vor'ackov'a F. AST to platelet ratio index (APRI) for the noninvasive evaluation of liver fibrosis. Ann Hepatol. 2008;7(4):350–7.
50. Chrysanthos N, Papatheodoridis G, Savvas S, et al. Aspartate aminotransferase to platelet ratio index for fibrosis evaluation in chronic viral hepatitis. Eur J Gastroenterol Hepatol. 2006;18(4):389–96.
51. Lok A, Ghany M, Goodman Z, et al. Predicting cirrhosis in patients with hepatitis C based on standard laboratory tests: results of the HALT-C cohort. Hepatology. 2005;42(2):282–92.
52. Toniutto P, Fabris C, Bitetto D, et al. Role of AST to platelet ratio index in the detection of liver fibrosis in patients with recurrent hepatitis C after liver transplantation. J Gastroenterol Hepatol. 2007;22(11):1904–8.
53. Toson SA, Shiha GE, El-Mezayen HA, El-Sharkawy AM. Diagnostic performance of T lymphocyte subpopulations in assessment of liver fibrosis stages in hepatitis C virus patients: simple noninvasive score. Eur J Gastroenterol Hepatol. 2016;28(8):931–9.
54. Croquet V, Vuillemin E, Ternisien C, et al. Prothrombin index is an indirect marker of severe liver fibrosis. Eur J Gastroenterol Hepatol. 2002;14:1133–41.
55. Pilette C, Oberti F, Aubé C, et al. Non-invasive diagnosis of esophageal varices in chronic liver diseases. J Hepatol. 1999;31:867–73.
56. Kim BK, Kim DY, Park JY, Ahn SH, Chon CY, et al. Validation of FIB-4 and comparison with other simple noninvasive indices for predicting liver fibrosis and cirrhosis in hepatitis B virus-infected patients. Liver Int. 2010;30:546–53.
57. Yang HR, Kim HR, Kim MJ, Ko JS, Seo JK. Noninvasive parameters and hepatic fibrosis scores in children with nonalcoholic fatty liver disease. World J Gastroenterol. 2012;18(13):1525–30.

58. Mallet V, Dhalluin-Venier V, Roussin C, et al. The accuracy of the FIB-4 index for the diagnosis of mild fibrosis in chronic hepatitis B. Aliment Pharmacol Ther. 2009;29(4):409–15.
59. Shiha G, Seif S, Eldesoky A, Elbasiony M, Soliman R, Metwally A. A simple bedside blood test (Fibrofast; FIB-5) is superior to FIB-4 index for the differentiation between non-significant and significant fibrosis in patients with chronic hepatitis C. Hepatol Int. 2017;11(3):286–91.
60. Angulo P, Hui J, Marchesini G, et al. The NAFLD fibrosis score: a noninvasive system that identifies liver fibrosis in patients with NAFLD. Hepatology. 2007;45:847–54.
61. Shah AG, Lydecker A, Murray K, et al. Comparison of noninvasive markers of fibrosis in patients with nonalcoholic fatty liver disease. Clin Gastroenterol Hepatol. 2009;7:1104–12.
62. Koda M, Matunaga Y, Kawakami M, et al. FibroIndex, a practical index for predicting significant fibrosis in patients with chronic hepatitis C. Hepatology. 2007;45(2):297–306.
63. Halfon P, Penaranda G, Renou C, et al. External validation of FibroIndex. Hepatology. 2007;46(1):280–1.
64. Poynard T, Imbert-Bismut F, Munteanu M, et al. Overview of the diagnostic value of biochemical markers of liver fibrosis (FibroTest, HCV FibroSure) and necrosis (ActiTest) in patients with chronic hepatitis C. Comp Hepatol. 2004;3:8.
65. Poynard T, Munteanu M, Deckmyn O, et al. Validation of liver fibrosis biomarker (FibroTest) for assessing liver fibrosis progression: proof of concept and first application in a large population. J Hepatol. 2012;2012(57):541–8.
66. Cales P, Veillon P, Konate A, et al. Reproducibility of blood tests of liver fibrosis in clinical practice. Clin Biochem. 2008;41:10–8.
67. Poynard T, Munteanu M, Imbert-Bismut F, et al. Prospective analysis of discordant results between biochemical markers and biopsy in patients with chronic hepatitis C. Clin Chem. 2004;50:1344–55.
68. Rockey DC, Bissell DM. Noninvasive measures of liver fibrosis. Hepatology. 2006;43:S113–20.
69. Salkic NN, Jovanovic P, Hauser G, Brcic M. FibroTest/Fibrosure for significant liver fibrosis and cirrhosis in chronic hepatitis B: A meta-analysis. Am J Gastroenterol. 2014;109(6):796–809.
70. Munteanu M, Ratziu V, Morra R, et al. Noninvasive biomarkers for the screening of fibrosis, steatosis and steatohepatitis in patients with metabolic risk factors: FibroTest-FibroMax experience. J Gastrointestin Liver Dis. 2008;17:187–91.
71. Mousa N, Abdel-Razik A, Sheta T, Shabana W, Zakria Z, Awad M, et al. Serum Leptin and Homeostasis Model Assessment-IR as a novel predictor of early liver fibrosis among patients with chronic hepatitis B virus infection. Br J Biomed Sci. 2018;75(4):192–6.
72. Abdel-Razik A, Mousa N, Besheer TA, Eissa M, Elhelaly R, Arafa M, El-Wakeel N, Eldars W. Neutrophil to lymphocyte ratio as a reliable marker to predict insulin resistance and fibrosis stage in chronic hepatitis C virus infection. Acta Gastroenterol Belg. 2015;78(4):386–92.
73. Poynard T, Aubert A, Bedossa P, et al. A simple biological index for detection of alcoholic liver disease in drinkers. Gastroenterology. 1991;100(5):1397–402.
74. Nguyen-Khac E, Chatelain D, Tramier B, et al. Assessment of asymptomatic liver fibrosis in alcoholic patients using FibroScan: prospective comparison with seven non-invasive laboratory tests. Aliment Pharmacol Ther. 2008;28:1188–98.
75. Oberti F, Valsesia E, Pilette C, et al. Noninvasive diagnosis of hepatic fibrosis or cirrhosis. Gastroenterology. 1997;113:1609–16.
76. Forns X, Ampurdanes S, Llovet J, Aponte J, Quinto L, Martinez-Bauer E, et al. Identification of chronic hepatitis C patients without hepatic fibrosis by a simple predictive model. Hepatology. 2002;36:986–92.
77. Adams LA, Bulsara M, Rossi E, et al. Hepascore: an accurate validated predictor of liver fibrosis in chronic hepatitis C infection. Clin Chem. 2005;51:1867–73.
78. Huang Y, Adams LA, Joseph J, Bulsara MK, Jeffrey GP. The ability of Hepascore to predict liver fibrosis in chronic liver disease: a meta-analysis. Liver Int. 2017;37:121–31.
79. Abdel-Razik A, Mousa N, Shabana W, Refaey M, El Mahdy Y, Elhelaly R, Elzehery R, Zalata K, Arafa M, Elbaz S, Hafez M, Awad M. A novel model using mean platelet volume and neutrophil to lymphocyte ratio as a marker of nonalcoholic steatohepatitis in NAFLD patients: multicentric study. Eur J Gastroenterol Hepatol. 2016;28(1):e1–9.
80. Calès P, Boursier J, Oberti F, Hubert I, Gallois Y, Rousselet M, et al. FibroMeters: a family of blood tests for liver fibrosis. Gastroenterol Clin Biol. 2008;32(6 Suppl 1):40–51.
81. Munteanu M, Tiniakos D, Anstee Q, Charlotte F, Marchesini G, Bugianesi E, et al. Diagnostic performance of FibroTest, SteatoTest and ActiTest in patients with NAFLD using the SAF score as histological reference. Aliment Pharmacol Ther. 2016;44(8):877–89.
82. Poynard T, Ratziu V, Naveau S, Thabut D, Charlotte F, Messous D, et al. The diagnostic value of biomarkers (SteatoTest) for the prediction of liver steatosis. Compar Hepatol. 2005;4:Article 10.
83. Lassailly G, Caiazzo R, Hollebecque A, Buob D, Leteurtre E, Arnalsteen L, et al. Validation of noninvasive biomarkers (FibroTest, SteatoTest, and NashTest) for prediction of liver injury in patients with morbid obesity. Eur J Gastroenterol Hepatol. 2011;23(6):499–506.
84. Callewaert N, Vlierberghe HV, Hecke AV, Laroy W, Delanghe J, Contreras R. Noninvasive diagnosis of liver cirrhosis using DNA sequencer-based total serum protein glycomics. Nat Med. 2004;10:429–34.
85. Younossi ZM, Baranova A, Stepanova M, Page S, Calvert VS, Afendy A, Goodman Z, Chandhoke V, Liotta L, Petricoin E. Phosphoproteomic biomarkers predicting histologic nonalcoholic steatohepatitis and fibrosis. J Proteome Res. 2010;9(6):3218–24.
86. Baranova A, Lal P, Birerdinc A, Younossi Z. Noninvasive markers for hepatic fibrosis. BMC Gastroenterol. 2011;11:Article 92.
87. Castera L. Noninvasive methods to assess liver disease in patients with hepatitis B or C. Gastroenterology. 2012;142:1293–302.
88. Tamura H, Matsuda A, Kidoguchi N, Matsumura O, Mitarai T, Isoda K. A family with two sisters with collagenofibrotic glomerulonephropathy. Am J Kidney Dis. 1996;27(4):588–95.
89. Kalluri R. Basement membranes: structure, assembly, and role in tumour angiogenesis. Nat Rev Cancer. 2003;3:422–33.
90. Takahashi H. Type IV collagen 7S domain is an independent clinical marker of the severity of fibrosis in patients with nonalcoholic steatohepatitis before the cirrhotic stage. J Gastroenterol. 2007;42:375–81.
91. Kropf J, Gressner AM, Negwer A. Efficacy of serum laminin measurement for diagnosis of fibrotic liver diseases. Clin Chem. 1988;34:2026–30.
92. Li F, Zhu CL, Zhang H, Huang H, Wei Q, Zhu X, Cheng XY. Role of hyaluronic acid and laminin as serum markers for predicting significant fibrosis in patients with chronic hepatitis B. Braz J Infect Dis. 2012;16:9–14.
93. Leroy V. Other non-invasive markers of liver fibrosis. Gastroenterol Clin Biol. 2008;32(6 Suppl):52–7.
94. Halfon P, Bourlière M, Pénaranda G, et al. Accuracy of hyaluronic acid level for predicting liver fibrosis stages in patients with hepatitis C virus. Comp Hepatol. 2005;4:6.
95. Körner T, Kropf J, Gressner AM. Serum laminin and hyaluronan in liver cirrhosis: markers of progression with high prognostic value. J Hepatol. 1996;25(5):684–8.
96. Geramizadeh B, Janfeshan K, Saberfiroozi M. Serum hyaluronic acid as a noninvasive marker of hepatic fibrosis in chronic hepatitis B. Saudi J Gastroenterol. 2008;14(4):174–7.
97. Montazeri G, Estakhri A, Mohamadnejad M, et al. Serum hyaluronate as a non-invasive marker of hepatic fibrosis and inflammation in HBeAg-negative chronic hepatitis B. BMC Gastroenterol. 2005;5:32.

98. Guéchot J, Laudat A, Loria A, Serfaty L, Poupon R, Giboudeau J. Diagnostic accuracy of hyaluronan and type III procollagen amino-terminal peptide serum assays as markers of liver fibrosis in chronic viral hepatitis C evaluated by ROC curve analysis. Clin Chem. 1996;42:558–63.
99. Montazeri G, Estakhri A, Mohamadnejad M, et al. Serum hyaluronate as a non-invasive marker of hepatic fibrosis and inflammation in HBeAg-negative chronic hepatitis B. BMC Gastroenterol. 2005;5:Article 32.
100. Vizzutti F, Arena U, Nobili V, et al. Non-invasive assessment of fibrosis in non-alcoholic fatty liver disease. Ann Hepatol. 2009;8(2):89–94, 2009
101. Naveau S, Raynard B, Ratziu V, et al. Biomarkers for the prediction of liver fibrosis in patients with chronic alcoholic liver disease. Clin Gastroenterol Hepatol. 2005;3(2):167–74.
102. Lausen M, Lynch N, Schlosser A, Tornoe I, Saekmose SG, et al. Microfibril-associated protein 4 is present in lung washings and binds to the collagen region of lung surfactant protein D. J Biol Chem. 1999;274:32234–40.
103. Schlosser A, Thomsen T, Shipley JM, Hein PW, Brasch F, et al. Microfibril-associated protein 4 binds to surfactant protein A (SP-A) and colocalizes with SP-A in the extracellular matrix of the lung. Scand J Immunol. 2006;64:104–16.
104. Molleken C, Sitek B, Henkel C, Poschmann G, Sipos B, et al. Detection of novel biomarkers of liver cirrhosis by proteomic analysis. Hepatology. 2009;49:1257–66.
105. Molleken C, Sitek B, Henkel C, Poschmann G, Sipos B, Wiese S, et al. Detection of novel biomarkers of liver cirrhosis by proteomic analysis. Hepatology. 2009;49(4):1257–66.
106. Takahara T, Furui K, Yata Y, Jin B, Zhang LP, Nambu S, et al. Dual expression of matrix protease −2 and membrane type I-matrix proteinase in fibrotic human livers. Hepatology. 1997;26:1521–9.
107. Walsh KM, Timms P, Campbell S, MacSween RN, Morris AJ. Plasma levels of matrix metalloproteinase-2 (MMP-2) and tissue inhibitors of metalloproteinases-1 and -2 (TIMP-1 and TIMP-2) as non invasive markers of liver disease in chronic hepatitis C: comparison using ROC analysis. Dig Dis Sci. 1999;44:624–30.
108. Pinzani M, Marra F. Cytokine receptors and signalling in hepatic stellate cells. Semin Liver Dis. 2001;21(3):397–416.
109. Harada KI, Shiota G, Kawasaki H. Transforming growth factor α and epidermal growth factor receptor in chronic liver disease and hepatocellular carcinoma. Liver. 1999;19(4):318–25.
110. Nelson DR, Gonzalez PRP, Qian K, et al. Transforming growth factor-β1 in chronic hepatitis C. J Viral Hepat. 1997;4(1):29–35.
111. Kanzler S, Baumann M, Schirmacher P, et al. Prediction of progressive liver fibrosis in hepatitis C infection by serum and tissue levels of transforming growth factor-β. J Viral Hepat. 2001;8(6):430–7.
112. Manning DS, Afdhal NH. Diagnosis and quantitation of fibrosis. Gastroenterology. 2008;134(6):1670–81.
113. Gressner OA, Gressner AM. Connective tissue growth factor: a fibrogenic master switch in fibrotic liver diseases. Liver Int. 2008;28:1065–79.
114. Pinzami M, Milani S, Herbst H, et al. Expression of platelet-derived growth factor and its receptors in normal human liver and during active hepatic fibrogenesis. Am J Pathol. 1996;148:785–800.
115. Ikura Y, Morimoto H, Ogami M, et al. Expression of platelet-derived growth factor and its receptor in livers of patients with chronic liver disease. J Gastroenterol. 1997;32:496–501.
116. Zhou J, Deng Y, Yan L, Zhao H, Wang G. Serum platelet derived growth factor BB levels: a potential biomarker for the assessment of liver fibrosis in patients with chronic hepatitis B. Int J Infect Dis. 2016;49:94–9.
117. Yoshida S, Ikenaga N, Liu SB, et al. Extra hepatic platelet-derived growth factor-beta, delivered by platelets, promotes activation of hepatic stellate cells and biliary fibrosis in mice. Gastroenterology. 2014;147:1378–92.
118. Susanne GS, Belinda M, Peer BC, et al. Microfibrillar associated protein 4: a potential biomarker for screening for liver fibrosis in a mixed patient cohort. PLoS One. 2015;10(10):e0140418.
119. Molleken C, Sitek B, Henkel C, Poschmann G, Sipos B, Wiese S, Warscheid B, et al. Detection of novel biomarkers of liver cirrhosis by proteomic analysis. Hepatology. 2009;49(4):1257–66.
120. Christian M, Barbara S, Corinna H, et al. Detection of novel biomarkers of liver cirrhosis by proteomic analysis. Hepatology. 2009;49:1257–66.
121. Chu PG, Weiss LM. Keratin expression in human tissues and neoplasms. Histopathology. 2002;40:403–39.
122. Yilmaz Y, Dolar E, Ulukaya E, et al. Soluble forms of extracellular cytokeratin 18 may differentiate simple steatosis from non-alcoholic steatohepatitis. World J Gastroenterol. 2007;13: 837–44.
123. Yang M, Xu D, Liu Y, et al. Combined serum biomarkers in non-invasive diagnosis of non-alcoholic steatohepatitis. PLoS One. 2015;10(6):e0131664.
124. Feldstein A, Alkhouri N, De Vito R, Alisi A, Lopez R, Nobili V. Serum cytokeratin-18 fragment levels are useful biomarkers for nonalcoholic steatohepatitis in children. Am J Gastroenterol. 2013;108:1526–31.
125. Juran BD, Lazaridis KN. Genomics and complex liver disease: challenges and opportunities. Hepatology. 2006;44:1380–90.
126. Chalasani N, Guo X, Loomba R, et al. Genome-wide association study identifies variants associated with histologic features of non-alcoholic Fatty liver disease. Gastroenterology. 2010;139:1567–76. e1561–1566
127. Thomasson HR, Crabb DW, Edenberg HJ, Li TK, Hwu HG, Chen CC, Yeh EK, Yin SJ. Low frequency of the ADH2∗2 allele among atayal natives of Taiwan with alcohol use disorders. Alcohol Clin Exp Res. 1994;18:640–3.
128. Huang H, Shiffman ML, Friedman S, et al. A 7 gene signature identifies the risk of developing cirrhosis in patients with chronic hepatitis C. Hepatology. 2007;46:297–306.
129. Huang H, Shiffman ML, Cheung RC, Layden T, Friedman S, Abar OT, et al. Identification of two gene variants associated with risk of advanced fibrosis in patients with chronic hepatitis C. Gastroenterology. 2006;130:1679–87.
130. Powell EE, Edwards-Smith CJ, Hay JL, Clouston AD, Crawford DHG, Shorthouse C, Purdie DM, Jonsson JR. Host genetic factors influence disease progression in chronic hepatitis. Hepatology. 2000;31:828–33.
131. Gewaltig J, Mangasser-Stephan K, Gartung C, Biesterfeld S, Gressner AM. Association of polymorphisms of the transforming growth factor-1 gene with the rate of progression of HCV-induced liver fibrosis. Clin Chim Acta. 2002;316:83–94.
132. Tag CG, Mengsteab S, Hellerbrand C, Lammert F, Gressner AM, Weiskirchen R. Analysis of the transforming growth factor-beta1 (TGF-beta1) codon 25 gene polymorphism by Light Cycler-analysis in patients with chronic hepatitis C infection. Cytokine. 2003;24:173–81.
133. Wang H, Mengsteab S, Tag CG, Gao CF, Hellerbrand C, Lammert F, Gressner AM, Weiskirchen R. Transforming growth factor-beta1 polymorphisms are associated with progression of liver fibrosis in Caucasians with chronic hepatitis C infection. World J Gastroenterol. 2005;11:1929–36.
134. Osterreicher CH, Datz C, Stickel F, Hellerbrand C, Penz M, Hofer H, Wrba F, Penner E, Schuppan D, Ferenci P. TGF-[beta]1 codon 25 gene polymorphism is associated with cirrhosis in patients with hereditary hemochromatosis. Cytokine. 2005;31:142–8.
135. Hall RA, Liebe R, Hochrath K, et al. Systems genetics of liver fibrosis: identification of fibrogenic and expression quantitative

trail loci in the BXD murine reference population. PLoS ONE. 2014;9(2):e89279.
136. Lopez-Rodriguez R, Hernandez-Bartolome A, Borque MJ, et al. Interferon-related genetic markers of necroinflammatory activity in chronic hepatitis C. PLoS One. 2017;12(7):e0180927.
137. Ambros V. The functions of animal microRNAs. Nature. 2004;431:350–5.
138. Kren BT, Wong PY, Sarver A, Zhang X, Zeng Y, Steer CJ. Micro RNAs identified in highly purified liver-derived mitochondria may play a role in apoptosis. RNA Biol. 2009;20:65–72.
139. Lanford RE, Hildebrandt-Eriksen ES, Petri A, et al. Therapeutic silencing of microRNA-122 in patients with chronic hepatitis C virus infection. Science. 2010;327:198–201.
140. Szabo G, Shashi B. MicroRNAs in liver disease. Nat Rev Gastroenterol Hepatol. 2013;10(9):542–52.
141. Smith BC, Grove J, Guzail MA, Day CP, Daly AK, Burt AD, et al. Heterozygosity for hereditary hemochromatosis is associated with more fibrosis in chronic hepatitis C. Hepatology. 1998;27:1695–9.
142. Erhardt A, Maschner-Olberg A, Mellenthin C, Kappert G, Adams O, Donner A, et al. HFE mutations and chronic hepatitis C: H63D and C282Y heterozygosity are independent risk factors for liver fibrosis and cirrhosis. J Hepatol. 2003;38:335–42.
143. Geier A, Reugels M, Weiskirchen R, Wasmuth HE, Dietrich CG, Siewert E, et al. Common heterozygous hemochromatosis gene mutations are risk factors for inflammation and fibrosis in chronic hepatitis C. Liver Int. 2004;24:285–94.
144. Cal'es P, Lain'e F, Boursier J, et al. Comparison of blood tests for liver fibrosis specific or not to NAFLD. J Hepatol. 2009;50(1):165–73.
145. Cal'es P, Oberti F, Michalak S, et al. A novel panel of blood markers to assess the degree of liver fibrosis. Hepatology. 2005;42(6):1373–81.
146. Rosenberg WM, Voelker M, Thiel R, Becka M, Burt A, Schuppan D, Hubscher S, Roskams T. Serum markers detect the presence of liver fibrosis: a cohort study. Gastroenterology. 2004;127:1704–13.
147. Valva P, Casciato P, Diaz Carrasco JM, Gadano A, Galdame O, Galoppo MC, et al. The role of serum biomarkers in predicting fibrosis progression in pediatric and adult hepatitis C virus chronic infection. PLoS One. 2011;6:e23218.
148. Valva P, Casciato P, Carol Lezama C, Galoppo M, Gadano A, Galdame O, et al. Serum apoptosis markers related to liver damage in chronic hepatitis c: sfas as a marker of advanced fibrosis in children and adults while m30 of severe steatosis only in children. PLoS One. 2013;8(1):e53519.
149. Patel K, Gordon S, Jacobson I, et al. Evaluation of a panel of non-invasive serum markers to differentiate mild from moderate-to-advanced liver fibrosis in chronic hepatitis C patients. J Hepatol. 2004;41:935–42.
150. Kelleher TB, Mehta H, Bhaskar R, et al. Prediction of hepatic fibrosis in HIV/HCV coinfected patients using serum fibrosis markers: The SHASTA index. J Hepatol. 2005;43(1):78–84.
151. Rosenberg WM, Voelker M, Thiel R, Becka M, Burt A, Schuppan D, et al. Serum markers detect the presence of liver fibrosis: a cohort study. Gastroenterology. 2004;127:1704–13.
152. Guha IN, Parkes J, Roderick P, Chattopadhyay D, Cross R, Harris S, et al. Non-invasive markers of fibrosis in nonalcoholic fatty liver disease: validating the European liver fibrosis panel and exploring simple markers. Hepatology. 2008;47(2):455–60.
153. Toson EA, Shiha GE, Abdelgaleel AE. Fibrogenic/angiogenic linker for non-invasive assessment of hepatic fibrosis staging in chronic hepatitis C among Egyptian patients. Ann Hepatol. 2017;16(6):862–73.
154. Shiha G, Ibrahim A, Helmy A, Sarin S, Omata M, Kumar A, et al. Asian-Pacific Association for the Study of the Liver (APASL) consensus guidelines on invasive and non-invasive assessment of hepatic fibrosis: a 2016 update. Hepatol Int. 2017;11:1–30.
155. European Association for the Study of the Liver, Asociacion Latinoamericana para el Estudio del Higado. EASL-ALEH clinical practice guidelines: non-invasive tests for evaluation of liver disease severity and prognosis. J Hepatol. 2015;63:237–64.

Peritoneal Fluid Analysis

37

Giulia Tosetti and Vincenzo La Mura

Key Concepts
- Ascites is pathological fluid accumulation in peritoneum. Cirrhosis is the most common cause and portal hypertension is the main pathogenic driver of this complication, however, it can be also the consequence of not liver-related diseases.
- Differential diagnosis through ascitic fluid analysis is mandatory to guide clinical management and treatment.

37.1 Introduction

Peritoneal fluid is the liquid which covers and lubricates the surface of the organs into the superior and inferior abdominal cavity. The abnormal increase of peritoneal fluid volume is called ascites which is the most frequent first complication of cirrhosis occurring in more than 50% of patients within 10 years from the diagnosis and is a hallmark of poor outcome with 5-year mortality up to 50% [1]. Cirrhosis with portal hypertension accounts for up to 85% of patients presenting with ascites, with the remaining 15% being due to malignancy, infections (among them tuberculosis), pancreatitis, malnutrition or malabsorption or other rare inflammatory conditions [2]. Differential diagnosis between ascites due to cirrhosis or other causes is crucial to start the best therapeutic approach and correctly define the prognosis.

At the onset, diagnosis is mainly based on clinical history and physical examination. Ultrasound often confirms fluid presence, especially in obese patients or in case of modest amount of abdominal fluid not detectable with physical examination. For etiological diagnosis, paracentesis with ascitic fluid analysis is the first recommended approach to differentiate between portal-hypertension from other potential etiologies. The preferred site for paracentesis is the left lower quadrant of the abdomen, 3 cm higher up and medial to the anterior superior iliac spine. During paracentesis, care should be taken to avoid visible collateral vessels and inferior epigastric artery that runs longitudinally between the pubic symphysis and the anterior superior iliac spine; doppler-ultrasonography can be used to identify the optimal site for needle insertion avoiding spleen and other vascular structures.

Paracentesis is considered a safe procedure since serious adverse events such as bowel perforation or hemoperitoneum occur in less than 0.5% paracentesis [3, 4]; overall complication rate is less than 1% even in patients with impaired traditional coagulation tests such as patients with cirrhosis who, by definition, have abnormal prothrombin time [3]. At this respect, if the suspect of cirrhosis is high or is a well-known condition, it has been demonstrated that neither the coagulation tests (i.e. prothrombin time), neither the platelet count reflect the procedural-associated bleeding risk. Therefore, at today, there is not a pre-defined cut-off in any of these parameters which can reliably guide a prophylactic transfusion policy of fresh frozen plasma or platelet before paracentesis in patients with cirrhosis. In this clinical setting an international normalized ratio over 1.5–1.8 and/or a platelet count below 50,000 units/mm^3 are the recommended thresholds for a transfusion policy [2, 5]. In our experience, paracentesis should be avoided only when coagulopathy is clinically evident with hyperfibrinolysis (evidence of hematoma) or evident disseminated intravascular coagulation.

G. Tosetti
CRC "A.M. and A. Migliavacca" Center for liver disease, Division of Gastroenterology and Hepatology, Fondazione IRCCS Cà Granda Ospedale Maggiore Policlinico, Università degli studi di Milano, Milan, Italy

V. La Mura (✉)
CRC "A.M. and A. Migliavacca" Center for liver disease, Division of Gastroenterology and Hepatology, Fondazione IRCCS Cà Granda Ospedale Maggiore Policlinico, Università degli studi di Milano, Milan, Italy

Fondazione IRCCS Cà Granda, Ospedale Maggiore Policlinico, U.O.C. Medicina Generale Emostasi e Trombosi, Dipartimento di Scienze Biomediche per la Salute, Università degli studi di Milano, Milan, Italy
e-mail: vincenzo.lamura@unimi.it

F. Radu-Ionita et al. (eds.), *Liver Diseases*, https://doi.org/10.1007/978-3-030-24432-3_37

37.2 Ascitic Fluid Analysis: "When and How"

All patients with first evidence of ascites should undergone paracentesis, even when cirrhosis is already *known*. Ascitic fluid analysis defines liquid characteristics, evaluates potential infections and neoplastic/inflammatory nature as resumed in Table 37.1. Macroscopic fluid aspect could vary from water-clear to frankly purulent, bloody, or chylous. Traditionally, as it occurs for any biological fluid, the biochemical nature of ascites can be divided into transudates or exudates according to fluid protein concentration lower or higher than 2.5 g/dL, respectively. Moreover, in cirrhotic patients, determination of ascitic protein concentration is necessary to identify patients at increased risk for the development of spontaneous bacterial peritonitis (SBP), since a protein concentration below 1.5 g/dL is a risk factor for the development of SBP [2].

Afterwards, serum-ascites albumin gradient (SAAG) has been proved to be more specific and sensitive at defining ascites type and etiology in relation or not with portal hypertension. Calculating the SAAG involves measuring the albumin concentration of serum and ascitic fluid specimens obtained on the same day and subtracting the ascitic fluid value from the serum value. If the SAAG is greater than or equal to 1.1 g/dL, the patient has portal hypertension, with approximately 97% accuracy [6]. In patients with cirrhosis, ascitic fluid should be examined to ruling out spontaneous bacterial peritonitis (SBP): an ascitic fluid neutrophil count of 250 polymorphonuclear cells/mm^3 or more is diagnostic of SBP. The appearance of fever, abdominal pain, or unexplained encephalopathy or liver function worsening, acute kidney injury or acidosis, suggest ascitic fluid infection. In these cases, bacterial culture of the fluid in aerobic and anaerobic blood culture bottles inoculated at bed-side should be performed before antibiotics since also a single dose of effective antibiotic may lead to negative cultures and the delay in paracentesis has been associated with a reduced chance of successful therapy [7]. This is true even for patients without cirrhosis suffering from a secondary bacterial peritonitis (i.e. after surgical intervention, cholecystitis) as microbiological analysis of any fluid in patients with infection increases the odds of the earliest and most appropriate antibiotic therapy. Unfortunately, bacterial isolation during infection is not always possible since up to 50% of ascites in cirrhosis can be culture negative even in patients with cirrhosis and neutrophil count over 250 cells/mm^3. Additional tests, such as lactate dehydrogenase, and glucose can be performed to differentiate spontaneous from secondary bacterial peritonitis. Only patients at high risk of tuberculosis associated-peritonitis should be tested for mycobacteria on the first ascitic fluid specimen. In this specific case, high levels of lactate dehydrogenase in comparison with serum levels are highly suggestive of this etiology.

If malignant ascites is suspected fluid should be sent to cytology even though the probability of achieving a positive results is high only for peritoneal carcinomatosis. The sensitivity of cytology in detecting peritoneal carcinomatosis is 96.7% if three samples (from different paracentesis procedures) are sent and processed promptly. Patients with peritoneal carcinomatosis usually have a history of a breast, colon, gastric, or pancreatic primary carcinoma [8].

Table 37.1 Most common ascitis fluid laboratory tests

Routine mandatory tests	Additional tests
– Cell count (polymorphonuclear leukocyte/mm^3) – Albumin in ascites and serum for SAAG – Total protein in ascites	– Aerobic and anaerobic blood culture bottles – Glucose – Lactate dehydrogenase – Amylase – Triglyceride – Cytology – Polymerase chain reaction for mycobacteria

37.3 Ascites in Cirrhosis vs. Other Conditions: Differential Diagnosis

The majority of patients with ascites has cirrhosis; however, in up to 15% of cases, the cause is different and the pathological mechanism of formation and retention of ascitic fluid is different from portal hypertension. Unusually, patients with ascites may have two or more causes of ascites formation, the so called "mixed" ascites; they are cirrhotic patients with another cause, e.g., peritoneal carcinomatosis or peritoneal tuberculosis.

37.3.1 Ascites with SAAG ≥1.1 g/dL

Ascites in liver disease has typically a SAAG ≥1.1 g/dL when it is consequence of clinically significant portal hypertension. This is true whatever the etiology of portal hypertension: prehepatic (i.e. extrahepatic portal vein obstruction), intrahepatic (i.e. cirrhosis) post-hepatic level (i.e. Budd Chiari syndrome or right cardiac failure) (Table 37.2). Typically in patients

Table 37.2 Causes of ascites with SAAG >1.1 g/dL: ascites due to portal hypertension

Pre-hepatic portal hypertension	– Extrahepatic portal vein obstruction – Arterio-venous fistula
Hepatic portal hypertension	– ***Pre-sinusoidal***: schistosomiasis, idiopathic portal hypertension – ***Sinusoidal***: cirrhosis – ***Post-sinusoidal:*** sinusoidal obstructive disease (SOS)
Post-hepatic portal hypertension	– Budd-Chiari syndrome – Membranes vena cava obstruction – Right cardiac failure

with post-hepatic portal hypertension the SAAG ≥1.1 g/dL is accompanied by a high content of proteins close to the biochemical threshold of exudate (around 2.5 g/dL). Signs and symptoms related with cardiac failure, abnormal levels of brain-natriuretic peptide can help physicians for the diagnosis [9]. Recently, it has been described a group of patients with cirrhosis, without heart failure, who presented with a SAAG ≥1.1 g/dL and high protein content in the ascitic fluid close to the cut-off of 2.5 g/dL [10]. It is an open question whether or not this subgroup of patients (18% in the series) have a different hemodynamic and/or evolution compared to patients with lower protein content in the peritoneal fluid.

37.3.2 Ascites with SAAG <1.1 g/dL

In case of SAAG <1.1 g/dL ascitic fluid is not related to portal hypertension and can be with a high or a low protein content. The typical condition of ascites with SAAG <1.1 g/dL and with scarce proteins is anasarca in nephrotic syndrome. Other rare conditions associated with ascites not due to portal hypertension and protein poor fluid are related to gastrointestinal loss of proteins such as malabsorption or exudative enteropathy; also malnutrition can lead to severe hypoprotidemia with ascites with scarce proteins and anasarca. Rarely even benign tumors can be associated with ascites poor in proteins: one example is the "Meigs syndrome" a rare benign ovarian tumor with low-protein ascites that solves after tumor removal [11] (Table 37.3).

Malignancies represent the second most frequent cause of ascites. In these cases, ascites is generally a protein-rich fluid with SAAG <1.1 g/dL. Malignant solid tumors of the ovary, colon and stomach with peritoneal carcinosis or infiltration are frequently associated with neoplastic ascites that typically has hematic aspect [8]. Even mesothelioma, a primitive malignant neoplasia of the peritoneum, is diagnosed after neoplastic ascites occurrence in more than 50% of cases [12].

In the rare condition of mucosecernent malignant tumor of the appendix, generally adenocarcinoma slow-growing, ascites has a mucinous appearance: this condition is known as "pseudomyxoma peritonei" [13].

Table 37.3 Causes of ascites with SAAG <1.1 g/dL

Low proteins (below 2.5 g/dL)	– Nephrotic syndrome – Enteropathy with malabsorption – Malnutrition – Rare ovarian benign tumors (Meigs syndrome) – Desmoid tumors
High proteins (over 2.5 g/dL)	– Malignant ascites – TBC or infections – Hypothyroidism – Gynecological diseases – Pancreatic ascites – Lymphatic obstruction ascites (Chylous)

In developing countries a relatively frequent cause of non cirrhotic ascites are infections such as tuberculosis although peritoneum is an unusual tubercular localization: in most cases it is due to diffusion from lung localization, less frequently it is due to a direct involvement of an abdominal organ as intestine; typical tubercular ascitic fluid is rich in proteins and lymphocytes with a SAAG lower than 1.1 g/dL.

In some conditions ascites development is a rare but not negligible complication. Infectious diseases such as Filariasis, Trachomatis Chlamydia infection and rarely Salmonellosis and Brucellosis may cause ascites.

During severe and protracted hypothyroidism ascites is possible to occur [14]. Gynecological conditions such as diffuse endometriosis or ovarian hyperstimulation syndrome during medically assisted procreation treatments are associated with mild ascites, less frequently clinically relevant ascites. Serositis in systemic connective diseases, such as lupus, may exceptionally develop ascites.

Pancreatic ascites is due to an accumulation of pancreatic fluid at the abdominal cavity for pancreatic ducts lesion or for pseudocyst rupture that may occur during necrotic pancreatitis or for abdominal trauma [15]. Medical history, clinical aspects and significant amylase increase on the ascitic fluid make the diagnosis of pancreatic ascites.

A peculiar and uncommon form of ascites is chylous ascites: fluid has milky aspect and typical high proteins and triglycerides (>2 g/L) concentrations. It is due to obstruction of a lymphatic duct by external compression or traumatic injury; also post-radiotherapy ascites on abdominal organs may have a chylous appearance for fibrosis and obstruction of lymphatic channels [16].

37.4 Conclusion/Summary

The analysis of peritoneal fluid is mandatory to differentiate the etiology of ascites. Often ascites is the manifestation of hepatic decompensation and is associated with cirrhosis or other conditions of portal hypertension: in this setting fluid is a transudate with a typical serum-ascites albumin gradient greater than 1.1 g/dL. High protein content and/or a serum-ascites albumin gradient <1.1 g/dL call for important comorbidities or other etiologies that should be accurately explored by complementary diagnostic tools.

Exercises

Case 1

Sixty-eight years old man, recent 5 kg weight gain and abdominal distension. In medical history: diabetes mellitus for 3 years, hypothyroidism treated, no history of liver disease.

- Blood Tests: AST 87 U/L; ALT 56 U/L; total bilirubin 1.4 mg/dL; **albumin 3 g/dL**; pCHE 1388 U/L, INR 1.31, creatinine 0.65 mg/dL. **Anti HCV Ab positive**, **HCVRNA positive**, normal TSH test.
- Abdominal US: Ascitic fluid, small-sized liver, no focal lesions, portal vein 17 mm, splenomegaly (15 cm).
- Diagnostic paracentesis:
  - Clear fluid
  - Liquid analysis: WBC 110/mm^3, **albumin 0.8 g/dL**, total protein 1.1 g/dL, amylase 38 mg/dL, LDH 73 U/L, glucose 10 mg/dL ➔ **SAAG 2.2 g/dL**
  - Aerobic and anaerobic fluid culture: negative

  Diagnosis: ascites in previously unknown HCV-related cirrhosis.

Case 2

Fifty-one years old woman, abdominal distension and pain. In medical history: breast cancer 8 years before (surgery, radiotherapy and chemotherapy).

- Blood Tests: AST 14 U/L; ALT 12 U/L; total bilirubin 0.2 mg/dL; **albumin 3.9 g/dL**; pCHE 6974 U/L, INR 1.03, creatinine 0.76 mg/dL. Anti HCV Ab negative; HBsAg negative, **CA 15.3 1287 U/mL (<34 U/mL)**.
- Abdominal US: Ascitic fluid, regular liver, no focal lesions, portal vein 9 mm, spleen regular.
- Total body CT scan: lymphadenomegaly (chest and abdomen, diameter max 4 cm) abundant ascites, suspected peritoneal carcinomatosis
- Diagnostic paracentesis:
  - Blood fluid
  - Liquid analysis: WBC 192/mm^3, **albumin 3.1 g/dL**, amylase 47 mg/dL, LDH 106 U/L ➔ **SAAG 0.8 g/dL**
  - Aerobic and anaerobic fluid culture: negative
  - Cytology: positive for atypical cell (suspected malignant cells)

  Diagnosis: malignant ascites in metastatic breast cancer.

References

1. Runyon BA, AASLD Practice Guidelines Committee. Management of adult patients with ascites due to cirrhosis: update 2012. Hepatology. 2013;57(4):1651–3.
2. European Association for the Study of the Liver. EASL clinical practice guidelines for the management of patients with decompensated cirrhosis. J Hepatol. 2018;69(2):406–60.
3. Wong F. Management of ascites in cirrhosis. J Gastroenterol Hepatol. 2012;27(1):11–20.
4. De Gottardi A, Thévenot T, Spahr L, et al. Risk of complications after abdominal paracentesis in cirrhotic patients: a prospective study. Clin Gastroenterol Hepatol. 2009;7(8):906–9.
5. Hemostatic balance in patients with liver cirrhosis: Report of a consensus conference. Under the auspices of the Italian Association for the Study of Liver Diseases (AISF) and the Italian Society of Internal Medicine (SIMI). Dig Liver Dis. 2016;48:455–67.
6. Uddin MS, Hoque MI, Islam MB, et al. Serum-ascites albumin gradient in differential diagnosis of ascites. Mymensingh Med J. 2013;22(4):748–54.
7. Kim JJ, Tsukamoto MM, Mathur AK. Delayed paracentesis is associated with increased in-hospital mortality in patients with spontaneous bacterial peritonitis. Am J Gastroenterol. 2014;109(9):1436–42.
8. Cavazzoni E, Bugiantella W, Graziosi L, et al. Malignant ascites: pathophysiology and treatment. Int J Clin Oncol. 2013;18:1–9.
9. Farias AQ, Silvestre OM, Garcia-Tsao G, et al. Serum B-type natriuretic peptide in the initial workup of patients with new onset ascites: a diagnostic accuracy study. Hepatology. 2014;59(3):1043–51.
10. Guillaume M, Robic MA, Péron JM, et al. Clinical characteristics and outcome of cirrhotic patients with high protein concentrations in ascites: a prospective study. Eur J Gastroenterol Hepatol. 2016;28(11):1268–74.
11. Riker D, Goba D. Ovarian mass, pleural effusion, and ascites: revisiting Meigs syndrome. J Bronchol Interv Pulmonol. 2013;20(1):48–51.
12. Field Z, Zori A, Khullar V. Malignant peritoneal mesothelioma presenting as mucinous ascites. ACG Case Rep J. 2018;5:e23.
13. Chauhan A, Patodi N, Ahmed M. A rare cause of ascites: pseudomyxoma peritonei and a review of the literature. Clin Case Rep. 2015;3(3):156–9.
14. Khalid S, Asad-Ur-Rahman F, Abbass A, et al. Myxedema ascites: a rare presentation of uncontrolled hypothyroidism. Cureus. 2016;8(12):e912.
15. Karlapudi S, Hinohara T, Clements J, et al. Therapeutic challenges of pancreatic ascites and the role of endoscopic pancreatic stenting. BMJ Case Rep. 2014; https://doi.org/10.1136/bcr-2014-204774.
16. Lizaola B, Bonder A, Trivedi HD, et al. Review article: The diagnostic approach and current management of chylous ascites. Aliment Pharmacol Ther. 2017;46(9):816–24.

Measurement of the Hepatic Venous Pressure Gradient (HVPG)

38

Thomas Reiberger

Key Concepts

- The measurement of the hepatic venous pressure gradient (HVPG) represent the gold standard for the evaluation of portal hypertension in patients with advanced chronic liver disease.
- Despite HVPG measurement is invasive, it is well tolerated by patients and holds only a low risk of complications.
- An HVPG of ≥10 mmHg defines clinically significant portal hypertension (CSPH) that indicates an increased risk for subsequent hepatic decompensation.
- A decrease in HVPG after intravenous non-selective betablocker (NSBB) by 10% from baseline or to absolute values <12 mmHg indicates a hemodynamic response.
- Patients with varices achieving a hemodynamic response to NSBB have a decreased risk for variceal (re-)bleeding and for subsequent development of ascites.

38.1 Introduction

Patients with advanced chronic liver disease (ACLD) are at risk for development of complications (i.e. decompensating events, such as ascites or variceal bleeding) or subsequently for further decompensation [1, 2]. Portal hypertension (PHT) represents a main driver of decompensation and further decompensation, and thus for mortality in patients with ACLD [3].

T. Reiberger (✉)
Hepatic Hemodynamic Laboratory, Division of Gastroenterology & Hepatology, Department of Medicine III, Medical University of Vienna, Vienna, Austria
e-mail: thomas.reiberger@meduniwien.ac.at

Measurement of the hepatic venous pressure gradient (HVPG) represents the diagnostic gold standard for PHT in patient with ACLD. An HVPG of 6–9 mmHg indicates mild portal hypertension, while an HVPG ≥10 mmHg defines clinically significant portal hypertension (CSPH).

The main clinical indications for HVPG measurements include:

1. to establish the diagnosis of intrahepatic portal hypertension,
2. to identify patients at risk for hepatic decompensation by diagnosing CSPH (HVPG ≥10 mmHg),
3. to guide pharmacological therapy in primary or secondary prophylaxis of variceal bleeding and
4. to assess the risk of hepatic failure after hepatectomy.

In interventional studies, HVPG measurement is used as an established surrogate marker for improvement and/or worsening of liver disease, since a decrease in HVPG has been shown to translate into a clinically meaningful benefit [4].

Based on observations on changes in HVPG in patients under non-selective beta-blocker (NSBB) therapy, a decrease in HVPG of 10% is considered to be clinically relevant [5, 6].

38.2 How and Why to Perform HVPG Measurements

Importantly, HVPG measurements should be performed using a balloon catheter to maximize the assessed amount of liver parenchyma [7]. Although HVPG measurement is invasive and resource-intensive, requires interventional skills and expertise in interpreting the reliability and plausibility of pressure readings, the method is the current gold standard for diagnosing and monitoring portal hypertension in patients with cirrhosis [8].

F. Radu-Ionita et al. (eds.), *Liver Diseases*, https://doi.org/10.1007/978-3-030-24432-3_38

Simple laboratory values, such as the platelet count may help to estimate the likelihood for CSPH, however, the accuracy of the platelet count alone (or combined scores) for the non-invasive prediction of portal hypertension is limited [9].

Imaging modalities showing splenomegaly or portosystemic collaterals in patients with cirrhosis might also hint towards the presence of CSPH but are not helpful for quantifying the actual degree of portal hypertension [10, 11]. Novel non-invasive imaging tools, such as elastography of the liver and/or of the spleen are useful for ruling-in or ruling-out the presence of CSPH [12, 13]. Still, none of the available methods is able to directly measure changes in portal pressure.

A landmark study by Garcia-Tsao et al. [14] examined the correlation of hepatic venous pressure gradient (HVPG) measurements with the presence and size of esophagogastric varices and the occurrence of variceal bleeding in 93 patients with alcoholic cirrhosis: All patients with varices on endoscopy had an HVPG of >12 mmHg, HVPG was also significantly higher in patients with a history of variceal bleeding. Interestingly, this study provided the hemodynamic data for the risk concept for variceal bleeding depending on size of varices, wall thickness and transmural pressure [14].

The prognostic value of HVPG has been underlined by several clinical studies, showing that an HVPG ≥10 mmHg (i.e. CSPH) is predictive for the formation of varices [6] and for the development of complications related to portal hypertension [3], while a (pharmacologically-induced) decrease of HVPG modulates the respective risk of variceal growth [15] and decompensation [16]. HVPG-response is the only established surrogate for the effectiveness of NSBBs in preventing (recurrent) variceal bleeding [5]. If HVPG decreases to a value of ≤12 mmHg or is reduced by ≥10–20% during NSBB treatment, patients are protected from variceal bleeding and survival is increased. Similarly, achieving an HVPG-response also decreases the incidence of ascites and related complications in patients with compensated cirrhosis [3].

Several studies provide evidence supporting the use of HVPG-guided therapy. Thus, in centers with sufficient experience, HVPG measurements should be used to guide treatment decisions in patients with ACLD and portal hypertension [2].

Moreover, measuring of HVPG might serve as a surrogate endpoint for proof-of-concept studies assessing the effectiveness of novel treatments for cirrhosis and/or portal hypertension being translated from bench to bedside, such as sorafenib [17] or simvastatin [18]. Ultimately, measurements of HVPG can also provide important prognostic information about the risk for development of HCC [19] and for post resection liver failure [20].

A hemodynamic response to non-selective betablocker therapy (e.g. with carvedilol 12.5 mg once daily) is defined as an HVPG decrease of at least ≥10% compared to baseline, or as a decrease to absolute values <12 mmHg: Here it has been shown, that the achievement of a hemodynamic response in primary prophylaxis does not only prevent rebleeding but also reduced the risk of decompensation and of mortality as compared to endoscopic band ligation [21].

It has already been demonstrated that HVPG-guided pharmacological therapy is more effective than ‘uncontrolled’ combined therapy of NSBB plus endoscopic band ligation in secondary prophylaxis and even improves survival [22].

38.3 Methodological Considerations

HVPG measurements requires considerable resources and trained personal with interventional skills and expertise in the reading of pressure tracings [23]. Importantly, HVPG improves prognostication and helps to guide treatment decisions [24]. In addition, the opportunity to safely obtain liver biopsy specimens via the transjugular route in the same session is another argument in favour of implementing hepatic hemodynamic laboratories at tertiary care centers [25]. The infrastructure to measure HVPG should be readily available at secondary and tertiary care centers. Sufficient expertise for HVPG measurement can be obtained after 50–100 supervised measurements.

Indeed, guidelines support the use of HVPG measurements in centers with adequate expertise and resources [2]. The safety of the procedures is largely related to the vascular access to the internal jugular vein. Once correctly placed, the risk of the remaining procedure is negligible and patient’s comfort is mostly limited by the duration of the procedure, if placement of the balloon catheter in the hepatic vein takes longer as expected.

Importantly, a recently published study on patient-reported outcomes demonstrated that the HVPG procedure is well-tolerated [26]. Nevertheless, low dose midazolam (0.02 mg/kg body weight) can be used in anxious patients in order to relief anxiety and improve patient comfort [27]. However, the most critical part of HVPG measurements is the correct recording of the pressure tracings for a sufficient amount of time while the balloon is insufflated and deflated to allow an accurate acquisition of WHVP and FHVP.

Very high values of FHVP and IVC may hint to incorrect calibration of the pressure transducer but might also indicate right heart failure or tricuspid valve insufficiency. A difference of more than ≥4 mmHg between the FHVP and the IVC pressure indicates an outflow obstruction/stenosis of the hepatic vein. Additionally, in case of severe Budd-Chiari Syndrome with complete thrombotic obstruction of the hepatic veins, the insertion of the balloon catheter is usually not possible. Thus, in case Budd-Chiari Syndrome or other causes of hepatic outflow obstruction are suspected, a Doppler ultrasound examination of the hepatic veins is recommended.

In case veno-venous shunts are observed during dye injection while the balloon is inflated, the HVPG is typically underestimated. However, while in this case the absolute value of HVPG cannot be used to estimate prognosis or guide pharmacological therapy, the diagnosis of CSPH can still be made if the HVPG is recorded at ≥10 mmHg in the presence of veno-venous vascular communications.

Certain liver diseases (e.g. nodular regenerative hyperplasia) might also affect presinusoidal resistance which impacts on the severity of portal hypertension but is not adequately reflected by HVPG. Furthermore, HVPG is also not able to detect the presence of (additional) prehepatic portal hypertension, as caused by portal vein thrombosis or mechanical compression of the portal vein. Thus, abdominal imaging with a special focus on the splenoportal vascular axis, on the mesenteric veins, as well as on spleen size and the presence of ascites should be performed in unclear cases and whenever a prehepatic component of portal hypertension is suspected.

38.4 Summary and Conclusions

The four main indications for HVPG measurements include (1) to ensure a correct diagnosis of intrahepatic/sinusoidal portal hypertension, (2) to evaluate the risk for hepatic decompensation in patients with compensated cirrhosis, (3) to guide NSBB treatment in primary or secondary prophylaxis of variceal bleeding, and (4) to estimate the risk of liver failure after liver surgery. While CSPH diagnosis and risk stratification might also be performed by imaging/laboratory studies or by endoscopy, currently, there are no adequate alternative means to monitor the response to NSBB therapy. While some patients might be readily excluded from major hepatic surgery by considering signs of hepatic impairment (i.e. ascites or jaundice), measurement of HVPG represents an important predictor of postoperative complications and mortality in patients without overt signs or symptoms of compromised liver function. In order to provide a personalized treatment approach to patients with ACLD, pharmacological therapy should be monitored by HVPG and more invasive treatment options (such as TIPS) may be considered in patients not achieving hemodynamic response, especially in patients that have already experienced variceal bleeding or other events of hepatic decompensation, such as ascites. Clinical trials evaluation potential treatment options for patients. With ACLD will likely include HVPG measurements as an integrative readout of pharmacological effects on fibrosis (static component) and on vascular function (functional component) in portal hypertension.

Self Study

Questions

1. *Which statement(s) are true?*
   (a) Normal portal pressure is present at an hepatic venous pressure gradient (HVPG) of maximum 5 mmHg.
   (b) Clinically significant portal hypertension (CSPH) is defined as HVPG of ≥10 mmHg.
   (c) Variceal bleeding is mainly observed in patients with HVPG values between 5 and 10 mmHg
   (d) Development of ascites only occurs if HVPG has risen to values of ≥15 mmHg
   (e) A hemodynamic response is defined a decrease in HVPG to normal values.
2. *Which of the following treatments does not decrease portal pressure?*
   (a) Non-selective betablockers propranolol and nadolol
   (b) L-ornithine L-aspartate
   (c) Carvedilol
   (d) Nitrates, such as ISMN
   (e) Somatostatin
3. *Which of the following statements related to the description of an accurate measurement of HVPG is not correct?*
   (a) Measurement of HVPG should be performed under fastened conditions
   (b) Balloon catheters rather than straight catheters should be used for measurement of HVPG
   (c) HVPG can be measured under general anesthesia and ventilation to increase patient comfort
   (d) Correct position of the catheter should be confirmed by X-ray and dye injection
   (e) Jugular veins and femoral veins can be used for venous access for HVPG measurements

Answers

1. *Which statement(s) are true?*
   Statements (a) and (b) are true.
2. *Which of the following treatments does not decrease portal pressure?*
   Option (b) L-ornithine L-aspartate does not decrease portal pressure, but is used to treat hepatic encephalopathy.
3. *Which of the following statements related to the description of an accurate measurement of HVPG is not correct?*
   Answer (c) is wrong, since most drugs used for general anesthesia affect portal pressure and thus, prevent a correct measurement of "awake" = "true" HVPG. Ventilation induced pressure thoracic pressure changes that affect both abdominal pressure and

venous pressures and also impact on HVPG. Thus, HVPG should be measured either under local anesthesia or should only used low-dose midazolam (0.02 mg/kg bodyweight) sedation.

References

1. Reiberger T, Püspök A, Schoder M, et al. Austrian consensus guidelines on the management and treatment of portal hypertension (Billroth III). Wien Klin Wochenschr. 2017;129:135–58. http://www.ncbi.nlm.nih.gov/pubmed/29063233. Accessed 25 Aug 2018.
2. De Franchis R, Abraldes JG, Bajaj J, et al. Expanding consensus in portal hypertension Report of the Baveno VI Consensus Workshop: Stratifying risk and individualizing care for portal hypertension. J Hepatol. 2015;63(3):743–52.
3. Ripoll C, Groszmann R, Garcia-Tsao G, et al. Hepatic venous pressure gradient predicts clinical decompensation in patients with compensated cirrhosis. Gastroenterology. 2007;133(2):481–8.
4. Mandorfer M, Kozbial K, Schwabl P, et al. Sustained virologic response to interferon-free therapies ameliorates HCV-induced portal hypertension. J Hepatol. 2016;65(4):692–9.
5. Abraldes JG, Tarantino I, Turnes J, et al. Hemodynamic response to pharmacological treatment of portal hypertension and long-term prognosis of cirrhosis. Hepatology. 2003;37(4):902–8.
6. Groszmann RJ, Garcia-Tsao G, Bosch J, et al. Beta-blockers to prevent gastroesophageal varices in patients with cirrhosis. N Engl J Med. 2005;353(21):2254–61.
7. Ferlitsch A, Bota S, Paternostro R, et al. Evaluation of a new balloon occlusion catheter specifically designed for measurement of hepatic venous pressure gradient. Liver Int. 2015;35(9):2115–20.
8. Abraldes JG, Sarlieve P, Tandon P. Measurement of portal pressure. Clin Liver Dis. 2014;18(4):779–92.
9. Berzigotti A, Seijo S, Reverter E, et al. Assessing portal hypertension in liver diseases. Expert Rev Gastroenterol Hepatol. 2013;7:141–55.
10. Simón-Talero M, Roccarina D, Martínez J, et al. Association between portosystemic shunts and increased complications and mortality in patients with cirrhosis. Gastroenterology. 2018;154(6):1694–1705.e4.
11. Vilgrain V, Lebrec D, Menu Y, et al. Comparison between ultrasonographic signs and the degree of portal hypertension in patients with cirrhosis. Gastrointest Radiol. 1990;15(3):218–22.
12. Procopet B, Berzigotti A, Abraldes JG, et al. Real-time shear-wave elastography: applicability, reliability and accuracy for clinically significant portal hypertension. J Hepatol. 2015;62:1068–75.
13. Colecchia A, Colli A, Casazza G, et al. Spleen stiffness measurement can predict clinical complications in compensated HCV-related cirrhosis: a prospective study. J Hepatol. 2014;60:1158–64.
14. Garcia-Tsao G, Groszmann RJ, Fisher RL, et al. Portal pressure, presence of gastroesophageal varices and variceal bleeding. Hepatology. 1985;5(3):419–24.
15. Merkel C, Marin R, Angeli P, et al. A placebo-controlled clinical trial of nadolol in the prophylaxis of growth of small esophageal varices in cirrhosis. Gastroenterology. 2004;127(2):476–84.
16. Hernández-Gea V, Aracil C, Colomo A, et al. Development of ascites in compensated cirrhosis with severe portal hypertension treated with β-blockers. Am J Gastroenterol. 2012;107(3):418–27.
17. Pinter M, Sieghart W, Reiberger T, et al. Effects of sorafenib on the portal hypertensive syndrome in patients with liver cirrhosis and hepatocellular carcinoma - a proof of concept study. Hepatology. 2011; https://doi.org/10.1111/j.1365-2036.2011.04896.x.
18. Abraldes JG, Albillos A, Bañares R, et al. Simvastatin lowers portal pressure in patients with cirrhosis and portal hypertension: a randomized controlled trial. Gastroenterology. 2009;136(5):1651–8.
19. Ripoll C, Groszmann RJ, Garcia-Tsao G, et al. Hepatic venous pressure gradient predicts development of hepatocellular carcinoma independently of severity of cirrhosis. J Hepatol. 2009;50(5):923–8.
20. Stremitzer S, Tamandl D, Kaczirek K, et al. Value of hepatic venous pressure gradient measurement before liver resection for hepatocellular carcinoma. Br J Surg. 2011;98(12):1752–8.
21. Reiberger T, Ulbrich G, Ferlitsch A, et al. Carvedilol for primary prophylaxis of variceal bleeding in cirrhotic patients with haemodynamic non-response to propranolol. Gut. 2013;62(11):1634–41.
22. Villanueva C, Graupera I, Aracil C, et al. A randomized trial to assess whether portal pressure guided therapy to prevent variceal rebleeding improves survival in cirrhosis. Hepatology. 2017;65(5):1693–707.
23. Silva-Junior G, Baiges A, Turon F, et al. The prognostic value of hepatic venous pressure gradient in patients with cirrhosis is highly dependent on the accuracy of the technique. Hepatology. 2015;62(5):1584–92.
24. Kumar A, Sharma P, Sarin SK. Hepatic venous pressure gradient measurement: time to learn! Indian J Gastroenterol. 2008;27(2):74–80.
25. Kalambokis G, Manousou P, Vibhakorn S, et al. Transjugular liver biopsy - indications, adequacy, quality of specimens, and complications - a systematic review. J Hepatol. 2007;47(2):284–94.
26. Casu S, Berzigotti A, Abraldes JG, et al. A prospective observational study on tolerance and satisfaction to hepatic haemodynamic procedures. Liver Int. 2015;35(3):695–703.
27. Steinlauf AF, Garcia-Tsao G, Zakko MF, et al. Low-dose midazolam sedation: an option for patients undergoing serial hepatic venous pressure measurements. Hepatology. 1999;29(4):1070–3.

39 Liver Biopsy for Histopathology

Horst Kinkel and Francisca Blanca Călinescu

> **Key Concepts**
> - Liver biopsy is indicated when the expected amount of information obtained exceeds the risks related to the procedure, when the diagnosis required for establishing a prognosis cannot be obtained without pathological examination of the liver, and finally, when the treatment decision depends on pathological results [1].
> - Liver biopsy is an uncomplicated and safe method in the hands of an experienced examiner.
> - The ultrasound-assisted liver biopsy is inexpensive and consumes the least resources compared to CT and MRI. Therefore, ultrasound-assisted liver biopsy should be the method of choice.
> - For liver biopsy, written consent should be obtained from the patient and the patient should be monitored for at least 6 h after biopsy. Reduced physical effort is recommended after biopsy for at least 10–14 days.

39.1 Introduction

Liver biopsy is the most common procedure performed in clinical hepatology, being in effect for many years. Paul Ehrlich is credited with performing the first percutaneous liver biopsy in 1883 in Germany [2]. Schüpfer [3] in 1907 published the first liver biopsy series.

Due to technological advancements and the widespread use of diagnostic imaging modalities in current clinical practice focal liver lesions are increasingly being discovered. Differentiation of these lesions is considered to be critical for determining treatment options. In this regard, histological assessment of the liver, liver biopsy remains a cornerstone in the evaluation and management of patients with liver disease. Despite that sensitive and relatively accurate blood tests used to detect and diagnose liver disease have now become widely available, liver biopsy will remain a valuable diagnostic tool. It has currently three major roles: (1) diagnosis, (2) assessment of prognosis (disease staging), and/or (3) to assist in making therapeutic management decisions.

Several techniques may be used to obtain liver tissue. These include a percutaneous method, a transvenous (transjugular or transfemoral), an endoscopic (transgastric) approach as well as intra-abdominal biopsy (laparoscopic or laparotomic). While in case of percutaneous approach ultrasound guidance is the favored modality, computed tomography (CT), magnetic resonance (MR) and fusion imaging techniques have all been used [4].

The purpose of this chapter is to summarize the current practice of liver biopsy with an emphasis on the indications, contraindications, technique and risk of complications.

39.2 Indications

The utility of routine liver biopsy has been the subject of debate in the last years. Until recently, liver biopsy played a key role in the evaluation of chronic liver disease, but now due to the development of sensitive and specific tests for diagnosis of several chronic liver diseases (serology, genetic screening), development of non-invasive assessment of fibrosis using serum tests and/or by physical methods such as pulsed elastography [5], its role has to be re-evaluated.

In order either to differentiate liver diseases, quantify disease activity or the fibrotic or cirrhotic changes, biopsy is useful in the following setting (Table 39.1).

For more detailed information on specific liver diseases, see Table 39.2.

H. Kinkel (✉)
Department of Internal Medicine 2, Municipal Hospital Düren, Düren, Germany

F. B. Călinescu (✉)
Rolf Dammrau Vascular and Thorax Surgery Clinic, Merzenich, Germany

F. Radu-Ionita et al. (eds.), *Liver Diseases*, https://doi.org/10.1007/978-3-030-24432-3_39

39.2.1 Parenchymal Liver Diseases

For parenchymatous liver disease, histological evaluation in primary diagnosis and follow-up is crucial (Tables 39.1 and 39.2). Neither imaging techniques nor serological parameters can reliably quantify disease activity and the patient's prognosis that depends on the extent of the remodeling process (fibrosis, cirrhosis).

In acute viral hepatitis, the diagnosis is usually serological (anti-HAV-IgM, anti-HEV-IgM; HbsAg, if positive anti-HBc-IgM and HBV-DNA; anti-HCV, if positive HCV-RNA; anti-DHV IgM in acute B hepatitis; EBV-IgM by clinical suspicion as well as CMV-Ak and CMV-DNA in immunosuppression). Histological validation is only in exceptional cases necessary, when beside acute viral hepatitis is another cause of liver damage suspected (for example, previously known chronic hepatitis with suspected superinfection, known alcohol abuse, autoimmune hepatitis). However, if there is a fulminant course with impending liver failure, the timely puncture may be important for estimating the prognosis, as liver transplantation remains the only therapeutic option in the, albeit rare, necrotizing form. In case of increasing jaundice, rapid decrease of transaminases, hepatic encephalopathy and devastating clinical picture, transcutaneous puncture is contraindicated due to the risk of bleeding (Table 39.3). For histological necrosis assessment, a transjugular puncture can then be selected, as the risk of relevant bleeding is significantly lower.

In hematochromatosis, the diagnosis can be made serologically. The low gene penetrance requires liver biopsy in suspected other cause of liver damage (e.g., non-alcoholic steatohepatitis NASH). The suspicion of higher-grade fibrosis or cirrhosis should be histologically clarified. This also applies to hepatic porphyria and α1-antitrypsin deficiency. In Wilson's disease, the diagnosis must be histologically confirmed in case of doubt. In advanced stages, a new puncture may be necessary to determine cirrhosis, especially before transplantation.

Table 39.1 Indications for liver biopsy

Indications	
For diagnostic purposes	• Multiple parenchymal liver diseases • Abnormal liver tests of unknown etiology • Focal or diffuse abnormalities on imaging studies
For prognostic purposes	• Staging of known parenchymal liver disease
Therapeutic conduit	• Developing treatment plans based on histologic analysis

Table 39.2 Main advantages of liver biopsy with respect to the etiology of liver disease

	Diagnosis	Staging	Prognosis	Treatment
Hepatitis B	---	++++	+	+
Hepatitis C	---	++	+	---
Acute viral hepatitis in case of fulminating clinical course and impending liver failure	++	---	++	+
Autoimmune hepatitis	++++	++++	+	++++
Primary biliary cirrhosis	++	++++	++	++
Primary sclerosing cholangitis	+	+	---	+
Overlap Syndrome	++++	++++	+	++
Caroli Syndrome	+++	---	+	---
Vanishing bile duct syndrome	+++	---	+	---
Veno-occlusive disease	++++	+	---	---
Budd–Chiari syndrome	---	---	---	---
Porphyria	+++	---	++	++
Alpha1-anti-trypsin deficiency	+++	++	++	---
Glycogen storage disease	+++	+++	+	---
Wilson's disease	+++	+++	++	---
Iatrogenic/toxic injury	+++	++	+	+
Non-alcoholic steatohepatitis	++++	+++	++	++
Alcoholic steatohepatitis	+	+++	++	+
Osteomyelofibrosis	+++	---	---	---
Hemochromatosis	+	+	---	---
Focal lesions				
• Hepatocellular carcinoma	+++	---	+	+
• Liver-cell adenoma	+	---	---	---
• Metastases	+++	---	---	+
Post-orthotopic liver transplantation	++++	+++	++	+++

--- irrelevant; + occasionally relevant; ++ usually relevant; +++ in most cases relevant; ++++ highly relevant

Table 39.3 Contraindications to percutaneous liver biopsy

Absolute
• Severe coagulopathy
• Infection of the hepatic bed
Relative
• Ascites
• Morbid obesity
• Infection in the right pleural cavity or below the right hemidiaphragm
• Suspected hemangioma or other vascular tumor
• Hydatid disease (Echinococcal cysts)
• Unavailability of blood transfusion support
• Uncooperative patient
• Extrahepatic biliary obstruction

Primary biliary cirrhosis (PBC) is diagnosed serologically (AMA); the histological evaluation of the activity and the stage of the disease has additional prognostic significance (extension of medicamentous therapy, preparation for transplantation), so that a liver puncture is justified. Autoimmune hepatitis should be punctured before start of therapy then regularly for the evaluation of therapy efficiency. Histological evaluation is also recommended before end of therapy.

While in Budd-Chiari syndrome, the occlusion of the great hepatic veins can be adequately assessed with Doppler sonography, the diagnosis of a veno-occlusive disease can only be made histologically.

In chronic hepatitis C and B, the histological staging of viral hepatitis (for example, according to the Desmet-Scheuer-Score) provides an additional decision criterion in treatment planning, as higher-grade fibrosis causes a poorer response to interferon therapy. Assessment by an experienced pathologist will also reveal aspects that may be important in the clinical management of patients. (e.g., changes due to frequent additional NASH with the need for weight reduction).

In non-alcoholic steatohepatitis (NASH), we routinely use transcutaneous liver biopsy for differential diagnosis and staging (Table 39.2). Alcohol-induced hepatitis is usually revealed by the patient's history and does not require regular biopsy.

39.2.2 Focal Liver Lesions

Focal liver changes are a common puncture reason not least because of the question of metastasis of different tumor entities in the liver. Due to the high diagnostic accuracy of contrast ultrasound [6], however, the proportion of biopsies has decreased (estimated at 5–10%).

39.2.2.1 Benign Lesions

Hemangiomas and focal nodular hyperplasia (FNH) are the most common benign liver tumors that occur more frequently in women [7]. Most of these are sufficiently clear and they do not require a biopsy, differentiation however between focal nodular hyperplasia and fibrolamellar liver carcinoma can be difficult. Puncture is indicated only in patients with a history of tumors and unclear imaging findings. This also applies to the much rarer liver adenoma. For larger adenomas, the indication for resection is due to the risk of rupture of up to 30% [8]. Here, in consultation with the surgeon, a preoperative biopsy could be decided.

39.2.2.2 Malignant Lesions

Metastases

Cytological fine needle aspiration of metastases in patients with known tumor disease is often sufficient to confirm malignant histology. However, if no primary tumor is known or if a primary liver tumor is assumed, histology must be performed, possibly by a coarse needle puncture.

If liver metastases are initially diagnosed without the knowledge of the primary tumor (CUP syndrome), biopsy of the metastases may be a therapy guiding finding and should therefore be used generously and early. The immunohistological differentiation is extremely helpful.

Primary Liver Tumors

Sonographic imaging of cholangiocellular carcinoma (CCC) is difficult and often only possible with the use of echo contrast enhancers. A cytological-histological examination can be carried out in the context of the endoscopic examination (ERCP: endoscopic retrograde cholangiopancreatography) when the bile duct system is invaded. In the palliative situation, a transcutaneous biopsy of a CCC can also be performed [9, 10], whereby we usually perform a fine needle biopsy.

In the cirrhotic liver the incidence of hepatocellular carcinomas (HCC) is high in comparison with metastases. Due to the friable structure of the cirrhotic liver tissue, obtaining a good punch cylinder is difficult, but particularly important for the pathologist in this situation, since the differentiation of regenerative nodules, dysplastic nodules and highly differentiated hepatocellular carcinomas is already difficult [8].

Contrast-enhanced ultrasound assures a better visualization of the cirrhotic liver allowing a better differentiation of focal lesions. If a HCC with potential resectability is suspected, in particular in the case of positive Alpha-fetoprotein (AFP) biopsy [11, 12] may be considered.

CEUS guided Biopsy allows a better differentiation of necrotic poorly perfused areas within a focal lesion. In principle, a puncture should be performed from the marginal area of a lesion, and the puncture of strongly vascularized areas in larger lesions should be avoided.

Key Concepts

- Despite improvements in serological and radiological techniques, liver biopsy is still the most reliable way to diagnose diffuse hepatic disease and hepatic nodules.
- Liver biopsy should be considered in patients in whom diagnosis is in question, and when knowledge of a specific diagnosis is likely to alter the management plan.
- Liver histology is an important adjunct in the management of patients with known liver disease, particularly in situations where information about fibrosis stage may guide subsequent treatment; the decision to perform liver biopsy in these situations should be closely tied to considerations of the risks and benefits of the procedure.
- Liver biopsy can be used to assess the degree of activity of an inflammatory process and the extent of fibrosis.
- Liver biopsy is very important as a means of securing the initial diagnosis of autoimmune diseases affecting the liver, including autoimmune hepatitis (AIH), primary sclerosing cholangitis(PSC), mixed forms with features of both AIH and PSC "overlap syndrome", and primary biliary cirrhosis (PBC).
- Among all diagnostic methods for hepatic nodules, liver biopsy has the greatest sensitivity and specificity with respect to the determination of malignancy.

39.3 Contraindications

Specifying contraindications to liver biopsy is difficult, considering the scarcity of data in this area. It depends on the biopsy approach, operator/physician experience and available local expertise. For this reason, most of the listed contraindications are considered to be relative (Table 39.3).

Key Concepts

- Uncooperative patients should undergo the procedure under general anesthesia or via the transvenous approach.
- In patients with clinically evident ascites a transvenous approach should be opted.
- Real time image guidance or CEUS guidance should be used in patients with identified vascular lesions.
- The decision to perform liver biopsy in the setting of abnormal hemostasis parameters should be evaluated at the local practice, considering that there are no specific PT/INR and platelet count cutoff values above which potentially adverse bleeding can be reliably predicted [13].

39.4 Biopsy Technique

There are different approaches for obtaining liver tissue: percutaneous, transjugular, laparoscopic and intraoperative, each having advantages and disadvantages. The biopsy technique is chosen on the basis of the indication, risks and benefits in the individual patient.

39.4.1 Percutaneous Liver Biopsy (PLB)

The most common approach for collecting a liver sample is percutaneous LB.

A variety of needles are available for percutaneous LB; they are classified into suction needles (Menghini, Klatskin, Jamshidi), cutting needles (Tru-cut, Vim-Silverman) and spring loaded needles that have a triggering mechanism. The choice of a specific needle type depends in part on local practice. Cutting needles usually produce a larger sample and are less likely to result inadequate specimens than are suction needles, but they present a higher complication rate [4]. Recently developed shark core needles are used with superior results compared to classical needles [14].

In order to justify risks of the procedure, care must be taken to ensure specimen adequacy. The size of the specimen is extremely important for accurate diagnosis and some pathologists recommend up to 11 complete portal triads for adequacy [15–17]. The American Association for Study of liver diseases (AASLD) recommends a 16-gauge biopsy of 2–3 cm in length for the diagnosis, grading and staging of diffuse, non-neoplastic parenchymal disease [13]. Due to the ease of penetration, we prefer ultrasound-assisted puncture technique with the Menghini needle (Hepafix Luer Lock, Braun 18 Gauge/1.2 mm, needle length 88 mm, 45° bevel angle).

Percutaneous liver biopsy may be undertaken in one of three ways, namely palpation/percussion guided, image guided (US, CEUS, MRT, CT), and real-time image guided (fusion technique).

39.4.1.1 Ultrasound-Guided Percutaneous LB

Ultrasound-assisted and ultrasound-guided liver puncture is the most cost-effective puncture method and requires the least resources. The advantage of sonography is that the needle path can be continuously monitored and controlled.

In the ultrasound-assisted puncture technique, a puncture mark is set on the skin after sonographic mapping of the liver. Thereafter, the biopsy needle is inserted without US control. The ultrasound-assisted puncture has replaced the blind liver puncture. This method is suitable for biopsy in parenchymatous liver diseases.

For focal liver lesions and difficult puncture conditions, an ultrasound-guided puncture should be performed. In the so-called freehand technique, the needle is guided with one hand and the transducer with the other. Under sonographic control, the needle is directed into the focal lesion to be punctured (Fig. 39.1a).

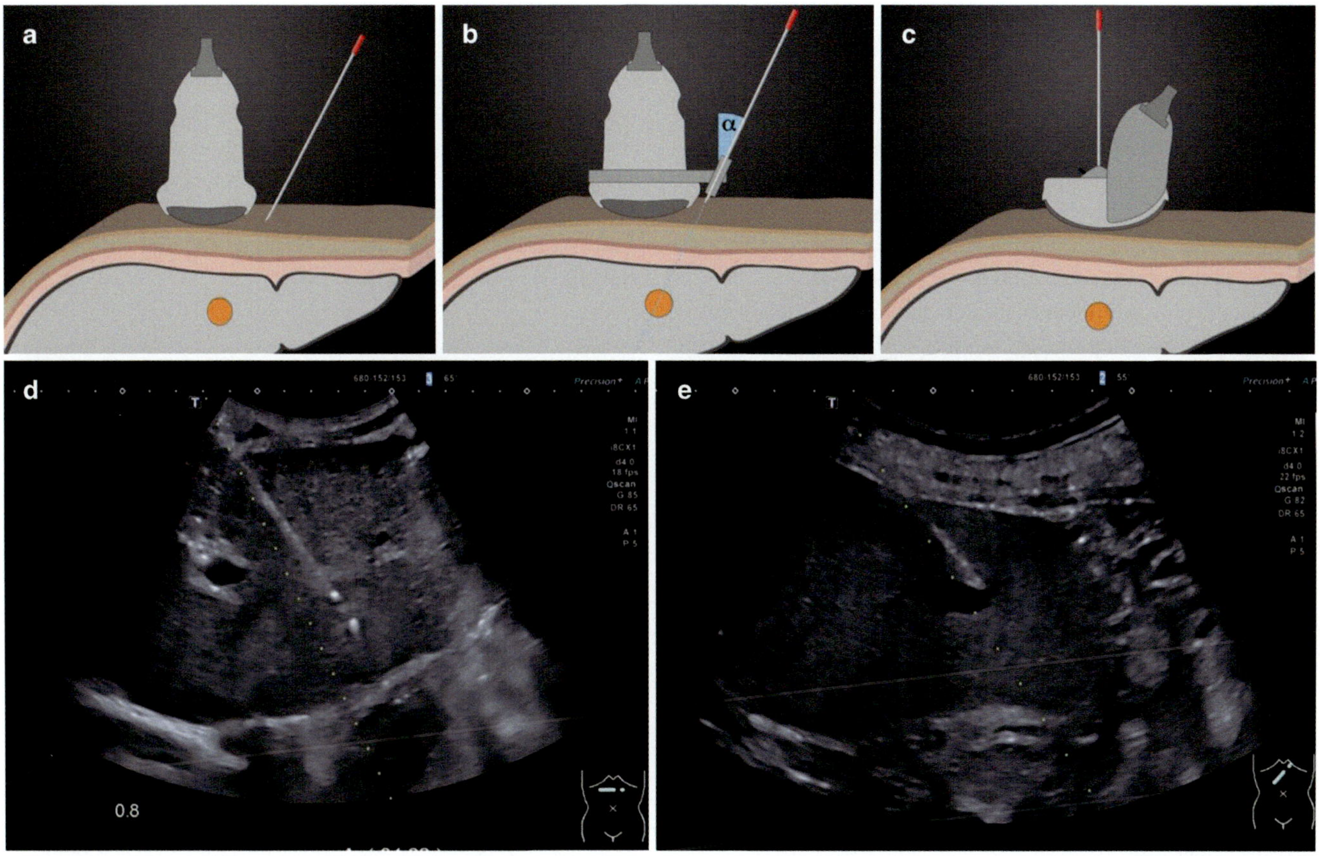

Fig. 39.1 Punction techniques. (**a**) Freehand; (**b**) mounted needle guide; (**c**) puncture transducer; (graphic by S. Tugendheim); (**d**) biopsy of diffuse parenchymal lesion; (**e**) puncture of a focal liver lesion

In the needle-guided puncture, the needle is mounted in a needle holder attached to the ultrasound probe (Fig. 39.1b). At a predetermined variable angle, which is visible in the ultrasound monitor, the needle is guided into the target region under continuous visualization. Alternatively, a puncture probe can be used (Fig. 39.1c). Here, the needle is inserted through the transducer itself under continuous visualisation.

39.4.1.2 CT-Guided and MRT-Guided Percutaneous LB

Computed tomography (CT)- and Magnetic-resonance-tomography (MRT)-guided biopsies are less frequently performed in current practice. This is because they are more time consuming, CT is associated with radiation exposure, and they tie up resources being more expensive.

Both CT and MRT offer a very good anatomical resolution and are recognized methods for guiding punctures. The problem, however, is that many of the lesions can be better detected only over a short period of time and then become isointense to the surrounding liver parenchyma, whereby only a short time window is suitable for a puncture.

The localization and puncture of liver lesions, especially in the liver segments 7, 8 and 4a, by means of ultrasound is in many cases difficult. Among other things, this localization may be challenging due to superimposition of intestinal gas or ribs. CT-guided puncture can overcome these limitations. By means of fluoroscopy, continuous visualization of the needle is also possible in CT. A major disadvantage of CT-guided interventions, however, is the radiation exposure for the radiologist and patient.

Since MRT offers a very good tissue differentiation and good vascular visualization, it makes possible to safely puncture subphrenic or upper retroperitoneal located lesions.

A problem with MRI-controlled punctures is the tubular design of MRI devices, which severely limits access to the patient. Although the first open MRI systems have been in clinical use since 1987, they are still not widely available.

39.4.1.3 Fusion Technique

Fusion imaging is an exciting new application in US-guided Liver biopsy. It is a technique that fuses two different imaging modalities. In the field of hepatic intervention, real-time US is usually fused with other imaging modalities such as CT, MRT or PET-CT in order to enhance US soft tissue differentiation. This allows direct comparison of volumetric data from prior imaging (CT/MRT/PET) with real-time US images to evaluate specific areas of interest [18–20].

Limitations of the technique are that it requires technical training for the user and is operator dependent, requires US-machines to be compatible with fusion techniques and can be time consuming.

Although results are promising further studies and more widespread training with this technique are necessary.

39.4.2 Transjugular Liver Biopsy (TJLB)

TJLB eliminates the need to traverse the peritoneal cavity and puncture the liver capsule. It offers a safer biopsy option in a number of specific situations: massive ascites, coagulopathy (prothrombin time greater than 3 s over the control value, thrombocytopenia <50,000/m^3, INR >1.5), morbid obesity, a small cirrhotic liver, suspected vascular tumor as well as patients in whom PLB has failed [21].

TJLB as any other method can be followed by particular complications, including hemorrhage, subcapsular or neck hematoma and ventricular arrhythmia. The complications rate ranges between 0% and 20% [22]. The major drawback of TJLB is the size of the biopsy specimens obtained; they are generally smaller and more fragmented than those obtained by PLB. With regard to technical success rate there is no significant difference between TJLB and other techniques [23].

TJLB should be attempted only by a skilled interventional radiologist or physician due to its more time-consuming nature, use of intravenous contrast and the need for a dedicated fluoroscopy suite.

39.4.3 Surgical/Laparoscopic biopsy (SLB)

In many circumstances, a surgical or laparoscopic approach is applied because the liver is noted to be abnormal in appearance prior to planned surgery or at the time of surgery. Biopsy can be performed either with typical needle devices or by wedge resection. While intraoperatively obtained liver biopsies have the added advantage of obtaining adequate tissue sampling under direct vision, with immediate control of bleeding, they are suboptimal for assessment of liver fibrosis and inflammation. Other advantages are the ability to evaluate for potential extrahepatic spread of malignancy. The major disadvantages are cost and the added risk of anesthesia.

39.5 Post-biopsy Monitoring

Several studies indicate that most major complications occur within 2 h post procedure [24, 25]. While most major complications present acutely, delayed hemorrhage may occur later. In our institution, the current practice post procedure (Fig. 39.2) includes observation in the subacute care unit (SACU) for 6 h with assessment of vital signs every 15 min in the first hour, then every 30 min for 2 h and every hour for further 4 h. Beside vital signs and blood pressure, Hb values are determined minimum two times until discharge. We strongly recommend a 24 h surveillance.

39.6 Complications

As an invasive procedure, LB can cause complications that may present intra- as well as early or late post-procedural, and are due to the needle insertion in the hepatic area of interest (Table 39.4). Among these, the most common is pain, occurring in up to 84% of patients [26]. Hemorrhage (intrahepatic, intraperitoneal or intrapleural-hemothorax)

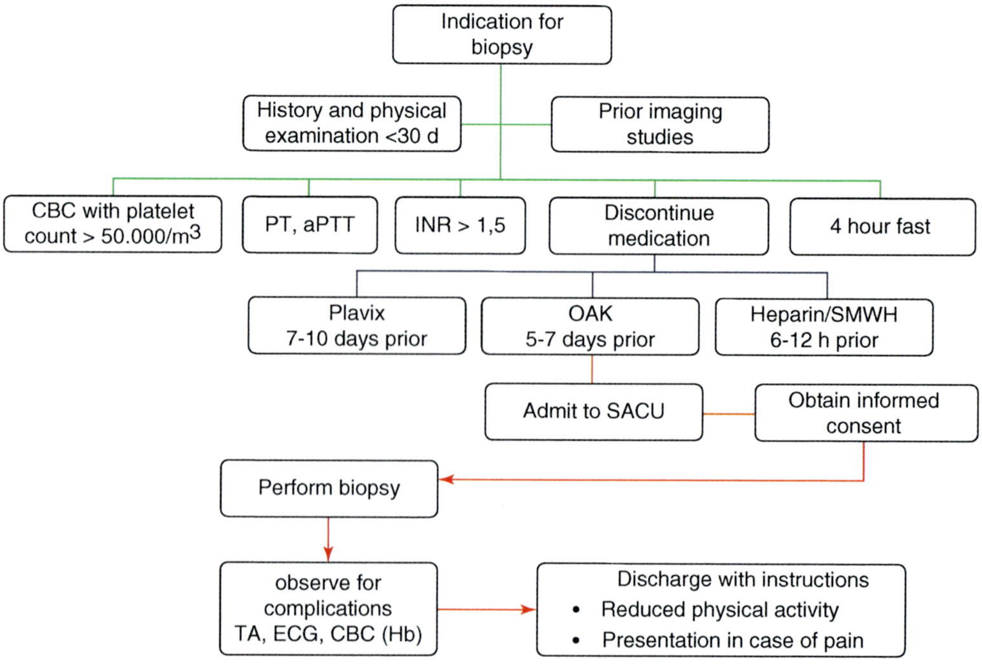

Fig. 39.2 Algorithm for performance of PLB followed at our institution

Table 39.4 Complications of percutaneous liver biopsy

Major	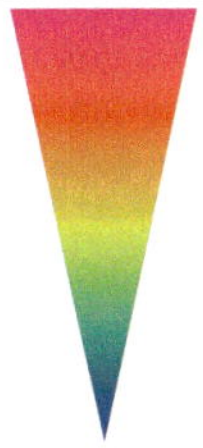 • Haemorrhage (intraperitoneal, intrahepatic, haemothorax) • Perforation of the gallbladder or of the bowel • Pneumothorax, haemothorax • Intrahepatic arterio-venous fistula • Bile peritonitis • Death
Minor	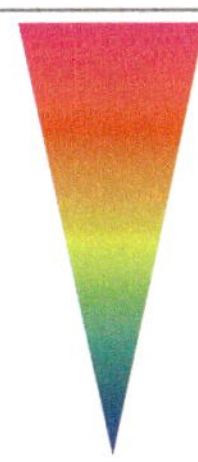 • Pain (biopsy site, right upper quadrant and right shoulder pain) • Transient hypotension (vasovagal response) • Pneumoperitoneum • Hemobilia • Infection (bacterial sepsis, local abscess) • Intrahepatic and subcapsular hematoma

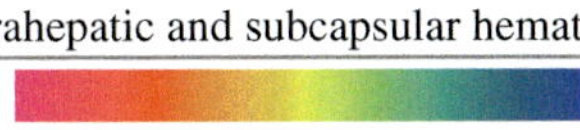

occurs less frequently, but is the most important complication. Severe bleeding is usually evident within 2–4 h post-procedural, but late hemorrhage can occur even one week after biopsy. The results of a prospective study have shown that the overall risk of major bleeding and death due to percutaneous US-guided intra-abdominal procedures is very low, 0.43% and 0.05% respectively [27]. Rare complications are also hemobilia, pneumoperitoneum and infection.

Self Study

Questions

1. When is there an indication for liver puncture?
   (a) Liver biopsy should be performed to exclude parenchymal damage in every case of elevated liver function tests
   (b) Biopsy is useful only for chronic liver disease
   (c) The method of choice is CT-guided hepatic puncture
   (d) Hepatic puncture is associated with a relatively high risk and should therefore be limited.
   (e) If hepatic metastases are suspected by an unknown primary tumor, a liver biopsy should be carried out early.
2. Which statement is wrong?
   (a) Written patient consent should be obtained prior to liver biopsy.
   (b) The diagnosis of Budd-Chiari syndrome requires a liver biopsy.
   (c) A liver biopsy can be performed while taking ASA.
   (d) The most common complication of liver biopsy is pain.
   (e) In the hands of an experienced examiner, sonographic liver biopsy is a low complication method.

Answers

1. When is there an indication for liver puncture?
   e. By histological confirmation and, in particular, immunohistochemical support, the pathological finding can in the majority of cases either delimit or definitively differentiate the primary tumor.
2. Which statement is wrong?
   b. Atresia of the large liver veins can be clearly diagnosed by sonography or CT imaging. Liver biopsy is not required.

References

1. Taltavull TC. Rethinking the role of liver biopsy in the era of personalized medicine. In: Tagaya N, editor. Liver biopsy. Rijeka: IntechOpen; 2012. https://doi.org/10.5772/53120. Available from: https://www.intechopen.com/books/liver-biopsy-indications-procedures-results/rethinking-the-role-of-liver-biopsy-in-the-era-of-personalized-medicine.
2. Dahiya N, Middleton WD, Menias CO. Ultrasound-guided visceral biopsies: renal and hepatic. Ultrasound Clin. 2012;7:363–75.
3. Schüpfer F. De la possibilite de faire "intra vitam" un diagnostic histo-pathologique precis des maladies due foie et de la rate. Sem Med. 1907;27:229.
4. Randazzo C, Licata A, Almasio PL. Liver biopsy - indications, procedures, results. In: Tagaya N, editor. Liver biopsy. Rijeka: IntechOpen; 2012. https://doi.org/10.5772/52616. Available from: https://www.intechopen.com/books/liver-biopsy-indications-procedures-results/liver-biopsy-indications-procedures-results.
5. Cadranel J-F, Nousbaum J-B. Current trends in liver biopsy indications for chronic liver diseases. In: Tagaya N, editor. Liver biopsy. Rijeka: IntechOpen; 2012. https://doi.org/10.5772/52618. Available from: https://www.intechopen.com/books/liver-biopsy-indications-procedures-results/current-trends-in-liver-biopsy-indications-for-chronic-liver-diseases.
6. Strobel D, et al. Contrast-enhanced ultrasound fort the characterisation of focal liver lesions – diagnostic accuracy in clinical practice (DEGUM multicenter trial). Eur J Ultrasound. 2008;59:499–505.
7. Nufer M, Stuckmann G, Decurtins M. Benigne Tumoren der Leber: Diagnostik und Therapie – eine Übersicht. Schweiz Med Wochenschr. 1999;129:1257–64.
8. Schirmacher P, Longerich T. Hochdifferenzierte Lebertumore Neue Entwicklungen und ihre diagnostische Relevanz. Pathologe. 2009;30(Suppl 2):200–6.
9. Khan SA, et al. Guidelines for the diagnosis and treatment of cholangiocarcinoma: consensus document. Gut. 2002;51(Suppl VI):vi1–9.

10. Anderson CD, Pinson CW, Berlin J, Chari RS. Diagnosis and treatment of cholangiocarcinoma. Oncologist. 2004;9:43–57.
11. Caselmann WH, et al. Leitlinie der Deutschen Gesellschaft für Verdauungs- und Stoffwechselkrankheiten zur Diagnostik und Therapie des hepatozellulären Karzinoms. Z Gastroenterol. 1999;37:353–65.
12. Bruix J, Sherman M. AASLD practice guideline: management of hepatocellular carcinoma. Hepatology. 2005;42:1208–36.
13. Rockey DC, Caldwell SH, Goodman ZD, Nelson RC, Smith AD. AASLD position paper: Liver biopsy. Hepatology. 2009;49:1017–44.
14. Huang JY. Role of EUS-guided liver biopsy in benign parenchymal disease (with video). Endosc Ultrasound. 2018;7(4):236–9.
15. Vijayaraghavan GR, David S, Bermudez-Allende M, Sarwat H. Imaging-guided parenchymal liver biopsy: how we do it. J Clin Imaging Sci. 2011;1(2):30.
16. Colloredo G, Guido M, Sonzogni A, Leandro G. Impact of liver biopsy size on histological evaluation of chronic viral hepatitis: the smaller the sample, the milder the disease. J Hepatol. 2003;39:239–44.
17. Crawford AR, Lin XZ, Crawford JM. The normal adult human liver biopsy: a quantitative reference standard. Hepatology. 1998;28:323–31.
18. Park HJ, et al. Fusion imaging-guided percutaneous biopsy of focal hepatic lesions with poor conspicuity on conventional sonography. J Ultrasound Med. 2013;32:1557–64.
19. Ewersten C, et al. Real-time image fusion involving diagnostic ultrasound. AJR. 2013;200:249–55.
20. Lee MW. Fusion imaging of real-time ultrasonography with CT or MRI for hepatic intervention. Ultrasonography. 2014;33(4):227–39.
21. Tagaya N, Makino N, Saito K, Okuyama T, Sugamata Y, Oya M. Types of liver biopsy. In: Tagaya N, editor. Liver biopsy. Rijeka: IntechOpen; 2012. https://doi.org/10.5772/52914. Available from: https://www.intechopen.com/books/liver-biopsy-indications-procedures-results/types-of-liver-biopsy.
22. Meng HC, et al. Transjugular liver biopsy: comparison with percutaneous liver biopsy. J Gastroenterol Hepatol. 1994;9(5):457–61.
23. Keshava SN, et al. Transjugular liver biopsy: what to do and what not to do. Indian J Radiol Imaging. 2008;18:245–8.
24. Bravo AA, Sheth SG, Chopra S. Liver biopsy. N Engl J Med. 2001;344:495–500.
25. Zaman A, Ingram K, Flora KD. Diagnostic liver biopsy. Available from: http://emedicine.medscape.com. Last updated on 18 Nov 2009.
26. Alswat KA, Mumtaz K, Jafri W. Liver biopsy for histological assessment: the case in favor. Saudi J Gastroenterol. 2010;16(2):133–9.
27. Strobel D, et al. Incidence of bleeding in 8172 percutaneous ultrasound-guided intraabdominal diagnostic and therapeutic interventions - results of the prospective multicenter DEGUM interventional ultrasound study (PIUS Study). Ultraschall Med. 2015;36:122–31.

Liver Ultrasonography

40

Laura Iliescu

Key Concepts
- The frequency used in liver ultrasonography is 3–7 MHz
- Low frequency sounds are used for deep tissues (such as large livers), while high frequency sounds are used for high resolution images of superficial structures
- Liver size over 16 cm is considered hepatomegaly
- Ultrasonography is the first imagistic approach in patients with focal liver lesions

40.1 Principles of Liver Ultrasonography

Ultrasonography uses sounds of frequencies ranging from 1 to 20 MHz, which are transmitted as pulses inside the body, echoing back to the transducer; further processing transforms these pulses into images [1]. The transducer is responsible for converting electrical energy into sound waves and then re-converting the echoes into electrical signals. The depths of the tissues analyzed is determined by the amount of time the waves take to return to the transducer. By sending repeated pulses, a two-dimensional image is generated [2].

The echoes are generated by acoustic interfaces which reflect the sound waves. These interfaces appear at the contact zone between two surfaces with different acoustic impedances (proportional to the density of the tissue and the velocity of the waves within the tissue). As the acoustic impedance difference between two tissues grows, the quantity of sound waves reflected (and the echo) is higher. In case of bones or gases, the acoustic impedance difference related to other tissues is so high, that all the waves are reflected and thus tissues beyond that surface are not visible on ultrasonography [1].

L. Iliescu (✉)
Internal Medicine and Gastroenterology, Institutul Clinic Fundeni, University of Medicine and Pharmacy (UMF) Carol Davila, Bucharest, Romania

The amplitude of the echoes given by different structures is transformed into a scale from white to black, where whiter shades represent higher amplitude echoes. The whiter the images, the more dense the tissue. Terms used to describe this “density” are anechoic (echo-free structures), isoechoic, hypo and hyperechoic [1]. The larger the distance the sound waves travel in the tissue until they are reflected, the more the waves are weakened (attenuated). Doppler sonography is used to evaluate dynamic structures (such as blood flow) in real time. Color Doppler sonography superimposes a color-code flow on top of the grey-scale imaging, showing flow direction and estimating flow velocity [1].

An important disadvantage of ultrasonography is the presence of artifacts, due to the interaction of sound waves and tissue, such as acoustic shadowing, multipath reflection artifacts or comet-tail artifacts. Using non-linear sound in tissue harmonic imaging is a newly developed ultrasonography technique resulting in less artifacts [2].

New technical advances have led to the development of small, portable ultrasound machines that can be used anywhere; thus ultrasonography can become an extension of the clinical examination [2]. Table 40.1 summarizes the advantages and disadvantages of using ultrasonography in the evaluation of the liver.

Frequency selection in ultrasonography is a key aspect in obtaining high quality images. Low frequency sounds are used for deep tissues (such as large livers), while high

Table 40.1 Advantages and disadvantages of ultrasonography

Advantages	Disadvantages
Cost-effective	Operator-dependent
Accessible	Possible artifacts due to: – Superimposed structures – Inadequate preparation for the examination
Real-time evaluation	Poor images for deep structures
High resolution images when using new techniques	Poor quality images in obese patients or with deposit diseases
Non-invasive, non-irradiant, non-toxic	Inaccessible in patients with cutaneous lesions

F. Radu-Ionita et al. (eds.), *Liver Diseases*, https://doi.org/10.1007/978-3-030-24432-3_40

frequency sounds are used for high resolution images of superficial structures. In general, the frequency used in liver ultrasonography is 3–7 MHz [2].

For a good quality image, the patient must have fasted for a minimum of 6 h prior to the investigation, in order to avoid emptying of the gall bladder and artifacts due to intestinal gases. The patient needs to be positioned supine and in left lateral decubitus for better visualization [3]. Difficult to see areas are those above the costal margin, the lateral segment of the left lobe and the anterior subdiaphragmatic regions [4]. The most commonly used acoustic window is subcostal, with intercostal windows used complementarily. Generally, the large curved linear transducer is used, with small sector transducers used for supplemental imaging in difficult-to-access areas.

The evaluation protocol of the liver includes assessment of size, capsular contour, parenchymal echogenicity, vascularization, biliary tree, potential masses or collections [3].

40.2 Normal Liver Ultrasonography

Due to its dimensions and location, the liver requires several incidences to perform a complete ultrasonographic evaluation (Fig. 40.1). For an extensive view, the incidences used are subcostal and intercostal, with the left lateral decubitus and left posterior oblique positions for supplemental access. Points of interest in liver ultrasonography are the size, echo texture and surface [3].

40.2.1 Liver Size

Liver volume is poorly estimated by diameter measuring. However, comparison to previous examinations is always helpful in assessing the evolution of liver diseases. The typical measurement of the liver is from the liver dome (under the right hemi diaphragm) to the tip of the right lobe, with the probe placed in a mid-clavicular position. While normal values range depending on age, body size and congenital variations of liver segmentation, a dimension of over 16 cm is considered hepatomegaly [5]. Another sign of liver enlargement is the blunting of the inferior liver edge (best seen in the right lobe), which is normally sharp.

40.2.2 Liver Echostructure

To determine the normal aspect of the liver, a comparison to the renal cortex is required. Normally, the liver is isoechoic or slightly hyperechoic compared to the renal cortex. If there appears to be an abnormal mass or a diffuse liver disease, a comparative split screen image of Liver/Kidney and Spleen/Kidney should be obtained, as the standard assessment of the liver echotexture [6].

40.2.3 Liver Surface

The integrity and regularity of the liver capsule is highly relevant in the diagnosis of liver disease. This is evaluated by placing a high frequency linear probe intercostally, thus obtaining images of the anterior surface of the right lobe. The normal capsule appears as a fine continue hyperechoic line surrounding the liver. Occasionally, one can opt for a left lateral decubitus or left posterior oblique position to obtain better images [7].

40.2.4 Liver Vascularization

Particular sites of interest in evaluating liver vascularization are the liver hilum and the drainage of hepatic veins into the inferior vena cava. The images for porta hepatis are acquired from a subcostal position, while the patient is inhaling deeply, with the transducer placed parallel to the portal vein

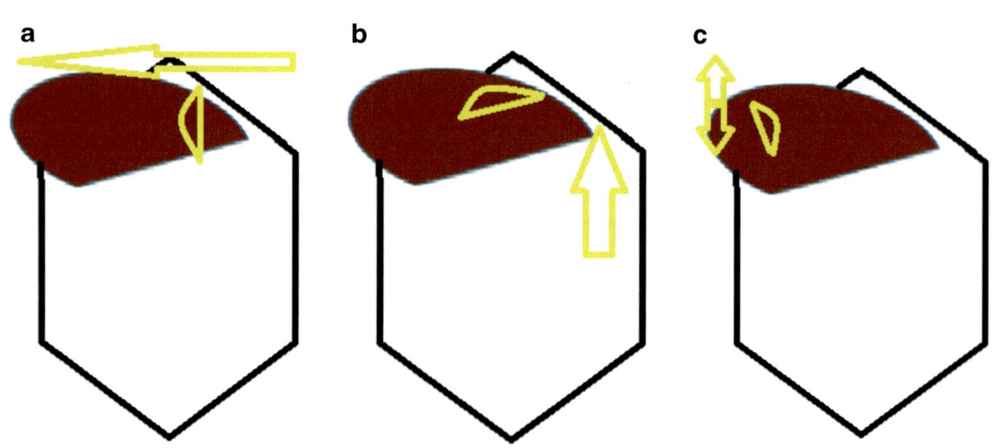

Fig. 40.1 Position of the transducer (drawn in yellow) in liver ultrasonography. (**a**) The transducer is moved longitudinally from the xiphoid process to the right. (**b**) Transverse scan in the epigastrium. (**c**) Intercostal scans

(parallel to the left costal arch) [7]. The portal vein and its branches have hyperechoic walls and can easily be distinguished in the parenchyma [8].

If the transducer is angled cranial, the confluence of the splenic vein and superior mesenteric vein appear in the image. From this position, three hypoechoic structures can be identified. The inferior vena cava is obliquely sectioned, and anterior to it the portal vein can be visualized. More anteriorly, the common bile duct and the hepatic artery are seen (Fig. 40.2). Normal diameters of structures measured from this position are:

- Portal vein: less than 13 mm.
- Common bile duct: less than 6 mm.
- Hepatic veins (peripheral): less than 6 mm.

Dilatation of the portal vein is suspected when the diameter (measured perpendicular to the longitudinal axis) is over 15 mm. This is a clear sign of portal hypertension. The hepatic artery needs to be visualized from the bifurcation to the celiac axis and the portal vein to the porto-splenic confluence [3].

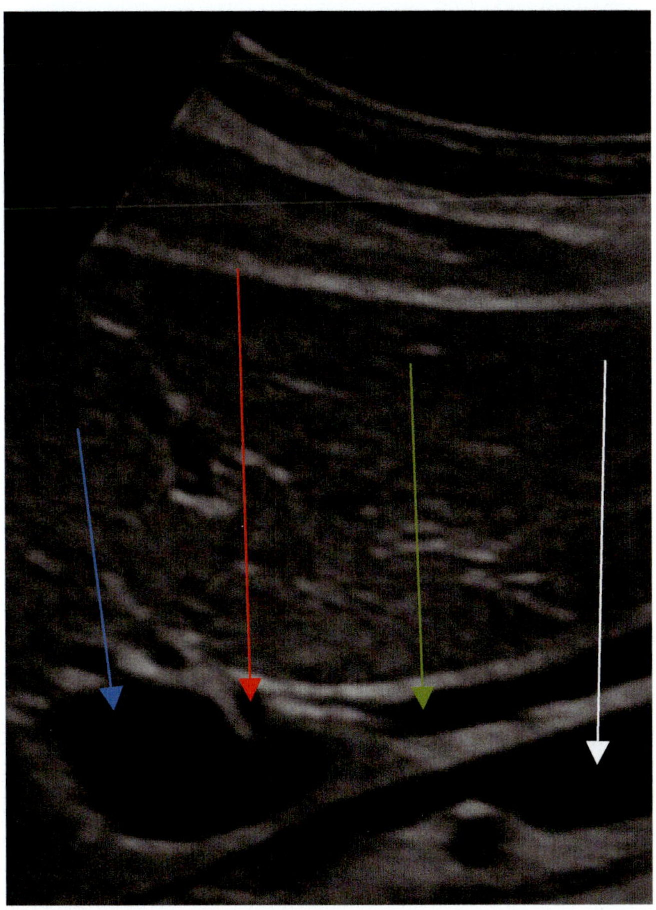

Fig. 40.2 Structures in the hepatic hilum: portal vein (blue arrow), hepatic artery (red arrow), common bile duct (green arrow), inferior vena cava (white arrow)

After cholecystectomy, the common bile duct party acts a new bile reservoir; due to this, its diameter increases, reaching up to 9 mm (in normal cases). A dilated bile duct can no longer be recognized by possessing the smallest caliber, but only by its location (directly anterior of portal vein). It is important to analyze the entire length of the common bile duct to visualize any potential intraductal gallstones, proximally until the porta hepatis and distally until the duodenal ampulla [5].

After the liver hilum has been evaluated, the examination of the liver should continue from transverse and subcostal oblique images (parallel to the right costal arch). This position is preferable for the exploration of hepatic veins and their confluence with the inferior vena cava. The normal value of the diameter of a hepatic vein is less than 6 mm. The measurement needs to be taken under caval collapse while the patient forces inspire [3]. However, anatomic variants and the proximity to the vena cava can lead to false measurements. The typical example is in patients with right-sided heart failure, with dilated vena cava and dilated proximal hepatic veins, who have normal diameters of the peripheral hepatic veins [7]. Another aspect to consider is the presence of vascularization in the liver periphery. Normally, the vasculature is constantly present throughout the liver parenchyma, except in patients with cirrhosis, who have diminished peripheral vascularization. Also, normal hepatic veins have a straight course, are joined at an acute angle and can be traced distally to the periphery of the liver [7].

If there are abnormalities in the liver echostructure or if there is a clinical suspicion of hepatitis or cirrhosis, Doppler analysis of the portal and hepatic veins is required. Parameters to monitor are the peak velocity and flow direction in the portal vein and the waveform pattern in the hepatic arteries. The normal flow velocity in the portal vein ranges from 12 to 25 cm/s [3]. In liver transplant recipients, a velocity of over 40 cm/s may indicate vessel stenosis. The normal waveform in the hepatic veins is triphasic; if the wave is mono or biphasic, it is a sign of low liver compliance, associated with cirrhosis but also other causes. Otherwise, if there are highly pulsatile waveforms, they may be a sign of right-sided heart failure [9].

40.3 Pathologic Aspects in Liver Ultrasonography

40.3.1 Diffuse Liver Disease

Diffuse liver diseases have a large variety of causes, from fatty liver disease and acute or chronic hepatitis, to deposit disorders leading to fibrosis and cirrhosis [10].

Table 40.2 summarizes the potential ultrasonography aspects in different diffuse hepatopathies.

Table 40.2 Short presentation of diffuse liver disease

Diffuse disease	Ultrasonography aspect
Fatty liver disease	Hyperechoic liver with fatty infiltration Accentuated posterior attenuation
Acute and chronic hepatitis	Possibly hypoechoic Signs of portal hypertension in fulminant hepatitis Lymph nodes in the hepato-duodenal ligament
Acute and chronic hepatic congestion	Distended hepatic veins Ascites
Vascular disorders	Budd Chiari syndrome – Hyperechoic nonhomogeneous areas – Enlargement of the caudate lobe Osler's disease – Ectatic vessels
Fibrosis	Coarse and uneven internal echoes
Cirrhosis	Irregular surface Signs of portal hypertension

Fig. 40.3 Ultrasonography aspect of fatty liver disease, showing a hyperechoic parenchyma with posterior attenuation

40.3.1.1 Fatty Liver

Fatty liver disease is one of the most frequent hepatopathies worldwide, with a growing incidence. Risk factors for fatty liver disease include the metabolic syndrome, use of birth control pills, use of steroids, and abuse of alcohol. It has been proven recently that patients with fatty liver disease are prone to the development of liver cirrhosis and hepatocellular carcinoma, non-alcoholic fatty liver disease representing about 10% of all indications for liver transplant in the USA [11].

The histologic definition of fatty liver disease is based on a minimum of 30% fatty infiltration of hepatocytes. However, the diagnosis can be made by non-invasive evaluations, including serologic evaluation of liver cytolysis, Fibroscan® or ultrasonography. For long, ultrasonography has proven its sensitivity and specificity in the diagnosis of fatty liver [12–14].

Technically, the liver is first evaluated on transverse and subcostal incidences, in deep inspiration, then sagittally. Due to the prolonged duration of the investigation, several breathing pauses are required. The suggested technique is to evaluate the left liver lobe with a continuous scan up to the inferior vena cava during deep inspiration, followed by a normal breathing period during which the transducer is moved from the midline to the right middle clavicle line. Afterwards, the patient is again asked to take a deep breath and the evaluation of the right liver lobe is performed. Measurement of the liver is done during inspiration; for enlarged livers, the transducer should be angled superiorly and inferiorly to encompass the entire liver [3].

Ultrasonography reveals a "bright" liver parenchyma (as compared to the renal echogenicity), with increased reflectivity and usually an enlarged liver (Fig. 40.3). As such, there is a loss of acoustic signal in the deep segments [7]. The aspect is homogenous throughout the liver, however, there may be small areas of focal sparing, which may resemble focal liver lesions [15]. Areas of fatty sparing are more often found anterior to the right portal vein and superior to the gallbladder; other locations are atypical and may require contrast-enhanced imaging techniques for proper evaluation. On the other hand, there may be areas of focal steatosis; these appear more echogenic and may form geographic configurations. Importantly, adjacent vessels are not displaced—this is useful in the differential diagnosis to focal liver lesions [16]. Another important aspect encountered in fatty liver disease is the loss of prominence of intrahepatic portal vein branch walls. Furthermore, due to the high echogenicity of the liver parenchyma, the diaphragm may not be visualized [17].

40.3.1.2 Acute Hepatitis

Acute hepatitis can be caused by viral or bacterial infections, or by toxic ingestion (including medication). Ultrasonography in this case reveals a hypoechoic liver, typically described as "dark liver" or "starry sky" [16]. The reduced reflectivity of the liver causes the portal tracts to be more enhanced than normal. Furthermore, the liver is enlarged, with rounded margins and there may appear edema of the gallbladder wall. Occasionally, in fulminant hepatitis, there may be ascites. This appears as an intense hypoechoic mass, without clear delimitations, mobile with the patient's position. If there is supra-infection, the ascites may have hyperechoic structures within, suggesting fibrin deposits [18].

The presence or absence of fatty liver disease influences the ultrasonographic aspect of acute hepatitis. A liver with low fat content may appear hypoechoic (like in acute hepatitis), but there are no secondary signs; the correlation to clinical and biological parameters is very important in this case. On the other hand, fatty liver disease already appears hyperechoic on ultrasonography, therefore superimposed acute hepatitis may not be directly visualized and associated signs should be assessed.

40.3.1.3 Chronic Hepatitis

In chronic hepatitis, there is increased liver echogenicity, coarsely heterogenous throughout the parenchyma. Occasionally, enlarged lymph nodes may appear in the liver hilum or periportal [16]. Areas of periportal fibrosis may be translated into an increased periportal reflectivity. Advanced cases may present regenerative nodules, hypertrophy of the left lobe with atrophy of the posterior right lobe and a patent para-umbilical vein.

40.3.1.4 Hepatic Congestion

The hallmark sign for liver congestion, both acute and chronic, is the distension of the inferior vena cava accompanied by the distension of hepatic veins. The inferior vena cava is noncollapsing during inspiration. With the progression to cirrhosis, slow and undulating flow in the portal vein is observed in color Doppler assessment. Also, the inferior edge of the liver may be blunted. Late in the evolution, ascites is nearly always present [5] (Fig. 40.4).

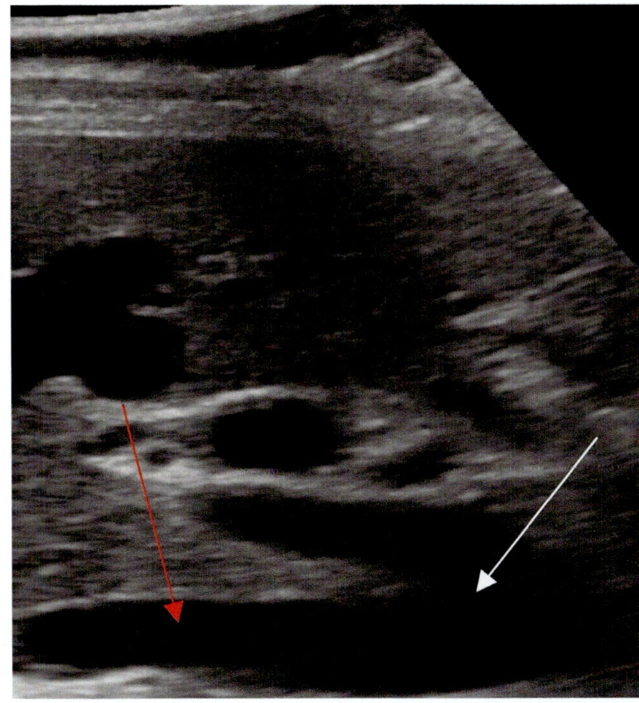

Fig. 40.4 Ultrasonography aspect of dilated hepatic vein (red arrow) and dilated inferior vena cava (white arrow), signs of hepatic congestion

40.3.1.5 Fibrosis and Cirrhosis

Liver cirrhosis may appear in the evolution of all chronic liver disease. The most common causes include chronic hepatitis B and C, alcoholic and non-alcoholic fatty liver disease, metabolic disorders (hemochromatosis, Wilson's disease); some causes of cirrhosis may remain cryptogenic despite extensive evaluation [19]. The diagnosis of cirrhosis is based on serologic signs (signs of impaired liver function like hypoalbuminemia, hypofibrinogenemia, increased coagulation times, thrombocytopenia) and imagistic findings. Liver biopsy is still the gold standard for the diagnosis of cirrhosis, especially in early stages or in patients without relevant risk factors [20]. Several histology scores have been validated for the staging of fibrosis (Table 40.3).

The ultrasonography aspect of cirrhosis is characteristic, comprising elements of liver parenchyma, portal circulation and associated organ anomalies. Nevertheless, these elements may vary according to the degree of liver damage and are quite subtle in the early stages, with more obvious and severe changes in the late stages [22].

In the early stages, ultrasonography reveals hepatomegaly with a rounded inferior edge and coarse hyperechogenicity, similar to that seen in fatty liver disease. However, in the late stages, the liver may have reduced dimensions, appearing as "shrunken liver". Also, the fourth segment appears narrower and the caudate lobe is enlarged. Normally the transverse diameter of the fourth segment is 43 ± 8 mm in non-cirrhotic patients, while cirrhotic patients have a diameter of 28 ± 9 mm [23]. The echo-structure is non-homogenous and coarse, and regeneration nodules may appear, which give the irregularity of the liver surface (Fig. 40.5). The intrahepatic portal vein branches have irregular caliber and the hepatic veins appear compressed by fibrosis, while the hepatic arteries are prominent and have a pseudo double barrel aspect. The peripheral vasculature becomes rarefied. The gallbladder wall is thickened (by portal hypertension) and frequently gallstones are visible. A wall thickness of over 4 mm is

Table 40.3 Histological classification systems for evaluating the stage of fibrosis [21]

Stage of fibrosis	HAI (Knodell)	Ishak	Metavir[a]
0	No fibrosis	No fibrosis	No fibrosis
1	Portal fibrosis	Fibrosis of isolated portal areas with or without short septa	Portal fibrosis
2	n. d.	Increased fibrosis in most portal areas with or without short septa	Portal fibrosis with scattered septa
3	Portoportal or portocentral septa	Portal fibrosis with portoportal septa	Numerous septa without cirrhosis
4	Cirrhosis	Portal fibrosis Cirrhosis with marked porportoportal or portocentral septa	Cirrhosis
5	n. d.	Marked septum formation (portoportal or portocentral) with some nodule formation (incomplete cirrhosis)	n. d.
6	n. d.	Probable or definite cirrhosis	n. d.

n. d. not defined

[a]Only validated in chronic hepatitis C

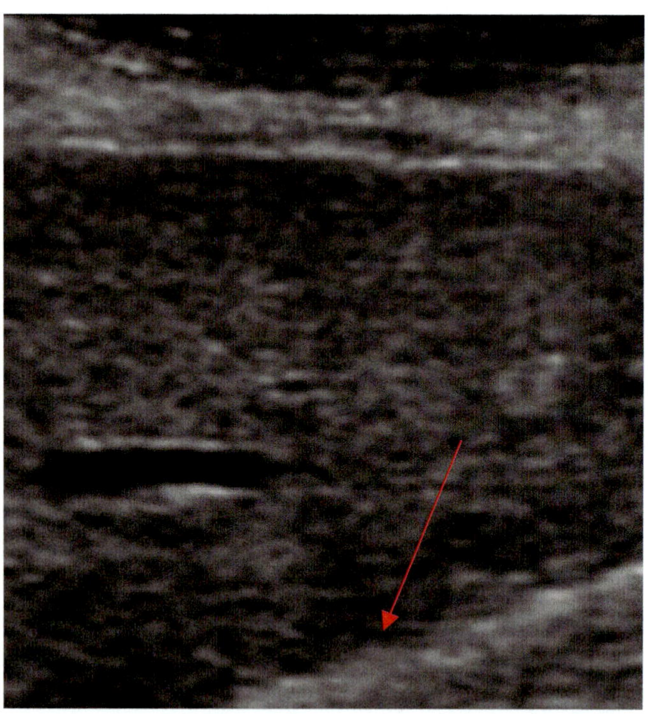

Fig. 40.5 Ultrasonography aspect of cirrhotic liver: reduced dimensions and nodular structure, irregular contour (red arrow)

highly suggestive of cirrhosis and correlates well to the Child Pugh score [24]. Further signs of cirrhosis are given by the portal hypertension, which will be discussed in Sect. 40.3.3.

Ultrasonography is also the imagistic method of choice in the diagnosis of ascites, a frequent sign of cirrhosis decompensation. It can detect small volumes of ascites as narrow echo-free spaces located perihepatic or perisplenic (as opposed to abdominal percussion, which detects moderate to large volumes of ascites) [19]. If hyperechoic structures appear within the echo-free space, this is a sign of spontaneous bacterial peritonitis; the definitive diagnosis is made by paracentesis and cell count of the ascites. Yet again, ultrasonography can be used to determine compartments of ascites (formed after peritonitis, surgery or repeated paracentesis) and to guide the paracentesis to the place most accessible and suitable.

40.3.2 Focal Liver Lesions

Ultrasonography is usually the primary method of detection of focal liver lesions whether benign or malignant, and it is also the method of choice for screening in patients with risk factors for developing liver masses. Usually, finding a liver lesion frequently opens a large range of differential diagnosis, which take into account imagistic aspects, serology markers and the risk factors for specific medical conditions [25].

Histologically, focal liver lesions can be divided into malignant or benign lesions, each with its own cellular content and aspect. Frequently, contrast enhanced imaging techniques (ultrasonography, computer tomography or magnetic resonance) and even biopsies are required for a clear diagnosis (Table 40.4).

Table 40.4 Types of focal liver lesions

Benign	Malignant
Liver cysts – Simple cysts – Traumatic cysts – Echinococcal cysts – Abscesses – Biliary cysts	Rare tumors – Embryonal sarcoma – Hepatoblastoma – Fibrolamellar carcinoma – Hemangioendothelioma – Rhabdomyosarcoma
Calcifications	Hepatocellular carcinoma
Focal fatty infiltration/fatty sparing[a]	Cholangiocarcinoma
Hemangioma	Carcinoid tumors
Focal nodular hyperplasia	Liver metastases
Lipoma	
Angiomyolipoma	
Hamartoma	
Hepatocellular adenoma	
Hemangioendothelioma	
Hematoma	
Liver infarction	

[a]See previous section

The following will discuss the ultrasonography aspects of the most common focal liver lesions.

40.3.2.1 Benign Focal Liver Lesions

Liver Cysts

Incidental liver cysts are found in 3% of performed ultrasonographies. The imagistic criteria for defining a cyst are: spherical configuration, with a smooth outline, clearly defined from the surrounding parenchyma, with echo-free interior and distal acoustic enhancement. Finding of over 10–15 cysts defines a polycystic liver [26]. If cysts are present in other organs (kidneys, spleen, pancreas), this may raise the suspicion of a genetic condition (for example the Hippel-Lindau syndrome). Large cysts of over 5–10 cm can be associated with a cholestatic syndrome and treatment may be required.

The differential diagnosis for simple cysts comprises the rare early cystic metastases, from melanoma, lymphoma, carcinoid tumors, carcinomas of the ovary or esophagus, cystadenocarcinomas. A definite diagnosis frequently requires diagnostic aspiration.

The hydatid cyst is a particular case, where several daughter cysts are found within a large cyst with a hyperechoic rim [27] (Fig. 40.6). In some cases, the membranes of the daughter cysts rupture and flow within the main cyst, forming a honeycomb structure.

Liver abscesses can appear secondary to prolonged immune suppressive therapy, in patients undergoing interventions such as biliary drainage, liver biopsy, transarterial chemoembolization, or as septic metastases from other sites, mainly abdominal (for example diverticulitis). The lesion is difficult to observe in early stages (an important posterior

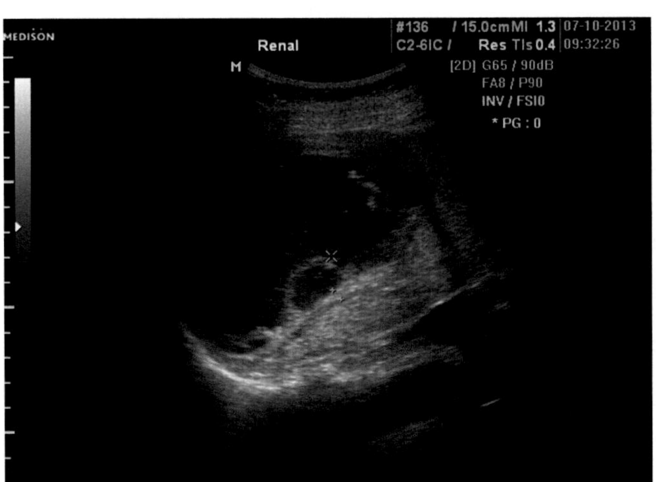

Fig. 40.6 Hydatid cyst in the posterior liver segments 6 and 7, underneath the diaphragm, measuring 9/10 cm, with liquid content, delimited by a 5 mm wall with decollated internal membrane and multiple daughter cysts

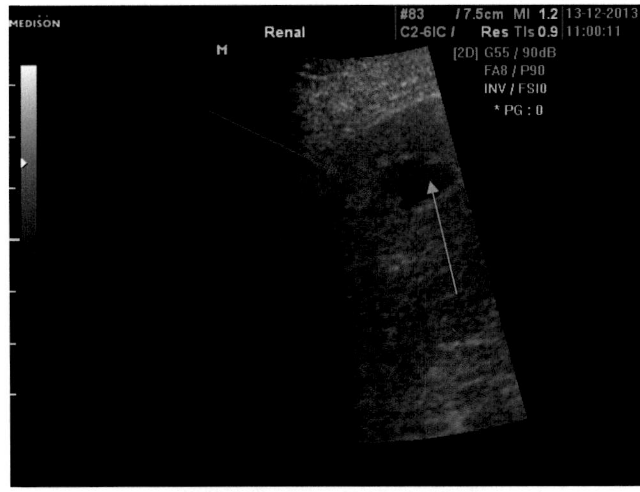

Fig. 40.7 Liver abscess (red arrow) in the right liver lobe, with a hypoechoic center (green arrow) suggesting necrosis

enhancement associated with clinical signs of infection). As the disease progresses, the lesion is hypoechoic, better defined and may contain gas, depending on the causative microorganism [28]. The evolution may be complicated by portal vein thrombosis (Fig. 40.7).

Hemangiomas

These are the most common type of benign liver nodules, consisting of distended capillaries, with a lacuna-like aspect, with slow blood flow. There are five times more cases described in women, possibly in relation to hormonal imbalances.

The typical aspect is of an intensely echogenic tumor with smooth margins, compared to a snowball. An inflow or outflow vessel is usually observed. If hypoechoic structures are seen within, there may be thrombosis or fibrosis of the vessels. Calcifications can also be present. There is a rim of normal hepatic tissue between the liver surface and the hemangioma [29] (Fig. 40.8).

Liver Cell Adenoma

Adenomas are epithelial tumors, also affecting preponderantly women, with a clear connection to the use of steroids. They contain hepatocytes, portal areas and bile ducts and they can be difficult to distinguish histologically from normal liver parenchyma or hepatocellular carcinoma. The ultrasonographic aspect is variable, ranging from hypoechoic (usually) to complex echostructure or without any delimitation from the surrounding normal tissue. Contrast imagistic methods and biopsy are required for diagnosis [25].

Focal Nodular Hyperplasia (FNH)

FNH is a benign hepatic tumor, also influenced by the use of corticoid therapy. It appears frequently in women between

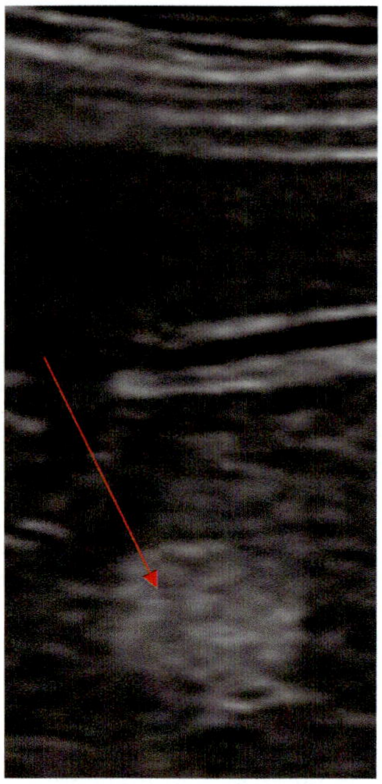

Fig. 40.8 Liver hemangioma (red arrow): a hyperechoic homogenous structure

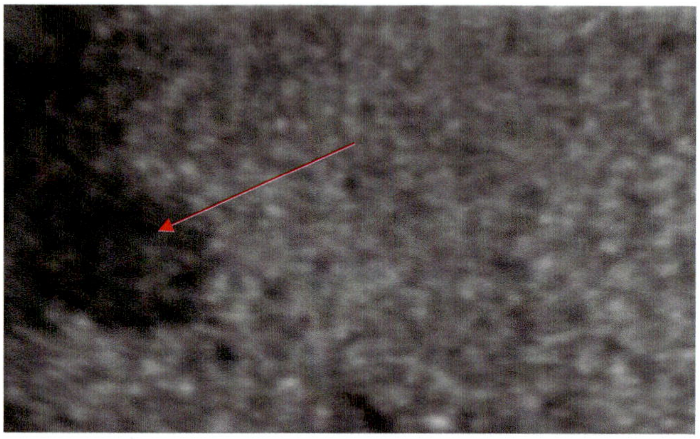

Fig. 40.9 Focal nodular hyperplasia (red arrow)

the ages of 20 and 50 years old. The ultrasonographic aspect is non-specific; small lesions are homogenous, while lesions larger than 3 cm can present a stellate scar; Doppler ultrasonography may reveal a wheel spoke pattern, given by the arteries present in the connective tissue septa [30] (Fig. 40.9).

40.3.2.2 Malignant Focal Liver Lesions

Hepatocellular Carcinoma (HCC)

HCC is one of the most common malignant tumors worldwide, due to its causality related to chronic viral hepatitis. It frequently appears in cirrhotic patients, but cases on normal liver parenchyma have been described. High-risk patients are those with chronic hepatitis B and C, alcoholic cirrhosis, non-alcoholic fatty liver disease and hemochromatosis [31]. Many international guidelines have specific recommendations for the screening and monitoring of these patients (Fig. 40.10 and Table 40.5).

HCC may appear as a solitary or multifocal lesion, without calcifications, often ill-defined. Correlation between tumor markers (chiefly alpha-fetoprotein) and contrast enhanced imaging techniques can replace biopsy in some cases (Table 40.5). On ultrasonography, HCC has echo free and echo-rich areas, with a mosaic pattern. Color Doppler can reveal signals at the periphery or in the interior of the tumor [33]. If the internal flow signals are pulsatile, there is a high probability of HCC (a continuous spectrum in the interior suggests more likely regenerative nodules or adenomas). Portal vein thrombosis can accompany an HCC nodule, but thrombosis of the hepatic veins is rare (Fig. 40.11) [34].

Cholangiocarcinoma (CCC)

CCCs are classified according to localization, as peripheral and hilar tumor. Tumors located in the liver hilum often appear just indirectly, as congestion of the bile ducts [35]. Most tumors appear a single, homogenous, hypoechoic mass, with ill-defined margins and poorly reflective (Fig. 40.12). It is surrounded by dilated bile ducts, which end abruptly in the tumor. Occasionally, a tumor is intraluminal or causes focal thickening of the bile duct wall, resulting in stenosis in the absence of a mass. Generally, portal vein thrombosis is rare [36].

Liver Metastases

Metastases are some of the most common etiologies of liver tumors. Depending on the origin, they have a variety of aspects [3]. Nodular micro metastases and diffuse infiltration of the parenchyma are invisible on ultrasonography. Nodular normoechoic metastases can be differentiated due to liver surface irregularity or displacement or compression of vessels. Patients may also present map-like infiltration. Focal liver metastases may appear as:

- Anechoic with posterior enhancement
- Hypoechoic with or without a rim
- Echogenic with or without a rim
- Complex echo-structures
- With scars or calcifications or necrosis.

The detection of an echo-free rim surrounding a slightly more echogenic center is highly suggestive for a metastasis. Liver determination of lymphomas usually appear diffusely infiltrative or localized and echo-poor (which can be confused with a metastasis from melanoma or from breast cancer). Hyperechoic metastases may appear in gastrointestinal primary tumors; a "bull's eye" aspect has been described in this case, with an echo-poor rim, echogenic ring and echo-poor interior.

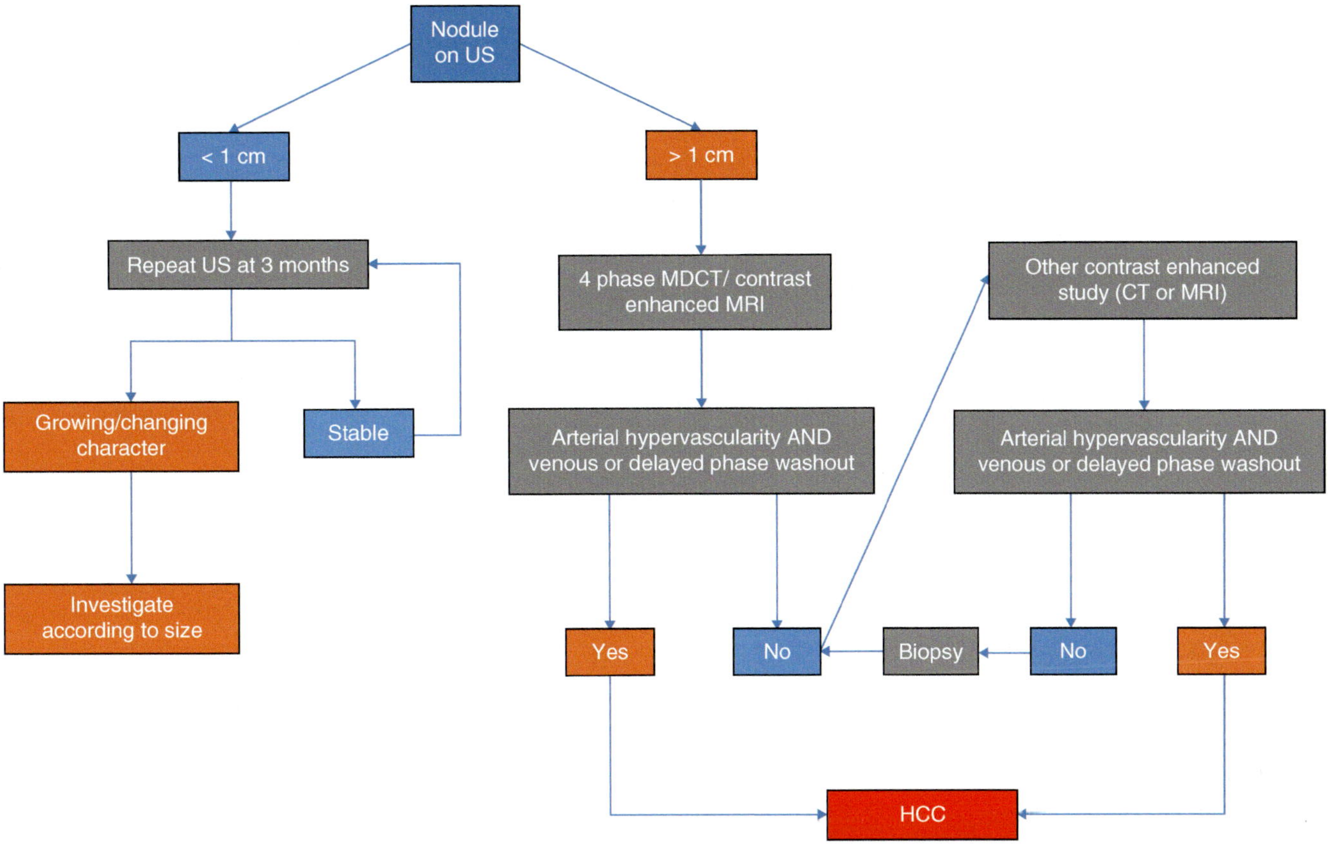

Fig. 40.10 Diagnostic algorithm of AASLD guideline for nodule in patients at risk of HCC [32]. (© 2017 The Author(s). Licensee IntechOpen. This chapter is distributed under the terms of the Creative Commons Attribution 3.0 License, which permits unrestricted use, distribution, and reproduction in any medium, provided the original work is properly cited)

40.3.3 Vascular Related Pathologies of the Liver

40.3.3.1 Portal Hypertension and Portal Thrombosis

Portal hypertension frequently appears in association with the progression of liver disease, but it can also be related to other conditions, such as Budd Chiari syndrome, extrinsic compression, myeloproliferative disorders.

The most important sign of portal hypertension is the enlargement of the portal vein diameter over 15 mm, measured before the bifurcation [2]. There are several other signs of portal hypertension found on abdominal ultrasonography (Fig. 40.13) [7]. In late stages, the portal vein undergoes a cavernomatous transformation, which is a counter-indication for several therapeutic procedures in patients with HCC.

Portal vein thrombosis can appear in the evolution of liver cirrhosis (as a complication of portal hypertension) or in association with abdominal malignancies, mainly hepatocellular carcinoma. The ultrasonography in this case reveals hyperechoic material in the portal lumen, with the absence of color on Doppler interrogation [37] (Fig. 40.14). Contrast-enhanced ultrasonography can be useful to distinguish between a malignant and benign thrombosis, a very important aspect in the prognosis of the patients (see Chap. 42).

40.3.3.2 Budd-Chiari Syndrome

Budd Chiari syndrome defines an obstruction of the hepatic venous outflow. Primary causes include pro-coagulant states (myeloproliferative disorders, Factor V Leyden mutation, genetic deficit of protein C and S, hormonal factors) resulting in venous thrombosis, while secondary Budd Chiari syndrome appears in conditions associated with extrinsic compression of hepatic veins or tumor invasion. In order for the disease to become clinically manifest, two or more hepatic veins must be occluded [38].

Ultrasonography reveals absence of imaging of the hepatic veins and tumor-like parenchymal non-homogenicity (Fig. 40.15). Progression of the disease causes portal hypertension, with its specific signs.

40.3.3.3 Veno-Occlusive Disease

This is a disease of the small intrahepatic veins, occurring usually after chemotherapy but also as a result of pro-coagulant states [9]. In the acute phase there is no out-flow in the hepatic veins, they remain patent but the blood only

Table 40.5 Comparison of EASL, AASLD, APASL guidelines, and LI-RADS [32]

	EASL	AASLD	APASL	JAPAN	LI-RADS
Target population	Cirrhosis	Hep B carriers, cirrhosis	Cirrhosis only with Hep B or Hep C	All patients at high risk of HCC	All patients at high risk of HCC
Targeted lesion	Detected nodule by US	Detected nodule by US	Detected nodule by US and elevated AFP	Detected nodule by US and elevated AFP, AFP-L3, DCP	All nodules
Imaging modality	4-phase MDCT, CE-MRI	4-phase MDCT, CE-MRI	CT, CEUS, SPIO-MRI	CT, CEUS, Gd-EOB-DTPA-enhanced MRI, CT angiography	CT, MRI with extracellular and hepatobiliary agent
Diagnostic criteria	Larger than 1 cm	Larger than 1 cm	Washout on PVP, DP or	AP enhancement	AP enhancement
	AP enhancement	AP enhancement	High SPIO-MR signal or	Washout on DP	Washout on PVP, DP
	Washout on PVP, DP	Washout on PVP, DP	Defect in KP on CEUS	Larger than 1 or 1.5 cm	Capsule appearance
			Regardless of the size		
Number of required exam	≥2 cm: one exam	One exam	One exam	One exam	One exam
	1–2 cm: two exams				
Serum marker	N/A	N/A	Only for small nodules (<1 cm)	Yes	N/A
Category of diagnosis	HCC	HCC	HCC	HCC	LR-1 definitely benign
	Not HCC	Not HCC	Not HCC	Not HCC	LR-2 probably benign
	Indeterminate	Indeterminate	Indeterminate	Indeterminate	LR-3 indeterminate
					LR-4 probably HCC
					LR-5 definitely HCC
					LR-5V definitely tumor invading vein
					LR-M probably malignancy but not specific for HCC
Diagnosis of subcentimetre HCC without biopsy	No	No	Yes (tumor marker + imaging)	No	Yes (probably HCC)
Biopsy required	Yes	Yes	No	Yes	Yes (LR-4, LR-M)

AASLD Association for the Study of Liver Diseases, *AFP* alpha-fetoprotein, *AP* arterial phase, *CHB* chronic hepatitis B, *CHC* chronic hepatitis C, *DP* delayed phase, *EASL* European Association for the Study of the Liver, *4-phase MDCT* +phase multidetector computerized tomography, *CE-MRI* contrast-enhanced magnetic resonance imaging, *HCC* hepatocellular carcinoma, *KLCSG-NCC* Korean Liver Cancer Study Group-National Cancer Center, *LC* liver cirrhosis, *LI-RADS* Liver Imaging Reporting and Data System, *N/A* not applicable, *PVP* portal venous phase, *TP* transitional phase, *US* ultrasonography, *KP* Kupfer

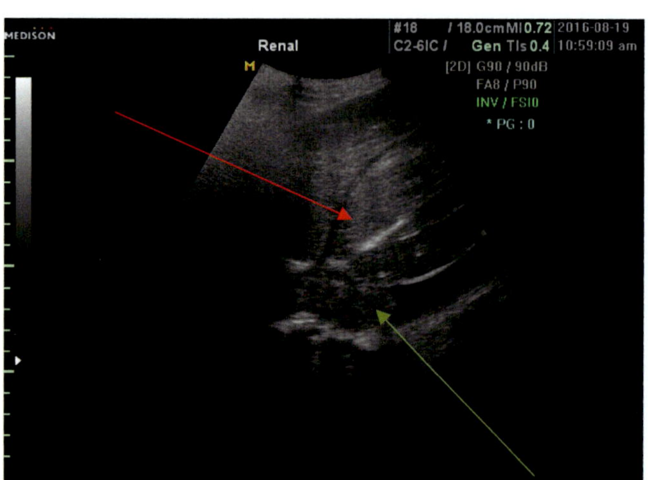

Fig. 40.11 Hepatocellular carcinoma (red arrow) with malignant thrombus extending from the right hepatic vein to the inferior vena cava (green arrow)

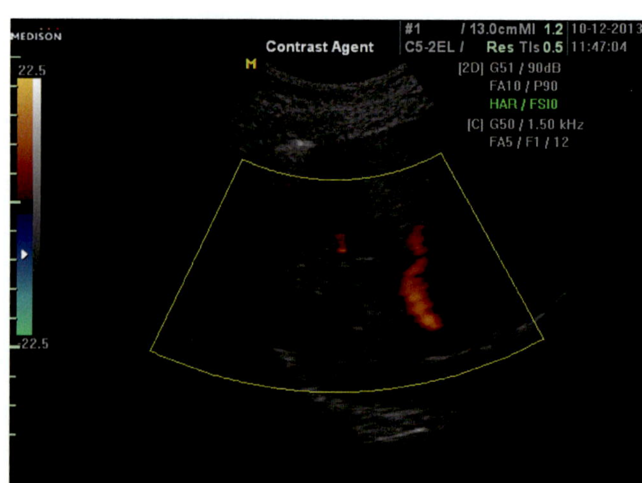

Fig. 40.12 Intrahepatic cholangiocarcinoma, Doppler interrogation

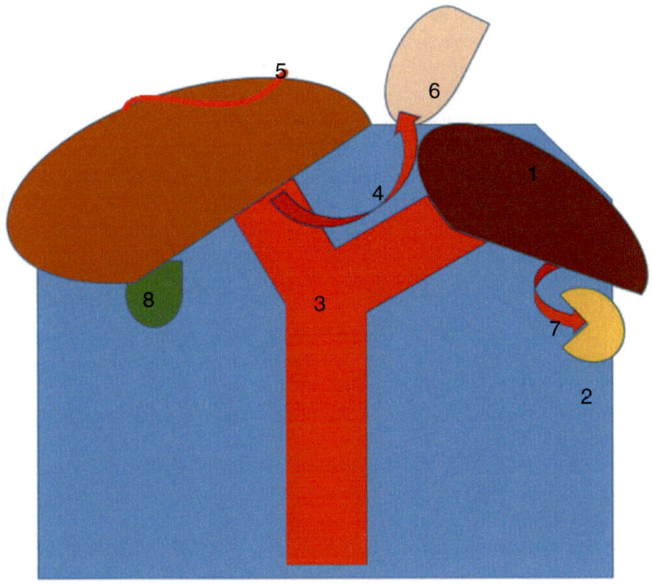

Fig. 40.13 Ultrasonography signs of portal hypertension: (1) Splenomegaly; (2) Ascites; (3) Distension of the portal vein and drainage veins (splenic, superior mesenteric); (4) Porto-systemic collaterals; (5) Patent umbilical vein; (6) Thickening of the gastric wall; (7) Spontaneous spleno-renal shunt; (8) Thickening of the gallbladder wall

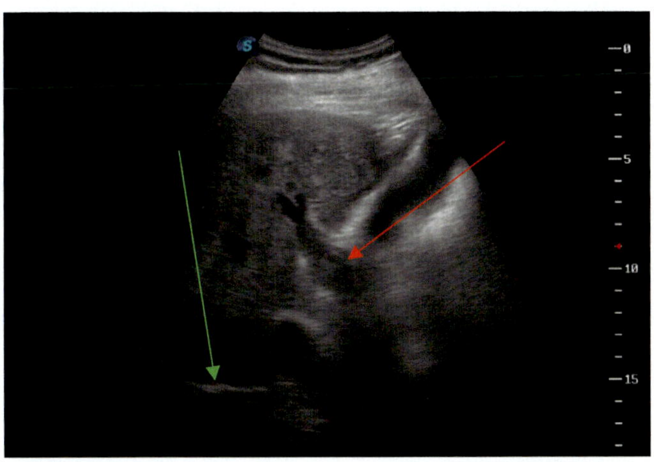

Fig. 40.14 Large portal vein thrombosis (red arrow) in a patient with thrombophilia and liver cirrhosis. Note the non-homogenous aspect of the liver parenchyma, with important posterior attenuation and irregular contour of the liver (green arrow)

oscillates during respiration. The portal flow reverses and there is ascites and splenomegaly. The liver becomes fatty. As the patient improves the hepatic vein flow re-establishes and the portal flow returns to anterograde flow.

40.3.3.4 Osler-Weber-Rendu Disease

This is a rare hereditary disorder characterized by the development of multiple angiodysplasias. Ultrasonography of the liver reveals large corkscrew-like vascular malformation, with a hepatic artery tipically larger than 1 cm [9].

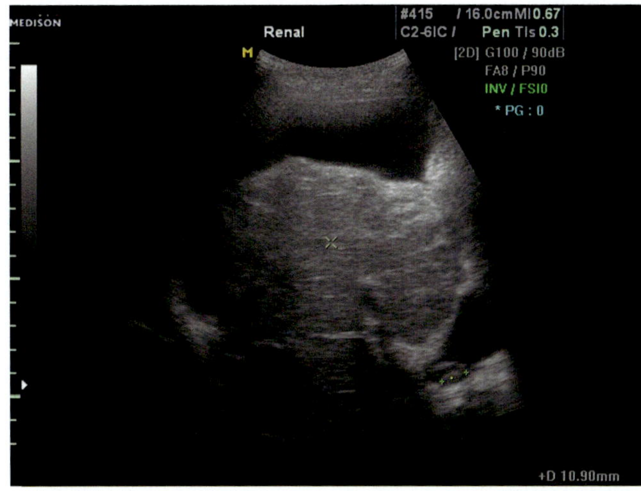

Fig. 40.15 Budd Chiari syndrome in a patient with myeloproliferative disorder, with chronic alterations in the hepatic veins, as seen from longitudinal section of the right and caudate lobe

Complications include heart failure associated to large arterio-venous shunts and cirrhosis.

Self Study

Questions

1. Which statement is true:
   (a) The patient must fast for a minimum of 6 h prior to the investigation.
   (b) Low frequency sounds are used for deep tissues (such as large livers).
   (c) High frequency sounds are used for high resolution images of superficial structures.
   (d) The frequency used in liver ultrasonography is 3–7 MHz.
2. Which statement is true:
   (a) Renal cortex is a reference for normal aspect of the liver echostructure.
   (b) The normal capsule appears as a fine continue hyperechoic line surrounding the liver.
   (c) The normal flow velocity in the portal vein ranges from 12 to 25 cm/s.
   (d) The hallmark sign for acute/chronic liver congestion is the distension of the inferior vena cava accompanied by the distension of hepatic veins.
3. Which statement is true about ultrasonography in liver cirrhosis:
   (a) The liver appears hypoechoic.
   (b) The liver contour is irregular.
   (c) The portal vein has a diameter of over 15 mm.
   (d) The intrahepatic portal vein branches have irregular caliber.

Answers

1. Which statement is true:
   (a) CORRECT
   (b) CORRECT
   (c) CORRECT
   (d) CORRECT
2. Which statement is true:
   (a) CORRECT
   (b) CORRECT
   (c) CORRECT
   (d) CORRECT
3. Which statement is true about ultrasonography in liver cirrhosis:
   (a) FALSE
   (b) CORRECT
   (c) CORRECT
   (d) CORRECT

References

1. Hassani S. Principles of ultrasonography. J Natl Med Assoc. 1974;66(3):205–8.
2. Ralls PW, Jeffrey RB Jr, Kane RA, Robbin ML. Diagnostic sonography. In: Yamada T, editor. Textbook of gastroenterology. 5th ed. Hoboken, NJ: Blackwell Publishing Ltd; 2009. p. 3083–113.
3. Hofer M. Ultrasound teaching manual - the basics of performing and interpreting ultrasound scans. Stuttgart: Thieme; 1999. p. 23–33.
4. Kudo M, Hirasa M, Takakuwa H, et al. Small hepatocellular carcinomas in chronic liver disease: detection with SPECT. Radiology. 1986;159:697.
5. Penny S. Examination review for ultrasound: abdominal & obstetrics and gynecology. Philadelphia: Wolters Kluwer; 2018.
6. Borges VF, Diniz AL, Cotrim HP, Rocha HL, Andrade NB. Sonographic hepatorenal ratio: a noninvasive method to diagnose nonalcoholic steatosis. J Clin Ultrasound. 2013;41(1):18–25.
7. Choi BI, Lee JY. The liver, Chapter 7. In: Lutz H, Buscarini E, editors. WHO manual of diagnostic ultrasound, vol. 1. 2nd ed. Malta: Gutenberg Press Ltd.; 2011. p. 139–67.
8. Guidelines for professional ultrasound practice. Society and College of Radiographers and British Medical Ultrasound Society, Revision 3; 2018.
9. EASL. EASL Clinical practice guidelines: vascular diseases of the liver. J Hepatol. 2015; https://doi.org/10.1016/j.jhep.2015.07.040.
10. Grant EG. Parenchymal disease of the liver. In: Rifkin MD, Charboneau JW, Laing FC, editors. Ultrasound 1991 syllabus: special course. Oak Brook, IL: Radiological Society of North America; 1991. p. 281.
11. Browning JD, Szczepaniak LS, Dobbins R, Nuremberg P, Horton JD, Cohen JC, Grundy SM, Hobbs HH. Prevalence of hepatic steatosis in an urban population in the United States: impact of ethnicity. Hepatology. 2004;40(6):1387–95.
12. Petritsch W, Pristautz H, Eber B. Is sonography superior to enzyme diagnosis in the detection of hepatic steatosis? Wien Klin Wochenschr. 1987;99(5):153–6.
13. Ricci C, Longo R, Gioulis E, Bosco M, Pollesello P, Masutti F, et al. Noninvasive in vivo quantitative assessment of fat content in human liver. J Hepatol. 1997;27(1):108–13.
14. Ahima RS. Insulin resistance: cause or consequence of nonalcoholic steatohepatitis? Gastroenterology. 2007;132(1):444–6.
15. White EM, Simeone JF, Mueller PR, et al. Focal periportal sparing in hepatic fatty infiltration: a cause of hepatic pseudomass on US. Radiology. 1987;162:57.
16. Forsberg L, Floren CH, Hederstrom E, et al. Ultrasound examination in diffuse liver disease. Clinical significance of enlarged lymph nodes in the hepatoduodenal ligament. Acta Radiol. 1987;28:281.
17. Quinn SF, Gosink BB. Characteristic sonographic signs of hepatic fatty infiltration. AJR Am J Roentgenol. 1985;145:753.
18. Gerstenmaier JF, Gibson RN. Ultrasound in chronic liver disease. Insights Imaging. 2014;5:441–55. https://doi.org/10.1007/s13244-014-0336-2.
19. Harbin WP, Robert NJ, Ferrucci JT Jr. Diagnosis of cirrhosis based on regional changes in hepatic morphology. Radiology. 1980;135:273.
20. Choong CC, Venkatesh SK, Siew EP. Accuracy of routine clinical ultrasound for staging of liver fibrosis. J Clin Imaging Sci. 2012;2:58.
21. Macarini L, Stoppino LP. Radiologic assessment of liver fibrosis – present and future, practical management of chronic viral hepatitis, Gaetano Serviddio. IntechOpen. https://doi.org/10.5772/55164. 2013. https://www.intechopen.com/books/practical-management-of-chronic-viral-hepatitis/radiologic-assessment-of-liver-fibrosis-present-and-future.
22. Hess CF, Schmiedl U, Koelbel G, et al. Diagnosis of liver cirrhosis with US; receiver-operating characteristic analysis of multidimensional caudate lobe indexes. Radiology. 1989;171:349.
23. Lafortune M, Matricardi L, Denys A, Favret M, Dery R, Pomier-Layrargues G. Degment 4 (the quadrate lobe): a barometer of cirrhotic liver disease at US. Radiology. 1998;206:157–60.
24. Wang TF, Hwang SJ, Lee EY, Tsai YT, Lin HC, Li CP, et al. Gall-bladder wall thickening in patients with liver cirrhosis. J Gastroenterol Hepatol. 1997;12(6):445–9.
25. EASL. EASL clinical practice guidelines on the management of benign liver tumours. J Hepatol. 2016;65:386–98.
26. D'Onofrio M, Crosara S, De Robertis R, Canestrini S, Mucelli RP. Contrast enhanced ultrasound of focal liver lesions. AJR Am J Roentgenol. 2015;205:W56–66.
27. Richter J, Hatz C, Häussinger D. Ultrasound in tropical and parasitic diseases. Lancet. 2003;362(9387):900–2.
28. Kuligowska E, Connors SK, Shapiro JH. Liver abscess: sonography in diagnosis and treatment. Am J Roentgenol. 1982;138(2):253–7.
29. Quaia E, Bertolotto M, Dalla Palma L. Characterization of liver hemangiomas with pulse inversion harmonic imaging. Eur Radiol. 2002;12:537–44.
30. Buetow PC, Pantongrag-Brown L, Buck JL, Ros PR, Goodman ZD. Focal nodular hyperplasia of the liver: radiologic-pathologic correlation. Radiographics. 1996;16:369–88.
31. EASL. EASL clinical practice guidelines: management of hepatocellular carcinoma. J Hepatol. 2018;69:182–236.
32. Kefeli A, Basyigit S, Yeniova AO. Diagnosis of hepatocellular carcinoma, updates in liver cancer. Hesham Mohamed Abdeldayem. IntechOpen. https://doi.org/10.5772/64992. 2017. https://www.intechopen.com/books/updates-in-liver-cancer/diagnosis-of-hepatocellular-carcinoma.
33. Forner A, Vilana R, Ayuso C, Bianchi L, Sole M, Ayuso JR, et al. Diagnosis of hepatic nodules 20 mm or smaller in cirrhosis:

prospective validation of the noninvasive diagnostic criteria for hepatocellular carcinoma. Hepatology. 2008;47:97–104.
34. Bolondi L, Sofia S, Siringo S, Gaiani S, Casali A, Zironi G, et al. Surveillance programme of cirrhotic patients for early diagnosis and treatment of hepatocellular carcinoma: a cost effectiveness analysis. Gut. 2001;48:251–9.
35. Choi BI, Lee JH, Han MC, Kim SH, Yi JG, Kim CW. Hilar cholangiocarcinoma: comparative study with sonography and CT. Radiology. 1989;172:689–92.
36. Kurtz AB, Middleton WD. Ultrasound: the requisites. St Louis, MO: Mosby-Year Book; 1996. p. 55–73.
37. Harding DJ, Perera M, Chen F, Olliff S, Tripathi D. Portal vein thrombosis in cirrhosis: controversies and latest developments. World JGastroenterol. 2015;21:6769–84.
38. Aydinli M, Bayraktar Y. Budd-Chiari syndrome: etiology, pathogenesis and diagnosis. World J Gastroenterol. 2007;13(19):2693–6. https://doi.org/10.3748/wjg.v13.i19.2693.

41 Endoscopy in Hepatic Diseases

Nitin Jagtap and D. Nageshwar Reddy

Key Concepts

- Endoscopy plays vital role in management of liver diseases; it is not limited to management of varices.
- Capsule endoscopy and device assisted enteroscopy have shown to be effective in treating patients with obscure GI bleed including ectopic varices in patients with portal hypertension.
- ERCP in liver cirrhosis is safe and effective as compared to surgical alternative in patients having pancreatobiliary diseases.
- Metabolic and bariatric endoscopy can be utilized to achieve required weight loss for management of NASH.

41.1 Introduction

Endoscopy plays a vital role in the management of patients with hepatobiliary diseases. In recent time, endoscopy has undergone extensive improvement that expanded its role in the diagnosis and therapeutic interventions. This chapter will highlight role in endoscopy in management of hepatobiliary diseases.

41.2 Gastro Esophageal Varices

Portal hypertension is the initial and main consequence of cirrhosis which is responsible for majority of complications [1]. The gastroesophageal junction is the main site of formation of the varices, esophageal varices develop when hepatic vein pressure gradient (HVPG) is greater than or equal to 10 mmHg [2]. All patients diagnosed with liver cirrhosis should be screened for esophageal varices [3]. Upper gastrointestinal endoscopy (UGIE) is most commonly used method to diagnose varices, as it provides direct visualization and enables to decide therapy by assessing the size and stigmata of recent bleed [3]. Current guidelines recommends repeat UGIE in 2–3 years if no varices are seen and in 1–2 years or earlier if patients shows any decompensation [1]. Esophageal varices are examined during endoscope withdrawal, with esophagus maximally inflated with air and stomach air completely aspirated [3]. The Baveno consensus and AASLD recommended that esophageal varices to be classified as small (<5 mm) and large (>5 mm) [1, 4]. Patients with large varices, CTP class C and red color signs on the varices carry highest risk for bleeding within 1 year [5].

Gastric varices are classified as Sarin's classification (Fig. 41.1) [6, 7]:

- GOV1: Gastric varices extending 2–5 cm below the GE junction and in continuity with esophageal varices;
- GOV2: Gastric varices in the fundus and in continuity with esophageal varices;
- IGV1: Isolated gastric varices in fundus in absence of esophageal varies and
- IGV2: isolated gastric varices in body, antrum or pylorus of stomach.

41.3 Primary Prophylaxis

The incidence of formation of new varices is <5% per year, while varices increases in size with time at rate from 5% to 30% per year depending on HVPG and ongoing liver injury [8]. The incidence of formation of new varices can be reduced with non-selective beta blockers compared to placebo [9]. Current guidelines do not recommend beta blockers for prevention of the development of new varices; such patients should undergo screening EGD every 2–3 years [1, 4].

N. Jagtap, MD, DNB (✉) · D. N. Reddy, MD, DM
Asian Institute of Gastroenterology, Hyderabad, India

F. Radu-Ionita et al. (eds.), *Liver Diseases*, https://doi.org/10.1007/978-3-030-24432-3_41

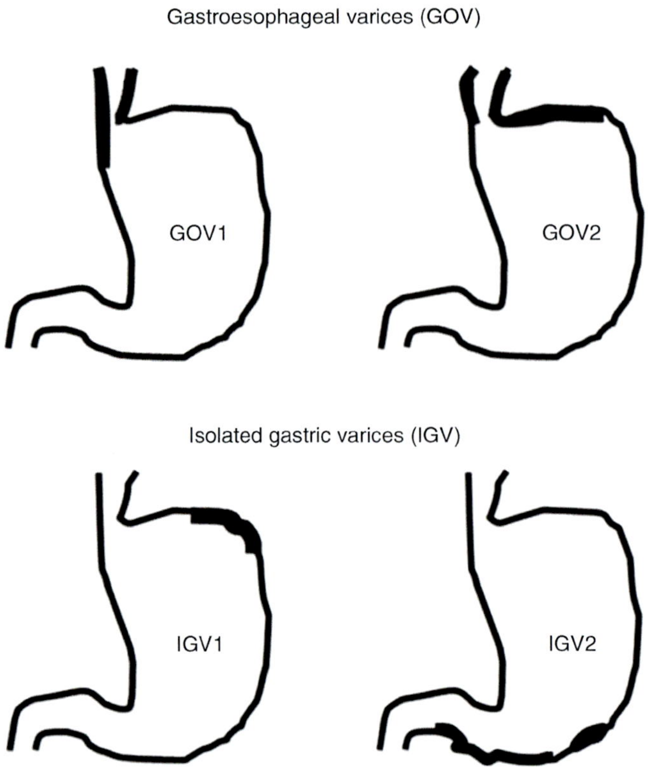

Fig. 41.1 Classification of gastric varices. (Adapted from Sarin classification [6]). Gastric varices in the presence of esophageal varices are defined as gastroesophageal varices (GOVs). Types 1 GOV (GOV1) are gastric varices that occur along the lesser curvature, whereas GOVs present along the fundus are defined as type 2 GOV (GOV2). Gastric varices with no concurrent esophageal varices as called isolated gastric varices (IGVs). IGVs are further classified into type 1 (IGV1) when they are present in the gastric fundus or type 2 (IGV2) if present elsewhere in the stomach or first portion of the duodenum. GOV2 and IGV1 are sometimes grouped together and referred to as 'fundic varices'. *GOV* gastroesophageal varies, *IGV* isolated gastric varices. (From Kapoor et al. [7] with **permission**)

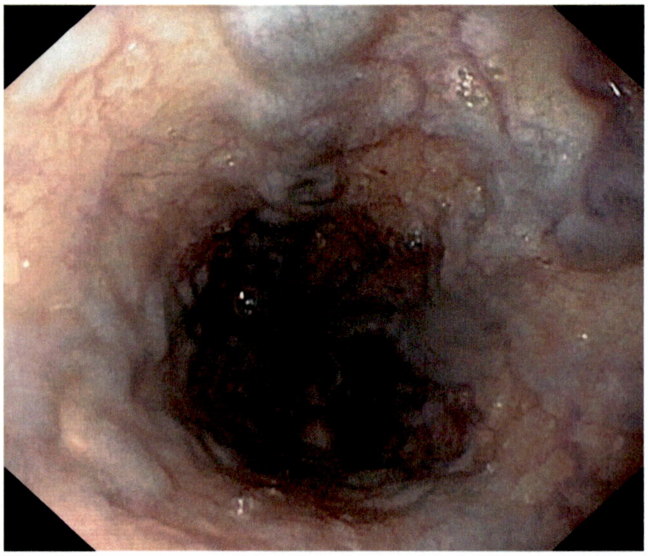

Fig. 41.2 Small esophageal varices

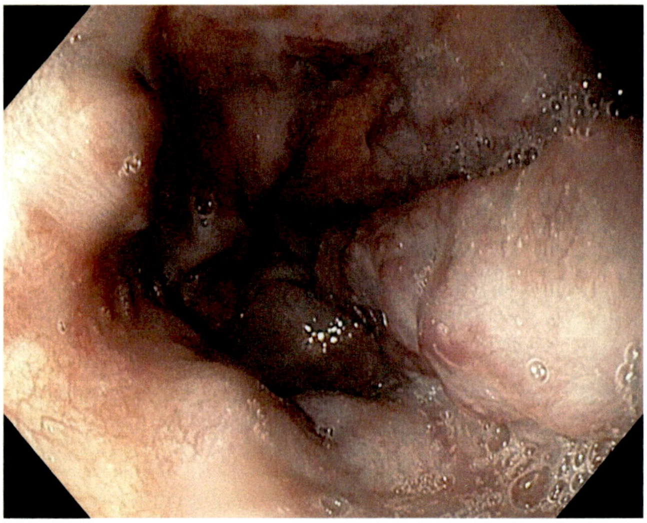

Fig. 41.3 Large esophageal varices

Patients with compensated cirrhosis with small esophageal varices (Fig. 41.2) without high risk features at EGD should undergo repeat EGD in 1–2 years [1, 4]. It is recommended that patients with small esophageal varices with advanced liver disease (Child-Pugh class B or C) should be treated with non-selective beta-blockers and should undergo EGD yearly [10]. For patients with large esophageal varices (Fig. 41.3) and high risk features, endoscopic band ligation (EBL) is an alternative to NSBBs for primary prophylaxis in whom NSBBs are contraindicated or not tolerated due to adverse events. Several studies compared EBL with NSBBs for primary prophylaxis; meta-analysis of these studies showed that EBL is superior in reducing bleeding episode without survival benefits [11]. EBL requires several sessions at interval between 2 and 4 weeks and may result is post-EBL ulcers bleeding [1].

Similar to esophageal varices, annual bleeding risk from gastric varices depends on size, presence of red signs and degree of liver dysfunction which ranges from 4% in compensated cirrhosis with small varices to 65% in patients with advanced liver diseases with red signs [12]. For prevention of first variceal bleed from gastric varices (GOV2 and IGV1), NSBBs can be used. Endotherapy is not recommended for primary prevention in gastric varices (GOV2 and IGV1), however for GOV1 recommendations of esophageal varices can be followed.

41.4 Acute Variceal Bleeding

Acute variceal bleeding (AVB) is a life threatening complication of portal hypertension and is a leading cause of death in patients with liver cirrhosis [1]. The therapeutic strategies should be directed towards reducing portal inflow, reducing portal pressure or compressing or obliterating the varices [1]. Variceal hemorrhage is defined as (a) active bleeding from esophageal or gastric varix (b) the presence of varices with an clot or fibrin plug or (c) the presence of large esophageal and/or gastric varices with blood in the stomach without any other recognizable cause of bleeding during EGD.

Management of AVB includes hemodynamic resuscitation, prevention and treatment of complications and endoscopic therapy to control bleeding. Resuscitation, management of complications and pharmacotherapy will be described in other topics, in this topic details of endotherapy will be described.

EGD is the gold standard for diagnosis and treatment of variceal hemorrhage. EGD should be performed within 12 h of admission and once the patient is hemodynamically stable [1, 4]. There are two principal methods for management of esophageal varices—endoscopic sclerotherapy (EST) and endoscopic variceal band ligation (EBL).

EST, first described by Crafood and Frenckner in 1939 is a technique which uses flexible catheter with needle to inject a sclerosing agent either into the varix (intravariceal) or adjacent to the varix (paravariceal). Various sclerosant such as sodium morrhuate, sodium tetradecyl sulfate, ethanolamine oleate, polidocanol and absolute alcohol have been used. EST can achieve hemostasis by variceal thrombosis and/or tamponade due to surrounding edema. EST is cheap and easy to use. EST is associated with various adverse events which includes fever, chest pain, bacteremia, pleural effusion, dysphagia due to esophageal stricture, post-EST ulcerations. Post EST mortality is usually due to recurrent bleeding, perforation or sepsis [1].

EST is more effective than balloon tamponade or placebo and not superior to vasoactive agents. Due to major adverse events EST has been superseded by EBL.

EBL was first described by Stiegmann and Goff in 1989 with 88% success rate in controlling AVB. This technique involves suction of a varix into hollow cylinder attached to end of the endoscope followed by placement of rubber band which ligates and strangulates the varix. Currently available devices can deploy multiple bands making procedure faster and simple. Esophageal intubation with ligation device can achieved with flexion of neck, gentle pressure and slight torque of shaft of scope. Once scope is passed up to varix, tip of the scope is pointed towards it and continuous suction is applied to red out appears inside the cap and at this point the band is applied. As the varix blood supply originate from gastro-esophageal junction (GEJ), EBL should be performed at GEJ first then upwards in circular fashion. The most common adverse events are chest pain and post banding ulcers.

EBL (Fig. 41.4) should be considered as gold standard endoscopic therapy for AVB from esophageal varix and

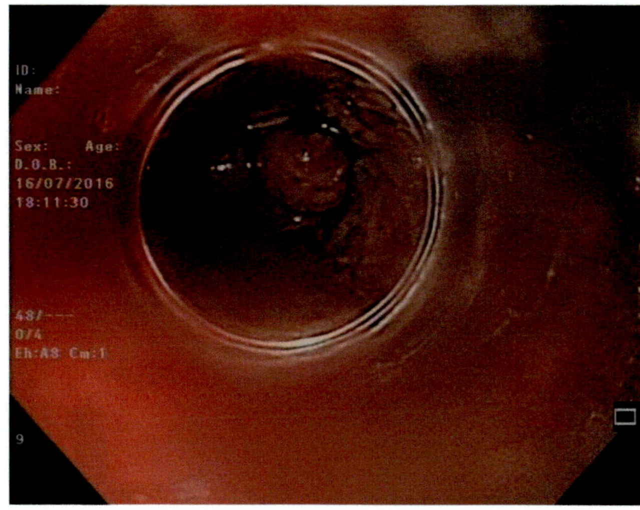

Fig. 41.4 Endoscopic band ligation for active esophageal variceal hemorrhage

EST should be reserved where EBL is technically unsuccessful [1, 4].

Ten to twenty percent of patients with AVB will experience treatment failure or early rebleeding. Any bleeding that occurs >48 h after initial admission for variceal hemorrhage represents rebleeding. Rebleeding that occurs within 6 weeks of the onset of active bleeding is considered early rebleeding and later is called late rebleeding [1, 4]. Treatment options in setting of rebleeding include a second endoscopy, balloon tamponade, esophageal stent tamponade, trans-jugular intrahepatic porto-systemic shunt (TIPS) or a surgical shunt [1]. A recent systemic review and meta-analysis showed endoscopic esophageal SEMS placement for acute refractory esophageal variceal bleeding is 97% technically successful with 96% clinical success within 24 h [13].

41.5 Endoscopic Therapy for Gastric Varices

Gastric variceal bleed is less common than esophageal bleed. It develops in 20% of patients with portal hypertension. Gastric variceal bleed is generally more severe and is associated with higher morbidity and mortality than esophageal varices [1, 4]. GV should be classifies as per Sarin classification which is described before. Risk of gastric variceal bleed is higher is IGV1 than GOV2 and GOV1 [6]. The therapeutic options for acute GVB include balloon tamponade, endoscopic therapies (cyanoacrylate glue, thrombin, EBL), radiological therapies (TIPS and BRTO) and surgical procedures.

Endoscopy remains the initial treatment of choice. EBL in acute GVB is indicated for GOV1, which have shown similar rates of hemostasis and rebleeding to EBL for esophageal varices [14]. Endoscopic glue injection (Fig. 41.5) uses tissue

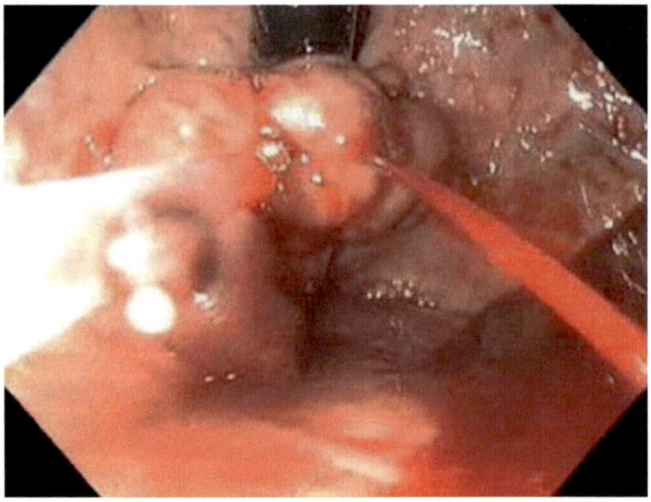

Fig. 41.5 Active gastric variceal hemorrhage being treated with endoscopic cyanoacrylate glue injection

adhesive such as n-butyl-2-cyanoacrylate which rapidly polymerizes when comes in contact with blood. In this technique, a disposable sclerotherapy needle is passed through working channel to puncture the varix. Cyanoacrylate is then injected into the varix in 1–2 ml aliquots followed by flush of saline as needle is withdrawn. Following injection, the needle should be withdrawn immediately to prevent adherence to the varix. Successful injection results in hardened feel of varix with blunt palpation. One to three injection are usually required to achieve variceal obliteration.

The major adverse events include thromboembolic events such as pulmonary embolism, cerebral stroke, portal vein embolization even deaths in rare cases [1]. Other adverse events includes needle entrapment in the varix, bacteremia or sepsis. Endosonography guided insertion of cyanoacrylate and/or coils is emerging therapy as an alternative to standard endotherapy which may have better safety [15].

If initial endoscopic therapy for acute GVB is failed or rebleeding occurs, then second attempt should be considered. If endoscopic attempts fail to control bleeding, rescue therapy with TIPS or BRTO should be done [1].

41.6 Secondary Prophylaxis

It is prevention of variceal rebleeding in patients who have survived an initial episode of variceal hemorrhage. The risk of rebleeding is high during the first 6 weeks; at about 20% between day 5 and day 42 [1, 4]. After this period, the risk of recurrent bleeding decreases to approximately the same as in patients on primary prophylaxis.

The available treatment options for secondary prevention includes pharmacotherapy, endotherapy, combination of pharmacotherapy and endotherapy, TIPS and surgical shunts. Current guidelines suggest combination of EBL plus NSBBs as the best available first line treatment for secondary prophylaxis [1].

41.7 PHG and GAVE

Portal hypertensive gastropathy (PHG) and gastric antral vascular ectasia (GAVE) are other EGD findings in patients with liver diseases. Both can either remain asymptomatic or result in anemia from blood loss. It is essential to differentiate between two as both can present in similar ways but having different treatment options.

Portal hypertension is essential for development of PHG. The prevalence of PHG ranges from 20% to 80% depending on severity of liver disease and previous EBL [1]. Pathologically PHG consists of vascular dilatation in the mucosa and submucosa without inflammation. The characteristic findings on EGD include a snake-skin mosaic mucosal pattern with or without red spots mainly involving proximal stomach. PHG can be categorized as mild or severe depending upon extent of red spots on mosaic mucosa. Variceal eradication has been associated with the development or worsening of PHG. Before establishing PHG as cause of iron deficiency anemia, other causes must be ruled out. The mainstay therapy for PHG involves NSBBs and endoscopic therapy is of limited value.

GAVE (Fig. 41.6) typically causes chronic blood loss resulting into iron deficiency anemia. Apart from portal

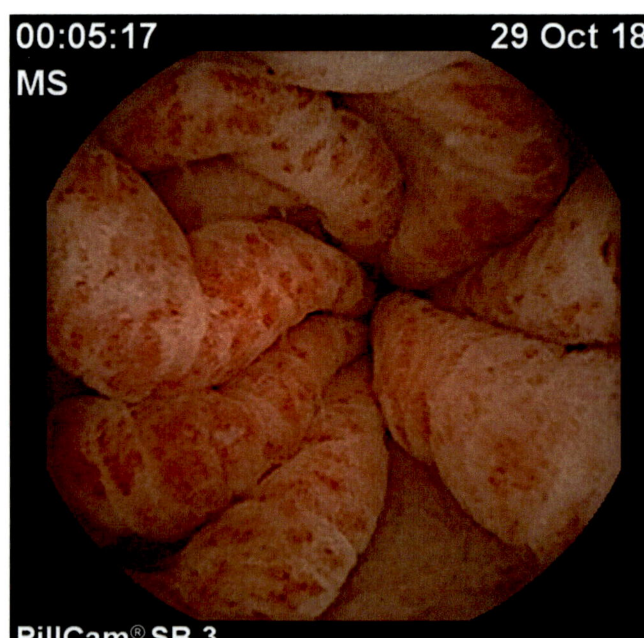

Fig. 41.6 Video capsule endoscopy showing gastric vascular antral ectasia

hypertension other conditions such as connective tissue disorders, bone marrow transplantation and chronic renal failure can have GAVE. GAVE can be diagnosed endoscopically which typically involves antral region as angioectatic red spots in the absence of mosaic mucosa. The longitudinal strips of red spots called as watermelon stomach. Histological findings include dilated vessels with smooth muscle hyperplasia and fibrin thrombi. Symptomatic GAVE is primarily treated with endotherapy which includes argon plasma coagulation (APC), laser therapy using Nd:YAG, radiofrequency ablation (RFA), cryotherapy and band ligation.

41.8 Capsule Endoscopy and Enteroscopy

The introduction of capsule endoscopy (CE) and enteroscopy has revolutionized evaluation of small bowel for obscure gastrointestinal bleed. CE can detect mucosal changes of portal hypertensive enteropathy (PHE) in two third of cirrhotic patients. PHE related small bowel mucosal changes can be classified into four main types; red spots, angioectasias, small bowel varices (Fig. 41.7) and inflammatory like lesions [16]. Double balloon enteroscopy in portal hypertension showed mucosal edema (73%), mucosal atrophy (40%), reddening of villi (47%), angioectasias (67%), dilated vessels (93%) and varices (7%) [17]. Balloon assisted enteroscopy can be used as therapeutic modality to manage ectopic varices.

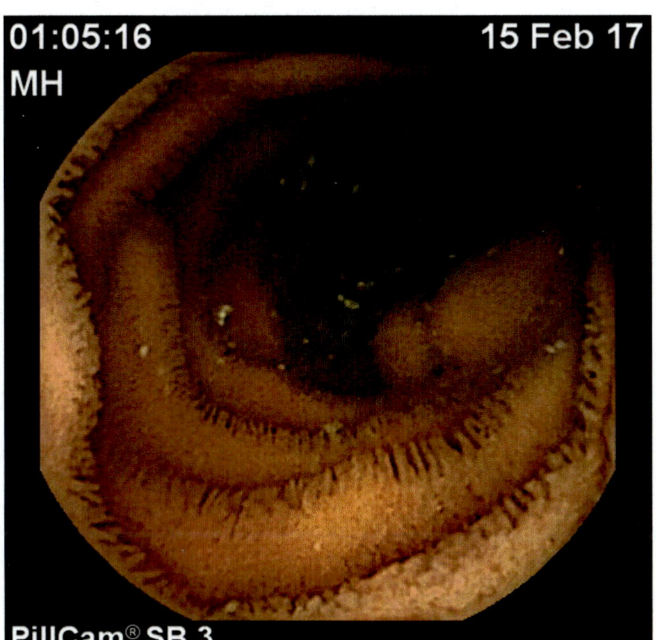

Fig. 41.7 Video capsule endoscopy showing ectopic small bowel varices

41.9 Endoscopic Retrograde Cholangiopancreatography

ERCP is one of the main treatment modality for management of pancreatobiliary diseases. The safety and efficacy of ERCP in patients with liver cirrhosis is studied in few studies. Adler et al. demonstrated in 539 ERCPs that ERCP related adverse events were higher in CTP class B and C compared to CTP class A [18]. Endoscopic sphincterotomy might be safe for the patients with cirrhosis undergoing ERCP; advanced liver cirrhosis may be independent risk factor for post-ERCP adverse events [19]. ERCP can be considered for diagnosis of primary sclerosing cholangitis if MRCP plus liver biopsy is equivocal or contraindicated in patients with suspected PSC. Current guidelines suggested performing endoscopic treatment with ductal sampling of significant stricture identified at MRCP in PSC who have symptoms like to improve following endotherapy. It is recommended that cholangiocarcinoma should be suspected in any patient with worsening cholestasis, weight loss, raised serum CA 19-9 and/or progressive dominant stricture [20].

41.10 Biliary Complications After Liver Transplantation

Biliary complications remain a major source of morbidity in liver transplant patients. Post liver transplant biliary complications include strictures (anastomotic and non-anastomotic), leaks, stones, recurrence of PSC [21]. For biliary leak, ERCP with stenting of bile duct has shown treatment success rate in 85–100%. Similarly, anastomotic biliary strictures can be treated with ERCP and biliary stenting (single or multiple plastic stents or covered metal stents) with or without balloon dilatation of stricture [22]. Non-anastomotic strictures are difficult to manage but treated similar to anastomotic stricture [21].

41.11 Metabolic and Bariatric Endoscopy for NASH

As weight loss is primary treatment of NASH, minimally invasive endoscopic bariatric procedures are being widely used for the same. Intra-gastric balloons have shown improvement in liver enzymes and histology [23]. The duodenal-Jejunal bypass liner improves biochemical parameters of NASH. Further studies in this area are warranted.

41.12 Conclusions

Without a doubt, the role of endoscopy in management of gastroesophageal varices, in prevention of bleeding and control of active bleeding is well established. Capsule endoscopy and device assisted enteroscopy has revolutionized concepts of small bowel evaluation for obscure GI bleed. Furthermore, ERCP can be used to treat post liver transplant biliary complications with safety and efficacy. Though, there are higher adverse events of ERCP in patients with advanced liver diseases, it is more safe than surgical alternative in patients with cirrhosis having pancreatobiliary diseases.

Self Study

Questions

1. Which of the following patients will have higher risk of variceal bleed?
   (a) Large varices
   (b) Presence of red wale sign
   (c) High CTP score
   (d) HVPG >20 mmHg
   (e) All of the above
2. Which statement is true?
   (a) EST should be preferred to EBL
   (b) IGV1 can be managed with EBL
   (c) EST is reserved where EBL is not feasible or failed
   (d) Cyanoacrylate glue injection is not associated with pulmonary embolism

Answers

1. Which of the following patients will have higher risk of variceal bleed?

   Answer is all of the above.

   The risk of variceal bleed is higher in patients with larger varices, presence of red wale signs, cherry red spots, higher CTP class and HVPG more than 20 mmHg. These patients can be treated with primary prevention.
2. Which statement is true?

   Answer is EST is reserved where EBL is not feasible or failed.

   EBL is preferred over EST as it is more safe and efficacious. EST is reserved for cases where EBL is not feasible due to small varices or poor visibility owning to active bleed and when EBL is failed to control bleed. Cyanoacrylate glue injection is associated with major thromboembolic events, even death.

References

1. Garcia-Tsao G, Abraldes JG, Berzigotti A, et al. Portal hypertensive bleeding in cirrhosis: risk stratification, diagnosis, and management: 2016 practice guidance by the American Association for the study of liver diseases. Hepatology. 2017;65:310–35.
2. Vianna A, Hayes PC, Moscoso G, et al. Normal venous circulation of the gastroesophageal junction. A route to understanding varices. Gastroenterology. 1987;93:876–89.
3. Coelho-Prabhu N, Kamath PS. Current staging and diagnosis of gastroesophageal varices. Clin Liver Dis. 2010;14:195–208.
4. de Franchis R, Baveno VIF. Expanding consensus in portal hypertension: Report of the Baveno VI Consensus Workshop: Stratifying risk and individualizing care for portal hypertension. J Hepatol. 2015;63:743–52.
5. North Italian Endoscopic Club for the Study and Treatment of Esophageal Varices. Prediction of the first variceal hemorrhage in patients with cirrhosis of the liver and esophageal varices. A prospective multicenter study. N Engl J Med. 1988;319:983–9.
6. Sarin SK, Lahoti D, Saxena SP, et al. Prevalence, classification and natural history of gastric varices: a long-term follow-up study in 568 portal hypertension patients. Hepatology. 1992;16:1343–9.
7. Kapoor A, Dharel N, Sanyal AJ. Endoscopic diagnosis and therapy in gastroesophageal variceal bleeding. Gastrointest Endosc Clin N Am. 2015;25(3):491–507. https://doi.org/10.1016/j.giec.2015.03.004.
8. Abraldes JG, Sarlieve P, Tandon P. Measurement of portal pressure. Clin Liver Dis. 2014;18:779–92.
9. Groszmann RJ, Garcia-Tsao G, Bosch J, et al. Beta-blockers to prevent gastroesophageal varices in patients with cirrhosis. N Engl J Med. 2005;353:2254–61.
10. Merkel C, Marin R, Angeli P, et al. A placebo-controlled clinical trial of nadolol in the prophylaxis of growth of small esophageal varices in cirrhosis. Gastroenterology. 2004;127:476–84.
11. Gluud LL, Krag A. Banding ligation versus beta-blockers for primary prevention in oesophageal varices in adults. Cochrane Database Syst Rev. 2012;(8):CD004544.
12. Kim T, Shijo H, Kokawa H, et al. Risk factors for hemorrhage from gastric fundal varices. Hepatology. 1997;25:307–12.
13. McCarty TR, Njei B. Self-expanding metal stents for acute refractory esophageal variceal bleeding: a systematic review and meta-analysis. Dig Endosc. 2016;28:539–47.
14. Girotra M, Raghavapuram S, Abraham RR, et al. Management of gastric variceal bleeding: role of endoscopy and endoscopic ultrasound. World J Hepatol. 2014;6:130–6.
15. Binmoeller KF, Weilert F, Shah JN, et al. EUS-guided transesophageal treatment of gastric fundal varices with combined coiling and cyanoacrylate glue injection (with videos). Gastrointest Endosc. 2011;74:1019–25.
16. Abdelaal UM, Morita E, Nouda S, et al. Evaluation of portal hypertensive enteropathy by scoring with capsule endoscopy: is transient elastography of clinical impact? J Clin Biochem Nutr. 2010;47:37–44.
17. Kodama M, Uto H, Numata M, et al. Endoscopic characterization of the small bowel in patients with portal hypertension evaluated by double balloon endoscopy. J Gastroenterol. 2008;43:589–96.
18. Adler DG, Haseeb A, Francis G, et al. Efficacy and safety of therapeutic ERCP in patients with cirrhosis: a large multicenter study. Gastrointest Endosc. 2016;83:353–9.
19. Nitin Jagtap, Zaheer Nabi, Manu Tandan, Mohan Ramchandani, Mithun Sharma, Sundeep Lakhtakia, P.N. Rao, Rajesh Gupta, Rakesh Kalapala, Jahangeer Basha, Santosh Darishetty, G.V. Rao, D.N. Reddy, (2019) Is It Safe to Perform Endoscopic Retrograde Cholangiopancreatography in Decompensated Cirrhosis?. Journal of Clinical and Experimental Hepatology
20. European Society of Gastrointestinal Endoscopy and European Association for the Study of the Liver. Role of endoscopy in primary sclerosing cholangitis: European Society of Gastrointestinal Endoscopy (ESGE) and European Association for the Study of the Liver (EASL) clinical guideline. J Hepatol. 2017;66:1265–81.
21. Kochhar G, Parungao JM, Hanouneh IA, et al. Biliary complications following liver transplantation. World J Gastroenterol. 2013;19:2841–6.
22. Morelli J, Mulcahy HE, Willner IR, et al. Long-term outcomes for patients with post-liver transplant anastomotic biliary strictures treated by endoscopic stent placement. Gastrointest Endosc. 2003;58:374–9.
23. Lee YM, Low HC, Lim LG, et al. Intragastric balloon significantly improves nonalcoholic fatty liver disease activity score in obese patients with nonalcoholic steatohepatitis: a pilot study. Gastrointest Endosc. 2012;76:756–60.

Dynamic and Multi-phase Contrast-Enhanced CT Scan

42

Piero Boraschi, Gaia Tarantini, Federica Pacciardi, and Francescamaria Donati

Key Concepts
- Imaging of liver disease represents the diagnostic tool useful for guiding and confirming the clinical suspicion
- Multiphasic CT has a central role in the diagnosis of liver diseases
- CT scanning protocol should be optimized in order to answer to a specific clinical question
- For the diagnosis of liver diseases, it is essential to know what are the most common CT imaging features
- CT imaging usually allows to differentiate the most common benign and malignant liver diseases

42.1 Introduction

Imaging actually plays a pivotal role in the diagnosis of liver diseases. Ultrasound (US), Computed Tomography (CT), and MR imaging (MRI) are daily used in the management of patients with liver abnormalities. Although contrast-enhanced US (CEUS) and MRI with hepato-biliary contrast media and diffusion-weighted sequences are increasingly used in the evaluation of hepatic diseases, CT remains the workhorse in this field [7, 20].

Over the last years substantial developments have been mapped out. In fact, with the advent of the spiral technology and multi-slice CT, there has been an exponential use of this technique. It may provide a large number of acquisition parameters and reconstruction modes. Furthermore multiphasic and multiplanar capabilities of multislice CT represent the added power of this modality [7].

P. Boraschi (✉) · G. Tarantini · F. Pacciardi · F. Donati
Department of Diagnostic Imaging, Pisa University Hospital, Pisa, Italy
e-mail: p.boraschi@do.med.unipi.it

CT plays a very important role in the diagnosis, staging, preoperative planning and follow-up of patients with hepatic diseases.

CT is associated with higher radiation exposure than conventional radiography so, for each patient, exposure to ionizing radiation must be justifiable on the basis of the likely benefit.

The liver scanning protocol usually provides for a non-enhanced scan followed by enhanced acquisitions (acquired at different time-points after the intravenous administration of the iodine-based contrast medium) [7].

42.2 CT Technology Developments

Since the introduction of CT in a clinical scenario in 1974, this modality underwent a progressive and rapid improvement in terms of both acquisition time and spatial resolution. CT provided sequential acquisition of axial slices until the advent of spiral technology at the end of 1980s. So, CT evolved from two-dimensional to three-dimensional technique. A further revolution happened when multi-slice or multi-detector CT (MDCT) was appeared on medical scene in 1992 ("dual slice" scanner) and in 1998 ("four slice" scanner). From then the number of detectors has progressively increased: from 8-, 16-, 32-slices in the early 2000s until to 64-, 128-, 256-, 320-, 512-, etc. slices in the last years. This continuous technological evolution caused a progressive reduction in acquisition time and an ever better spatial resolution. With MDCT technology larger volume coverage can be obtained within one breath-hold time of the patient. Due to the increased number and reduced thickness of slices generated by MDCT, images should be evaluated by the radiologist on a dedicated workstation. This offers the opportunity to create reconstructed images with different algorithms (Multiplanar Reformation, Maximum Intensity Projection, Volume Rendering), that are particularly useful for the surgical planning. In this way diagnostic capability of the radiologist is also strengthened [11, 20].

F. Radu-Ionita et al. (eds.), *Liver Diseases*, https://doi.org/10.1007/978-3-030-24432-3_42

On the other hand, with MDCT there was a significant increase in radiation dose. For this reason various strategies to reduce dose have been employed modifying scanning parameters—such as tube potential (kV) and tube current (mA)—or personalizing protocols for individual patients or specific clinical questions. Moreover, for multiphasic CT examinations there are new ways to reduce radiation exposure such as adaptive statistical iterative reconstruction (ASiR); it helps reducing patient dose while maintaining image quality [7, 20].

Further advances were obtained with the more recent introduction of Dual-energy CT. It is based on the appearance of different substances (calcium, iodine and so on) at two separates energy sets. It can generate virtual unenhanced images allowing a reduction in radiation dose. It also helps to distinguish iodine, calcium and acid uric crystal from soft tissues. This technique proved to be useful in the evaluation of hypervascular liver lesions, such as hepatocellular carcinoma especially after treatment.

42.3 Hounsfield Units

Hounsfield units (HUs) are a unit without dimension universally used in CT to express CT numbers in a standardised form. HUs derive from a linear transformation of the measured attenuation coefficients. The mathematical transformation is based on the arbitrary definitions of air and water: radio density of distilled water at standard temperature and pressure (STP) is 0 HU, while radio density of air at STP is −1000 HUs. HUs are measured and utilised in a variety of clinical applications by the radiologists. For example the cysts demonstrate a content with attenuation values similar to water, approximately from 0 to +20 HUs. On the other hand, bone and all types of calcification show strong positive values of HUs (bone ranging from +400 to +3000) [7].

42.4 Liver Scanning Protocol

The use of iodinated contrast medium (ICM) is essential for diagnosis of liver diseases. Current guidelines recommend the use of a minimal dose of ICM necessary to obtain adequate images for diagnosis. Theoretically, a complete liver examination should include a non-enhanced acquisition followed by contrast-enhanced multi-phasic scans [11].

Non-enhanced acquisition is useful in detecting different component of liver lesions with high attenuation (calcifications, bleed, glycogen, iron, etc.) and with low attenuation (cystic lesions, fat, oedema, necrosis, air and so on). It is also useful for evaluating contrast-enhancement of hepatic lesions compared to hepatic parenchyma [7].

The use of contrast-enhanced CT with ICM has significantly improved the accuracy of imaging diagnosis. The rapid development of CT technologies has led to an increase in worldwide usage of ICM. With the contrast-enhanced CT it is possible to localize a lesion increasing the contrast between the lesion and the surrounding hepatic parenchyma [7, 20].

The CT protocols must be established on the basis of the clinical question and of the diagnostic suspicion.

An hepatic mass will be hypodense, isodense or hyperdense in relation to the surrounding hepatic tissue in a specific phase of enhancement. Hypodense is defined when the density of the lesion is lower than that of surrounding hepatic parenchyma; isodense when the density is equal or very similar, and hyperdense when the density is higher than that of hepatic parenchyma. So, it is important to understand the principal CT phases to answer the clinical question or to deepen a radiological finding [2, 13].

Important parameters are: volume and iodine concentration of the ICM, the injection rate (3–5 mL/s) and the scanning delay from the intravenous injection of ICM [13].

Individual variations (body weight, heart rate, circulation time) can influence the time window, so we can use contrast agent bolus timing methods (bolus tracking or bolus test) in order to correct for differences them. Iodine dose should be increased with increasing body weight (BW) of individual patient. This can be assessed by multiplying the body weight with a constant amount of contrast per kg of BW keeping the iodine flow rate constant.

The rate of iodine injection and timing of contrast bolus primarily influence hepatic arterial enhancement; instead, venous phase enhancement is conditioned by total administered dose of iodine.

Following the main enhanced CT phases are reported:

- **Early arterial phase** starting 15–20 s post intravenous administration of ICM or immediately after bolus tracking;
- **Late arterial phase** starting 35–40 s post intravenous administration of ICM or 15–20 s after bolus tracking;
- **Portal-venous phase** is performed 70–80 s post intravenous administration of ICM or 50–60 s after bolus tracking;
- **Delayed/equilibrium phase** is performed 180–300 s after ICM injection or 160–280 s after bolus tracking;
- **Ultra-delayed phase** starting after 5–10 min after ICM injection.

However, in the daily clinical activity, all the six phases (non-enhanced, early arterial, late arterial, portal-venous phase, delayed/equilibrium and ultra-delayed) are not performed in each patient, first of all for radiation exposure and uselessness in diagnosis.

In the early arterial phase the contrast is prevalently confined in the arteries and has not well enhanced the liver. The early arterial phase allows to explore the arterial anatomy of the patient and shows possible arterial anatomical variants that are information helpful for the surgeons. This phase is useful for patients who are candidates for liver transplantation, for complex hepatobiliary surgery, for trans-catheter arterial chemo or radio-embolization [7, 13].

With the late arterial phase all anatomical structures and lesions that have arterial supply enhance; in particular, all hypervascular lesions such as hepatocellular carcinoma (HCC), hypervascular liver metastasis, hemangioma (typical peripheral enhancement starting in this phase), adenoma and focal nodular hyperplasia are typically hyperdense. However, the usefulness of performing the early arterial phase and the late arterial phase is debated in the diagnosis of HCC; some authors report that the difference in sensitivity between the late arterial phase and the double arterial phase is not statistically significant in detecting HCC [15].

In the portal-venous phase there is the maximal difference in attenuation between the lesion and the enhanced surrounding liver parenchyma. With this phase most of primary and secondary malignant liver lesions are identified. They appear as hypodense lesions compared to the liver parenchyma. In fact, malignant tumours are vascularised by arterial system instead of liver parenchyma, predominantly ensured by portal venous system [13].

The delayed/equilibrium phase is characterized by a reduction in attenuation between lesions and liver parenchyma. So, it is helpful in detecting and diagnosing liver lesions with prevalent fibrous component, such as cholangiocarcinoma, cavernous hemangioma and diffuse liver fibrosis. These disease entities show a prolonged contrast enhancement due to their fibrous tissue, appearing hyperdense compared to liver parenchyma. For these entities it may be important to obtain an ultra-delayed phase in order to highlight the progressive enhancement of the lesion and improve the diagnostic confidence [7, 13].

42.5 Benign Focal Liver Lesions

42.5.1 Hepatic Cystic Lesions

Simple hepatic cysts represent one of the commonest lesions involving the liver. They are developmental lesions without communication with the biliary tree, generally unilocular. They are benign entities, without malignant potential. They can be isolated or multiple. They are more often diagnosed in women and are usually asymptomatic. Their size is variable from few millimeters to several centimeters. They tend to grow in number and size with age. Rarely, due to regressive phenomena, they may decrease in volume [14, 20].

On non-enhanced CT scan the hepatic cysts appear as round or ovoid and have well-defined margins, with no evident wall. They demonstrate hypoattenuating content with attenuation values similar to water (less than 20 HUs). On enhanced CT scans (arterial, portal-venous, delayed phases), their density doesn't change and their wall doesn't show any enhancement (Fig. 42.1) [14, 20].

Polycystic Liver Disease is a hereditary condition characterised by development of several cysts involving the liver, often found in association with renal polycystic disease. The cysts are generally large and multiple and determine a significant enlargement of the organs involved. Spontaneous intracystic hemorrhage, infection and rupture may occur. On unenhanced CT scan some cysts can be hyperdense because of hemorrhagic content. Their density does not significantly increase after ICM injection [2, 13].

Caroli disease is a rare congenital autosomal recessive disorder. It belongs to group of entities resulting from abnormal development of the ductal plates. The simple type of Caroli disease affects the large bile ducts, instead Caroli syndrome involve both the central intrahepatic bile ducts and the ductal plates of the smaller peripheral bile ducts. It can be diffuse, lobar or segmental. In 95% of the cases there are calculi in the cysts. Pre-contrast CT shows hypoattenuating cystic structures (generally do not exceed 2–3 cm in diameter) that communicate with dilated intrahepatic biliary tree. A sign considered very suggestive of Caroli disease is the "central dot sign"; it consists in small dots within the dilated intrahepatic bile ducts with evident contrast enhancement, representing portal radicles. In 7% of cases it degenerates into cholangiocarcinoma [2].

Peribiliary cysts are multiple retention cysts of peribiliary glands. They appear as multiple cystic formations at the level of the periportal spaces (often at the level of biliary confluence) that do not show communication with the biliary tree. Most of them are found in patients with chronic liver disease and are benign. On CT continuous small cysts are typically identified along the portal veins reflecting the periportal collar (Fig. 42.2) [2].

42.5.2 Benign Hepatic Tumors

Hepatic haemangioma is the most frequent benign hepatic tumour, much more common in women (F:M = 5:1). Usually, it is an incidentally detected lesion since the patient is nearly always asymptomatic. It has a congenital origin and it is prevalently of cavernous subtype. It can be solitary or multiple; it can have dimensions ranging from a few millimetres up to over 10 cm (giant haemangioma) [3, 12].

The imaging features of the typical cavernous haemangioma are the following:

On non-contrast CT scan it is generally hypoattenuating relative to the surrounding liver parenchyma, whereas during

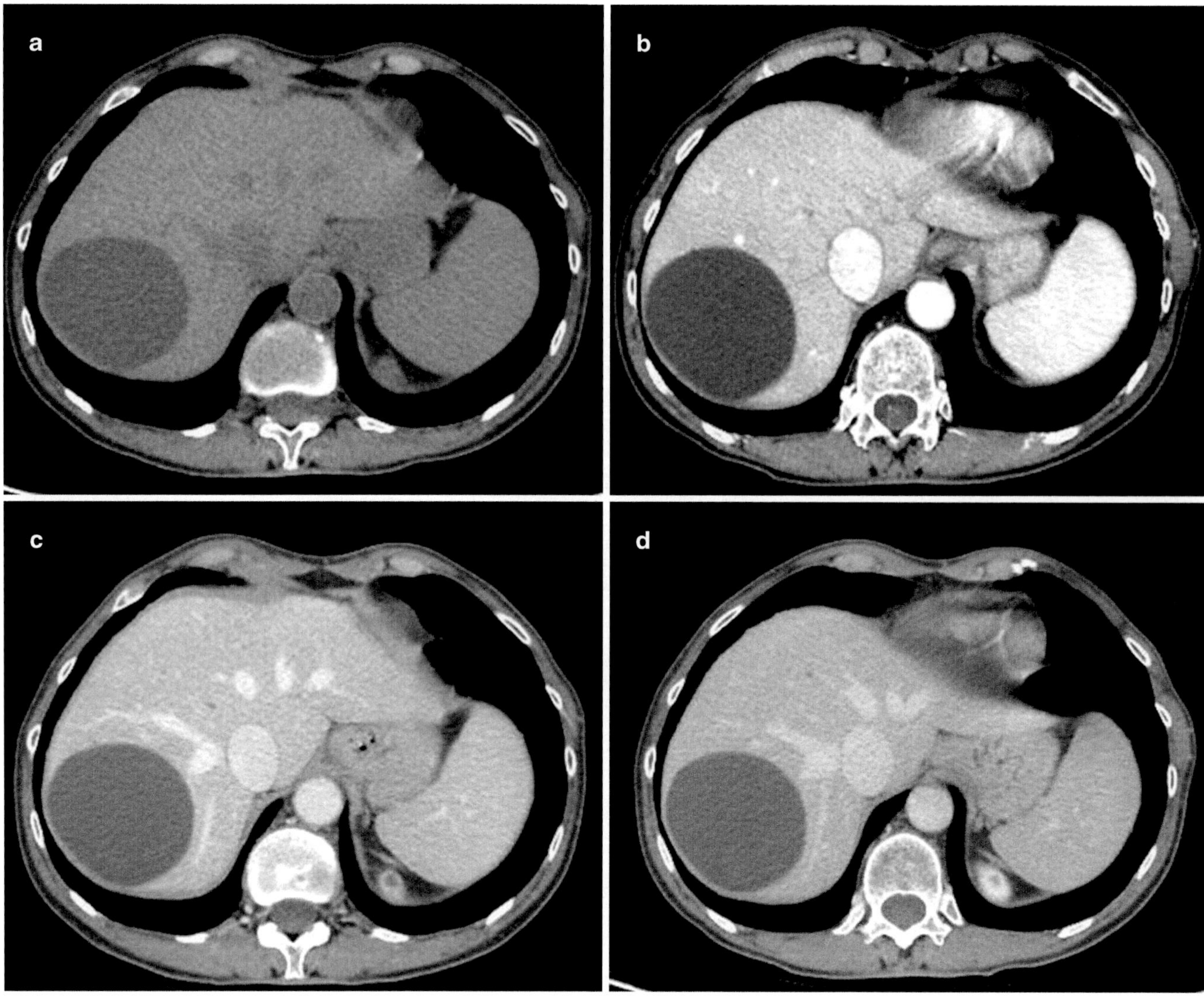

Fig. 42.1 (**a–d**) Simple cyst in the right hepatic lobe. CT shows a round-oval lesion in the VII–VIII segment with homogeneous hypoattenuation on unenhanced scan (**a**). The wall is imperceptible and the cyst does not enhance after intravenous administration of ICM on the arterial (**b**), portal-venous (**c**) and delayed (**d**) phases

the arterial phase it shows peripheral globular enhancement with *wreath-like* appearance. On portal-venous phase a progressive centripetal enhancement of the lesion is observed and a complete filling is generally appreciable on delayed/ultradelayed phase (Fig. 42.3).

In the case of the so-called "atypical" haemangioma these peculiar imaging CT features are not so easily recognizable. In the case of giant haemangioma we can have an incomplete filling of the lesion by ICM due to its fibrosis and/or necrotic component or to thrombotic phenomena [12].

Another type of haemangioma is the capillary haemangioma. It is usually iso-/hypodense on unenhanced CT scan. On arterial phase it appears like a fleeting brilliant focus of enhancement (similar to the aortic enhancement in the arterial phase), whereas on the portal-venous and delayed acquisitions it retains the contrast and remains isodense or slightly hyperdense to the surrounding liver parenchyma (Fig. 42.4) [12].

Focal nodular hyperplasia (FNH) is the second most common benign liver lesion after haemangioma and it is usually treated conservatively. It is found mostly in young women. Typically it is an asymptomatic lesion. On unenhanced CT scan it commonly appears isodense or sometimes hypodense respect to the surrounding hepatic parenchyma. A hypoattenuating central scar can be seen in the lesion, especially in larger ones. On arterial phase FNH demonstrates a vivid contrast enhancement except for the central scar which doesn't enhance (it remains hypodense). On the following phases it becomes hypo/isoattenuating respect to the liver. On ultradelayed phase the central scar shows contrast enhancement becoming isodense and not recognizable (Fig. 42.5) [10, 13].

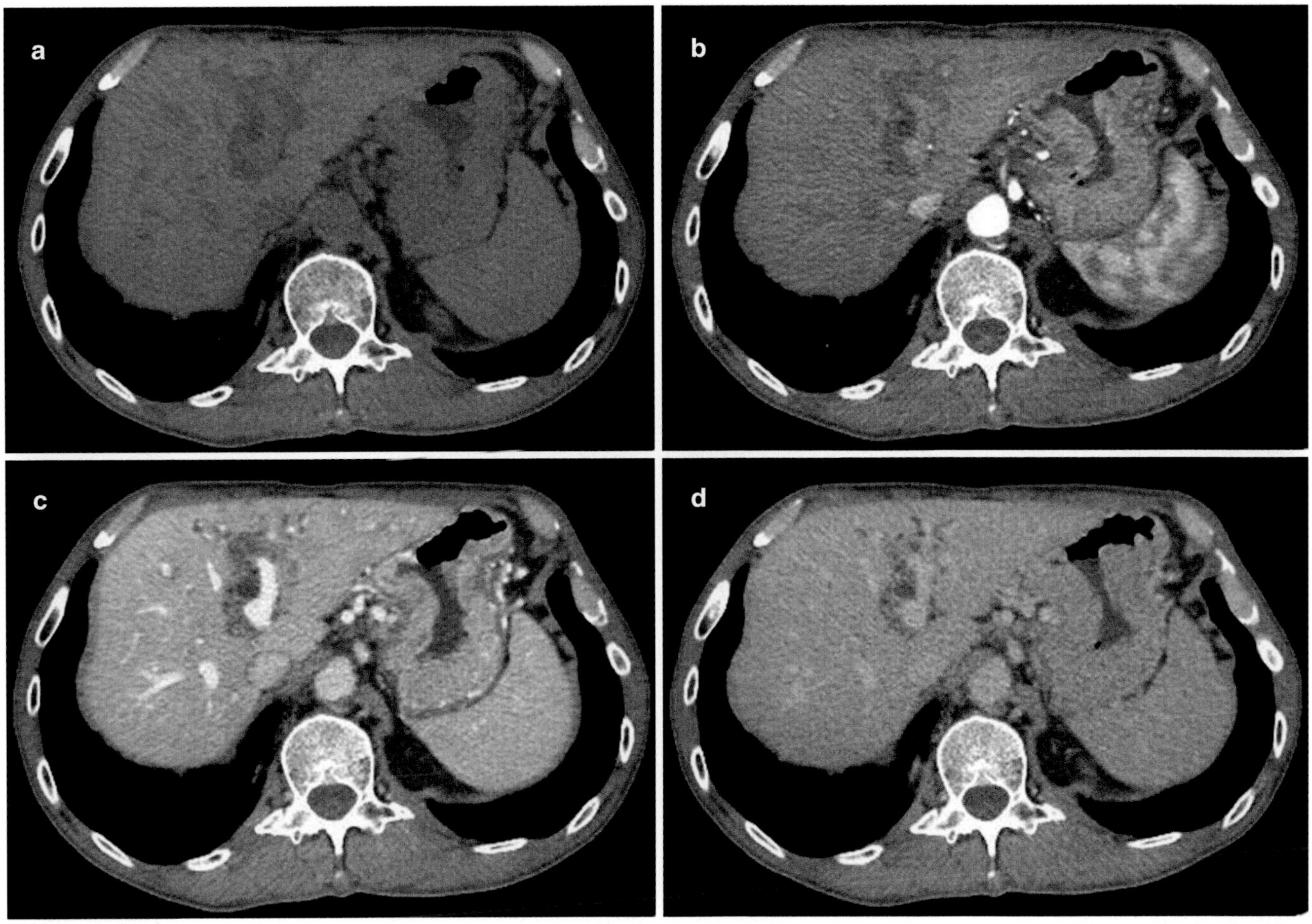

Fig. 42.2 (**a**–**d**) Multiple hepatic peribiliary cysts. Fluid density, well-defined intrahepatic structures are appreciable at the level of the peri-portal spaces around the liver hilum. They appear hypodense on unenhanced CT scan (**a**) with no significant enhancement on the arterial (**b**), portal-venous (**c**) and delayed (**d**) phases

Hepatic adenoma is a rare benign tumour of the liver with a strong prevalence in women, generally hormone-induced (mostly related to prolonged use of oral contraceptives). It can bleed (causing hemoperitoneum) or can rarely degenerate into hepatocarcinoma. It is usually solitary (80%), larger than 5 cm at the time of diagnosis, more frequently located in the right hepatic lobe. The surgical resection can be indicated in specific cases for the risk of hemorrhage and possible malignant transformation. On unenhanced CT scan it may be clearly hypodense due to its fatty component; sometimes it can present hyperdense areas inside for the presence of calcifications and/or hemorrhages. After ICM injection it shows a transient vivid enhancement, with reduction of density on the portal-venous and delayed phases (becoming isodense). The differential diagnosis of this lesion with FNH can be very difficult on multiphasic CT and it is indicated the use of MR imaging with hepato-biliary contrast agents [10, 13].

42.6 Malignant Hepatic Tumours

42.6.1 Hepatocellular Carcinoma (HCC)

HCC is the most common primary malignant hepatic tumour (80–90% of cases) and occurs predominantly in patients with underlying chronic liver disease and cirrhosis. It develops from a regenerative nodule to a carcinoma through a dysplastic phase [9, 10, 13, 20].

The risk of tumour formation is higher in patients with chronic viral hepatitis, but nowadays there is an increased HCC incidence in patients with NAFLD (Non Alcoholic Fatty Liver Disease) associated with metabolic syndrome, diabetes and obesity. Other causes of liver cirrhosis are chronic alcohol abuse and genetic hemochromatosis.

Three main subtypes of HCC are reported:

1. Nodular type (the most common), often characterized by multiple lesions;

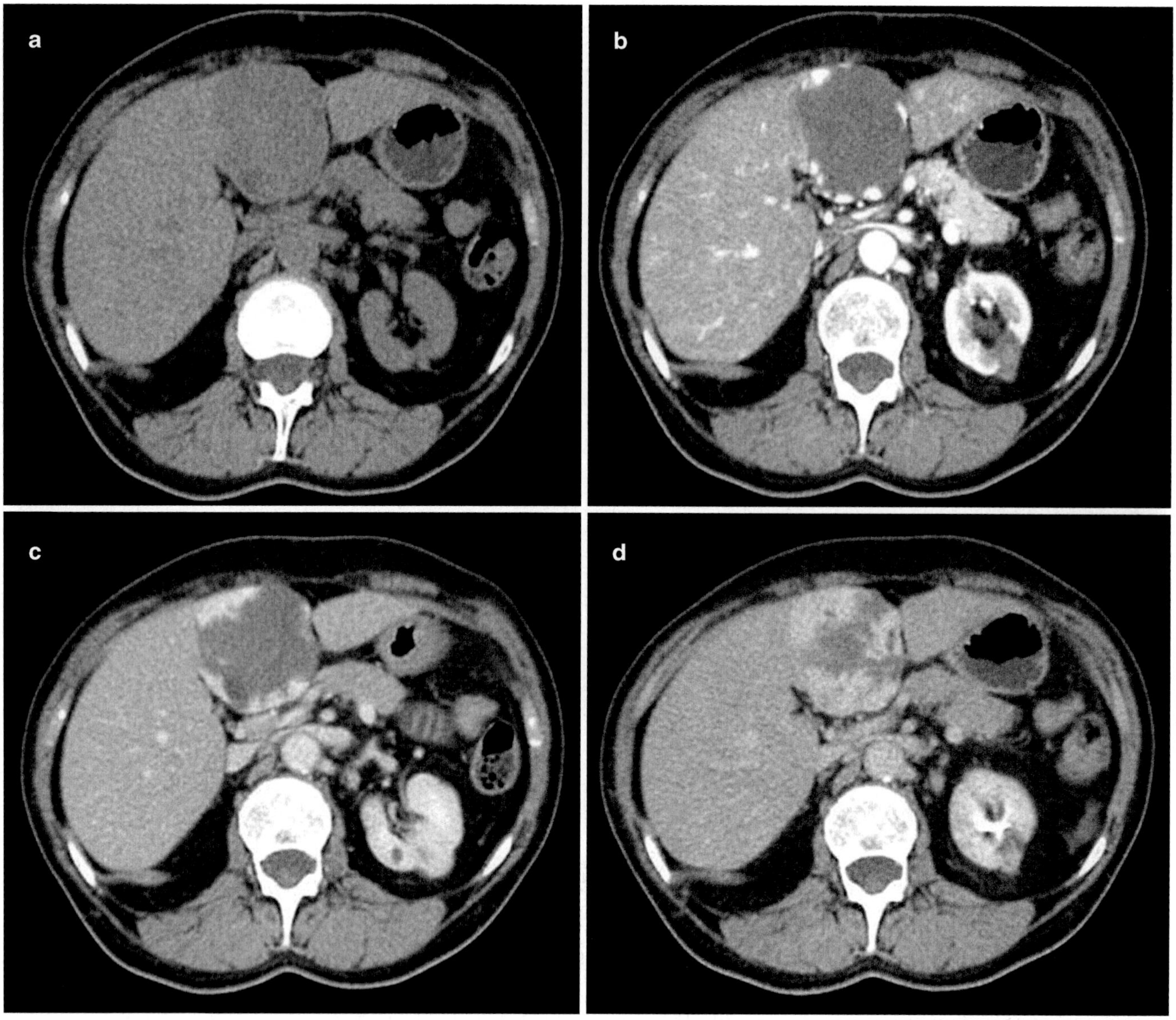

Fig. 42.3 (**a**–**d**) Cavernous haemangioma in the left hepatic lobe. Unenhanced CT scan (**a**) shows a 7-cm-in-size lesion with smooth margins that is slightly hypodense respect to the surrounding parenchyma. On arterial (**b**), portal-venous (**c**) and delayed (**d**) phases the lesion demonstrates a characteristic progressive globular and centripetal enhancement that is isoattenuating to the vessels

2. Macronodulary type (often fibrolamellar type) occurring on healthy liver, usually single or with satellite malignant nodules, and often diagnosed late when they reach large dimensions;
3. Diffuse or infiltrating type, characterized by multiple micronodules (<1 cm) scattered throughout the liver parenchyma with a cirrhotic-like appearance [5, 20].

Furthermore, small satellite HCC nodules can be identified near to the main tumour (representing intrahepatic metastases) and show the same CT appearance of the main lesion.

At the baseline CT scan nodular and macronodular types of HCC are well defined and appear hypodense respect to the surrounding hepatic parenchyma, sometimes with a central necrotic portion or focal adipose degeneration (with negative density values). Hyperdense foci are also present in case of calcifications and/or haemorrhage. On the other hand, the infiltrative type has poorly defined margins. This type is sometimes isodense and is only visible for the dislocation of intrahepatic vessels and/or deformation of the hepatic margins [7, 13, 20].

After ICM administration late arterial, portal-venous and delayed phases are usually acquired. In late arterial phase there is a typical arterial enhancement; so, vital neoplastic tissue (sometimes with a central necrotic hypodense portion) is clearly hyperdense for the rapid wash-in of contrast medium due to arterial neoangiogenesis. Early-stage HCCs might fail to enhance and cannot be distinguished on the arterial phase due to the lack of adequate vascular supply [7, 13].

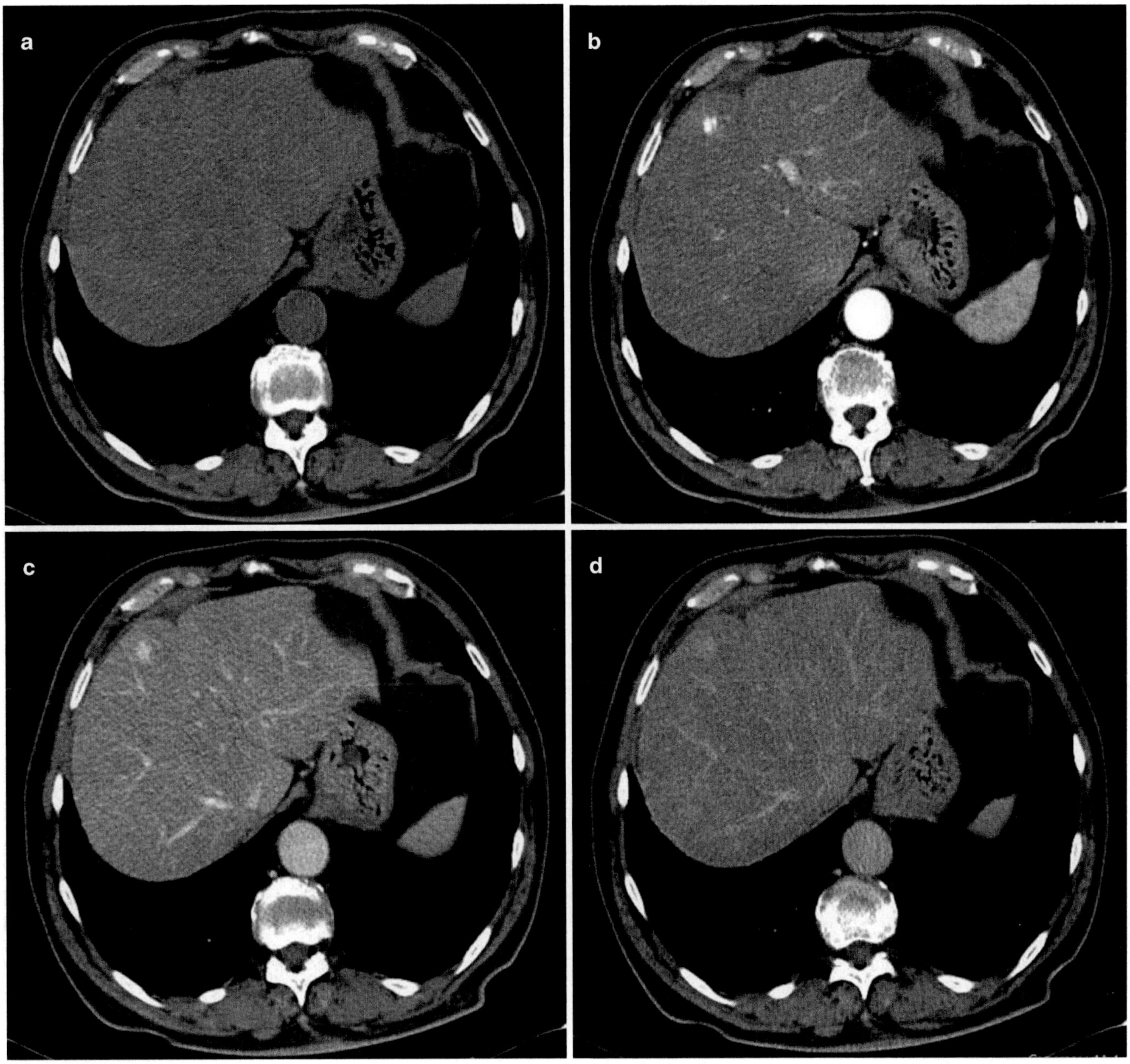

Fig. 42.4 (**a**–**d**) Capillary "flash-filling" haemangioma in the right hepatic lobe. Unenhanced CT scan (**a**) demonstrates a centimetric subcapsular hypodense lesion in the IV segment. On arterial phase (**b**) the lesion shows homogeneous vivid enhancement similar to the aortic one. It maintains slightly hyperdense respect to the surrounding liver parenchyma on portal-venous (**c**) and delayed (**d**) phases, remaining isoattenuating to the vessels ("blood-pool" features of the lesion)

As just mentioned in the text, the early arterial phase is useful to map the arterial anatomy of the patient; the presence of possible anatomical variants is helpful for the surgeon and interventional radiologist.

In the portal-venous and delayed phases HCC is characterized by a rapid contrast wash-out and so it becomes hypodense. Huge tumours can present a peripheral hyperdense fibrous capsule on delayed phases (Fig. 42.6).

The presence of tumour thrombi within the main branches of portal vein is crucial for the staging of HCC and represents a prognostic factor for the therapeutic management. Neoplastic thrombi show the same CT pattern of the main lesion appearing as solid masses with a characteristic wash-in and wash-out [4, 16].

Moreover, CT plays a pivotal role in tumour response assessment after surgery and loco-regional therapy (such as Radiofrequency ablation, TransArterial ChemoEmbolization and Selective Internal Radiation Therapy). Dynamic CT studies are able to detect persistent or residual tumour by identifying a nodular enhancing area within or peripherally

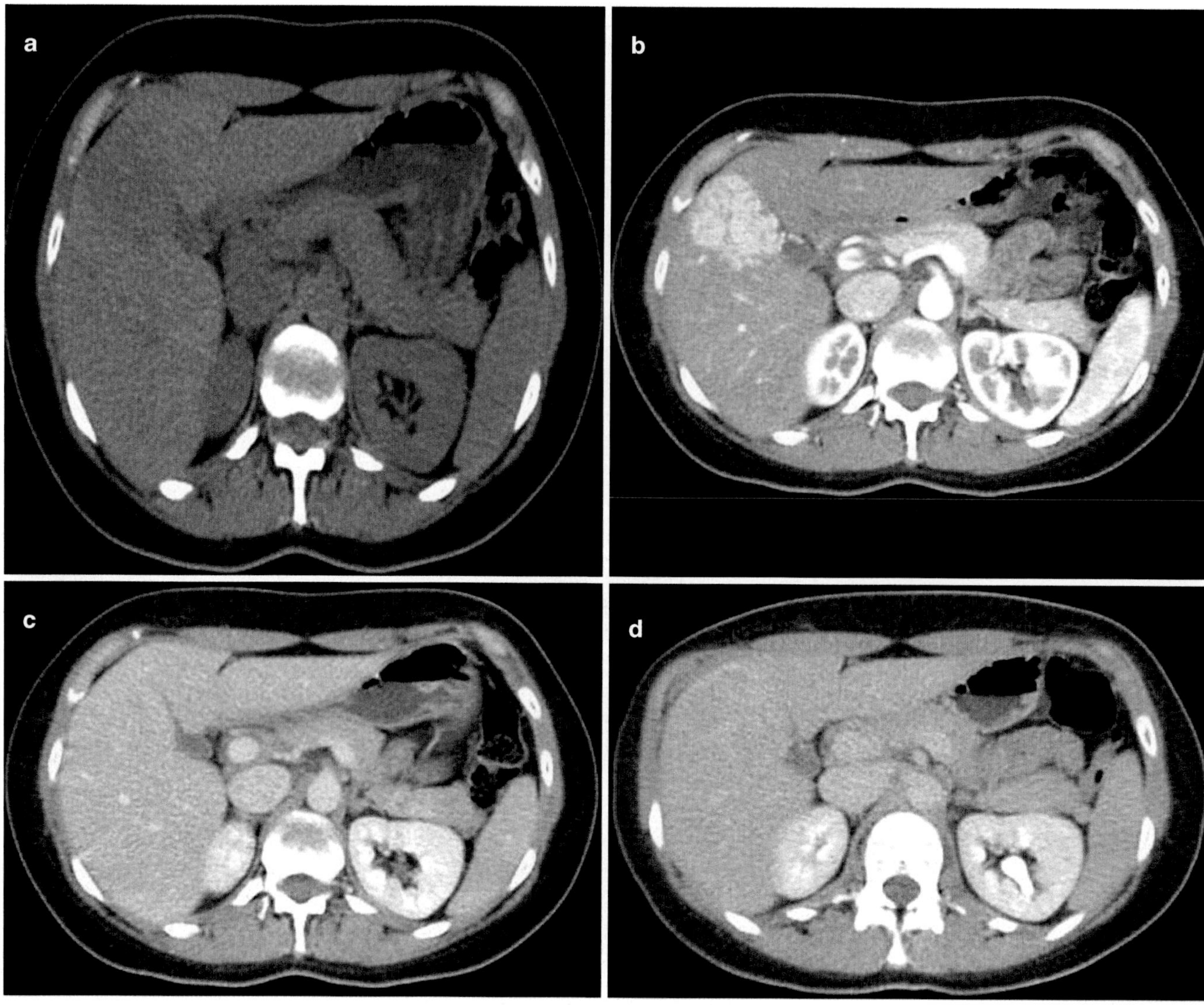

Fig. 42.5 (**a**–**d**) Focal nodular hyperplasia in the right hepatic lobe. A round-oval slightly hypodense area is present in the V segment on unenhanced CT scan (**a**). The lesion is markedly hyperdense except for the central scar which doesn't enhance on arterial phase (**b**). It becomes isodense respect to the surrounding liver parenchyma on portal-venous phase (**c**). The central scar is slightly hyperdense on delayed phase (**d**)

to the treated lesion, with the same pattern of the native HCC. At least, CT is also useful in identifying extrahepatic spread of the disease (lung, adrenal glands, lymph nodes, and bone are the most common sites) [8, 19].

42.6.2 Cholangiocarcinoma

Cholangiocarcinoma is the second most common primary malignant hepatic tumour and originates from the epithelium of the intra and extrahepatic bile ducts. It often develops in people aged 50–60 with chronic calculi of the biliary tract, Carolì disease and primary sclerosing cholangitis [13, 18].

Cholangiocarcinoma can be divided into intra- or extrahepatic form and it includes three types:

1. Mass-forming type, predominantly intrahepatic (originating from small intrahepatic peripheral bile ducts);
2. Periductal-infiltrating type, predominantly intrahepatic, central or hilar (the most common type); it often originates at the confluence of the right, left and common hepatic ducts (Klatskin tumour); obstructive jaundice is the usual clinical manifestation;
3. Intraductal-growing type, intra or extrahepatic; it is characterized by small polypoid projections often confined into the biliary lumen, without infiltration of the hepatic parenchyma; this subtype grows slowly, and has a relatively favourable prognosis [1, 2, 6].

Intrahepatic cholangiocarcinoma seldom includes the hepatocellular-cholangiocellular carcinoma subtype.

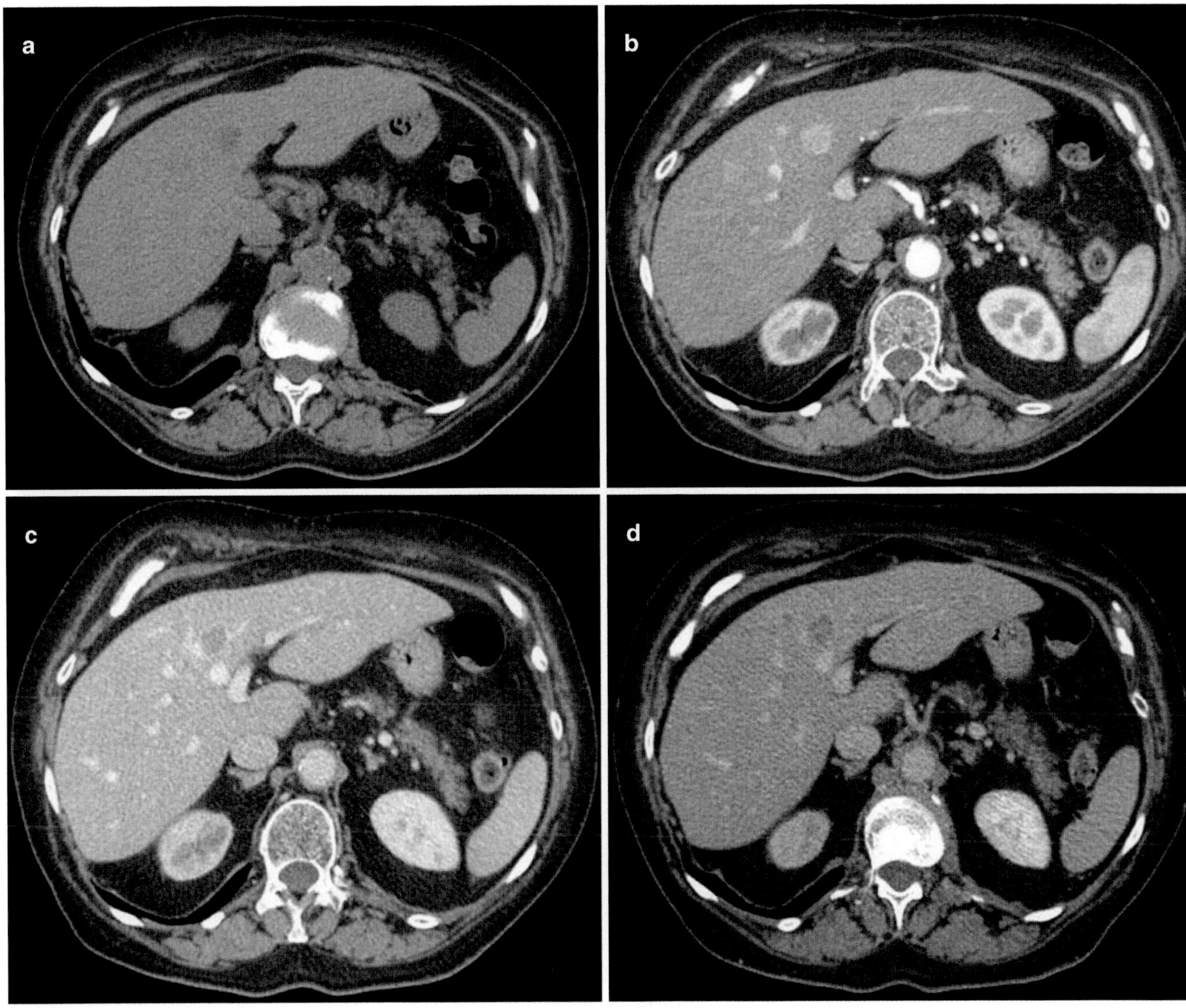

Fig. 42.6 (**a**–**d**) Hepatocellular carcinoma in the right hepatic lobe. Unenhanced CT scan (**a**) shows a 2.5-cm-in-size hypodense lesion in the IV hepatic segment. On late arterial phase (**b**) the lesion appears hyperdense, due to contrast medium wash-in. It becomes clearly hypodense on portal-venous (**c**) and delayed (**d**) phases for typical wash-out of contrast agent. These features are diagnostic for HCC

CT is often helpful for a reliable diagnosis and staging in patients with disease entity. This technique is also very useful for depicting a vascular roadmap in order to establish arterial and venous invasion.

CT protocol for cholangiocarcinoma usually includes a non-enhanced acquisition (in order to detect intraductal lithiasis) and a three-phase acquisition: late arterial (for arterial anatomy evaluation), portal-venous and delayed phases.

Mass-forming type is tenuously hypodense compared to the normal liver parenchyma at non-enhanced CT scan. It shows inhomogeneous enhancement in the arterial and venous phase with a progressive uptake of the contrast medium from the periphery to the centre of the lesion. Signs of vascular encasement and infiltration of the contiguous intrahepatic venous vessels can be present. The lesion typically appears inhomogeneously hyperdense on delayed phases, in particular at the level of central portion. An ultra-delayed phase can be also performed in order to assess a persistent tumour enhancement compared to the surrounding liver parenchyma, due to the significant fibrous component of the tumour (Fig. 42.7) [6, 18].

Biliary tract dilation upstream of the lesion can be reported. In the more advanced stages, lobar or segmental atrophy of the involved hepatic territories with capsular retraction may be present due to the abundant desmoplastic reaction. Hepatic hilar lymphadenopathies and peritoneal nodules are identified whenever lymphatic metastatic diffusion is present [13, 14].

Periductal infiltrating type results in an irregular bile stricture growing along the bile duct (involving mucosa and serosa). It

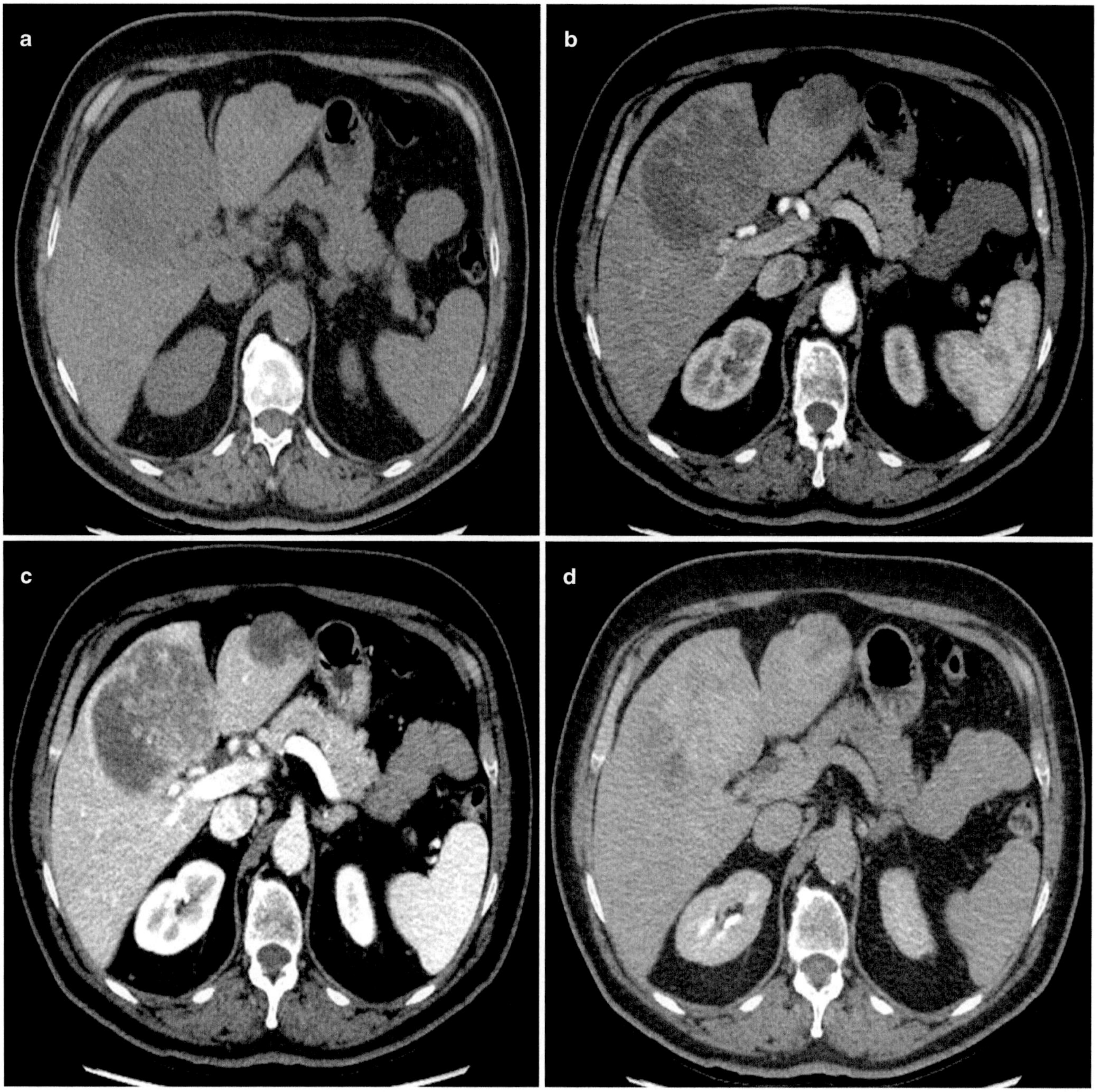

Fig. 42.7 (**a**–**d**) Multifocal peripheral mass-forming cholangiocellular carcinoma. Unenhanced CT scan (**a**) shows a large, heterogeneously hypodense mass with lobulated margins in the IV–V–VIII hepatic segments and another smaller one with analogous CT appearance in the III segment. After ICM administration both lesions well exhibit inhomogeneous progressive enhancement from the late arterial phase (**b**) to the portal-venous (**c**) and delayed (**d**) ones. The lesions result slightly and inhomogenously hyperdense on delayed phase

appears as a concentric thickening of the biliary wall, hyperenhancing in delayed phase, without forming a nodular mass. It is often associated to upstream biliary dilation. Differential diagnosis of these malignant strictures from the benign ones (inflammatory or post-traumatic) is always difficult [2, 6].

Intraductal type includes a variety of imaging features. CT can demonstrate diffuse and marked duct ectasia with or without a grossly visible mass, that appears hypodense on unenhanced CT scan and shows progressive enhancement on the subsequent post-contrastographic phases. These lesions tend to grow within the biliary tract [6].

42.6.3 Hepatic Metastases

Metastatic lesions originate throw a sequential process which favours the survival of a small population of metastatic cells in the context of the primary tumour. Liver is the second most common site of metastasis in the human body, after lymph nodes, due to its double blood supply: portal vein for intra-abdominal primary tumour and arterial system for extra-abdominal malignancies. Less frequently, there are liver metastases by continuity, via the lymphatic vessels or by intra-peritoneal spread [7].

Most frequently, liver metastases originate from primary carcinoma of the colon, stomach, pancreas, breast and lung. Usually metastatic lesions are multiple with different diameter and bilobar involvement [2].

CT is useful to identify focal liver lesions, their number, localization, and characterization. Furthermore, CT provides information in order to assess surgical or loco-regional treatment [17].

Before ICM administration, CT appearance of hepatic metastases is variable: isodense, hypodense (the most frequent) or hyperdense respect to the surrounding liver parenchyma. Isodense lesions are often visible only for indirect signs such as vascular dislocation or capsular deformation. Metastases appear hyperdense when are detected in diffuse hepatic steatosis or when contain haematic or calcific component inside (such as colorectal or mucinous metastases). After ICM injection, CT features of metastases are dictated by their vascularity because, differently to liver parenchyma, hepatic metastases get their blood supply almost exclusively by the hepatic artery [17].

Also for the detection and characterization of liver metastases late arterial, portal-venous and delayed phases are needed on CT.

Most of hepatic metastases are generally hypovascular because they receive only minimal arterial and portal-venous blood supply due to confluent dense cellularity, fibrosis or necrosis. On late arterial and portal-venous phases these metastases often show a continuous hyperdense peripheral rim enhancement that is the most specific sign for a positive diagnosis of metastasis. As the size of the lesions increases, only its peripheral part continues to be adequately vascularized and hyperdense, while the central part becomes necrotic or replaced by fibrosis. Hypovascular lesions usually originate from gastrointestinal tract adenocarcinomas, lung and breast tumours and are better visualized during the portal-venous phase as hypodense lesions. In the delayed phase peripheral rim may become isodense to surrounding liver parenchyma and the lesion appears smaller than it is in reality (Fig. 42.8) [13, 17].

Hypervascular metastases, frequently found in neuroendocrine tumours of pancreatic or enteric origin, renal cell carcinoma, and thyroid cancer (more rarely in melanoma, sarcomas, and ovarian choriocarcinoma), show a rapid diffuse enhancement during late arterial phase and rapid washout during the portal-venous and delayed phases [7].

Cystic degeneration may be evident in liver metastases from head and neck squamous cell carcinoma and after chemotherapy treatment, mainly with new antiangiogenic drugs.

42.7 Conclusions

In conclusion, CT has a crucial role in the diagnosis, staging, preoperative planning and follow-up of patients with hepatic diseases. CT scanning protocol should be optimized on the basis of the clinical question and of the diagnostic suspicion. For the diagnosis of liver diseases, it is essential to know what are the most common CT imaging features in order to differentiate the most common benign and malignant disease entities.

Self Study

Questions

1. Which statement is true?
   (a) The arterial phase is helpful in detecting and diagnosing liver lesions with prevalent fibrous component.
   (b) In the daily clinical activity, all the six CT phases (non-enhanced, early arterial, late arterial, portal-venous phase, delayed/equilibrium and ultra-delayed) are performed in each patient.
   (c) On the portal-venous phase there is the maximal difference in attenuation between the lesion and the enhanced surrounding liver parenchyma.
   (d) With ultra-delayed phase all anatomical structures and lesions that have arterial supply enhance.
2. Which statement is true?
   The typical cavernous haemangioma after ICM injection:
   (a) On arterial phase it appears like a fleeting brilliant focus of enhancement whereas on the portal-venous and delayed acquisitions it retains the contrast.
   (b) On arterial phase it shows peripheral globular enhancement and on portal-venous phase it shows a progressive centripetal enhancement.
   (c) On arterial phase it shows a transient vivid enhancement, with reduction of density on the portal-venous and delayed phases.
   (d) Its density doesn't change compared to non-enhanced CT scan.

Answers

1. Which statement/statements is/are true?
   (a) The DELAYED/EQUILIBRIUM phase is helpful in detecting and diagnosing liver lesions with prevalent fibrous component. This phase is characterized by a reduction in attenuation between lesions and liver parenchyma.
   (b) In the daily clinical activity, all the six CT phases (non-enhanced, early arterial, late arterial, portal-venous phase, delayed/equilibrium and ultra-

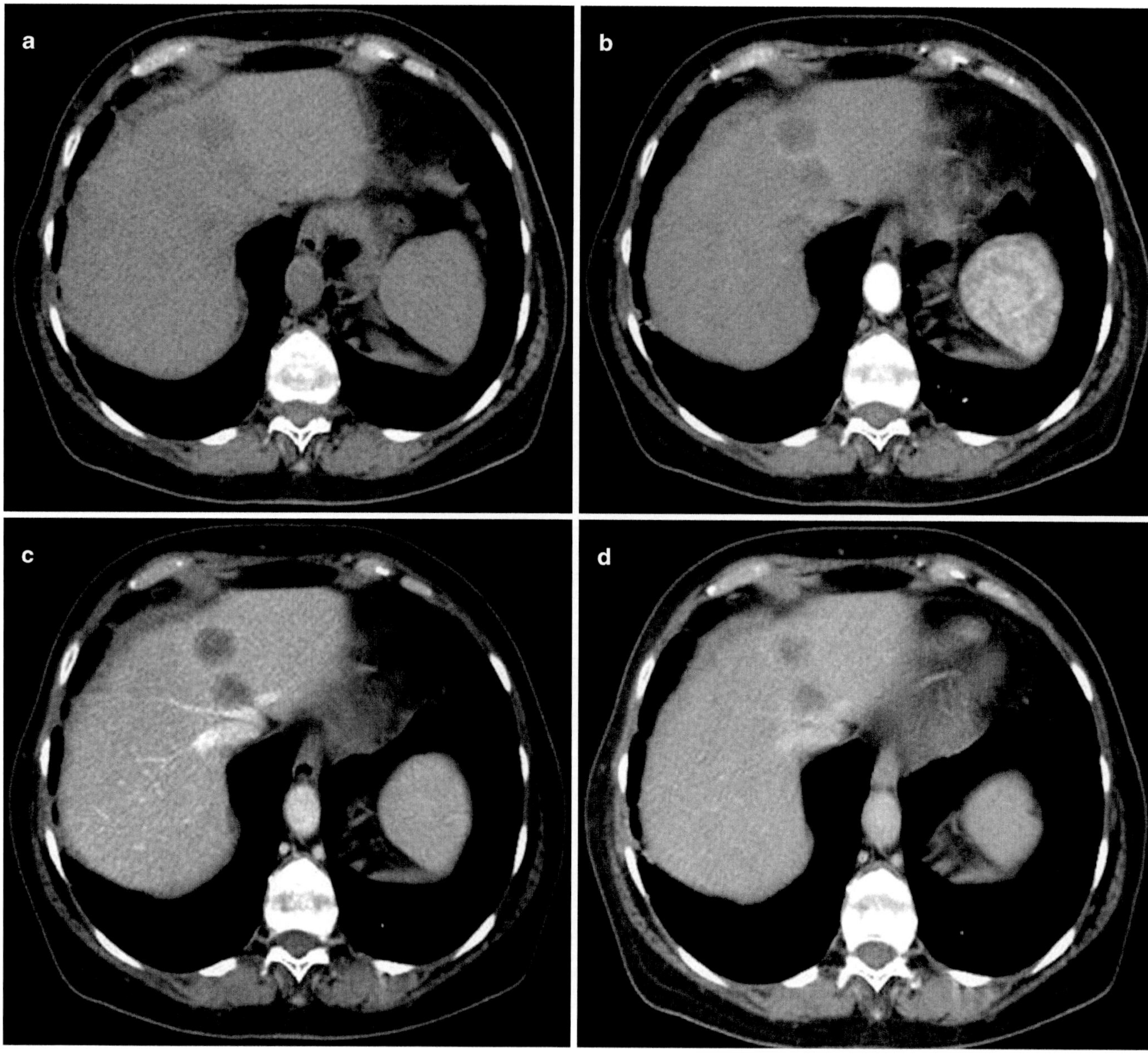

Fig. 42.8 (**a**–**d**) Colorectal cancer liver metastases. Unenhanced CT scan (**a**) shows two hypodense lesions in the IV–II hepatic segments. On arterial (**b**) and portal-venous (**c**) phases these lesions show a typical hyperdense peripheral rim enhancement with a hypodense central portion. On delayed phase (**d**) metastatic lesions appear inhomogeneously hypodense and smaller than the previous ones, with an isodense peripheral rim

delayed) are NOT performed in each patient due to the radiation exposure and due to uselessness in diagnosis.

(c) On the portal-venous phase there is the maximal difference in attenuation between the lesion and the enhanced surrounding liver parenchyma. **CORRECT.** In fact with this phase most of primary and secondary malignant liver lesions are identified. They appear as hypodense lesions compared to the liver parenchyma.

(d) With LATE ARTERIAL phase all anatomical structures and lesions that have arterial supply enhance. In fact all hypervascular lesions are typically hyperdense on late arterial phase.

2. Which statement is true?

The typical cavernous haemangioma after ICM injection:

(a) On arterial phase it appears like a fleeting brilliant focus of enhancement whereas on the portal-venous and delayed acquisitions it retains the contrast. This is the appearance of the capillary haemangioma.

(b) On arterial phase it shows peripheral globular enhancement and on portal-venous phase it shows a progressive centripetal enhancement. **CORRECT.** These are the CT imaging features typical of a cavernous hemangioma.

(c) On arterial phase it shows a transient vivid enhancement with reduction of density on the portal-venous and delayed phases. This is the appearance of a hypervascular lesion such as hepatic adenoma.

(d) Its density doesn't change compared to non-enhanced CT scan. This is the appearance of a cystic-like lesion.

References

1. Bartella I, Dufour JF. Clinical diagnosis and staging of intrahepatic cholangiocarcinoma. J Gastrointestin Liver Dis. 2015;24(4):481–9.
2. Bernd H, Ros PR, editors. Abdominal imaging. Berlin: Springer; 2013.
3. Boland GW, editor. Gastrointestinal imaging: the requisites (requisites in radiology). 4th ed. Philadelphia: Elsevier Saunders; 2014.
4. Chan SL, Chong CCN, Chan AWH, et al. Management of hepatocellular carcinoma with portal vein tumor thrombosis: review and update at 2016. World J Gastroenterol. 2016;22(32):7289–300.
5. Choi JY, Lee JM, Sirlin CB. CT and MR imaging diagnosis and staging of hepatocellular carcinoma: Part I. Development, growth, and spread: key pathologic and imaging aspects. Radiology. 2014;272(3):635–54.
6. Chung YE, Kim MJ, Park YN, et al. Varying appearances of cholangiocarcinoma: radiologic-pathologic correlation. Radiographics. 2009;29:683–700.
7. Dal Pozzo G. Compendio di Tomografia Computerizzata e TC multistrato. Torino: UTET Scienze Mediche; 2007.
8. European Association for the Study of the Liver EASL. Clinical practice guidelines: management of hepatocellular carcinoma. J Hepatol. 2018;69(1):182–236.
9. Ganeshan D, Szklaruk J, Kundra V, et al. Imaging features of fibrolamellar hepatocellular carcinoma. Am J Roentgenol. 2014;202(3):544–52.
10. Horton KM, Bluemke DA, Hruban RH, et al. CT and MR imaging of benign hepatic and biliary tumors. Radiographics. 1999;19(2):431–51.
11. Kagawa Y, Okada M, Yagyu Y, et al. Optimal scan timing of hepatic arterial-phase imaging of hypervascular hepatocellular carcinoma determined by multiphasic fast CT imaging technique. Acta Radiol. 2013;54(8):843–50.
12. Klotz T, Montoriol PF, Da Ines D, et al. Hepatic haemangioma: common and uncommon imaging features. Diagn Interv Imaging. 2013;94(9):849–59.
13. Lencioni R, Cioni D, Bartolozzi C, editors. Focal liver lesions - detection, characterisation, ablation. Berlin: Springer; 2005.
14. Levy AD, Mortele KJ, Yeh BM, editors. Gastrointestinal imaging. Oxford: Oxford University Press; 2015.
15. Pozzi Mucelli RM, Como G, Del Frate C, et al. Multidetector CT with double arterial phase and high-iodine-concentration contrast agent in the detection of hepatocellular carcinoma. Radiol Med. 2006;111(2):181–91.
16. Reynolds AR, Furlan A, Fetzer TD, et al. Infiltrative hepatocellular carcinoma: what radiologists need to know. Radiographics. 2015;35:371–86.
17. Sica GT, Ji H, Ros PR. CT and MR imaging of hepatic metastases. Am J Roentgenol. 2000;174:691–8.
18. Sureka B, Bansal K, Arora A. Imaging of perihilar cholangiocarcinoma. Am J Roentgenol. 2015;205(3):W385.
19. Willatt J, Ruma JA, Azar SF, et al. Imaging of hepatocellular carcinoma and image guided therapies - how we do it. Cancer Imaging. 2017;17(1):9.
20. Zech CJ, Bartolozzi C, Baron R, Reiser MF, editors. Multislice CT of the abdomen. Berlin: Springer; 2012.

Patient-Specific 3D Printing in Liver Disease

43

Zhonghua Sun

> **Key Concepts**
> - 3D printed liver models show advantages in improving understanding of hepatic anatomy and pathology when compared to conventional image visualizations
> - 3D printed liver models can be used to assist preoperative planning and simulation of surgical procedures for malignant hepatic tumour treatment
> - Costs associated with 3D printing should be addressed in future studies
> - Large clinical trials should be the future research focus in this area

43.1 Introduction

Three-dimensional (3D) printing shows great promise in medicine with increased applications in a variety of diseases, ranging from orthopaedics to cardiovascular and cerebral vascular diseases [1–12]. Individual case reports, case series, systematic reviews and randomised controlled studies have shown that 3D printed realistic models based on medical imaging data are able to replicate complex anatomy and pathology with high accuracy, improve understanding of the spatial relationship between anatomical structures and pathological changes, and assist surgical planning and simulation, especially in difficult cases [13–15].

Application of 3D printing technique in liver disease has been proved to be superior to conventional image visualisations mainly because of complex hepatic anatomy which is difficult to be appreciated on 2D or 3D diagnostic image visualisations [16–18]. 3D printed liver models created from patient's imaging data have been shown to improve understanding of variable anatomic structures of the liver and assist clinical decision-making in patient treatment [19–35]. Despite promising results from these studies, generation of patient-specific liver models is challenging which is represented by two main areas: a time-consuming process involved in post-processing and segmentation of imaging data for 3D printing purpose, and high cost associated with 3D printed liver models. However, clinical value of 3D printed liver models is promising with future development and application of bioprinting technology. This chapter covers different aspects of 3D printing in liver disease, ranging from the initial step of image processing and segmentation to clinical application of 3D printed models.

43.2 Image Post-processing and Segmentation

Similar to other 3D printing applications, the first step to generate a patient-specific 3D printed model is to conduct image post-processing and segmentation from volume data, either obtained with computed tomography (CT) or magnetic resonance imaging (MRI) imaging modalities. Ideally an imaging dataset should be acquired with thin slice thickness (less than 1 or 2 mm for liver imaging, while for cardiac imaging, slice thickness is preferred to be less than 1 mm) to enable generation of high-quality 3D printed models.

The two-dimensional (2D) axial images, saved in the format of Digital Imaging and Communications in Medicine (DICOM) are converted into 3D volumetric data. The purpose of segmentation is to divide the volume data into several parts with the aim of separating regions of interest such as hepatic structures including tumours from surrounding structures including bony structure or soft tissues. The commonly used approach of CT number thresholding technique works well in CT angiographic data such as CT angiography of cardiovascular disease because contrast-enhanced vessels can be easily differentiated or separated

Z. Sun (✉)
Discipline of Medical Radiation Sciences, School of Molecular and Life Sciences, Curtin University, Perth, WA, Australia
e-mail: z.sun@curtin.edu.au

F. Radu-Ionita et al. (eds.), *Liver Diseases*, https://doi.org/10.1007/978-3-030-24432-3_43

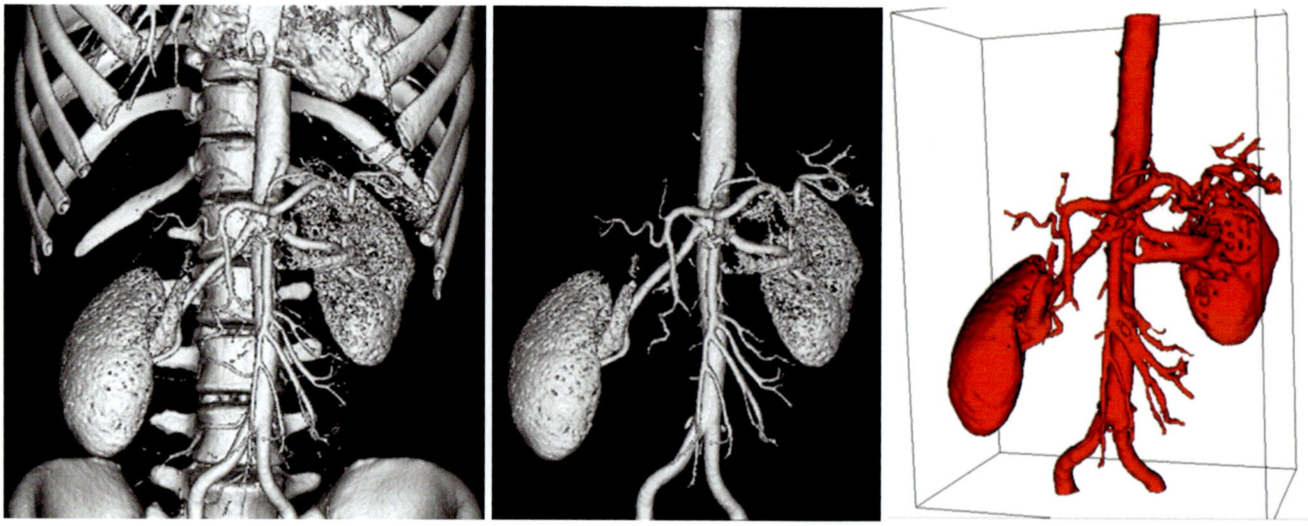

Fig. 43.1 Image segmentation of contrast-enhanced abdominal aorta and its arterial branches using CT number thresholding technique. Minimum CT attenuation of 150 HU is applied to the volume data to segment the contrast-enhanced vessels and kidneys from the surrounding soft tissue structures. Bones are still kept in the initial segmented data (left image). After applying object separation to differentiate bony structures from the aorta and kidneys, lumbar spine and ribs are removed (middle image). The segmented data are saved in stl (standard tessellation language) format for 3D printing (right image)

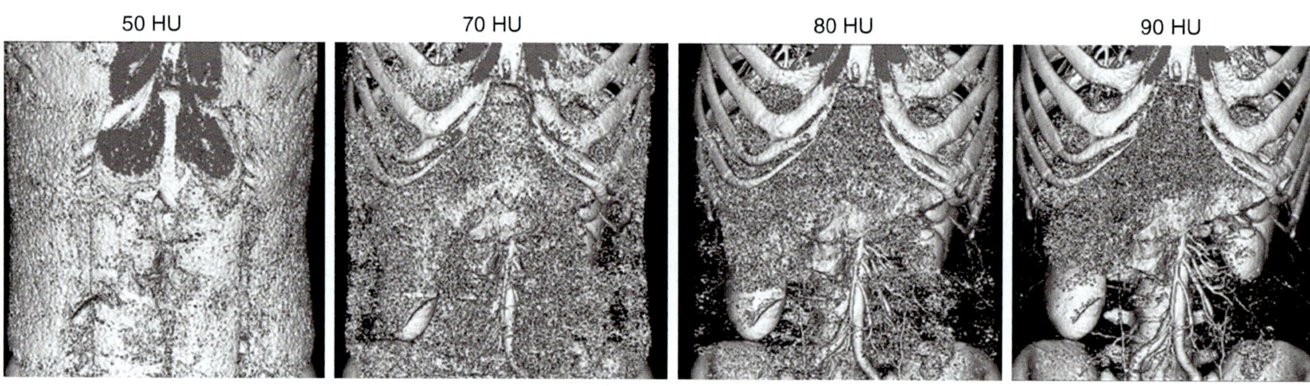

Fig. 43.2 Image segmentation of hepatic anatomy using CT number thresholding technique. After applying the minimum CT attenuation of 50 HU, 70 HU, 80 HU and 90 HU to the volume data, hepatic anatomy cannot be clearly visualised in the segmented data due to its attenuation overlap with surrounding soft tissues. This indicates that use of CT number thresholding technique alone is inappropriate to segment hepatic structures

from the low-attenuating adjacent structures. Figure 43.1 is an example of demonstrating the segmentation of contrast-enhanced abdominal aorta and arterial branches from surrounding structures when applying the CT thresholding technique. However, for hepatic anatomy segmentation, semi-automatic or manual editing is necessary since there is overlap in CT attenuation between hepatic anatomy and adjacent structures, which makes it difficult to achieve good segmentation by using CT thresholding technique as shown in Fig. 43.2. Figure 43.3 is another example of showing segmentation process through semi-automatic and manual editing of images based on multi-phasic CT scans of the liver.

When segmentation process is complete, the digital 3D model is saved as Standard Tessellation Language (STL) format which is recognised by 3D printers for printing the physical models. The STL file usually undergoes some further editing or smoothing process to fix some small 'openings' which are likely to result from converting the 3D virtual model into STL format. Figure 43.3 shows the editing of STL file using a commercially available software tool, Geomagic Wrap. This process is performed to further remove or eliminate small 'openings' that might be present in the STL file so that high-quality 3D printed models can be produced with excellent visualization of anatomical structures and pathologies.

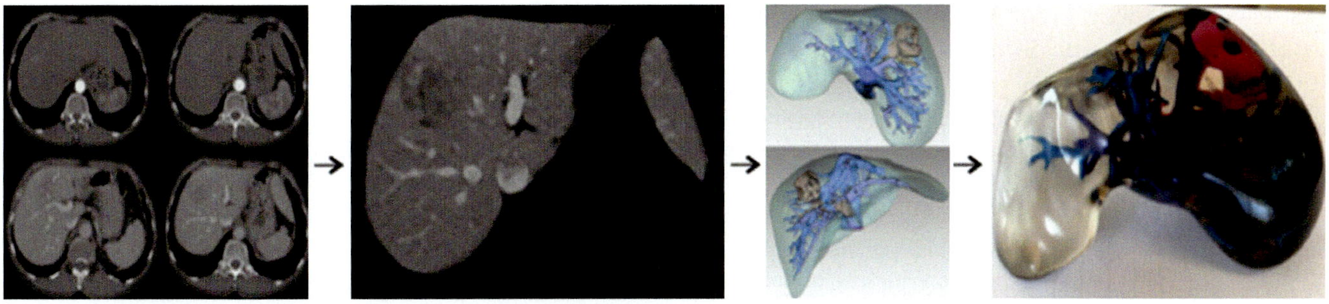

Fig. 43.3 Flow diagram showing the workflow of performing image segmentation using semi-automatic and manual editing approach. Both liver and hepatic anatomic structures are segmented with stl files saved differently to allow visualisation of these structures in a single model. Further editing is needed to remove small openings in the stl files so as to create excellent 3D printed models. (Reprinted with permission under the open access from Perica and Sun [33])

43.3 3D Printed Liver Models: Dimensional Accuracy

3D printed physical models should accurately replicate anatomy and pathology to allow them being accepted as a reliable tool in clinical diagnosis and guiding patient treatment. Studies have reported high accuracy of 3D printed models in cardiovascular diseases with excellent correlation between 3D printed models and original source images [10, 13]. However, 3D printed model accuracy in liver disease was reported to be variable according to studies and systematic reviews. There is a lack of quantitative assessment of accuracy of 3D printed liver models as very few studies reported the dimensional accuracy according to the current literature.

There are three systematic review articles available with analysis of application of 3D printed models in liver disease [36–38]. Soon et al. reported the first systematic review of six studies on 3D printing related to the liver application [36]. Of six studies in their analysis, authors only described one study providing details of model accuracy in delineating vascular structure, with accuracy to ±1.3 mm, and the whole liver to ±4 mm when compared to the recipient's liver [39]. Witowski et al. analysed 14 studies of 3D printed liver models in their recent systematic review, with very general information provided on model accuracy [37]. Of 14 studies in their analysis, 10 studies provided observers' opinion (qualitative assessment) on whether the model was accurate (yes or possibly), and 1 study stated no or not accurate enough. In the remaining 3 studies, model accuracy was not specified.

Detailed analysis of 3D printed model accuracy was reported in a recently published systematic review article with inclusion of 19 studies [38]. This review article analyses the largest number of studies so far on 3D printing in liver disease when compared to the previous two systematic reviews. Further, both qualitative and quantitative assessments of 3D printed liver models were performed in the analysis, thus providing insight into the clinical value of 3D printed models in liver disease. Of 19 studies, quantitative assessment of accuracy of 3D printed liver models was provided in 5 studies with 4 of them focusing on dimensional accuracy between 3D model and original CT or MRI images. Two studies compared model accuracy in terms of liver volume (one of the studies compared both dimensional and volume accuracy) between 3D printed models and CT images [26, 39]. The analysis shows that 3D printed models are highly accurate in replicating hepatic structures and pathologies with mean difference between 1.30% and 5.08% as shown in 3 studies, while in the remaining study, large differences were reported when comparing 3D printed liver model with original CT and STL files, ranging from 7.4% in measurement difference between 3D printed model and STL image, to 20.80% between 3D printed model and CT images [38].

Witowski and colleagues in their recent study further reported the accuracy of 3D printed models when compared to original CT images [40]. Fifteen patient-specific 3D liver models were printed in a 1-1 scale with inclusion of liver, tumour and hepatic vessels using the developed cost-effective approach. These 3D printed models were CT scanned with measurements of hepatic diameters and volume analysis of liver parenchyma and tumours compared to the original CT images. No significant bias was found in the measurements of liver volume and hepatic structures as well as tumour location. Based on this one of the largest studies (with inclusion of 15 models), authors confirmed the accuracy of 3D printed models in liver disease and suggested the future research should focus on clinical trials for assessment of clinical outcomes with incorporation of 3D printing into presurgical planning.

43.4 3D Printed Liver Models: Pre-surgical Planning and Simulation

One of the main applications of 3D printed models lies in the pre-surgical planning and simulation of hepatic surgeries. Although most of the current studies are based on case reports, patient-specific 3D printed models are shown to play an important role in preoperative planning and simulation of malignant hepatic tumour treatment as indicated by the summary of a recent systematic review [38]. These applications are demonstrated in the following areas.

43.4.1 3D Printed Liver Models in Pre-surgical Planning of Hepatic Tumours

CT and MRI images are routine visualization tools for planning of hepatic surgeries. Due to difficulty in demonstrating complex hepatic anatomy and pathology by traditional 2D or 3D image visualisations, 3D printed physical models can overcome these limitations by providing comprehensive assessment of hepatic anatomy and pathology which are essential for hepatic resections of malignant tumours (Figs. 43.4 and 43.5). Takagi et al. first reported the usefulness of 3D printing model in preoperative simulation of surgical resection [41]. They created a 3D printed model of perihilar cholangiocarcinoma from 3D CT angiographic data containing hepatic vasculature and the main tumour. 3D printed model shows the similar resected line when compared to the resected specimen, indicating the potential value of using 3D printed model for preoperative simulation of surgical resection. This was confirmed by a recent study [32] with creation of a 3D printed model comprising the hepatic tumour and hepatic structures such as hepatic veins. The model was used to simulate the resection line prior to surgery and the simulated resection was successful during operation. These studies further highlight the benefit of 3D printed

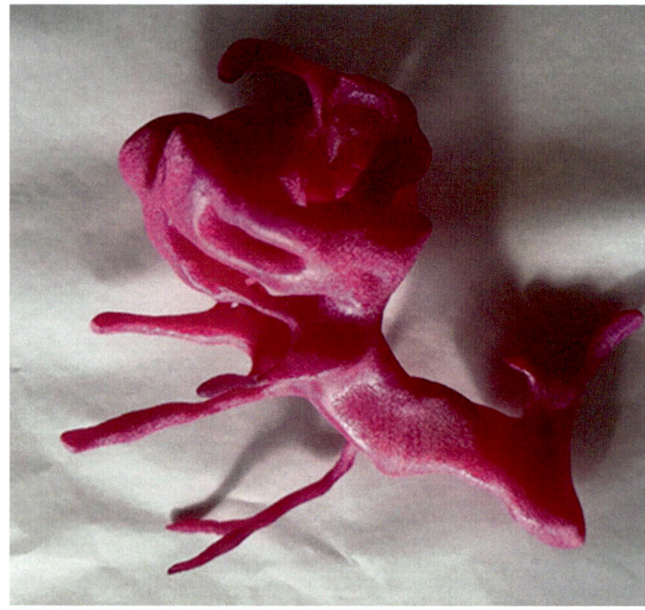

Fig. 43.5 Anterior view of the full size 3D printed tumour model demonstrating the arterial phase enhancement characteristics of the tumour and associated hepatic arterial branches. (Reprinted with permission under the open access from Perica and Sun [33])

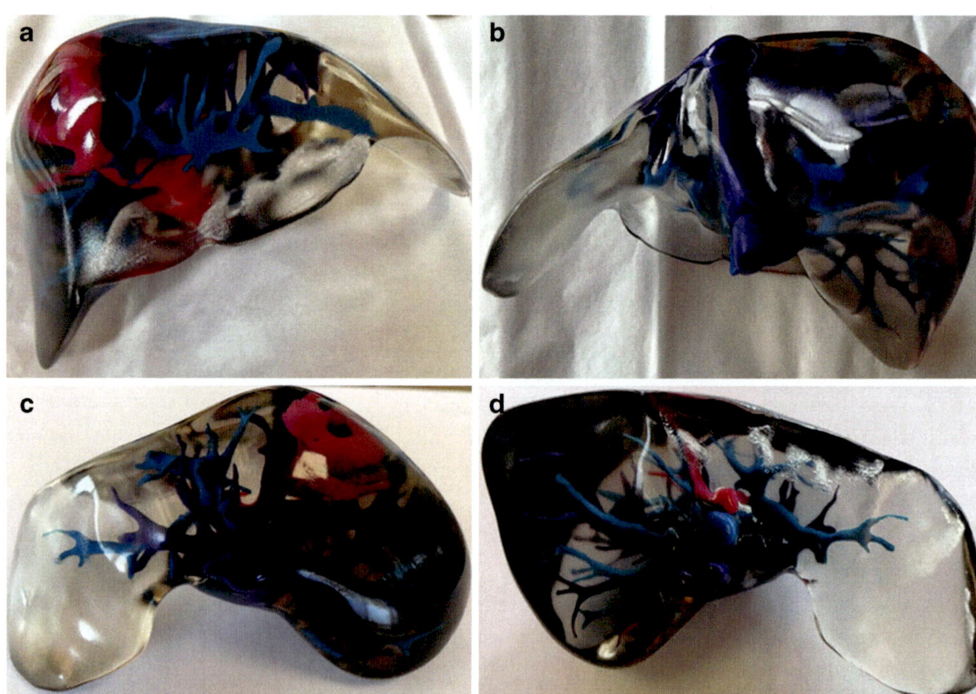

Fig. 43.4 Anterior (**a**), posterior (**b**), superior (**c**), and inferior (**d**) views of the 3D printed liver model generated from CT images, demonstrating the liver parenchyma (transparent), inferior vena cava and hepatic veins (purple), portal veins (blue), the tumour, and hepatic arterial supply (pink). (Reprinted with permission under the open access from Perica and Sun [33])

models in planning hepatectomy of liver tumours, especially improving visibility of small tumours when compared to traditional image visualizations.

In addition to simulation of surgical procedures, 3D printed models can be used to simulate interventional procedures for treating hepatobiliary diseases. Zeman and colleagues [28, 29] developed realistic 3D printed hepatic and biliary models based on graphic designs. Hepatic parenchyma, hollow structures including hepatic vessels and biliary components as well as tumours and abscesses were simulated in the 3D printed models to allow simulation of stent placement or other percutaneous procedures. These results need to be confirmed by patient-specific 3D printed models for replicating actual clinical situations.

43.4.2 3D Printed Liver Models in Pre-surgical Planning of Liver Transplantation

Living donor liver transplantation (LDLT) is an established and effective approach to treat patients with end-stage liver diseases. Inaccurate preoperative assessment and characterization of anatomical structures and volume estimation will lead to donor morbidities [34]. 3D printing is able to address these challenges by providing a direct visualisation and assessment of livers from both recipients and donors.

A number of studies have reported the usefulness of 3D printing for LDLT [24, 34, 39]. Zein et al. in their study [39] created six 3D printed liver models from three donor and three recipients. They compared the volume of the liver between 3D printed models and donor and recipient's livers, as well as anatomical accuracy in terms of length, width, height, portal vein and hepatic vein diameters in these three cases. The mean volume and standard deviation between 3D printed models and recipient and donor's livers were 6.90% ± 0.06 and 4.70% ± 0.02. The corresponding values between 3D printed models and recipient and donor's livers in the above-defined hepatic diameter measurements were 11.62% ± 0.06 and 7.66% ± 0.08, 1.90% ± 0.02 and 2.64% ± 0.04, 3.80% ± 0.01 and 2.88% ± 0.01 for cases 1, 2 and 3, respectively. These 3D printed liver models were found to be highly accurate with small mean dimensional errors, and results were validated against the actual livers during surgery. Later case reports confirm the clinical value of 3D printed model in preoperative simulation of LDLT.

Baimakhanov et al. [24] made a 3D solid model of portal vein tree and portal vein graft from 3D imaging data and found it to be a useful tool for preoperative simulation by assisting selection of an appropriate surgical strategy. Since 3D printed model offers details of the complex anastomosis in LDLT, authors also concluded that it could be used to train young surgeons. Soejima et al. in [34] their case report provided further evidence of 3D printed models in LDLT for paediatric patients. They generated a 3D printed model from CT imaging data of an 11-year-old girl diagnosed with biliary atresia following Kasai procedure. A real-sized 3D printed model of the left lateral segment graft of the donor was created along with the recipient abdominal cavity with the aim of simulating the transplant. The 3D printed prototype graft and the abdominal cavity represent realistic liver graft and the abdomen, which are found to be very helpful for surgeons to perform simulation of donor surgery. Another advantage of the 3D printed model over conventional 3D imaging lies in the model texture which is soft and transparent, with hepatic vasculature clearly visualised, as shown in their study. 3D printed realistic liver models could contribute to technical accuracy and extend applications to complex cases of liver and biliary diseases, although this needs to be confirmed by further studies.

43.5 3D Printed Liver Models: Medical Education

3D printing serves as a valuable tool for education of medical students, healthcare professionals and patient-doctor communication. This has been demonstrated by a number of studies focusing on the 3D printed models in cardiovascular disease, according to recent systematic reviews [11, 13]. Similarly, 3D printed liver models have been shown to assist education of medical students according to some studies [28, 30, 42, 43]. Watson in their case series [42] showed that low-cost 3D printed models created from CT or MRI data (less than $100) served as a useful tool for education of junior residents and medical students in terms of practicing surgical procedures of hepatic operations. Javan et al. [28] also designed low-cost 3D printed models of hepatic anatomy (costs between 40 and $100) using graphic design approach. These 3D printed models are able to demonstrate complex anatomical structures of the liver anatomy when compared to conventional 2D or 3D visualisations.

Kong et al. [30] in their randomized controlled studies further confirmed the value of 3D printed models in medical education. In their first report, authors developed a 3D printed liver model based on CT data of a healthy candidate. Six experts (four were professors of Anatomy and two were consultant surgeons) assessed the 3D printed models and 3D visualisation of virtual hepatic segmental model regarding demonstration of anatomical structures and overall satisfaction of these models as a teaching tool. Further, 61 first year medical students were randomly assigned to three groups for evaluating the effects of 3D printed models, 3D virtual model and traditional method of using anatomical atlases on hepatic anatomy teaching. 3D printed models of hepatic segments with partition (Fig. 43.6) and without hepatic parenchyma (Fig. 43.7) were successfully generated with realistic

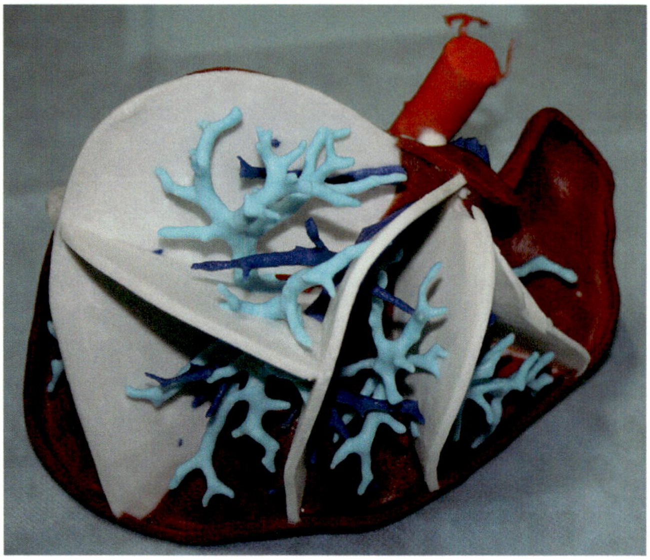

Fig. 43.6 3D printed model of hepatic segments partition. (Reprinted with permission from Kong et al. [30])

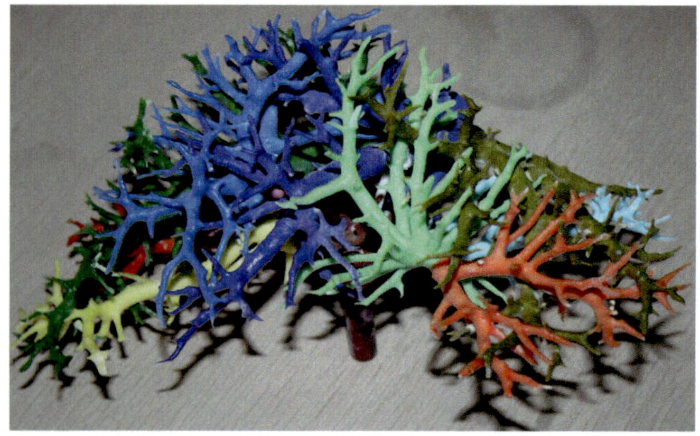

Fig. 43.7 3D printed model of hepatic segments without the liver parenchyma. (Reprinted with permission from Kong et al. [30])

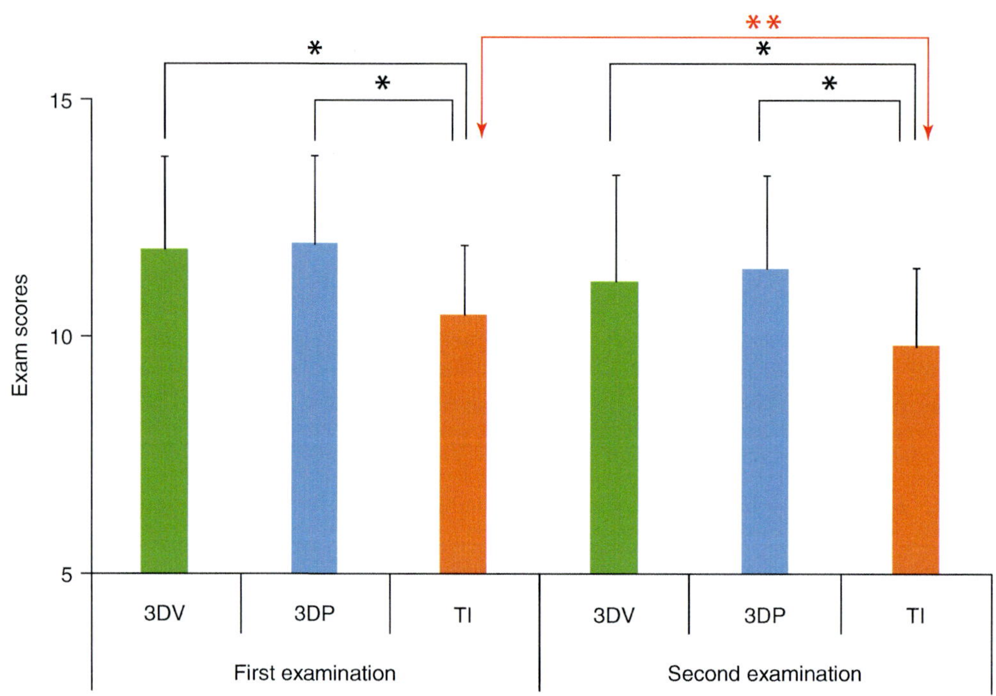

Fig. 43.8 Medical student examinations cores. * Significant differences between three groups with post hoc tests in the first and second examinations, respectively. ** Significant differences between the two examinations (the second questionnaire examination was conducted 5 days later to ask the same groups of medical students) in each group with paired-sample t tests. *3DP* 3D printing, *3DV* 3D visualization, *TI* traditional imaging. (Reprinted with permission from Kong et al. [30])

visualisation of hepatic anatomy as assessed by all experts. Both 3D printed models and 3D virtual model received similar scores by the experts with no significant differences ($p > 0.05$). Results from medical students' evaluation showed that 3D printed models and 3D virtual model were found to be significantly better than traditional teaching method ($p < 0.05$) (Fig. 43.8).

The same group conducted another randomized controlled study with a focus on investigation of the effect of 3D printed models with or without hepatic parenchyma on teaching hepatic segments [42]. Apart from the same 6 experts who were invited in their previous study, 92 first year medical students were randomly assigned to four groups, namely, 3D printed models of hepatic segments with and without transparent parenchyma, hepatic vessels with segmental partition and traditional method using atlas. The 3D printed models were created from CT data of a human liver cadaver without any disease. Results from experts' assessment showed that the 3D printed model with hepatic segment partition was found to be significantly better than the other two types of models in terms of anatomical condition ($p < 0.05$), and better than the model without parenchyma in overall satisfaction ($p < 0.05$). The models with and without transparent parenchyma were found to be significantly better than the one with segment partition in tactility ($p < 0.05$). The students' tests showed that all of these three types of 3D printed models were significantly better than traditional anatomy teaching ($p < 0.05$). Authors concluded that the 3D printed model with hepatic segment partition is the optimal one due to its simple design and offering sufficient information for teaching hepatic anatomy. Since 3D virtual models are also useful for teaching medical students based on these studies, further studies are necessary to look into the comparative effects of 3D printed models versus virtual models.

43.6 3D Printed Liver Models: Limitations and Future Directions

There are some limitations that need to be addressed before 3D printing is widely used in clinical practice. First, high cost associated with 3D printing is a main issue when printing 3D liver models with high-quality materials. Low-cost 3D printed models are reported in some studies with less than USD100, however, creation of high-quality realistic 3D printed models of replicating hepatic anatomy and pathology comes at high cost, which could be as high as USD 2000, according to a recent systematic review [38]. Due to this reason, most of the current models are printed with scaled down to 50% and 70% of the full-size liver models. Reduction in printing costs represents the direction of future development to improve feasibility of 3D printed liver models.

Another limitation associated with 3D printing in liver disease is relatively long segmentation time. Although most of the studies did not report time taken for 3D printed liver models, the reported duration of 3D printing is between 11 and 100 h. It could take up to 2 weeks when delivery or shipping time is considered [38]. The average duration of 3D printing for liver models is much longer than that for 3D printing of heart and kidney models [13, 44]. Shortening 3D printing process is absolutely necessary to ensure that 3D printed models can be used in daily clinical practice for patient's planning and treatment.

Bioprinting represents the future development in 3D printing in medicine. In recent years, tissue engineering in combination with 3D printing technology has been shown to be the most useful and promising tools for creating scaffold structures which play an important role in regeneration of tissues and organs, in particular, 3D printing of liver tissues for liver transplantation [45–50]. Bioprinting of hepatic cells, structures and liver constructs seems to be feasible according to these studies, thus, creating great opportunities for reducing surgical complications and developing personalized medicine in the near future (Fig. 43.9). Research in this area is still at its infancy, thus requiring more studies to be conducted in the near future.

43.7 Summary

3D printing has attracted increasing attention in medical applications, and patient-specific 3D printed models have seen successful applications in liver disease. This chapter provides an overview of the applications of 3D printed realistic liver models, which include delineation of normal hepatic anatomy and pathology, accuracy of 3D printed

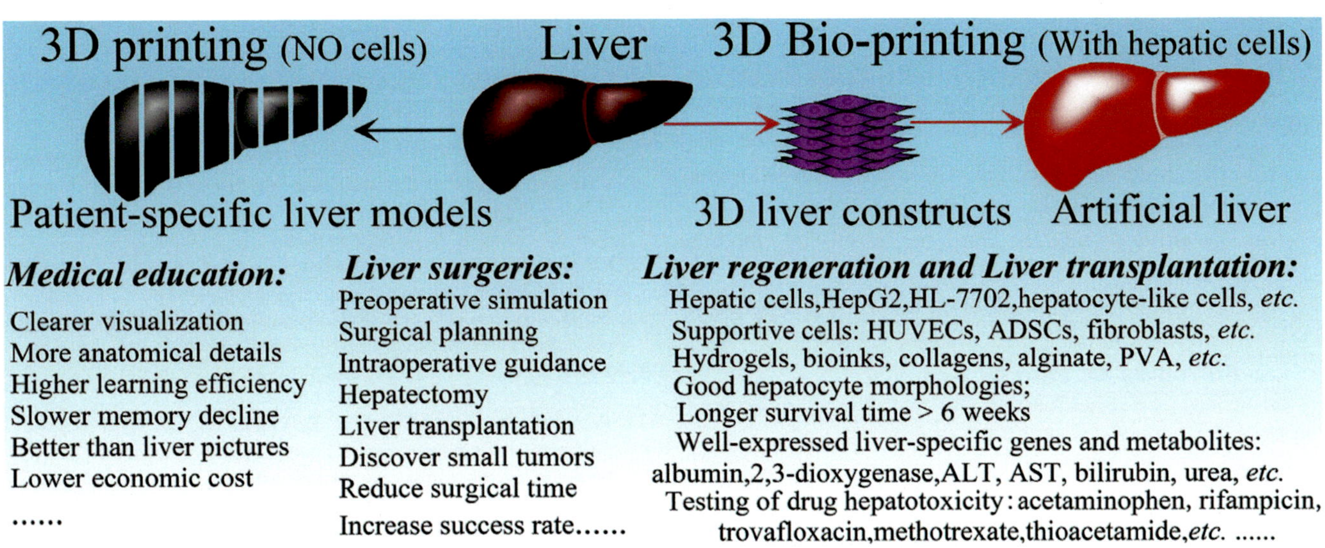

Fig. 43.9 3D-printing (no cells) and 3D Bioprinting (with hepatic cells) facilitate liver anatomy, liver surgery, liver regeneration, liver transplantation and drug hepatotoxicity testing. *ADSCs* adipose tissue-derived stem cells, *ALT* alanine aminotransferase, *AST* aminotransferase, *HUVECs* human umbilical vein endothelial cells, *PVA* polyvinyl alcohol. (Reprinted with permission from Wang et al. [45])

models, pre-surgical planning and simulation of complex surgical procedures for treating liver disease and education of medical students. 3D printed liver models continue to show its impact on current clinical practice and may lead to paradigm shift in managing liver disease.

Glossary

3D printing A process to produce a solid 3D object from a 3D digital model using different materials enabling creation of customizable or patient-specific geometries or shapes.

Hepatocellular carcinoma Most common type of primary malignant liver cancer.

Liver transplantation Treatment option for a diseased liver by replacing it with a healthy liver from another person (donor).

Tumour An abnormal mass of tissue growth resulting in swelling or enlargement of a part of the organ or body.

Self Study

Questions

1. Which statement/s is/are true?
   (a) 3D printed liver models can be produced using CT data
   (b) 3D printed liver models can be produced using MRI data
   (c) 3D printed liver models can be produced using Ultrasound data
   (d) 3D printed liver models can be producing using angiographic data
2. Which statement/s is/are true?
   (a) 3D printed liver models can be generated with high accuracy
   (b) 3D printed models can be used for pre-surgical planning and simulation
   (c) 3D printed models can be used for medical education
   (d) 3D printed models can be used for assisting patient-doctor communication
   (e) All of them are correct

Answers

1. Which statement/s is/are true? **a and b are correct.**
   CT and MR imaging data are commonly used to generate 3D printed liver models.
   Ultrasound or angiographic imaging modalities do not provide volume data, thus are not used for 3D printing in liver disease.
2. Which statement/s is/are true? **e is correct.**
   Despite reported discrepancy in diameter measurements between original source images and 3D printed liver models, 3D printed liver models are shown to be accurate with applications in different areas ranging from pre-surgical planning and simulation to education.

References

1. Farooqi KM, Sengupta PP. Echocardiography and three-dimensional printing: sound ideas to touch a heart. J Am Soc Echocardiogr. 2015;28:398–403.
2. Sumida T, Otawa N, Kamata YU, Kamakura S, Misushita T, Kitagaki H, Mori S, Sasaki K, Fujibayashi S, Takemoto M, Yamaguchi A, Sohmura T, Nakamura T, Mori Y. Custom-made titanium devices as membranes for bone augmentation in implant treatment: clinical application and the comparison with conventional titanium mesh. J Craniomaxillofac Surg. 2015;43:2183–8.
3. Aranda JL, Jimenez MF, Rodriguez M, Varela G. Tridimensional titanium-printed custom-made prosthesis for sternocostal reconstruction. Eur J Cardiothorac Surg. 2015;48:e92–4.
4. Kim GB, Lee S, Kim H, Yang DH, Kim YH, Kyung YS, Kim CS, Choi SH, Kim BJ, Ha H, Kwon SU, Kim N. Three-dimensional printing: basic principles and applications in medicine and radiology. Korean J Radiol. 2016;17:182–97.
5. Choi JY, Choi JH, Kim NK, Kim Y, Lee JK, Kim MK, Lee JH, Kim MJ. Analysis of errors in medical rapid prototyping models. Int J Oral Maxillofac Surg. 2002;31:23–32.
6. Chang PS, Parker TH, Patrick CW Jr, Miller MJ. The accuracy of stereolithography in planning craniofacial bone replacement. J Craniofac Surg. 2003;14:164–70.
7. Vukicevic M, Mosadegh B, Min JK, Little SH. Cardiac 3D printing and its future directions. JACC Cardiovasc Imaging. 2017;10:171–84.
8. Giannopoulos AA, Steigner ML, George E, Barile M, Hunsaker AR, Rybicki FJ, Mitsouras D. Cardiothoracic applications of 3-dimensional printing. J Thorac Imaging. 2016;31:253–72.
9. Giannopoulos AA, Mitsouras D, Yoo SJ, Liu PP, Chatzizisis YS, Rybicki FJ. Applications of 3D printing in cardiovascular diseases. Nat Rev Cardiol. 2016;13:701–18.
10. Sun Z, Lee SY. A systematic review of 3-D printing in cardiovascular and cerebrovascular diseases. Anatol J Cardiol. 2017;17:423–35.
11. Sun Z, Squelch A. Patient-specific 3D printed models of aortic aneurysm and aortic dissection. J Med Imaging Health Inf. 2017;7:886–9.
12. Ho D, Squelch A, Sun Z. Modelling of aortic aneurysm and aortic dissection through 3D printing. J Med Radiat Sci. 2017;64:10–7.
13. Lau I, Sun Z. Three-dimensional printing in congenital heart disease: a systematic review. J Med Radiat Sci. 2018;65:226–36.
14. Preece D, Williams SB, Lam R, Weller R. 'Let's get physical': advantages of a physical model over 3D computer models and textbooks in learning imaging anatomy. Anat Sci Educ. 2013;6:216–24.
15. Waran V, Narayanan V, Karuppiah R, Pancharatnam D, Chandran H, Raman R, Rahman ZA, Owen SL, Aziz TZ. Injecting realism in surgical training - initial simulation experience with custom 3D models. J Surg Educ. 2014;71:193–7.

16. Zheng Y, Yu D, Zhao J, Wu Y, Zheng B. 3D printout models vs. 3D rendered images: which is better for preoperative planning? J Surg Educ. 2016;73:518–23.
17. Witowski JS, Pędziwiatr M, Major P, Budzyński A. Cost-effective, personalized, 3D-printed liver model for preoperative planning before laparoscopic liver hemihepatectomy for colorectal cancer metastases. Int J Comput Assist Radiol Surg. 2017;12:2047–54.
18. Madurska MJ, Poyade M, Eason D, Rea P, Watson AJM. Development of a patient-specific 3D-printed liver model for preoperative planning. Surg Innov. 2017;24:145–50.
19. Xiang N, Fang C, Fan Y, Yang J, Zeng N, Liu J, Zhu W. Application of liver three-dimensional printing in hepatectomy for complex massive hepatocarcinoma with rare variations of portal vein: preliminary experience. Int J Clin Exp Med. 2015;8:18873–8.
20. Alkhouri N, Zein NN. Three-dimensional printing and pediatric liver disease. Curr Opin Pediatr. 2016;28:626–30.
21. Oshiro Y, Ohkohchi N. Three-dimensional liver surgery simulation: computer-assisted surgical planning with three-dimensional simulation software and three-dimensional printing. Tissue Eng Part A. 2017;23:474–80.
22. Yao R, Xu G, Mao SS, Yang HY, Sang XT, Sun W, Mao YL. Three-dimensional printing: review of application in medicine and hepatic surgery. Cancer Biol Med. 2016;13:443–51.
23. Fang CH, Tao HS, Yang J, Fang ZS, Cai W, Liu J, Fan YH. Impact of three-dimensional reconstruction technique in the operation planning of centrally located hepatocellular carcinoma. J Am Coll Surg. 2015;220:28–37.
24. Baimakhanov Z, Soyama A, Takatsuki M, Hidaka M, Hirayama T, Kinoshita A, Natsuda K, Kuroki T, Eguchi S. Preoperative simulation with a 3-dimensional printed solid model for one-stop reconstruction of multiple hepatic veins during living donor liver transplantation. Liver Transpl. 2015;21:266–8.
25. Bucking TM, Hill E, Robertson JL, Maneas E, Plumb AA, Nikitichev DI. From medical imaging data to 3D printed anatomical models. PLoS One. 2017;12:e0178540.
26. Choi YR, Kim JH, Park SJ, Hur BY, Han JK. Therapeutic response assessment using 3D ultrasound for hepatic metastasis from colorectal cancer: application of a personalized, 3D-printed tumor model using CT images. PLoS One. 2017;12:e0182596.
27. Igami T, Nakamura Y, Hirose T, Ebata T, Yokoyama Y, Sugawara G, Mizuno T, Mori K, Nagino M. Application of a three-dimensional print of a liver in hepatectomy for small tumors invisible by intraoperative ultrasonography: preliminary experience. World J Surg. 2014;38:3163–6.
28. Javan R, Herrin D, Tangestanipoor A. Understanding spatially complex segmental and branch anatomy using 3D printing: liver, lung, prostate, coronary arteries, and circle of Willis. Acad Radiol. 2016;23:1183–9.
29. Javan R, Zeman M. A prototype educational model for hepatobiliary interventions: unveiling the role of graphic designers in medical 3D printing. J Digit Imaging. 2018;31:133–43.
30. Kong X, Nie L, Zhang H, Wang Z, Ye Q, Tang L, Li J, Huang W. Do three-dimensional visualization and three-dimensional printing improve hepatic segment anatomy teaching? A randomized controlled study. J Surg Educ. 2016;73:264–9.
31. Leng S, Chen B, Vrieze T, Kuhlman J, Yu L, Alexander A, Matsumoto J, Morris J, McCollough CH. Construction of realistic phantoms from patients images and a commercial three-dimensional printer. J Med Imag (Bellingham). 2016;3:033501.
32. Oshiro Y, Mitani J, Okada T, Ohkohchi N. A novel three-dimensional print of liver vessels and tumors in hepatectomy. Surg Today. 2017;47:521–4.
33. Perica E, Sun Z. Patient-specific three-dimensional printing for pre-surgical planning in hepatocellular carcinoma treatment. Quant Imaging Med Surg. 2017;7:668–77.
34. Soejima Y, Taguchi T, Sugimoto M, Hayashida M, Yoshizumi T, Ikegami T, Uchiyama H, Shirabe K, Maehara Y. Three-dimensional printing and biotexture modeling for preoperative simulation in living donor liver transplantation for small infants. Liver Transpl. 2016;22:1610–4.
35. Souzaki R, Kinoshita Y, Ieiri S, Hayashida M, Koga Y, Shirabe K, Hara T, Maehara Y, Hashizume M, Taguchi T. Three-dimensional liver model based on preoperative CT images as a tool to assist in surgical planning for hepatoblastoma in a child. Pediatr Surg Int. 2015;31:593–6.
36. Soon DSC, Chae MP, Pilgrim CHC, Rozen WM, Spychal RT, Hunter-Smith DJ. 3D hepatic modelling for preoperative planning of hepatic resection: a systematic review. Ann Med Surg (Lond). 2016;10:1–7.
37. Witowski JS, Coles-Black J, Zuzak TZ, Pedziwiatr M, Chuen J, Major P, Budzyriski A. 3D printing in liver surgery: a systematic review. Telemed J E Health. 2017;23:943–7.
38. Perica ER, Sun Z. A systematic review of three-dimensional printing in liver disease. J Digit Imaging. 2018; https://doi.org/10.1007/s10278-018-0067-x.
39. Zein NN, Hanouneh IA, Bishop PD, Samaan M, Eghtesad B, Quintini C, Miller C, Yerian L, Klatte R. Three-dimensional print of a liver for preoperative planning in living donor liver transplantation. Liver Transpl. 2013;19:1304–10.
40. Witowski J, Wake N, Grochowska A, Sun Z, Budzyriski A, Major P, Jan Popiela T, Pedziwiatr M. Investigating accuracy of 3D printed liver models with computed tomography. Quant Imaging Med Surg. 2019;9(1):43–52.
41. Takagi K, Nanashima A, Abo T, Arai J, Matsuo N, Fukuda T, Nagayasu T. Three-dimensional printing model of liver for operative simulation in perihilar cholangiocarcinoma. Hepatogastroenterology. 2014;61:2315–1216.
42. Watson RA. A low-cost surgical application of additive fabrication. J Surg Educ. 2014;71:14–7.
43. Kong X, Nie L, Zhang H, Wang Z, Ye Q, Tang L, Huang W, Li J. Do 3D printing models improve anatomical teaching about hepatic segments to medical students? A randomized controlled study. World J Surg. 2016;40:1969–76.
44. Sun Z, Liu D. A systematic review of clinical value of three-dimensional printing in renal disease. Quant Imaging Med Surg. 2018;8:311–25.
45. Wang JZ, Xiong NY, Zhao LZ, Hu JT, Kong DC, Yuan JY. Review fantastic medical applications of 3D-printing in liver surgeries, liver regeneration, liver transplantation and drug hepatotoxicity testing: a review. Int J Surg. 2018;56:1–6.
46. Lewis PL, Green RM, Shah RN. 3D-printed gelatin scaffolds of differing pore geometry modulate hepatocyte function and gene expression. Acta Biomater. 2018;69:63–70.
47. Lee JW, Choi YJ, Yong WJ, Pati F, Shim JH, Kang KS, Kang IH, Park J, Cho DW. Development of a 3D cell printed construct considering angiogenesis for liver tissue engineering. Biofabrication. 2017;8:015007.
48. Faulkner-Jones A, Fyfe AC, Cornelissen DJ, Gardner J, King J, Courtney A, Shu W. Bioprinting of human pluripotent stem cells and their directed differentiation into hepatocyte-like cells for the generation of mini-livers in 3D. Biofabrication. 2015;7:044102.
49. Jeon H, Kang K, Park SA, Kim WD, Paik SS, Lee SH, Jeong J, Choi D. Generation of multilayered 3D structures of HepG2 cells using a bio-printing technique. Gut Liver. 2017;11:121–8.
50. Murphy SV, Atala A. 3D bioprinting of tissues and organs. Nat Biotechnol. 2014;32:773–85.

Dynamic Contrast-Enhanced Ultrasonography of the Liver

44

Laura Iliescu

Key Concepts

- Contrast-enhanced ultrasonography is highly sensitive and sensible in differentiating between benign and malignant focal liver lesions.
- CEUS can establish the diagnosis of hepatocellular carcinoma by the typical aspect (hyperenhancement in the arterial phase and wash out in the late phase) in 97% of the cases.
- CEUS can differentiate between malignant and benign portal vein thrombosis.

44.1 Introduction

44.1.1 General Considerations

While conventional grayscale ultrasonography is an important means of diagnosis, used to acquire anatomical data, and Doppler ultrasound examination is highly valuable in offering information concerning the blood flow, their role remains limited, as they cannot be used for the evaluation of micro-vessels and tissue perfusion. Contrast-enhanced ultrasonography, also referred to as CEUS, is an ultrasound examination technique that overcomes these limitations. The procedure involves the use of microbubble contrast agents, in order to obtain a better visualization of the organs and blood vessels [1].

The microbubbles can be described as gas-filled particles, with a supporting shell, having a diameter of several micrometers—a particularity that prevents their passage through the vascular endothelium into the interstitial space [2]. Depending on the type of gas within the microbubbles, the contrast media classifies as either first or second generation.

L. Iliescu (✉)
Internal Medicine and Gastroenterology, Institutul Clinic Fundeni, University of Medicine and Pharmacy (UMF) Carol Davila, Bucharest, Romania

The first-generation contrast agent, known under the name of Levovist (Bayer Schering Pharma, Berlin, Germany) was introduced in 1996 and consisted of air, surrounded by a shell of galactose microparticles (99.9%) and palmic acid (0.1%). The main use was for echocardiography, vascular ultrasonography and Doppler exploration, while the abdominal applications were limited [3]. Due to a high mechanical index technique and early destruction of the microbubbles, only intermittent scanning was possible. Later-on, in 2001, with the development of second-generation contrast agents, came the possibility of a more accurate real-time evaluation and, therefore, the interest in using CEUS increased significantly [3]. The effort to stabilize the microbubbles led to the use of a more slowly diffusing gas, such as sulfur hexafluoride or perfluorobutane, instead of air. Second-generation contrast agents include: SonoVue (Bracco, Milan, Italy), Definity/Luminity (Lantheus Medical Imaging, North Billerica, USA), Sonazoid (GE Healthcare, Oslo, Norway) and Optison (GE Healthcare, Princeton, USA). Their efficacy relies on a low mechanical index technique (<0.3), with continuous scanning [3].

SonoVue is characterized by a phospholipid shell, containing sulfur hexafluoride. During the procedure, destruction of the microbubbles is followed by the excretion of gas solely through the lungs. In the European Union, it has been approved and recognized as a means to evaluate the heart, macrovasculature (cerebral arteries, extracranial carotid, peripheral arteries, portal vein assessment), as well as microvascular structures (such as focal lesions of the liver or breast) [3, 4].

Sonazoid contains perfluorobutane microspheres, stabilized by a monomolecular membrane of hydrogenated egg phosphatidylserine. Its chemical structure allows Sonazoid to be used for Kupffer phase imaging, unlike other second-generation contrast agents. The microbubbles within is structure are phagocytized by the Kupffer cells, leading to the amplification of ultrasound waves and respectively, to a homogeneous enhancement of the normal functioning liver parenchyma. Therefore, Sonazoid can be used in the

F. Radu-Ionita et al. (eds.), *Liver Diseases*, https://doi.org/10.1007/978-3-030-24432-3_44

diagnosis and evaluation of focal liver lesions, as well as in guiding surgical or radiological interventions, in Japan and Korea [5, 6].

When administered into the vasculature, the ultrasound contrast agent acts as an enhancer of the ultrasound waves, resulting in an important amplification of the signals from the blood flow.

44.1.2 Safety Considerations

Following the destruction of the microspheres, all contrast agents are excreted through the lungs. Therefore, they are not nephrotoxic and can be safely used in individuals with renal failure, that cannot benefit from computerized tomography or magnetic resonance imaging [2, 7]. Moreover, the contrast agents used in ultrasound exploration do not affect the thyroid, since they are iodine-free.

Hypersensitivity reactions are possible, with an incidence that has been reported to approximately 0.002% in large-scale abdominal application studies. However, compared to iodine contrast agents used in computerized tomography, the overall incidence of hypersensitivity reactions during CEUS is lower and reportedly comparable to that encountered when using gadolinium chelate as a contrast agent in magnetic resonance imaging [7, 8].

Both SonoVue and Sonazoid are contraindicated in patients with adult respiratory distress syndrome, acute coronary syndrome, ischemic cardiac disease, right-to-left shunts or pulmonary hypertension [4]. There is not enough evidence concerning the use of contrast agents during pregnancy or lactation.

Contrast-enhanced ultrasonography may induce microvascular lesions, hemolysis, increased heating of the tissue or death of the cells that have phagocytized the microbubble, although these effects have not yet been demonstrated in vivo, on human subjects [9]. In vivo animal studies showed that the aforementioned harmful biological effects are enhanced in the presence of a mechanical index higher than 0.4. Therefore, for safety purposes, this parameter should be kept as low as possible during the procedure [8, 9].

44.1.3 Terminology

When characterizing a lesion or a region of interest, during the contrast-enhanced ultrasonography exploration of the liver, it is important to describe it using the following terms: the degree of enhancement and the timing (phase). The contrast behavior of the lesion and of the liver parenchyma depends on the liver status (healthy liver vs. steatosis, fibrosis or cirrhosis).

Enhancement reflects the vascularity of the region, by referring to the intensity of the signal by comparison to the adjacent parenchyma: it can either be equal to (isoenhancing), higher than (hyperenhancing) or lower than (hypoenhancing) the parenchyma. Sustained enhancement describes the persistence of enhancement in the lesion/region, over time; the terms applies only to those lesions that are iso- or hyperenhancing in the arterial phase. The absence of enhancement in a liver area can be characterized as nonenhancing [8, 10].

The aforementioned enhancement pattern should be described for each of the CEUS phases. When referring to a region of interest, the period of progressive enhancement, from the arrival of microbubbles in the investigator's field of view until reaching the "peak enhancement", is described using the term "wash-in phase". Similarly, the "wash-out phase" describes the enhancement lowering, after the peak enhancement [8, 10].

The mechanical index (MI) can be defined as an estimation of the maximum amplitude of the pressure pulse within the tissue, thus being an indicator of the power in the system. A higher MI is associated with a more rapid disruption of the microbubbles, therefore low MI techniques are recommended [8].

44.1.4 CEUS Phases: Examination Technique

One of the main advantages of CEUS examination is that it offers the possibility of real-time exploration, evaluating both wash-in and wash-out phases of the contrast agent, during several minutes [10].

Owing to the dual blood supply of the liver, from the portal vein (70–75%) and from the hepatic artery (25–30%), there are three CEUS vascular phases (Table 44.1). The arterial phase (AP) begins within approximately 10–20 s following the contrast injection, and continues to 30–45 s, offering valuable information about the degree and pattern of the arterial supply; as it is a very rapid phase, it is often better assessed during a slow replay of the stored video. The portal venous phase (PVP) usually ends at 120 s. The late phase (LP), also known as the sinusoidal phase ends with the microbubble clearance from the blood (usually 4–6 min after injection) [8, 11]. Furthermore, some ultrasound contrast agents have an extended late phase, also called postvascular

Table 44.1 Vascular phases in CEUS of the liver postinjection (adapted from Claudon et al. [8])

Phase	Start	End
Arterial	10–20	30–45
Portal venous	30–45	120
Late	>120	Microbubble clearance (approx. 4–6 min)

phase or Kupffer phase, due to their ability to persist for several hours in both liver and spleen [12, 13].

The importance of the late and postvascular phases reside in their ability to provide important information, such as distinguishing between malignant and benign lesions. On CEUS, most benign lesions are characterized by either an iso- or hyperenhancing pattern, when compared to the adjacent normal liver parenchyma, while malignant lesions usually appear as hypoechoic [3].

Owing to the low incidence of adverse effects and to the excellent safety profile, the assessment of liver or kidney function is not necessary before beginning the CEUS examination. Before commencing the exploration, the patient should be placed in the best position for him and for the examiner. Usually, the left arm of the patient is chosen for injection, with a preference for the antecubital vein, for minimal interaction of the injector with the right-sided examiner. The venous line diameter should be large enough to avoid microbubble destruction during passage (minimum 20 G); a length as short as possible is also indicated. Central venous lines and portal system may be used, with a decrease in contrast arrival time. However, their use should be averted if a peripheral vein is accessible [8, 10].

It is recommended that the investigation starts with conventional B-mode ultrasonography and Doppler techniques. After identifying the targeted lesion, as well as the most appropriate scanning plane along the axis of the respiratory movements, the transducer should be held still, while switching the scanner to low MI contrast-specific imaging. For anatomical guidance purposes, a dual screen format (with both B-mode and contrast-enhanced image) can and should be used, especially in the case of small lesions. There are also devices that overlay conventional and CEUS images with different colour scales, instead of using the split-screen method [8, 10].

The contrast agent is administered in bolus, followed by 5–10 ml of saline solution 0.9%, and a stopwatch is started at the moment of injection [8]. Choosing the proper dose for the examination is very important, as elevated doses may lead to artefacts, especially during the early phases, such as: acoustic shadowing, over-enhancement of small structures or signal saturation. Low dosage may result in wash-out issues. If the wash-out occurs too early there are two possible scenarios: either the contrast dose was too low, or intrahepatic shunting is present, thus preventing a longer enhancement time. For a proper evaluation of difficult cases, a second contrast agent dose can be administered, with limited scanning during the first phases, in order to diminish the destruction of microbubbles. Choosing the right dose for the CEUS examination depends on the contrast agent that is utilized, device (including software and transducer), target lesion, as well as constitution and age of the patient. For example, if wanting to characterize a liver lesion using SonoVue, a dose of 2.4 ml is recommended [10].

Multiple injections of contrast agent may be necessary in case of insufficient data, if the initial dosage couldn't completely characterize the target lesion or in the presence of additional lesions that also require characterization. In these situations, there should be a variable waiting time before reinjecting, so that the bubbles from the previous injection may have enough time to disappear (usually 10–15 min for SonoVue and Definity). In order to evaluate the arterial enhancement of a wash-out region that is not visible on B-mode imaging, the examiner should have the contrast reinjected *before* the disappearance of the bubbles, so that visibility of the wash-out area may be maintained [10].

44.2 Characterization of Focal Liver Lesions

CEUS has demonstrated the ability to accurately differentiate between malignancies and benign focal liver lesions, having a high sensitivity and specificity. Its diagnosis capacity is comparable to that of contrast-enhanced computerized tomography (CECT) and contrast-enhanced magnetic resonance (CEMR) (Table 44.2) [3, 13, 14]. CEUS has also been reported to offer definitive diagnosis for focal liver lesions found on conventional ultrasonography. Moreover, CEUS is able to improve diagnostic accuracy for lesions considered to be inconclusive on CECT [15].

The Liver Imaging Reporting and Data System (LI-RADS) was created in order to standardize the CT and MRI data, for patients at risk for hepatocellular carcinoma (HCC) [16]. As CEUS has become more widely used in clinical practice, the American College of Radiology (ACR) developed a new means of lesion standardization—CEUS LI-RADS, which provides a diagnostic algorithm, classifying observations in the liver from LR-1 (definitely benign) to LR-5 (definitely HCC), by size and enhancement patterns (Table 44.3). The term "observation" defines a distinct region within the hepatic parenchyma, with imaging characteristics that are different from the adjacent liver parenchyma (either lesion/nodule or pseudolesion) [17].

LR-5 nodules should be treated as HCC, without performing biopsy and without further imaging, while for LR-4 nodules biopsy is typically necessary; if neither biopsy, nor

Table 44.2 Sensibility and specificity of CT, MRI, CEUS (adapted from [3, 13, 14])

	CT	MRI	CEUS
Sensibility	80%	90%	80%
Specificity	93%	79%	100%

Table 44.3 CEUS diagnostic table in LI-RADS v2017

Arterial phase hyperenhancement (APHE)	No APHE		APHE (not rim or peripheral globular discontinous enhancement)	
Nodule size (mm)	<20	≥20	<10	≥10
No wash-out of any type	CEUS LR-3	CEUS LR-3	CEUS LR-3	CEUS LR-4
Late and mild wash-out	CEUS LR-3	CEUS LR-4	CEUS LR-4	CEUS LR-5

Table 44.4 CEUS and 2D ultrasonographic features in most frequent benign liver lesions (adapted from Badea and Ioanitescu [18])

Tumor	Arterial phase	Portal phase	Delayed phase	2D feature
Cyst	No uptake	No uptake	No uptake	Transsonic
Hemangioma	"Ring-like" peripheral uptake	Centripetal enhancement resembling "buds"	Complete uptake	Hyperechoic Well-defined Compressibility "Mirror" effect
Focal nodular hyperplasia	Central enhancement with a "spoked wheel" distribution of the CA	Complete enhancement with an isoechoic appearance compared with liver parenchyma	Isoechoic aspect when compared with the liver parenchyma	Echoic scar in the centre of the lesion Arterial signal in the centre of the tumor
Adenoma	Inhomogeneous uptake	Discrete wash-out Iso or hypoechoic aspect compared to liver parenchyma	Discrete wash-out Iso or hypoechoic aspect compared to liver parenchyma	Hypoechoic nodule Non-cirrhotic liver

specific therapy is performed immediately, imaging follow-up is required. The LR-3 lesions are considered to have intermediated probability of malignancy and can be further investigated using alternative imagistic methods, but may require biopsy in some cases (multidisciplinary discussion is needed). LR-M define nodules that are probably or definitely malignant (and can be either HCC, intrahepatic cholangiocarcinoma or metastases), being characterized by a rim arterial phase hyperenhancement, early wash-out (in less than 60 s) or marked wash-out. These lesions usually stand in need for biopsy. LR-NC is the term used if the observation is not categorizable. The term LR-TIV (tumor in vein) is used when certain enhancement is observed within the portal or hepatic vein, during the arterial phase, followed by washout [7, 17].

44.2.1 Benign Liver Lesions

Not all benign liver masses have characteristic features, when examined by CEUS. However, some of the lesions (such as hemangiomas, hepatocellular adenomas, focal nodular hyperplasia or cysts) develop specific circulatory patterns, that allow a more rapid recognition by the investigator (Table 44.4).

44.2.1.1 Hemangioma

Hemangiomas are the most frequently encountered benign liver lesions. Being asymptomatic, they are usually discovered incidentally during conventional ultrasonography, especially within the female population. Usually, the conventional ultrasonography examination is able to clearly characterize and diagnose the lesion as hemangioma, with no need for additional exploration. However, there are several situations when CEUS is needed, like in the presence of severe steatosis, chemotherapic treatment or for extremely large hemangiomas [18].

In CEUS examination, hemangiomas are typically characterized by nodular peripheral enhancement during arterial phase, with centripetal progression during portal venous and late phases, until partial or complete filling is observed. The filling occurs more rapidly in smaller lesions (Fig. 44.1).

One particular situation is the encounter of high flow (or shunt) hemangiomas, which can be described by a rapid homogeneous hyperenhancement in the arterial phase, thus leading to a possible diagnosis confusion with focal nodular hyperplasia (FNH), or even with hepatocellular adenomas or carcinomas. Thrombosed hemangiomas can also be difficult to differentiate from malignant lesions, since the lack of enhancement in the thrombosed areas may be misread as wash out [10].

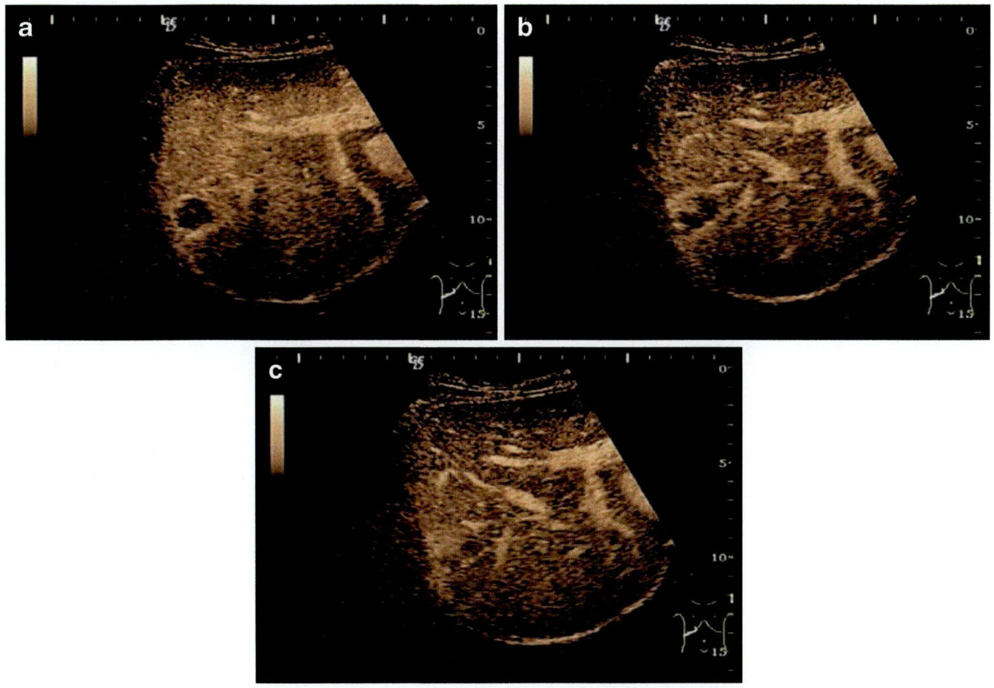

Fig. 44.1 CEUS examination of liver hemangioma: (**a**) arterial phase reveals well-defined peripheral enhancement; (**b**) centripetal progression of the contrast; (**c**) complete enhancement of the lesion

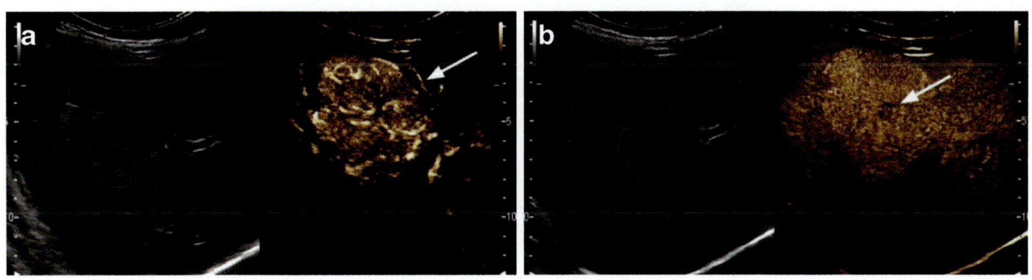

Fig. 44.2 CEUS examination of focal nodular hyperplasia: (**a**) spoked wheel appearance; (**b**) sustained enhancement, revealing a central scar, during the late phase

44.2.1.2 Focal Nodular Hyperplasia

Focal nodular hyperplasia (FNH) is the second most common benign tumor of the liver, after hemangioma. It is also more frequently encountered in women, usually asymptomatic and discovered incidentally. An important anatomic particularity of focal nodular hyperplasia is the abundant portal circulatory bed.

On CEUS, focal nodular hyperplasia lesions exhibit a central "spoked wheel" shaped hyperenhancement during early arterial phase (accelerated uptake in the middle of the mass, with a radial distribution), that rapidly becomes homogeneous in the late arterial phase. They maintain the hyperenhancing pattern or can become isoenhancing during portal venous and late phases and may present with a hypoechoic central area, in the late phase [10, 19] (Fig. 44.2).

If the lesion is small, switching to color Doppler exploration may prove itself to be a valuable solution, since the remaining microspheres can be used to improve the Doppler effect, in order to obtain a better visualization of the typical "spoked wheel" image.

If using Sonazoid, the postvascular phase describes either iso- or hyperenhancement [10].

44.2.1.3 Hepatocellular Adenoma

Hepatocellular adenoma (HCA), a benign estrogen-dependent focal lesion, is characterized by the ability to become very large in size, thus possibly leading to intratumoral bleeding. The tumor also has a 5% risk of malignant transformation. There are no portal vessels within its structure, only arteries.

On CEUS, they are characterized by arterial hyperenhancement (either homogeneous or heterogeneous, when intratumoral bleeding is present). The enhancement pattern begins in the peripheral region of the tumoral mass, followed by a very rapid centripetal filling, in the opposite direction to that seen in FNH. However, this feature is not pathognomonic for hepatocellular adenomas, as it can also be found in hepatocellular carcinoma or in metastatic lesions. At the beginning of the portal venous phase, the mass transitions from hyper- to isoenhanced [10, 19].

44.2.1.4 Focal Fatty Change

Both focal fat infiltration and fatty sparing can have nodular appearance, thus mimicking the aspect of focal liver masses in conventional ultrasonography. Therefore, CEUS examination is vital for differential diagnosis, showing homogeneous enhancement similar to that of the surrounding liver parenchyma during all phases. Moreover, visualization of normal portal veins within the lesion confirms its benign character [10, 20].

44.2.1.5 Liver Abscess

Liver abscess is a potentially lethal condition, most often caused by bacteria, that requires immediate recognition, in order to ensure adequate therapeutic measures. In conventional ultrasonography, liver abscesses may appear as hypoechoic masses with contorted wall and internal septa, but for a rapid positive diagnosis, a contrast-enhance ultrasonography is required. There are several types of enhancement patterns, when describing a liver abscess by using CEUS. The most common features include rim enhancement in the arterial phase (with the absence of central enhancement, due to perilesional hyperemia), honeycomb appearance (due to the enhancement of the septa, with variable areas of no uptake), no enhancement in the liquid areas, as well as venous hypoenhancement. Sometimes, the surrounding edema can lead to the presence of a hypoenhanced peripheral region [10, 21].

44.2.1.6 Liver Cyst

Liver cysts can be defined as serous collections delimited by cuboidal epithelium. Hepatic cystic lesions, which usually tend to remain asymptomatic, are found as a mere coincidence on abdominal imaging techniques. In spite of their mostly benign appearance, identification of potentially harmful cysts (such as echinococcosis, cystadenoma and cystadenocarcinoma) is vital [22].

Simple cysts are nonenhancing on CEUS in all vascular phases [10] (Fig. 44.3). Complex cysts show septal and nodular enhancement in the arterial phase, followed by hypoenhancement in the portal phase.

44.2.1.7 Other Benign Liver Lesions

Hepatic angiomyolipoma represents a rare benign mesenchymal tumor, describing heterogeneous echogenicity on conventional ultrasound. CEUS exploration reveals arterial hyperenhancement [10].

Cholangiocellular adenoma (CCA or bile duct adenoma) is a rarely encountered lesion, usually presenting as a small mass (90% of them have less than 1 cm in diameter). On CEUS, cholangiocellular adenomas demonstrate strong arterial enhancement, as well as an early wash out in the portal and late phases, due to the lack of portal veins [10].

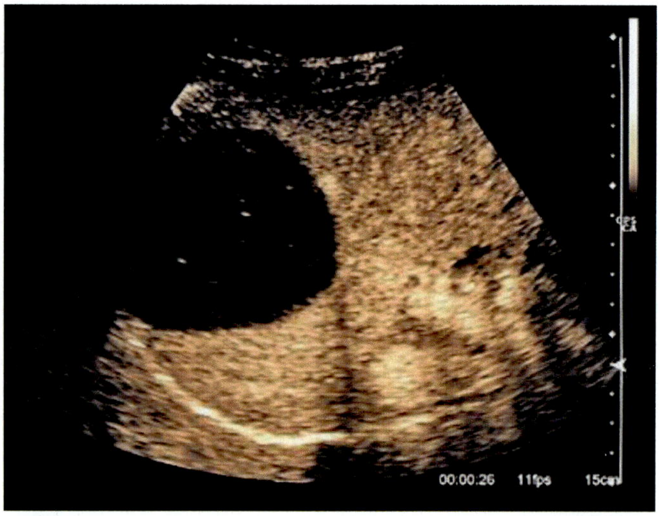

Fig. 44.3 CEUS examination of a cystic lesion within the liver, showing nonenhancing pattern

Hepatic hematoma, most commonly caused by blunt abdominal trauma, show no enhancement during all CEUS phases.

44.2.2 Malignant Liver Lesions

On CEUS exploration, malignancies are usually characterized by hypoenhancement during the late and postvascular phases, corresponding to the wash out of the contrast agent (Table 44.5).

44.2.2.1 Hepatocellular Carcinoma

Hepatocellular carcinoma is known to be the most frequent primary tumor of the liver. In more than 80% of the cases, HCC appears on a cirrhotic liver, due to a multistep pathway that begins with the process of hepatic fibrosis and reorganization. As a consequence of liver reorganization, variable-sized nodules start to develop, involving the whole liver parenchyma, transforming sequentially into dysplastic nodule and further into hepatocellular carcinoma [10, 18]. During this transformation process, a decrease in normal arterial and portal circulation occurs and, at the same time, there is a progressive increase in the arterial blood supply due to neo-angiogenetic tumor vessels. This explains the hyperenhancement pattern that characterizes the arterial phase of CEUS in HCC [10].

Apart from the changes in vascularity, the hepatocellular carcinomas tend to lack reticuloendothelial (Kupffer) cells. This particular feature explains the enhancement defect of HCC in the postvascular phase of CEUS. Also, the probability of a nodule to be HCC highly depends on its size: those having less than 1 cm are rarely malignant [10].

Table 44.5 CEUS and 2D ultrasonographic features of malignant liver masses (adapted from Badea and Ioanitescu [18])

Tumor	Arterial phase	Portal venous phase	Late phase	"Grey scale" ultrasound (2D)
Hepatocellular carcinoma	Intense enhancement Hyperechoic aspect	Moderate/intense wash-out Hypoechoic or isoechoic aspect	Moderate/intense wash-out Hypoechoic aspect	Solid tumor Inhomogeneous structure "Basket-like" appearance of the CFM vascular pattern Arterialized circulation Portal invasion
Cholangiocarcinoma	Moderate, inhomogeneous uptake Hyperechoic/isoechoic aspect	Moderate wash-out Hypoechoic aspect	Moderate or intense wash-out Hypoechoic aspect	Solid tumor located in the hilum or subcapsulary Bile ducts dilations oriented towards the tumor
Hypovascular metastases	Peripheral uptake Hypoechoic aspect	Peripheral wash-out Hypoechoic aspect	Intense wash-out Hypoechoic aspect	Multiple, solid masses Involvement of all liver lobes
Hypervascular metastases	Intense uptake Hyperechoic aspect	Moderate wash-out Hypoechoic aspect	Intense wash-out Hypoechoic aspect	

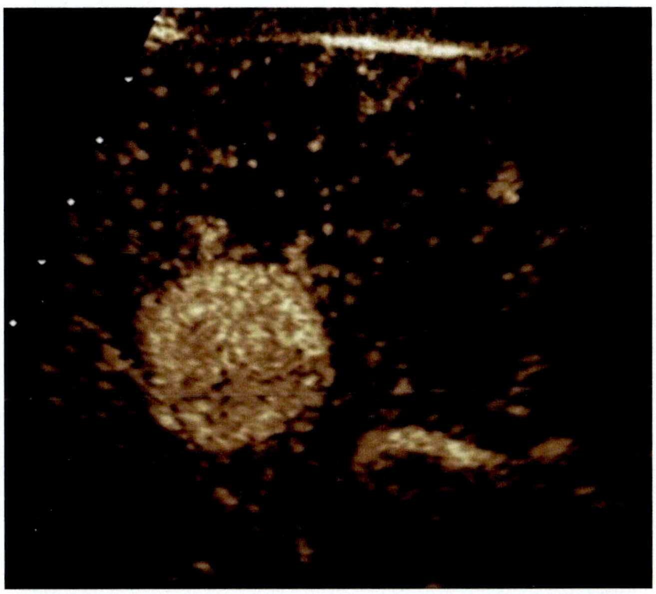

Fig. 44.4 CEUS examination of hepatocellular carcinoma during arterial phase, showing hyperenhancement

The key element for CEUS diagnosis of HCC is represented by the hyperenhancement occurring in the arterial phase and wash out in the late phase. This enhancing pattern is associated with the presence of HCC in more than 97% of the cases. The remaining 1–3% of cases consist of peripheral cholangiocarcinoma and hepatic lymphoma.

Typical for HCC is the homogeneity and intensity that depict the arterial hyperenhancement (Fig. 44.4). However, HCC nodules may appear inhomogeneous if larger than 5 cm (due to the presence of necrotic areas). Rim enhancement is not considered a typical feature of HCC.

Contrast wash-out is more often observed in hepatocellular carcinomas with lower differentiation degrees, while well-differentiated HCCs tend to be isoechoic in the late phase. Comparing to other malignant tumors, the late phase hypoenhancement is usually less obvious in HCC and the wash out process starts later in HCC (after about 60 s post injection). Furthermore, in approximately a quarter of the cases, the wash-out begins after 180 s. This explains the importance of observing the nodules in cirrhotic patients until very late (>4 min), in order to enhance sensitivity for the diagnosis of HCC. Poorly differentiated HCC may show early wash out (<60 s). Arterial hyperenhancement, but with no following wash-out, also raises the suspicion of a HCC nodule (well-differentiated variants may show this pattern) [10].

If CEUS is inconclusive, further imagistic investigation must be performed (CT or MRI) and, in the case their results are ambiguous as well, biopsy is required. If the biopsy turns out as negative, the hepatic nodule should be followed up every 3 months (for at least 2 years) and, if changes in size or enhancement pattern are noted, imagistic investigations should be continued [10].

44.2.2.2 Cholangiocarcinoma

Cholangiocarcinoma is a relatively rare primary malignant tumor, representing 3–7% of all hepatic malignancies. It usually appears on a non-cirrhotic liver, originating in the small biliary ducts, but its development may be induced by several conditions, such as: primary sclerosing cholangitis, choledochal cysts, Caroli disease, intrahepatic biliary lithiasis.

During the arterial phase of CEUS, cholangiocarcinomas may present various types of patterns, but all characterize by late phase wash-out [10–18].

44.2.2.3 Liver Metastases

The liver is the second most frequent localization for secondary malignancies, most of them originating in the digestive tract, lungs, breast and head of the pancreas [18]. CEUS has an important role in detecting and characterizing hepatic metastases smaller than 10 mm in diameter, playing an important part when assessing the efficacy of oncologic treatment.

During the arterial phase of CEUS, liver metastases may appear as either hypo- or hyperenhancing masses. When hypervascular, hepatic metastatic lesions are associated with carcinoid tumors, melanomas, sarcomas, thyroid or renal cancers.

The diagnosis of liver metastases however relies on revealing a hypoenhancement pattern, during the portal venous and late phases, with very few exceptions (Fig. 44.5). The metastatic lesions usually have an early and marked wash-out, that begins within the portal venous phase. This pattern explains their appearance as punched-out "black foci" against the background of the normal parenchyma. Large vessels may sometimes be visible, presenting as enhancing lines. The late phase of CEUS allows even the detection of very small metastatic lesions, that remained hidden during conventional ultrasonography [10].

44.2.2.4 Lymphoma

Lymphomas of the liver usually have variable arterial enhancement, but they show typical wash-out during the portal venous and late phases, predictive of malignancy [10].

44.3 Characterization of Portal Vein Thrombosis

Portal vein thrombosis (PVT) is characterized by the complete or incomplete obstruction of the portal vein lumen, due to the development of solid material, that may appear within any portion of the vein. In evolution, the normal vascular structure can be replaced by the presence of multiple tortuous neo-formation vessels, characterized by a hepatopetal flow, a condition that can be described by the term "cavernomatous transformation" or "cavernoma". The thrombotic process can either evolve in the intra- or extrahepatic tract and may involve the superior mesenteric vein and/or the splenic vein [23].

Portal vein thrombosis may be bland (appositional), represented by a simple clot within the vein, or malignant, which usually appears as a complication of hepatocellular carcinomas [10].

When explored by CEUS, the bland thrombus shows no signs of enhancement and can be described as a gap within the enhancing liver parenchyma, during all phases (Fig. 44.6). A malignant thrombus, however, shows the

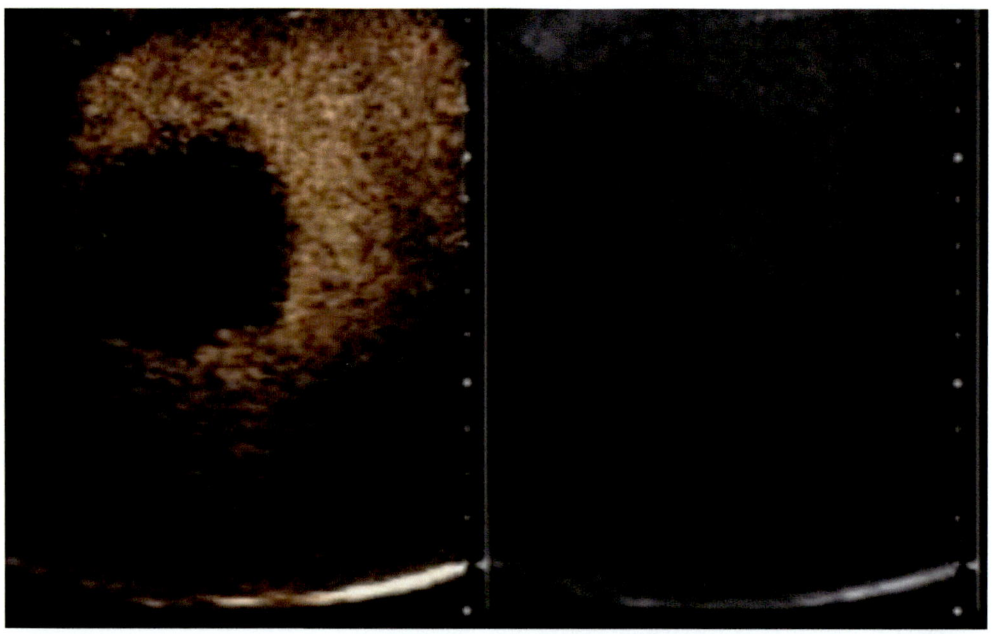

Fig. 44.5 CEUS examination of liver metastasis showing washout in the portal phase

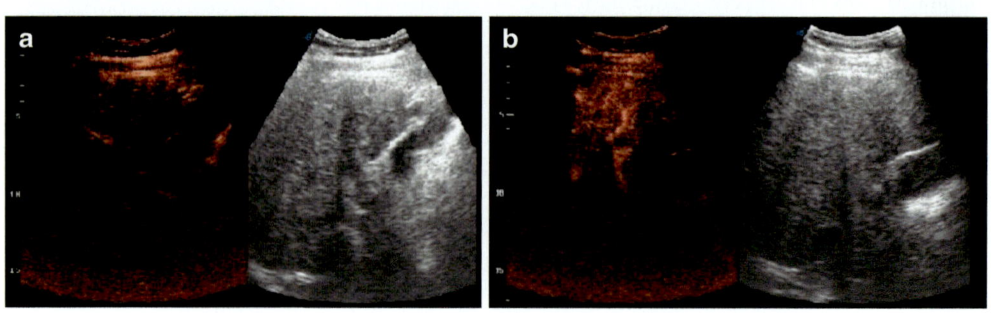

Fig. 44.6 CEUS examination of the liver showing benign portal vein thrombosis (no enhancement of the thrombus in the arterial phase)

same enhancement pattern as the source tumor, including rapid hyperenhancement in the arterial phase. The wash-out usually occurs rapidly, although in some cases slow wash-out during the portal venous phase can be described. The thrombotic material should be examined during the wash-in process of the contrast agent. In tumoral thrombi, the vascularization should parallel the arrival of the microspheres in the hepatic artery [10].

The primary tumor from which the thrombus originated may remain undetectable on ultrasound, even when using CEUS. In these cases, sweeping through the liver may help the investigator in the identification of the lesion.

Self Study

Questions

1. **Which statement is true:**
   (a) The arterial phase of CEUS lasts from the first 10 s to 30–45 s.
   (b) The portal phase of CEUS last from 30–45 s to 120 s.
   (c) The late phase of CEUS last from 120 s to 4–6 min, until the gas bubbles are fully eliminated.
   (d) CEUS should not be performed in patients with renal impairment.
2. **Which statement is true:**
   (a) Hepatocellular carcinoma appears hyperenhanced in the arterial phase of CEUS.
   (b) Malignant thrombus in the portal vein appears hyperenhanced in the arterial phase of CEUS.
   (c) Liver metastases typically have rapid wash-out and appear hypoenhanced in the portal phase.
   (d) Liver hemangiomas have nodular peripheral enhancement during arterial phase, with centripetal progression during portal venous and late phases.

Answers

1. Which statement is true:
   (a) CORRECT
   (b) CORRECT
   (c) CORRECT
   (d) FALSE
2. Which statement is true:
   (a) CORRECT
   (b) CORRECT
   (c) CORRECT
   (d) CORRECT

References

1. Wilson SR, Greenbaum LD, Goldberg BB. Contrast-enhanced ultrasound: what is the evidence and what are the obstacles? Am J Roentgenol. 2009;193:55–60. https://doi.org/10.2214/AJR.09.2553.
2. Jo PC, Jang HJ, Burns PN, Burak KW, Kim TK, Wilson SR. Integration of contrast-enhanced US into a multimodality approach to imaging of nodules in a cirrhotic liver: how I do it. Radiology. 2017;282(2):317–31.
3. Chung YE, Kim KW. Contrast-enhanced ultrasonography: advance and current status in abdominal imaging. Ultrasonography. 2014;34:3–18.
4. SonoVue. Assessment Report. European Medicines Agency; 2017.
5. Park JH, et al. Contrast-enhanced US with Perfluorobutane (Sonazoid) used as a surveillance test for hepatocellular carcinoma (HCC) in cirrhosis (SCAN): an exploratory cross-sectional study for a diagnostic trial. BMC Cancer. 2017;17(1):279. https://doi.org/10.1186/s12885-017-3267-8.
6. Zhang XY, et al. Contrast-enhanced ultrasound: improving the preoperative staging of hepatocellular carcinoma and guiding individual treatment. World J Gastroenterol. 2014;20(35):12628–36.
7. Kim TK, et al. Contrast-enhanced ultrasound (CEUS) liver imaging reporting and data system (LI-RADS) 2017 - a review of important differences compared to the CT/MRI system. Clin Mol Hepatol. 2017;23(4):280–9.
8. Claudon M, Dietrich CF, et al. Guidelines and good clinical practice recommendations for contrast enhanced ultrasound (CEUS) in the liver – update 2012 a WFUMB-EFSUMB initiative in cooperation with representatives of AFSUMB, AIUM, ASUM, FLAUS and ICUS. Ultraschall in Med. 2013;34:11–29.
9. ter Haar G. Safety and bio-effects of ultrasound contrast agents. Med Biol Eng Comput. 2009;47:893–900.
10. Dietrich CF, Averkiou M, Nielsen MB, et al. How to perform contrast-enhanced ultrasound (CEUS). Ultrasound Int Open. 2018;4(1):E2–E15.
11. Ferraioli G, Franca Meloni M. Contrast-enhanced ultrasonography of the liver using SonoVue. Ultrasonography. 2018;37(1):25–35. https://doi.org/10.14366/usg.17037.
12. Yanagisawa K, Moriyasu F, Miyahara T, et al. Phagocytosis of ultrasound contrast agent microbubbles by Kupffer cells. Ultrasound Med Biol. 2007;33:318–25.
13. Friedrich-Rust M, Klopffleisch T, Nierhoff J, Herrmann E, Vermehren J, Schneider MD, et al. Contrast-enhanced ultrasound for the differentiation of benign and malignant focal liver lesions: a metaanalysis. Liver Int. 2013;33:739–55.
14. Xie L, Guang Y, Ding H, Cai A, Huang Y. Diagnostic value of contrast-enhanced ultrasound, computed tomography and magnetic resonance imaging for focal liver lesions: a meta-analysis. Ultrasound Med Biol. 2011;37:854–61.
15. Quaia E, De Paoli L, Angileri R, Cabibbo B, Cova MA. Indeterminate solid hepatic lesions identified on non-diagnostic contrast-enhanced computed tomography: assessment of the additional diagnostic value of contrast-enhanced ultrasound in the noncirrhotic liver. Eur J Radiol. 2014;83:456–62.
16. Chernyak V, Santillan CS, Papadatos D, Sirlin CB. LI-RADS(R) algorithm: CT and MRI. Abdom Radiol. 2018;43(1):111–26.
17. Piscaglia F, Wilson SR, Lyshchik A, Cosgrove D, Dietrich CF, Jang HJ, et al. American College of Radiology contrast enhanced ultrasound liver imaging reporting and data system (CEUS LI-RADS) for the diagnosis of hepatocellular carcinoma: a pictorial essay. Ultraschall Med. 2017;38:320–4.

18. Badea R, Ioanitescu S. Contrast-enhanced ultrasonography (CEUS) of liver masses—principles, clinical applications, drawbacks. Liver Tumors Epidemiol Diagn Prev Treat. 2013; https://doi.org/10.5772/55500.
19. Thakur S, Jhobta A, Dhiman DS, Sood RG, Chauhan A, Thakur CS. Role of contrast enhanced ultrasound in characterization of focal liver lesions. Egyptian J Radiol Nucl Med. 2014;45:7–17.
20. Kim TK, Jang HJ. Contrast-enhanced ultrasound in the diagnosis of nodules in liver cirrhosis. World J Gastroenterol. 2014;20(13):3590–6.
21. Kunze G, Staritz M, Köhler M. Contrast-enhanced ultrasound in different stages of pyogenic liver abscess. Ultrasound Med Biol. 2015;41:952–9.
22. Lantinga MA, Gevers TJ, Drenth JP. Evaluation of hepatic cystic lesions. World J Gastroenterol. 2013;19(23):3543–54.
23. Margini C, Berzigotti A, et al. Portal vein thrombosis: the role of imaging in the clinical setting. Dig Liver Dis. 2017;49(2):113–20.

Ultrasound Elastography

45

Woo Kyoung Jeong

Key Concepts

- Ultrasound elastography is useful to estimate parenchymal stiffness of internal organs such as the liver.
- There are several representative methods of ultrasound elastography: transient elastography, point shear wave elastography, and 2D shear wave elastography.
- Ultrasound elastography is generally used for estimation of the hepatic fibrosis stage in chronic liver diseases including viral hepatitis and non-alcoholic fatty liver disease and the severity of portal hypertension in cirrhosis.
- There are remaining issues about ultrasound elastography: limitation of ultrasound beam penetration, the unit of elasticity, and comparability of data between the different shear wave technologies.
- Ultrasound elastography is still emerging for a non-invasive diagnostic tool for diffuse liver disease because of its economic merit and safety. Especially it can be used as a monitoring tool for chronic liver disease patients.

45.1 Introduction

Ultrasound elastography (USE) is not only useful to discriminate a malignant tissue in the breast [1] and thyroid [2], but also to estimate parenchymal fibrosis of the liver [3]. In order to diagnose the stage of hepatic fibrosis, the patient with chronic hepatitis should have undergone liver biopsy before development of transient elastography (TE), a kind of USE. However, liver biopsy has intrinsic limitations such as a risk of bleeding, expensiveness, and sampling error caused by a small specimen [4]. During a recent decade, various types of USE have been developed: TE is a frontier of non-invasive method to diagnose liver fibrosis; several different methods of USE including acoustic radiation force impulse (ARFI) imaging, point shear wave elastography (pSWE), and two dimensional shear wave elastography (2D-SWE), are following [3, 5, 6]. The clinical indication of USE initiated from diagnosis of liver fibrosis in hepatitis C patients [7], and expanded into predicting liver-related complications, development of HCC, clinical decompensation of the patients, and patients' survival [8, 9].

In this chapter, we addressed the principle of USE including basic technique of elastography, clinical use of USE including diagnostic and prognostic roles, emerging issues during liver stiffness measurement including standard technique and quality criteria of USE, and practically important things to know to avoid its limitation.

45.2 Basic Technology of Ultrasound Elastography

Elastography is a method to evaluate the displacement of tissue (deformation) using imaging modalities, such as ultrasonography and magnetic resonance imaging [10]. Therefore, in order to know the elasticity, it is necessary to apply a force that can be deformed. In the case of the liver, it is located in a place where it is difficult to directly apply force. For this reason, specific equipment using ultrasound or MRI was developed to reveal the elasticity of the deep tissues such as the liver and to visualize the difference in elasticity.

There are several elastographic techniques using ultrasonography: displacement or strain imaging, shear wave speed measurement, and shear wave speed imaging [5] (Table 45.1). Strain imaging consists of strain elastography and ARFI imaging, and it is also introduced as a hepatic elastography. However, most of hepatic elastography shows quantitative results using shear wave speed measurement or mapping (shear wave speed imaging), and there are three representa-

W. K. Jeong (✉)
Department of Radiology and Center for Imaging Science, Samsung Medical Center, Sungkyunkwan University School of Medicine, Seoul, South Korea

F. Radu-Ionita et al. (eds.), *Liver Diseases*, https://doi.org/10.1007/978-3-030-24432-3_45

Table 45.1 Classification of ultrasound elastography

Classification	Method	Type of force	Applied force	Measured property	Qualitative or quantitative	Commercial implementation
Strain imaging	Strain elastography	Quasi-static	Mechanical	Strain/strain rate	Qualitative	Many vendors
	ARFI imaging		Focused acoustic beam	Displacement on imaging	Qualitative	Siemens
SWS measurement	TE		Mechanical	SWS	Quantitative	Echosens
	pSWE		Focused acoustic beam	SWS	Quantitative	Siemens Philips Hitachi-Aloka Samsung
SWS imaging	2D-SWE		Focused acoustic beam	SWS	Qualitative/ quantitative	Siemens Toshiba Philips Mindray Zonare GE Supersonic imagine

2D-SWE two dimensional-shear wave elastography, *ARFI* acoustic radiation force impulse, *pSWE* point shear wave elastography, *SWS* shear wave speed, *TE* transient elastography

tive shear wave methods: transient elastography (TE), point shear wave elastography (pSWE), and 2D- and 3D-shear wave elastography (SWE) (Fig. 45.1).

Shear wave technique is generally used for hepatic elastography including transient elastography and SWE. Shear deformation is caused by forces applied across the body surface. It will propagate transiently as shear waves [5]. The shear wave occurs in an elastic medium when it is subject to periodic shear effect, which is defined as morphological change generated by a pair of equal forces acting in opposite directions along two sides of the layer. Shear waves which propagate serially into adjacent tissue and make it deformed can be observed by ultrasound technique such as Doppler, and shear modulus to calculate by using the function between the shear wave velocity and the elasticity (Fig. 45.2).

45.2.1 Transient Elastography

TE, which is most used in clinical practice, is a method of measuring the elasticity by measuring the shear wave velocity after applying a mechanical vibrator. The shear wave velocity is measured by the amplitude modulation-mode ultrasound probe mounted on the axis of the vibrator. The stiffer the liver is, such as advanced fibrosis, the faster the shear waves are. The range of observation in TE is between 25 and 65 mm using the standard (M-) probe. To overcome the limitation of the obese, a new (XL-) probe with 35–75 mm of observational range was developed. It should be paid attention that measured stiffness on XL probe is usually lower than that on M probe.

45.2.2 Point SWE

Point SWE applies force using focused acoustic impulse instead of mechanical vibrator and then measure shear wave velocity like TE. These methods have the advantage of being integrated in conventional ultrasonography system. It means that the operator can obtain the elasticity adding to anatomic information using conventional ultrasonography. Unlike TE, the operator can position the region of interest (ROI) for measuring elasticity on the ultrasonogram, avoiding from a large vessel and gallbladder.

45.2.3 2D-SWE

Basically, the principle of 2D-SWE is very similar to pSWE; however, it enables to calculate the shear wave speed in large ROI, and display it with a color map which shows distribution of elasticity of the target tissue. In 2D-SWE, multiple, high-frequency (hundreds of Hz) of shear waves induced by repeated focused acoustic impulse make a single or real-time large ROI possible.

45.2.4 Strain Elastography

Strain elastography, which is mainly used in superficial organs such as the breast or thyroid, is a method of measuring the elastic ratio after applying an intrinsic force such as the heartbeat, and is less utilized than the shear wave methods.

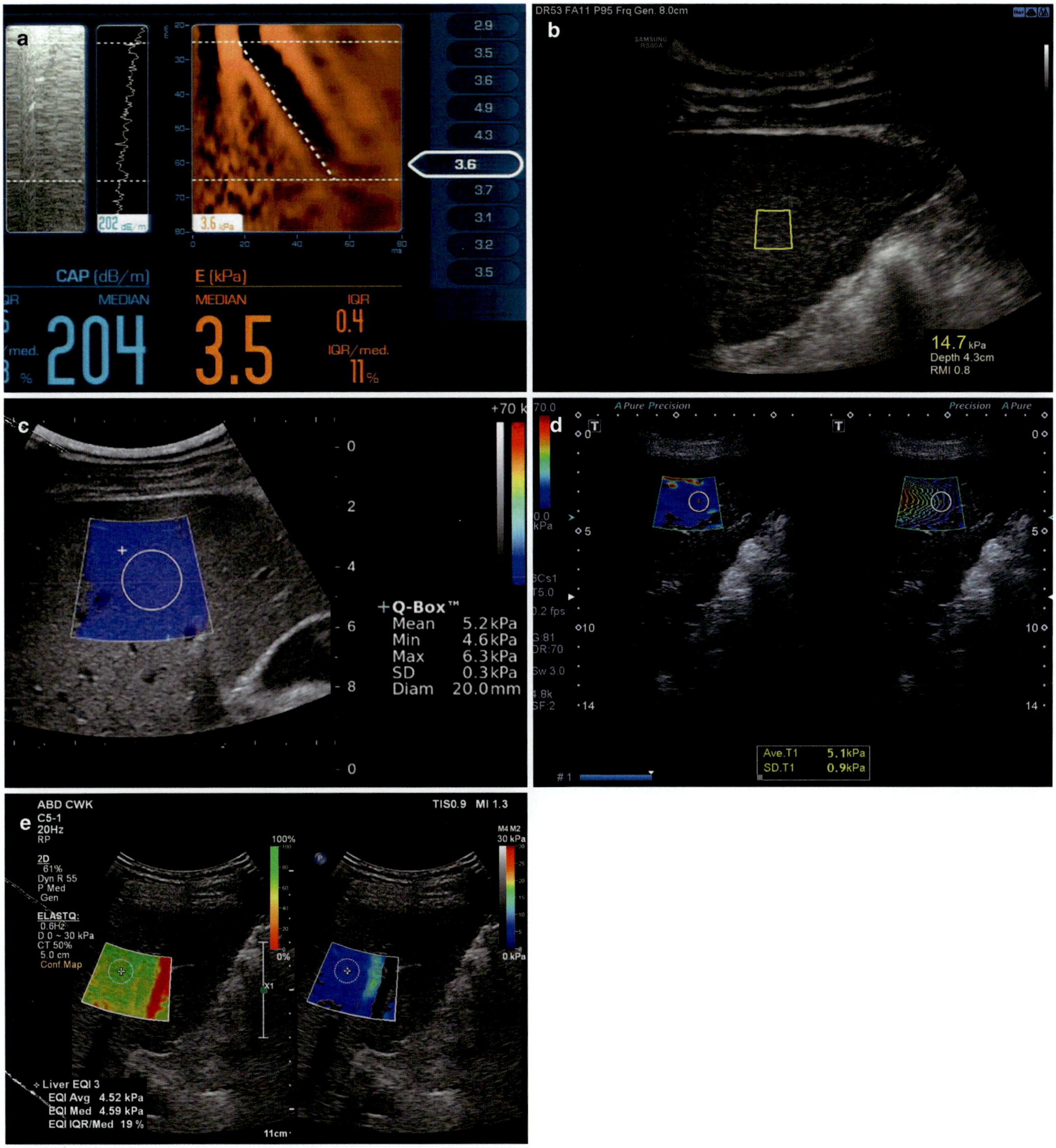

Fig. 45.1 Various types of US elastography. Transient elastography (Echosens) (**a**); Point shear wave elastography (pSWE; Samsung Medison) (**b**); two dimensional shear wave elastography. Supersonic Imagine (**c**); Canon Medical (**d**); and Philips Healthcare (**e**)

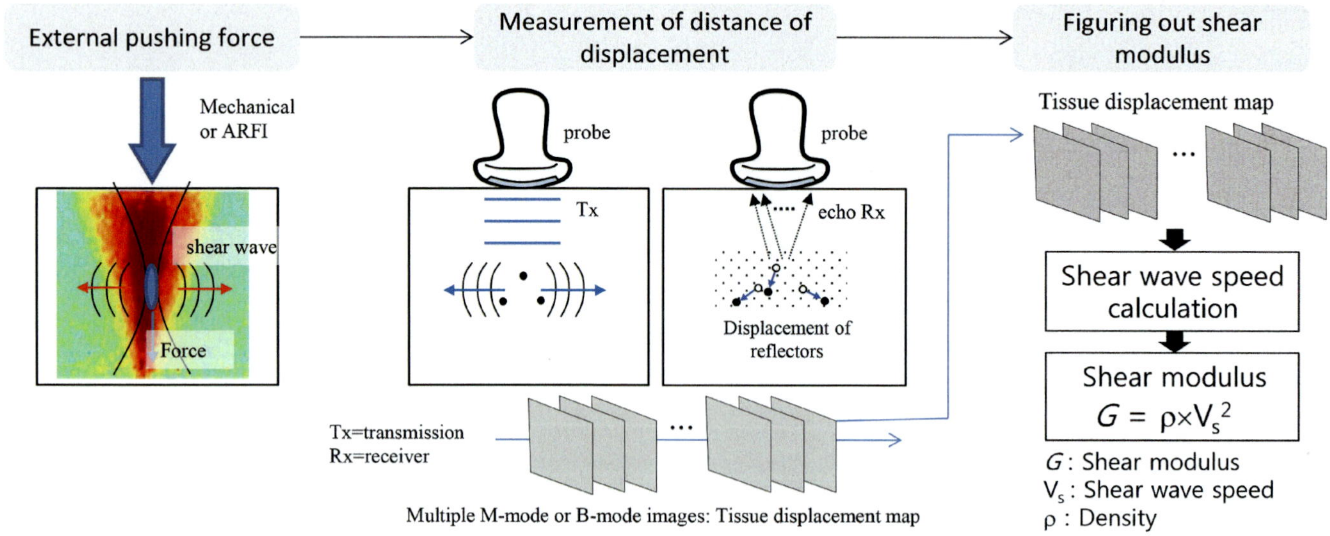

Fig. 45.2 Three steps of making shear wave elastography. USE is divided three steps: making shear wave by pushing pulse; estimating shear wave velocity observed from tissue displacement by propagation of shear wave; figuring out elastic modulus from shear wave velocity. (Modified and reprinted from Jeong et al. [3] with permission from Korean Society of Ultrasound in Medicine)

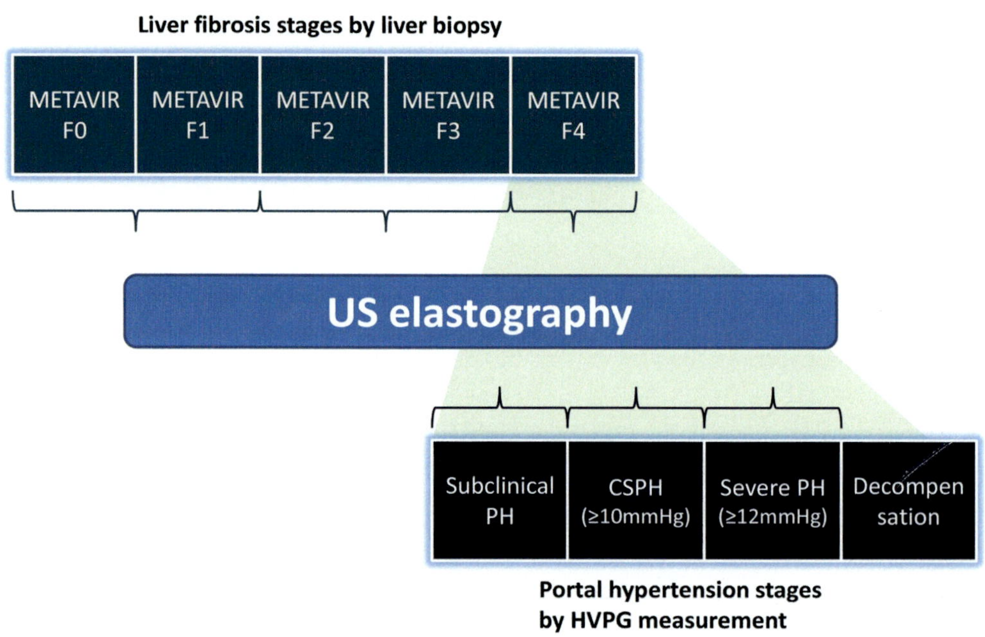

Fig. 45.3 Practical usefulness of US elastography. USE is generally used for two parts of clinical practices: estimation of the hepatic fibrosis in the chronic liver diseases and estimation of the severity of portal hypertension. USE cannot only discriminate no fibrosis, significant fibrosis for observation of cirrhosis development, and overt cirrhosis, but also subclinical portal hypertension, clinically significant portal hypertension (CSPH), and severe portal hypertension instead of liver biopsy and HVPG measurement

45.3 Clinical Studies of Ultrasound Elastography

Looking at the published researches, the USE is generally used for two parts of clinical practices: estimation of the hepatic fibrosis in the chronic liver diseases and estimation of the severity of portal hypertension (Fig. 45.3).

There are several meta-analyses of diagnostic performance of TE to estimate hepatic fibrosis (Table 45.2) [11–16]. According to these papers, the estimated cut-off values for significant fibrosis (≥F2 on METAVIR score system) were suggested of 7.0–7.65 kPa with a sensitivity of 78–84% and specificity of 78–80%. In the case of cirrhosis (F4 on METAVIR score system), the results of TE showed a cut-off of 11.3–15.3 kPa with a sensitivity of 80–84.6% and specificity of 81.5–90%. In terms of pSWE and 2D-SWE, the diagnostic performance was also comparable to that of TE. The areas under the curves for diagnosis of significant fibrosis and cirrhosis were 0.85–0.87 and 0.91–0.94, respectively. In addition, these meta-analyses showed that TE could be used as a good screening test for cirrhosis, but could not be used for accurately diagnosing less serious fibrotic stages. According to the underlying diseases, the hepatic stiffness could be different; the value of liver stiffness measurement in hepatitis B virus (HBV) patients could be lower than that of hepatitis C virus (HCV) because HBV-associated liver cirrhosis includes large cirrhotic nodules

Table 45.2 Summary of meta-analyses: pooled diagnostic performance of US elastography for significant fibrosis (F2) and cirrhosis (F4)

Author	Modality	Number of studies	Underlying diseases	Fibrosis stage ≥F2				Fibrosis stage ≥F4			
				Cut-off (kPa)	AUC	Sn	Sp	Cut-off (kPa)	AUC	Sn	Sp
Friedrich-Rust et al. [16]	TE	50	Variable	7.65	0.84			13.01	0.94		
Chon et al. [14]	TE	18	CHB	7.0		78	80	11.7		84.6	81.5
Tsochatzis et al. [15]	TE	14	CHC	7.6		78	80	15.3		83	90
		6	CHB	7.0		84	78	11.3		80	89
Friedrich-Rust et al. [13]	ARFI/Point SWE	8	Variable	1.34*	0.87	79	85	1.80*	0.91	92	86
Bota et al. [12]	ARFI/Point SWE	13	Variable	1.30*	0.85	74	83	1.80*	0.93	87	87
Jiang et al. [11]	2D-SWE	13	Variable		0.87	84	83		0.94	89	88

Reprinted from Park et al. [8] with permission from Korean Association of Study of Liver

2D-SWE two dimensional shear wave elastography, *ARFI* acoustic radiation force impulse, *AUC* area under curve, *CHB* chronic hepatitis B, *CHC* chronic hepatitis C, *Sn* sensitivity, *Sp* specificity, *TE* transient elastography

*The unit of values is m/sec

with relatively sparse fibrotic bands. On the contrary, increased liver stiffness value in the patients with acute exacerbation on chronic hepatitis with HBV infection should be carefully interpreted because alanine aminotransferase (ALT) flares can lead to overestimate the fibrosis grade [17].

In the non-alcoholic fatty liver disease (NAFLD), USE can be used for two purposes: estimation of hepatic fibrosis and estimation of the quantity of hepatic steatosis. Controlled attenuation parameter (CAP) driven in TE has been used for the purpose of fat quantification. The principle of CAP is that ultrasonic attenuation coefficient could be estimated in the sample of which stiffness was assessed by TE and expressed in dB/m for quantification [18]. According to the recent paper which performed a meta-analysis of several biopsy-proven studies, the areas under the curves for diagnose each steatosis stage was about 0.82–0.88 [19]. Other USE does not include a quantification tool for steatosis, but the degree of ultrasonic attenuation has been basically a diagnostic criterion of ultrasonography from the past, as well as increase in echogenicity. There is a study of evaluation about hepatorenal index and ultrasound attenuation index using conventional ultrasonography, and these parameters were useful to diagnose higher than 5% of hepatic steatosis [20]. According to a diagnostic algorithm introduced by a review article [21], TE could be useful for reducing NAFLD patients who are at indeterminate risk (liver stiffness was ranged 7.9–9.6 kPa) that liver biopsy is required for diagnosis. Thus, the number of liver biopsy can be decreased, leading to reduced incidence of biopsy-induced complications.

Portal hypertension is a common clinical syndrome associated with liver cirrhosis. Most of the cases with portal hypertension were associated with cirrhosis, and it appears at the intrahepatic sinusoidal site, as a result of fibrotic disruption of hepatic architecture and dynamic component produced by vasoconstriction of intrahepatic vasculature [22]. It may affect the clinical course of cirrhotic patients due to significant complications. Clinically, there are two stages with different prognoses in the cirrhosis: compensated and decompensated cirrhosis. To predict development of clinical events in cirrhotic patients, hepatic venous pressure gradient (HVPG) is considered as a surrogate marker of portal hypertension. When HVPG is same or higher than 10 mmHg, clinically significant portal hypertension is present. The other exam for monitoring of cirrhotic patients is gastroscopy. It is used to diagnose esophageal and gastric varices and to manage them with endoscopic variceal ligation and sclerotherapy as a prophylactic purpose before variceal bleeding, or as a bleeding control after variceal bleeding [23, 24]. For the cirrhotic patients, elastography is useful for non-invasive diagnostic method to discriminate subclinical, clinically significant, and severe portal hypertension groups; therefore it could replace a specific role of invasive diagnostic methods such as HVPG measurement and gastroscopy. As a prediction of hepatic fibrosis, liver stiffness by USE well correlates with HVPG value, especially up to 10–12 mmHg [25], and it can predict the presence and size of varices [26]. And it is also useful to find a responder of non-selected beta blocker to decrease portal hypertension in decompensated cirrhotic patients [27, 28]. Recently, splenic stiffness measurement is highlighted because it showed a closer correlation with HVPG than liver stiffness although some limitations still remain (e.g. splenic size, range limitation of measured stiffness, etc.) [29].

45.4 US Elastography Is Reliable?: Quality Criteria of Ultrasound Elastography

According to the result of previous studies, the accuracy of liver stiffness is high for liver fibrosis staging under the optimized condition, e.g. fasting, unforced expiration, and without necroinflammation of hepatocytes. Thus, the precision of USE is an emerging issue for liver fibrosis estimation.

The distribution of measured liver stiffness values should be considered as quality criteria because it represents the precision and reproducibility of measurement. In many studies which dealt with USE, mean and median values were mixed as the representative value of measurement. And interquartile range with median value or standard deviation with mean value was appeared in the papers. In the case of TE, standard protocol and quality criteria for measurement of liver stiffness had been already established. The validity of liver stiffness measurement is determined by the success rate and the interquartile range divided by the median (IQR/M) of correct measurements. The success rate is the ratio of the number of correct measurements to the total attempts of measurements, and must be greater than 60%; the IQR/M of successive ten measurements should be lower than 30% [30].

On the other hand, there is neither generally accepted standard protocol nor quality criteria for pSWE and 2D-SWE. Like TE, an IQR/M ≤30% is widely used for quality criterion of pSWE and 2D-SWE [31–35]. The other group used coefficient of variance (CV) of liver stiffness measurement by 2D-SWE, and they suggested <20% of the CV would be more reliable, which was better than IQR/M [36]. Also according to the consensus report by the Society of Radiologists in Ultrasound (SRU), the report for USE should provide the median value, as well as the IQR/M value as a measure of quality [6]. In the most of the studies, right hepatic lobe was preferred to measure via intercostal sonic window because left lobe is vulnerable to erroneous measurement by a motion artifact due to heartbeat, and manual compression with transducer, and poor sonic window. The number of measurement was ranged from three to ten. The number of measurement in 2D-SWE was smaller than pSWE, and it may be reasonable because the stiffness value on the monitor of 2D-SWE machine is average of three successive elasticity maps; so three or four measurements of 2D-SWE can be comparable to ten measurements of TE or pSWE [37]. According to another study using 2D-SWE, the result of five-time repetition was nearly coincident to that of ten-time repetition except the condition with fatty liver or high liver stiffness [38].

On contrary, the reliability of single measurement is also important. The measured value in elastography could be changed by positioning of region of interest (ROI). Thiele et al. introduced a new concept for valid measurement of 2D-SWE [36, 39]. Reliability criteria defined as standard deviation divided by mean value of stiffness within a single ROI should be lower than 10% for high accuracy to diagnose liver cirrhosis and clinically significant portal hypertension [40]. For interobserver agreement, a standard deviation of single ROI is also important. The author recommended that mean value of standard deviations in single ROIs should be less than 1.4 to avoid significant interobserver discrepancy in fibrosis stage [41]. In addition, the ROI should be set to at least 10 mm, preferably 15 mm or more. Temporal stability of the elastogram for 3 s or more during breath hold, in combination with placement of the analysis box in a homogeneous area with complete filling results in high accuracy, high reliability and low variance of measurements [39, 42, 43].

Recently, various reliability parameters are equipped in the USE machines, such as reliability measurement index (RMI) by Samsung Medison, stability index (SI) of Aixplorer system by Supersonic imagine, confidence map by Philips, and propagation map by Toshiba. RMI is a quantitative parameter calculated by the weighted sum of the residual of the wave equation and the magnitude of the shear wave. It is ranged from 0 to 1, and higher than 0.5 can be considered as a reliable value. Confidence map and propagation map can guide the operator locate the measurement ROI into the proper area in which shear waves propagate homogeneously.

45.5 US Elastography: Limitations and Promises

Although the role of USE as a non-invasive method to diagnose hepatic fibrosis and to predict a clinical outcome of the patients is emerging, several critical issues are remained.

First, US-based technique has an important issue regarding to ultrasound beam penetration. In TE, very low frequency of shear waves are needed because shear waves are attenuated rapidly [44], and they should propagate longitudinally from surface to target liver tissue. In contrast, pSWE and 2D-SWE uses ARFI technique, and ultrasound beam penetrates and makes shear waves in target depth of liver tissue [3]. These shear waves don't need to penetrate through long distance and even though the shear wave may then travel only a short distance, another shear wave may easily be generated at a new source position using another ARFI beam [5]. The second technical issue is which unit of elasticity should be chosen. Several machines can display two types of units: kPa as an elastic modulus and ms^{-1} as shear wave speed. It is preferable to report results in units of ms^{-1} rather than kPa. Because many assumptions should be needed to make for conversion of speed to elastic modulus, and these are generally not valid. Thus, shear wave speed can be measured directly; an elastic modulus cannot be, but calculated indirectly with many assumptions which are not generally proven in real situation [5] Moreover, it could be misunderstood as shear modulus which has the same unit, kPa. It is measured by MR elastography directly. Conversion using the relation Young modulus (E) = 3 × shear modulus (G) is possible, which need the prerequisite assumption that the tissue is incompressible. Third, there is an issue for comparability of data between the different SWE technologies.

Because there are several important factors to affect shear wave speed such as shear wave frequency and bandwidth, stiffness thresholds for clinical use known for specific equipment should not be utilized for other equipment. Higher frequencies generate shear waves that travel faster. The 'dispersion error' could render results from different studies incomparable. According to the studies by the Radiological Society of North America/Quantitative Imaging Biomarker Alliance (RSNA/QIBA), there was a statistically significant difference in the shear wave speed estimates among systems and depth of measurement in the phantom [45, 46].

45.6 Need to Know When Doing US Elastography

As Doppler examination is dependent to operator's skill, patients' status, and ultrasound machine, USE is also affected by various factors. Generally, USE is a highly reproducible and user-friendly technique, and a learning curve is not required so long. However, several factors can affect the result of liver stiffness measurement: location of measurement, patient's position, respiratory status, and postprandial status [47, 48]. Measuring liver stiffness in the left hepatic lobe could be different from that in the right lobe, so left liver stiffness is not appropriate to apply reference values of USE for liver stiffness [49]. Upright position, deep inspiration and postprandial status are also increasing factors of liver stiffness. Therefore, a standard protocol of liver stiffness measurement should be given to reduce operator- or protocol-dependent factors [3].

Patient-dependent factors are also important factors not to be ignored. Because USE uses basically ultrasonic pulse to make and measure shear waves, the pulse is attenuated by soft tissue, especially fat. In the case of TE, a low frequency pushing pulse made by external vibration theoretically do not propagate through liquid, displacement of liver tissue may not appear, and liver stiffness measurement is not accurate under the ascites [50]. Thus, the accuracy and reproducibility could be compromised in the obese patients, patients with severe fatty liver, and patients with ascites [38, 51]. Necroinflammation of hepatocytes which appears in active phase of viral hepatitis also can affect accuracy. Nevertheless, USE can be used for a good method of longitudinal follow-up to perform the tailored management strategies by providing more detailed prognostic information. In this situation, cut-off values of liver stiffness which are important levels of cross-sectional assessment of the patient may be less important, and the quality of serial measurements may be more emphasized [27, 52].

For the best practice for elastography for diffuse liver disease, there was a panel discussion by specialists from radiology, hepatology, pathology, and basic science and physics in the SRU with regards of the use of USE in the assessment of liver fibrosis in chronic liver disease [6]. According to the report of the panel discussion, a stepwise approach to the diagnosis of liver fibrosis would be helpful, and the literature has been suggested that TE and pSWE techniques are at least equivalent so far. Also it is clinically useful to discriminate patients who underwent elastography into three categories: those with a low likelihood of cirrhosis (category I; equivalent to METAVIR F0 or F1 in pathologic finding), those with a high likelihood of cirrhosis (category III; equivalent to METAVIR F4), and those in between two categories (category II; equivalent to METAVIR F2 or F3). The patients who belong to the category I, they do not need any follow-up study to observe the progression of liver fibrosis. On the contrary, the category II patients require close observation about the progression to liver cirrhosis, and the category III patients should be observed whether development of life-threatening complication is imminent.

45.7 Conclusion

USE is still emerging for a non-invasive diagnostic tool for diffuse liver disease. Because it is safe and cheap, it can be used as a monitoring tool for the patients with chronic liver disease. As many ultrasound machines equip the USE function, examiners can perform USE as well as B-mode ultrasonography without patients' inconvenience. Moreover, the accuracy and reliability of USE have been proven, and it is included in the clinical practice guideline.

As mentioned former, although some limitations still remain, there are many attempts for merging the knowledge about USE and for publishing guidelines for its technical and clinical applications. Finally, USE would be more widely used for a basic follow-up method for the patient with chronic liver diseases, and most of clinicians would believe the well-qualified result of USE and utilize it for patient management.

Self Study

Questions

1. Which statement is true?
   (a) The cut-off level of liver stiffness of cirrhosis (F4) is same regardless of etiology of liver disease.
   (b) The velocity of shear wave in a firm medium is faster than that in a soft medium.
   (c) Young modulus is equivalent to shear modulus.
   (d) The value of liver stiffness measurement is comparable regardless of center frequency of transducer.

2. Which one is different from others?
   (a) Transient elastography
   (b) Point shear wave elastography
   (c) Two-dimensional shear wave elastography
   (d) Strain elastography

Answers

1. Which statement is true?
   (a) The cut-off level of liver stiffness is different among the etiology of liver disease. According to a meta-analysis of liver stiffness measurement using transient elastography, the cut-off level of cirrhosis by hepatitis B viral infection was 11.3 kPa, which was slightly lower than that by hepatitis C viral infection (15.3 kPa).
   (b) It is CORRECT.
   (c) Young modulus is about three-times of shear modulus, but it needs the prerequisite assumption that the tissue is incompressible.
   (d) The shear wave speed depends on the frequency and bandwidth of shear waves, which is affected by center frequency of transducer.
2. Which one is different from others?
   (a) Transient elastography is one of shear wave technique.
   (b) Point shear wave elastography is one of shear wave technique.
   (c) Two-dimensional shear wave elastography is one of shear wave technique.
   (d) Strain elastography is a qualitative method, which doesn't use shear wave propagation. It is CORRECT.

References

1. Youk JH, Gweon HM, Son EJ. Shear-wave elastography in breast ultrasonography: the state of the art. Ultrasonography. 2017;36:300–9.
2. Kwak JY, Kim EK. Ultrasound elastography for thyroid nodules: recent advances. Ultrasonography. 2014;33:75–82.
3. Jeong WK, Lim HK, Lee HK, Jo JM, Kim Y. Principles and clinical application of ultrasound elastography for diffuse liver disease. Ultrasonography. 2014;33:149–60.
4. Bedossa P, Dargere D, Paradis V. Sampling variability of liver fibrosis in chronic hepatitis C. Hepatology. 2003;38:1449–57.
5. Dietrich CF, Bamber J, Berzigotti A, et al. EFSUMB guidelines and recommendations on the clinical use of liver ultrasound elastography, update 2017 (short version). Ultraschall Med. 2017;38:377–94.
6. Barr RG, Ferraioli G, Palmeri ML, et al. Elastography assessment of liver fibrosis: Society of Radiologists in Ultrasound Consensus Conference Statement. Radiology. 2015;276:845–61.
7. Ziol M, Handra-Luca A, Kettaneh A, et al. Noninvasive assessment of liver fibrosis by measurement of stiffness in patients with chronic hepatitis C. Hepatology. 2005;41:48–54.
8. Park SH, Kim SY, Suh CH, et al. What we need to know when performing and interpreting US elastography. Clin Mol Hepatol. 2016;22:406–14.
9. Friedrich-Rust M, Poynard T, Castera L. Critical comparison of elastography methods to assess chronic liver disease. Nat Rev Gastroenterol Hepatol. 2016;13:402–11.
10. Sarvazyan AP, Skovoroda AR, Emelianov SY, et al. Biophysical bases of elasticity imaging. In: Jones JP, editor. Acoustical imaging, vol. 21. Boston, MA: Springer; 1995. p. 223–40.
11. Jiang T, Tian G, Zhao Q, et al. Diagnostic accuracy of 2D-shear wave elastography for liver fibrosis severity: a meta-analysis. PLoS One. 2016;11:e0157219.
12. Bota S, Herkner H, Sporea I, et al. Meta-analysis: ARFI elastography versus transient elastography for the evaluation of liver fibrosis. Liver Int. 2013;33:1138–47.
13. Friedrich-Rust M, Nierhoff J, Lupsor M, et al. Performance of acoustic radiation force impulse imaging for the staging of liver fibrosis: a pooled meta-analysis. J Viral Hepat. 2012;19:e212–9.
14. Chon YE, Choi EH, Song KJ, et al. Performance of transient elastography for the staging of liver fibrosis in patients with chronic hepatitis B: a meta-analysis. PLoS One. 2012;7:e44930.
15. Tsochatzis EA, Gurusamy KS, Ntaoula S, Cholongitas E, Davidson BR, Burroughs AK. Elastography for the diagnosis of severity of fibrosis in chronic liver disease: a meta-analysis of diagnostic accuracy. J Hepatol. 2011;54:650–9.
16. Friedrich-Rust M, Ong MF, Martens S, et al. Performance of transient elastography for the staging of liver fibrosis: a meta-analysis. Gastroenterology. 2008;134:960–74.
17. Oliveri F, Coco B, Ciccorossi P, et al. Liver stiffness in the hepatitis B virus carrier: a non-invasive marker of liver disease influenced by the pattern of transaminases. World J Gastroenterol. 2008;14:6154–62.
18. Sasso M, Beaugrand M, de Ledinghen V, et al. Controlled attenuation parameter (CAP): a novel VCTE guided ultrasonic attenuation measurement for the evaluation of hepatic steatosis: preliminary study and validation in a cohort of patients with chronic liver disease from various causes. Ultrasound Med Biol. 2010;36:1825–35.
19. Karlas T, Petroff D, Sasso M, et al. Individual patient data meta-analysis of controlled attenuation parameter (CAP) technology for assessing steatosis. J Hepatol. 2017;66(5):1022–30.
20. Kwon HJ, Kim KW, Jung JH, et al. Noninvasive quantitative estimation of hepatic steatosis by ultrasound: a comparison of the hepato-renal index and ultrasound attenuation index. Med Ultrason. 2016;18:431–7.
21. Festi D, Schiumerini R, Marzi L, et al. Review article: The diagnosis of non-alcoholic fatty liver disease—availability and accuracy of non-invasive methods. Aliment Pharmacol Ther. 2013;37:392–400.
22. Sanyal AJ, Bosch J, Blei A, Arroyo V. Portal hypertension and its complications. Gastroenterology. 2008;134:1715–28.
23. D'Amico G, Garcia-Pagan JC, Luca A, Bosch J. Hepatic vein pressure gradient reduction and prevention of variceal bleeding in cirrhosis: a systematic review. Gastroenterology. 2006;131:1611–24.
24. Garcia-Tsao G, Abraldes JG, Berzigotti A, Bosch J. Portal hypertensive bleeding in cirrhosis: risk stratification, diagnosis, and management: 2016 practice guidance by the American Association for the study of liver diseases. Hepatology. 2017;65:310–35.
25. Vizzutti F, Arena U, Romanelli RG, et al. Liver stiffness measurement predicts severe portal hypertension in patients with HCV-related cirrhosis. Hepatology. 2007;45:1290–7.
26. Shi KQ, Fan YC, Pan ZZ, et al. Transient elastography: a meta-analysis of diagnostic accuracy in evaluation of portal hypertension in chronic liver disease. Liver Int. 2013;33:62–71.
27. Choi SY, Jeong WK, Kim Y, Kim J, Kim TY, Sohn JH. Shear-wave elastography: a noninvasive tool for monitoring changing hepatic venous pressure gradients in patients with cirrhosis. Radiology. 2014;273:917–26.

28. Reiberger T, Ferlitsch A, Payer BA, et al. Non-selective beta-blockers improve the correlation of liver stiffness and portal pressure in advanced cirrhosis. J Gastroenterol. 2012;47:561–8.
29. Berzigotti A. Non invasive evaluation of portal hypertension using ultrasound elastography. J Hepatol. 2017;67(2):399–411.
30. Kim SU, Seo YS, Cheong JY, et al. Factors that affect the diagnostic accuracy of liver fibrosis measurement by Fibroscan in patients with chronic hepatitis B. Aliment Pharmacol Ther. 2010;32:498–505.
31. Gerber L, Kasper D, Fitting D, et al. Assessment of liver fibrosis with 2-D shear wave elastography in comparison to transient elastography and acoustic radiation force impulse imaging in patients with chronic liver disease. Ultrasound Med Biol. 2015;41:2350–9.
32. Cassinotto C, Lapuyade B, Ait-Ali A, et al. Liver fibrosis: noninvasive assessment with acoustic radiation force impulse elastography—comparison with FibroScan M and XL probes and FibroTest in patients with chronic liver disease. Radiology. 2013;269:283–92.
33. Sporea I, Sirli R, Bota S, Popescu A, Sendroiu M, Jurchis A. Comparative study concerning the value of acoustic radiation force impulse elastography (ARFI) in comparison with transient elastography (TE) for the assessment of liver fibrosis in patients with chronic hepatitis B and C. Ultrasound Med Biol. 2012;38:1310–6.
34. Ferraioli G, Maiocchi L, Lissandrin R, et al. Accuracy of the ElastPQ technique for the assessment of liver fibrosis in patients with chronic hepatitis C: a "Real Life" single center study. J Gastrointestin Liver Dis. 2016;25:331–5.
35. Bota S, Sporea I, Sirli R, Popescu A, Jurchis A. Factors which influence the accuracy of acoustic radiation force impulse (ARFI) elastography for the diagnosis of liver fibrosis in patients with chronic hepatitis C. Ultrasound Med Biol. 2013;39:407–12.
36. Lim S, Kim SH, Kim Y, et al. Coefficient of variance as quality criterion for evaluation of advanced hepatic fibrosis using 2D shear-wave elastography. J Ultrasound Med. 2018;37:355–62.
37. Ferraioli G, Tinelli C, Dal Bello B, et al. Accuracy of real-time shear wave elastography for assessing liver fibrosis in chronic hepatitis C: a pilot study. Hepatology. 2012;56:2125–33.
38. Choi SH, Jeong WK, Kim Y, et al. How many times should we repeat measuring liver stiffness using shear wave elastography?: 5-repetition versus 10-repetition protocols. Ultrasonics. 2016;72:158–64.
39. Thiele M, Madsen BS, Procopet B, et al. Reliability criteria for liver stiffness measurements with real-time 2D shear wave elastography in different clinical scenarios of chronic liver disease. Ultraschall Med. 2017;38(6):648–54.
40. Procopet B, Berzigotti A, Abraldes JG, et al. Real-time shear-wave elastography: applicability, reliability and accuracy for clinically significant portal hypertension. J Hepatol. 2015;62:1068–75.
41. Yoon KJ, Jeong WK, Kim Y, Kim MY, Kim TY, Sohn JH. 2-Dimensional shear wave elastography: interobserver agreement and factors related to interobserver discrepancy. PLoS One. 2017;12(4):e0175747.
42. Cassinotto C, de Ledinghen V. Reply to: "New imaging assisted methods for liver fibrosis quantification: is it really favorable to classical transient elastography?". J Hepatol. 2015;63:767.
43. Cassinotto C, Charrie A, Mouries A, et al. Liver and spleen elastography using supersonic shear imaging for the non-invasive diagnosis of cirrhosis severity and oesophageal varices. Dig Liver Dis. 2015;47:695–701.
44. Madsen EL, Sathoff HJ, Zagzebski JA. Ultrasonic shear wave properties of soft tissues and tissuelike materials. J Acoust Soc Am. 1983;74:1346–55.
45. Palmeri M, Nightingale K, Fielding S, et al. RSNA QIBA ultrasound shear wave speed Phase II phantom study in viscoelastic media. Taipei, Taiwan: IEEE; 2015. p. 1–4.
46. Hall TJ, Milkowski A, Garra B, et al. RSNA/QIBA: Shear wave speed as a biomarker for liver fibrosis staging. Prague, Czech Republic: IEEE; 2013. p. 397–400.
47. Goertz RS, Egger C, Neurath MF, Strobel D. Impact of food intake, ultrasound transducer, breathing maneuvers and body position on acoustic radiation force impulse (ARFI) elastometry of the liver. Ultraschall Med. 2012;33:380–5.
48. Mederacke I, Wursthorn K, Kirschner J, et al. Food intake increases liver stiffness in patients with chronic or resolved hepatitis C virus infection. Liver Int. 2009;29:1500–6.
49. Goertz RS, Zopf Y, Jugl V, et al. Measurement of liver elasticity with acoustic radiation force impulse (ARFI) technology: an alternative noninvasive method for staging liver fibrosis in viral hepatitis. Ultraschall Med. 2010;31:151–5.
50. Sandrin L, Fourquet B, Hasquenoph JM, et al. Transient elastography: a new noninvasive method for assessment of hepatic fibrosis. Ultrasound Med Biol. 2003;29:1705–13.
51. Fraquelli M, Rigamonti C, Casazza G, et al. Reproducibility of transient elastography in the evaluation of liver fibrosis in patients with chronic liver disease. Gut. 2007;56:968–73.
52. Kim BK, Fung J, Yuen MF, Kim SU. Clinical application of liver stiffness measurement using transient elastography in chronic liver disease from longitudinal perspectives. World J Gastroenterol. 2013;19:1890–900.

46 MR Elastography and Functional MRI of the Liver

Ioana G. Lupescu, Mugur Cristian Grasu, and Radu Lucian Dumitru

Key Concepts

- Magnetic Resonance Elastography (MRE) is a noninvasive MRI technique for quantitatively assessing the mechanical properties of the tissues in vivo in our case the liver parenchyma.
- There is a strong correlation between MRE-measured hepatic stiffness and the stage of fibrosis at histology demonstrated by multiple studies.
- MRE is a safer, less expensive, and accurate alternative to invasive liver biopsy which is currently considered the gold standard for diagnosis and staging of liver fibrosis.
- Multiparametric MRI of the liver, combining morphologic and functional informations, represent an essential tool for radiologists and include in the functional part of the MR protocol diffusion weighted imaging, multiphase dynamic 3D T1 weighted GRE (Gradient Echo) imaging evaluation with hepato-specific contrast agents, and qualitative and quantitative analysis of the liver parenchyma particularly in the hepatobiliary phase.

46.1 Magnetic Resonance Elastography

46.1.1 Introduction

Hepatic fibrosis and cirrhosis represent an important health public problem worldwide. Liver biopsy is necessary for the diagnosis and staging of liver fibrosis. However, it is an invasive method with risk and potential complications [1]. MR elastography (MRE) techniques and automated analysis, permits a more accurate assessment of liver fibrosis especially in cases in which fibrosis is not uniform [1–3]. Even if MRE cannot differentiate fibrosis distribution as histopathologic examination does, it may distinguish the various degrees of tissue stiffness by drawing a ROI (region of interest) on each of four liver axial images acquired, and by measuring the mean stiffness [1]. The degree of fibrosis quantified by MRE are classified into: F1: mild fibrosis, F2: moderate fibrosis, F3: severe fibrosis and F4: cirrhosis [1, 4].

I. G. Lupescu (✉) · M. C. Grasu · R. L. Dumitru
Radiology, Medical Imaging and Interventional Radiology Department, Fundeni Clinical Institute, University of Medicine and Pharmacy "Carol Davila", Bucharest, Romania

Definitions

MR elastography is a noninvasive medical imaging technique by means of which it can be appreciated the mechanical properties of a soft tissue such as elasticity, corresponding to the deformation resistance of a tissue on which was applied a stress [1–7].

46.1.2 Principles

MRE uses a modified phase-contrast method to image the propagation characteristics of the shear wave in the liver [1–7]. Elasticity is quantified by MRE (expressed in kPa-KiloPascal) using a formula that determines the shear modulus [7]. The normal liver stiffness range is between 1.54 and 2.87 kPa [4]. The theoretical advantages of MRE include its ability to analyze almost the entire liver and its good applicability in patients with obesity or ascites [1–6]. Liver stiffness measurement using MRE is reproducible, operator independent and has a good consistency across vendor platforms [7, 8].

46.1.3 Technical Aspects

Elastography techniques may be classified according to the source (static, quasistatic, or dynamic) and duration (transient or continuous) of tissue deformation and the modality

F. Radu-Ionita et al. (eds.), *Liver Diseases*, https://doi.org/10.1007/978-3-030-24432-3_46

used for tracking (ultrasound or MRI). Techniques also may be classified according to the device type (stand alone or adjunct to an imaging scanner), wave generation method (external vibrator or internally focused acoustic radiation force), inversion algorithm (1D, 2D, or 3D), reported parameters (shear-wave speed, magnitude of complex shear modulus, and the Young modulus), or output display (purely numeric, M-mode image, or parametric imaging map) [2, 8]. MRE techniques use continuous waves and requires five components: a driver system to generate oscillatory mechanical waves continuously at a fixed frequency, a phase-contrast multiphase pulse sequence with motion-encoding gradients that are synchronized to the mechanical waves, processing of phase-sensitive MR images to depict wave amplitudes (shear-wave displacement images or, simply, wave images), further postprocessing (using an inversion algorithm) to generate elastograms and analysis of the elastograms [2–7]. In MRE, images are acquired with a modified phase-contrast technique that generates both magnitude and phase images. The total acquisition time in liver MRE is about 1 min, typically divided into four separate approximately 15-s breath-holds (one for each slice liver location), acquired in end expiration if possible. Images at each phase offset are acquired through color maps and are typically applied to these wave images, in which red and blue hues indicate opposite wave polarity and color saturation indicates wave amplitude. The color elastograms represent the shear modulus with scales of 0–8 kPa [1–6].

In clinical practice, the patient is placed in supine position with a pneumatic driver placed over the liver on the anterior abdominal wall. The pneumatic driver generates mechanical waves by vibrating at low frequencies. The waves propagating into the liver are measured using a 2D gradient-echo sequences and cyclic motion-encoding gradients (MEG). Specialized computer-based algorithms analyse these mechanical waves [7].

Fibrosis leads to increased liver stiffness (Fig. 46.1). As shear waves travel through a tissue, the speed of the wave depends on the tissue stiffness [1–6]. In stiffer tissues, the shear-wave speed is greater, enabling estimation of the degree of liver fibrosis from measuring the speed of a shear wave [2]. In MRE, increased wavelength is evident in stiffer tissues. An obstacle to direct comparison between techniques is the frequency dependence of biologic tissue. Higher frequency shear waves produce higher stress and strain rates, resulting in higher stiffness measurements [2–4, 6, 9].

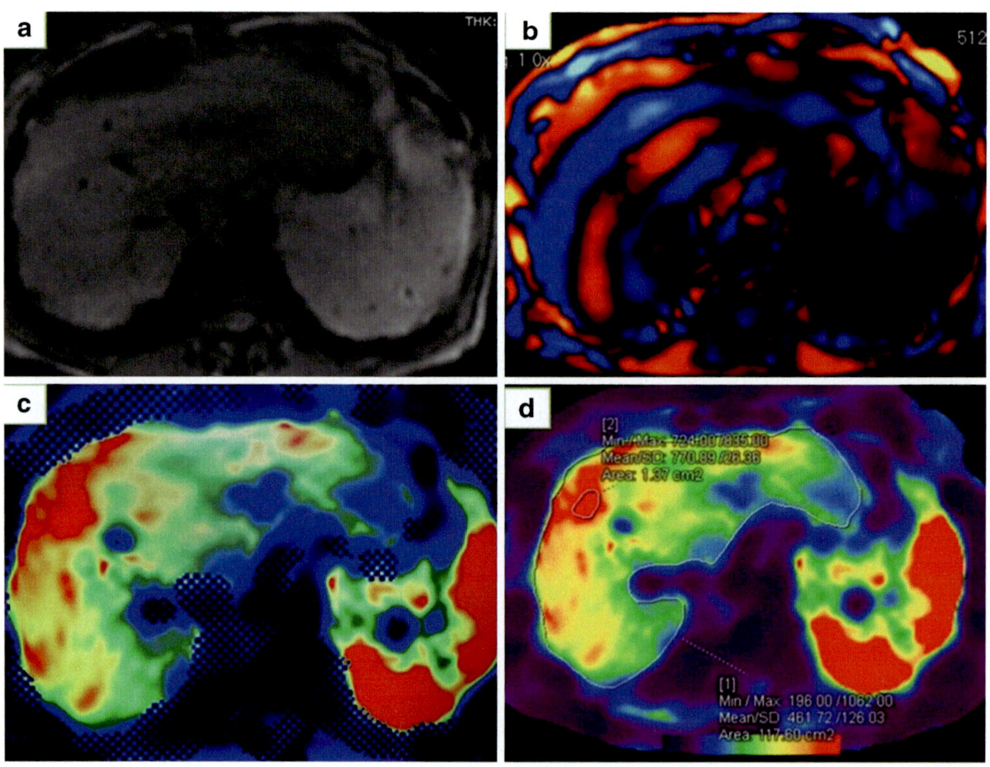

Fig. 46.1 MRE. (**a**) *Magnitude image*—image quality is lower compared to standard imaging due to the acquisition technique, but is sufficient to visualize the anatomy; (**b**) *wave image*—the unwrapped and corrected wave displacements are displayed in this series; (**c**) *relative stiffness 95% Map*—stiffness map with checkered areas for low confidence areas standard; (**d**) *elastogram* or *relative stiffness map*—contains the magnitude of the complex shear modulus, providing reliable data about liver stiffness. By applying a ROI that includes the hepatic contour it is possible to calculate the mean value of the hepatic elasticity, and at the level of the area corresponding to the color map with an increased fibrosis, by overlapping an ROI circumscribing the respective area, the value corresponding to the degree of maximal fibrosis

46.2 Clinical Applications of MRE

46.2.1 MRE in Staging of Liver Fibrosis

Chronic HBV and HCV infections. Knowledge of liver fibrosis stage in chronic HBV and HCV infections is beneficial for prognosis, follow-up, and treatment decisions [3, 8–14]. From the published studies in chronic HCV or HBV infections, 2D GRE MRE has shown excellent accuracy in diagnosing liver fibrosis or cirrhosis, with AUC (area under the curve) for the diagnosis of fibrosis stages F2–F4, F3–F4, and F4 of 0.95–0.99, 0.94–1, and 0.92–1, respectively [3, 9, 14]. Several studies also showed that necroinflammation may increase liver stiffness [9, 15–19].

46.2.2 Nonalcoholic Steatohepatitis (NASH) and Nonalcoholic Fatty Liver Disease (NAFLD)

Liver fibrosis has been shown to be the strongest predictor of complications in NAFLD patients, which motivates the need for reliable noninvasive techniques for detection of liver fibrosis and will be of major interest for clinicians and in terms of public health perspective. A meta-analysis of nine studies with 232 patients [15] reported AUCs of 0.90 or greater for the diagnosis of fibrosis stages F3–F4 and F4, with associated cutoffs of 3.77 kPa and 4.09 kPa, respectively [15]. In patients with NAFLD MRE is highly accurate, for liver fibrosis staging, and is not significantly influenced by age, sex, obesity or by the degree of inflammation [15].

There is also evidence that MRE may be able to differentiate NASH and simple steatosis in NAFLD patients with a reported AUC of 0.93, but this needs further confirmation [9]. In steatohepatitis or NASH, liver stiffness (LS) measured by MRE increase, even before the onset of fibrosis [4]. MRE is more accurate than acoustic radiation force impulse (ARFI) for diagnosing any fibrosis in all NAFLD patients and obese NAFLD patients [16–18]. Both 2D and 3D-MRE at the standard shear-wave frequency, are highly accurate in diagnosing NAFLD advanced fibrosis [18]. Patients with steatosis had lower liver inflammation and fibrosis compared to patients with non-alcoholic steatohepatitis [19].

46.2.3 Primary Sclerosing Cholangitis

MRE may be useful in detection of early fibrosis in primary sclerosing cholangitis (PSC) especially when there are no other morphological signs of disease; in these cases, stiffness measurement at baseline and longitudinal changes has been shown to be a useful biomarker for monitoring and prognostication [20].

46.2.4 MRE Potential Role in Liver Tumors

Other potential clinical application of MRE is to add more information to the classical appearance of a liver nodule on T2, diffusion weighted images, and on unenhanced and dynamic enhancement T1 features of the nodule after bolus injection of a gadolinium-based contrast agent. Malignant liver tumors had significantly greater mean shear stiffness (10.1 kPa); than benign tumors (2.7 kPa), also significantly greater shear stiffness than normal liver parenchyma. Cholangiocarcinoma and HCC had greater stiffness than fibrotic liver, benign tumors, and normal liver parenchyma. MRE can stratify the risk for development of HCC during follow-up in patients with chronic liver disease [21, 22]. The LS value can be used as a predictive factor for occurrence of hepatocellular carcinoma [22].

Obese patients can be reliably examined by MRE and no observer variability exists [23]. *MR elastography is preferable to US elastography* because an acoustic window is not needed and the entire liver can be assessed compared with US elastography in which only small regions of interest can be explored [16, 17, 24].

46.2.5 Limitations and Pitfalls of MRE

The most common technical limitation of MRE is liver hemochromatosis [1, 3]. In patients with moderate to severe hepatic iron overload (the short $T2^*$ time of the affected liver) the signal intensity of the liver is so low that the shear waves cannot be visualized on the phase-contrast 2D gradient-echo (GRE) image. There is conflicting evidence on the effect of body mass index on MRE measurements. A recent study found that body mass index was not a contributing factor in failure but found waist circumference to be a significant factor of failure. In contrast, a recent large retrospective study investigating the cause of MRE failure using a 2D GRE sequence found that body mass index, iron deposition, massive ascites, and use of 3 T were significantly associated with MRE failure. This limitation can be suppressed using Short echo time (TE) 2D spin echo echoplanar imaging (SE-EPI)-based MRE which may allow measurement of stiffness in the iron loaded liver [25]. In context of biliary system dilatation, the elevated liver stiffness is nonspecific and does not indicate fibrosis (this is a false positive MRE). Sarcoidosis, amyloidosis or sinusoidal obstruction syndrome (SOS) are other examples of false positive MRE [9, 12].

The actual trend, is to combine MRE with lipid and iron quantification sequences, which allows a so called multiparametric MR approach to diffuse liver disorders [1, 5, 8, 19, 26].

46.3 Functional MRI of the Liver

46.3.1 Introduction

In the last decade, the MRI evaluation of the liver, include outside the conventional morphological MRI sequences, *functional techniques* such as diffusion weighted imaging (DWI), perfusion weighted imaging (PWI) and dynamic 3D GRE T1 multiphase acquisition with hepato-specific Gadolinium based contrast agents allowing both vascular and interstitial distribution, but also a specific hepatocyte uptake during the "hepatobiliary" phase (HBP), which improves detection and characterization of nodular liver lesions. DWI sequences are important to characterize nodular lesions developed into a cirrhotic liver, but also in oncological patients which are suspected to have secondary hepatic nodules and take an important place in the evaluation of tumor functional response [26–32].

46.3.2 DWI Definition

DWI gives information's about the movement of water molecules at the microscopic scale. In water, the diffusion of the water molecules is free compared with the tissues DWI in which is restricted, because restriction of diffusion in biological tissues is correlated with tissue cellularity, cell membrane integrity, and tissue vascularization [26, 31, 32].

46.3.3 Principles and Applications of DWI

The factor b called "diffusion constant" is expressed in s/mm^2 and corresponds to the combination of the amplitude, the duration and the time separating the two gradient pulses. The optimal values of b for the evaluation of liver focal lesions ranged from 100 to 800 s/mm^2. For interpretation, it is important to calculate the apparent diffusion coefficient (ADC) value in addition to the qualitative approach. In current practice, DWI sequence is performed with multiple b values: 0, 50, 500 and 800 s/mm^2 allowing the calculation of the ADC. Small values of b are particularly interesting for the detection of liver lesions but not for characterization, being superior to a T2 fast-spin echo (FSE) sequence for tumor detection due to a best contrast-to-noise ratio of the DWI and the absence of the endovascular signal [31]. The persistence of the hypersignal at high b values reflects a restriction of the diffusion while a drop of the signal reflects a freer diffusion. A tumor signal intensity that is higher than that of the surrounding liver on high b DW value, and correspond to low ADC values on quantitative maps, has a "diffusion restriction" [32]. Simplifying, in clinical practice, protonic movements into a cyst are free without "restriction of diffusion" and the intracystic signal decreases as the b factor value increases (cysts have a high ADC). Conversely, in hepatic malignant lesions (primary and secondary lesions), protonic movements are constrained due to increased intratumoral cellularity, and the ADC is low [30]. But, the characterization of liver focal lesions only on the basis of DWI is impossible. The current data published in the literature shows an overlap of the ADC values, for example between hepatocellular carcinoma (HCC) and benign solid liver tumors such adenoma or focal nodular hyperplasia [30]. Several studies have shown statistically higher ADC values in benign lesions than in malignant lesions [31–33]. In the cirrhotic liver compared with the normal liver it has been known for several years that there is a restriction of diffusion; the decrease of ADC values in cirrhotic patients is found in all studies and the assumption is increased of the collagenous weft associated with a fall in hepatic perfusion [34]. The ADC values of patients with moderate to severe fibrosis (F2–F4) were lower than those measured in cases of minimal or no fibrosis (F0–F1). DWI may be superior to Fibroscan and serum tests for patient identification of F3–F4 stage [34].

DWI is a simple aid for the liver MRI interpretation and is integrated into the classification and characterization algorithms for nodular liver lesions. Li-RADS (Liver Imaging Reporting and Data System) developed by the American College of Radiology (ACR), integrates DWI as an ancillary criterion of liver lesion malignancy appeared into a cirrhotic liver.

Moreover, DWI is very sensitive to show the appearance of necrosis into a tumor (passage from restricted diffusion to free diffusion due to necrosis), allowing to appreciate the tumoral response under treatment [30]. Numerous articles have evaluated the value of diffusion imaging for measuring the therapeutic response (chemotherapy, radiotherapy or local ablation) in experimental studies. Pre-treatment ADC may be a predictor of successful chemotherapy for hepatic metastases [32–34].

46.4 Liver-Specific Gadolinium (Gd) Based Contrast Agents

46.4.1 Introduction

Liver-specific Gadolinium (Gd) based contrast agents or hepato-biliary (HB) contrast agents include Gd-EOB-DTPA, Gadoxetic Acid (Primovist®, Bayer Schering Pharma, Berlin, Germany) 0.25 mol/l and Gd-BOPTA (Multihance®, Bracco, Italy) 0.5 mol/l, both being positive T1 weighted image (wi) contrast agents, with a higher T1 relaxivity compared to the conventional extracellular agents [35].

46.4.2 Definition and Mechanism

These two specific liver contrast agents are capable to provide vascular and interstitial enhancement images identical to extracellular Gadolinium chelates, but have an additional property represented by the hepatocyte uptake via OATP receptors expressed on the hepatocyte surface before being partially excreted into the bile through MRP2 canalicular ducts. The hepatobiliary phase, which reflects at the cellular level the concentration balance between input OATP receptors and MRP2 output, is observed 20 min after the intra venous (i.v.) injection of Gd-EOB-DTPA, and 1 h after i.v. injection of Gd-BOPTA. Approximately 3–5% of the intravenous injected dose of Gd-BOPTA (0.05–0.1 mmol/kg bodyweight (bw) or 0.1–0.2 ml/kg; flow rate: 2 ml/s) is taken up by functioning hepatocytes and excreted via the biliary system, the hepatocytic uptake given at the normal liver parenchyma a strong enhancement on delayed T1-weighted images that is maximal between 1 and 2 h after i.v. administration. Gd-EOB-DTPA is injected manually or using a power injector through an intravenous route in a dose of 0.025 mmol/kg bw or 0.1 ml/kg, flow rate—1 ml/s, it is taken up by hepatocytes and has a double excretion: hepatobiliary (50%) and renal (50%). In patients with severe hepatic impairment (>3 mg/dl serum bilirubin levels) the elimination half-life of Primovist increase, the hepatobiliary excretion substantially decrease, and the hepatic signal enhancement is reduced [28–30, 35–39].

46.4.3 Contrast MR Acquisitions

Two type of MR acquisitions after i.v. injection of HB contrast agents can be performed: *"classical"* ***dynamic multiphase 3DT1*** *wi sequence* and ***dynamic contrast-enhanced (DCE) MR perfusion (MRP)***. DCEMRP is a particular MRI sequence also known as permeability MRI, which calculates perfusion parameters by evaluating T1 shortening induced by a gadolinium-based contrast bolus passing through tissue. Liver perfusion MRI gives information about microcirculation and microenvironment of liver tumors and the underlying hepatic parenchyma [35, 37–39].

In cases of HCC evaluate by DCEMRP there is an increased of the: arterial flow, of the total blood flow as well as early contrast arrival time. The early contrast arrival is related to angiogenesis of the tumor caused by branches with direct supply from the hepatic artery. Tumor vascularity (fractional intravascular volume) is in general higher and portal venous flow is decreased [30, 31].

DCEMRP is indicated also to improve detection of liver metastases; to assess the efficacy of anti-angiogenic therapy and the viable HCC after intraarterial chemotherapy or postablation; to evaluate cirrhosis and its severity. Gd-EOB-DTPA-enhanced MRI associated with DW-MRI is the best combination for detection and follow-up of liver metastasis [33].

46.4.4 Indications

These two hepato-specific contrast agents are particularly interesting for the following indications [30, 32–39]:

- Characterization of certain liver lesions, in particular to delineate between lesions with increased expression of OATPs (such as focal nodular hyperplasia-HNF) and lesions free of overexpression of OATP (such as moderately or poorly differentiated HCC or hepatocellular adenomas);
- Non-invasive assessment of hepatic function, with a lack of hepatocyte uptake correlating with loss of hepatic function observed in metabolic/toxic steatohepatitis, in chronic liver disease, or after chemotherapy especially Oxaliplatin-based treatments [40–43].

46.4.5 Advantage

The main advantage of the selective uptake by functioning hepatocytes is that the normal liver enhances (normal hepatic parenchyma exhibit T1 shortening in the longitudinal relaxation time), while tumors of non-hepatocytic origin (e.g. metastases and cholangiocarcinoma as well as non-functioning hepatocytic tumors) are unable to take up HB contrast agents, remaining unenhanced, getting an optimal liver-lesion contrast-to-noise ratio (CNR) and increasing the ability to detect supplementary liver lesions [30, 32]. Also, the use of hepato-specific Gd based agents allow to optimize the liver fibrosis assessment using a qualitative approach (Fig. 46.2). In oncological patients who received Oxaliplatin-based chemotherapy or in a context of hematopoietic stem-cell transplantation, it is possible to observe in the HBP using Gd-EOB-DTPA, a patchy or diffuse reticular T1 wi hypointensity associated with hepatocyte dysfunction related to sinusoidal obstruction syndrome (SOS) or heterogenous liver enhancement, FHN-like lesions (which appears because of vascular injury induced by chemotherapy and represent benign hyperplasia of hepatic parenchyma due to increased arterial perfusion in area with reduced portal blood flow), marked periportal hyperintensity (due to increased liver function) and fat spare liver areas mimicking metastasis (Fig. 46.3). Liver function recovery following interruption of chemotherapy may be monitored with by Gd-EOB-DTPA MRI. The literature reported that Gd-EOB-DTPA-enhanced liver MRI could identify SOS with high specificity and good interobserver agreement [40–43].

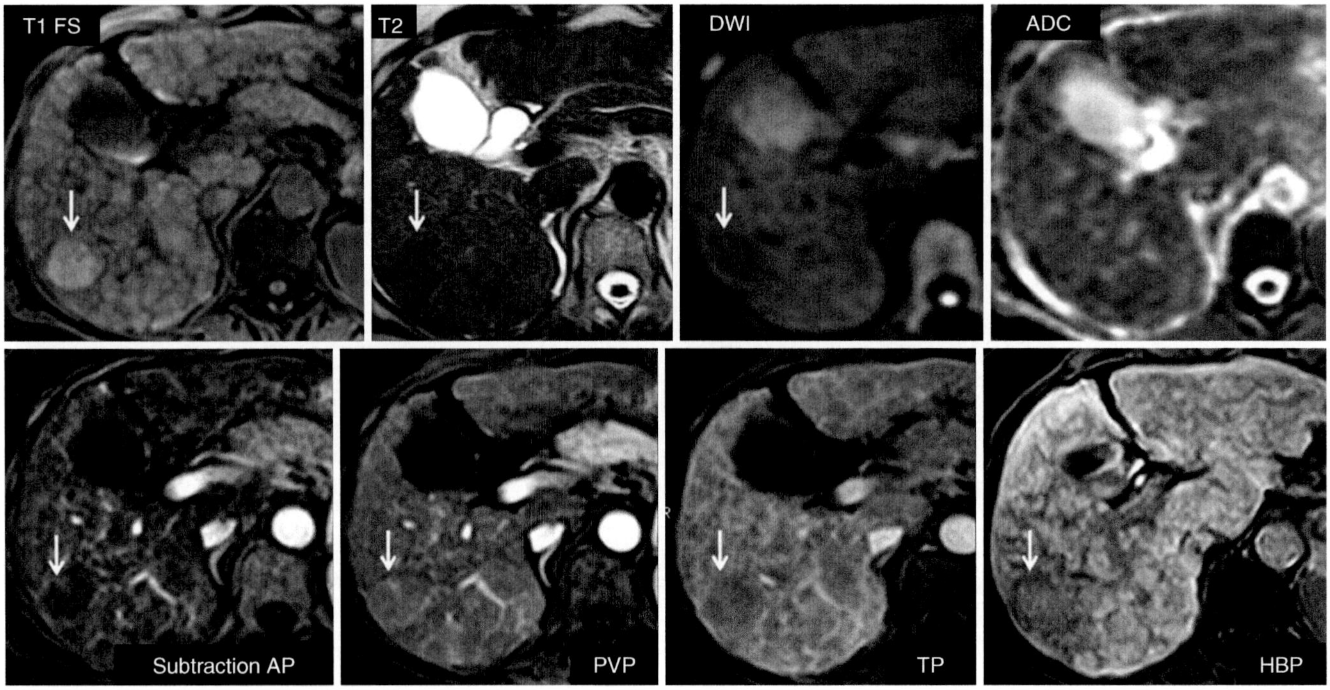

Fig. 46.2 Multiparametric MRI evaluation of the liver in a cirrhotic patient—T1 Fat Sat, T2 wi, DWI and ADC, dynamic 3D T1 FatSat acquisition with Gd-EOB-DTPA in arterial phase (subtraction), portal venous phase, transitional phase and hepato-biliary phase: important liver fibrosis in association with multiple regenerative nodules and a dysplastic nodule (white arrow)

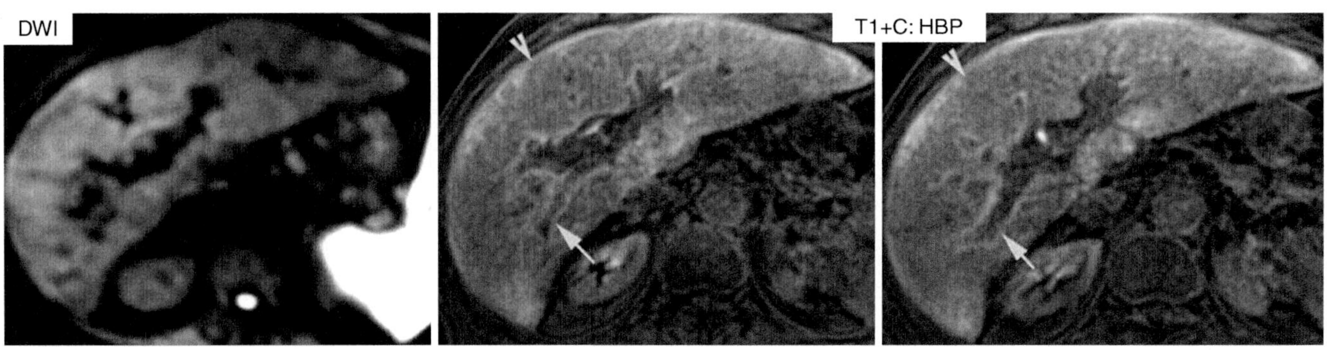

Fig. 46.3 Liver MP MRI evaluation in a patient with hepatocyte dysfunction related to SOS after chemotherapy: comparison between DWI and hepato-biliary phase after Gd-EOB-DTPA i.v. injection: periportal T1 hyperintensity (arrow) associated with large and confluent hypointense T1 liver areas (arrowhead) visible in HBP

Based on T1 shortening effects of hepatocellular Gd-EOB-DTPA uptake, the quantitative evaluation allows for the direct measurement of liver function, with the possibility to correlate the liver function evaluated by Gd-EOB-MRI with MELD (Model for End Stage Liver Disease)/or Child-Pugh score [30, 44]. Measurement of T_1 relaxation time on Gd-EOB-DTPA-enhanced MR imaging is accurate in evaluating liver function in patients with HBV-related HCC and can be used as a biomarker for estimating the remnant liver functional reserve [32, 37, 45]. Histogram analyses of the HBP after gadoxetic acid-enhanced MRI may be used as a biomarker for liver function assessment, liver fibrosis, and necro-inflammation.

Primovist MRI protocol: multiphased array coil, locator 3 plans, T1 dual GRE (TE-Echo Time in/out of phase), MRCP (Magnetic Resonance Cholangiopancreatography) ssFSE (single shot Fast Spin Echo) long TE; 3D T1 FAME/VIBE unenhanced and enhanced dynamic multiphase acquisition with Gd-EOB-DTPA (late arterial phase, portal venous phase and transitional phase); ssFSE with short TE; DWI and ADC (b: 50, 500, 800); T2 FSE (+/−FatSat); T2 GR (T2*); 3D T1 axial/coronal in hepatobiliary (HBP) phase 20 min after contrast material (CM) i.v. injection; 3D T1—MRCP (Magnetic Resonance Cholangio-Pancreatography) T1 wi in the HBP permit an optimal evaluation of the biliary tree. *Optimal window for Primovist®* in patients without cholestasis using T1 wi acquisition is 20 min after CM i.v. injection and in patients with cholestasis 40–60 min after CM i.v. injection.

46.4.6 Pitfalls Using Primovist

Lesions such as hemangiomas and hepatic fibrosis, and also areas of altered liver perfusion, may be mistaken for malignancy due to their hypointense T1 wi signal on the HBP.

The principles and recommendations for the use of HB contrast agents were the subject of expert recommendations in 2015 [29]. An expert position of the European Society of Abdominal and Digestive Radiology (ESGAR) recalled four major applications [28]:

- Optimizing the characterization of benign hepatocellular (HC) nodules [30, 32]. HB contrast agents allow a significant improvement in diagnostic performance of focal nodular hyperplasia (FNH) and propose to perform an MRI with HB contrast agents for the characterization of indeterminate atypical hepatocyte lesions on conventional MRI sequences with a reduction of the number of biopsies or monitoring of these benign lesions.
- Optimization of the detection of secondary liver lesions [33]. The combination of HB imaging after injection of Gd-EOB-DTPA and DWI represents the best MR modality for evaluating oncological patients, the HBP making possible to optimize the identification of infracentimetric metastatic liver lesions.
- Optimization of the characterization of primary HC lesions [29–34]. The presence of hypersignal lesions in T2 wi and DWI (with low ADC) correlated with hyposignal in the HBP would be in favor of high-grade dysplastic lesions or beginning HCC whatever their vascular profile [30]. In some recommendations, HB contrast agents are recommended as first-line tool to evaluate patients with chronic hepatopathy [37].
- Optimization of the biliary imaging; because HB contrast agents are excreted by the bile ducts after their hepatocyte capture, they allow positive enhancement of the biliary tree; this allows a positive contrast imaging of the bile ducts, but also allows the detection of biliary leakage by showing the presence of contrast agent outside the bile ducts [30].

46.4.7 Limitations

Even if Gd-EOB-DTPA is now integrated in the algorithms for characterization of nodules developed into a chronic liver disease, its use poses some difficulties because there exists a rapid competition between the interstitial enhancement of the lesion and the specific capture: the tumors enhancement beyond 90 s after injection is no longer the same as that seen with extracellular gadolinium chelates. The "wash-out" observed conventionally in the portal or late phase after injection of extracellular gadolinium chelates is then no longer specific for HCC after injection of Gd-EOB-DTPA and it can also be observed in case of cholangiocarcinoma [30]. So, the use of HB contrast agents tends to increase the sensitivity of HC nodules detection at the expense of limiting specificity regarding characterization [32]. In addition, the interpretation of the HBP signal intensity may require quantitative measurements, especially when the liver contrast is modified (e.g. in liver steatosis).

In summary, DW imaging is validated as a cellularity-/architecture biomarker; hepatospecific MR contrast agents represents biomarkers of the hepatocellular functions, and molecular imaging of tumors biology.

46.5 Conclusions: Future Perspectives

Liver MR-elastography represents a field of research in continuous evolving and refining. Beyond liver fibrosis assessment, liver MR-elastography has been proposed for liver stiffness monitoring, assessment of liver cirrhosis, detection of inflammation, to obtain additional information's concerning portal hypertension, liver tumors, and for the hepatic complications' prognosis [14–25].

Concerning liver functional MRI, there are several important issues [26–40]:

- DWI sequences are now systematically performed in the exploration of nodular liver lesions, adding also information's regarding liver fibrosis.
- DWI sequences are essential to explore patients with suspicion of secondary liver lesions and for monitoring the effectiveness of oncology therapies.
- DCEMRP together with DWI, contribute to a multiparametric functional assessment of the liver pathology improving the diagnosis.
- MRI with liver-specific contrast agents allows optimization for characterization of hepatocellular lesions and to detect supplementary liver nodules. They are useful for the evaluation of benign hepatocellular nodules particularly for small FNH and for the characterization of HCC.
- Hepatobiliary contrast agents appear to be useful to evaluate liver diffuse pathology such as fibrosis and steatohepatitis, and to give information about liver function considering that functioning areas of the hepatic parenchyma exhibit shortening of the T1 relaxation time, with the possibility to make a qualitative and quantitative analysis.
- In oncological patients treated by chemotherapy, after liver transplantation, in biliary cirrhosis, in primary sclerosing cholangitis, or in other biliary tree malformations or tumors, Gd-EOB MRI add more information's allowing also to have a mapping of hepatocytes function, correlated with specific lab data and MELD/or Child-Pugh score.

Self Study

Questions

1. Which are the incorrect answers concerning the use of Gd-EOB-DTPA (Primovist) in liver evaluation?
   (a) Primovist is an extracellular contrast agent
   (b) In liver cirrhosis with a multinodular pattern the MRI protocol include obligatory DWI and multiphase dynamic 3DT1 wi acquisition with Gd-EOB-DTPA
   (c) Around 3–5% of the i.v. injected dose is uptake by functioning hepatocytes and excreted via the biliary tree
   (d) The 3D T1 acquisition for the hepatobiliary phase is made in a nonicteric patient after 20 min
   (e) Liver fibrosis is better delineated in HBP compared to the nonenhanced 3D T1 MRI acquisition
2. Which answers are incorrect?
   (a) MR-elastography (MRE) is optimal to detect liver hemochromatosis
   (b) In liver fibrosis there is a decrease of stiffness
   (c) DWI correlated with ADC values can be used as biomarkers in monitoring the effectiveness of oncology therapies
   (d) ADC values doesn't allow to evaluate patients with moderate or severe liver fibrosis
   (e) MRE stiffness is different in liver solid tumors compared with the normal liver parenchyma

Answers

1. Which are the incorrect answers concerning the use of Gd-EOB-DTPA (Primovist) in liver evaluation?
   Incorrect answers: a, c because:
   (a) Primovist is a hepato-specific contrast agent
   (c) About 50% of the i.v. injected dose is uptake by functioning hepatocytes and excreted via the biliary tree
2. Which answers are incorrect?
   Incorrect answers: a, b, d because:
   (a) MRE is not indicate in liver hemochromatosis. In patients with moderate to severe hepatic iron overload (the short $T2^*$ time of the affected liver) the signal intensity of the liver is so low that the shear waves cannot be visualized on the phase-contrast 2D GRE acquisition
   (b) In liver fibrosis there is an increase of stiffness
   (d) ADC values of patients with moderate to severe fibrosis are lower than those measured in cases of minimal or no fibrosis.

References

1. Babu AS, Wells ML, Teytelboym OM, et al. Elastography in chronic liver disease: modalities, techniques, limitations, and future directions. Radiographics. 2016;36:1987–2006.
2. Tang A, Cloutier G, Szeverenyi NM, Sirlin CB. Ultrasound elastography and MR elastography for assessing liver fibrosis: Part 1, Principles and techniques. Am J Roentgenol. 2015;205(1):22–32.
3. Tang A, Cloutier G, Szeverenyi NM, Sirlin CB. Ultrasound elastography and MR elastography for assessing liver fibrosis: Part 2, Diagnostic performance, confounders, and future directions. Am J Roentgenol. 2015;205(2):33–40.
4. Venkatesh SK, Yin M, Ehman RL. Magnetic resonance elastography of liver: technique, analysis and clinical applications. J Magn Reson Imaging. 2013;37(3):544–55.
5. Venkatesh SK, Ehman RL. Magnetic resonance elastography of abdomen. Abdom Imaging. 2015;40:745–59.
6. Venkatesh SK, Yin M, Takahashi N, Glockner JF, Talwalkar JA, Ehman RL. Non-invasive detection of liver fibrosis: MR imaging features vs. MR elastography. Abdom Imaging. 2015;40(4):766–75.
7. Serai SD, Yin M, Wang H. Cross-vendor validation of liver magnetic resonance elastography. Abdom Imaging. 2015;40:789–94.
8. Faria SC, Ganesan K, Mwangi I, et al. MR imaging of liver fibrosis: current state of the art. Radiographics. 2009;29(6):1615–35.
9. Kennedy P, Wagner M, Castéra L, Hong C-W, et al. Quantitative elastography methods in liver disease: current evidence and future directions. Radiology. 2018;286(3):738–63.
10. Afdhal N, Bedossa P, Friedrich-Rust M, Han K-H, Pinzani M. EASL-ALEH clinical practice guidelines: non-invasive tests for evaluation of liver disease severity and prognosis. J Hepatol. 2015;63(1):237–64.
11. Yin M, Glaser KJ, Talwalkar JA, Chen J, Manduca A, Ehman RL. Hepatic MR elastography: clinical performance in a series of 1377 consecutive examinations. Radiology. 2016;278(01):114–24.
12. Wagner M, Corcuera-Solano I, Lo G, et al. Technical failure of MR elastography examinations of the liver: experience from a large single-center study. Radiology. 2017;284(02):401–12.
13. Shiha G, Ibrahim A, Helmy A, et al. Asian-Pacific Association for the Study of the Liver (APASL) consensus guidelines on invasive and non-invasive assessment of hepatic fibrosis: a 2016 update. Hepatol Int. 2017;11(01):1–30.
14. Singh S, Venkatesh SK, Wang Z, et al. Diagnostic performance of magnetic resonance elastography in staging liver fibrosis: a systematic review and meta-analysis of individual participant data. Clin Gastroenterol Hepatol. 2015;13(03):440–51.
15. Singh S, Venkatesh SK, Loomba R, et al. Magnetic resonance elastography for staging liver fibrosis in non-alcoholic fatty liver disease: a diagnostic accuracy systematic review and individual participant data pooled analysis. Eur Radiol. 2016;26(5):1431–40.
16. Cui J, Heba E, Hernandez C, et al. Magnetic resonance elastography is superior to acoustic radiation force impulse for the diagnosis of fibrosis in patients with biopsy-proven nonalcoholic fatty liver disease: a prospective study. Hepatology. 2016;63:453–61.
17. Imajo K, Kessoku T, Honda Y, et al. Magnetic resonance imaging more accurately classifies steatosis and fibrosis in patients with nonalcoholic fatty liver disease than transient elastography. Gastroenterology. 2016;150:626–37.
18. Loomba R, Cui J, Wolfson T, et al. Novel 3D magnetic resonance elastography for the noninvasive diagnosis of advanced fibrosis in NAFLD: a prospective study. Am J Gastroenterol. 2016;111:986–94.

19. Pavlidea M, Banerjee R, Tunnicliffe EM, et al. Multiparametric magnetic resonance imaging for the assessment of non-alcoholic fatty liver disease severity. Liver Int. 2017;37:1065–73.
20. Bookwalter CA, Venkatesh SK, John E, Eaton JE, et al. MR elastography in primary sclerosing cholangitis: correlating liver stiffness with bile duct strictures and parenchymal changes. Abdom Radiol. 2018;43:3260–70.
21. Ichikawa S, Motosugi U, Enomoto N, Onishi H. Magnetic resonance elastography can predict development of hepatocellular carcinoma with longitudinally acquired two-point data. Eur Radiol. 2019;29:1013–21.
22. Lee DH, Lee M, Chang W. Prognostic role of liver stiffness measurements using magnetic resonance elastography in patients with compensated chronic liver disease. Eur Radiol. 2018;28:3513–21.
23. Chen J, Yin M, Talwalkar JA, et al. Diagnostic performance of MR elastography and vibration-controlled transient elastography in the detection of hepatic fibrosis in patients with severe to morbid obesity. Radiology. 2017;283(2):418–28.
24. Yin M, Venkatesh SK. Ultrasound or MR elastography of liver: which one shall I use? Abdom Radiol. 2018;43:1546–51.
25. Serai SD, Trout AT. Can MR elastography be used to measure liver stiffness in patients with iron overload? Abdom Radiol. 2018; https://doi.org/10.1007/s00261-018-1723-9.
26. Donato H, França M, Candelária I, Caseiro-Alves F. Liver MRI: from basic protocol to advanced techniques. Eur J Radiol. 2017;93:30–9.
27. Van Beers BE, Daire J-L, Garteiser P. New imaging techniques for liver diseases. J Hepatol. 2015;62:690–700.
28. Neri E, Bali MA, Ba-Ssalamah A, et al. ESGAR consensus statement on liver MR imaging and clinical use of liver-specific contrast agents. Eur Radiol. 2016;26:921–31.
29. Jhaveri K, Cleary S, Audet P, et al. Consensus statements from a multidisciplinary expert panel on the utilization and application of a liver-specific MRI contrast agent (gadoxetic acid). Am J Roentgenol. 2015;204:498–509.
30. Luciani A, Frédéric Pigneur F. Séquences de diffusion et produits de contraste hépatobiliaires en IRM du foie: les évolutions en cours. POST'U 2017, pp 49–54.
31. Lewis S, Dyvorne H, Cui Y, Taouli B. Diffusion-weighted imaging of the liver: techniques and applications. Magn Reson Imag Clin N Am. 2014;22:373–95.
32. Ronot M, Clift AK, Vilgrain V, Frilling A. Functional imaging in liver tumours. J Hepatol. 2016;65:1017–30.
33. Vilgrain V, Esvan M, Ronot M, et al. A meta-analysis of diffusion-weighted and gadoxetic acid-enhanced MR imaging for the detection of liver metastases. Eur Radiol. 2016;26:4595–615.
34. França M, Martí-Bonmatí L, Alberich-Bayarri A, et al. Evaluation of fibrosis and inflammation in diffuse liver diseases using intravoxel incoherent motion diffusion-weighted MR imaging. Abdom Radiol. 2017;42(2):468–77.
35. Schalkx HJ, van Stralen M, Coenegrachts K, et al. Liver perfusion in dynamic contrast-enhanced magnetic resonance imaging (DCE-MRI): comparison of enhancement in Gd-BT-DO3A and Gd-EOB-DTPA in normal liver parenchyma. Eur Radiol. 2014;24:2146–56.
36. Ricke J, Seidensticker M. Molecular imaging and liver function assessment by hepatobiliary MRI. J Hepatol. 2016;65:1081–2.
37. Nilsson H, Blomqvist L, Douglas L, Nordell A, Janczewska I, Naslund E, et al. Gd-EOB-DTPA-enhanced MRI for the assessment of liver function and volume in liver cirrhosis. Br J Radiol. 2013;86:20120653.
38. Kukuk GM, Schaefer SG, Fimmers R, et al. Hepatobiliary magnetic resonance imaging in patients with liver disease: correlation of liver enhancement with biochemical liver function tests. Eur Radiol. 2014;24:2482–90.
39. Truhn D, Kuhl CK, Ciritsis A. A new model for MR evaluation of liver function with gadoxetic acid, including both uptake and excretion. Eur Radiol. 2019;29:383–91.
40. Yoneda N, Matsui O, Ikeno H, et al. Correlation between Gd-EOB-DTPA-enhanced MR imaging findings and OATP1B3 expression in chemotherapy-associated sinusoidal obstruction syndrome. Abdom Imaging. 2015;40:3099–103.
41. Lee NK, Kim S, Kim GH, et al. Significance of the "delayed hyperintense portal vein sign" in the hepatobiliary phase MRI obtained with Gd-EOB-DTPA. J Magn Reson Imaging. 2012;36:678–85.
42. Han NY, Park BJ, Sung DJ, et al. Chemotherapy-induced focal hepatopathy in patients with gastrointestinal malignancy: gadoxetic acid-enhanced and diffusion-weighted MR imaging with clinical-pathologic correlation. Radiology. 2014;271:416–20.
43. Unal E, Karaosmanoğlu AD, Ozmen MN, et al. Hepatobiliary phase liver MR imaging findings after Oxaliplatin-based chemotherapy in cancer patients. Abdom Radiol. 2018;43(9):2321–8.
44. Zhou Z-P, Long L-L, Qiu W-J, et al. Evaluating segmental liver function using T1 mapping on Gd-EOB-DTPA-enhanced MRI with a 3.0 Tesla. BMC Med Imaging. 2017;17:20.
45. Ding Y, Rao S-X, Chen C, et al. Assessing liver function in patients with HBV-related HCC: a comparison of T1 mapping on Gd-EOB-DTPA-enhanced MR imaging with DWI. Eur Radiol. 2015;25:1392–8.

Contrast Enhanced MR imaging of Liver

47

Ran-Chou Chen, Chen-Te Chou, and Yung-Liang Wan

Key Concepts

- Contrast enhanced MR imaging is the image of choice for the diagnosis of focal hepatic lesions. Gd-DTPA is currently the most frequently used contrast medium in clinical practice. The dynamic phases include arterial, venous and delayed phases.
- The hepatocyte-specific Gd-EOB-DTPA is another widely used contrast medium nowadays. GD-EOB-DTPA enhanced MR provides additional tumor information in the hepatobiliary images. Therefore, the sensitivity and specificity of hepatic tumor diagnosis are increased. It also provides quantitative liver and biliary functional information, and helps in staging liver fibrosis.
- The characteristic contrast enhanced MR images of focal nodular hyperplasia (FNH) are isointense in both T1-weighted image (T1WI) and T2-weighted image (T2WI), have dense enhancement in arterial phase, rapidly return to isointensity in venous phase, and then occasionally have delayed enhancement of central scar. Gd-EOB-DTPA-enhanced hepatobiliary phase showed typically hyperintense/isointense to adjacent liver parenchyma with a hypointense central scar. MR is better than contrast enhanced CT in the diagnosis of FNH.
- The typical MR contrast enhancing patterns of HCC are arterial enhancement and washout phenomenon in venous and/or delayed phases. The specificity is 96–100%. However, the sensitivity is 60%. Most HCCs showed hypointense in the hepatobiliary phase of Gd-EOB-DTPA enhanced MR, which is helpful in increasing the diagnostic sensitivity and specificity.

47.1 Introduction

A variety of imaging modalities are currently used in evaluating patients with liver disease; these include ultrasonography (US), computed tomography (CT), magnetic resonance imaging (MRI), nuclear medicine, and angiography. Among these modalities, contrast enhanced dynamic MRI is one of the best noninvasive imaging techniques. Recent progress of the MR scanner hardware, software techniques and new contrast agents have increased the effectiveness and accuracy in detecting and characterizing liver disease, especially focal hepatic lesions [1]. The progress in MR machines include

Ran-Chou Chen and Chen-Te Chou contributed equally to this work.

R.-C. Chen (✉)
Commissioner, Department of Health, New Taipei City Government, New Taipei City, Taiwan

Department of Biomedical Imaging and Radiological Sciences, National Yang-Ming University, Taipei City, Taiwan

C.-T. Chou
Department of Biomedical Imaging and Radiological Sciences, National Yang-Ming University, Taipei City, Taiwan

Department of Radiology, Changhua Christian Hospital, Changhua City, Taiwan

School of Medicine, Kaohsiung Medical University, Kaohsiung, Taiwan

Department of Molecular Biotechnology, College of Biotechnology and Bioresources, Dayeh University, Changhua City, Taiwan

Y.-L. Wan
Department of Medical Imaging and Radiological Sciences, College of Medicine, Chang Gung University, Taoyuan City, Taiwan

Department of Medical Imaging and Intervention, Linkou Chang Gung Memorial Hospital, Taoyuan City, Taiwan
e-mail: ylw0518@cgmh.org.tw

F. Radu-Ionita et al. (eds.), *Liver Diseases*, https://doi.org/10.1007/978-3-030-24432-3_47

3-T MRI, high performance gradient coils, advanced phased-array torso coils, parallel-acquisition imaging (a powerful gradient system with increased speed), a new 3D gradient-echo sequence with increased resolution, dynamic contrast enhanced (DCE) MR imaging and a variety of new or faster MR imaging techniques [2]. The new contrast media such as hepatocyte-specific Gd-EOB-DTPA provide quantitative functional information, help in staging liver fibrosis and provide additional tumor information in hepatobiliary images [3]. Therefore, the contrast enhanced MRI is widely used in the diagnosis of diffuse liver disease and focal hepatic lesions.

Using the most common hepatic malignant tumor hepatocellular carcinoma (HCC) as an example, dynamic studies, including CT and MR, are the images of choice and are accepted as the final diagnostic methods for HCC in all the clinical practices guidelines around the world. The typical vascular patterns of the dynamic images consist of enhancement in arterial phase and hypointense signals in the venous/delayed phases. This has a sensitivity of 60% and a specificity of 96–100% [4]. With the use of hepatocyte-phase imaging of Gd-EOB-DTPA enhanced MR, the diagnostic accuracy would be higher [5]. Furthermore, Gd-EOB-DTPA enhanced MRI can replace the role of CT during hepatic arteriography (CTHA) and the role of CT during arterial portography (CTAP) in the diagnosis of HCC [3].

In this chapter, we will present the currently used MR techniques and contrast mediums used during contrast enhanced MRI of liver diseases.

47.2 Contrast Medium

The contrast agents used for liver MRI include extracellular agents (e.g., Gd-DTPA), reticuloendothelial agents (e.g. ferucarbotran), hepatobiliary agents (e.g. mangafodipir), blood pool agents, and combined agents.

47.2.1 Extracellular Agents

After intravenous (IV) administration, the extracellular agents are distributed within the extracellular interstitial space. Gadolinium chelates are formed from the chelation of gadolinium to organic ligands. Structurally, the extracellular gadolinium-based contrast agents can be divided into two subgroups according to the type of ligand—linear agents and macrocyclic agents. Linear agents have an elongated organic ligand that wraps around the gadolinium ion. Macrocyclic agents form a cage-like ligand structure with the gadolinium ion wrapped in a preformed circle. Gadolinium has seven unpaired electrons, which can be used as high paramagnetic agents. Gadolinium chelates, such as gadolinium diethylenetriamine-pentaacetate (Gd-DTPA) and gadolinium tetraazacyclododecane-tetraacetate (Gd-DOTA), were the first contrast agents available for clinical use in hepatic imaging. High paramagnetic gadolinium ions could shorten the T1 (spin-lattice) and T2 (spin-spin) relaxation times of adjacent water protons. These effects cause an increase in signal intensity of post contrast T1-weighted images (T1WI) [6]. The T1 shortening effect predominates at low concentrations of gadolinium, and the T2 shortening effect predominates at high gadolinium concentrations. After the administration of gadolinium chelates in clinically approved doses, the T1 shortening effect is observed in essentially all tissues. Therefore, T1 is the imaging property that is routinely evaluated after the administration of extracellular agents. Subsequent to the administration, these agents are initially distributed in the intravascular space and rapidly filtered through the capillaries into the extracellular space, producing contrast enhancement in the T1WI and providing dynamic-enhanced information [7].

47.2.1.1 Toxic Effects

Gadolinium chelates in high doses might cause more nephrotoxic injury than that of iodinated contrast agents [8]. In recent reports, an association between the gadolinium-based contrast agents and the development of nephrogenic systemic fibrosis (NSF) has been identified in patients with severe renal impairment, inflammatory burden, and exposure to high doses of contrast agents [9]. This has led to modifications in clinical practices to reduce the incidence of NSF development. The more recent reports have also demonstrated that gadolinium accumulates in various tissues (e.g. bone and brain) of patients who have normal renal function [10]. Despite the observations of gadolinium accumulation in tissues regardless of renal function, there have been very limited clinical data regarding the potential effects for patient health.

Subsequent to the gadolinium agent administration, the potential adverse effects include transient headache, nausea, and emesis. Other reactions have been reported, but only at a frequency of 1% or less. Anaphylaxis is exceedingly rare; only one anaphylaxis death related to a gadolinium-based agent has been reported [11]. Because the gadolinium-based contrast agents cross the placenta and their long-term effects are unknown, the contrast agents should be avoided in the first trimester and breast-feeding should be suspended for 48 h after contrast administration.

47.2.1.2 MR Technical Considerations

MR protocols need to be carefully designed to obtain high quality images as well as to shorten the examination time. Basic pulse sequences of liver MR protocol include T1- and T2-weighted imaging, together with a dynamic series following intravenous administration of a gadolinium-based contrast agent. Standard protocols on the high performance MR gradient system with phased-array body coils are as follows: (1) coronal T2-weighted with SSFSE sequence, (2) T2-weighted FSE with fat suppression and respiratory trigger, (3) T1-weighted dual echo GRE images, (4) diffusion weighted imaging (5) heavily T2-weighted SSFSE for lesion characterization when high-intensity nodules are depicted on T2-weighted FSE images, and (6) 3D fast spoiled gradient-echo T1W sequence with fat suppression before and after the administration of contrast material in a dynamic fashion [12]. Gadolinium-enhanced MR imaging has been used in lesion detection and in characterization and depiction of hepatic vessels. On the dynamic contrast enhancement, the arterial-dominant phase is the most important for lesion characterization; various types of liver lesions have distinctive arterial enhancement patterns. This arterial phase is obtained in most patients by initiating a 3D spoiled GRE sequence approximately 16–17 s after the start of injection. The portal venous phase or early hepatic venous phase is acquired at 45–60 s after initiation of the gadolinium-based agent injection. On this phase, the hepatic parenchyma is maximally enhanced so that hypovascular lesions are most clearly shown as regions of zero or diminished enhancement. Hepatic venous phase or interstitial phase is acquired 90 s to 5 min after initiation of the contrast agent injection. Late enhancement features of focal liver lesions are shown on this phase [13].

47.2.1.3 Dosage

The recommended dosage of an extracellular gadolinium-based contrast agent for liver imaging is 0.1 mmol/kg of body weight. The recommended injection rate is 2–3 mL/s followed by a 20 mL saline flash. There are three methods available in determining the acquisition delay time to obtain images during the late hepatic arterial phase: a best-guess, fluoroscopic triggering, and timing with a test bolus [14]. In our opinion, the use of fluoroscopic triggering is recommended.

47.2.2 Reticuloendothelial Agents

These contrast agents are targeted to the reticuloendothelial system (RES) of the liver and spleen to improve detection and characterization of focal liver lesions. These particles are absorbed by phagocytic Kupffer cells in the reticuloendothelial system (RES). In contrast, the contrast agent is not retained in lesions lacking Kupffer cells. Consequently, there are significant differences in T2/T2* relaxation between normal tissue and focal lesions, resulting in improvement of lesion conspicuity and detectability [15]. Two SPIO agents have been clinically approved: ferumoxides (Feridex in the USA, Endorem in Europe) with a particle size of 120–180 nm, and ferucarbotran (Resovist) with a particle size of 60 nm. The principal effect of the SPIO particles is on T2* relaxation, and thus MR imaging is usually performed using T2*-weighted sequences or EPI sequences in which the tissue signal loss is due to the susceptibility effects of the iron oxide core. Enhancement on T1-weighted images can also be seen with the smaller particle agent (Resovist) and can be administered as a rapid bolus (can be used for both dynamic and delayed imaging).

47.2.2.1 MR Technical Considerations

For pre-enhanced imaging, the MR protocol was similar to standard protocols mentioned above for extracellular agents. Contrast-enhanced MR imaging with the use of SPIO particles should be performed with T2*-weighted sequences. Ferumoxide-enhanced imaging is typically performed 1–4 h after infusion. Ferucarbotran-enhanced imaging is typically performed 10 min after ferucarbotran administration.

47.2.2.2 Dosage

The recommended dose of ferumoxides is 0.05 mL/kg. The manufacturer recommends dilution of the dose in 100 mL of a 5% dextrose solution and intravenous infusion over 30–60 min. The ferucarbotran consists of SPIO microparticles coated with carboxydextran, and this was preloaded into 1.4 mL (>50 kg body weight) syringe using a connecting intravenous tube.

47.2.3 Hepatobiliary Agents

Hepatobiliary agents are paramagnetic compounds that are absorbed by hepatocytes and excreted into bile ducts. This contrast agent increases the signal intensity of the liver parenchyma, bile ducts, and hepatocyte-containing lesions in post-enhanced T1-weighted imaging. Manganese is chelated to dipyridoxyl diphosphate to produce the prototype hepatobiliary agent known as mangafodipir trisodium (Teslascan; Nycomed Amersham, Oslo, Norway). The agent shortens the T1 and T2 relaxation times of water protons. Low manganese concentrations resulted in high signal intensity on T1-weighted images; and high concentrations resulted in low signal intensity on T2-weighted images. Dipyridoxyl diphosphate has a chemical structure similar to that of vitamin B6 and is taken up by functioning hepatocytes [14]. Hepatic enhancement begins at approximately 1 min after administration; enhancement peaks at approximately 15 min and persists for several hours. Biliary excretion is usually visible at 5 min after contrast agent administration. Complete delineation of the biliary system might require more than 15 min. One use of mangafodipir is to characterize lesions as hepatocellular or nonhepatocellular in contrast-enhanced cholangiography [16].

47.2.3.1 MR Technical Considerations

For pre-enhanced study, the MR protocol was similar to standard protocols mentioned above for extracellular agents. Contrast-enhanced 3D spoiled GRE T1W imaging at 3–10 minutes (for detection and characterization of the focal liver lesion) and at 20 min (for biliary evaluation) after the administration of mangafodipir has recommended [17].

47.2.3.2 Dosage

The recommended adult dose of mangafodipir is 5 mol/kg body weight. The dose is administered with a relatively slow injection over 10–20 min.

47.2.4 Blood Pool Agents

Blood pool agents are retained in the intravascular space much longer than extracellular agents. As a result, blood pool agents are currently under active investigation for MR angiography, which could be performed in the equilibrium phase. These agents may be divided into three subgroups: ultrasmall SPIO particles, agents that reversibly bind to plasma proteins, and macromolecules [18]. Only limited clinical data are available for these blood pool agents, particularly in liver imaging scenarios.

47.2.5 Combined Agents

The contrast agent gadolinium ethoxybenzyl diethylenetriamine pentaacetic acid (Gd-EOB-DTPA) was developed to improve the detection and characterization of focal liver lesions in hepatic magnetic resonance imaging. Gd-EOB-DTPA is a gadolinium-based contrast agent with approximately 50% uptake by hepatocytes and subsequent biliary excretion [19]. After IV administration, it is distributed into the vascular and extravascular spaces, allowing for dynamic study (arterial, portal venous, and late phases). This contrast-enhanced dynamic imaging is similar to nonspecific extracellular gadolinium contrasts in lesion detection and characterization. The contrast also provides hepatocyte information during the hepatobiliary phases. Approximately 50% of the injected dose is absorbed into the functional hepatocyte and is excreted into the biliary system. The contrast enhancement of liver parenchyma peaks at about 20 min and persists for more than 2 h. The elimination pathway of Gd-EOB-DTPA is unique compared to other extracellular gadolinium agents. The renal and hepatobiliary systems both eliminate half of the Gd-EOB-DTPA [19]. Because of this property, Gd-EOB-DTPA also has the potential to be a biliary contrast agent and an aid in predicting liver function reserve. Gd-EOB-DTPA-enhanced MR cholangiography could be effective in the evaluation of biliary anatomy, the assessment of bile duct obstruction, and the detection of bile duct injuries, including leakage and stricture.

47.2.5.1 MR Technical Considerations

For pre-enhanced imaging and dynamic enhanced study, the MR protocol for Gd-EOB-DTPA was similar to standard protocols mentioned above for extracellular agents. Hepatobiliary phase imaging using the same 3D fast spoiled gradient-echo T1W sequence with fat suppression was obtained at 20 min after the administration of contrast material. For patients with impaired liver function, extra delay time might be needed [20]. Additional high-resolution 3D T1W imaging with respiration trigger might be helpful in detection of small focal liver lesions [21].

Dynamic contrast-enhanced MRI (DCE-MRI) can be performed either by extracellular agent or by Gd-EOB-DTPA. The dual blood supply, the portal vein and the hepatic artery, of the liver presents opportunities for DCE-MR imaging. The sequence allows us to produce pharmacokinetic parameters that can quantify endothelial permeability (Ktrans) and fractional blood plasma volume in focal liver lesions and liver parenchyma. These parameters can provide more information about micro-vascularity than conventional multi-phase enhancements in the abdomen and have potentially important clinical values for diagnosing disease and therapeutic planning [22]. The DCE-MRI protocol was composed of two parts, a pre-contrast multi-flip angle sequence for T1 mapping and a dynamic sequence to monitor contrast media flow in and out. It has been applied to quantify perfusion changes in the liver parenchyma observed in hepatic fibrosis and cirrhosis, and to quantify the angiogenic activity in malignant focal liver lesions [23].

47.2.5.2 Dosage

Gd-EOB-DTPA is approved at a dose of 0.1 mL/kg to 0.025 mmol/kg body weight. Because transient-apnea was frequently found in the arterial phase for patients with 2 mL/s injection rates. The recommended injection rate is 1 mL/s according to some reports demonstrating that the transient-apnea could be reduced with a lower injection rate [24]. A newly developed MR protocol (compressed sensing technique) for dynamic study under free breathing was introduced. It might resolve the transient apnea during arterial phase for Ga-EOB-DTPA-enhanced MRI [25].

Gadobenate dimeglumine is another combined agent with extracellular and hepatobiliary behavior. In contrast to 50% of Gd-EOB-DTPA being absorbed by hepatocyte, only 5% of Gadobenate dimeglumine was absorbed by hepatocyte. A longer delay time might be needed for Gadobenate dimeglumine-enhanced hepatobiliary phase imaging [26].

47.3 Diagnosis of Diffuse Liver Diseases with Contrast Enhanced MR

Gd-EOB-DTPA-enhanced MRI can be used to evaluate diffuse liver diseases. Approximately 50% of the injected dose undergoes specific OATP1B1/B3-dependent hepatocyte uptake with consecutive biliary excretion via multidrug resistance protein 2 (MRP2) at the canalicular membranes of hepatocytes. Using the OATP1B1/B3—MRP2 pathway, Gd-EOB-DTPA and indocyanine green (ICG) are dependent on the same transport mechanisms; therefore, like ICG clearance, Gd-EOB-DTPA-enhanced MR imaging could provide information for quantitative evaluation of liver function and allow for anatomic delineation of hepatic function [27].

Patients with impaired liver function presenting with decreased liver parenchymal enhancement on hepatobiliary phase has been demonstrated. Signal intensity of liver parenchyma on hepatobiliary phase showed a negative correlation to the patient's Child-Pugh score.

The evaluation of T1 relaxation time with Gd-EOB-DTPA-enhanced MRI is an alternative approach to the direct measurement of SI and has recently been reported as a diagnostic tool for quantitative evaluation of liver function.

47.4 Diagnosis of Focal Liver Lesions with Contrast Enhanced MR

Gd-DTPA and Gd-EOB-DTPA are widely used in clinical practice. The dynamic enhancement for both Gd-DTPA and Gd-EOB-DTPA were similar. Besides the above dynamic phases, the Gd-EOB-DTPA enhanced MR provides additional information in the hepatobiliary phase. The characteristics of contrast enhanced MRI of common focal hepatic lesions (Table 47.1) are shown as follows.

47.4.1 Hemangiomas

Hemangioma is the most common benign liver tumor. The majority of lesions show low signals on T1-weighted images and very high signals on T2-weighted images as compared with liver parenchyma. The characteristic enhancing patterns are peripheral nodule-like enhancement in the arterial phase, with slow centripetal fill-in and persistent enhancement on delayed images. Some atypical hemangiomas showed rapid, strong homogenous enhancement in arterial phase and an iso to mildly high signal in venous or delayed phases. However, the diagnosis of hemangioma can be usually achieved with the combination of a very high signal (as a light bulb appearance) in T2WI and enhancement on contrast enhanced images (Fig. 47.1).

In Gd-EOB-DTPA-enhanced MR, hemangioma showed hypointense to adjacent liver parenchyma on hepatobiliary phase imaging.

47.4.2 Focal Nodular Hyperplasia (FNH)

The majority of FNHs have similar signal intensities on both T1WI and T2WI. A typical display was early circumscription, strong enhancement, rapid return to isointensity, and then occasionally a delayed enhancement of the central scar. MRI is better than contrast enhanced CT in the diagnosis of FNH; the vascularity pattern alone cannot make a definite diagnosis in atypical cases. The characteristic signal intensity in T1WI and T2WI helps in the diagnosis of such cases.

On Gd-EOB-DTPA-enhanced MRI, FNH showed typically hyperintense/isointense to adjacent liver parenchyma on hepatobiliary phase imaging with a hypointense central scar. This additional information plays an important role in the diagnosis (Fig. 47.2).

Table 47.1 Contrast enhanced MRI for the focal liver lesions

	Extracellular agents Gd-DTPA			Gd-EOB-DTPA
Liver tumor	Dynamic study			Hepatobiliary phase
	Arterial phase	Portal venous phase	Delayed phase	
Hemangioma	Peripheral nodular	Centripetal fill-in	Persistent stain hyperintense	Hypointense
Focal nodular hyperplasia	Hypervascularity with hypointense central scar	Hypervascularity with hypointense central scar	Hyper-/iso-intense with delayed central scar enhancement	Hyperintense with hypointense central scar
Simple cyst	No enhancement	No enhancement	No enhancement	No enhancement
Adenoma	Hypervascularity	Hypervascularity	Hypo-/iso-intense	Hypointense
Hepatocellular carcinoma	Hypervascularity	Hypointense to isointense	Hypointense	Hypointense
Cholangiocarcinoma	Hypervascular rim enhancement	Heterogenous hyper/hypointense	Heterogenous central delayed enhancement	Hypointense
Metastasis	Hypervascular rim or hypovascularity	Hypointense	Hypointense	Hypointense

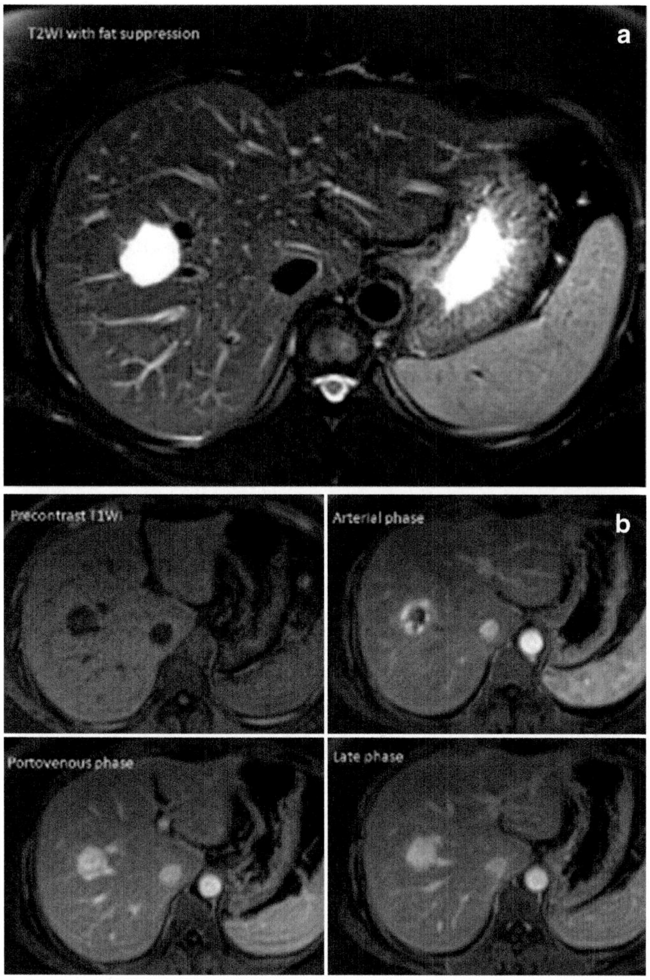

Fig. 47.1 A 56-year-old female with hemangioma at S8 of liver underwent Gd-DTPA-enhanced MR imaging. (**a**) The tumor depicted bright signal intensity on T2W images. (**b**) The tumor showed hypointense on precontrast T1W imaging, peripheral nodular enhancement on arterial phase, centripetal fill-in with homogenous enhancement on portovenous/late phase images

47.4.3 Hepatic Cyst

Simple hepatic cysts showed low signals on T1WI and very high signals in T2WI, and do not enhance after the contrast administration.

47.4.4 Hepatocellular Adenoma

Hepatocellular adenoma is a rare benign neoplasm that is usually seen in young women with a history of oral contraceptive usage; about 70–80% of them are solitary. Under the MR imaging, adenomas are heterogeneous in appearance due to areas of increased signal intensity resulting from fat (36–77% of cases in different series) or hemor-

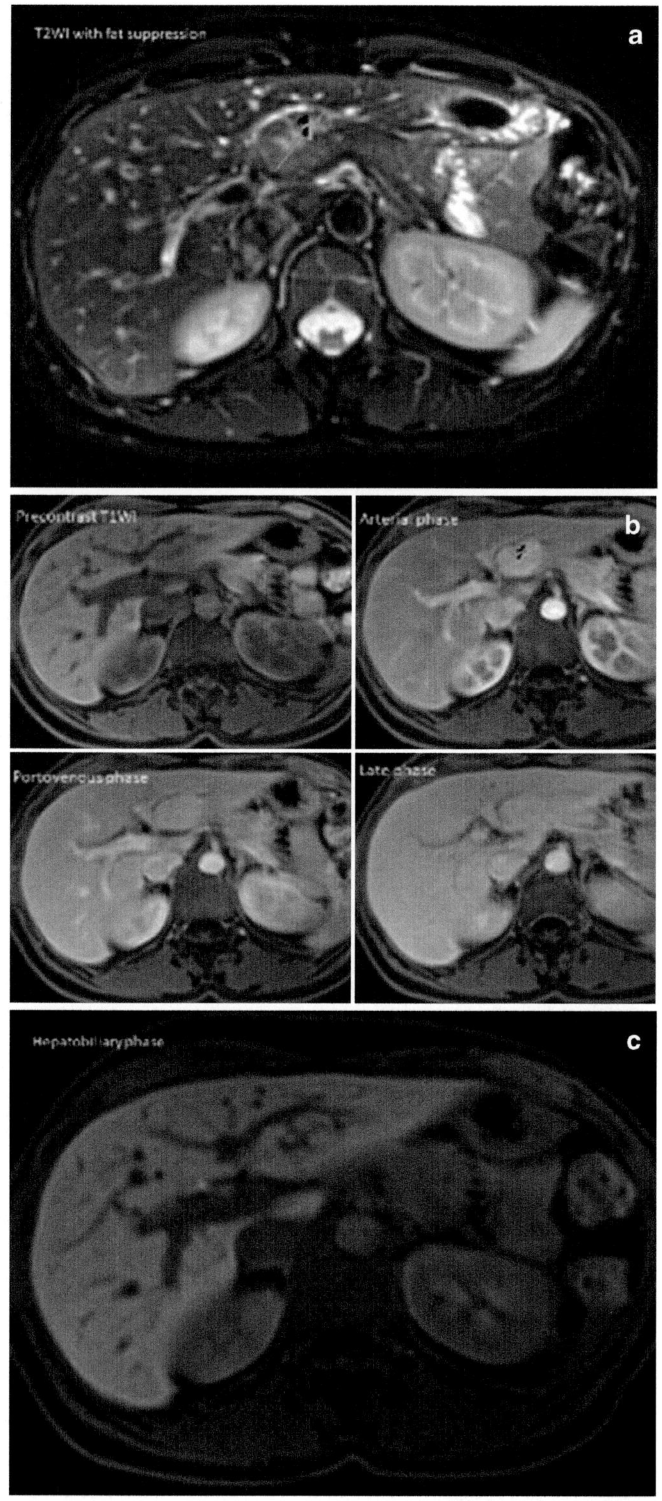

Fig. 47.2 A 50-year-old female with focal nodular hyperplasia at S2 of liver underwent Gd-EOB-DTPA-enhanced MR imaging. (**a**) The tumor shows mild hyperintense with bright signal central scar on T2WI. (**b**) The tumor is hypointense on precontrast T1W imaging, heterogenous and hypervascular on arterial phase, homogenous enhancement on late phase images. (**c**) The tumor features hyperintense with dark central scar on hepatobiliary phase

rhages (52–93%); and areas of low signal-intensity corresponding to necrosis, old hemorrhages or calcifications. On T1WI, the tumors showed various signal intensities, about 35–77% of them showed high signals. The presence of fat areas showed signal drops on opposed-phase dual T1 imaging. On T2WI, they demonstrated a combined hyper- and hypo signal intensity; these may be related to hemorrhages and necrosis. Contrast enhanced MRI demonstrated early arterial homogenous enhancement. However, they sometimes showed atypical features such as heterogeneous enhancement. The tumors became nearly isointense on late or delayed images [28].

On Gd-EOB-DTPA-enhanced MR imaging, hepatocellular adenoma showed hypointense to adjacent liver parenchyma on hepatobiliary phase imaging.

47.4.5 Malignant Metastatic Tumors

The liver is a common site of metastatic tumors. The appearance of a hepatic metastatic tumors can vary; it depends on the origin of the malignancy. The colon, breast, and lung comprise the majority of the primary sites. Most of the tumors showed hypointensity on T1WI and hyperintensity on T2WI and enhanced heterogeneously. A large number of liver metastases are hypovascular and are best imaged during the portal venous phase; they occasionally show central non-enhancing areas that represent necrosis (Fig. 47.3) [29].

On Gd-EOB-DTPA-enhanced MR imaging, metastatic tumors showed hypointense to adjacent liver parenchyma on hepatobiliary phase imaging.

47.4.6 Hepatocellular Carcinoma (HCC)

HCC is the most common of the malignant primary hepatic tumors. These tumors frequently appeared in patients with underlying liver disease. The liver parenchyma showed heterogeneous appearance in the diffuse liver disease. Furthermore, it demonstrated nodular appearance in the cirrhotic liver. The hepatic and renal functions may also lead to different contrast uptakes of the liver parenchyma. The contrast uptake of the background liver parenchyma affects the appearance of hepatic tumors. HCCs against a background of cirrhosis are diagnostically challenging in daily practices. According to the American Association for the Study of Liver diseases (AASLD) and the European Association for the Study of the Liver (EASL) guidelines, the recognition of a hepatic nodule larger than 10 mm by US in patients at high risk for HCC should be followed by diagnostic contrasted enhanced dynamic CT or MR.

On MR images, it usually shows a heterogeneous signal on T1WI and a high signal on T2WI. Diffusion-weighted imaging (DWI) is currently a standard sequence of the protocol of liver MR, and it improves the detection of small focal liver lesions, including HCC. The majority of HCC showed mild to moderate signal hyperintensity compared to the surrounding liver parenchyma on the DWI. The mean apparent diffusion coefficient (ADC) value is usually low in malignant tumors. However, there are debates about the effectiveness of DWI and ADC among different studies [4].

The performance in contrast enhanced MR is crucial in the diagnosis of HCC. The typical enhancing patterns are

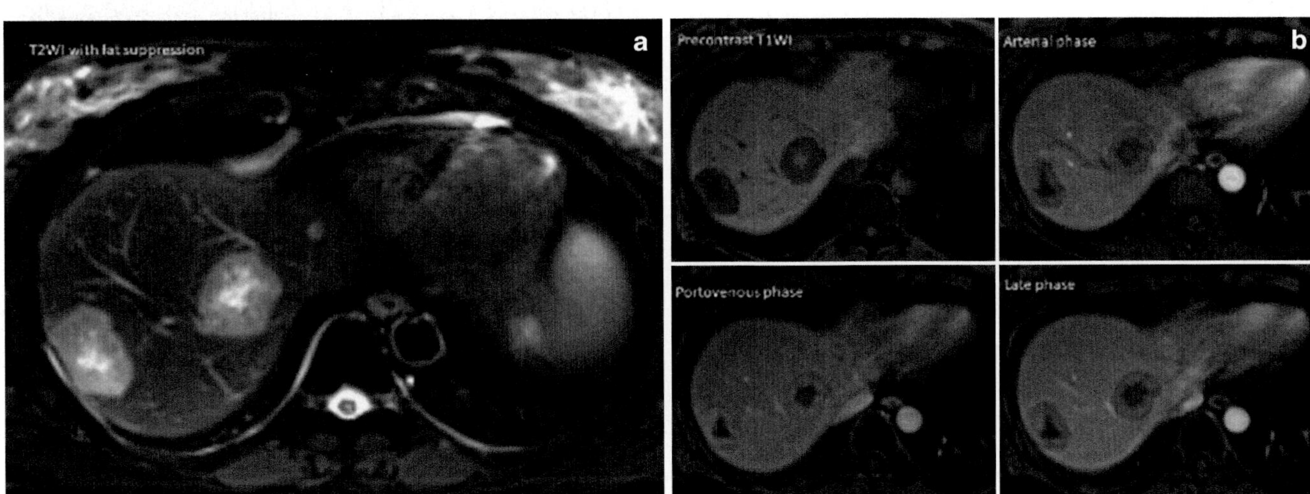

Fig. 47.3 A 46-year-old female with breast carcinoma and multiple liver metastases underwent Gd-DTPA-enhanced MR imaging. (**a**) The tumor is hyperintense on T2WI. (**b**) The tumor features hypointense on pre-enhanced T1W imaging, rim enhancement in arterial phase, and hypointense with target appearance on late phase images

consistent on arterial enhancement, are more than that of the surrounding liver parenchyma (wash-in), and have hypo-signal intensity compared to the surrounding liver (wash-out) in the venous phase. According to the AASLD/EASL and other guidelines, if the above typical images appears on an MR profile, the diagnosis of HCC is established. The specificity can reach to 96–100%. However, there are lesions with atypical presentations; for example, an early HCC (the small well-differentiated HCC) usually features diminished enhancement in the arterial and venous phases of contrast enhanced MRI [30]. Therefore, the sensitivity is only 60% [4].

It is sometimes difficult to differentiate benign cirrhotic nodules from HCC since there are atypical presentations and overlapping appearances in the conventional Gd-DTPA enhanced MR images. The Gd-EOB-DTPA enhanced hepatobiliary phase imaging can show cellular function of focal hepatic lesions. Therefore, it can help in the differentiation of functional benign hepatic nodules from HCCs with no hepatocellular functions. HCC is typically homogenous and hypointense to adjacent liver parenchyma on hepatobiliary phase imaging. However, a few HCCs (5–10%) might depict heterogeneous hyperintensity instead of hypointensity on hepatobiliary phase imaging. This may be a result of expression of organic anion transporter in HCCs, rather than tumor differentiation. Using quantitative evaluation, the liver-to-lesion contrasts of HCC showed a significant increase in the mean value on the hepatobiliary phase T1WI in comparison with adjacent liver parenchyma. In contrast, the liver-to-lesion contrasts of dysplastic nodules were only slightly increased on hepatobiliary phase T1WI. Thus, the differences in the CNR change provide useful diagnostic clues in the differentiation of benign nodules from HCC in cirrhotic livers.

On the Gd-EOB-DTPA enhanced MR imaging, both dynamic and hepatobiliary phase imaging contribute to characterization of focal hepatic lesions. The typical HCC features arterial enhancement followed by washout in dynamic study, and hypointense on hepatobiliary phase (Fig. 47.4).

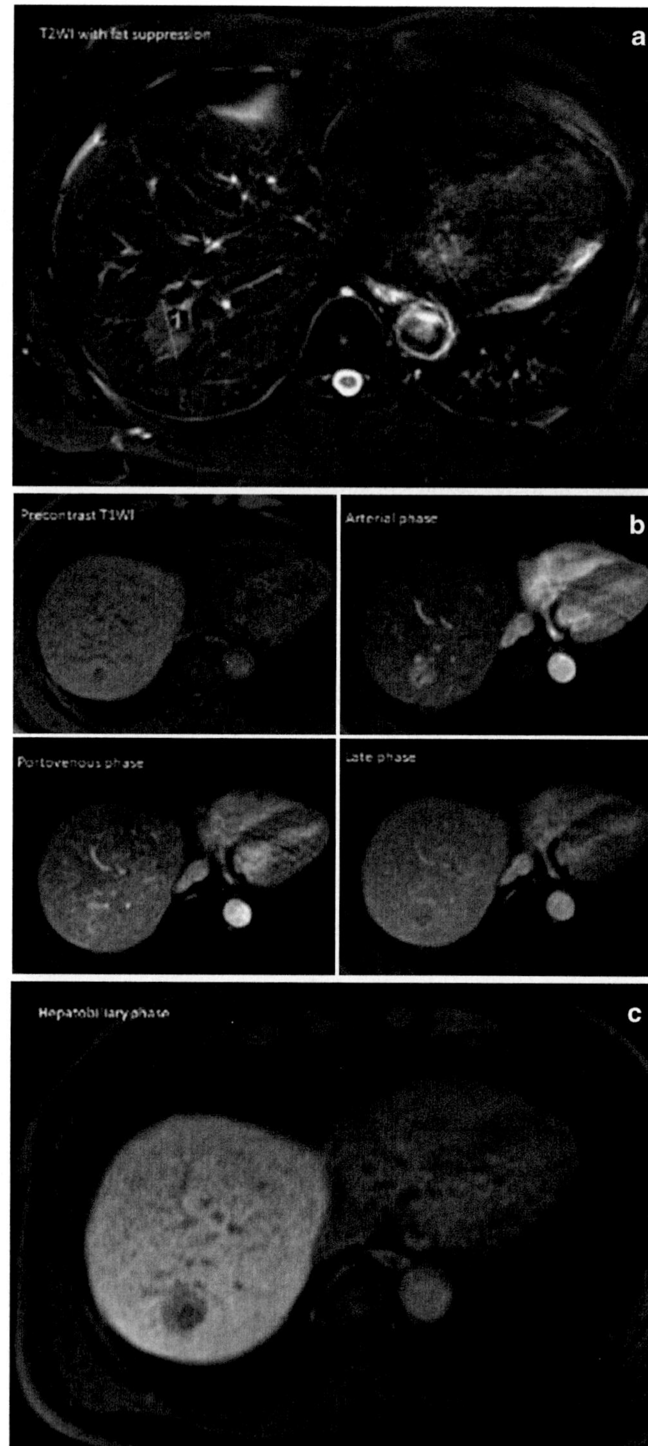

Fig. 47.4 A 78-year-old male with chronic B hepatitis and HCC at S7 of liver underwent Gd-EOB-DTPA-enhanced MR imaging. (**a**) The tumor is hyperintense on T2WI. (**b**) The tumor appears isointense with focal hypointense on pre-enhanced T1W imaging, it is heterogenous and hypervascular in arterial phase, and contrast washout on late phase images. (**c**) The tumor is heterogenously hypointense on hepatobiliary phase image

47.4.7 Intrahepatic Cholangiocarcinoma (ICC)

ICC is the second most common malignancy arising from the liver. MR imaging rarely identifies any pathognomonic features of ICC compared with other liver lesions. The majority of MR imaging showed hypointensity on T1WI and high intensity on T2WI, peripheral enhancement, progressive concentric filling, and contrast pooling on delayed images.

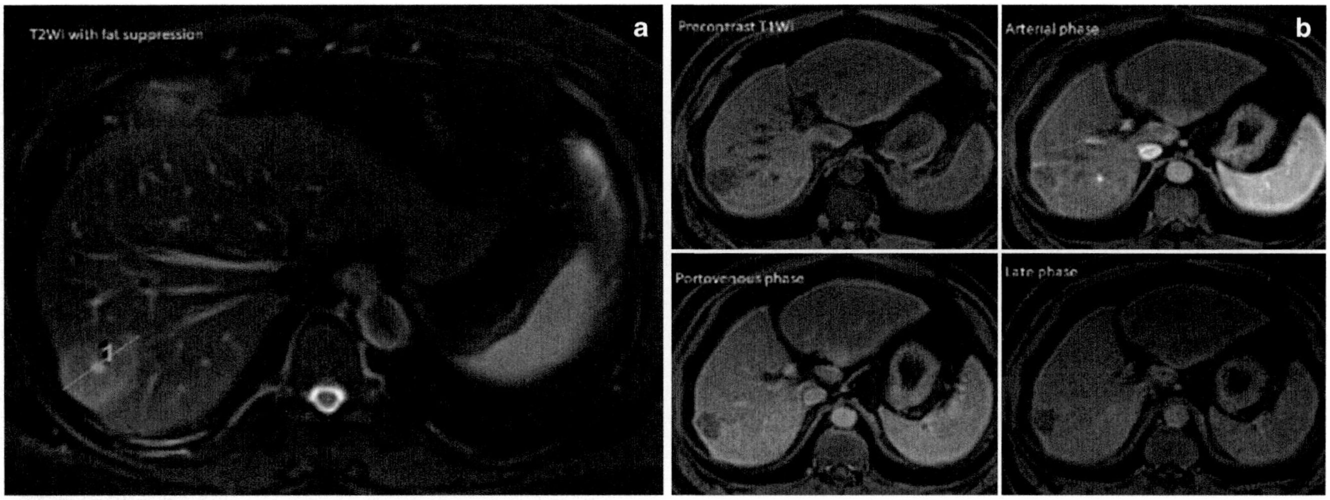

Fig. 47.5 A 57-year-old male with cholangiocarcinoma at S7 of liver underwent Gd-DTPA-enhanced MR imaging. (**a**) The tumor is hyperintense on T2WI. (**b**) The tumor features hypointense on pre-enhanced T1W imaging, peripheral enhancement in arterial phase, and is mildly enhanced on late phase images

The T2W-MR cholangiopancreatogram (MRCP) was introduced in 1990; it depicts static fluid as high signal intensity in heavily T2 weighted sequences. MRCP has been proven to be an effective and noninvasive method in the characterization of both extrahepatic and intrahepatic biliary abnormalities. In ICC, MRCP depicts biliary involvement of the tumors, and therefore, it plays an important role in the diagnosis (Fig. 47.5).

On Gd-EOB-DTPA-enhanced MRI, ICC is hypointense to adjacent liver parenchyma on hepatobiliary phase imaging.

47.4.8 Diagnostic Pitfalls of Focal Hepatic Disease

Many of the above statements overlap among focal hepatic lesions. Some of the authors had reported up to 5–7% of intrahepatic cholangiocarcinoma (ICC) demonstrated similar enhancement patterns to HCC [31]. Various enhancement patterns in liver parenchyma are also demonstrated on hepatic arterial–dominant phase images. One of the most common perfusion abnormalities observed is the transient increase in segmental enhancement in liver segments with compromised portal venous flow due to compression or thrombosis. These are the challenges of diagnosing focal liver lesions by contrast enhanced MR imaging.

47.5 Conclusions/Summary

Contrast enhanced dynamic MRI is one of the best noninvasive imaging modalities in both detection and diagnosis of liver lesions. Currently, the extracellular contrast agent Gd-DTPA and the combined agent Gd-EOB-DTPA are the most frequently used contrast media in clinical practice. Different focal liver lesions show distinct enhancement patterns in the dynamic arterial, venous or delayed phases of Gd-DTPA enhanced MR images. The different signal appearance in the hepatobiliary phase of Gd-EOB-DTPA enhanced MR helps in further differentiating diagnoses among these lesions and plays a role in diagnosing diffuse liver disease. However, there are challenges because of the overlaps among the lesions and atypical presentations of some tumors. Diagnosis of liver diseases has been improving continuously over the past decades with imaging technology advances and new contrast mediums. However, future studies are still needed to continuously improve the diagnostic accuracy.

Self Study

Questions

1. Which of the following are true for the Gd-DTPA enhanced MR images of liver lesions with typical presentations?
   (a) Hepatic hemangioma showed peripheral nodular enhancement in arterial phase and centripetal fill-in and persistent enhancement on delayed images.
   (b) HCC features arterial enhancement and washout phenomenon on venous and/or delayed phases.
   (c) FNH is hypovascular in arterial and portal venous phases.
   (d) ICC showed no enhancement in all the dynamic phases.

2. Which of the followings are true for the Gd-EOB-DTPA enhanced MR images of liver lesions?
   (a) Most HCCs are hyperintense on hepatobiliary phase.
   (b) The enhancement patterns in dynamic phases are similar to Gd-DTPA.
   (c) A typical FNH is hyperintense/isointense to adjacent liver parenchyma on hepatobiliary phase imaging with a hypointense central scar.
   (d) Metastatic tumors showed hyperintense to adjacent liver parenchyma on hepatobiliary phase imaging.

Answers to the Questions

1. Which of the following are true for the Gd-DTPA enhanced MR images of liver lesions with typical presentations?
   (a), (b) Correct.
   (c) FNH showed dense arterial enhancement, rapidly returned to isointensity in venous phase, and occasionally showed delayed enhancement of its central scar.
   (d) Most ICC showed peripheral enhancement in arterial phase, progressive concentric filling, and contrast pooling on delayed images.
2. Which of the followings are true for the Gd-EOB-DTPA enhanced MR images of liver lesions?
   (a) Most HCC showed hypointense on hepatobiliary phase.
   (b), (c) Correct.
   (d) Most metastatic tumors showed hypointensity on hepatobiliary phase.

References

1. Lee JM, Yoon JH, Joo I, Woo HS. Recent advances in CT and MR imaging for evaluation of hepatocellular carcinoma. Liver Cancer. 2012;1(1):22–40.
2. Fahlenkamp UL, Wagner M, Nickel D, et al. Novel dynamic hepatic magnetic resonance imaging strategy using advanced parallel acquisition, rhythmic breath-hold technique, and gadoxetate disodium enhancement. Investig Radiol. 2016;51(1):33–40.
3. Chen BB, Murakami T, Shih TT, et al. Novel imaging diagnosis for hepatocellular carcinoma: consensus from the 5th Asia-Pacific Primary Liver Cancer Expert Meeting (APPLE 2014). Liver Cancer. 2015;4(4):215–27.
4. Ayuso C, Rimola J, Vilana R, et al. Diagnosis and staging of hepatocellular carcinoma (HCC): current guidelines. Eur J Radiol. 2018;101:72–81.
5. Wang YC, Chou CT, Lin CP, Chen YL, Chen YF, Chen RC. The value of Gd-EOB-DTPA-enhanced MR imaging in characterizing cirrhotic nodules with atypical enhancement on Gd-DTPA-enhanced MR images. PLoS One. 2017;12(3):e0174594.
6. Brown JJ, vanSonnenberg E, Gerber KH, Strich G, Wittich GR, Slutsky RA. Magnetic resonance relaxation times of percutaneously obtained normal and abnormal body fluids. Radiology. 1985;154(3):727–31.
7. Kenney PJ, Sobol WT, Smith JK, Morgan DE. Computed model of gadolinium enhanced MRI of breast disease. Eur J Radiol. 1997;24(2):109–19.
8. Prince MR, Arnoldus C, Frisoli JK. Nephrotoxicity of high-dose gadolinium compared with iodinated contrast. J Magn Reson Imaging. 1996;6(1):162–6.
9. Sadowski EA, Bennett LK, Chan MR, et al. Nephrogenic systemic fibrosis: risk factors and incidence estimation. Radiology. 2007;243(1):148–57.
10. Murata N, Murata K, Gonzalez-Cuyar LF, Maravilla KR. Gadolinium tissue deposition in brain and bone. Magn Reson Imaging. 2016;34(10):1359–65.
11. Prince MR, Zhang H, Zou Z, Staron RB, Brill PW. Incidence of immediate gadolinium contrast media reactions. AJR Am J Roentgenol. 2011;196(2):W138–43.
12. Neri E, Bali MA, Ba-Ssalamah A, et al. ESGAR consensus statement on liver MR imaging and clinical use of liver-specific contrast agents. Eur Radiol. 2016;26(4):921–31.
13. Semelka RC, Helmberger TK. Contrast agents for MR imaging of the liver. Radiology. 2001;218(1):27–38.
14. Gandhi SN, Brown MA, Wong JG, Aguirre DA, Sirlin CB. MR contrast agents for liver imaging: what, when, how. Radiographics. 2006;26(6):1621–36.
15. Wang YX. Superparamagnetic iron oxide based MRI contrast agents: current status of clinical application. Quant Imaging Med Surg. 2011;1(1):35–40.
16. Sahani DV, O'Malley ME, Bhat S, Hahn PF, Saini S. Contrast-enhanced MRI of the liver with mangafodipir trisodium: imaging technique and results. J Comput Assist Tomogr. 2002;26(2):216–22.
17. Rofsky NM, Earls JP. Mangafodipir trisodium injection (Mn-DPDP). A contrast agent for abdominal MR imaging. Magn Reson Imaging Clin N Am. 1996;4(1):73–85.
18. Hope MD, Hope TA, Zhu C, et al. Vascular imaging with ferumoxytol as a contrast agent. AJR Am J Roentgenol. 2015;205(3):W366–73.
19. Zech CJ, Herrmann KA, Reiser MF, Schoenberg SO. MR imaging in patients with suspected liver metastases: value of liver-specific contrast agent Gd-EOB-DTPA. Magn Reson Med Sci. 2007;6(1):43–52.
20. Cruite I, Schroeder M, Merkle EM, Sirlin CB. Gadoxetate disodium-enhanced MRI of the liver: Part 2, Protocol optimization and lesion appearance in the cirrhotic liver. AJR Am J Roentgenol. 2010;195(1):29–41.
21. Hopkinson G, Lockwood P, Dolbear G. Evaluation of an equilibrium phase free-breathing dynamic contrast-enhanced MRI prototype sequence compared to traditional breath-held MRI acquisition in liver oncology patients. Radiography. 2018;24(3):211–8.
22. Materne R, Smith AM, Peeters F, et al. Assessment of hepatic perfusion parameters with dynamic MRI. Magn Reson Med. 2002;47(1):135–42.
23. Taouli B, Johnson RS, Hajdu CH, et al. Hepatocellular carcinoma: perfusion quantification with dynamic contrast-enhanced MRI. Am J Roentgenol. 2013;201(4):795–800.
24. Haradome H, Grazioli L, Tsunoo M, et al. Can MR fluoroscopic triggering technique and slow rate injection provide appropriate arterial phase images with reducing artifacts on gadoxetic acid-DTPA (Gd-EOB-DTPA)-enhanced hepatic MR imaging? J Magn Reson Imaging. 2010;32:334–40.
25. Chandarana H, Feng L, Ream J, et al. Respiratory motion-resolved compressed sensing reconstruction of free-breathing radial acquisition for dynamic liver MRI. Investig Radiol. 2015;50(11):749–56.
26. Thian YL, Riddell AM, Koh DM. Liver-specific agents for contrast-enhanced MRI: role in oncological imaging. Cancer Imaging. 2013;13(4):567–79.

27. de Graaf W, Häusler S, Heger M, et al. Transporters involved in the hepatic uptake of (99m)Tc-mebrofenin and indocyanine green. J Hepatol. 2011;54(4):738–45.
28. Grazioli L, Federle MP, Brancatelli G, Ichikawa T, Olivetti L, Blachar A. Hepatic adenomas: imaging and pathologic findings. Radiographics. 2001;21(4):877–92.
29. Sica GT, Ji H, Ros PR. CT and MR imaging of hepatic metastases. AJR Am J Roentgenol. 2000;174(3):691–8.
30. Choi J-Y, Lee J-M, Sirlin CB. CT and MR imaging diagnosis and staging of hepatocellular carcinoma: Part I. Development, growth, and spread: key pathologic and imaging aspects. Radiology. 2014;272(3):635–54.
31. Li R, Cai P, Ma KS, Ding SY, Guo DY, Yan XC. Dynamic enhancement patterns of intrahepatic cholangiocarcinoma in cirrhosis on contrast-enhanced computed tomography: risk of misdiagnosis as hepatocellular carcinoma. Sci Rep. 2016;6:26772.

Transient Elastography in Chronic Liver Diseases

48

Gamal El-Sayed Shiha and Nasser Mousa

48.1 Introduction

Appraisal of the degree of liver fibrosis is crucial in deciding for patients with CLD [1]. Albeit, liver biopsy has been considered as the perfect technique for assessment of liver fibrosis to date, several problems such as sampling errors, intra- and inter-observer variability, and potential life-threatening complications have averted wide utilization of liver biopsy in clinical practice [2, 3]. In addition, the capacity to screen the dynamic process of liver fibrosis is incomprehensible. In this way, the requirement, for a non-invasive method of liver fibrosis evaluation has increased. Liver stiffness measurement using transient elastography which is an ultra-sound dependent modality for quantitative appraisal of liver fibrosis, has been introduced and has been increasing consideration all around [4].

Transient elastography (TE) using FibroScan presently takes into consideration a fast estimation of liver stiffness, by methods of an ultrasound transducer probe (FibroScan(R), Echosens, Paris, France), which measures the speed of slight amplitude and a low-frequency (50 Hz). This result in elastic shear wave that are propagated through the underlying liver parenchyma. This velocity is directly related to tissue stiffness and correlates with fibrosis. The stiffer the tissue, the faster the shear wave propagates [5].

TE is done while the patient is requested to lie in the dorsal decubitus position with the right arm in maximal abduction. The tip of the probe is reached to the intercostal skin with connector gel in the (9th to 11th) intercostal space at a similar site of liver biopsy. The administrator, helped by ultrasound time motion and A-mode images, places the probe upon the liver, finds a liver part at least 6 cm thick and free of large vascular structures. The administrator at that point presses the probe button and vibration starts toward the liver ("potshots"). TE measures is between 25 and 65 mm under the skin surface (an area at least one hundred times > the common liver biopsy). When a shot is unsuccessful, the machine does not return a value. The whole procedure is considered to have failed when no value is obtained after ten shots. The final result of a TE sitting can be regarded as valid if the following criteria are fulfilled: (1) at least ten valid shots; (2) a success rate equal to the ratio of number of valid measurements to the total number of measurements is ≥60%, and (3) an interquartile range (IQR, reflecting the variability of measurements) less than 30% of the median value of liver stiffness measurements (LSM). LSM measurement using TE is failed when no value is obtained after ten shots of measurement or more [6, 7]. The results are expressed in kilopascals (kPa), and range from 1.5 to 75 kPa with usual values around 5 kPa, greater in men also, in patients with low or high body mass index (U-shaped distribution) [8–11].

48.2 Advantages of Transient Elastography

A speedy procedure time (<5 min), painless, the results are present at the same setting, and simple to complete even in outpatient clinic. Simple learning of the technique. Even so, the clinical interpretation of TE results should always be in the hands of a specialist clinician and should be made with full information of patient Clinical-demographic data [12].

48.3 Limitations of Transient Elastography

Transient elastography measurements can be confused by both pathologic and normal factors. TE indeed measures the shear wave speed via the liver giving an idea about liver stiffness and not necessarily the true degree of fibrosis in the

G. E.-S. Shiha (✉)
Department of Internal Medicine, Mansoura University, Mansoura, Egypt

Egyptian Liver Research Institute and Hospital (ELRIH), Sherbin, El-Mansoura, Egypt

N. Mousa
Department of Tropical Medicine, Mansoura University, Mansoura, Egypt

F. Radu-Ionita et al. (eds.), *Liver Diseases*, https://doi.org/10.1007/978-3-030-24432-3_48

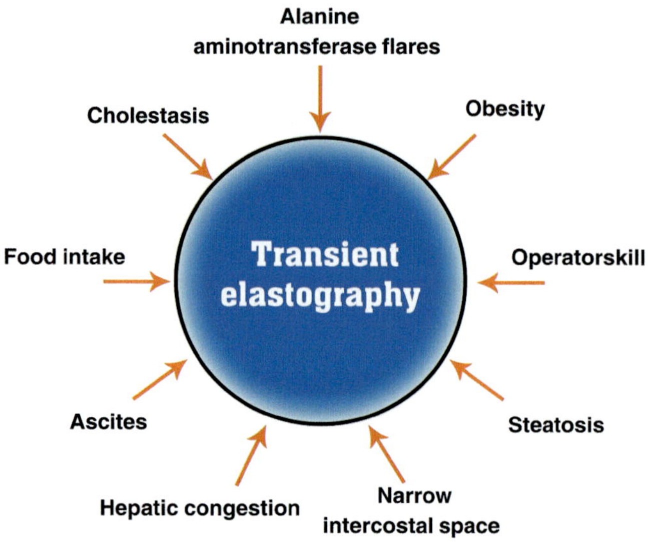

Fig. 48.1 Limitation of elastography of liver

liver. Therefore, situations in which stiffness of the liver increases independent of fibrosis will result in an increased LSM and falsely giving a higher estimate of fibrosis degree (Fig. 48.1).

48.3.1 Operator Skill

TE to a certain degree depends on operator skill. Consequently, there may be some inter-observer variability in results may reach up to 98% among operators of TE [13]. Moreover, a enormous review about TE examinations revealed that unsuccessful rate is 3.1% and unreliable measurements are 15.8%. Yet, both were associated with higher body mass index (BMI) > 30 kg/m^2 and operator skill of less than 500 examinations [14].

48.3.2 Obesity

Unfortunately, estimations by standard M test can't generally be made in obese patients and they can have higher outcomes and higher failure rate (5–22%) in patients with high BMI (>30 kg/m^2) [13, 14]. Numerous clarification of this disadvantages in light of disabled transmission of shear waves through the liver parenchyma, e.g. thick subcutaneous fat tissue [15], and expanded subcutaneous thoracic fat that upsurge the distance between the skin and liver capsule [16]. Hence, XL probes were introduced for obese patients. The XL probe reaches a lower frequency with a extra sensitive transducer, longer length, abroad vibration amplitude, and greater depth under the skin surface. This probe is beneficial in obese subjects [17].

48.3.3 Cholestasis

Extrahepatic cholestasis apart from fibrosis degree increase the liver stiffness estimates. Reports demonstrated a high degree of correlation of liver stiffness measurements with total bilirubin values and these measurements declines after successful biliary drainage [18, 19]. Explanations for higher stiffness in cholestasis are uncertain but may possibly be attributed to tissue swelling, inflammation, edema, and increased intracellular pressure due to obstructed bile drainage. Furthermore, the increased hydrostatic pressure alone appears to add to increased liver stiffness during extrahepatic cholestasis [18].

48.3.4 Alanine Aminotransferase Flares

Initial reports revealed that severe necroinflammation with >10-folds increase in Alanine aminotransferase (ALT), might lead to an increase in liver stiffness overestimating degree of fibrosis [20]. Later investigations demonstrated that even in lesser grades of necroinflammation, liver stiffness might be overestimated. In patients with chronic hepatitis B having the same fibrosis stage by liver biopsy, those with ALT levels ≥2 times ULN had higher TE outcomes compared to those with normal transaminases (9.5 versus 4.7 kPa) [21]. The stiffness measurements generally return to baseline along with the normalization of liver enzymes. Hence, it is advisable not to use TE in the presence of elevated transaminases [22].

48.3.5 Narrow Intercostal Space

Greater failure rates were reported in children and lean patients with narrow intercostal spaces, leading to development of newer pediatric S2 probes to improve reliability in these situations [23].

48.3.6 Hepatic Congestion

Liver stiffness estimations were significantly higher in patients with heart failure which return to baseline after hospitalization and control of cardiac disease [24]. Additionally, liver stiffness was higher in patients with right-sided heart failure versus healthy controls [25]. These results can be explained by deterioration of cardiac function that increase the hepatic vein pressure and producing intrahepatic blood stasis and higher liver stiffness. It is vital for clinicians to avoid use of TE in patients with heart failure and those with tricuspid regurgitation as it will overestimate degree of liver fibrosis.

48.3.7 Food Intake

It is established that, the food ingestion will significantly increase liver stiffness estimation. Arise in liver stiffness was observed discovered 15–45 min once the start the start of the meal with come to baseline levels before meal within 2 h. Hence, it is recommended to use TE after 120–180 min of fasting state [26].

48.3.8 Steatosis

The impact of steatosis on TE measurements is still a matter of debate. Up till now, no available well-controlled studies of TE in patients with NAFLD. Kim et al. reported that hepatic steatosis doesn't influence liver stiffness. But it's probably that, different cutoff values are going to be needed for patients with nonalcoholic steatohepatitis [27].

48.3.9 Ascites

It is nearly impossible to use TE in patients with ascites due to its infeasibility in patients with ascites [5, 28].

48.3.9.1 Validation of Transient Elastography in Liver Fibrosis Assessment

TE has been broadly investigated for determination of fibrosis degree in different chronic liver diseases especially HCV, HBV and non-alcoholic liver disease. Many researches revealed that, the hepatic stiffness measurements correlated with fibrosis stages detected by liver biopsy in studied patients [29]. TE revealed practically high area under the receiver operating characteristic curves (AUROCs) in the HCV group (AUROC: F≥2 0.89, F≥3 0.92, F4 0.92) and in the HBV group (F≥2 0.73, F≥3 0.83, F4 0.90), supporting previous results demonstrating that, TE permits staging of significant fibrosis [29, 30]. Furthermore, studies demonstrated value of TE in estimation of hepatic stiffness in NAFLD [31]. Additional meta-analysis of 50 studies in patients with different causes of CLD (n = 518) utilizing liver biopsy as the reference standard demonstrated that, 1D-TE was more precise in diagnosing F4 fibrosis than F2 or F3 fibrosis (AUROCF4 0.93 vs. F≥2 0.87, F≥3 0.91), irrespective of the underlying etiology of liver disease [10]. Generally, 1D-TE is considered useful to identify cirrhosis (F4 fibrosis) as well as for discriminating significant (≥F2) from non-significant (F0 and F1) fibrosis. Yet, discrimination between individual fibrosis stages is still not well validated [28].

48.4 Normal Values of Liver Stiffness on TE

In really healthy individuals, reports revealed that, the normal range of liver stiffness measurements on TE is between (4.8 and 6.9 kPa). These estimations were not affected by age, but higher measurements were obtained in the presence of steatosis or components of metabolic syndrome [8, 10].

48.5 Transient Elastography in Chronic Liver Diseases

A study conducted by Rajakannu et al., 2018 validated the Baveno VI criteria for non-invasive evaluation of Compensated advanced chronic liver disease (cACLD) and cirrhosis using TE, taking explants liver after surgery as a reference, in different etiologies of chronic liver diseases (CLD), with confirmation of its value even in obese patients having steatotic liver. Four hundred and ten patients (63.7% men) with variable degrees of underlying liver disease (liver tumors without liver disease [53.7%], viral [14.9%], alcohol [12.9%], non-alcoholic fatty liver disease [7.3%], and others [11.2%]) were included with valid LSM. All TE measurements were compared with the stage of fibrosis in resected liver specimen using the METAVIR scoring system by two expert pathologists. Agreeing with Baveno VI criteria, a cut-off of 10 kPa would confirm cACLD [AUROC: 0.95; 95%(CI) 0.923–0.973; sensitivity 86.1%; specificity 90.1%]. LSM ≥15 kPa would prove or exclude cirrhosis with 94.5% positive and 91.4% negative predictive values. In the earlier stages of fibrosis, TE seemed to have a better ability to rule in, with a cut-off of 6 kPa for F≥1 and 8 kPa for F≥2 stages with a positive predictive value of approximately 90% [32].

48.6 Transient Elastography and HCV

The first validation studies of TE and correlation with liver biopsy were performed in CHC. Sandrin et al. in 2003, revealed a study during which he analyzed 91 CHC patients underwent liver biopsy in additionally to TE. TE was (99%) effective in identifying cirrhosis and (88%) effective in identifying fibrosis [33]. Evaluation of the data on TE, principally in patients with CHC, shows that the liver stiffness measurement (LSM) does correlate strongly with the METAVIR fibrosis stage. Several studies have validated TE in CHC, and a meta-analysis of 50 studies showed characteristic area under the receiver operator curves (AUROCs) of 0.84, 0.89, and 0.94 for significant fibrosis (F≥2), F3–F4, and F4, respectively [34]. Similarly, in genotype 4 CHC patients, a significant hepatic fibrosis, advanced hepatic fibrosis and cirrhosis have a good validated cut-offs of (7.1, 9 and 12.2 kPa, respectively) in CHC patients with genotype 4 [35]. Rout et al., reported a reduction in liver stiffness measurement (LSM) by transient elastography, but increase in hepatic steatosis after completion of DAA therapy [36]. TE also is a useful tool to evaluate the severity of HCV recurrence after LT reducing the need of follow-up liver biopsies [37]. LSM perfectly predicts the existence of advanced fibrosis and portal hypertension (HTN) 1 year post-SVR in patient who had undergone liver transplantation [38]. In concordance with fibrosis progression rate, TE can predict time-to-cirrhosis. Erman et al., 2018 estimated time to cirrhosis using TE and comparing it with biopsy. They found it 39 and 38 years, respectively, [39]. Moreover, in pediatric study assessing the usefulness of TE (FibroScan) in liver fibrosis using the METAVIR score in a cohort of 30 chronic hepatitis C patients is from Egypt it was found that, the highest predictive performance of TE was detected for liver cirrhosis, followed by advanced fibrosis (F3). The accuracy for the discrimination of liver cirrhosis and advanced fibrosis was 96.7% and 85.3% at cut-off values of 9.5 kPa and 12.5 kPa, respectively [40].

48.7 Transient Elastography and CHB

TE can reliably assess degree of hepatic fibrosis in patients with CHB and therefore has been suggested by the American Association for the Study of Liver Diseases (AASLD) and European Association for the Study of the Liver (EASL) [41]. TE showed a good performance in both. Significant fibrosis (F2–4) and cirrhosis (F4) with pooled sensitivity of 78% and 84%, summary specificity of 81% and 87%. However, Qi et al. suggested that, TE is optimal in diagnosis of CHB-related cirrhosis (With cut-off value 12.4 kPa) but has a less accuracy in identifying significant fibrosis(With cut-off value 7.25 kPa) [42]. Some studies suggested liver(LS) stiffness cut-offs ranging from 5.2 to 8.7 kPa in diagnosing significant fibrosis (≥grade 2), with sensitivity (70–93%), specificity (38–92%). These studies suggested that, LS cut-off from 10.3 to 13.4 kPa, to diagnose cirrhosis (≥F4) with sensitivity 59–100% and specificity 79–94% [43, 44]. TE also provides a useful monitoring tool for evaluation of dynamic changes and response to treatment in CHB patients receiving antiviral therapy. After 3 years of follow up of patients receiving either entecavir or lamivudine, a significant reduction in LS measurements were reported (medians from baseline to 1, 2, and 3 years after treatment were 12.9 kPa, 7.5 kPa, 6.5 kPa, and 4.7 kPa, respectively; all $P < 0.05$) [45].

48.8 Transient Elastography and Portal Hypertension

The standard tools to detect PH in cirrhotic patients are invasive methods, they include, angiographic measurement of HVPG, upper gastrointestinal endoscopy to screen for esophageal varices [46]. TE with sensitivity ≥90% can define presence of portal hypertension in cirrhotic patients at cut-off values of 17.6 and 21.0 kPa, to detect hepatic venous pressure gradient (HVPG) above 10–12 mmHg [47]. The existence of varices could be excluded with a liver stiffness below 12.5–19.8 kPa [48]. LSM by TE cannot provide the precise value of HVPG, nor identify with high certainty which patients carry EV, but it can identify clinically significant portal hypertension. Even more importantly, LSM joint with platelet count has currently entered within the decision algorithm for patients with compensated ACLD, permitting patients at very low risk of varices needing treatment, to avoid endoscopy [49].

48.9 Transient Elastography and Autoimmune Hepatitis

Recent studies detected a significant correlation of LSM with stage of liver fibrosis in patients with autoimmune hepatitis (AIH), revealing a better performance, accuracy and reliability than non-invasive markers [50, 51]. LSM had significant correlation with fibrosis ($r = 0.752$, $P < 0.01$) and increased gradually with increasing fibrosis stages in AIH patients. AUROC values of LSM for stages F≥2, F≥3, and F4 were 0.878 (95% CI: 0.789–0.967), 0.883 (0.820–0.946), and 0.914 (0.852–0.976), respectively. The optimal cut-off values of LSM for fibrosis stages F≥2, F≥3, and F4 were 6.45, 8.75, and 12.50 kPa, respectively. LSM was better than APRI score and FIB-4 score in identifying advanced fibrosis (F≥3). Hepatic inflammatory activity and Serum ALT levels had no significant effect on LSM measurements [51]. Guo et al. confirm this better performance of TE more than other non-invasive markers in determination of fibrosis stages in patients with AIH. AUROC value of LSM was 0.885 for stage F2, 0.897 for stage F3, and 0.878 for stage F4. The optimal LSM cut-off value was 6.27 kPa for stage F2, 8.18 kPa for F3, and 12.67 kPa for F4 [52].

48.10 Transient Elastography and NAFLD

TE is an essential alternative for liver biopsy in NAFLD patients and it has a great value in ruling out liver cirrhosis. As the pathological fibrosis progresses, the sensitivity, specificity and NPV of TE in the diagnosis of fibrosis improves in NAFLD patients [53]. A meta-analysis of TE in patients with NAFLD suggests that, TE has brilliant diagnostic accuracy for cirrhosis, good accuracy for F3, however modest accuracy for F2 [54]. Despite this, TE can exclude cirrhosis with a high NPV (~90%). Clinicians may use various cut-offs for different stages of fibrosis in different situations depending whether they want to rule out or diagnose a fibrosis stage with high probability. In general, a cut-off of <8 kPa (or 7.2 kPa for the XL probe) reliably excludes a advanced fibrosis (F3–4) and a cut-off >9.6 kPa is suggestive of F3–4 [55]. A future meta-analysis revealed a pooled area under the receiver operating curve of (0.94) with 94% sensitivity and 95% specificity for advanced fibrosis [56]. Though, a chief disadvantage of this modality is its discrepancy in obtaining measurements in obese patients [57], and this was newly addressed by a study using a new XL probe, which has facilitate the examination in obese patients with comparable diagnostic accuracy to the standard probe [58].

48.11 Transient Elastography and Hepatocellular Carcinoma

TE can also be used in patients with CHB and CHC to predict the risk of development of hepatocellular carcinoma (HCC). Taking patients with LSM ≤10.0 kPa as a standard, the hazard ratios of developing HCC were (17, 21, 26 and 46) in patients with LSM at 10.1–15.0 kPa, 15.1–20.0 kPa, 20.1–25.0 kPa and higher than 25.0 kPa, respectively, in a study of 866 CHC patients [59]. TE, as well as FibroTest, may be useful in patients with CHC to predict 5-year survival rate; even after adjustments for age, degree of activity and treatment response degree of activity [60].

48.12 Transient Elastography and Acute Cellular Rejection Following Liver Transplantation

TE may be useful in assessing the severity of acute cellular rejection (ACR) after liver transplantation. A study on 33 patients with ACR by means of TE verified a cutoff point of >7.9 kPa to detect graft damage and < 5.3 kPa to rule out graft damage (receiver operating characteristic 0.93; $P < 0.001$). Another study showed elevated levels of liver stiffness in ACR patients. Yet, in this study, no cutoff point for ACR was definite. The latter study included 27 patients with ACR at liver biopsy. It suggests a Cutoff value of >8.5 kPa by TE to diagnose moderate to severe ACR, with a specificity of 100% and receiver operating characteristic curve of 0.924. The measurement of TE < 4.2 kPa rules out the opportunity of any ACR ($P = 0.02$) [61].

48.13 Transient Elastography and Alcoholic Liver Disease

TE may be used as a diagnostic tool to exclude high degrees of fibrosis (F3) and liver cirrhosis (F4) in persons with alcoholic liver disease. There is a debate about the best cut-off values for liver fibrosis in patients with alcoholic liver disease. By the most usually used cut-off value of 12.5 kPa, the sensitivity and specificity of transient elastography were 0.95 and 0.71 with LR+ 3.3 and LR− 0.07, which again confirms value of transient elastography in excluding cirrhosis, without need of liver biopsy [62].

48.14 Controlled Attenuation Parameter (CAP)

Controlled attenuation parameter is a physical parameter, applying the property that hepatic steatosis affects ultrasound propagation [63]. It measures ultrasound attenuation at the center frequency (expressed as dB/m) of the M probe. Ledinghen et al., 2012 conducted a study on 112 patients taking liver biopsy as a reference, concluding that CAP is a valuable tool in diagnosis of low grade steatosis [64]. A cut-off value of 215 dB/m has a sensitivity of 90% to detect S1 steatosis [64]. Studies have revealed that CAP can detect more than 5% hepatic steatosis exceeding the sensitivity of conventional ultrasound which can only detect greater than 30% steatosis [65, 66]. Furthermore, CAP is more reliable when the IQR of CAP is <30 dB/m. These findings support usefulness of CAP clinical evaluation of NAFLD [67].

48.15 Transient Elastography and Postoperative Outcomes

LSM is also an important prognostic device in patients with HCC. A study included one hundred and five HCC patients revealed that, a LSM cut-off of 12.0 kPa had a sensitivity of 86% and specificity of 72% concerning real post-operative complications. This cut-off would possibly recognize patients with more severe operative blood loss and higher transfusion rates [68]. An extra study of 133 HCC patients verified that, patients with LSM ≥13.4 kPa had an respecting dual rise in the risk of HCC recurrence, compared with those with LSM <13.4 kPa [69].

48.16 Conclusions/Summary

The accessibility of TE as noninvasive event for estimation of fibrosis and cirrhosis is a vital discovery within the clinical management of patients with chronic liver disease. It is a non-invasive, accurate and reproducible test alternative to biopsy for the assessment of liver fibrosis and possible steatosis. It has been valid during a wide spectrum of different liver diseases. There are still issues that require to be addressed with the utilization of FibroScan. In addition to technological restrictions (ascites and obesity), questions related to variable cutoffs based on disease etiology, clinical utility in management of NAFLD, clinical approach to longitudinal assessment, and frequency of repeated measurements must be addressed. Additional studies are necessary to investigate the reasonable cut-off values of newer **XL** and **S** probes; in addition those of the novel controlled attenuation parameter.

48.17 Future Perspectives for Liver FibroScan

Transient elastography has been shown to be a brilliant diagnostic means if strict quality criteria are applied, ensuring the reliability of the results. In spite of the lack of consensus guidelines concerning the use of liver stiffness measurements in clinical practice, transient elastography is already extensively used in many places. The main center now should be on the development of validated guidelines on the use of transient elastography, and to incorporate this new technology into current treatment guidelines.

Self Study

Questions

1. **Which statement is true?**
   (a) Liver fibrosis is a sign of progressive liver disease.
   (b) Transient elastography provides fast estimation of liver stiffness.
   (c) The stiffer the tissue, the slower the shear wave propagates.
   (d) TE is done while the patient is requested to lie on right side.
2. **Which statement/statements is/are true?**
   (a) Transient elastography is time consuming technique.
   (b) Transient elastography invasive maneuver.
   (c) Transient elastography is painless technique.
   (d) Transient elastography should be made with full information of patient Clinical-demographic data.
3. **Which statement/statements is/are true as regard Transient elastography?**
   (a) Standard M test can't generally be made in obese patients.
   (b) XL probes were ideal for obese patients.
   (c) Marked increase in Alanine aminotransferase, might lead to decrease in liver stiffness.
   (d) Liver stiffness estimations not exaggerated in patients with heart failure.
4. **Which statement/statements is/are true?**
   (a) TE has been suggested by the American Association for the Study of Liver Diseases and European Association for the Study of the Liver in patients with CHB.
   (b) TE is very well validated in NAFLD.
   (c) TE lacks a high-quality as noninvasive method for the measurement of liver stiffness.
   (d) Studies have shown non promising results in the use of TE in assessing fibrosis and disease progression in the setting of HIV-HCV co-infection.

Answers

1. **Which statement is true?**
   a
2. **Which statement/statements is/are true?**
   c and d
3. **Which statement/statements is/are true as regard Transient elastography?**
   a and b
4. **Which statement/statements is/are true?**
   a

References

1. Bruix J, Sherman M. Management of hepatocellular carcinoma. [J] Hepatology. 2005;42(5):1208–36.
2. Regev A, Berho M, Jeffers LJ, Milikowski C, Molina EG, Pyrsopoulos NT, et al. Sampling error and intraobserver variation in liver biopsy in patients with chronic HCV infection. Am J Gastroenterol. 2002;97(10):2614.
3. Bedossa P, Dargère D, Paradis V. Sampling variability of liver fibrosis in chronic hepatitis C. Hepatology. 2003;38(6):1449–57.
4. Jung KS, Kim SU. Clinical applications of transient elastography. Clin Mol Hepatol. 2012;18(2):163.
5. Sandrin L, Fourquet B, Hasquenoph JM, Yon S, Fournier C, Mal F, et al. Transient elastography: a new noninvasive method for assessment of hepatic fibrosis. Ultrasound Med Biol. 2003;29:1705–13.
6. Castera L, Forns X, Alberti A. Non-invasive evaluation of liver fibrosis using transient elastography. J Hepatol. 2008;48:835–47.
7. Castera L, Foucher J, Bernard PH, Carvalho F, Allaix D, Merrouche W, et al. Pitfalls of liver stiffness measurement: a 5-year prospective study of 13,369 examinations. Hepatology. 2010;51:828–35.
8. Roulot D, Czernichow S, Le Clesiau H, Costes L, Vergnaud C, Beaugrand M. Liver stiffness values in apparently healthy

subjects: influence of gender and metabolic syndrome. J Hepatol. 2008;48:606–13.
9. Kim U, Choi H, Han K, Kim K, Park Y, Kim DY, et al. What are 'true normal' liver stiffness values using FibroScan?: a prospective study in healthy living liver and kidney donors in South Korea. Liver Int. 2010;30:268–74.
10. Colombo S, Belloli L, Zaccanelli M, Badia E, Jamoletti C, Buonocore M, et al. Normal liver stiffness and its determinants in healthy blood donors. Dig Liver Dis. 2011;43:231–6.
11. Das K, Sarkar R, Ahmed M, Mridha R, Mukherjee S, Dhali GK, et al. Normal liver stiffness measure (LSM) values are higher in both lean and obese individuals: a population-based study from a developing country. Hepatology. 2012;55:584–93.
12. Boursier J, Konate A, Guilluy M, Gorea G, Sawadogo A, Quemener E, et al. Learning curve and interobserver reproducibility evaluation of liver stiffness measurement by transient elastography. Eur J Gastroenterol Hepatol. 2008;20:693–701.
13. Wong GL. Transient elastography: kill two birds with one stone? World Hepatol. 2013;5:264–74.
14. Castéra L, Foucher J, Bernard PH, Carvalho F, Allaix D, Merrouche W, Couzigou P, de Lédinghen V. Pitfalls of liver stiffness measurement: a 5-year prospective study of 13,369 examinations. Hepatology. 2010;51:828–35.
15. Wong GL, Wong VW, Chim AM, Yiu KK, Chu SH, Li MK, Chan HL. Factors associated with unreliable liver stiffness measurement and its failure with transient elastography in the Chinese population. J Gastroenterol Hepatol. 2011;26:300–5.
16. de Lédinghen V, Vergniol J. Transient elastography (FibroScan). Gastroenterol Clin Biol. 2008;32:58–67.
17. de Lédinghen V, Vergniol J, Foucher J, El-Hajbi F, Merrouche W, Rigalleau V. Feasibility of liver transient elastography with FibroScan using a new probe for obese patients. Liver Int. 2010;30:1043–8.
18. Millonig G, Reimann FM, Friedrich S, Fonouni H, Mehrabi A, Büchler MW, Seitz HK, Mueller S. Extrahepatic cholestasis increases liver stiffness (FibroScan) irrespective of fibrosis. Hepatology. 2008;48:1718–23.
19. Trifan A, Sfarti C, Cojocariu C, et al. Increased liver stiffness in extrahepatic cholestasis caused by choledocholithiasis. Hepat Mon. 2011;11(5):372–5.
20. Arena U, Vizzutti F, Corti G, et al. Acute viral hepatitis increases liver stiffness values measured by transient elastography. Hepatology. 2008;47(2):380–4.
21. Fung J, Lai C, Chan C, et al. Correlation of liver stiffness and histological features in healthy persons and in patients with occult hepatitis B, chronic active hepatitis B, or hepatitis B cirrhosis. Am J Gastroenterol. 2010;105(5):1116–22.
22. Coco B, Oliveri F, Maina AM, et al. Transient elastography: a new surrogate marker of liver fibrosis influenced by major changes of transaminases. J Viral Hepat. 2007;14(5):360–9.
23. Pradhan F, Ladak F, Tracey J, Crotty P, Myers RP. Feasibility and reliability of the FibroScan S2 (pediatric) probe compared with the M probe for liver stiffness measurement in small adults with chronic liver disease. Ann Hepatol. 2013;12(1):100–7.
24. Colli A, Pozzoni P, Berzuini A, et al. Decompensated chronic heart failure: increased liver stiffness measured by means of transient elastography. Radiology. 2010;257(3):872–8.
25. Hopper I, Kemp W, Porapakkham P, et al. Impact of heart failure and changes to volume status on liver stiffness: non-invasive assessment using transient elastography. Eur J Heart Fail. 2012;14(6):621–7.
26. Arena U, Platon M, Stasi C, et al. Liver stiffness is influenced by a standardized meal in patients with chronic hepatitis C virus at different stages of fibrotic evolution. Hepatology. 2013;58(1):65–72.
27. Kim KM, Choi WB, Park SH, et al. Diagnosis of hepatic steatosis and fibrosis by transient elastography in asymptomatic healthy individuals: a prospective study of living related potential liver donors. J Gastroenterol. 2007;42:382–8.
28. Shiha G, Ibrahim A, Helmy A, Sarin S, Omata M, Kumar A, et al. Asian-Pacific Association for the Study of the Liver (APASL) consensus guidelines on invasive and non-invasive assessment of hepatic fibrosis: a 2016 update. Hepatol Int. 2017;11:1–30.
29. Ziol M, Handra-Luca A, Kettaneh A, Christidis C, Mal F, Kazemi F, et al. Noninvasive assessment of liver fibrosis by measurement of stiffness in patients with chronic hepatitis C. Hepatology. 2005;41(1):48–54.
30. Castéra L, Vergniol J, Foucher J, Le Bail B, Chanteloup E, Haaser M, et al. Prospective comparison of transient elastography, Fibrotest, APRI, and liver biopsy for the assessment of fibrosis in chronic hepatitis C. Gastroenterology. 2005;128(2):343–50.
31. Petta S, DiMarco V, Cammà C, Butera G, Cabibi D, Craxì A. Reliability of liver stiffness measurement in non-alcoholic fatty liver disease: the effects of body mass index. AlimentPharmacol Ther. 2011;33:1350–60.
32. Rajakannu M, Coilly A, Adam R, Samuel D, Vibert E. Prospective validation of transient elastography for staging liver fibrosis in patients undergoing hepatectomy and liver transplantation. J Hepatol. 2018;68(1):199–200.
33. Sandrin L, Fourquet B, Hasquenoph JM, et al. Transient elastography: a new noninvasive method for assessment of hepatic fibrosis. Ultrasound Med Biol. 2003;29(12):1705–13.
34. Friedrich-Rust M, Ong MF, Martens S, et al. Performance of transient elastography for the staging of liver fibrosis: a meta-analysis. Gastroenterology. 2008;134(4):960–74.
35. Elsharkawy A, Alboraie M, Fouad R, Asem N, Abdo M, Elmakhzangy H, et al. Establishing ultrasound based transient elastography cutoffs for different stages of hepatic fibrosis and cirrhosis in Egyptian chronic hepatitis C patients. Arab J Gastroenterol. 2017;18(4):210–5.
36. Rout G, Nayak B, Patel AH, Gunjan D, Singh V, Kedia S. Therapy with oral directly acting agents in hepatitis C infection is associated with reduction in fibrosis and increase in hepatic steatosis on transient elastography. J Clin Exp Hepatol. 2019;9(2):207–14.
37. Carrión JA, Navasa M, Bosch J, Bruguera M, Gilabert R, Forns X. Transient elastography for diagnosis of advanced fibrosis and portal hypertension in patients with hepatitis C recurrence after liver transplantation. Liver Transpl. 2006;12(12):1791–8.
38. Mauro E, Crespo G, Montironi C, Londoño MC, Hernández-Gea V, Ruiz P, et al. Portal pressure and liver stiffness measurements in the prediction of fibrosis regression after sustained virological response in recurrent hepatitis C. Hepatology. 2018;67(5):1683–94.
39. Erman A, Sathya A, Nam A, Bielecki J, Feld J, Thein HH, et al. Estimating chronic hepatitis C prognosis using transient elastography-based liver stiffness: a systematic review and meta-analysis. J Viral Hepat. 2018;25(5):502–13.
40. Awad M-D, Shiha GE, Sallam FA, Mohamed A, El Tawab A. Evaluation of liver stiffness measurement by fibroscan as compared to liver biopsy for assessment of hepatic fibrosis in children with chronic hepatitis C. J Egypt Soc Parasitol. 2013;43:805–19.
41. Qi X, Liu F, Li Z, et al. Insufficient accuracy of computed tomography-based portal pressure assessment in hepatitis B virus-related cirrhosis: an analysis of data from CHESS-1601 trial. J Hepatol. 2017;68(1):210–1.
42. Qi X, An M, Wu T, Jiang D, Peng M, Wang W, et al. Transient elastography for significant liver fibrosis and cirrhosis in chronic hepatitis B: a meta-analysis. Can J Gastroenterol Hepatol. 2018;2018:3406789, 13 pages.
43. Verveer C, Zondervan PE, ten Kate FJ, Hansen BE, Janssen HL, de Knegt RJ. Evaluation of transient elastography for fibrosis assessment compared with large biopsies in chronic hepatitis B and C. Liver Int. 2012;32(4):622–8.

44. Cardoso AC, Carvalho-Filho RJ, Stern C, Dipumpo A, Giuily N, Ripault MP, et al. Direct comparison of diagnostic performance of transient elastography in patients with chronic hepatitis B and chronic hepatitis C. Liver Int. 2012;32(4):612–21.
45. Osakabe K, Ichino N, Nishikawa T, Sugiyama H, Kato M, Kitahara S, et al. Reduction of liver stiffness by antiviral therapy in chronic hepatitis B. J Gastroenterol. 2011;46(11):1324–34.
46. Castera L, Pinzani M, Bosch J. Non invasive evaluation of portal hypertension using transient elastography. J Hepatol. 2012;56(3):696–703.
47. Bureau C, Metivier S, Peron JM, et al. Transient elastography accurately predicts presence of significant portal hypertension in patients with chronic liver disease. Aliment Pharmacol Ther. 2008;27:1261–8.
48. Castera L, Le Bail B, Roudot-Thoraval F, et al. Early detection in routine clinical practice of cirrhosis and oesophageal varices in chronic hepatitis C: comparison of transient elastography (FibroScan) with standard laboratory tests and non-invasive scores. J Hepatol. 2009;50:59–68.
49. Berzigotti A. Non-invasive evaluation of portal hypertension using ultrasound elastography. J Hepatol. 2017;67(2):399–411.
50. Li Y, Cai Q, Zhang Y, et al. Development of algorithms based on serum markers and transient elastography for detecting significant fibrosis and cirrhosis in chronic hepatitis B patients: significant reduction in liver biopsy. Hepatol Res. 2016;46:1367–79.
51. Xu Q, Sheng L, Bao H, et al. Evaluation of transient elastography in assessing liver fibrosis in patients with autoimmune hepatitis. J Gastroenterol Hepatol. 2017;32:639–44.
52. Guo L, Zheng L, Hu L, Zhou H, Yu L, Liang W. Transient elastography (FibroScan) performs better than non-invasive markers in assessing liver fibrosis and cirrhosis in autoimmune hepatitis patients. Med Sci Monit. 2017;23:5106–12.
53. Hashemi S, Alavian S, Fesharaki M. Assessment of transient elastography (FibroScan) for diagnosis of fibrosis in non-alcoholic fatty liver disease: a systematic review and meta-analysis. Caspian J Intern Med. 2016;7(4):242–52.
54. Kwok R, Tse YK, Wong GH, Ha Y, Lee A, Ngu M, et al. Systematic review with meta-analysis: non-invasive assessment of non-alcoholic fatty liver disease–the role of transient elastography and plasma cytokeratin-18 fragments. Aliment Pharmacol Ther. 2014;39(3):254–69.
55. Hardy T, McPherson S. Imaging-based assessment of steatosis, inflammation and fibrosis in NAFLD. Curr Hepatol Rep. 2017;16(4):298–307.
56. Musso G, Gambino R, Cassader M, Pagano G. Meta-analysis: natural history of non-alcoholic fatty liver disease (NAFLD) and diagnostic accuracy of non-invasive tests for liver disease severity. Ann Med. 2011;43(8):617–49.
57. Wong VW, Vergniol J, Wong GL, Foucher J, Chan HL, Le Bail B, et al. Diagnosis of fibrosis and cirrhosis using liver stiffness measurement in nonalcoholic fatty liver disease. Hepatology. 2010;51(2):454–62.
58. Friedrich-Rust M, Hadji-Hosseini H, Kriener S, Herrmann E, Sircar I, Kau A, Zeuzem S, Bojunga J. Transient elastography with a new probe for obese patients for non-invasive staging of non-alcoholic steatohepatitis. Eur Radiol. 2010;20(10):2390–6.
59. Masuzaki R, Tateishi R, Yoshida H, et al. Prospective risk assessment for hepatocellular carcinoma development in patients with chronic hepatitis C by transient elastography. Hepatology. 2009;49:1954–61.
60. Vergniol J, Foucher J, Terrebonne E, et al. Noninvasive tests for fibrosis and liver stiffness predict 5-year outcomes of patients with chronic hepatitis C. Gastroenterology. 2011;140:1970–9.
61. Nacif L, Gomes C, Mischiatti M, Kim V, Paranaguá-Vezozzo D, Reinoso G, et al., editors. Transient elastography in acute cellular rejection following liver transplantation: systematic review. Transplantation Proceedings. Amsterdam: Elsevier; 2018.
62. Pavlov CS, Casazza G, Nikolova D, Tsochatzis E, Burroughs AK, Ivashkin VT, Gluud C. Transient elastography for diagnosis of stages of hepatic fibrosis and cirrhosis in people with alcoholic liver disease. Cochrane Database Syst Rev. 2015;1:CD010542.
63. Sasso M, Tengher-Barna I, Ziol M, et al. Novel controlled attenuation parameter for noninvasive assessment of steatosis using Fibroscan: validation in chronic hepatitis C. J Viral Hepat. 2012;19:244–53.
64. de Ledinghen V, Wong VW, Vergniol J, et al. Diagnosis of liver fibrosis and cirrhosis using liver stiffness measurement: comparison between M and XL probe of FibroScan (R). J Hepatol. 2012;56:833–9.
65. Kumar M, Rastogi A, Singh T, Behari C, Gupta E, Garg H, Kumar R, et al. Controlled attenuation parameter for non-invasive assessment of hepatic steatosis: does etiology affect performance? J Gastroenterol Hepatol. 2013;28:1194–201.
66. Chon YE, Jung KS, Kim SU, Park JY, Park YN, Kim DY, Ahn SH, Chon CY, Lee HW, Park Y, et al. Controlled attenuation parameter (CAP) for detection of hepatic steatosis in patients with chronic liver diseases: a prospective study of a native Korean population. Liver Int. 2014;34:102–9.
67. Caussy C, Alquiraish M, Nguyen P, Hernandez C, Cepin S, Fortney L. Optimal threshold of controlled attenuation parameter with MRI-PDFF as the gold standard for the detection of hepatic steatosis. Hepatology. 2018;67:1348–59.
68. Wong JS, Wong GL, Chan AW, et al. Liver stiffness measurement by transient elastography as a predictor on post-hepatectomy outcomes. Ann Surg. 2013;257(5):922–8.
69. Jung KS, Kim SU, Choi GH, et al. Prediction of recurrence after curative resection of hepatocellular carcinoma using liver stiffness measurement (FibroScan). Ann Surg Oncol. 2012;19:4278–86.

Portal Venography

49

Haokang Wei, Vishnu Chandra, Faisal Shah, and Sohail G. Contractor

Key Concepts
- Imaging modalities to evaluate portal venous system include ultrasonography, computed tomography, magnetic resonance imaging, spleno-portography, wedged hepatic venography, and splenic or superior mesenteric artery angiography with delayed venous phase imaging.
- Ultrasonography is the initial modality for evaluation.
- Computed tomography provides better global images of portal circulation when compared to ultrasound, but it does not provide functional status of the circulation
- Magnetic resonance imaging (MRI) provides excellent global images of the portal venous system. Four-dimensional flow MRI has the potential to be used to evaluate the hemodynamics of portal venous system.
- Catheter angiography is the "gold standard" to evaluate portal venous system.

49.1 Introduction

Evaluating and establishing an understanding of the portal venous system is helpful in vascular disorders of the liver and splanchnic circulation and also vital in planning and following-up on procedures such as liver transplantations, hepatic resections, and trans-jugular intrahepatic portosystemic shunt (TIPS) placements. Portal venography provides valuable information regarding the anatomy, patency, and nature of collateral circulations of the portal venous system.

H. Wei · V. Chandra · F. Shah · S. G. Contractor (✉)
Department of Radiology, Rutgers New Jersey Medical School, Newark, NJ, USA
e-mail: contrasg@njms.rutgers.edu

The portal venous system can be studied in both noninvasive and invasive approaches. The noninvasive modalities include ultrasonography (US) with duplex and color Doppler imaging, computed tomography (CT) venography, and magnetic resonance imaging (MRI). The invasive modalities include hepatic venography, trans-hepatic portography, percutaneous spleno-portography, and arterial portography.

49.2 Noninvasive Imaging of the Portal System

49.2.1 Ultrasonography (US)

Ultrasound is one of the most commonly utilized noninvasive imaging modalities to evaluate liver anatomy and pathology. Easy accessibility, low cost, favorable safety profile, and high sensitivity and specificity make ultrasound the first line study of choice for many liver diseases.

Using grey scale (B-mode) US, hepatic parenchyma, intrahepatic structures, and peri-hepatic structures can be differentiated by the echogenicity of the structures. This mode is preferred to outline and differentiate vessels, ducts, and lesions. Signs of portal hypertension, such as a dilated portal vein more than 13 mm diameter, can sometimes be seen, although it has a poor sensitivity for this. Similarly, US can also be used to assess the patency of the vessels and evaluate TIPS function. Portal vein thrombi are identified as hyperechoic material within the lumen. Contrast enhanced ultrasound might allow for the differentiation of a bland thrombus from a malignant thrombus, and has a sensitivity of 94% and specificity of 96% for this purpose [1, 2]. A bland thrombus is avascular and shows up as a void within the enhancing liver in all phases, whereas a malignant thrombus has the same enhancement characteristics as a tumor from which it originates [3–5].

Color doppler ultrasound allows visualization of body fluid movement and its velocity relative to the probe, allowing for functional evaluation of the portal venous system.

F. Radu-Ionita et al. (eds.), *Liver Diseases*, https://doi.org/10.1007/978-3-030-24432-3_49

Vascular anomalies in the portal circulation can be assessed with color Doppler evaluation. A fistula between the portal vein and the hepatic vein or hepatic artery is an infrequent finding on liver ultrasound. While a fistula between the portal vein and hepatic vein is usually asymptomatic due to the low resistance in both veins, while a fistula between the hepatic artery and portal vein is a high resistance connection and generates turbulent and flow reversal within the portal vein [6]. Color doppler can also be useful in determining if a thrombus is occlusive or nonocclusive. Similarly, reduced or reversal of flow in portal vein can be observed in patients with portal hypertension, with low velocity flow sometimes appearing stagnant under US.

These findings however are only found in a portion of the patients with portal hypertension, and thus US is not a sensitive study to evaluate for portal hypertension. While TIPS stenosis may be identified on grey scale US, TIPS dysfunction can also be identified by a decrease or increase in peak shunt velocity and further supported by a decrease in portal vein velocity and reversal of flow direction (Fig. 49.1) [7]. Although, there is no consensus in the criteria to diagnose shunt dysfunction, ultrasound and color doppler is often the primary tool to screen for TIPS dysfunction.

49.2.2 Computed Tomography

Intravenous iodinated contrast enhanced CT (CECT), specifically during portal venous phase of contrast enhancement, is another noninvasive imaging modality used to evaluate the portal venous system. Similar to US, CT is widely available, has a relatively low cost and a short procedure time. Moreover, CT is not operator dependent and offers a global view of the abdominal structures. This feature allows for the identification of liver volume, characteristics of liver disease, vascular variants, and portosystemic collateral vessels which can be helpful for preoperative evaluation for liver transplantation [8].

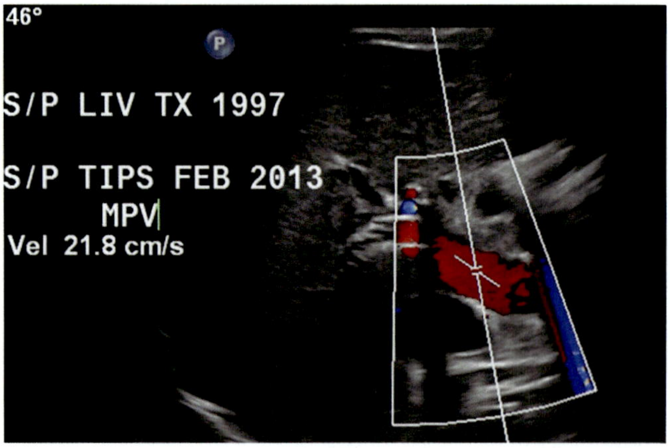

Fig. 49.1 Main portal vein. Color doppler US of the liver post TIPS shows of a patent TIPS shunt with main portal vein velocities slightly decreased compared with previous examination

The capability of using CT to assess the presence of a portal venous thrombus has also been well established. Focal high attenuation and venous enlargement in a nonenhanced CT scan is suggestive of an acute thrombus, whereas linear areas of calcification are seen in chronic thrombosis. In a CECT, thrombi are identified by the presence of a filing defect with partial or total occlusion of the lumen and rim enhancement of the vessels. Once a thrombus is identified, CT texture analysis and attenuation values can aid in differentiating malignant thrombus from bland thrombus [9]. The use of multi-detector CT with iodine quantification can further improve sensitivity and specificity in differentiating malignant and bland thrombi, with a sensitivity of 100%, specificity 95.2%, PPV 92.9%, NPV 100%, and an overall accuracy 97%, which is significantly better than conventional enhancement measurement ($p < 0.001$) [10].

CT imaging can also point towards a diagnosis of portal hypertension, although imaging findings of portosystemic collaterals and splenomegaly are sometimes not seen in a small portion of patients with clinically significant portal hypertension. The disadvantage of this modality is that it does not allow for quantification of portal venous flow or provide functional status of the structure, but a few studies have evaluated the reliability of using imaging finding indicative of portal hypertension to estimate portal pressure [11–13]. Currently, even though CT is a useful tool to evaluate TIPS stenosis, there is a lack of evidence to recommend using CT to evaluate shunt dysfunction (Figs. 49.3, 49.4 and 49.6) [14].

49.2.3 Magnetic Resonance Imaging

MRI is another imaging study that can provide a global image of abdominal structures. MRI with contrast allows for excellent evaluation of the liver anatomy, collateral circulation, portal venous system, and thrombus just like CT. But unlike CT, phase contrast MR angiography is capable of evaluating directional flow and velocity within the portal venous system. While MRI has this advantage over both CT and US, it is expensive, requires longer imaging time and is inaccessible to certain patient populations. Further, it is difficult to evaluate stagnant flow, and artifact from surgical clips and ascites making it less desirable compared to other noninvasive imaging modalities.

Recent advances in MRI technology have reduced imaging time to 8–12 min with four-dimensional (4D) flow MRI. Studies of 4D flow MRI to obtain quantitative measurements of the hemodynamic parameters in the hepatic and splanchnic system have been promising, with low inter-observer variability, and this technique can potentially be used to evaluate portal hypertension and TIPS function [15–18].

49.3 Invasive Imaging of the Portal System

Catheter angiography is the gold standard to evaluate the portal venous system. It can evaluate the portal venous system anatomy and hemodynamics and identify collaterals. However, angiography is invasive, has a longer procedural time and can be more expensive compared to noninvasive imaging modalities.

49.3.1 Wedged Hepatic Venography

Wedged hepatic venography has numerous applications but is most commonly used to visualize the portal vein during the TIPS procedure and evaluate hepatic hemodynamics, specifically the portosystemic pressure gradient. To perform wedged hepatic venography, one of the hepatic veins, usually the right hepatic vein, an angled vascular catheter is used from a jugular venous, or less commonly, a femoral approach. A hepatic venogram is first performed with the catheter floating free in the vein ("free hepatic venogram") with pressure measurements taken. Subsequently, the catheter is advanced further into the vein till the end hole of the catheter is wedged against the liver parenchyma ("wedged hepatic"), and a venogram and pressure measurements are performed. This yields a wedged hepatic venogram that pushes the contrast across the hepatic sinusoids into the portal circulation. In general, the higher the viscosity of the contrast used, the more force is required to get the contrast across the sinusoids. This exposes the patient to a risk of liver and capsular perforation, especially if excessive force is required to push contrast across (Fig. 49.2). As a result of this potential complication, either a diluted solution of contrast, or alternatively, carbon dioxide gas (CO_2) is used as the contrast agent (Fig. 49.3). CO_2 has low viscosity and hence a lower risk of capsular perforation. The portal venous pressure is indirectly determined by subtracting the free hepatic vein (FHV) pressure from the wedged hepatic venous (WHV) pressure. This is then regarded as the portal venous pressure (WHV-FHV). The right atrial pressure is then subtracted from this to yield the porto-systemic gradient. A gradient of less than 12 is considered normal.

The venograms and pressure measurements can also be performed using a balloon occlusion catheter. The free hepatic venogram is first performed as with the end hole catheter, subsequently, the balloon is inflated and the venous outflow obstructed. This yields a more predictable and repeatable wedged venogram and pressure measurement as the wedge measurements are averaged over multiple segments. When comparing CO_2 to contrast, CO_2 is preferred over contrast because of its low viscosity, cost, and toxicity. Renal function of the patient should be considered when using contrast.

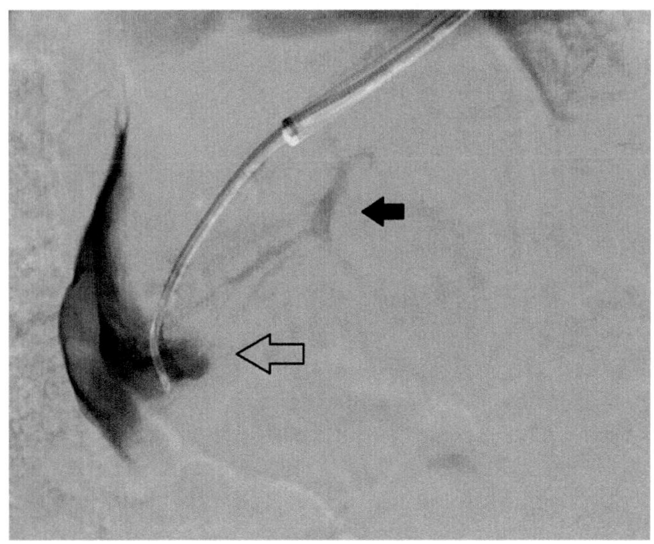

Fig. 49.2 Wedged hepatic venography using iodinated contrast performed prior to TIPS procedure showing portal vein (solid arrow) and a ruptured liver capsule (hollow arrow)

Fig. 49.3 CT (left) and wedged CO_2 hepatic venography (right) for TIPS and embolization on a 61-year-old male patient with portal hypertension and upper gastrointestinal bleeding showing a coronary vein varix (hollow arrow) and splenic vein varices (solid arrow)

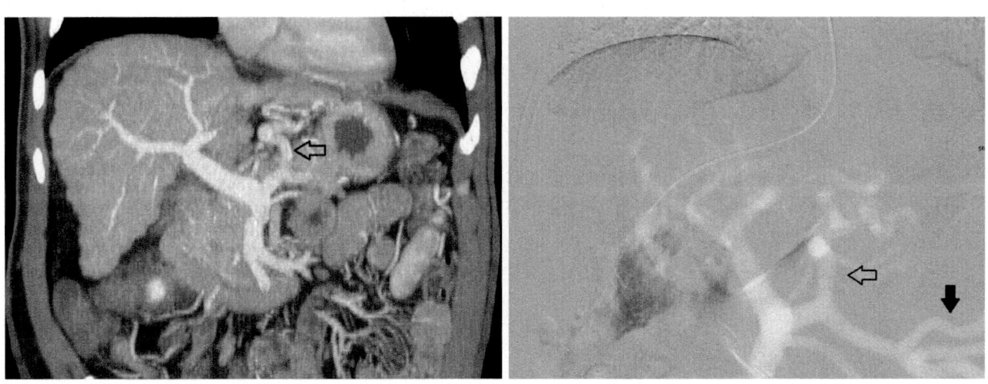

49.3.2 Percutaneous Splenoportography

In patients with an occluded main portal vein or intrahepatic portal vein branches, a percutaneous trans-splenic approach may be warranted to visualize the portal circulation. This is reserved for only those patients when noninvasive and other invasive studies are inconclusive, or when an intervention is planned, given that this method has a relatively increased risk of parenchymal hematoma, pseudo-aneurysm formation, and intraperitoneal hemorrhage [19].

To perform spleno-portography, the spleen is located using an ultrasound and is accessed from a mid-posterior axillary line between the eighth and ninth ribs. The needle is inserted at a 45° angle toward the dome of the diaphragm 3–4 cm into the spleen. The intra-splenic position of the needle is confirmed by aspiration of blood and the splenic vein is catheterized. A portal venography can then be performed after advancing the catheter into the main portal vein and injecting iodinated contrast or CO_2 [20] (Fig. 49.4).

This method is especially useful in patients with main portal venous thrombosis (PVT) in whom either portal thrombolysis is being considered; or in those with PVT and varices where antegrade embolization of bleeding varices is to be performed.

49.3.3 Transhepatic Portography

Percutaneous trans-hepatic portography is performed by directly accessing a portal venous branch under ultrasound and fluoroscopic guidance from a subxiphoid approach or low right intercostal approach under ultrasound guidance. Once portal venous access is acquired, iodinated contrast or CO_2 can be injected for the venogram (Fig. 49.5). Direct portal venous pressure measurements are also taken and therapeutic interventions like portal venous embolization or variceal embolizations performed. At the end of the procedure, the catheter tract is embolized with coils or gelatin sponge pellets to reduce the risk of hemorrhage.

The trans-hepatic approach carries similar risks and complications as the trans-splenic approach, and thus is reserved for those patients in whom noninvasive and other invasive methods have failed. When performing trans-hepatic portography, special attention should be paid to the proximity of biliary tracts to hepatic vasculature since there is a potential for formation of an arterial-portal fistula, biliary injury and infection.

49.3.4 Arterial Portography

Arterial portography is an indirect method to evaluate the portal system. Splenic or superior mesenteric arterial portography and wedged hepatic venography can usually provide a complete view of the portal venous system.

To perform an arterial portography, the superior mesenteric artery or splenic artery is usually selected. Nitroglycerin maybe administered in the catheterized artery immediately

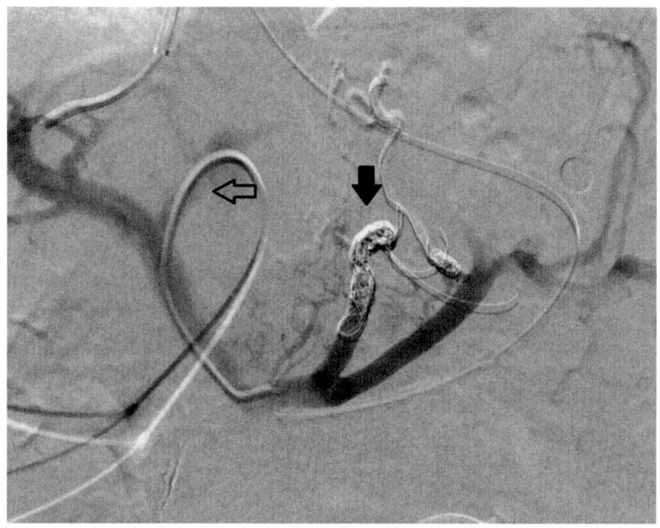

Fig. 49.5 Percutaneous trans-hepatic portography of a 29-year-old female patient with nonalcoholic steatohepatitis with bleeding esophageal varix showing embolized esophageal varices (solid arrow) via percutaneous trans-hepatic access of the left portal vein (open arrow)

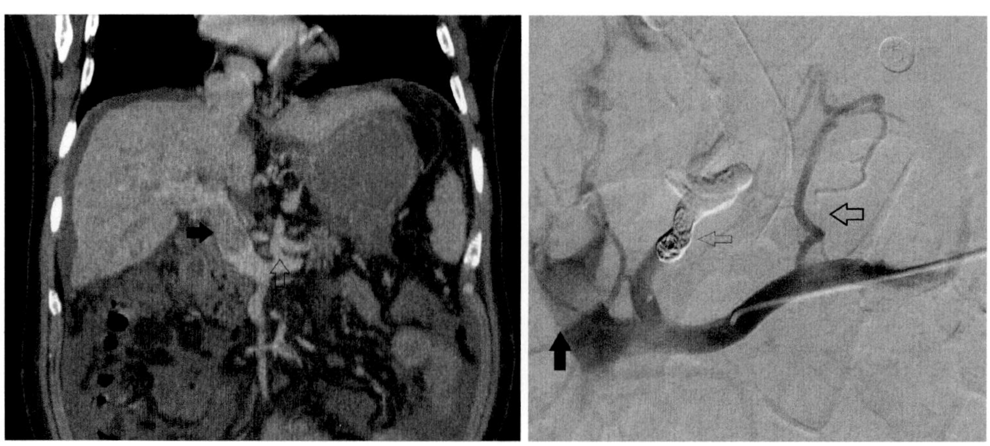

Fig. 49.4 CT (left) and percutaneous spleno-portography (right) of a 58-year-old male patient with bleeding esophageal varices showing a thrombosis in the main portal vein (solid arrow). CT image shows esophageal varix, Splenoportography demonstrates embolized esophageal varix (thin open arrow), and a gastric varix (thick open arrow)

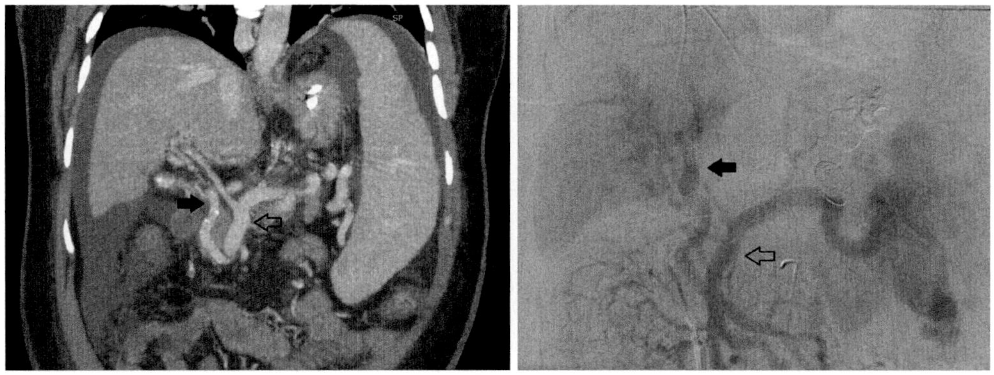

Fig. 49.6 CT (left) and superior mesenteric artery portography (right) of a 32-year-old female with chronic portal vein thrombosis with bleeding gastric varices showing a prominent superior mesenteric venin (open arrow) with numerous collateral vessels supplying the intrahepatic portal circulation (solid arrow)

prior to contrast injection. A contrast angiography is performed with imaging followed through in the venous phase to delineate the portal venous system. The portal veins and collateral circulation are usually well seen 5–15 s following contrast administration (Fig. 49.6).

49.4 Conclusion

There are many clinical situations that require an evaluation of the portal venous system. Selection of the appropriate imaging modality depends on the consideration multiple factors including the risks and benefits, invasiveness, cost, availability, and accuracy of all available modalities.

Though noninvasive, US is the most operator dependent test. But due to its accessibility, short imaging duration, accuracy, and safety profile, it is the modality of choice for evaluation of the portal venous system, especially after liver transplantation or TIPS placement. CT and MRI are both noninvasive tests and have the advantage of being the least operator dependent. These modalities are excellent for preprocedural planning and mapping the portal venous system and its collaterals. Angiography is considered the gold standard imaging modality to evaluate portal venous system, but due to its invasive nature, it is often reserved when noninvasive imaging studies are inadequate to evaluate the venous system, or the results are inconclusive for the clinical presentation.

Self Study

Questions

1. Which statement is true?
   (a) US can reliably diagnose portal hypertension.
   (b) Biopsy is the only way to differential malignant and benign thrombus.
   (c) MRI can be used to evaluate the hemodynamics of portal venous system.
   (d) US is the gold standard to evaluate portal venous system.
2. Which statement is true?
   (a) Iodinated contrast is the preferred contrast agent when performing wedged hepatic venography.
   (b) Percutaneous splenoportography can only be done with iodinated contrast.
   (c) Arterial portography is most concerning for significant post procedural infection.
   (d) Wedged hepatic venography is the most reliable to way diagnose portal hypertension.

Answers

1. Which statement is true?
   (a) US findings of portal hypertension include reversed, decreased or increased venous flow, splenomegaly, or dilated veins. But these findings are not always seen in patients with portal hypertension.
   (b) Recent studies have shown that CT texture analysis and attenuation values are reliable in differentiating malignant thrombus from bland thrombus.
   (c) CORRECT ANSWER. Recent studies have shown that 4D flow MRI can acquire quantitative measurement of the hemodynamic parameters in liver and splanchnic system with low inter-observer variability.
   (d) Angiography is the gold standard to evaluate portal venous system.
2. Which statement is true?
   (a) CO_2 is preferred contrast agent because its low viscosity, low cost, low toxicity.
   (b) Portal venography can then be done with iodinated or CO_2 contrast.
   (c) The proximity of biliary tract to vasculatures increased concern for the potential of arterial portal fistula, biliary injury and infection.
   (d) CORRECT ANSWER. Hepatic venous pressure, which is the difference between wedged hepatic pressure and free hepatic pressure, is the best available method to diagnose portal hypertension.

References

1. Tarantino L, Francica G, Sordelli I, Nocera V. Contrast-enhanced US: a simple, quick and sensitive tool in the differential diagnosis of benign and malignant portal vein thrombosis in cirrhotic patients with hepatocellular carcinoma. J Hepatol. 2008;48:S12.
2. Raza SA, Jang HJ, Kim TK. Differentiating malignant from benign thrombosis in hepatocellular carcinoma: contrast-enhanced ultrasound. Abdom Imaging. 2014;39(1):153–61.
3. Rossi S, Rosa L, Ravetta V, Cascina A, Quaretti P, Azzaretti A, Scagnelli P, Tinelli C, Dionigi P, Calliada F. Contrast-enhanced versus conventional and color Doppler sonography for the detection of thrombosis of the portal and hepatic venous systems. AJR Am J Roentgenol. 2006;186:763–73.
4. Sorrentino P, D'Angelo S, Tarantino L, Ferbo U, Bracigliano A, Vecchione R. Contrast-enhanced sonography versus biopsy for the differential diagnosis of thrombosis in hepatocellular carcinoma patients. World J Gastroenterol. 2009;15:2245–51.
5. Piscaglia F, Gianstefani A, Ravaioli M, Golfieri R, Cappelli A, Giampalma E, Sagrini E, Imbriaco G, Pinna AD, Bolondi L. Criteria for diagnosing benign portal vein thrombosis in the assessment of patients with cirrhosis and hepatocellular carcinoma for liver transplantation. Liver Transpl. 2010;16:658–67.
6. Oguz B, Akata D, Balkanci F, Akhan O. Intrahepatic portosystemic venous shunt: diagnosis by colour/power Doppler imaging and three-dimensional ultrasound. Br J Radiol. 2003;76:487–90.
7. Moran DE, Bennett AE, Sheiman RG. Diagnostic radiology of transjugular intrahepatic portosystemic shunts. In: Seminars in ultrasound, CT and MRI, vol. 34(4). Philadelphia: WB Saunders; 2013. p. 352–64.
8. Dani G, Sun MR, Bennett AE. Imaging of liver transplant and its complications. In: Seminars in ultrasound, CT and MRI, vol. 2013, 34(4). Philadelphia: WB Saunders. p. 365–77.
9. Canellas R, Mehrkhani F, Patino M, Kambadakone A, Sahani D. Characterization of portal vein thrombosis (neoplastic versus bland) on CT images using software-based texture analysis and thrombus density (Hounsfield units). Am J Roentgenol. 2016;207(5):W81–7.
10. Ascenti G, Sofia C, Mazziotti S, Silipigni S, D'Angelo T, Pergolizzi S, Scribano E. Dual-energy CT with iodine quantification in distinguishing between bland and neoplastic portal vein thrombosis in patients with hepatocellular carcinoma. Clin Radiol. 2016;71(9):938–e1.
11. Iranmanesh P, Vazquez O, Terraz S, Majno P, Spahr L, Poncet A, Morel P, Mentha G, Toso C. Accurate computed tomography-based portal pressure assessment in patients with hepatocellular carcinoma. J Hepatol. 2014;60(5):969–74.
12. Lee JY, Kim TY, Jeong WK, Kim Y, Kim J, Kim KW, Kim YH, Sohn JH. Clinically severe portal hypertension: role of multi-detector row CT features in diagnosis. Dig Dis Sci. 2014;59(9):2333–43.
13. Kihira S, Kagen AC, Vasudevan P, Jajamovich GH, Schiano TD, Andrle AF, Babb JS, Fischman A, Taouli B. Non-invasive prediction of portal pressures using CT and MRI in chronic liver disease. Abdom Radiol. 2016;41(1):42–9.
14. Darcy M. Evaluation and management of transjugular intrahepatic portosystemic shunts. Am J Roentgenol. 2012;199(4):730–6.
15. Roldán-Alzate A, Frydrychowicz A, Niespodzany E, Landgraf BR, Johnson KM, Wieben O, Reeder SB. In vivo validation of 4D flow MRI for assessing the hemodynamics of portal hypertension. J Magn Reson Imaging. 2013;37(5):1100–8.
16. Stankovic Z, Jung B, Collins J, Russe MF, Carr J, Euringer W, Stehlin L, Csatari Z, Strohm PC, Langer M, Markl M. Reproducibility study of four-dimensional flow MRI of arterial and portal venous liver hemodynamics: influence of spatio-temporal resolution. Magn Reson Med. 2014;72(2):477–84.
17. Stankovic Z, Blanke P, Markl M. Usefulness of 4D MRI flow imaging to control TIPS function. Am J Gastroenterol. 2012;107(2):327.
18. Stankovic Z, Rössle M, Euringer W, Schultheiss M, Salem R, Barker A, Carr J, Langer M, Markl M, Collins JD. Effect of TIPS placement on portal and splanchnic arterial blood flow in 4-dimensional flow MRI. Eur Radiol. 2015;25(9):2634–40.
19. Zhu K, Meng X, Zhou B, Qian J, Huang W, Deng M, Shan H. Percutaneous transsplenic portal vein catheterization: technical procedures, safety, and clinical applications. J Vasc Interv Radiol. 2013;24(4):518–27.
20. Ali F, Mangi MA, Rehman H, Kaluski E. Use of carbon dioxide as an intravascular contrast agent: a review of current literature. World J Cardiol. 2017;9(9):715.

Minilaparoscopy and Conventional Laparoscopy

50

Guido Fiorentini, Francesca Ratti, Federica Cipriani, and Luca Aldrighetti

Abbreviations

MPL	Multiport laparoscopy
NOTES-LR	Natural Orifice Transluminal Endoscopic Surgery—Liver Resection
Sg	Segment
SILS	Single Incision Laparoscopic Surgery

Key Concepts

- Minilaparoscopy differs from conventional laparoscopy by the use of a single incision to gain access to the abdominal cavity.
- While the range of indications in multiport laparoscopic liver surgery is wide, only few procedures can be tackled in SILS.
- No specific superiority has emerged until now by experimenting SILS while comparing with MPL; nevertheless, few selected patients could benefit from SILS in terms of better aesthetics, without any significant advantage on intra-operative nor post-operative outcomes.

50.1 Introduction

The development of laparoscopic surgery has been aimed to decrease as much as possible the degree of invasiveness since its onset and development. In the last decade, a new approach was born, with the goal to reduce the number of incisions through a single mini-laparoscopic access (SILS—Single Incision Laparoscopic Surgery). This technique was initially applied to several gastroenteric procedures, encompassing cholecystectomy, splenectomy, appendectomy, colectomy, while the application to liver resections has occurred later, mainly because of the difficulty to achieve parenchymal hemostasis and to perform the parenchymal transection. Recently, few reports did show the feasibility of SILS in hepatic surgery [1–22], which slowly developed following the progresses of surgical skills and the implementation of new devices.

Aim of this chapter is to provide an overview on the most recent applications of SILS to liver resections, with notions on devices, indications and future perspectives. A literature review has been performed to investigate the state of the art of this technique in the clinical practice.

50.2 Indications

The applications of SILS to liver resections are not standardized and, until now, limited in comparison with conventional multi-access laparoscopic liver surgery. Actually, while conventional laparoscopy can theoretically be applied to multiple, bilobar, deep lesions, the difficulty in instrument triangulation with SILS limits indications to favourably localized, single lesions, preferentially located in laparoscopic segments (anterior and lateral—i.e. Sg 4b, 2, 3, 5) or in the left liver lobe (Sg 2 + 3), thereby reducing the pool of patients that could benefit from this technique.

50.3 Surgical technique

50.3.1 Access to the Abdominal Cavity, Pneumoperitoneum, Exposition of the Operative Field

While in conventional laparoscopic surgery (multiport laparoscopy, MPL) the minimum number of abdominal incision is 3 plus a service laparotomy for specimen retrieval, the aim of SILS is to gain access for all instruments through

G. Fiorentini (✉) · F. Ratti · F. Cipriani · L. Aldrighetti
Hepatobiliary Surgery Division, San Raffaele University Hospital, Milan, Italy
e-mail: fiorentini.guido@hsr.it; ratti.francesca@hsr.it; cipriani.federica@hsr.it; aldrighetti.luca@hsr.it

F. Radu-Ionita et al. (eds.), *Liver Diseases*, https://doi.org/10.1007/978-3-030-24432-3_50

a single 3–4 cm incision which is also used for specimen retrieval. Such incision has to be placed in an adequate location, providing a comfortable access to the target area. For instance, while a left lateral sectionectomy (i.e. the resection of the left hepatic lobe, Segments 2 + 3) will require a midline minilaparotomy, the approach to a postero-superior segment will require a more lateral access on the right flank.

After the incision and entry into the abdominal cavity, a dedicated port specifically designed for SILS access has to be adopted, which role is to work as platform both for instrument access and CO_2 insufflation. Several types are available on the market: Gelport® (Applied Medical); GelPoint® (Applied Medical); Gloveport® (Nelis Medical); SILSport® (Covidien); TriPort+® (Olympus); Octoport® (AFS Medical) (Fig. 50.1). Regardless of the manufacture, these devices contemporarily act as a wound retractor, as an interface for establishing and maintaining the pneumoperitoneum and inserting the instruments. Such devices are constituted of predefined ports for the direct insertion of instruments or, as an alternative, are provided with malleable membranes on the surface (like the Gelport®), which permit a customized insertion of trocars. Three accesses (one for the camera, two for the instruments) or four (one for the camera, two instruments for the first operator and one additional for the assistant, like in the TriPort®) are usually available on SILS devices. While in MPL trocars are positioned to obtain the triangulation of instruments with the camera, keeping adequate distances from each other, for SILS both instruments and the camera get close to each other, creating problems of sword fighting and clashing. Such difficulties have been partially overcome by curved shafts and the adoption of flip-top cameras; therefore, the need for specific devices has to be considered in institutions interested in the development of a program of SILS, requiring dedicated economic resources in addition to those already allocated for conventional laparoscopic surgery. In addition, the use of crooked instruments implies to work with crossed devices; therefore, the instrument appearing on the left of the screen will correspond to the

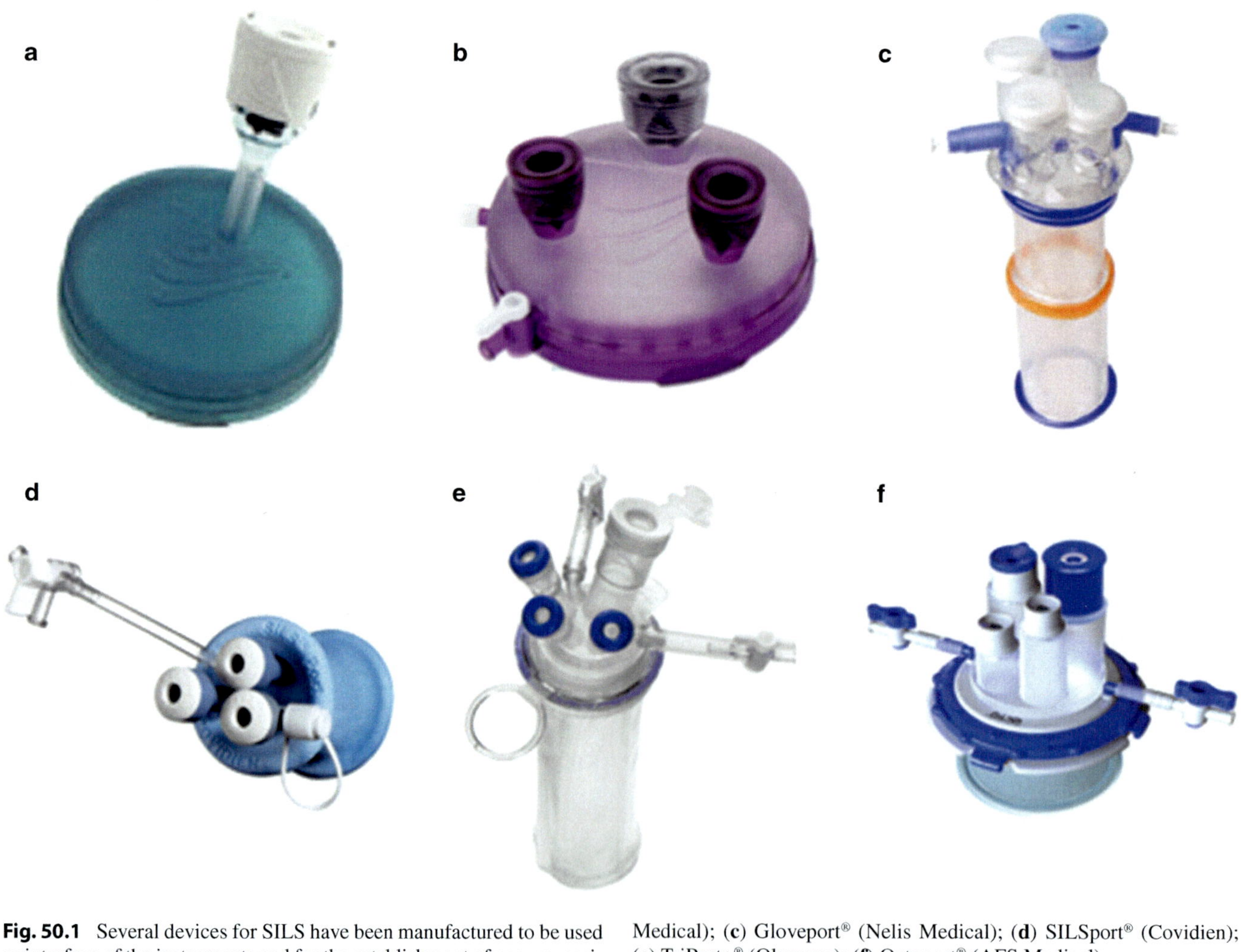

Fig. 50.1 Several devices for SILS have been manufactured to be used as interface of the instruments and for the establishment of pneumoperitoneum. (**a**) Gelport® (Applied Medical); (**b**) GelPoint® (Applied Medical); (**c**) Gloveport® (Nelis Medical); (**d**) SILSport® (Covidien); (**e**) TriPort+® (Olympus); (**f**) Octoport® (AFS Medical)

right hand of the operator and vice-versa. This difficulty requires a great adaptability from the operator, who actually finds himself working reverse on the screen.

50.3.2 Parenchymal Transection

One of the items actually limiting on a wide scale single incision liver surgery is the device used for parenchymal transection. Beside to angulated instruments like forceps and scissors, liver surgery requires use of instruments suitable for parenchymal division during hepatic transection. While articulating energy devices basing on radiofrequencies are available, there is no ultrasonic dissector yet. This particularity limits use of ultrasonic aspirator for cavitation, that can be used only in a straight approach to the area of resection. In fact, the vibration needed for the ultrasonic dissector function cannot be transmitted on a curved shaft, and this strongly limits the application when fine dissection is required. This can be partially overcome by moving the incision used for SILS in more comfortable positions, whereas devices could be in the straighter line as possible with the area of intervention (i.e. a midline supraumbilical incision for a left lateral sectionectomy vs. a right flank incision for gaining access to right areas of the liver).

A good alternative in substitution of ultrasonic aspirator is using energy devices based on the principles of radiofrequencies, which actually exist in articulating versions. Articulating devices allow unparalleled access to the field, conferring a greater freedom for manipulation. Nevertheless, articulating energy devices can be used mainly for most superficial layers while fine dissection of parenchyma close to major pedicles is more difficult.

Another choice for parenchymal transection is the use of linear staplers, which can be used, for instance, not just in left lateral sectionectomy for the interruption of the left hepatic vein, but also for the parenchymal transection and the stapling of sectorial pedicle. With this technique, accessing through the SILS device, one hand is used for exposure and traction, while the other operator's hand is used for stapling, allowing transecting liver parenchyma and sealing vascular structures at the same time. While left lateral sectionectomy is a suitable procedure for stapling technique, small wedge resections are more difficult due to the dimension of linear stapler's jaws.

Various devices based on the precoagulation principle exist, like the Habib®4x resection device for laparoscopy: basing on four radiofrequency needles, the probe is inserted through the resective perimeter. Once activated, it induces a precoagulation, sealing effectively the small vessels of the parenchyma, making the subsequent transection bloodless, even by cutting with cold forceps.

50.4 Procedures

Differently from MPL (see Chap. 62), where application of laparoscopy is wide, the indications to SILS are limited to wedge resections, segmentectomies of anterior and lateral segments and to left lateral sectionectomies. The main reason is the aforementioned technical difficulty represented by limited number of available ports, challenging exposition and need to work with crossed instruments.

Left lateral sectionectomy is the ideal procedure for SILS. Through a midline access, a frontal vertical transection plane is offered, that is suitable for stapling technique and for straight instruments like the ultrasonic aspirator or clip appliers.

Few authors reported their experience in SILS during last years. In the majority of experiences, anyway, retrospective, non-randomized, case reports and case series are present in literature, lacking with randomized clinical trial, and are principally aimed to demonstrate safety and reproducibility (Table 50.1).

Two prospective studies have been performed: Hu et al. [7] did enroll 38 patients in two cohorts equally representing SILS and MPL; all patients were affected by benign disease. They did not observe differences in operative time and blood loss, with no differences in the postoperative morbidity. Weiss et al. [18] enrolled 21 patients in their non-randomised trial, retrieving 33 segments (Segmentectomies 2–6); the peculiarity of their experience was adopting the precoagulation technique through a radiofrequency device, showing feasibility even for lateral segments like Sg6 by moving the access to the right flank.

As evidenced in Table 50.1, SILS was adopted mainly for minor resections, encompassing left lobectomies. About this, Aldrighetti et al. [2] conducted a single center case-matched analysis specifically investigating the role of SILS in left lateral sectionectomy. They retrospectively compared 13 patients receiving SILS left lateral sectionectomy with 13 multi-port procedures. No differences were found in operative time, blood loss, conversion to open rate, R0 margin, requirements of post-operative pain medications. This series furtherly validate the possible role for standardization in SILS applied to left lateral sectionectomy, even if SILS can result in higher costs due to ports and specifically designed instruments, potentially raising the costs of a minimally-invasive program.

Limited experiences exist on major hepatectomies (defined as the resection of three or more segments): Shetty et al. [14] in 2012 reported their series performed on 23 patients, which enclosed 1 left and 1 right hepatectomy. Beside this experience, there are no other reports on SILS for major hepatectomies, reasonably because of the technical challenges that this technique adds to an already difficult procedure.

Table 50.1 Review of the literature on recent single-institutional experience in single-incision liver surgery

Author	Cit.	Year	# of SILS cases	# Major resections	Type of resection	# Minor resections	Type of resection	Device	Conversion
Aikawa et al.	[1]	2012	8	–		8	Sg	SILS Port	–
Aldrighetti et al.	[2]	2012	13	–		13	LLS	TriPort	–
Belli et al.	[3]	2011	1	–		1	WR	TriPort	–
Camps-Lasa et al.	[4]	2014	5	–		5	WR; LLS	GelPoint	–
Chang et al.	[5]	2011	3	–		3	Sg; LLS	GelPort	–
Gaujoux et al.	[6]	2011	5	–		5	Sg	GelPort	–
Hu et al.	[7]	2014	19	–		19	Sg; LLS	TriPort	–
Karabicak et al.	[8]	2015	9	–		9	WR; Sg; LLS	SILSPort	–
Kim et al.	[9]	2014	3	–		3	Sg; LLS	GelPoint	–
Kobayashi et al.	[10]	2010	1	–		1	WR	None	–
Machado et al.	[11]	2014	8	–		8	LLS	GelPoint	–
Pan et al.	[12]	2012	8	–		8	WR; LLS	None	–
Patel et al.	[13]	2010	1	–		1	LLS	TriPort	–
Shetty et al.	[14]	2012	23	2	LH; RH	22	Sg; LLS	Gloveport	4 to open; 2 to MPL
Tan et al.	[15]	2012	7	–		7	Sg; LLS	GelPoint	–
Tayar et al.	[16]	2014	7	–		7	Sg	GelPoint, SILSPort	–
Tzanis et al.	[17]	2014	3	–		3	WR; LLS	QuadriPort; TriPort	–
Weiss et al.	[18]	2015	21	–		33	WR; Sg; LLS	GelPort, OctoPort, SILSPort	–
Wu et al.	[19]	2014	17	–		17	WR; LLS	None	–
Zhao et al.	[20]	2011	12	–		12	WR; LLS	TriPort	2 to MPL

LH left hepatectomy, *RH* right hepatectomy, *WR* wedge resection, *Sg* segmentectomy, *LLS* left lateral sectionectomy, *MPL* multiport laparoscopy

Benzing et al. [21] in 2015 performed a systematic review photographing the state of the art of this topic: among 345 studies identified, 15 resulted eligible for their purpose, globally accounting for 133 cases. Among these, left lateral sectionectomy was the most frequent procedure (49%), followed by wedge resections (41%). This experience furtherly sustains the role of SILS for minor resections, potentially being left lateral sectionectomy the ideal procedure for SILS.

50.5 Comparison of Single Incision and Multi Port Laparoscopic Surgery

The main technical difficulty in SILS is related to the capacity of achieve adequate exposure of the operative field and success in instruments triangulation. The introduction of instruments with angulated shaft and articulating devices partially solved this problem in SILS. On the contrary, in MPL triangulation is eased by customized ports positioning, minimizing the risk of clashing instruments only to limited situations.

As stated, SILS requires adaptability, as surgeon will find his right hand working with the instrument on the left of the screen and vice-versa, while one of the basic principle of MPL is never to cross the instruments.

According to two observational studies comparing the two techniques, no differences were detected in terms of blood loss, operative time, post-operative pain and radicality between SILS and MPL [2, 7], so there is no clear superiority of SILS over MPL that could justify the increased degree of challenge, beside to the aesthetic outcome with fewer scars in the SILS.

Similar items have been investigated also out of the field of liver resections. In a recent meta-analysis on available randomized and prospective studies for SILS in colorectal surgery [23], post-operative pain was addressed among the short-term outcomes investigated. Patients receiving SILS experienced less severe pain only at rest. Nevertheless, no differences were found in opioid consume in comparison with MPL, as a possible expression of similar pain in comparison to MPL once the patient is in activity and out of the bed. Furthermore, no specific studies have ever objectively proved a superiority in terms of cosmetic benefit. If, on one side, it can be assumed that the single incision required for SILS might result in fewer scars, on the other side it could be speculated that the shorter incisions of MPL can be less evident on a patient abdomen when associated with a Pfannenstiel's incision for specimen retrieval.

While benefits in reducing ascitic decompensation due to fewer collateral circles breakdown in the abdominal wall have been proved for MPL in comparison to open surgery, no studies have proved advantages for SILS in comparison to MPL in liver cirrhosis.

Eventually, further difference is related to patient selection: due to the technical difficulty imposed by SILS, application of mini-laparoscopy is limited to few, selected cases, characterized by singular lesions, superficial, or located in the left lateral sector. Contrarily, thc broad spectrum of procedures that can be tackled through MPL is potentially limited only by the evidence of major vascular invasion (like hepatic veins or inferior vena cava infiltration).

50.6 Future Perspectives

Some limitations of SILS can potentially be overcome by robotic surgery, as the software can restore intuitive control by associating the right hand to the corresponding instrument seen on the screen, despite of the crossing shafts. Nevertheless, the still elevated prices of robotic surgery strongly limit its diffusion.

Possible future perspectives on further developments of minimally-invasiveness is represented by Natural Orifice Transluminal Endoscopic Surgery Liver Resection (NOTES-LR). This technique makes use of natural orifices (per-oral trans-gastric; trans-anal; trans-vaginal) to gain access to the abdominal cavity. Katagiri et al. [24] collected the few existing experiences on this topic, which have been conducted mainly on animals. To our knowledge, even fewer experiences [25, 26] of hybrid trans-vaginal partial liver resection have been performed in human, with specimens retrieved trans-vaginally. Even if it is reasonable to imagine a future that is less and less invasive, while NOTES-LR could be implemented, an extensive application is difficult to be conceived in standardized fashions, especially for more complex procedures.

50.7 Conclusion

In conclusion, the rationale of SILS liver surgery is to use a single 3–4 cm incision to gain access to the abdominal cavity, establishing the pneumoperitoneum and inserting the instruments to perform hepatic resections. Due to clashing instruments and the vicinity of instruments to each other, technical limitations exist, which are mainly related to difficult exposure and triangulation with the camera. Therefore, only selected cases could benefit from SILS, like for small wedge resections and left lateral sectionectomies, even though specific instruments are needed, requiring additional expenses. In the end, literature lacks of randomized, non-inferiority, clinical trials, and is consistent with a low level of evidence that is limited to case series performed in high volume centers with expertise in the field of laparoscopic liver surgery.

Self Study

Questions

1. Which statement is true?
   (a) SILS is superior for better cosmesis, reduced post-operative pain and faster functional recovery.
   (b) There is no proved evidence of a superiority for SILS in comparison with MPL.
   (c) There are no additional technical limitations in single-port surgery in comparison to multiport laparoscopy as the two techniques can be used to approach any procedure at the same way.
   (d) SILS and MPL share the same instruments, thus costs are contained for programs developing both techniques.
2. Which statement is false?
   (a) Technical difficulties represented by the proximity of instruments, their curved shafts, and their crossing are reasons for limited exposure and triangulation.
   (b) SILS has been broadly applied for all liver procedures, encompassing wedge resections, segmentectomies and major hepatectomies.
   (c) Several devices have been designed and manufactured specifically for SILS, encompassing special interfaces for ports and articulating dissectors.
   (d) Future perspectives of minimally-invasiveness consider achieve access to the abdominal cavity through natural orifice, like per-oral trans-gastric and trans-vaginal access.

Answers

1. Which statement is true?
   (a) False. No studies have been conducted to assess superior intra-operative outcomes and functional recovery of SILS over MPL.
   (b) True. Several experiences assessing feasibility and safeness are present in terms of case series and case reports, even though randomized controlled trials lack on this topic.

(c) False. In SILS, exposure is poor and the range of procedures are limited.
(d) False. Specific instrumentary encompassing SILS devices, curved instruments and articulating dissector are required to achieve triangulation in SILS and avoid instrument clashing. Therefore, SILS requires specific additional costs.

2. Which statement is false?
(a) True. Working with crossing instruments requires adaptability from the surgeon.
(b) False. In only one case series two major resections were reported, embodying the significant limitations determined by SILS in major resections.
(c) True. Specific instrumentary is required.
(d) True. Even if performed mainly on experimental studies conducted on animals, new approaches on minimally-invasiveness see NOTES surgery as a potential branch for development in highly selected cases.

References

1. Aikawa M, Miyazawa M, Okamoto K, Toshimitsu Y, Okada K, Ueno Y, Yamaguchi S, Koyama I. Single-port laparoscopic hepatectomy: technique, safety, and feasibility in a clinical case series. Surg Endosc. 2012;26(6):1696–701. https://doi.org/10.1007/s00464-011-2095-1. Epub 2011 Dec 18.
2. Aldrighetti L, Ratti F, Catena M, Pulitanò C, Ferla F, Cipriani F, Ferla G. Laparoendoscopic single site (LESS) surgery for left-lateral hepatic sectionectomy as an alternative to traditional laparoscopy: case-matched analysis from a single center. Surg Endosc. 2012;26(7):2016–22. https://doi.org/10.1007/s00464-012-2147-1. Epub 2012 Jan 26.
3. Belli G, Fantini C, D'Agostino A, Cioffi L, Russo G, Belli A, Limongelli P. Laparoendoscopic single site liver resection for recurrent hepatocellular carcinoma in cirrhosis: first technical note. Surg Laparosc Endosc Percutan Tech. 2011;21(4):e166–8. https://doi.org/10.1097/SLE.0b013e3182207d3a.
4. Camps Lasa J, Cugat Andorrà E, Herrero Fonollosa E, García Domingo MI, Sánchez Martínez R, Vargas Pierola H, Rodríguez Campos A. Single-port laparoscopic approach of the left liver: initial experience. Cir Esp. 2014;92(9):589–94. https://doi.org/10.1016/j.ciresp.2014.05.009.
5. Chang SK, Mayasari M, Ganpathi IS, Wen VL, Madhavan K. Single port laparoscopic liver resection for hepatocellular carcinoma: a preliminary report. Int J Hepatol. 2011;2011:579203. https://doi.org/10.4061/2011/579203. Epub 2011 May 26.
6. Gaujoux S, Kingham TP, Jarnagin WR, D'Angelica MI, Allen PJ, Fong Y. Single-incision laparoscopic liver resection. Surg Endosc. 2011;25(5):1489–94. https://doi.org/10.1007/s00464-010-1419-x. Epub 2010 Oct 26.
7. Hu M, Zhao G, Wang F, Xu D, Liu R. Single-port and multi-port laparoscopic left lateral liver sectionectomy for treating benign liver diseases: a prospective, randomized, controlled study. World J Surg. 2014;38(10):2668–73. https://doi.org/10.1007/s00268-014-2610-3.
8. Karabicak I, Karabulut K, Yuruker S, Kesicioglu T, Ozen N. Single-port laparoscopic liver resection: largest Turkish experience. Indian J Surg. 2017;79(2):111–5. https://doi.org/10.1007/s12262-015-1435-0. Epub 2016 Jan 11.
9. Kim G, Lau AC, Chang SK. Single-incision laparoscopic hepatic resection in patients with previous hepatic resections: a mini case series. Asian J Endosc Surg. 2014;7(1):63–6. https://doi.org/10.1111/ases.12072.
10. Kobayashi S, Nagano H, Marubashi S, Wada H, Eguchi H, Takeda Y, Tanemura M, Sekimoto M, Doki Y, Mori M. A single-incision laparoscopic hepatectomy for hepatocellular carcinoma: initial experience in a Japanese patient. Minim Invasive Ther Allied Technol. 2010;19(6):367–71. https://doi.org/10.3109/13645706.2010.518731. Epub 2010 Oct 14.
11. Machado MA, Surjan RC, Makdissi FF. Intrahepatic glissonian approach for single-port laparoscopic liver resection. J Laparoendosc Adv Surg Tech A. 2014;24(8):534–7. https://doi.org/10.1089/lap.2013.0539. Epub 2014 Jun 13.
12. Pan M, Jiang Z, Cheng Y, Xu X, Zhang Z, Zhou C, He G, Xu T, Liu H, Gao Y. Single-incision laparoscopic hepatectomy for benign and malignant hepatopathy: initial experience in 8 Chinese patients. Surg Innov. 2012;19(4):446–51. https://doi.org/10.1177/1553350612438412. Epub 2012 Apr 2.
13. Patel AG, Belgaumkar AP, James J, Singh UP, Carswell KA, Murgatroyd B. Video. Single-incision laparoscopic left lateral segmentectomy of colorectal liver metastasis. Surg Endosc. 2011;25(2):649–50. https://doi.org/10.1007/s00464-010-1237-1. Epub 2010 Jul 22.
14. Shetty GS, You YK, Choi HJ, Na GH, Hong TH, Kim DG. Extending the limitations of liver surgery: outcomes of initial human experience in a high-volume center performing single-port laparoscopic liver resection for hepatocellular carcinoma. Surg Endosc. 2012;26(6):1602–8. https://doi.org/10.1007/s00464-011-2077-3. Epub 2011 Dec 17.
15. Tan EK, Lee VT, Chang SK, Ganpathi IS, Madhavan K, Lomanto D. Laparoendoscopic single-site minor hepatectomy for liver tumors. Surg Endosc. 2012;26(7):2086–91. https://doi.org/10.1007/s00464-011-2128-9. Epub 2012 Jan 11.
16. Tayar C, Subar D, Salloum C, Malek A, Laurent A, Azoulay D. Single incision laparoscopic hepatectomy: advances in laparoscopic liver surgery. J Minim Access Surg. 2014;10(1):14–7. https://doi.org/10.4103/0972-9941.124454. Erratum in: J Minim Access Surg. 2014 Apr;10(2):71.
17. Tzanis D, Lainas P, Tranchart H, Pourcher G, Devaquet N, Perlemuter G, Naveau S, Dagher I. Atypical as well as anatomical liver resections are feasible by laparoendoscopic single-site surgery. Int J Surg Case Rep. 2014;5(9):580–3. https://doi.org/10.1016/j.ijscr.2013.11.009. Epub 2014 Jul 12.
18. Weiss M, Mittermair C, Brunner E, Schirnhofer J, Obrist C, Pimpl K, Hell T, Weiss H. Inline radiofrequency pre-coagulation simplifies single-incision laparoscopic minor liver resection. J Hepatobiliary Pancreat Sci. 2015;22(12):831–6. https://doi.org/10.1002/jhbp.295. Epub 2015 Nov 18.
19. Wu S, Yu XP, Tian Y, Siwo EA, Li Y, Yu H, Yao D, Lv C. Transumbilical single-incision laparoscopic resection of focal hepatic lesions. JSLS. 2014;18(3):e2014.00397. https://doi.org/10.4293/JSLS.2014.00397.
20. Zhao G, Hu M, Liu R, Xu D, Ouyang C, Xu Y, Jiao H, Wang B, Gu X. Laparoendoscopic single-site liver resection: a preliminary report of 12 cases. Surg Endosc. 2011;25(10):3286–93. https://doi.org/10.1007/s00464-011-1706-1. Epub 2011 May 2.
21. Benzing C, Krenzien F, Atanasov G, Seehofer D, Sucher R, Zorron R, Pratschke J, Schmelzle M. Single incision laparoscopic liver resection (SILL) - a systematic review. GMS Interdiscip Plast Reconstr Surg DGPW. 2015;4:Doc17. https://doi.org/10.3205/iprs000076. eCollection 2015. Review.

22. Cipriani F, Catena M, Ratti F, Paganelli M, Ferla F, Aldrighetti L. LESS technique for liver resection: the progress of the mini-invasive approach: a single-centre experience. Minim Invasive Ther Allied Technol. 2012;21(1):55–8. https://doi.org/10.3109/13645706.2011.632013. Epub 2011 Nov 3.
23. Li HJ, Huang L, Li TJ, Su J, Peng LR, Liu W. Short-term outcomes of single-incision versus conventional laparoscopic surgery for colorectal diseases: meta-analysis of randomized and prospective evidence. J Gastrointest Surg. 2017;21(11):1931–45. https://doi.org/10.1007/s11605-017-3520-0. Epub 2017 Aug 3. Review.
24. Katagiri T, Otsuka Y, Horgan S, Sandler BJ, Jacobsen GR, Coker AM, Tsuchiya M, Maeda T, Kaneko H. Feasibility and technique for transvaginal natural orifice transluminal endoscopic surgery liver resection: a porcine model. Surg Laparosc Endosc Percutan Tech. 2017;27(1):e6–e11. https://doi.org/10.1097/SLE.0000000000000367.
25. Truong T, Arnaoutakis D, Awad ZT. Laparoscopic hybrid NOTES liver resection for metastatic colorectal cancer. Surg Laparosc Endosc Percutan Tech. 2012;22(1):e5–7. https://doi.org/10.1097/SLE.0b013e31823f7596.
26. Noguera JF, Dolz C, Cuadrado A, Olea JM, Vilella A. Transvaginal liver resection (NOTES) combined with minilaparoscopy. Rev Esp Enferm Dig. 2008;100(7):411–5.

Part III

Treatment

Medical Nutrition Therapy in Liver Disease

51

Anca Pantea Stoian, Andra Iulia Suceveanu, Adrian Paul Suceveanu, Laura Mazilu, and Irinel Raluca Parepa

Key Concepts

- Currently, Medical Nutrition Therapy has become more and more important as a part of the therapeutic attitude in both acute and chronic liver pathology.
- The Nutrition Care Process evaluate the nutritional status, prepare and implement recommendations for nutritional therapy, and comprises four steps: nutrition assessment, nutrition diagnosis, nutrition intervention and nutrition monitoring and evaluation.
- Nutritional intervention in acute liver disease aims the early recovery of the hepatic functional status without early denutrition.
- The nutritional attitude in chronic liver diseases or hepatic transplant requires long-term management of nutritional intervention, whose primary objective is the correction of malnutrition.

51.1 Introduction

Currently, Medical Nutrition Therapy (MNT) has become more and more important as a part of the therapeutic attitude in both acute and chronic pathology. The concept MNT is a general term which comprises the evaluation of the nutritional status, the preparation of personalized nutritional recommendations based on each pathology, and also an integrated nutritional education of the patient. Therefore, MNT may have a vital role in the therapeutic attitude, since the success or failure of the evolution and prognosis of each disease depends on the efficiency of its implementation. It has to be underlined that nutritional evaluation itself is a prognostic factor, used more and more often in the overall assessment of the patient and the morbimortality.

Certainly, acute or chronic hepatic pathology benefits, in such a context, from nutritional evaluation, but also from MNT implementation, having malnutrition as a primary objective. Even though clinical nutrition and nutritional intervention along with metabolic assessment are not generally implemented and there are no precise standards in this regard, ***malnutrition*** being an essential aspect of current medical practice concerning hepatic pathology, especially the chronic one. So far, no clinical trial has provided any consistent data, however the only consensus in the field being the one prepared by the European Society for Clinical Nutrition and Metabolism (ESPEN) [1].

51.1.1 General Principles of Nutritional Medical Intervention in Liver Diseases (LDs)

As a matter of fact, the Nutrition Care Process (NCP) is defined by the American Dietetic Associations (ADA). Briefly, it represents a global concept by which nutrition specialists evaluate the nutritional status, prepare and implement recommendations for nutritional therapy based on the available pathology, so that to ensure the safety and the quality of the optimal nutrition state of patients with both acute and chronic disorders [2]. Therefore, NCP consists of four steps: nutrition assessment, nutrition diagnosis, nutrition intervention and nutrition monitoring and evaluation, as it can be seen in Fig. 51.1 [1, 2].

A. P. Stoian (✉)
Diabetes, Nutrition and Metabolic diseases Department, Faculty of Medicine, UMF "Carol Davila", Bucharest, Romania

A. I. Suceveanu · A. P. Suceveanu
Internal Medicine Discipline—Gastroenterology Department, Faculty of Medicine, Ovidius University, Constanţa, Romania

L. Mazilu
Oncology Discipline, Faculty of Medicine, Ovidius University, Constanţa, Romania

I. R. Parepa (✉)
Internal Medicine—Cardiology Department, Faculty of Medicine, Ovidius University, Constanţa, Romania

F. Radu-Ionita et al. (eds.), *Liver Diseases*, https://doi.org/10.1007/978-3-030-24432-3_51

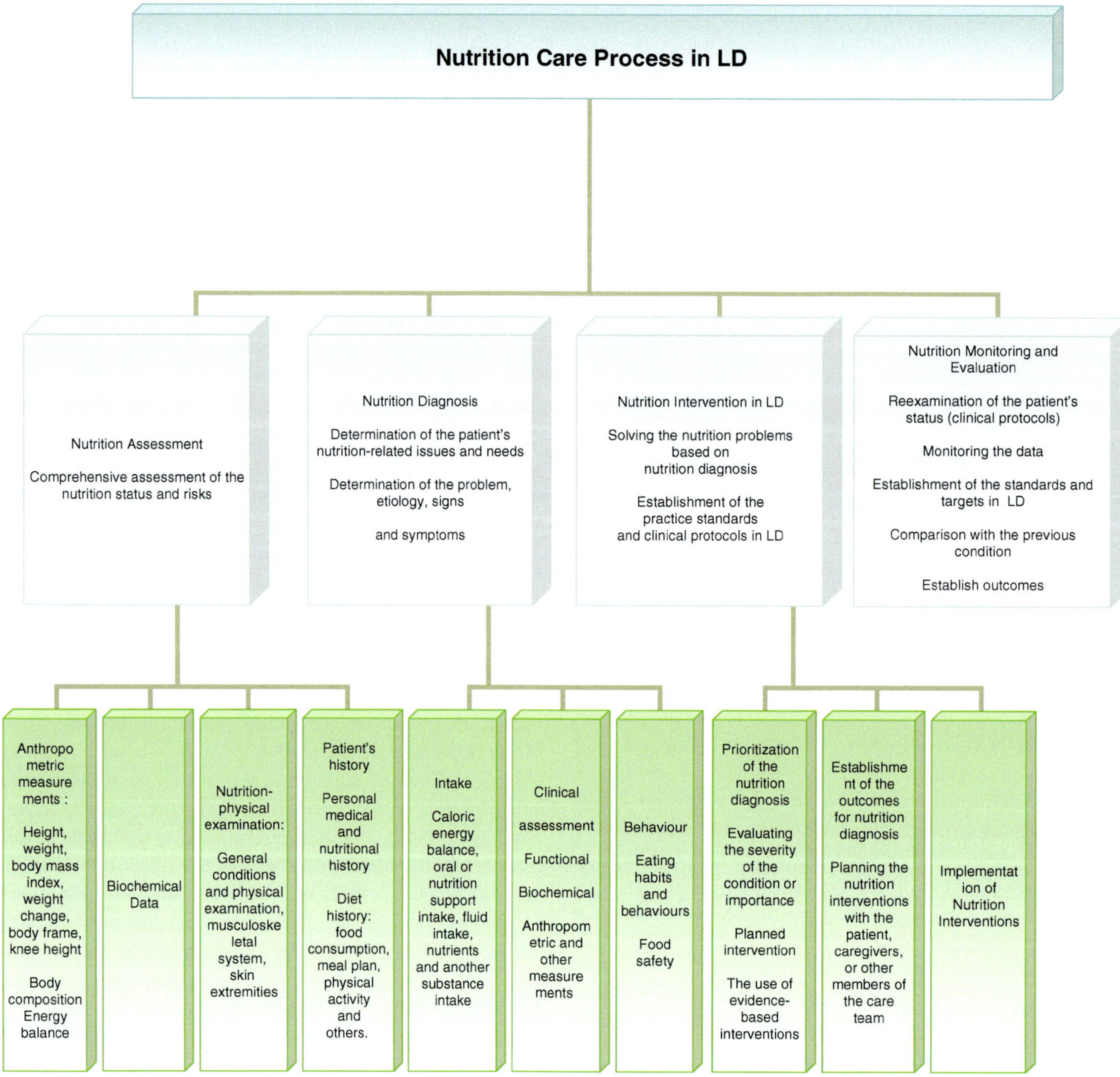

Fig. 51.1 Nutritional care process. The four steps

51.2 Nutrition Assessment

51.2.1 Anthropometric and Body Composition Assessment

Physical measurements such as the measurement of weight, height, skinfold thickness, girth measurements, and body composition have the purpose to evaluate the patients' state of underweight or overweight (obesity). Likewise, they have a major role in the subsequent monitoring and evaluation of the nutritional intervention. So far, we cannot say for sure that there is a consensus that the methods presented below are universally valid as appropriate techniques to all patients with liver disease. However, it is important to consider the **composite score**, this being used by the Veterans' Administration Study Group [3].

51.2.1.1 Measurement of Height and Weight

The height is calculated using the statiometer when condition of the patient permits. In case of immobilized patient to bed or wheelchair, the classical evaluation is no longer valid. In this situation, the knee height or demi-span (the measurement of the arm, preferably the right one) is evaluated. Depending on these evaluations, the height can be appreciated given the formula presented in Tables 51.1 and 51.2 [4, 5].

Body weight, especially body mass index, is not always a correct and coherent determination factor since it can be influenced by several factors such as oedema, ascites or diuretics.

The calculation of the actual body weight is done classically by using the scale, in the morning to a lightly dressed patient with emptied bladder. The ideal body weight (IBW) can be evaluated and is appreciated using the Metropolitan Life Insurance formula (the most used formula), Lorentz equation or Hamwi equation. Correspondingly, the usual body weight (UBW) is also a significant parameter, representing the stable weight in the last 6–12 months, stated by the patient. Based on each patient's situation, there can also be other weight estimation methods or formulas which we present below (obese, amputee, etc.), as it can be seen in Tables 51.3 and 51.4 [4–7].

(a) For obese people, the adjusted body weight (AdBW) is calculated using the formula [7–9]:

$$\text{AdBW} = 0.25(\text{ABW} - \text{IBW}) + \text{IBW}$$

where: ABW = actual body weight; IBW = ideal body weight.

(b) For amputees, the estimated IBW is calculated using the formula below and also Table 51.5:

$$\frac{100 - \%\ \text{amputation}}{100} \times \text{IBW for original height}$$

The **percentage** of weight loss/gain is an essential parameter in assessing the nutritional status especially in special conditions such as dehydration, water retention, acute inflammatory state, fever; a real indicator of disease severity and being positively correlated with morbidity and mortality. Blackburn Formula is usually applied to assess the severity of weight loss: %Weight Change = UBW − ABW/UBW × 100, where the percentage of weight loss of 1–2% × 1 week is significant, and >10% is considered severe [7].

51.2.1.2 Determination of Body Mass Index (BMI)

For calculation of the body mass index (BMI) is currently use Quetelet formula: BMI = W (kg)/H^2, where W = the weight measured in the morning, to a lightly dressed patient with emptied bladder, while H = height [3].

BMI is a quantitative method of evaluation, but it does not provide any information about the muscle mass, fat mass, and hydration degree of the patient. In some situations, BMI evaluation is not very precise i.e. cirrhotic patients with ascites, patients with morbid obesity, or athletes with very developed muscle mass. Depending on the determined BMI value, the nutritional status can be classified as presented in the next table.

A more accurate parameter in assessing fat mass, especially abdominal fat, is the determination of waist circumference (WC) and the waist-to-hip ratio (WHR). Both determinations are used in assessing the cardiovascular risk, blood pressure, type 2 diabetes mellitus and NAFLD, as it can be seen in Table 51.5.

Table 51.1 Calculating the estimated height with knee height [4, 5]

Sex	Calculating the estimated height with knee height
Females	84.88 − (0.24 × age in years) + (1.83 × knee height in cm)
Males	64.19 − (0.04 × age in years) + (2.02 × knee height in cm)

Table 51.2 Calculating the estimated height with demi span [4, 5]

Sex	Calculating the estimated height with demi span
Females	(1.35 × demi-span in cm) + 60.1
Males	(1.40 × demi-span in cm) + 57.8

Table 51.4 Amputation adjustments for calculating IBW

Percentage Body weight according to body part amputation	Percentage
Hand	0.7
Forearm	2.3
Arm	5
Foot	1.5
Lower leg below the knee	5.9
Leg	16

Table 51.3 IBW formulas

Type of equation	Male	Female
Metropolitan Life Insurance[a]	W (kg) = 50 + 0.75 × [H (cm) − 150] + (A − 20)/4	W (kg) = 50 + 0.75 [H (cm) − 150] + (A − 20)/4 × 0.9
Hamwi[b]	W (kg) = 48 kg + 2.7 kg for each inch over 5 ft	W (kg) = 45.5 kg + 2.2 kg for each inch over 5 ft
Lorentz formula	Male (kg) = Height (cm) − 100 − {(height (cm) − 150)/4}	Female (kg) = Height (cm) − 100 − {(height (cm) − 150)/2}

[a]Abbreviations: *W (kg)* ideal body weight calculated in kilograms, *H (cm)* height measured in centimeters, *A* actual age
[b]Note: 1 kg = 2.2 lb, 1 m = 3.28084 ft

Table 51.5 The nutritional status according to the BMI, WC and WHR, and also the assessment of CVD, HTN, T2D and NAFLD risk-classification

Nutrition/weight status	BMI (kg/m^2)	Waist circumference (cm) (WC)		Waist-to-hip ratio (WHR)		Health risk	Comorbidity risk CVD, HTN, T2D, NAFLD
	Non-Asian	Man	Women	Man	Woman		
Underweight	<18.5						Low but with other health problems
Healthy/normal	18.5–24.9	≤102	≤88	≤0.95	≤0.80	Low risk	Average
Overweight	25–29.9	≥102	≥88	0.96–1.0	0.81–0.85	Moderate risk	Increased
Obesity class I	30–34.9			≥1.0	≥0.85	High risk	Moderate
Obesity class II	35–39.9			≥1.0	≥0.85	Very high risk	Severe
Obesity class III	>40			≥1.0	≥0.85	Extremely high risk	High severity

Abbreviations: *BMI* body mass index, *WC* waist circumference, *CVD* cardiovascular disease, *HTN* hypertension, *T2D* type 2 diabetes, *NAFLD* non-alcoholic fatty liver disease [7, 8]

51.2.1.3 Other Anthropometric Evaluations

(a) Skinfold anthropometry is considered an indirect tool in assessing fat and muscle mass, especially in cirrhotic patients. It can be applied in more areas of the body so that the following can be determined: Biceps skinfold (the front side of the middle upper arm), Triceps skinfold (the back side of the middle upper arm), Subscapular skinfold (under the lowest point of the shoulder blade), Suprailiac skinfold (above the upper bone of the hip). This type of evaluation provides information about the body's reserve of adipose tissue, muscle mass, and accurate information about the malnutrition status. Depending on the obtained data, one can apply the table developed by Frisancho [10] to establish the nutritional status. In the presence of oedema or ascites, the triceps skinfold is an accurate parameter. Importantly, reassessment is applied whenever the nutritional status is changing or for periodic evaluation.

The most frequently method used in patients with chronic liver disease and especially in those with the alcoholic liver disease is the determination of muscle force through the handgrip test. Hand-grip evaluation with dynamometer is recognized as a good predictor of disease progression, but also an accurate parameter of malnutrition, being mainly indicated in fragile, elderly patients. It is a reproducible and repeatable method whenever necessary. Low grip strength correlates with early mortality, and it represents a negative prognostic factor in the evolution of complications, especially in middle-aged or elderly patients. It is interpreted according to the age and the sex of patient, given the already existing cartographic tables.

(b) The determination of body composition is also considered an indirect estimation method using total fat mass, visceral mass, body water, extracellular water and muscle mass. The determination of body composition through bioimpedance is controversial, especially in case of ascites. Therefore, it is not a recommended method.

(c) The determination of urinary creatinine or/and of potassium are techniques for the assessment of body cell mass in general, being precise and easy to apply them in patients with cirrhosis. Also, there are more accurate methods through bioimpedance, but not validated yet. The evaluation of total potassium load can be successfully used in body composition study since more than 90% of K + t exists in fat-free tissues. Its value ranges according to age, sex, weight (higher in obese) and it is achieved with a particular detector which displays gamma-ray interface.

(d) Sophisticated methods mainly used in the medical study of metabolism are the determination of total body nitrogen, total fat mass, visceral mass, water mass, muscle mass, skeletal mass, obtained by neutron activation analysis, dual-energy X-ray absorptiometry (DEXA), deuterium oxide dilution, air displacement plethysmography, ultrasound and magnetic resonance imaging, or underwater weighing.

51.2.1.4 Determination of the Energetic Balance

It can be determined by *conducting indirect calorimetry*, especially in patients with decompensated cirrhosis. If this method is not available, the **calorie requirement** can be calculated by Harris-Benedict or Mifflin-St. Jeor formulas as predictive equations for basal energy expenditure (BEE) and also resting energy expenditure (REE). After getting BEE or REE, the total energy expenditure (TEE) is estimated by adding the activity factor (AF) or the stress factor (SF). These determinations are still under discussion since errors appear in patients with ascites, where weight is masked by ascites. Practically, for a faster use, the daily energetic requirement (DER) is estimated by a shorter equation that uses the energy requirement factor (Erf) kcal/body kg and the current or ideal weight, as it can be seen in Table 51.6 [5, 11].

- Women: $BEE = 655 + 96W + 1.9H - 4.7A$
- Men: $BEE = 66.5 + 13.8W + 5H - 6.8A$

$\boxed{TEE = BEE \times AF}$ or $\boxed{DER = ABW(\text{or } IBW) \times Erf}$

W = weight in kg (use actual weight vs. ideal weight), H = height in cm, A = age in years

Table 51.6 Activity and stress factors necessary for TEE calculation [5]

Activity	Activity factor (AF)	Stress	Stress factor (SF)	Energy requirement factor (Erf) (kcal/kg)
Sedentary	1.2	Confined to bed	1.2	25–30
Lightly active (light exercise/sports 1–3 days/week)	1.375	Ambulatory	1.3	25–30
Moderately active (moderate exercise/sports 3–5 days/week)	1.55	Burns (depending on the % of burns)	1.5–2	30–35
Very active (hard exercise/sports 6–7 days a week)	1.725	Infections (mild to severe)	1.2–1.8	35–40
Extra active (very hard exercise/sports and physical job or 2× training)	1.9	Starvation	0.85	35–40
		Surgery (minor-major)	1.1–1.2	35–40
		Trauma	1.2–1.4	35–40

Once REE or DER are established, get the distribution of basic micro and macronutrients and of the total amount of liquids. It is recommended that a percentage of 45–60% from TEE to be represented by carbohydrates, respectively 25–30% lipids and 15–20% proteins, fibers 25–30 g/day and water 25–40 ml/kg [1, 5].

51.2.1.5 The Composite Score

This is a complex score that entirely estimates the caloric protein malnutrition, validated by the Veterans' Administration Study Group [12]. It reunites more variables such as skinfold thickness, mid-arm muscle determination, creatinine excretion, lymphocyte count, hand-grip determination corroborated with serum determinations of some proteins (albumin, prealbumin, retinol-binding protein) and IBW. Essentially, it is a complex score including the anthropometric assessment methods with the most accurate serum tests [1].

51.2.2 Biochemical Data

Laboratory data offers essential information regarding the nutritional and metabolic status, and about the severity of liver disease. In addition, they are useful in diagnosis, being a part of follow-up monitoring.

51.2.2.1 Biochemical Data Regarding the Nutritional Status

Practically, validated tests require collection of samples in morning usually after 8 h of food deprivation. They may be falsified by the coexistence of comorbidities or medication.

The most significant parameter is the proteins level, mainly albumin, prealbumin and transferrin. These hepatic proteins reflect the body's response to different acute injuries. Also, the total count of lymphocytes shows the protein status correlated with the immune system. Other parameters used for the evaluation of protein status are nitrogen balance, urea, hemoglobin, and lipid profile [5].

The nutritional risk index can be estimated using serum albumin. Similarly, the prognostic score can be obtained using the nutritional index and the inflammatory index.

Nutritional risk index (NRI) = (1.519 × albumin) + (41.7 × % IBW), where values below 97.5 indicate a high risk [5].

Nutritional risk index for prognosis (NRIP) = 158 − (16.6 × albumin) − (0.78 × triceps skinfold mm) − (0.2 × transferrin) − 5.8 (delayed skin sensibility), where all values ≥40 represent a severe prognosis [5].

Nutritional inflammatory risk index (NIRI) = C Reactive protein × alpha 1 acid-glycoprotein/prealbumin × albumin, where values ≥20 indicates a high risk [5, 13].

51.2.2.2 Specific Lab Determinations for Liver Disease

Specific Lab determinations for liver disease include tests of viral markers: HBsAg, HBeAg, Anti-HBS, Anti-HCV, etc., and direct parameters of hepatic liver function assessment: hepatic enzymes, serum lactic dehydrogenase, prothrombin time, partial thromboplastin time, ceruloplasmin, α-fetoprotein, α_1-antitrypsin, mitochondrial antibody, antinuclear antibodies, alkaline phosphatase (ALP), gamma-glutamyltranspeptidase (GGT), as well as amino acid dosage, and so on [1].

51.2.3 Nutrition: Physical Evaluation

Together with the anthropometric data, physical evaluation has high relevance in the assessment of the nutritional status, altogether being a part of the monitoring and revaluation stages. Physical exam provides data about poor nutritional status or even malnutrition. Nonetheless, different evaluation questionnaires including global questionnaires provide information not only about the nutritional status but also its evolution in time, eating habits etc.

There are several types of screening questionnaires, many of which validated and extremely useful in daily practice. Some of them are valuable elements in assessing malnutri-

Fig. 51.2 The Mini-Nutritional Assessment [14–18]. (*With Nestle's Nutrition Institute permission*)

Mini Nutritional Assessment
MNA®

Nestlé
NutritionInstitute

Last name: First name:

Sex: Age: Weight, kg: Height, cm: Date:

Complete the screen by filling in the boxes with the appropriate numbers. Total the numbers for the final screening score.

Screening

A Has food intake declined over the past 3 months due to loss of appetite, digestive problems, chewing or swallowing difficulties?
0 = severe decrease in food intake
1 = moderate decrease in food intake
2 = no decrease in food intake ☐

B Weight loss during the last 3 months
0 = weight loss greater than 3 kg (6.6 lbs)
1 = does not know
2 = weight loss between 1 and 3 kg (2.2 and 6.6 lbs)
3 = no weight loss ☐

C Mobility
0 = bed or chair bound
1 = able to get out of bed / chair but does not go out
2 = goes out ☐

D Has suffered psychological stress or acute disease in the past 3 months?
0 = yes 2 = no ☐

E Neuropsychological problems
0 = severe dementia or depression
1 = mild dementia
2 = no psychological problems ☐

F1 Body Mass Index (BMI) (weight in kg) / (height in m²)
0 = BMI less than 19
1 = BMI 19 to less than 21
2 = BMI 21 to less than 23
3 = BMI 23 or greater ☐

IF BMI IS NOT AVAILABLE, REPLACE QUESTION F1 WITH QUESTION F2.
DO NOT ANSWER QUESTION F2 IF QUESTION F1 IS ALREADY COMPLETED.

F2 Calf circumference (CC) in cm
0 = CC less than 31
3 = CC 31 or greater ☐

Screening score (max. 14 points)

12 - 14 points: Normal nutritional status
8 - 11 points: At risk of malnutrition
0 - 7 points: Malnourished ☐☐

References

1. Vellas B, Villars H, Abellan G, *et al.* Overview of the MNA® - Its History and Challenges. *J Nutr Health Aging*. 2006;**10**:456-465.
2. Rubenstein LZ, Harker JO, Salva A, Guigoz Y, Vellas B. Screening for Undernutrition in Geriatric Practice: Developing the Short-Form Mini Nutritional Assessment (MNA-SF). *J. Geront.* 2001; **56A**: M366-377
3. Guigoz Y. The Mini-Nutritional Assessment (MNA®) Review of the Literature - What does it tell us? *J Nutr Health Aging*. 2006; **10**:466-487.
4. Kaiser MJ, Bauer JM, Ramsch C, et al. Validation of the Mini Nutritional Assessment Short-Form (MNA®-SF): A practical tool for identification of nutritional status. *J Nutr Health Aging*. 2009; **13**:782-788.

For more information: www.mna-elderly.com

tion including liver disorders or other pathological circumstances. Out of these, Malnutrition Universal Screening Tool (MUST), Mini Nutritional Assessment (MNA), Geriatric Nutritional Risk Index (GNRI) and Subjective Global Assessment (SGA) are the most common [14].

Malnutrition Universal Screening Tool (MUST) developed by Straton [14] can rapidly identify malnutrition. It uses three criteria: actual weight and height under the form of the body mass index, the degree of unplanned weight loss in the last 3–6 months, and the acute disease score that also marks the therapeutic approach [14]. Another more complex score recommended to people older than 60 years of age is the Mini Nutritional Assessment (MNA-SF). It includes a questionnaire regarding the nutritional intake, the weight loss percentage over the last 3–6 months, the BMI, the mobility capacity, stress degree and neuro-psychic condition of the patient. This screening together with recommendations of nutritional intervention, were prepared by Kaiser et al. and implemented by Nestle Nutrition Institute, as it can be seen in Figs. 51.2 and 51.3 [14–18].

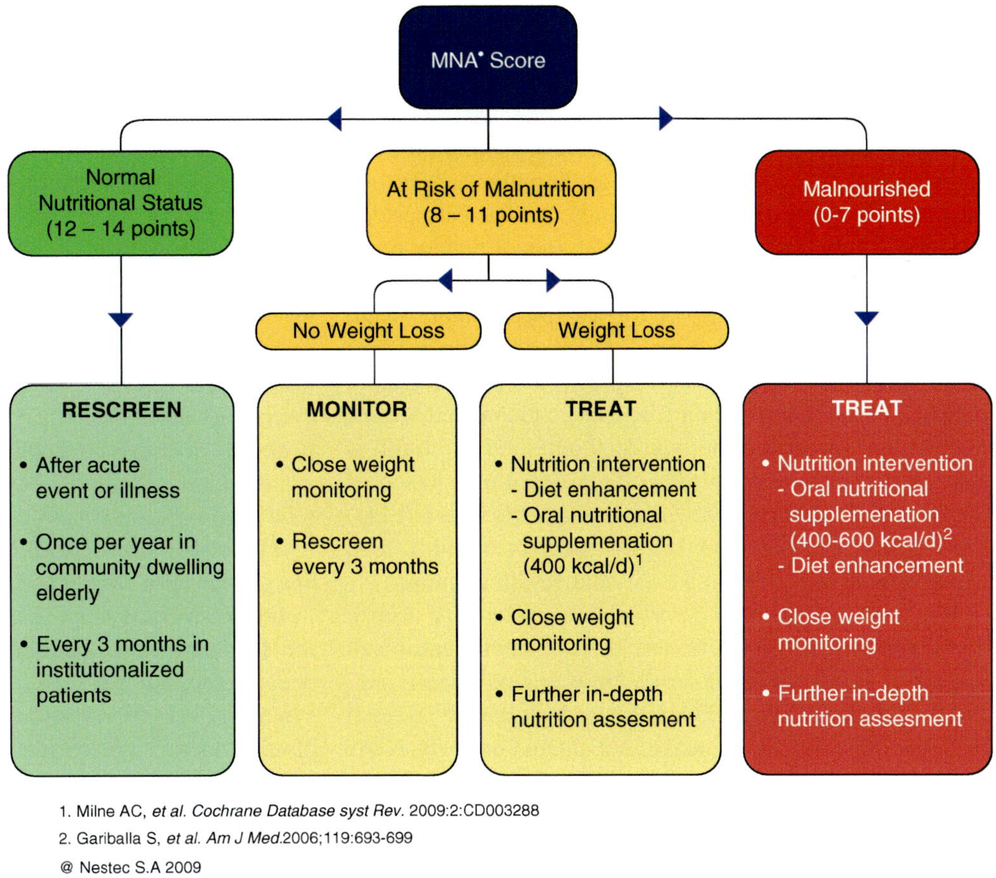

Fig. 51.3 The MNA score [14–18]. (*With Nestle's Nutrition Institute permission*)

A third screening instrument is the Geriatric Nutritional Risk Index (GNRI) score that includes both the actual and the ideal weight (according to Lorentz formula), but also serum albumin level; and it is calculated using the formula below [19–21].

GNRI = (1.489x albumin g/L) + (41.7 x ABW/IBW), where ABW = actual body weight, IBW = ideal body weight, calculated using Lorentz formula [21].

The score is assessed after calculating the result. It has four degrees: minimum = GNRI >98, low = GNRI between 92 and 98, moderate = GNRI between 82 and 92 and severe = GNRI <82. It is used in the evaluation of malnutrition or risk of malnutrition.

From all screening methods, subjective global assessment (SGA) is the most comprehensive. The subjective global assessment (SGA) method is currently accepted and validated, easy to apply, it can be repeated when needed, but it is not sensitive to modest changes in the nutritional status. It comprises data regarding weight and its variation, questions about diet, associated pathology, functional pathology, comorbidities and physical evaluation elements. The final score identifies nutritional state of the patient as being good, moderate or severely affected. It is also a screening and prognostic factor for malnutrition in all medical specialities After applying the SGA questionnaire, one gets a score that quantifies the patient's nutritional status, as next 0–1 points (a): *Well Nourish*, no interventions required, re-assessment on routine, 2–3 points (b): *Mild Nourish*, patient and family education by a clinician, re-assessment, 4–8 points (c): *Moderately Malnourished*, patient and family education by a clinician, requires nutrition intervention, and >9 points (d): *Severely Malnourished*, indicates a critical need to improve symptoms management and nutrition status [22–25].

51.2.4 Patient's History

Past medical history regarding both medical and nutritional history is extremely valuable in the management of nutritional intervention.

It includes a complete picture of the patient's diagnoses as well as the identification of all the factors that might affect his health (family medical history, surgical interventions, chronic diseases etc.). Typically, **nutritional history** identifies the factors which influence the nutritional state, starting from eating habits, preferences, nutritional education, duration and severity of some conditions (edentation, anorexia, bulimia, chronic or acute diseases, possible surgical interventions etc.), individual factors (genetics, age, sex, psychosocial factors etc.), current prescription/non-prescription medication or dietary supplements. Thus, the patterns of food consumption, predisposition or nutritional restraints are investigated.

The **diet history** cannot be achieved in patients with acute disorders, but it is essential to be performed in collaborating cooperative patients. In non-cooperative patients, diet history can be obtained from the family, attendants or from medical sources in case of hospitalized or institutionalized patient. It should provide data regarding the quality and quantity of consumed food consumed, and detect specific nutritional imbalances. From several forms of dietary questionnaires such as food diaries, the most commonly used are *the food frequency questionnaire* and *the 24-hour recall method*. Details about each type of food principle are provided (proteins, carbohydrates, lipids), about their quality (vegetal, animal), about their frequency, amount and way of preparation. Moreover, the type of food (solid or liquid) is also mentioned, as well as the artificial nutritional history if it exists. A simplified *food frequency questionnaire* (FFQ) can be rapidly applied and then assessed according to food composition tables to estimate the relative caloric intake.

The analysis of *relative caloric intake* can be done using a questionnaire that assesses the last 72 h to establish nutritional variations. If it cannot be done, the investigation extends until a complete picture of the FFQ can be made. It is analyzed each macronutrient, the caloric intake, and amount of fibers, water or other beverages. Micronutrients such as minerals and vitamins are determined based on quality of food and its type, using recommended tables for such a purpose. If it is possible, the phytonutrients and prebiotic consumption are estimated, as well as the oxygen radical absorbance capacity (ORAC) that can be determined based on the type and amount of ingested vegetables and fruits. This extensive food survey can also offer information about other details such as allergies/food intolerances, appetite status, diet issue aspects (chewing problems, dental problems, salivation issues etc.), eating habit influences (cultural, ethnic) [23–29].

51.3 Nutritional Intervention in LD

51.3.1 Related Issues Regarding Liver Physiopathology

Without a doubt, liver can be considered a central metabolic station, where more than 500 processes take place. It has a major metabolic role in the carbohydrate, protein and fat metabolism. Further, its function of storage and activation of several vitamins and minerals, the conversion of ammonia into urea, and its vital role from the steroid metabolism make it indispensable in the whole metabolic loop. **It should be noted that in chronic liver disease, insulin resistance is the central metabolic feature**. Thus, both glucose transport mechanisms and its storage in skeletal muscles are affected. Protein turnover is normal or high, and it is marked by increased catabolism, while lipids present impairment of the metabolic clearance and lipid oxidation in close relationship with the liver impairment degree.

To begin with, the first metabolic line, in the order of importance, is that of carbohydrates. It is well-known that liver is the "Gordian node" due to his role in the conversion of galactose and fructose into glucose at a hepatocyte level. On the other hand, liver actively stores glucose as glycogen through glycogenesis, which it subsequently releases into the bloodstream through glycogenolysis, when blood glucose level drops. On the other side, liver coordinates the main process of glucose formation from alternative sources (i.e. amino acids, lactic acid or intermediates of the tricarboxylic acid cycle) that takes place by gluconeogenesis. All above mentioned mechanisms are mainly altered in cirrhotic patients. As a consequence, cirrhosis is characterized by impaired glucose tolerance, hyperinsulinemia and insulin resistance [29].

The conversion of amino acids through transamination and oxidative deamination represents supports the liver role in protein metabolism. These amino acids are converted at the hepatic level, or more precisely their substrate will become alternative sources of energy production and glucose synthesis. The liver is also the main site where some blood-clotting factors are secreted: prothrombin, fibrinogen and serum proteins (α-globulin, β-globulin, albumin, transferrin and other lipoproteins). Chronic liver disease especially cirrhotic patients present increased protein turnover either due to excessive intake or to a decrease in protein synthesis. Accelerated protein catabolism influences amino acid balance and increase nitrogen level in liver with hyperammonemia. The plasma level of albumin evolves according to the degree of liver impairment [24].

Lipid metabolism with its central function in β oxidation in the liver, transforms **exogenous** (dietary) and **endogenous** (adipose tissue-related) **fatty acids** into a source of energy. Most important stages of synthesis and re-synthesis in case of triglycerides, cholesterol and phospholipids take place in the liver. Characteristically, in cirrhosis, essential and polyunsaturated fatty acids present low plasma levels, being directly correlated with both nutritional status of the patient and severity of liver impairment [25].

The activity of many micronutrients, minerals and vitamins depends on the hepatic function. Liver represents both storage and activation of micronutrients, thus actively intervening in their transportation process. It stores all fat-soluble vitamins: vitamin A, E, K; and plays an important role in the synthesis of vitamin D, being a central deposit of minerals such as iron, zinc, magnesium and copper [29].

The detoxifying function of liver is due to the process of ammonia conversion into urea in a proportion of 75% that is further excreted through the kidney [29]. Additionally, liver is a major detoxification station for most drugs, potentially toxic substances, alcohol; and for bacteria or debris through the intervention of Kupffer cells [29].

Aldosterone, glucocorticoids, estrogen, progesterone, testosterone are inactivated and excreted in the liver, the metabolism of steroids being directly correlated with functional status of the liver.

As already shown, liver has an essential role in the metabolism of nutritive factors, and food imbalances lead to adverse evolution of the underlying disease. Moreover, above aspects worsen in case of impaired hepatic function. There are at least two great nutritional attitudes regarding LD. On the one hand, nutritional intervention in acute liver disease (viral hepatitis) aims early restoration of the hepatic functional status with the avoidance of early denutrition. On the other site, nutritional attitude in chronic diseases (NAFLD, NASH, ALD, CH) or hepatic transplant require a long-term management of nutritional intervention, whose primary objective is the correction of malnutrition [23, 26].

51.3.2 Nutritional Intervention in Acute Liver Diseases

Acute viral hepatitis are contagious diseases with digestive or blood transmission and stage-evolution, from incubation phase to symptomatic stage and remission. Also, acute hepatitis can be toxic due to a toxic agent (alcohol, medication, food supplements or environmental agents), and acute hepatic inflammation characterizes them. However, there are many situations in which acute hepatitis (either toxic or viral) can develop asymptomatically. Usually, the clinical picture comprises the presence of anorexia, asthenia, muscle and articular pain, headache, nausea, bloating, constipation and, last but not least, jaundice and oedema. The attitude of nutritional intervention in such cases addresses three evolutionary phases: pre-jaundice period, intermediate period and remission. The primary aim of nutritional intervention is to promote liver regeneration and prevent relapses (especially in case of toxic hepatitis). Generally, nutritional attitude provides a caloric intake of 40–45 kcal/kg; where protein intake is the normal recommended one of 15–17% up to 20% of total caloric intake, with recommended restriction in case of hepatic comas. The amount of liquids does not undergo any particular restrictions, but fresh intake of liquids is advisable. The amount of carbohydrates, between 45% and 60% comprises fruits, vegetables, cereals, while concentrated sweets is avoided. Vitamin supplementation is not recommended if daily diet of the patient is right. If hypovitaminosis are detected, they should be corrected. The severe salt restriction is not recommended either, this being necessary only in case of hydro electrolytic imbalance with sodium retention. Meals are quantitatively reduced at every 2 h. This diet is also called the hepatic cleansing diet as it can be seen in Table 51.7 [26].

51.3.3 Nutritional Intervention in CLD

Firstly, nutritional approach in CLD is related to malnutrition. Caloric protein malnutrition as a physiological entity, is common in patients with CLD in about 60–90% cases [27]. Malnutrition can occur from the early stages of CLD (except in NAFLD), and there is a direct relation between the degree of hepatic impairment and the degree of malnutrition severity [28]. At the same time, severity of malnutrition is associated with the presence of CLD complications, such as hepatic-renal syndrome, encephalopathy, oesophageal varices, being associated with an adverse surgical prognosis and represent a valid predictor of morbi-mortality [28]. It is currently defined as a condition characterized by insufficient food intake with high mortality risk.

Several significant factors are incriminated in the onset and maintenance of **malnutrition**. Specifically, low food intake is associated with dysgeusia, early satiety, changes in taste and palatability, nausea, vomiting, bloating, dyspeptic syndrome, maldigestion and malabsorption, concomitant medication and anxiety. The most exposed patients are those who already have cirrhosis. Timely evaluation and nutritional screening of these patients can identify early deficiency of micro- and macronutrients; and their correction leads to risk lowering of complications and improving of hepatic function. As already stated, NCP should go through the four steps, and it should be applied to all patients with CLD.

From an etiological-pathological point of view, malnutrition is caused by increased catabolism, but other important factors are also involved, as it can be seen in Fig. 51.4 [29].

In the whole picture of investigations necessary for diagnosis and assessment of malnutrition, the nutritional screening completes the biochemical picture. The standard of nutritional evaluation is SGA, with re-assessment whenever required based on clinical situation. Biochemical evaluation includes the routine and hepatic functional samples as well as vitamin and mineral determinations, such as magnesium, iron etc., as illustrated in Fig. 51.5 [29].

After SGA score performing and diagnosis of malnutrition stage (low, mild or severe), the medical and nutritional managements are required, as presented in Fig. 51.6.

Determination of total energetic ratio is based on the previously presented formulas. Generally, higher total energetic ratio than determination per se is advisable, especially in the last stage of liver disease. Total energetic requirements range between 35 and 45 kcal/kg. In the case of ascites, it is advisable to calculate the dry body weight, to avoid overeating or overconsumption. The distribution of carbohydrates and lipids follows general recommendations previously presented. In patients with uncomplicated cirrhosis or stable chronic hepatitis, protein recommendation ranges between 0.8 and 1 g/kg body, to prevent nitrogen accumulation. Protein

Table 51.7 Dietary recommendations for acute liver disease

The stage of the disease	Symptoms	Caloric intake	Recommended food	Restriction food	Duration of the diet
The pre-jaundice period	Dyspeptic syndrome	40–45 kcal/kg Hypolipidemic, normoproteic, hyperglucidic, normal-sodium intake 30–40 ml liquids/kg	Soup/clear soup Mucilage, smoothies Milk/yoghurt incorporated in foods Egg white Breadcrumbs (1-day-old bread) Juices, jellies, fruit compotes Teas Non-spicy aromatic spices (parsley, lovage, rosemary, basil, tarragon, thyme, lemon juice, onion only used for boiling, then removed)	Thermally prepared fats Fat meat, caviar Vegetables and fruits rich in cellulose Concentrated sweets Fizzy drinks Alcohol Very spicy spices	7–10 days
The intermediate period	The jaundice syndrome	40–45 kcal/kg Normolipidemic, normoproteic, normoglycemic, normal-sodium intake 30–40 ml liquids/kg	Milk/yoghurt Light and fresh cheese (ricotta = a semi-soft white fresh cheese) Pasta (rice, 1-day-old white bread, dietetic biscuits) in soups/mucilage Pureed vegetables Juices, jellies, fruit compotes Teas Non-spicy aromatic spices (parsley, lovage, rosemary, basil, tarragon, thyme, lemon juice, onion only used for boiling, then removed)	Thermally prepared fats are forbidden Fat meat Vegetables and fruits rich in cellulose Concentrated sweets Fizzy drinks Alcohol Very spicy spices	As long as jaundice persists
The remission phase		40–45 kcal/kg Normolipidemic, normoproteic, normoglycemic, normal-sodium intake 30–40 ml liquids/kg	Light chow/steamed meat (chicken, fish) or as fresh dietetic mince 1–2 eggs/week (boiled, in soufflé) Fresh milk/yoghurts Pasta One-day-old white bread, breadcrumbs, crackers Oil Each type of food is gradually added to the jaundice phase diet after its tolerance has been tested	Thermally prepared fats, fried food Fat meat Fat/matured, mould cheese/dairy products, melted cheese, hard cheese Non-dietary sauces (roux, mayonnaise) Vegetables and fruits, cereals, bread rich in cellulose and fibers Hazelnuts, nuts, seeds Concentrated sweets Fizzy or icy drinks, coffee Alcohol Very spicy spices	12–18 months

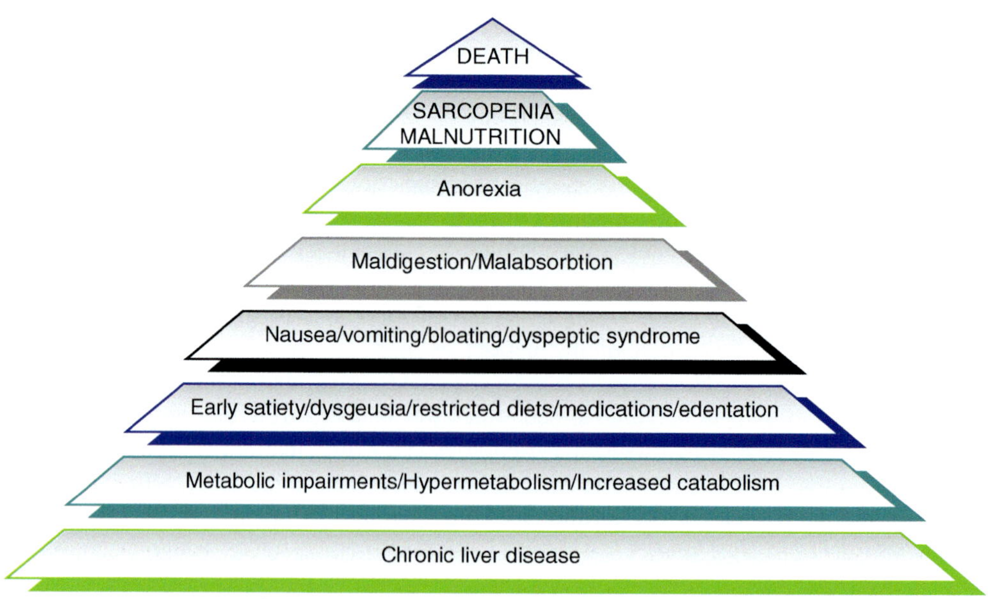

Fig. 51.4 Etiopathology of malnutrition [29]

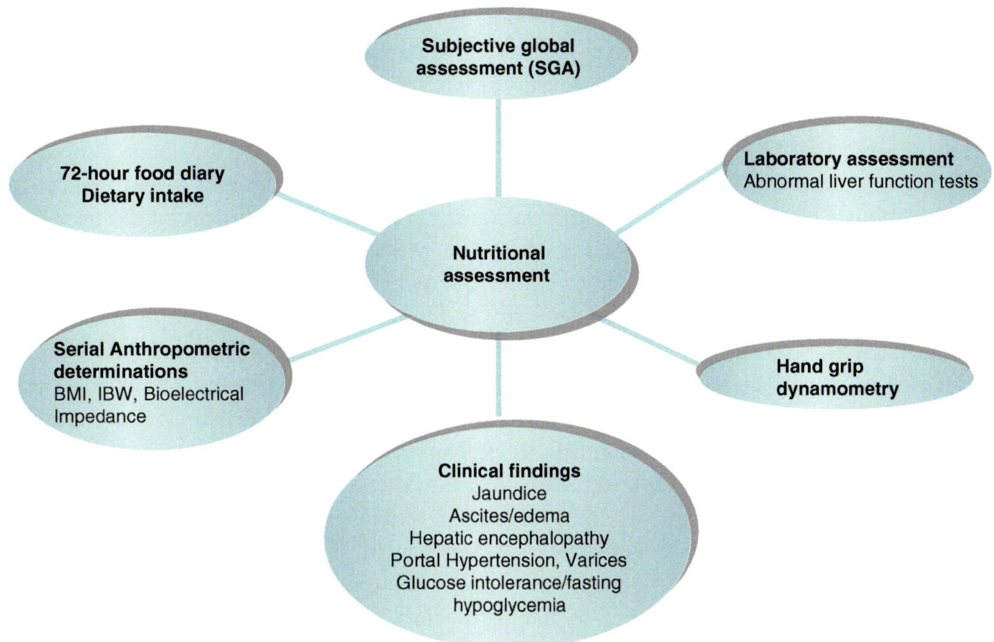

Fig. 51.5 The management of nutritional assessment in CLD [29]

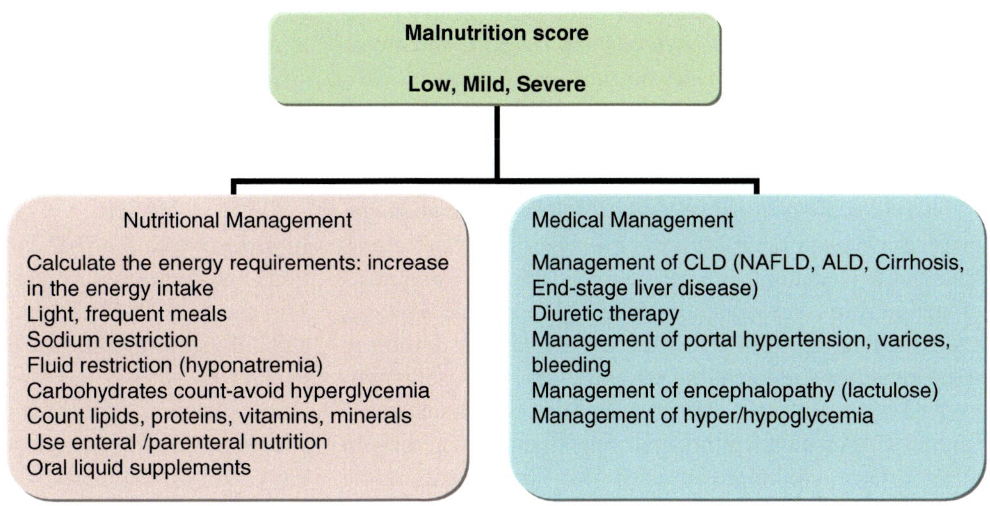

Fig. 51.6 The management of malnutrition in CLD [29]

restriction is indicated in fulminant hepatic failure. A significant amount of protein intake, between 1.2 and 1.5 g/kg is advisable in patients with ALD or decompensated disease (infections, sepsis, severe ascites) [29].

51.3.3.1 Nutritional Intervention in ALD

In ALD, malnutrition is the first expression of hepatic injury due to long-term excessive alcohol consumption. The initial alteration in more than 90% of chronic alcohol consumers, is fatty liver, while only 35% of them have concomitant liver inflammation, and 20% develop hepatic cirrhosis [30]. Several studies conducted on hospitalized patients with ALD have shown that the severity of protein-caloric malnutrition is associated with hepatic impairment degree, and increased mortality risk [31].

Due to the chronic alcohol consumption, patients with ALD have a caloric intake almost exclusively obtained from beverages to the detriment of food. Only 1 g of alcohol provides 7.1 kcal, while 1 g of carbohydrates only 4.1 kcal. Therefore, alcohol becomes the energetic source. Besides the direct hepatotoxic role, alcohol has also an adverse effect on the protein-caloric metabolism. Alcohol inhibits hepatic synthesis of proteins, protein synthesis related to skeletal muscles, protein synthesis with a role in immune defence, it increases intestinal permeability and enhances the muscle proteolysis induced by endotoxins/cytokines, it replaces other caloric sources in the diet but with reduced energetic efficiency compared to them. This is also the mechanism through which anorexia occurs, its severity developing according to duration and amount of alcohol consumption, as well as hepatic impairment degree. In this context, malabsorption and maldigestion of food principles accompany anorexia. Most often, there is an exocrine pancreatic alteration (pancreatic failure) at same time with liver impairment, fact that worsens malabsorption, especially of amino acids, folate and vitamin B12. The enzymatic deficiency, especially of lactase deficiency, alters digestion and metabolism of carbohydrates with their decreasing absorption. Insulin resistance is an obvious consequence of these processes. Lipid metabolism and lipid oxidation processes are altered, with increased fatty tissue deposits in liver and increased serum level of triglycerides. Protein synthesis decreases in liver with increased intestinal catabolism. The presence of steatorrhea completes all clinical picture and worsens the micro- and macronutrient deficiency. The level of fat-soluble vitamins is importantly affected. Vitamin A deficiency is the cause of early loss of night vision, and thiamin deficiency—for the occurrence of Wernicke encephalopathy. In advanced stages, there are deficiencies of vitamin B6; vitamin C, E, D, K; and hypocalcemia, hypomagnesaemia and hypokalemia accompany ALD [29, 32].

The benefits of nutritional intervention in these patients are available. About 15 studies have shown that early nutritional intervention could have benefits on both nutritional status and improvement of nutritional parameters [33]. However, optimal nutrition and recommended measures are not an universal treatment for ALD, but with direct benefits for the malnutrition prevention.

NCP is applied in patients with ALD, with the management previously detailed, and following the four steps. Nutritional evaluation is extremely valuable. The diagnosis of malnutrition subsequently dictates therapeutic attitude, and it is also the most relevant. Nutritional intervention in ALD aims to supplement the amount of nutrients, to administer nitrogenous substrates such as branched-chain amino acids (BCAA), deficient minerals and vitamins. The benefit of short-term administration of BCAA supplements is the positive nitrogen balance; but the long-term benefits are not clear yet [1, 34].

From the point of view of daily caloric ratio, recommended requirements are calculated according to above-presented equations, with an average between 35 and 45 kcal/kg and next distribution of nutritive principles: proteins 1.5–2.0 g/kg, supplementation with 0.3–0.5 g/kg BCAA especially in case of protein intolerance, carbohydrates 2.5–4.5 g/kg and lipids 1.5–5 g/kg with at least 50% medium-chain fatty acids (MCFA). Liquids are restricted to 2 l/day and sodium between 1 and 1.5 g/day, being recommended in case of advanced cirrhosis too. Supplementation with micronutrients, vitamins and minerals is also necessary, to correct possible deficiencies. Meal distribution is dictated by the presence of anorexia, which recommends small and frequent meals, rich in calories and enriched with oral solutions of nutritive principles [29, 34].

In patients with severe ALD, enteral feeding is an option, mainly when the nutritional status is severely altered, or oral feeding cannot be performed. It has been shown that artificial nutrition with pre-established solutions is more efficient than "ad lib" feeding, by improving survival prognosis and hepatic function. Currently data indicate that an optimal caloric requirement ranges from 30 to 40 kcal/kg with a protein ratio of 1.5 g/kg. Although this nutritional attitude is not fully accepted, especially in the presence of oesophageal varices, there is no study that contraindicate nasogastric tube [1, 29, 35]. Recommended enteral formula is hypercaloric with 1.5–2.4 kcal/ml, low in sodium (40 mmol/day) and enriched with BCAA (40–45%). Protein restriction in patients with ALD and cirrhosis is not advisable because of adverse effects, such as triggering of encephalopathy episodes.

Parenteral feeding is recommended to patients with ALD who cannot have oral feeding. The solution formulas respect indications of enteral nutrition, but supplementation with BCAA is not recommended [1]. Supplementation with vitamins such as vitamin B1, B6, PP, folic acid and fat-soluble vitamins is required in parenteral nutrition solution, but in case of the onset of Wernicke's encephalopathy, vitamin B1 is administered before glucose I.V. In patients with jaundice syndrome, supplementary administration of vitamin K is necessary [29].

51.3.3.2 Nutritional Intervention in NAFLD, NASH

In patients with NAFLD, NASH, the key to successful nutritional intervention is weight loss, especially in obese patients. The causes of NAFLD and NASH occurrence are obesity, alcohol consumption, type 2 diabetes mellitus, gastrointestinal bypass surgery, and long-term parenteral nutrition. As already known, NAFLD is a manifestation of the metabolic syndrome. It is characterized by excessive presence of triacylglycerol (TAG) deposits in the liver, caused by excessive red meat consumption, fructose, saturated fats, detrimental to the use of fibers- and omega-3-rich products, and due to a sedentary and unhealthy lifestyle (alcohol consumption, smoking). Once NAFLD is installed, there are alterations of carbohydrates metabolism with hyperglycemic state; of lipid metabolism through raise of free fatty acids and inflammatory cytokines from Kupffer cells; and of gut microbiome, due to increased level of gut-derived lipopolysaccharides which impair liver through insulin resistance, increased hepatic oxidative stress, acute inflammatory responses, metabolic deregulation and liver fibrosis. The evolution of NAFLD to NASH is due to the "double hit" mechanism, hypothesis which suggests that insulin resistance is the leading cause of fat accumulation in the hepatic cell and fatty liver, exposed to lipid peroxidation with inflammation due to the activity of pro-inflammatory cytokines with hepatic cellular apoptosis [5, 29].

Nutritional intervention in NAFLD and NASH is focused on the optimization of lifestyle, on balanced diet without smoking and alcohol consumption and increasing of physical activity, which brings real improvements in this patients. The Mediterranean diet or the Dietary Approach to Stop Hypertension (DASH) diet is the most recommended. The primary objective is weight loss, not more than 10% of the actual body weight in a year. Any of above mentioned diets should be included in a daily caloric requirement. In patients with NASH or NAFLD, the recommendation is an energetic intake of 30–35 kcal/kg, which can be adapted according to the physical activity of each patient. The intervention regarding macronutrients states that 45–55% of daily caloric ratio should be carbohydrates, usually obtained from unrefined sugar sources: whole grains, foods with low glycemic index. Moderate to low lipids amount is no longer strictly recommended, but the composition of these lipids is importantly. Between 20% and 30% lipids from daily energetic requirement should be composed of the so-called "healthy" fats, such as monounsaturated fatty acids (MUFA) and omega-3 polyunsaturated fatty acids (PUFA) which are abundantly found in olive oil, nuts, different seeds, oily fish, but *as little thermally processed as possible*. The recommended amount of protein is 10–15% to 20% of the daily energetic requirement, from both animal and vegetal in equal amounts. Fresh light meat, poultry, beef and fish is indicated at the expense of processed food. Dairy products and cheese should be skimmed or semi-skimmed. The amount of fibers and natural antioxidants are also a part of these recommendations; their daily consumptions should be increased, from fresh and unprocessed sources. Probiotics, abundantly found in fermented dairy products, especially in those containing *L. acidophilus*; along with a reasonable amount of prebiotics (fruits and vegetables) are recommended to be used from natural sources, and not from dietary supplements. The amount of liquids with an average of 33 ml/kg/day, as well as a moderate sodium restriction, have proven benefits [29, 36].

51.3.3.3 Nutritional Intervention in Cirrhosis

Nutritional interventions in liver cirrhosis have the roles of maintaining and improving nutritional state with good prognosis. Malnutrition, especially the protein-caloric one is present in most patients with liver cirrhosis. Improvement of the immunologic status and hepatic functions, stimulation of hepatic regeneration, reduction of infections, the increase of nitrate balance and the reduction of morbi-mortality are short- and medium-term benefits of the nutritional attitude. Studies also confirm the benefit of enteral and parenteral feeding especially in patients with advanced cirrhosis and complications (ascites, encephalopathy) [37].

NCP implementation in patients with cirrhosis is the first therapeutic and nutritional attitude. Patient assessment plays a central role in the management of cirrhosis. The four steps mentioned at the beginning of chapter should be followed as such for the final result to be the optimal health state of patient. At least, nutritional screening is recommended to be repeated whenever the nutritional state of patient and the biochemical picture indicate it. The most common and efficient assessment instrument remains SGA.

In general, nutritional measures include (1) the provision of the protein-caloric requirement, (2) the correction of vitamin and mineral deficiencies, (3) weight loss in case of obese patients (BMI $\geq$ 30 kg/m^2), (4) restriction of alcohol consumption and (5) nutritional interventions specific to complications (liver encephalopathy, ascites, alcoholic hepatitis, hyponatremia, and hyperglycemia).

The diet recommended for patients with hepatic cirrhosis should contain an adequate intake of calories, proteins, vitamins and minerals to ensure a positive nitrate balance and the correction of deficiencies. In patients with compensated liver cirrhosis, an intake of 25–35 kcal/kg body is necessary, as well as 1.0–1.2 g proteins/kg body. In malnourished patients or patients with advanced decompensated hepatic cirrhosis with complications, calories intake of 35–40 kcal/kg body is recommended as well as 1.5 g proteins/kg body, and supplementation with BCAA of 0.25 g/kg/day g/protein/kg. Carbohydrate ratio should range between 45% and 65% of daily caloric ratio from non-protein sources. Lipids represent between 25% and 40% of the energetic rate, with the mention that body prefers lipid source as energetic substratum in case of cirrhosis. In addition to the administration of deficient minerals and vitamins, use of anabolic hormones such as anabolic steroids—oxandrolone (40–80 mg/day) is only recommended in moderately nourished or malnourished patients. In case of severe malnutrition, this therapeutic attitude is no longer efficient. The IV administration of insulin growth factor (IGF) enhances protein anabolism and nutritional status of severely affected cirrhotic patients [1, 29, 38, 39].

The timing and composition of meals are also very important. Due to the presence of anorexia, of early satiety and malabsorption, 6–7 meals/day are recommended, in small amounts during day with 1–2 snacks of complex carbohydrates late in the evening or at night, so that intervals of dietary fasting longer than 6 h are avoided with a protein intake distributed during the day.

Oral feeding and administration of nutritional supplements are preferable whenever digestive tolerance permits it. Enteral feeding through a nasogastric tube or a nasojejunal tube can replace oral feeding in case of gastrointestinal tolerance reduction or impossibility of oral feeding. Parenteral nutrition is recommended in particular situations when nutritional requirements cannot be ensured orally/enterally: digestive bleeding, ileus, postoperatively.

Sodium Restriction in the Diet and the Management of Ascites

Renal retention of sodium, portal hypertension, hypoalbuminemia, and lymphatic obstruction represent central pathophysiological mechanisms which determine the formation of ascites in hepatic cirrhosis. Therefore, the key therapeutic principle to eliminate ascites is introduction of a negative balance of sodium. It is achieved by reducing sodium intake in the diet with concomitant increase of renal sodium excretion through diuretics. Renal sodium excretion in patients with hepatic cirrhosis and ascites, in the absence of the diuretic treatment, is reduced <20 mmol (mEq)/day, while non-renal sodium excretion is approximately 10 mmol/day. In case of a diet that contains 130–150 mmol sodium a day, such patients retain at least 100 mmol sodium per day, which leads to the accumulation of more than 10 l of ascites within 2 weeks (100 mmol/day × 14 days: 140 mmol/l = 10 l ascites). The International Ascites Club recommends the intake of 2 g sodium (88 mmol/day) in both inpatients and outpatients. A severe restriction (500 mg, respectively 22 mmol/day) makes the diet undesirable and therefore not respected [1, 29].

Determination of urinary sodium excretion/24 h represents an essential parameter for sodium balance and the treatment of ascites. On the other hand, sodium food intake represents an important source of sodium in absence of its iatrogenic administration (medication, saline infusions). Therefore, sodium intake and its urinary excretion are relatively equivalent in patients with stable weight. Patients who consume less than 88 mEq of sodium/day and excrete more than 78 mEq sodium/day progressively lose weight. Sodium excretion more than 78 mEq sodium/day associated with weight gain indicates an increased intake of sodium. Fluid restriction in patients with ascites is not recommended. Weight loss and ascites reduction are controlled through sodium restriction, water passively removing sodium. The elimination of ascites only through sodium restriction from diet with no concomitant administration of diuretics (furosemide, spironolactone) is possible in fewer than 10% of the cases, usually in patients with increased salt consumption in diet and urinary sodium excretion >78 mmol/day. In the context of diuretic administration, either separately or together, it is necessary to monitor potassium level [1, 5, 29].

Portal Hypertension

Portal hypertension is clinically manifested through occurrence of oesophageal varices, and it is due to collateral blood flow development. They are the leading cause of bleeding and secondary anaemia. During hemorrhagic episodes, the oral or enteral nutrition is not possible. Parenteral nutrition is the only one recommended, mainly if the patient has not been fed up more than 5 days [1].

Hepatic encephalopathy. Most cases of hepatic encephalopathy without any clinical manifestation do not require particular recommendations. In patients with hepatic encephalopathy and clinical signs (installed after digestive haemorrhage, hydro-electrolytic/acido-basic imbalance, constipation/diarrhoea), diet should include 1.5 g/kg/day of proteins (vegetal, based on casein and animals), protein restriction not being justified. In patients with protein intolerance, with recurrent episodes of encephalopathy, temporary protein restriction in the diet is recommended up to 0.5 g/kg body/day. In these patients, the additional nitrogen intake to achieve a favourable balance must be ensured through BCAA administration (36%) and aromatic amino acid (AAA) restriction, such as tryptophan, phenylalanine, tyrosine.

There are other theories which state that diet protein tolerance also varies according to the source; milk and dairy proteins are better tolerated than meat proteins, while vegetal proteins are better tolerated than animal proteins. Even proteins like casein seem to improve the mental state more than animal proteins. The increased tolerance to *diet vegetal proteins* reflects the increased dietary fibre content and their effect on the colon through the reduction of intestinal transit time, decrease of intraluminal pH, stimulation of fermentative bacterial flora, reduction of ammoniogenesis and increase of faecal excretion of ammonium. However, these protein types are poor in methionine and ammoniagenic amino-acids, but rich in BCAA. Each patient should be encouraged to consume the maximal percentage of vegetal proteins that can be tolerated; since plants have an intrinsic and modest content of salt, diet with 30–40 g vegetal proteins per day is relatively readily accepted organoleptically. A diet formed from casein (milk and dairy products) is beneficial and easily accepted. Except for these recommendations, an amount of probiotics and synbiotics added to the basic diet improve the ammonia concentration in blood and decrease the level of inflammation and oxidative stress at hepatocyte level [29].

Hyponatremia

Hyponatremia occurs due to the inability of body to excrete excessive fluids from various causes: sodium loss following repeated paracenteses, excessive diuretics and laxatives, severe sodium restriction, release of antidiuretic hormone. Under these conditions, fluid limitation to 1–1.5 l/day is required, according to the severity of ascites and presence of oedema. Severe sodium restriction (<2.5 g/day) is not indicated, and it is usually associated with significant reduction of the energetic and protein intake [1, 5, 29].

The nutritional management of patients with fluid retention (ascites or/and oedema) comprises, as well as in the case of hyponatremia, reduction of sodium and water intake. Within the hospital, severe restrictions of 250–500 mg sodium/day (0.63–1.3 g salt/day) can control ascites even in patients with minimal urinary excretion of sodium. In ambulatory patients, a sodium restriction of 2.5 g Na/day (6.3 g salt/day) is also useful and easily accepted organoleptically. A more severe limitation of sodium intake to 1 g Na/day (2.5 g salt/day) can be necessary as a temporary measure in patients with severe ascites. Fluid restriction (below 400–600 ml/day) is not needed in most patients with ascites. Alcohol intake is absolutely contraindicated to all patients with hepatic cirrhosis irrespective of its aetiology since it determines progression or decompensation of the liver disease and the enhancement of protein-caloric malnutrition [1, 5, 29].

Approximately 40% of the patients with non-alcoholic hepatic cirrhosis present *vitamin deficiencies* of liposoluble vitamins (A, E), 20% folic acid deficiency and 10% of them have deficiencies of vitamin B complex (nicotinic acid, thiamine, riboflavin, pyridoxine, vitamin B12). These deficiencies are more common and severe in patients with alcoholic cirrhosis. They are due to hepatic failure, decrease in hepatic reserves (folic acid, vitamin B12), dietary restriction and malabsorption. Hydrosoluble formulas are preferable. Vitamin A should not be administered excessively, as it is known, it has hepatotoxic potential. Dosages that exceed 40,000 IU/day are hepatotoxic. Usual dose of vitamin A 2500–500 UI/day is found in prepaid multivitamin complexes. Often, low serum level of vitamin A is due to zinc deficiency that determines the reduction of extrahepatic transport. Hydrosoluble vitamin supplements are administered as multivitamin preparations. The clinical manifestations associated with hepatic cirrhosis respond relatively well to vitamin deficiency corrections: macrocytic anaemia (folic acid, vitamin B12), neuropathy (pyridoxine, thiamine, vitamin B12), ataxia, and confusion (thiamine) [1, 29, 36].

Glucose Alteration

Glucose intolerance occurs in 10–30% of patients with cirrhosis, most of them developing diabetes. It occurs due to the presence of peripheral insulin resistance. On the other hand, hyperinsulinism is present as a consequence of increased insulin production, increased hepatic clearance and porto-hepatic shunt. Hyperglycemic state occurs primarily in fulminant hepatitis or in patients with end-stage liver disease. The nutritional attitude, in this case, is same one as in case of diabetes mellitus. In the presence of hypoglycemias, medication is reevaluated, and small and frequent meals which include complex carbohydrates are recommended [29].

Hepato-Renal Syndrome

Hepato-renal syndrome represents the association between renal failure and severe liver disease. It is diagnosed when sodium level in urine is lower than 10 mEq/l in the presence of oliguria. The nutritional and medical intervention aim to eliminate nephrotoxic therapy, monitoring intake-excretion of fluids and, in some cases, dialysis is recommended [5, 29].

Osteopenia

Many cirrhotic patients develop osteopenia or osteoporosis especially those who have benefited from long-term corticotherapy. From a nutritional point of view, it is recommended the consumption of low-fat dairy and calcium-rich products (yoghurt, cheese), supplementation of 1500 mg Ca/day, as well as administration of vitamin D, only after it has been biochemically determined [29].

In case of overweight and obese patients, caloric intake reduction with 500–1000 kcal/day is recommended (less than 30% of the daily intake), especially of saturated fats (less than 7–8% of the daily caloric intake); consumption of complex carbohydrates from plants, fruits and cereals (which should ensure ≥55% of daily caloric intake); proteins mainly vegetal and dairy sources (15% of the daily caloric intake), consumption of dietary fibers 20–30 g/day (fruits and vegetables, cereals—barley, oat, rye), an adequate intake of vitamins and minerals, calcium intake 1000–1500 mg/day for osteoporosis prevention [5, 29].

51.3.3.4 Nutritional Intervention in Liver Transplantation

Optimal nutritional status is recommended to patients with future liver transplant, its surgical outcome depending on it. Nutritional intervention is indicated before surgery. Therefore, most patients with liver transplant do not have an accentuated degree of malnutrition, if they have previously benefited from its correction. In such conditions, NCP begins by assessing the nutritional state achieved with help of SGA. If nutritional recommendations are implemented early, in the beginning of malnutrition, postoperative evolution is better, hospitalization in intensive care unit is limited, risk of postoperative complications decreases, and life expectancy prolongs. In addition to SGA assessment, the performance of composite score is also recommended for the identification of patients with risk. Most European transplant centres do not assess malnutrition "per se", and they do not consider it a major contraindication for the liver transplant. Nutritional indications are mostly those previously mentioned, with an optimal energetic requirement and a distribution of dietary principles within the limits of tolerance according to each condition. As already mentioned, oral feeding is preferable, but if it not possible, enteral nutrition is preferable to the parenteral one. Meals should be distributed at small time intervals, be rich in calories, and oral supplementation with mineral and vitamin supplements is recommended, as shown above [1, 29, 37].

In the acute post-transplantation phase, nutrient requirements and nitrogen substratum increase and the use of tube-feeding with pre-established solutions is recommended. Supplementation with BCAA as isotonic solutions and/or glucose solutions is also necessary. Between nasogastric tube and jejunal tube, as means of artificial feeding, the latter has more advantages, as also shown by Hasse and his colleagues [38]. The energetic requirement in acute post-transplantation phase is calculated given the Harris-Benedict formula, using the actual weight to which 30% of caloric requirements are added. In clinical practice, evaluation of the adequate use of energetic substratum is done by monitoring blood glucose levels, lactate and lipid profile. Carbohydrate metabolism is altered, with insulin resistance and hyperglycemia in most cases. In these situations, monitoring of glycemic profile and short-action insulin administration (in the infuser) is recommended to bring glycaemia within reasonable limits, especially in non-diabetic patients before transplant. Same recommendations are made in case of patients with diabetes mellitus diagnosed before transplantation, with the mention that insulin therapy is recommended [1, 29].

Patients with renal transplant develop a negative nitrogen balance in the following 25–30 days, and that is why early amino acid supplementation is indicated. An intake of 1–1.5 g/kg/day is recommended to normalize nitrogen values [39]. On a long-term, the recommendation of protein requirements is 1 g/kg/day. From micronutrients and electrolytes, there are no specific recommendations, only some related to severe hyponatremia (the cause of pontine myelinolysis) and serum magnesium level (its deficiency being the cause of using cyclosporine and tacrolimus). Regarding sodium restriction, it should range between 2–4 g sodium/day both in the acute post-transplant phase and also later [40, 41].

Unless corrections of the nitrogen balance are required, patients with an hepatic transplant are not different from patients who undergo any surgery [42]. If the patient is nutritionally correctly assessed before transplant and if nutritional intervention is implemented early, malnutrition is not a contraindication for surgery.

51.4 Conclusions

The nutritional intervention addresses each acute or chronic hepatic pathology, determines and implements the caloric requirements and even the composition of macro- and micronutrients necessary for the achievement of an optimal nutritional status, correct nutritional deficiencies and improves the life quality of patient with liver impairment.

Self Study

Questions

1. Concerning nutritional, medical intervention in acute liver disease, which of the following statements are false:
   (a) The daily calorie requirement for acute liver disease does not require significant adjustments.
   (b) The amount of protein must exceed 15% of the daily calorie requirement to prevent malnutrition.
   (c) The need for minerals and vitamins will be supplemented if their deficit is documented.
   (d) The nutritional attitude provides a caloric intake of 40–45 kcal/kg; the protein intake will be the normal recommended one of 15–17% up to 20% of the total caloric intake, the restriction is recommended in case of hepatic comas.
   Answer: b.
2. Concerning nutritional, medical intervention in chronic liver disease, which of the following statements are true:
   (a) Malnutrition can occur even from the early stages of the chronic liver disease, including NAFLD.
   (b) The severity of malnutrition is frequently associated with the presence of other complications such as hepatic, renal syndrome or encephalopathy in chronic liver disease.
   (c) The recommended amount of carbohydrates in NAFL or NASH is 40–55% of the recommended daily amount of energy, and they must come mostly from refined foods.
   (d) The recommended protein requirement in the patient's cirrhotic diet should be between 1 and 1.2 g/protein/kg/day, and in patients with decompensated cirrhosis this may increase to 1.5 g/protein/kg/day with an additional BCAA 0.25 g/protein/kg/day.
   Answer: b, d.

Answers

1. About nutritional, medical intervention in acute liver disease, which of the following statements are false:
   (b) **CORRECT ANSWER**: in the case of acute liver disease, malnutrition correction is not necessary because it is not yet installed. Therefore, protein supplementation is not recommended.
2. Concerning nutritional, medical intervention in chronic liver disease, which of the following statements are true:
   (b) **CORRECT ANSWER**: In chronic liver disease, malnutrition is almost exclusively due to excessive activation of anabolic processes. Any complication that accompanies the underlying liver disease aggravates the status of malnutrition in the sense of increasing its severity. Particularly hepato-renal syndrome, encephalopathy presenting ascites or oesophageal varices are the factors that hurt protein-calorie malnutrition.
   (d) **CORRECT ANSWER**: the recommended protein requirement in the patient's cirrhotic diet should be between 1 and 1.2 g/protein/kg/day, and in patients with decompensated cirrhosis this may increase to 1.5 g/protein/kg/day with an additional BCAA 0.25 g/protein/kg/day.

References

1. Plauth M, Merli M, Kondrup J, Weimann A, Ferenci P, Muller MJ. Espen guidelines for nutrition in liver disease and transplantation—Consensus Statement. Clin Nutr. 1997;16:43–5.
2. Lacey K, Pritchett E. Nutrition care process and model: ADA adopts road map to quality care and outcomes management. J Am Diet Assoc. 2003;103(8):1061–72.
3. National Institute of Health Clinical Guidelines on the identification, evaluation and treatment of overweight and obesity in adults. The evidence report. 1998. https://www.ncbi.nlm.nih.gov/books/NBK2003/. Accessed 18 July 2018.
4. National Heart, Lung, and Blood Institute. Clinical guidelines on the identification, evaluation, and treatment of overweight and obesity in adults - the evidence report. Bethesda, MD: National Heart, Lung, and Blood Institute; 1998. http://www.ncbi.nlm.nih.gov/books/NBK2003. Accessed 19 July 2018.
5. Width M, Reinhard T. The clinical dietitian's essential pocket guide. Philadelphia: Wolters Kluwer Health/Lippincott Williams & Wilkins; 2009. p. 3–30. ISBN 978-0-7817-8829-8.
6. Peterson M, Diana M, George B, Steven B. Universal equation for estimating ideal body weight and body weight at any BMI. Am J Clin Nutr. 2016;103:1197–203.
7. Peterson CM, Thomas DM, Blackburn GL, Heymsfield SB. Universal equation for estimating ideal body weight and body weight at any BMI. Am J Clin Nutr. 2016;103(5):1197–203.
8. Huffman GB. Evaluation and treating unintentional weight loss in elderly. J Fam Pract. 1998;47(1):19–25.
9. Garvey WT, Mechanick JI, Brett EM, et al. American Association of Clinical Endocrinologists and American College of Endocrinology comprehensive clinical practice guidelines for medical care of patients with obesity. Endocr Pract. 2016:22(Suppl 3):1–203.
10. Frisancho AR. New norms of upper limb fat and muscle areas for assessment of nutritional status. Am J Clin Nutr. 1981;34(11):2540–5.
11. Douglas CC, Lawrence JC, Bush NC, Oster RA, Gower BA, Darnell BE. Ability of the Harris-Benedict formula to predict energy requirements differ with weight history and ethnicity. Nutr Res. 2007;27(4):194–9. https://doi.org/10.1016/j.nutres.2007.01.016.
12. Mendenhall CL, Anderson CL, Weisner S, Robert E, et al. Protein-calorie malnutrition associated with alcoholic hepatitis. Am J Med. 1984;76(2):211–22.
13. Mackle TJ, Touger-Decker R, O'Sullivan Maillet J, Holland BK. Registered dietitians' use of physical assessment parameters in professional practice. J Am Diet Assoc. 2003;103(12):1632–8.
14. Stratton RJ, Hackston A, Longmore D, Dixon R, Price S, Stroud M, King CL, Elia M, et al. Br J Nutr. 2004;92(5):799–808.
15. Kaiser MJ, Bauer JM, Ramsch C, Uter W, Guigoz Y, Cederholm T, Thomas DR, Anthony P, Charlton KE, Maggio M, Tsai AC, Grathwohl D, Vellas B, Sieber CC, MNA-International Group. Validation of the mini nutritional assessment short-form (MNA-SF): a practical tool for identification of nutritional status. J Nutr Health Aging. 2009;13(9):782–8. With Nestle's Nutrition Institute permission.
16. Vellas B, Villars H, Abellan G, et al. Overview of the MNA® - its history and challenges. J Nutr Health Aging. 2006;10:456–65. With Nestle's Nutrition Institute permission.
17. Rubenstein LZ, Harker JO, Salva A, Guigoz Y, Vellas B. Screening for undernutrition in geriatric practice: developing the short-form mini nutritional assessment (MNA-SF). J Geront. 2001;56A:M366–77. With Nestle's Nutrition Institute permission.
18. Guigoz Y. The mini-nutritional assessment (MNA®) review of the literature - what does it tell us? J Nutr Health Aging. 2006;10:466–87. With Nestle's Nutrition Institute permission.
19. Bouillanne O, Morneau G, Dupont C, Coulombel I, Vincent JP, Nicolis I, Benazeth S, Cynobe L, Aussel C. Geriatric nutritional risk index: a new index for evaluating at-risk elderly medical patients. Am J Clin Nutr. 2005;82(4):777–83.
20. Abd-El-Gawad WM, Abou-Hashem RM, El Maraghy MO, Amin GE. The validity of Geriatric Nutrition Risk Index: simple tool for prediction of nutritional-related complication of hospitalised elderly patients. Comparison with mini nutritional assessment. Clin Nutr. 2014;33(6):1108–16. Epub 2013 Dec 28.
21. Tarnus E, Bourdon E. Anthropometric evaluations of body composition of undergraduate students at the University of La Re'union. Adv Physiol Educ. 2006;30:248–53.
22. Bauer JM, Vogl T, Wicklein S, et al. Comparison of the Mini Nutritional Assessment, Subjective Global Assessment, and Nutritional Risk Screening (NRS 2002) for nutritional screening and assessment in geriatric hospital patients. Z Gerontol Geriatr. 2005;38:322. https://doi.org/10.1007/s00391-005-0331-9.
23. https://ndb.nal.usda.gov/ndb/. Accessed 21 July 2018.
24. Ballmer PE, Walshe D, McNurlan MA, Watson H, Brunt PW, Garlic PJ, et al. Hepatology. 1993;18:292–7.
25. Cabre E, Nunez MC, Gonzalez-Huix F, et al. Clinical and nutritional factors predictive of plasma lipid unsaturation deficiency in advance liver cirrhosis: a logistic regression analysis. Am J Gastroenterol. 1993;88:1738–43.
26. Mincu I. Dietoterapia la inceputul mileniului II. Bucuresti: Fundatiei Romania de Maine; 2004. p. 290–1.
27. Campillo B, Richardet J-P, Scherman E, Bories PN. Evaluation of nutritional practice in hospitalised cirrhotic patients: results of a prospective study. Nutrition. 2003;19:515–21.
28. Silva M, Gomes S, Peixoto A, et al. Nutrition in chronic liver disease. GE Port J Gastroenterol. 2015;22(6):268–76. https://doi.org/10.1016/j.jpge.2015.06.004.
29. Mahan LK, Escott Stump S, Raymond JL. Krause's food and nutrition care process. 13th ed. Amsterdam: Elsevier; 2012. p. 646–65.
30. McCullough AJ, O'Connor JF. Alcoholic liver disease: proposed recommendations for the American College of Gastroenterology. Am J Gastroenterol. 1998;93(11):2022–36.
31. Mendenhall CL, Anderson S, Weesner RE, Goldberg SJ, Crolic KA. Protein-calorie malnutrition associated with alcoholic hepatitis. Am J Med. 1984;76:211–21.
32. Leevy CM, Moroianu SA. Nutritional aspects of alcoholic liver disease. Clin Liver Dis. 2005;9(1):67–81.
33. Griffith CM, Schenker S. The role of nutritional therapy in alcoholic liver disease. Alcohol Res Health. 2006;29(4):296–306.
34. Chao A, Waitzberg D, de Jesus RP, Bueno AA, Kha V, Allen K, Kappus M, Medici V. Malnutrition and nutritional support in alcoholic liver disease: a review. Curr Gastroenterol Rep. 2016;18(12):65.
35. Kearns PJ, Young H, Garcia G, et al. Accelerated improvement of alcoholic liver disease with enteral nutrition. Gastroenterology. 1992;102:200–2005.
36. Eslamparast T, Tandon P, Raman M. Dietary composition independent of weight loss in the management of non-alcoholic fatty liver disease. Nutrients. 2017;9:800. https://doi.org/10.3390/nu9080800.
37. Campillo B, Richardet JP, Bories PN. Enteral nutrition in severely malnourished and anorectic cirrhotic patients in clinical practice. Gastroenterol Clin Biol. 2005;29(6–7):645–51.
38. Hasse JM, Blue LS, Liepa GU, et al. Early enteral nutrition support in patients undergoing liver transplantation. J Parenter Enter Nutr. 1995;19:437–43.
39. Perumpail BJ, Li AA, Cholankeril G, Kumari R, Ahmed A. Optimizing the nutritional support of adult patients in the setting of cirrhosis. Nutrients. 2017;9:1114. https://doi.org/10.3390/nu9101114.

40. Lundbom N, Laurila O, Laurila S. Central pontine myelinolysis after correction of chronic hyponatraemia. Lancet. 1993;342(8865):247–8.
41. Plevak DJ, DiCecco SR, Wiesner RH, Porayko MK, Wahlstrom HE, Janzow DJ, Hammel KD, O'Keefe SJ. Nutritional support for liver transplantation: identifying caloric and protein requirements. Mayo Clin Proc. 1994;69(3):225–30.
42. Giusto M, Lattanzi B, Di Gregorio V, Giannelli V, Lucidi C, Merli M. Changes in nutritional status after liver transplantation. World J Gastroenterol. 2014;20(31):10682–90.

Molecular Targets in Liver Disease

52

Andrea Ferrigno, Laura Giuseppina Di Pasqua, and Mariapia Vairetti

Key Concepts
- Protein kinases are important mediators of cellular processes.
- Alterations of protein kinases are involved in carcinogenesis.
- Small-molecule multiple kinases inhibitors negatively modulate the downstream signaling of kinases involved in carcinogenesis.
- Nuclear receptors are involved in the control of several hepatic metabolic pathways.
- Farnesoid X receptor and peroxisome proliferator-activated receptors emerged as targets for cholestasis and non alcoholic steatosis/steatohepatitis.
- Selective agonists of farnesoid X receptors and peroxisome proliferator-activated receptors are promising medications against cholestasis and non alcoholic steatosis/steatohepatitis.

52.1 Protein Kinases

Protein kinases are enzymes that phosphorylate their substrates, which induces a functional modulation of the target by changing its activation state, cellular localization, or interactivity with other proteins. Kinases regulate the majority of cellular pathways, including those involved in cell growth, survival, angiogenesis, migration and differentiation. Protein kinases are highly regulated and mutations resulting in the loss of regulation are frequently associated with oncogenesis. Many protein kinases, especially surface receptor tyrosine kinases and intracellular serine/threonine kinases, are pharmacological targets of small-molecule multiple kinase inhibitors in hepatocellular carcinoma (HCC) therapy.

A. Ferrigno (✉) · L. G. Di Pasqua · M. Vairetti
Department of Internal Medicine and Therapeutics, Cellular and Molecular Pharmacology and Toxicology Unit, University of Pavia, Pavia, Italy
e-mail: andrea.ferrigno@unipv.it; lauragiuseppin.dipasqua01@universitadipavia.it; mariapia.vairetti@unipv.it

52.1.1 Receptor Tyrosine Kinases

Receptor tyrosine kinases (RTKs) are a vast family of cell surface receptors involved in the regulation of important cellular processes, such as differentiation, proliferation, migration, metabolism, survival and cell cycle control. The molecular structure of members of the RTK family is very well conserved from the nematode *Caenorhabditis elegans* to humans. All RTKs share a similar architecture: a ligand-binding region in the extracellular domain, a single α-helix as a transmembrane domain and a cytoplasmic domain, containing the tyrosine kinase protein's catalytic site and a C-terminal tail with regulatory functions. Because of their regulatory activity, many diseases originate from changes in RTK cellular expression or signaling. Mutations in the RTK genes and production of aberrant proteins have been causally linked to inflammation, cancer, bone disorders, diabetes, arteriosclerosis and angiogenesis.

As a general rule, RTK activation is mediated by ligand-induced receptor dimerization, even though a subclass of RTKs exists in a non-active dimeric or oligomeric form. However, the binding of the ligand is necessary to stabilize the interaction between the individual receptor molecules in their active form. Structural studies have shown that self-association of ligand-bound receptors occurs in the extracellular region, after which intracellular domains are driven into a dimeric conformation that activates tyrosine kinase domains. The phosphorylated tyrosine kinase site then serves as a site for activation of intracellular signaling proteins.

F. Radu-Ionita et al. (eds.), *Liver Diseases*, https://doi.org/10.1007/978-3-030-24432-3_52

52.1.1.1 Vascular Endothelial Growth Factor Receptors

Vascular endothelial growth factor (VEGF) is well known for its pivotal role in vasculogenesis, the *de novo* formation of vessels from hematopoietic precursors and angiogenesis, the formation of vessels from pre-existing vasculature. Today, angiogenesis is universally considered the biological process that supplies tumors with oxygen and VEGF is considered the factor that mediates this process by activating the VEGF receptor (VEGFR). Currently, VEGFR is considered one of the most important targets in HCC therapy and many VEGFR inhibitors such as apatinib, regorafenib, lenvatinib and cabozantinib, or monoclonal antibodies against VEGFRs such as ramucirumab, are already registered for use in HCC or under investigation in Phase 2 and Phase 3 clinical trials [1].

VEGFR structure and activation. There are four VEGF ligands in humans: VEGF (or VEGFA), VEGFB, VEGFC, VEGFD, and placenta growth factor (PlGF). Several splicing variants give rise to distinct isoforms, thus increasing the heterogeneity of the VEGF family, each member possessing specific functions as regards blood and lymph vessel formation and homeostasis. The members of the VEGF family bind with different affinity to three types of RTKs: VEGFR-1, VEGFR-2 and VEGFR-3 [2]. VEGFR-2 is the main endothelial VEGF signaling receptor and main pharmacological target for small-molecule multiple kinase inhibitors [3]. VEGFRs, like other Class V RTKs, are structured as follows: (1) a ligand-binding extracellular domain, consisting of approximately 750 amino acid residues organized in seven immunoglobulin (Ig)-like domains; (2) a single transmembrane domain; (3) a split tyrosine kinase domain; (4) a C terminal tail. As with many RTKs, the VEGFR monomer is inactive and the active form is dimeric. It should be noted, though, that VEGFR has a unique ligand-mediated mechanism of activation. In fact, VEGF is a bivalent molecule which interacts simultaneously with two receptor molecules, cross-linking them into an activated dimeric complex [2].

VEGFR2-mediated downstream signaling. The activation of VEGFR-2 triggers intracellular pathways crucial for endothelia. The most extensively studied pathways are the phospholipase Cγ (PLCγ)-ERK1/2 pathway and the SRC-AKT pathway. The PLCγ-ERK1/2 pathway regulates cell proliferation, cell migration and homeostasis in endothelial cells. After VEGF binding, a tyrosine phosphorylation internalizes VGFR2. The VEGFR-2 endosome activates PLCγ which catalyzes the hydrolysis of phosphatidylinositol 4,5-bisphosphate (PIP2), with the release of diacyl glycerol (DAG) and inositol 1,4,5-trisphosphate (IP_3). Phosphorylation of the tyrosine domain is crucial for receptor activation: the mutation of Y1173 into a phenylalanine has the same effect in mice as *Vegfr2* gene silencing. DAG activates a Ca^{2+}-dependent protein kinase that regulates the RAF1-MEK-ERK1/2 cascade. The opening of IP_3 channel receptors on the endoplasmic reticulum induces the release of Ca^{2+} from its intracellular stores, providing all the elements needed for pathway activation. Many transcription factors are upregulated by this pathway, such as the E26 transformation-specific (ETS) family, regulating many genes related to endothelial cell function, histone deacetylase 7 (HADC7) and nuclear factor of activated T-cells (NFAT) proteins (*via* calmodulin and calcineurin) regulating genes involved in endothelial proliferation and migration. The SRC-AKT pathway's activation depends on the phosphorylation of tyrosine pY949 (in mice; Y951 is the equivalent in humans), after which cytoplasmic SRC kinase is activated through the binding of a T cell-specific adaptor (TSAd). SRC substrates, including actin, focal adhesion kinase (FAK) and vascular endothelial (VE)-cadherin, regulate vascular permeability, vascular leakage, cell adhesion and cell shape. The SRC pathway also contributes to the activation of the PI3K-AKT pathway since VEGFR2 is not able to activate it directly. The PI3K-AKT pathway is involved in the regulation of cell survival, proliferation and apoptosis. In addition, VEGFR2 also activates the p38 MAPK pathway (angiogenesis, migration, permeability and survival) as well as signal transducers and activators of transcription (STAT) proteins in endothelial cells (cell cycle and apoptosis) [3].

Regulation of VEGF and VEGFR expression in hypoxia and in HCC. Mammalian embryos develop in a hypoxic environment relying on simple diffusion of oxygen and other nutrients, which persists after the onset of vascularization since rapidly expanding tissues increase their oxygen and nutrient demand, stimulating continuous growth of the circulatory system. In HCC, oxygen levels may be as low as 0.8% inducing a vast cellular response, often mediated by hypoxia inducible factors (HIFs). In hypoxic states, proteasome and prolyl hydroxylase-mediated HIF-1α degradation is inhibited. HIF1α is translocated into the nucleus where it forms heterodimers with HIF1β and binds to the hypoxia response element (HRE) located in the promoter of HIF-sensitive genes [1]. An oxygen-independent HIF stabilization has been also demonstrated. In osteosarcoma cells, tumor necrosis factor α (TNFα)-mediated upregulation of endogenous nuclear factor B (NF-κB) has been shown to induce NF-κB-dependent HIF-1α stabilization. Moreover, TNFα chronic administration induces faster growth and HIF1α upregulation in subcutaneous tumors from Hep1-6 cells implanted in mice; the upregulation of VEGF has also been observed. VEGF is considered a direct HIF target: the presence of an HIF1α binding site has been demonstrated in the 47 base pair hypoxia response element of the VEGF gene. As a result, VEGF mRNA and protein are upregulated in HCC and HCC is highly vascularized [1].

52.1.1.2 Platelet-Derived Growth Factor Receptors

Platelet-derived growth factor receptors (PDGFRs) are involved in the regulation of cell proliferation and survival, cell development and cell differentiation during embryonal development. They also play a role in tissue repair in adults. Mutations of the PDGFR genes causing hyperactivity or upregulation have been associated to tumorigenesis. In HCC and cholangiocarcinoma, upregulation of PDGFRα and PDGFRβ and their ligand PDGF-A has been observed. PDGFR signaling inhibitors have been shown to be promising tools for the treatment of HCC and small-molecule multikinase inhibitors such as sorafenib and lenvatinib, targeting PDGFR among other kinases, are recommended as first-line treatment for HCC [4].

PDGFR structure and activation. There are four isoforms of PDGFR ligands, PDGF A-, B-, C- and D, usually occurring as homodimers and the PDGF-AB heterodimer. PDGF dimers exert their effect by binding to PDGFRα and PDGFRβ. The structure of PDGFRs follows the general architecture of RTKs and includes: (1) a ligand binding Ig-like extracellular domain; (2) a single transmembrane domain; (3) a kinase domain and a C terminal tail with regulatory functions. Specifically, the PDGFR extracellular domain presents five Ig-like domains, two less than VEGFRs. Moreover, long kinase inserts in the kinase domain show a peculiar amino acidic sequence with no homology to other kinases. However, the motifs in PDGFR autophosphorylation sites have been shown to have good affinity for the VEGFR2 binding domain in PI3K [4]. Ligand binding promotes dimerization, occurring through further interactions among the intracellular parts of the receptors. The consequent closeness of the kinase domains induces reciprocal autophosphorylation between the receptors [4].

PDGFR-mediated downstream signaling. Autophosphorylation is essential for PDGFR activation since it induces a conformational change in the intracellular domain possibly by easing access to the catalytic cleft. After activation, the PDGFR intracellular domain interacts with a large series of SH2-domain-containing molecules thus triggering a wide range of downstream cascades. These downstream signaling mediators include the non-receptor kinases of the Src family, PLCγ and Rat sarcoma viral oncogene homolog (RAS)-specific GTPase activating protein. PDGFRs also activate STAT proteins promoting their translocation into the nucleus, where they act as transcription factors, upregulating many genes involved in immunity, proliferation, apoptosis and differentiation. Unlike VEGFRs, PDGFRs activate PI3K directly by binding the regulatory subunit p85; the RAS and Erk MAP-kinase pathways are activated by interaction with the regulatory Grb2. The activation of these downstream pathways promotes proliferation, survival and migration. Since the affected pathways are extensively intertwined, it is difficult to assign a specific response to each of them [4].

PDGF and PDGFR regulation. Originally found in platelets, PDGFs are also secreted by macrophages, endothelial cells and fibroblasts as a response to tissue damage. When injury occurs in mice, monocytes are recruited from the circulation to the liver where they differentiate into activated macrophages. These macrophages attract NK cells through the release of inflammatory cytokines and mediate the differentiation of hepatic stellate cells in collagen-producing myofibroblasts by secreting PDGF-bb and TGF-β1 [5]. As well as secreting PDGFs, macrophages also express PDGFRβs and proliferate in response to receptor activation. PDGFRβ expression is controlled by a transcription factor called Prox1. Prox1 silenced human dermal lymphatic endothelial cells have been shown to reduce PDGFRβ expression and decrease migratory potential [6]. JUN-mediated and JUNB-mediated transcriptional upregulation of PDGFRβ has also been demonstrated. Recently, evidence has emerged suggesting that PDGF and its receptors are regulated by micro RNAs; micro RNA miR-34a has been shown to inhibit the tumorigenic potential of stomach adenocarcinoma AGS cells by downregulation of PDGFR. Similarly, miR-34a downregulates PDGFRβ in rat mesangial cells. PDGFR gene silencing or overexpression of miR-34a has been shown to induce apoptosis in lung carcinoma cells [6].

52.1.1.3 Hepatocyte Growth Factor Receptor *c*-MET

c-MET is a membrane RTK for the hepatocyte growth factor (HGF) whose overexpression has been associated with increased invasiveness and poorer prognosis in HCC patients [7]. The relevance of this RTK is related to the fact that sorafenib-resistant HCC cells overexpress HGF. In these cells, the *c*-Met active form is increased but treatment with c-Met kinase inhibitors or anti-HGF monoclonal antibody reverses cellular metastatic potential [8].

52.1.1.4 *c*-MET Structure and Activation

c-MET is a single pass heterodimer with an extracellular region, a transmembrane region and an intracellular region. The extracellular region consists of three domains: (1) an N-terminal semaphorin domain; (2) a PSI domain (found in plexins, semaphorins and integrins) connected to the transmembrane helix via four immunoglobulin-like domains similar to those found in integrins, plexins and transcription factors; (3) an intracellular tyrosine kinase domain. After HGF binding, c-MET homodimerization occurs, promoting the autophosphorylation of residues Y1234 and Y1235 located in the catalytic loop of the tyrosine kinase domain, followed by phosphorylation of Y1349 and Y1356 in the C-terminal tail. These two tyrosines form a c-MET-specific SH2-motif recognized by a plethora of signaling effectors, including: growth factor receptor-bound protein 2 (GRB2), Src homology-2-containing phosphatase (SHP-2), PI3K,

PLCγ, v-src sarcoma viral oncogene homolog (SRC) and STAT-3. In addition, c-MET specifically associates with the adaptor protein GRB2-associated binding protein 1 (GAB1) which, once phosphorylated by c-MET, creates binding sites for more downstream adaptors. GAB1 can bind either directly to c-MET or indirectly, through GRB2 [8].

52.1.1.5 *c*-MET Downstream Signaling

The downstream response to c-MET activation relies on signaling modulators common to many RTKs. Via binding with SHC and GRB2, c-MET activates guanine nucleotide exchanger Son of Sevenless (SOS), which in turn activates the RAS. This leads to the indirect activation of rapid accelerated fibrosarcoma (RAF) kinases, which can subsequently activate the MAPK effector kinase (MEK), ultimately leading to the activation of the MAPK cascades. MAPK-activated transcription factors are responsible for the regulation of a large number of genes, resulting in increased cell motility, cell cycle progression and cell proliferation. PI3K binds c-MET directly or indirectly through GAB1 so activating AKT/protein kinase B axis, primarily responsible for cell survival. The activation of the CRK/JNK axis is responsible for transformation processes. After directly binding c-MET and undergoing dimerization, STAT3 is translocated to the nucleus, resulting in tubulogenesis and invasion. Cellular migration is also mediated by c-MET by indirect activation of focal adhesion kinase (FAK). FAK is indirectly activated by c-MET through SRCs. The c-MET–SRC–FAK axis is involved in cell migration and growth [8].

52.1.1.6 *c*-MET Regulation

Negative modulation of the c-MET receptor occurs through tyrosine Y1003, a specific regulatory site in the juxtamembrane domain, and various tyrosine phosphatases modulating c-MET signaling by dephosphorylation of either the tyrosines in the c-MET kinase domain or the tyrosines in the SH-2-motif. Finally, PKC and the increase in intracellular calcium levels can adversely regulate c-MET [8].

52.1.2 Intracellular Serine/Threonine Kinases: RAF Kinases

A-RAF, B-RAF, and C-RAF belong to the family of serine/threonine kinases. They are related to retroviral oncogenes like the sarcoma virus 3611, which enhances fibrosarcoma in mice. The first of these to be discovered was C-RAF, followed by A-RAF and B-RAF. Recently, it was discovered that RAF signaling is involved in HCC increased invasion and metastasis formation [9].

RAF kinases play an important role in the RAS-RAF-MEK-ERK signal pathway. This cascade regulates a plethora of processes from cell proliferation and differentiation, to cellular apoptosis and transformation into a cancerous state. RAF activation is a RAS-mediated multistep process. After dimerization, once activated RAF phosphorylates its own substrates, MEK1 and MEK2, which, in turn, activate ERK1/2, leading to the regulation of numerous cellular events. All the members of RAF family have structures similar to other protein kinases. They present a small ATP-binding N-terminal β-sheet-structured region also called P-loop, a catalytic site and a large C-terminal tail. Moreover, RAF presents three conserved cysteine-rich domains: (1) a phospholipid-binding domain (CR1); (2) a serine/threonine regulatory domain (CR2); (3) a protein kinase domain located near the C-terminus domain (CR3). The two protein domains move closer or further away, passing from a closed to an open conformation, to allow access to ATP. In the N-terminal region the αC-helix is involved in RAF activation and dimerization. In the inactivated form, a phenylalanine side-chain blocks the ATP-binding site; in the activated state, phenylalanine helps ATP positioning in its binding-pocket. The ATP-binding pocket is also the target for sorafenib, a small-molecule multiple kinase inhibitor which can prevent RAF dimerization and which has been registered for HCC therapy.

52.1.2.1 RAF Activation and Regulation

RAS-mediated phosphorylation is not sufficient to complete RAF activation. Other phosphorylating events are required, which occur in different serine residues, depending on the specific RAF isoform. Phosphorylation of Ser259 and Ser471 are required to bring about C-RAF's interaction with its substrates. Conversely, phosphorylation of Ser29, 43, 289, 296, 301 and 642 catalyzed by ERK are associated with feedback inhibition. Phosphorylation of Ser432 at the catalytic site is required for A-RAF and MEK1/2 interaction. In the same site, phosphorylation of serine 579 serves to activate B-RAF. B-RAF shows a higher inclination for mutation transforming it into a constitutively active kinase. This occurs in a great variety of tumors, while mutation in the two other isoforms is very rare. Recent studies have demonstrated that RAF kinases need dimerization to complete their activation; moreover, RAF kinases form homodimers or heterodimers. Rushworth and co-workers have demonstrated that Ser621 in the αC-helix region of C-RAF is essential for hetero-dimerization with B-RAF and that the heterodimer C-RAF-B-RAF is more active than the homodimer. To finalize RAF activation, ERK-catalyzed phosphorylation of threonine 753 is required.

52.1.2.2 RAF Signaling

After activation, RAF is translocated near the plasma membrane, where it interacts with phospholipids through its CR domains and recruits other kinases, such as Src family kinases and casein kinase 2 (CK2). MEK1/2 proteins are also recruited by RAF directly or through scaffolding proteins such as kinase suppressors of RAS (KSRs). KSRs hold together RAF, MEK and ERK in a dose-dependent manner. Until now, structural studies have shown that B-RAF-MEK1 and KSR2-MEK1 form a heterotetramer, in which two molecules of MEK1 associate with B-RAF and KSR2. However, in this configuration, RAF cannot phosphorylate MEK1, because this arrangement sequesters the MEK1 activation segment, preventing it from phosphorylating. Thus, a second RAF molecule in the tetramer is needed to reach the MEK1 phosphorylation site. Once activated, MEK1 recruits its own substrate, ERK1/2. At the end of signal transduction, the basal state is reached by dephosphorylation of specific residues of RAF such as Ser338, though, so far, not all the steps in this mechanism have been clarified. Another mechanism which turns the RAF signal off is ERK negative feedback, which phosphorylates specific B-RAF sites destroying the interaction between B-RAF and C-RAF, thus inhibiting RAS and ending the signalling cascade [10].

52.1.3 Drugs Targeting Protein Kinases in HCC

Sorafenib (4-[4-[[4-chloro-3-(trifluoromethyl)phenyl]carbamoylamino]phenoxy]-*N*-methylpyridine-2-carboxamide) was the first small-molecule kinase inhibitor approved for the management of HCC and is administered as first line treatment in HCC subjects [11]. *In vitro*, sorafenib inhibits HCC cell proliferation and induces apoptosis. In clinical trials, it is associated with a longer median overall survival with respect to placebo. Sorafenib targets include surface receptor tyrosine kinases (VEGFR, PDGFR, KIT, FLT-3, RET), intracellular serine/threonine kinases in the MAPK pathway (B-RAF, C-RAF) and other MAPK-unrelated proteins, such as p53-upregulated-modulator-of-apoptosis (PUMA) and Bcl-2 proteins. It has also been found that sorafenib enhances tumor-specific T cell activity. Numerous pathways are implicated in HCC growth and many selective tyrosine kinase inhibitors fail, suggesting that one possible reason for sorafenib efficacy is to be found in the number of molecular targets affected [12]. Sorafenib has 38–49% oral bioavailability; its plasmatic peak is reached in 3 h and its steady state blood concentration in 7 days. Oral bioavailability is affected when sorafenib is taken with fatty food. Sorafenib is highly protein-bound (99.5%). The drug has an elimination half-life of about 24–48 h. At steady state, 70–80% of sorafenib is present in plasma as the unchanged drug; 9–16% of the total drug is found as an N-oxide metabolite as a result of the action of CYP3A4. Most of the drug is excreted with the bile in the feces, the remaining 20% is eliminated in the urine, mostly as a glucuronidated metabolite [12]. Lenvatinib ([4-[3-chloro-4-(*N*′-cyclopropylureido)phenoxy]-7-methoxyquinoline-6-carboxamide-methanesulfonate]) is a multiple tyrosine kinase inhibitor recently added to first line treatments of HCC as, besides not being inferior to sorafenib, it has been shown to have higher progression-free survival and time to progression in a Phase 3 clinical trial [11]. Lenvatinib has been shown to be more potent than sorafenib in inhibiting a variety of kinases, including VEGFR (IC50: 5.2 and 20 nmol/l, respectively) and FGFR. Lenvatinib also inhibits RET, c-KIT, PDGFR. Its pharmacokinetic properties are similar to sorafenib, but with higher oral bioavailability [13]. Regorafenib is another small-molecule multikinase inhibitor affecting the same molecular targets as sorafenib and lenvatinib. It is currently recommended in patients with tumor progression under treatment with sorafenib. Cabozantinib was recently found to be effective when compared to placebos and is currently recommended for second- and third-line treatments. It is a tyrosine kinase inhibitor with a potent activity against *c*-MET, a HGF-activated protein kinase involved in cell growth, survival and motility found to be highly activated in sorafenib-resistant HCC [8]. Cabozantinib has also been shown to have a strong inhibitory activity against VEGFR2, to which *c*-MET is functionally linked [11, 14] (Fig. 52.1 and Table 52.1).

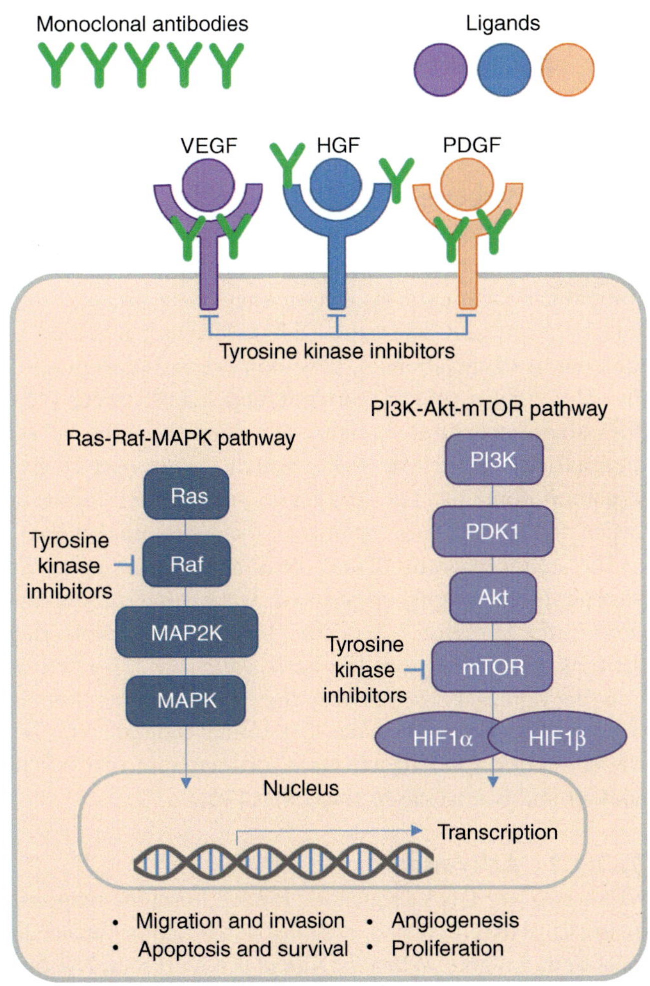

Fig. 52.1 Drug targets in HCC. Activation of receptor tyrosine kinases activates a plethora of downstream signaling pathways affecting cell survival, proliferation, angiogenesis, migration and invasion. Many small-molecule multiple kinase inhibitors inhibit these pathways. *VEGF* vascular endothelial growth factor, *PDGF* platelet-derived growth factor, *IGF* insulin-like growth factor, *MAPK* mitogen-activated protein kinase, *PI3K* phosphoinositide 3-kinase, *EGF* epidermal growth factor, *mTOR* mammalian target of rapamycin, *HIF* hypoxia-inducible factor, *SCF* stem cell factor. Image taken from [31]

Table 52.1 Drugs and molecular targets for the management of HCC

Compound	Classification	Molecular targets	Development stage
Sorafenib	Small-molecule multiple kinase inhibitors	VEGFR, KIT, PDGFR, RET, B-RAF, C-RAF	Licensed (2005)
Lenvatinib	Small-molecule multiple kinase inhibitors	VEGFR, FGFR, RET, KIT, PDGFR	Licensed (2018)
Regorafenib	Small-molecule multiple kinase inhibitors	VEGFR, FGFR, RET, KIT, PDGFR	Licensed (2015)
Cabozantinib	Small-molecule multiple kinase inhibitors	c-MET, HGF, VEGFR	Licensed (2018)
Nivolumab	Monoclonal antibody	Cell death checkpoint protein-1	Phase III

52.2 Nuclear Receptors

52.2.1 General Structure and Activation

52.2.1.1 Structure

Nuclear receptors (NRs) are a superfamily of ligand-regulated transcription factors activated by lipid soluble compounds such as steroid hormones, retinoic acid, thyroid hormone and bile acids (BAs). NRs are involved in the control of metabolism, development and reproduction and also play a role in hormone-dependent cancer [15]. NRs share structural domains classified in terms of six regions (called regions A–F), which correspond to five structural domains. The A/B region, called AF1 (for activation function 1) corresponds to the N-terminal domain (NTD) of the receptor. The C region, containing two Zn fingers, is the highly conserved DNA binding domain (DBD); the D region is a flexible hinge region connecting the DBD to the E region. The latter, called AF2 (for activation function 2), corresponds to the ligand-binding domain (LBD). The F Region, the C-terminal domain (CTD), whose function is still unknown, differs from one NR to another and is missing in some NRs [16].

52.2.1.2 Activation

NRs recognize DNA sequences, termed hormone response elements (HREs), which exist as homodimers, heterodimers or monomers. When the ligand is not present, NRs are frequently complexed on the chromatin with co-repressor proteins. When the ligand binds to the NR, the co-repressor complex dissociates, and co-activator proteins are recruited. The members of the NR superfamily can be divided into three classes. Hormone NRs belong to Class I located in the cytosol; they usually act as homodimers and, after activation, translocate to the nucleus. Metabolic NRs belonging to Class II are located in the nucleus; they bind to DNA as heterodimers with retinoid X receptors (RXRs) as obligate partners. Orphan NRs belong to Class III and act either as heterodimers or monomers; their natural ligands are unknown [15].

52.2.2 Farnesoid X Receptors

Farnesoid X receptors (FXRs), described in 1995 as a product of the NR1H4 gene and so named because of their ability to bind farnesol, were identified in 1999 as the receptor for BAs. FXRs, a member of NR Class II, are abundantly expressed in the liver, kidney and intestine, less expressed in adipose tissue, lungs, vascular walls and adrenal glands and have also been identified more recently in brain neurons [17]. In the liver, FXRs are involved in the regulation of bile acid synthesis and transport, modulation of lipid and glucose homeostasis and hepatic inflammation [18] (Table 52.2).

52.2.2.1 Structure and Activation

As a transcription factor, FXR binds to DNA either as a heterodimer with retinoid X receptors (RXR, NR2B1) or as a monomer; it regulates the expression of various FXR target genes involved in various biological processes. FXR shares structural domains comparable with those found in other NRs. After binding with the ligand, the conformational change in the LBD allows the release of corepressor proteins and subsequent recruitment of coactivator proteins. These events promote the initiation of transcription. In addition to the NR1H4 gene, which encodes FXRα, another gene has been found for the FXR receptor, the NR1H5 gene; this encodes FXRβ although its precise role is still unclear. The FXRα gene encodes FXRα1 or α2 and FXRα3 or α4 isoforms localized in a tissue-dependent manner: FXRα is mostly expressed in the liver. FXRα1 and FXRα2 are expressed respectively in the adrenal glands and ileum. FXRα3 and FXRα4 are predominantly expressed in the ileum, less in the kidney, and at low levels in the stomach, duodenum and jejunum. The physiological role of the FXR receptor is related to the control of whole body metabolism processes such as cholesterol/BA metabolism, gluconeogenesis/lipogenesis and inflammation. Thus, this receptor represents an attractive pharmacological target in liver diseases in which BAs and lipid accumulation occur such as cholestasis and non-alcoholic fatty liver disease (NAFLD), respectively.

BAs are endogenous ligands for FXR activation: both conjugated and unconjugated bile salts activate FXRs at physiological concentrations. The hydrophobic BA chenodeoxycholic acid (CDCA) is the most effective activator of FXRs. Deoxycholic acid (DCA) and lithocholic acid (LCA)

Table 52.2 FXR ligands, FXR activity, therapeutical indications and development stages

Compound	FXR EC50	Therapeutical indications	Development stage
OCA	99 nM	Primary biliary cirrhosis (PBC) Non-alcoholic steatohepatitis (NASH) Primary sclerosing cholangitis (PSC)	Licensed (2016) Phase III (REGENERETE) Phase II
INT-767	30 nM	Chronic liver diseases	Phase I
BAR704	950 nM	Hepatic fibrosis Liver disorders	Preclinical
Px-102	0.014 μM	NASH	Phase II
WAY362460	4 nM	Hypertriglyceridemia	Phase I

can both activate FXRs, but to a much lesser extent than CDCA. Cholic acid (CA) and ursodeoxycholic acid (UDCA) are markedly less potent than CDCA.

52.2.2.2 FXRs in Cholestasis

An alteration in the FXR pathway has been documented in progressive familiar intrahepatic cholestasis (PFIC), drug-induced cholestasis (DIC) and intrahepatic cholestasis of pregnancy (ICP). A downregulation of FXR target genes has been documented in ICP patients and FXR mutations have been found in PFIC patients. A NR1H4 gene mutation has been identified in the neonatal period associated with intra-lobular cholestasis leading to liver dysfunction and death. In line with these data, $FXR^{-/-}$ mice present a hereditary form of cholestasis associated with impaired canalicular bile salt (BS) secretion and control of BA synthesis, metabolism and transport. In animal models, the use of the semi-synthetic FXR agonist OCA reduces bile flow impairment and cholestasis. OCA is a strong FXR agonist and was approved by the FDA in May 2016 for PBC patients. In the POISE trial, the primary endpoint was reached after OCA treatment associated with UDCA administration: a reduction in serum alkaline phosphatase (ALP) and a normal bilirubin level after 12 months of therapy were obtained. In addition, in a separate Phase 2 trial, OCA monotherapy was also found to reduce serum ALP levels. The common adverse effect is dose-dependent pruritus. A recent FDA recommendation advises a low starting dose of OCA that can be increased after the evaluation of medication tolerability [19].

52.2.2.3 FXRs in Non-alcoholic Fatty Liver Disease (NAFLD)/Non-alcoholic Steatohepatitis (NASH)

Because the activation of FXRs improves lipid and glucose homeostasis, this receptor is a potential drug target for many metabolic syndromes such as non-alcoholic fatty liver disease (NAFLD). NAFLD is the principal cause of liver injuries worldwide affecting up to 20–30% of the human population. In about 10% of these individuals, NAFLD progresses to NASH, cirrhosis and HCC, which raises social, economic as well as medical and ethical issues. A specific pharmacological target has not yet been found. Several experimental models have reported the beneficial effects of the FXR agonist OCA against steatosis and fibrosis and recently its effectiveness in reducing the progression of fatty liver to NASH in a murine model with obesity and insulin resistance has been observed. The mechanism of action appears to be a reduction in p53 activation involved in hepatocyte death and liver fibrosis [20]. OCA is the first drug in Phase 3 clinical trials (REVERSE) under evaluation in NASH patients with compensated cirrhosis. The results of a previous multicenter, randomized, placebo-Phase 2b controlled trial (FLINT) reported the effects of OCA in non-cirrhotic, non-alcoholic steatohepatitis patients: in 283 subjects with NASH treated with OCA for 72 weeks, a decrease in the NAFLD fibrosis score (NAS) was obtained in 45% in the OCA group vs. 21% in the placebo group. OCA was associated with an improvement in hepatic steatosis, inflammation, ballooning and fibrosis, but did not lead to NASH resolution so that the evaluation of OCA long-term benefits and safety require further study [21].

52.2.2.4 Drugs Targeting FXRs

FXR ligands comprise steroidal agonists and non-steroidal agonists. Steroidal agonists are semisynthetic BA derivatives: chemistry changes in CDCA basic structure have produced several compounds that are in different developmental stages. The addition of an ethyl group in C6 produced 6-ECDA/INT-747/obeticholic acid/Ocaliva (OCA), the first-in-class ligand for FXR approved by the FDA in 2016 for the treatment of ECDA-resistant patients with primary biliary cirrhosis (PBC). INT-767, a second-generation agent with potent dual activity against FXRs and TGR5s (a G-protein coupled bile acid receptor), has entered Phase 1 clinical development for chronic liver diseases. Recently, the 3-deoxy-6-ethyl derivative of CDCA (BAR704) has been found to be a highly selective agonist for FXRs in preclinical studies for liver fibrosis. The first non-steroidal FXR agonist was GW4064, which demonstrated particular photolability that led to the addition of a trans-cyclopyl unit in a compound termed Px-102 (GS-9674), which is currently in a Phase 2 clinical trial for non-alcoholic steatohepatitis (NASH). In 2009, WAY362450 was identified as an innovative FXR agonist reducing hepatic inflammation and fibrosis in an experimental NASH model [21] (Fig. 52.2).

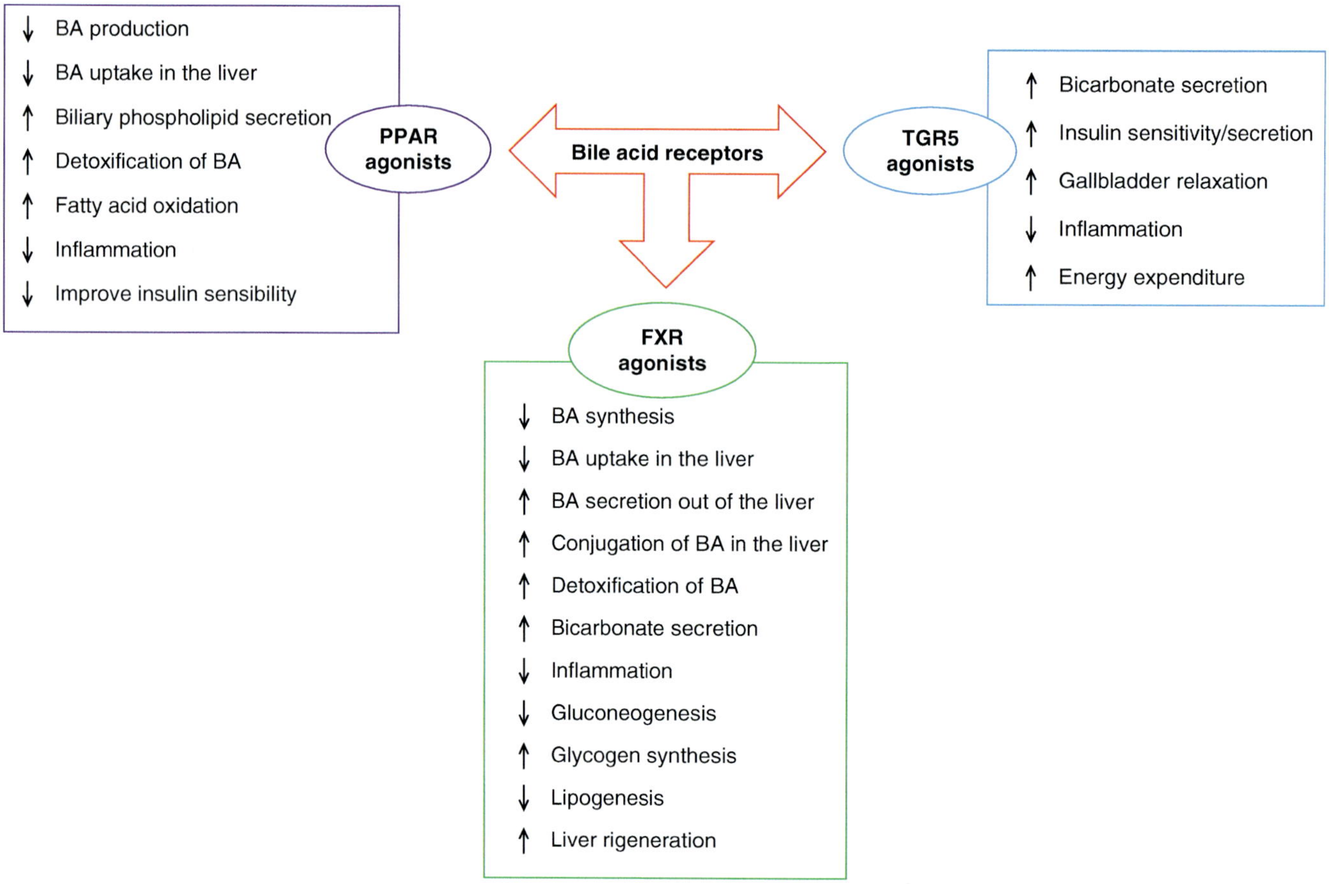

Fig. 52.2 Drug targets in primary biliary cirrhosis and NAFLD/NASH. PPAR, FXR and TGR5 are the most studied hepatic drug targets for the management of primary biliary cirrhosis and NAFLD/NASH. These receptors are important modulators of bile production, lipid metabolism, inflammation and insulin sensitivity

52.2.3 Peroxisome Proliferator-Activated Receptors

Peroxisome proliferator-activated receptors (PPARs) were identified in rodents in 1990. They belong to a Class II NR superfamily and act on DNA response elements as heterodimers with the RXRs. In particular, PPARs function with co-activator complex binding to DNA sequence named peroxisome proliferators response elements (PPREs) found in promoters of target genes involved both in the transactivation and in the transrepression of different genes.

52.2.3.1 Structure and Activation

The structural domains of PPARs are comparable to those found in other NRs: the amino-terminal AF-1 followed by a DBD, and LBD with a ligand-dependent function AF-2 located at the carboxy-terminal region. The LBD facilitates heterodimerization with RXRs and subsequently this heterodimer binds to PPREs with the recruitment of cofactors. The PPAR family plays a regulatory role in metabolic functions and energy homeostasis and has three isoforms: PPARα, PPARγ, and PPARβ/δ. The effects of PPAR activation depend on the specific isoform activated. In particular, activation of PPAR-α, principally identified in the liver, decreases triglyceride levels while activation of PPAR-γ, localized in the adipose tissue and immune cells, increases glucose metabolism and is involved in insulin sensitization. Activation of PPAR-β/δ, ubiquitously expressed, improves fatty acid metabolism.

52.2.3.2 Drugs Targeting PPARs

Several ligands have been identified with specific affinities for the three PPAR subtypes. Fenofibrate is a specific ligand for PPAR-α, while seladelpar selectively binds PPAR-β/δ. Bezafibrate similarly binds the three isoforms.

Although the beneficial effects of PPAR-α agonists have been demonstrated in several mouse models of NAFLD/NASH, the administration of clofibrate has produced no benefits in the treatment of patients affected by fatty liver disease [22].

Several small clinical trials have tested the efficacy of bezafibrate in PBC patients with sometimes controversial results. After 2 years of administration of bezafibrate/

UDCA versus placebo/UDCA, in the largest trial, BEZURSO, normalized ALP in 67% of patients compared to none in the placebo group [19]. Although a multicenter trial with Seladelpar in PBC patients was stopped for three patients with a high increase in aminotransferase, an ongoing Phase 2/3 trial has started using lower doses than those used previously. Recent results have reported no adverse side effects [19]. Elafibranor (GFT505), a dual PPAR-α and PPAR-γ agonist, appears to have antifibrotic activity and this drug is under evaluation in NAFLD and in PBC [19].

52.2.4 Glucocorticoid Receptors

Glucocorticoids (GCs) are liposoluble molecules freely diffusing across cell membranes and binding to a cytoplasmic GC receptor (GR). GRs exist in two forms: (1) a predominant GRα isoform and (2) the rare, non-functional splicing variant GRβ [23]. The binding of GRs with their ligands results in a dissociation of chaperone proteins and nuclear translocation of the active GR-ligand complex. In the nucleus, the GR-ligand complex binds to GC response elements (GREs) present in the promoter region of many GR-inducible genes, which respond by enhancing their transcription rate [23]. These genes encode anti-inflammatory proteins such as secretory leukoprotease inhibitors (SLPIs), mitogen activated protein kinase phosphatase-1 (MKP-1) and GC-induced leucine zipper (GILZ), which inhibits the activity of pro-inflammatory transcription factors such as NF-κB and activator protein-1 (AP-1), these last two also inhibited by GR direct binding to NF-κB and AP-1. This GR-driven inhibition could slow down the inflammatory process, since NF-κB is a pivotal mediator of inflammation and stimulates the expression of multiple genes encoding cytokines, chemokines, enzymes and receptors involved in the pathogenesis of multiple diseases [24]. GCs can also interfere with the binding of NF-κB and AP-1 to their consensus nucleotide sequences located in proinflammatory genes by activating histone deacetylase-2 (HDAC2). The activation of HDAC2 results in a tight winding of genomic DNA around core histones, thereby converting nuclear chromatin in a very compact and repressed molecular structure that impedes access to the DNA binding sites of NF-κB, AP-1, RNA polymerase and associated factors indispensable for DNA transcription. GRs are recommended in various liver diseases. Budesonide, a highly potent GR ligand, is administered together with ursodeoxycholic acid to reduce fibrotic progression in primary biliary cholangitis (currently an off-label prescription) [25] and to reduce inflammatory responses in autoimmune hepatitis [26].

52.3 Novel Therapeutic Targets

52.3.1 Takeda G Protein-Coupled Receptor 5 (TGR5, Gpbar-1, M-BAR)

Small and large cholangiocytes express several G protein-coupled receptors (GPCRs) responsive to bile salts (BSs) such as the Takeda G protein-coupled receptor 5 (TGR5, Gpbar-1, M-BAR) localized in the apical plasma membrane. Although TGR5 is not found in hepatocytes, it has also been identified in sinusoidal endothelial cells, Kupffer cells and hepatic stellate cells. The activation of these receptors results in an increase in the basal metabolism and anti-inflammatory properties. In cholangiocytes, TGR5 is involved in the increase of bicarbonate secretion and this event protects against bile cytotoxicity. A reduced TGR5 expression may be involved in the beginning of the progression of cholangiopathies given that a decrease in TGR5-dependent cell-protective mechanisms such as bicarbonate secretion renders cholangiocytes more susceptible to BS toxicity. On the other hand, an overexpression of TGR5 in mice dorsal root neurons has been associated with spontaneous itching and an increase or continuous activation of TGR5 promotes cholangiocyte proliferation or progression of cholangiocarcinoma. In addition, BA effects on immune cells are mediated by TGR5 activation. Based on these results, potential therapeutic approaches for different types of biliary diseases may include, blocking of TGR5 signaling by antagonists as well as the activation of TGR5-mediated pathways by TGR5 agonists [27]. Due to the ability of TGR5 agonists as anti-apoptotic and proliferative compounds in cholangiocytes, these drugs could promote the development of cholangiocarcinoma and may thus not be indicated in patients affected with primary sclerosing cholangitis (PSC). Instead, these ligands could be an emerging drug against NAFLD/NADH [19].

52.3.2 Cell Death Protein-1 Checkpoint Inhibitors

Since the beginning of the twentieth century, it has been postulated that the immune system is continuously involved in the eradication of clinically undetectable carcinomas. Immunological and cancer research has recently elucidated how subpopulations of malignant cells escape the immune system and establish clinically evident colonies, suggesting that effective cancer therapies depend on the blockade of these immune-escape mechanisms. Immune checkpoints are regulators of T lymphocytes. Their function is crucial for self-tolerance, which prevents autoimmune reactions. Programmed cell death protein-1 (PD-1) is an immune checkpoint protein expressed on the surface of cells that promotes self-tolerance by suppressing T cell activity. When PD-1 is expressed on the surface of cancer cells, it can also prevent the immune system from attacking them [28]. PD-1 exerts its defence against autoimmune reactions by two mechanisms: (1) by promoting regulatory T cell (Treg) development and inhibiting their apoptosis and (2) by directly inducing apoptosis in potentially pathogenic T cells. PD-1-induced Treg cells help to maintain immune homeostasis, keeping the T cell activation threshold sufficiently high and protecting against autoimmunity. PD-1 inhibitors, a new class of drugs suppressing immune control on T cells, have been increasingly considered as new target for cancer immunotherapy due to their potential for use in multiple types of cancer. The recent results from clinical trials testing the efficacy of checkpoint inhibitors in different tumors has encouraged the realization of similar clinical trials in HCC. The most promising, a large Phase 2 study, has shown nivolumab's superiority over a placebo in HCC patients. On this basis, nivolumab has received FDA approval for HCC second-line treatment. A Phase 3 clinical trial is currently ongoing [11].

52.3.3 Metabotropic Glutamate Receptors

The Metabotropic Glutamate Receptor Type 5 (mGluR5) is a Group I mGlu receptor coupled to the inositol trisphosphate/diacylglycerol pathway. It contains an extracellular orthosteric binding site and an allosteric binding site on the heptahelical transmembrane domain. It plays a crucial role in many conditions affecting the central nervous system and allosteric positive and negative modulators are currently under evaluation in clinical trials for the treatment of fragile X syndrome, addiction, Parkinson disease and other CNS conditions. It is also involved in pathologies affecting peripheral organs such as the gastrointestinal tract and accessory digestive organs such as tongue, liver and pancreas. In the liver, mGluR5s have shown a permissive role in the onset of ischemic damage in hepatocytes isolated from mice and rats. On the other hand, hepatocytes treated with mGluR5 negative allosteric modulators and mGluR5 knockout mice are less sensitive to ischemic injury. In an *in vivo* mouse model of acetaminophen intoxication, inducible nitric oxide synthase (iNOS) expression was upregulated by acetaminophen administration; the mGluR5 blockade neutralized iNOS induction and reduced free radical injury and inflammation [29]. Moreover, in a model of cold ischemic liver injury, mGluR5 KO mice showed reduced warm reperfusion injury in association with a decreased expression and release of TNF-α and iNOS, possibly by a PKC-mediated suppression of NF-kB [30]. Very little preclinical research has been carried out on this particular receptor. However, considering mGluR5's ability to modulate inflammatory mediators that are important in liver conditions including HCC, NASH, primary cholangitis and autoimmune hepatitis, further studies are needed to evaluate its potential as a pharmacological target in different animal models and to elucidate the downstream pathways involved in inflammation.

52.4 Summary

The number of molecular targets in the management of liver disease has increased consistently in the last decades. Small-molecule protein kinases inhibitors such as sorafenib, regorafenib, lenvatinib and cabozantinib are revolutionizing the management of HCC. Ocaliva, an FXR agonist, has been recently adopted in the management of primary cholangitis and is under evaluation for the treatment of NAFLD/NASH in Phase III studies. Fibrates such as bezafibrate and fenofibrate are considered potent regulators of lipid metabolism in the liver; however, as many nuclear receptor agonists, they modulate many different genes; moreover they showed an antifibrotic activity and are used in primary biliary cholangitis and NAFLD/NASH progression. Novel therapeutic targets such as the Takeda G protein-coupled receptor 5 and immune checkpoint proteins are currently being studied. The Takeda G protein-coupled receptor 5 is a newly discovered mediator of inflammatory processes in Kupffer cells and hepatic stellate cells. Immune checkpoint proteins promote self-tolerance suppressing the activity of the immune system and checkpoint inhibitors such as nivolumab amplified the immune response against HCC in Phase II studies.

The knowledge about molecular processes involved in cellular proliferation, development and survival as well as new insights in the modulation of inflammatory processes and cell metabolism have increased constantly, driving toward the discovery of new drug targets that are changing the management of hepatic disease. In the near future, an increase in survival rate of patients with HCC will be possible with the use of new small-molecule multiple kinase inhibitors; moreover, a more specific treatment of NAFLD will prevent the progression to NASH and cirrhosis.

Self Study

Questions

1. Which of these molecular targets are useful in cancer therapy?
   (a) Farnesoid X receptor (FXR)
   (b) Metabotropic glutamate receptor 5 (mGluR5)

(c) Vascular endothelial growth factor (VEGFR)
(d) Peroxisome proliferator activated receptors (PPARs)
(e) Platelet derived growth factor receptors (PDGFRs)

2. FXR receptor is a membrane protein.
   (a) True
   (b) False
3. Which of these targets are directly modulated by hypoxia inducible factor?
   (a) Farnesoid X receptor (FXR)
   (b) Metabotropic glutamate receptor 5 (mGluR5)
   (c) Vascular endothelial growth factor (VEGF)
   (d) Peroxisome proliferator activated receptors (PPARs)
   (e) Platelet derived growth factor receptors (PDGFRs)
4. Which of these drugs is useful in the therapy of primary biliary cirrhosis?
   (a) Ocaliva
   (b) Budesonide
   (c) Sorafenib
   (d) Fenofibrate

Answers

1. Which of these molecular targets are useful in cancer therapy?
   (a) FXR is an important regulator of biliary acid synthesis. It has also a role in lipid metabolism.
   (b) mGluR5 has showed a role in hepatic ischemia in preliminary preclinical studies.
   (c) Since growing tumors require oxygen, VEGFR is constantly activated to promote the formation of new vasculature. VEGFR and VEGF are considered among the most important targets in cancer therapy.
   (d) Hepatic PPAR has a pivotal role in regulating triglyceride levels, glucose metabolism and insulin response. Fibrates, targeting PPAR, are used in primary biliary cirrhosis and in NAFLD/NASH.
   (e) PDGFR is involved in cell proliferation, survival and differentiation and it is the target of many small-molecule kinase inhibitors used in cancer therapy.
2. FXR receptor is a membrane protein.

   FXR receptor, as well as PPAR and GR, is a nuclear receptor. Nuclear receptors are located in the cytoplasm and they translocate into the nucleus after interacting with its substrates.
3. Which of these targets are directly modulated by hypoxia inducible factor?

   Among the enlisted targets, VEGF is very sensitive to hypoxia and HIF. In response to the presence of high concentration of intact HIF, VEGF expression increases, activating VEGFR and ultimately leading to angiogenesis.
4. Which of these drugs is useful in the therapy of primary biliary cirrhosis?
   (a) Ocaliva has been recently included in the guidelines for the management of primary biliary cholangitis.
   (b) Budesonide, a glucocorticoid receptor inhibitor, is a potent anti-inflammatory glucocorticoid that has been shown to reduce fibrotic progression in clinical trials for primary biliary cholangitis.
   (c) Sorafenib is a serine kinase inhibitor targeting VEGFR and PDGFR used in hepatocellular carcinoma.
   (d) Fenofibrate is a PPAR inhibitor with antifibrotic activity.

References

1. Chen C, Lou T. Hypoxia inducible factors in hepatocellular carcinoma. Oncotarget. 2017;8:46691–703.
2. Sia D, Alsinet C, Newell P, Villanueva A. VEGF signaling in cancer treatment. Curr Pharm Des. 2014;20:2834–42.
3. Simons M, Gordon E, Claesson-Welsh L. Mechanisms and regulation of endothelial VEGF receptor signalling. Nat Rev Mol Cell Biol. 2016;17:611–25.
4. Heldin C-H. Targeting the PDGF signaling pathway in the treatment of non-malignant diseases. J Neuroimmune Pharmacol. 2014;9:69–79.
5. Tacke F. Targeting hepatic macrophages to treat liver diseases. J Hepatol. 2017;66:1300–12.
6. Farooqi AA, Siddik ZH. Platelet-derived growth factor (PDGF) signalling in cancer: rapidly emerging signalling landscape. Cell Biochem Funct. 2015;33:257–65.
7. Gramantieri L, Granito A, Guidetti E. c-MET receptor tyrosine kinase as a molecular target in advanced hepatocellular carcinoma. J Hepatocell Carcinoma. 2015;2:29.
8. Firtina Karagonlar Z, Koc D, Iscan E, Erdal E, Atabey N. Elevated hepatocyte growth factor expression as an autocrine c-Met activation mechanism in acquired resistance to sorafenib in hepatocellular carcinoma cells. Cancer Sci. 2016;107:407–16.
9. Wu X, Yang Y, Xu Z, Li J, Yang B, Feng N, Zhang Y, Wang S. Raf kinase inhibitor protein mediated signaling inhibits invasion and metastasis of hepatocellular carcinoma. Biochim Biophys Acta. 2016;1860:384–91.
10. Lavoie H, Therrien M. Regulation of RAF protein kinases in ERK signalling. Nat Rev Mol Cell Biol. 2015;16:281–98.
11. Galle PR, Forner A, Llovet JM, Mazzaferro V, Piscaglia F, Raoul J-L, Schirmacher P, Vilgrain V. EASL clinical practice guidelines: management of hepatocellular carcinoma. J Hepatol. 2018;69:182–236.
12. Keating GM. Sorafenib: a review in hepatocellular carcinoma. Target Oncol. 2017;12:243–53.
13. Oikonomopoulos G, Aravind P, Sarker D. Lenvatinib: a potential breakthrough in advanced hepatocellular carcinoma? Future Oncol. 2016;12:465–76.
14. Yakes FM, Chen J, Tan J, et al. Cabozantinib (XL184), a novel MET and VEGFR2 inhibitor, simultaneously suppresses metastasis, angiogenesis, and tumor growth. Mol Cancer Ther. 2011;10:2298–308.
15. Gadaleta RM, Magnani L. Nuclear receptors and chromatin: an inducible couple. J Mol Endocrinol. 2014;52:R137–49.

16. Lazar MA. Maturing of the nuclear receptor family. J Clin Invest. 2017;127:1123–5.
17. Huang C, Wang J, Hu W, Wang C, Lu X, Tong L, Wu F, Zhang W. Identification of functional farnesoid X receptors in brain neurons. FEBS Lett. 2016;590:3233–42.
18. Massafra V, Pellicciari R, Gioiello A, van Mil SWC. Progress and challenges of selective Farnesoid X Receptor modulation. Pharmacol Ther. 2018; https://doi.org/10.1016/j.pharmthera.2018.06.009.
19. Goldstein J, Levy C. Novel and emerging therapies for cholestatic liver diseases. Liver Int. 2018; https://doi.org/10.1111/liv.13880.
20. Goto T, Itoh M, Suganami T, Kanai S, Shirakawa I, Sakai T, Asakawa M, Yoneyama T, Kai T, Ogawa Y. Obeticholic acid protects against hepatocyte death and liver fibrosis in a murine model of nonalcoholic steatohepatitis. Sci Rep. 2018;8:8157.
21. Sepe V, Distrutti E, Fiorucci S, Zampella A. Farnesoid X receptor modulators 2014-present: a patent review. Expert Opin Ther Pat. 2018;28:351–64.
22. Tanaka N, Aoyama T, Kimura S, Gonzalez FJ. Targeting nuclear receptors for the treatment of fatty liver disease. Pharmacol Ther. 2017;179:142–57.
23. Pelaia G, Vatrella A, Busceti MT, Fabiano F, Terracciano R, Matera MG, Maselli R. Molecular and cellular mechanisms underlying the therapeutic effects of budesonide in asthma. Pulm Pharmacol Ther. 2016;40:15–21.
24. Liu T, Zhang L, Joo D, Sun S-C. NF-κB signaling in inflammation. Signal Transduct Target Ther. 2017;2:17023.
25. Hirschfield GM, Beuers U, Corpechot C, Invernizzi P, Jones D, Marzioni M, Schramm C. EASL clinical practice guidelines: the diagnosis and management of patients with primary biliary cholangitis. J Hepatol. 2017;67:145–72.
26. European Association for the Study of the Liver. EASL clinical practice guidelines: autoimmune hepatitis. J Hepatol. 2015;63:971–1004.
27. Deutschmann K, Reich M, Klindt C, Dröge C, Spomer L, Häussinger D, Keitel V. Bile acid receptors in the biliary tree: TGR5 in physiology and disease. Biochim Biophys Acta. 2018;1864:1319–25.
28. Syn NL, Teng MWL, Mok TSK, Soo RA. De-novo and acquired resistance to immune checkpoint targeting. Lancet Oncol. 2017;18:e731–41.
29. Ferrigno A, Berardo C, Di Pasqua LG, Siciliano V, Richelmi P, Vairetti M. Localization and role of metabotropic glutamate receptors subtype 5 in the gastrointestinal tract. World J Gastroenterol. 2017;23:4500.
30. Ferrigno A, Berardo C, Di Pasqua LG, Siciliano V, Richelmi P, Nicoletti F, Vairetti M. Selective blockade of the metabotropic glutamate receptor mGluR5 protects mouse livers in in vitro and ex vivo models of ischemia reperfusion injury. Int J Mol Sci. 2018; https://doi.org/10.3390/ijms19020314.
31. Kudo M. Signaling pathway/molecular targets and new targeted agents under development in hepatocellular carcinoma. World J Gastroenterol. 2012;18:6005.

Further Reading

Barnes PJ. Biochemical basis of asthma therapy. J Biol Chem. 2011;286:32899–905.

Brennan DF, Dar AC, Hertz NT, Chao WCH, Burlingame AL, Shokat KM, Barford D. A Raf-induced allosteric transition of KSR stimulates phosphorylation of MEK. Nature. 2011;472:366–9.

Davies H, Bignell GR, Cox C, et al. Mutations of the BRAF gene in human cancer. Nature. 2002;417:949–54.

Demoulin J-B, Montano-Almendras CP. Platelet-derived growth factors and their receptors in normal and malignant hematopoiesis. Am J Blood Res. 2012;2:44–56.

Derendorf H, Nave R, Drollmann A, Cerasoli F, Wurst W. Relevance of pharmacokinetics and pharmacodynamics of inhaled corticosteroids to asthma. Eur Respir J. 2006;28:1042–50.

Dougherty MK, Müller J, Ritt DA, Zhou M, Zhou XZ, Copeland TD, Conrads TP, Veenstra TD, Lu KP, Morrison DK. Regulation of Raf-1 by direct feedback phosphorylation. Mol Cell. 2005;17:215–24.

Francisco LM, Sage PT, Sharpe AH. The PD-1 pathway in tolerance and autoimmunity. Immunol Rev. 2010;236:219–42.

Ito K, Yamamura S, Essilfie-Quaye S, Cosio B, Ito M, Barnes PJ, Adcock IM. Histone deacetylase 2-mediated deacetylation of the glucocorticoid receptor enables NF-κB suppression. J Exp Med. 2006;203:7–13.

Jing Y, Ma N, Fan T, et al. Tumor necrosis factor-alpha promotes tumor growth by inducing vascular endothelial growth factor. Cancer Investig. 2011;29:485–93.

Laimer D, Dolznig H, Kollmann K, et al. PDGFR blockade is a rational and effective therapy for NPM-ALK-driven lymphomas. Nat Med. 2012;18:1699–704.

Leach DR, Krummel MF, Allison JP. Enhancement of antitumor immunity by CTLA-4 blockade. Science. 1996;271:1734–6.

Lemmon MA, Schlessinger J. Cell signaling by receptor tyrosine kinases. Cell. 2010;141:1117–34.

Leonard TA, Hurley JH. Regulation of protein kinases by lipids. Curr Opin Struct Biol. 2011;21:785–91.

Makishima M, Okamoto AY, Repa JJ, Tu H, Learned RM, Luk A, Hull MV, Lustig KD, Mangelsdorf DJ, Shan B. Identification of a nuclear receptor for bile acids. Science. 1999;284:1362–5.

Organ SL, Tsao M-S. An overview of the c-MET signaling pathway. Ther Adv Med Oncol. 2011;3:S7–S19.

Roskoski R. RAF protein-serine/threonine kinases: structure and regulation. Biochem Biophys Res Commun. 2010;399:313–7.

Rushworth LK, Hindley AD, O'Neill E, Kolch W. Regulation and role of Raf-1/B-Raf heterodimerization. Mol Cell Biol. 2006;26:2262–72.

Sakurai Y, Ohgimoto K, Kataoka Y, Yoshida N, Shibuya M. Essential role of Flk-1 (VEGF receptor 2) tyrosine residue 1173 in vasculogenesis in mice. Proc Natl Acad Sci U S A. 2005;102:1076–81.

Trusolino L, Bertotti A, Comoglio PM. MET signalling: principles and functions in development, organ regeneration and cancer. Nat Rev Mol Cell Biol. 2010;11:834–48.

Tyagi S, Gupta P, Saini AS, Kaushal C, Sharma S. The peroxisome proliferator-activated receptor: a family of nuclear receptors role in various diseases. J Adv Pharm Technol Res. 2011;2:236–40.

van Uden P, Kenneth NS, Rocha S. Regulation of hypoxia-inducible factor-1alpha by NF-kappaB. Biochem J. 2008;412:477–84.

Wang Y-D, Chen W-D, Moore DD, Huang W. FXR: a metabolic regulator and cell protector. Cell Res. 2008;18:1087–95.

Zebisch A, Troppmair J. Back to the roots: the remarkable RAF oncogene story. Cell Mol Life Sci. 2006;63:1314–30.

Zhu J, Balan V, Bronisz A, Balan K, Sun H, Leicht DT, Luo Z, Qin J, Avruch J, Tzivion G. Identification of Raf-1 S471 as a novel phosphorylation site critical for Raf-1 and B-Raf kinase activities and for MEK binding. Mol Biol Cell. 2005;16:4733–44.

Specific Medications for Chronic Viral Hepatitis

53

Daniela Gabbia and Sara De Martin

Key Concepts
- Despite the vaccination policies and the effectiveness of nucleos(t)ide analogues (NAs) and interferon (IFN), the eradication of HBV still represents an unmet goal.
- The goal of new HBV treatments is a combination therapy, targeting multiple pathways of the virus and restoring immune response.
- Direct-acting antivirals (DAAs) opened a new era in HCV therapeutic management, achieving the goal of obtaining sustained virologic response in most patients with limited adverse effects.
- New techniques for testing and diagnosis and global access to expensive therapies represent future goals in HCV therapy.

53.1 Introduction

Infections caused by hepatitis viruses will probably increase at least until 2020 and represent one of the major causes of the development of chronic liver diseases, including fibrosis, cirrhosis and hepatocellular carcinoma (HCC) [1]. Although showing the same hepatotropism, hepatitis viruses can be divided into five different families, according to their biological features, i.e. hepatitis A (HAV) and hepatitis E (HEV) viruses, causing almost exclusively acute self-limiting infections; hepatitis B (HBV) and hepatitis C (HCV) viruses, which are frequently causing chronic infections, and finally hepatitis D virus (HDV), a satellite virus whose replication depends on HBV presence. HAV and HEV infections do not cause chronic liver disease and are rarely fatal [2]. Although the majority of the hepatic diseases associated with HBV, HCV and HDV are chronic infections, the acute infections due to these viruses can be severe, and occasionally fulminant. According to the World Health Organization (WHO), HCV causes about 130 million cases of chronic infection and HBV about 240 millions, 15–20 millions of which due to HBV-HDV co-infection [3].

D. Gabbia (✉) · S. De Martin (✉)
Department of Pharmaceutical and Pharmacological Sciences, University of Padova, Padova, Italy
e-mail: daniela.gabbia@unipd.it; sara.demartin@unipd.it

53.2 Hepatitis B Virus (HBV) Infection

Chronic HBV infection represents a global health concern due to its still significant morbidity and mortality [4]. Despite the vaccination policies adopted in the last three decades, leading to a slight decrease of the global prevalence from 4.2% to 3.7%, the absolute number of chronically infected patients has grown from 223 million in 1990 to 240 million in 2005. In the United States, it has been estimated that 730,000 US residents may have chronic HBV infection, and this number can probably rise to about 2.2 million if high prevalence groups deriving from immigration from endemic countries are included [5].

Chronic HBV infection can be classified into five phases:

(I) HBeAg-positive chronic infection or immune tolerant phase
(II) HBeAg-positive chronic hepatitis
(III) HBeAg-negative chronic infection or 'inactive carrier' phase
(IV) HBeAg-negative chronic hepatitis
(V) HBsAg-negative phase.

The HBeAg-positive chronic infection is characterized by very high levels of HBV DNA (usually over 20,000 IU/mL), presence of HBeAg and persistently normal alanine aminotransferase (ALT) levels, which are increased in HBeAg-positive chronic hepatitis, as a marker of active hepatic inflammation.

F. Radu-Ionita et al. (eds.), *Liver Diseases*, https://doi.org/10.1007/978-3-030-24432-3_53

In HBeAg-negative chronic infection, patients usually show absent HBeAg, normal ALT, and undetectable or low levels of HBV DNA, generally below 2000 IU/mL. ALT values increase in HBeAg-negative chronic hepatitis, with liver necroinflammation and fibrosis. The HBsAg-negative phase, also known as "occult HBV infection", is characterized by absence of HBsAg and presence of anti-HBcAg antibodies, with or without detectable anti-HBsAg antibodies. It should be noticed that the evolution of chronic infection does not necessarily pass through every phase of the disease and the immune responses to each phase have not been fully characterized. However, the above reported classification of chronic HBV infection can be useful for finding more appropriate pharmacological treatments. Since the chronic infection is associated with an increased risk of developing cirrhosis and HCC, drug therapy is focused on improvement of survival and quality of life and also on prevention of disease progression, and consequently HCC development. The primary goal of current treatment strategies is the long-term suppression of HBV replication, although HBsAg loss represents a good surrogate end-point.

53.2.1 Treatment Strategies for HBV

Currently, two classes of drugs are approved for the treatment of chronic HBV infection: nucleos(t)ide analogues (NAs) and interferon (IFN) and its derivatives.

Although these drugs are effective in both suppressing viral replication and reducing hepatic inflammation, the eradication of HBV still represents an unmet goal. Generally, IFN therapy has a limited duration, whereas nucleos(t)ide analogues often need a life-long administration. This prolonged treatment is associated with a high risks of adverse reactions, drug resistance, nonadherence, and elevated cost. Nevertheless, the gold standard treatment is the long-term administration of a potent nucleos(t)ide analogue with high barrier to resistance, such as entecavir, tenofovir disoproxil or tenofovir alafenamide. However, in mild-to-moderate chronic HBV hepatitis, IFN treatment can also be considered. Since HCC remains the major concern for treated chronic patients, therapy response, adherence and risk of disease progression should be monitored. It should be noted that most current literature focuses only on the immune active phases of chronic HBV infection and, as a consequence, the therapy choice in both common and challenging clinical settings is based on indirect evidence and should consider individual patient preference and available resources.

53.2.1.1 Interferon (IFN)

Two formulations (standard and pegylated) of interferon (IFN and PegIFN-α) are available; PegIFN-α is generally better tolerated. In chronic HBV patients, IFN treatment produces the loss of HBV DNA and HBeAg and the development of anti-HBe antibody, together with an improvement of the biochemical and histological parameters of the liver. To achieve a lasting response and a long-term immunological control, PegIFN-α is used at moderate-to-high doses (5 or 10 MU/day) and with a limited duration treatment (typically a 4–6 weeks-course). The two main drawbacks of PegIFN-α are the high variability of response and the unfavorable safety profile, so that a significant number of patients are ineligible or unwilling to use this drug [6].

The prediction of individual responses can be assessed on the basis of several patient characteristics, such as disease activity, HBV genotype, stage of the disease, as well as levels of HBV DNA, HBsAg and HBeAg status [6]. Following these indications, PegIFN-α can be early discontinued in patients with a low probability of long-term response.

Theoretically, a combined therapy with NAs and PegIFN-α may provide advantages due to the synergistic antiviral effects of the two drugs [6–8]. However, evidence of the superiority of such an approach is lacking, and many questions regarding patient selection, timing and duration of the combination strategy are still unresolved. For these reasons, the combined therapy with NAs and PegIFN-α is not generally recommended.

53.2.1.2 Nucleos(t)ide Analogues (NAs)

Five NAs are approved for chronic HBV treatment: lamivudine, adefovir, entecavir, telbivudine and tenofovir (Fig. 53.1). These compounds can be classified into two classes: those having a low barrier (lamivudine, adefovir dipivoxil, telbivudine) and those with high barrier to HBV resistance (entecavir, tenofovir) [5, 6].

Usually, the NAs with high barrier to resistance (i.e., entecavir, tenofovir disoproxil fumarate, tenofovir alafenamide) are used as a first-line choice, since, besides a low risk of drug resistance, they have a desirable safety profile and a potent long-term antiviral activity leading to undetectable HBV DNA levels in the majority of adherent patients [5, 6]. For these reasons, these compounds can be safely used in all HBV infected patients, representing the only treatment option for several patient subgroups (decompensated liver disease, liver transplants, extrahepatic manifestations, or severe chronic HBV exacerbation) [5, 9]. Moreover, NAs are successfully used to prevent HBV reactivation in patients under immunosuppression. Common adverse reactions of entecavir include headache, fatigue, dizziness, and nausea. Lactic acidosis and hepatomegaly with steatosis are possible complications for decompensated cirrhotic patients (Child-Pugh B and C). The main adverse effects of tenofovir are impairment of renal function, with renal tubular dysfunction (Fanconi syndrome), and decreased bone mineral density. Despite the high antiviral efficacy of entecavir and tenofovir, a

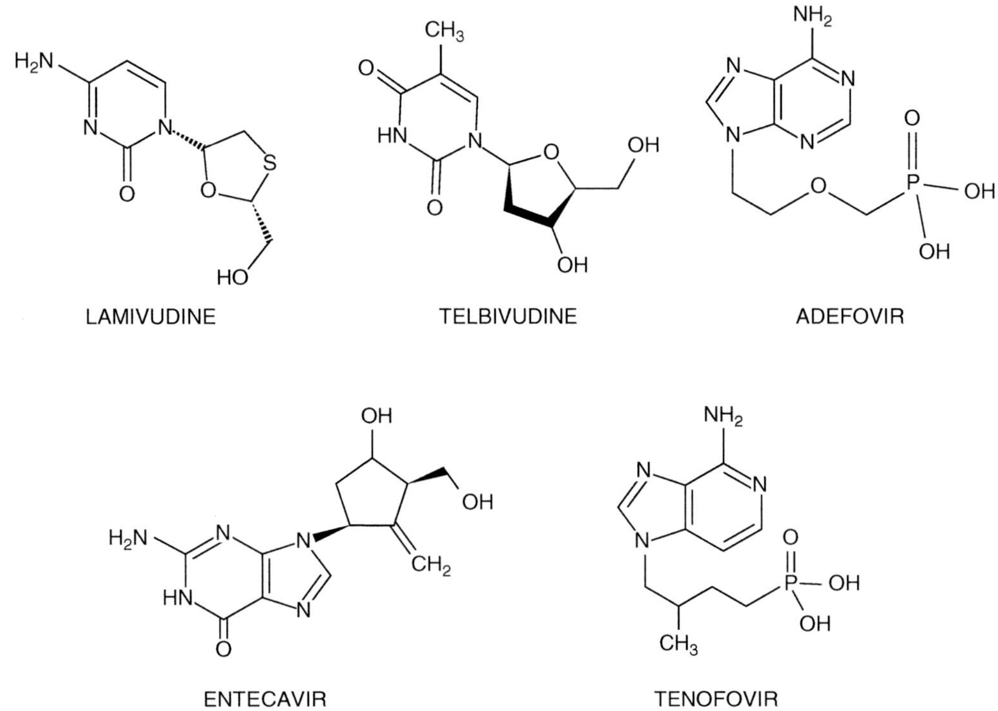

Fig. 53.1 NAs used in chronic HBV treatment

persistent viremia can be observed in some patients, particularly among HBeAg-positive ones with high baseline serum HBV DNA. Whether the association of a second antiviral agent increases the efficacy in patients with persistent viremia has not yet been tested.

The main characteristics (posology, pharmacokinetic profiles and possible drug-drug interactions) of the five NAs approved for HBV treatment are listed in Table 53.1.

53.2.1.3 HBV in Pregnancy

One of the major risk factors of chronic HBV infection is the perinatal or mother-to-child transmission (MTCT) of HBV in many high-prevalence areas [10]. In the absence of prophylaxis, MTCT may occur in up to 90% of HBsAg-positive and HBeAg-positive mothers. However, the administration of antiviral drugs during pregnancy is controversial, and precise guidelines on the risk-benefit balance are still unavailable. Although the highest risk of MTCT occurs during the immune tolerant phase, the benefit of antiviral therapy in preventing MTCT in this phase still awaits demonstration. Moreover, women in the immune active phase who have compensated liver disease can postpone antiviral treatment until delivery [10]. Additionally, it has been demonstrated that HBV infection can be prevented in approximately 90% of infants with post-delivery neonatal combined immune-prophylaxis. Unfortunately, in women presenting high levels of viremia (serum HBV DNA >10^6 copies/mL), neonatal immune-prophylaxis can have unacceptably high rates of failure (9%) [10].

Based primarily on in vivo preclinical data, FDA currently rates telbivudine and tenofovir as pregnancy category B ("Animal reproduction studies have failed to demonstrate a risk to the fetus and there are no adequate and well-controlled studies in pregnant women"), and lamivudine as pregnancy category C ("Animal reproduction studies have shown an adverse effect on the fetus and there are no adequate and well-controlled studies in humans, but potential benefits may warrant use of the drug in pregnant women despite potential risks"). However, in HIV-infected pregnant women, the use of tenofovir and lamivudine to prevent HIV transmission has not been linked to any significant safety concerns for either the mother or the newborn.

In conclusion, in pregnant women with chronic HBV infection, the administration of lamivudine, telbivudine, and tenofovir reduces the rate of MTCT and, although limited, safety data of clinical practice suggest no increased risk of adverse maternal or fetal outcomes. Larger-scale randomized controlled trials using tenofovir are ongoing, and their results are eagerly awaited. In the meantime, the treatment of HBeAg positive women with high HBV DNA level (>10^6 copies/mL; 200,000 IU/mL) with antiviral agents in the third trimester is recommended to prevent MTCT.

53.2.1.4 HBV in Children

In children and adolescents, all the currently approved therapeutic agents for chronic HBV show acceptable safety profiles and oral antivirals are safe and well tolerated. The side effects of IFN are similar to that reported for adults,

Table 53.1 Nucleo(s)tide analogues for HBV treatment

	Dosage	Pharmacokinetic tips	Route of drug elimination	Adverse reactions	Drug-drug interactions
High barrier to resistance					
Entecavir	• 0.5 mg once daily for naïve patients • 1 mg once daily for patients with lamivudine or telbivudine resistance or with decompensated cirrhosis	• Terminal $t_{1/2}$ 128–149 h • Slightly bound to serum proteins (13%)	Renally excreted	• Headache, fatigue, dizziness, and nausea	
Tenofovir	• 300 mg once daily	• $t_{1/2}$ of 17 h			• Drugs that inhibit or induce OAT1, MRP, Pgp and BCRP Transporters may affect tenofovir exposure • Sofosbuvir, ledipasvir, and velpatasvir increase tenofovir exposures
Tenofovir Alafenamide (TDF)	• 25 mg once daily			• Fewer adverse effects on BMD and kidney function (CLCr, eGFR, proteinuria) than tenofovir	
Low barrier to resistance					
Lamivudine	• 100 mg once daily				
Adefovir dipivoxil	• 10 mg once daily	• $t_{1/2}$ of 5–7.5 h	Renally excreted	• Dose-related nephrotoxicity and tubular dysfunction, manifested by azotemia and hypophosphatemia, acidosis, glycosuria, and proteinuria • Headache, abdominal discomfort, diarrhea, and asthenia	
Telbivudine	• 600 mg once daily	• $t_{1/2}$ of 40–49 h	Renally excreted	• Increased creatine kinase, nausea, diarrhea, fatigue, myalgia, and myopathy	

although transient effects on body weight and growth have been observed. In children, the development of viral resistance to lamivudine and adefovir is observed at least as often as in adults, whereas is less common with entecavir [11].

The decision of starting the pharmacological treatment in children depends on the patient's characteristics (persistently abnormal ALT levels, active disease on liver biopsy) and on the probability of obtaining appropriate therapeutic goals. In some cases, the treatment can improve chronic HBV infection, at least as far as HBV DNA suppression and HBeAg seroconversion are concerned, although the efficacy in preventing chronic liver diseases, e.g. cirrhosis and HCC in young adult life, remains to be demonstrated.

Generally, children in the immune-tolerant phase (ALT levels less than 1.5–2 times the normal upper limit and HBeAg-positivity with high HBV DNA levels) are not typical candidates for pharmacological treatment, because HBeAg seroconversion cannot be obtained. Children with ALT values 10 times over the upper normal range may undergo spontaneous HBeAg seroconversion, and the pharmacological treatment can be started only after several months of observation.

New therapeutic options for chronic HBV infection in childhood will be available in the next future, since entecavir has recently been shown to be safe and effective in children, and data regarding the safety of pegylated IFN and tenofovir are expected soon. Children in the immune-tolerant phase have not experienced substantial benefit from prolonged treatment with nucleos(t)ide analogues, moreover the risk of developing antiviral drug resistance to the drug used and structurally-related analogues should be considered. The only exception could be represented by those immune-tolerant children undergoing immunosuppressive therapy and chemotherapy, or receiving stem cell or solid organ transplantation [11]. In conclusion, the selection and timing of patient treatment is very critical in childhood and adolescence.

53.3 Hepatitis C Virus (HCV) Infection

Hepatitis C virus (HCV) infection is one of the major causes of chronic liver disease [12], with a very variable long-term course, ranging from minimal histological changes to extensive fibrosis, cirrhosis and HCC.

The number of chronically infected individuals is about 71 million worldwide [12, 13], but it should be noticed that many patients are unaware of their infection.

Clinical care for patients with HCV-related liver disease has advanced dramatically in recent years as a result of a better understanding of HCV pathophysiology, and the consequent improvement of prevention, diagnosis, and especially pharmacological therapy.

The principal end-point of HCV therapy is to cure the infection with a very low chance of relapse, thus obtaining a sustained virological response (SVR). SVR can be defined an undetectable HCV RNA after 12 weeks (SVR12) or 24 weeks (SVR24) of treatment completion. In patients without cirrhosis, this goal is generally associated with improvement or disappearance of liver necroinflammation and fibrosis and normalization of liver enzymes, whereas in patients with advanced fibrosis or cirrhosis, the risk of life-threatening complications still exists. Moreover, SVR is associated to reversal of a number of extra-hepatic manifestations related to HCV infection and to a significant reduction of all-cause mortality [14].

53.3.1 Treatment Strategies for HCV

HCV has been treated for many years with a prolonged regimen of IFN-α (or PegIFN-α) with or without ribavirin. Nevertheless, both efficacy and tolerability of these therapeutic regimens were not satisfactory. Recently, several orally administered antivirals, directly targeting HCV life cycle (the so-called direct antiviral agents-DAAs) have been approved for HCV treatment, and can be used alone or in combination to enhance their efficacy. They are characterized by a favorable toxicological profile, and can be taken for a limited period of time to achieve SVR rates of at least 90% in most patients. In some cases, ribavirin is still used with DAAs to improve their therapeutic efficacy.

Three are the major targets of available DAAs:

- The non-structural (NS) protein 3 protease, molecular target of paritaprevir, grazoprevir, voxilaprevir and glecaprevir
- The NS5B polymerase, molecular target of sofosbuvir and dasabuvir
- NS5A, molecular target of ledipasvir, velpatasvir, ombitasvir, elbasvir and pibrentasvir.

53.3.1.1 Ribavirin

Ribavirin is a purine nucleoside analogue that inhibits viral replication. The mechanism(s) of action are still unknown in vivo, but several immunomodulatory and antiviral effects have been observed *in vitro* (e.g. inhibition of HCV RNA-dependent RNA polymerase, depletion of GTP through inhibition of inosine 5′-monophosphate dehydrogenase, increase in viral mutagenesis, conversion of the T-helper cell from phenotype 2 to 1, induction of IFN-stimulated genes, and modulation of natural killer cells). Currently, ribavirin is not administered in monotherapy, but in combination with other direct-acting antivirals (DAAs) for treating chronic HCV infection only in specific clinical conditions. The possible associations between ribavirin and DAAs are described in details below.

53.3.1.2 Direct-Acting Antivirals (DAAs)

This paragraph discusses the DAAs which are available in Europe in 2018 [14]. Their posology, pharmacokinetic profiles and possible drug-drug interactions are listed in Table 53.2.

Sofosbuvir

Sofosbuvir, a nucleotide analog potently inhibiting NS5B polymerase in HCV, has shown high efficacy in combination with several other drugs against HCV. Generally, a sofosbuvir-based regimen ranging from 12 to 24 weeks is well tolerated. In urine, the major sofosbuvir metabolite is GS-331007, its dephosphorylated nucleoside (78%), while 3.5% is recovered as unmodified drug. Sofosbuvir is transported by P-gp, whereas cytochrome P450 is not involved in its metabolism. Since no potential drug-drug interactions with other antiviral agents are reported, sofosbuvir can be used in association with such drugs.

The main concern for drug-drug interactions is related to amiodarone. Patients taking this drug should not be treated with sofosbuvir-based regimens since the risk of life-threatening arrhythmias may not be excluded. The risk of cardiac toxicity of sofosbuvir when used in monotherapy is still controversial.

Combination Regimens

Sofosbuvir and Ledipasvir

Patients with mild-to-moderate renal impairment do not require dose adjustment of this combination regimen, whereas in case of severe renal impairment (eGFR <30 mL/min/1.73 m^2) or end-stage renal disease, no dose adjustment has yet been proposed. Co-administration with P-gp substrates (e.g. digoxin and dabigatran) and drugs transported by both P-gp and BCRP proteins (e.g. aliskiren, amlodipine, buprenorphine, carvedilol, cyclosporine) require patient strict monitoring. As for sofosbuvir, the coadministration

Table 53.2 DAAs for HCV treatment

	Dosage	Pharmacokinetic tips	Route of drug elimination	Adverse reactions	Drug-drug interactions
Pangenotypic drugs and combinations					
Sofosbuvir	Tablets containing 400 mg of sofosbuvir—one tablet once daily	Time-independent, near-linear pharmacokinetics across a range of doses	80% renally excreted as metabolite GS-331007, 15% eliminated in feces	• Fatigue and headache • Slight elevations of creatine kinase, amylase and lipase in combination with ribavirin	• Inducers of P-gp (rifampicin, carbamazepine, phenytoin or St. John's wort) significantly decrease plasma concentrations with rifabutin, rifapentine and modafinil • Amiodarone (risk of life-threatening arrhythmias)
Sofosbuvir/ velpatasvir	Tablets containing 400 mg of sofosbuvir and 100 mg of velpatasvir—one tablet once daily	Terminal $t_{1/2}$ of velpatasvir approximately 15 h Velpatasvir: 99.5% protein bound	Biliary excretion of velpatasvir parent drug	• Headache, fatigue and nausea	• P-gp or CYP inducers decrease in sofosbuvir and/ or velpatasvir exposure • Antacids, H2-receptor antagonists and proton pump inhibitors • Efavirenz, etravirine and nevirapine
Sofosbuvir/ velpatasvir/ voxilaprevir	Tablets containing 400 mg of sofosbuvir, 100 mg of velpatasvir and 100 mg of voxilaprevir—one tablet once daily		Biliary excretion of voxilaprevir parent drug	• Headache, diarrhoea and nausea • Risk of gastrointestinal side effects greater than with the combination sofosbuvir/velpatasvir	• Substrates of P-gp, BCRP, OATP1B1 and OATP1B3 transporters may increase the exposure of the co-medications • Rosuvastatin • Methotrexate, mitoxantrone, imatinib, irinotecan, lapatinib, sulfasalazine and topotecan • OATP1B inhibitors • OATP1B substrates • Dabigatran • Pgp and/or CYP inducers • Ethinylestradiol-containing contraception
Glecaprevir/ pibrentasvir	Tablets containing 100 mg of glecaprevir—three tablets once daily and 40 mg of pibrentasvir	$t_{1/2}$ approximately 6 and 23 h, respectively	Biliary excretion	• Fatigue and headache	• Co-administration with glecaprevir/pibrentasvir may increase the concentration of comedications that are substrates of P-gp, BCRP and OATP1B1/3 • Strong P-gp and CYP3A inducers • Pgp, BCRP and OATP1B1/3 inhibitors • Ethinylestradiol-containing contraception
Genotype-specific drugs and combination					
Sofosbuvir/ ledipasvir	Tablets containing 400 mg of sofosbuvir and 90 mg of ledipasvir—one tablet once daily	$t_{1/2}$ of ledipasvir 47 h		• Fatigue and headache	• P-gp inducers decrease both sofosbuvir and ledipasvir plasma concentrations • Amiodarone (risk of fatal bradycardia or asystole) • Rosuvastatin (potential inhibition of hepatic OATP by ledipasvir) • Statins • Antacids, H2-receptor antagonists, proton pump inhibitors decrease concentrations of ledipasvir

Paritaprevir/ ombitasvir/ ritonavir	Tablets containing 75 mg of paritaprevir, 12.5 mg of ombitasvir and 50 mg of ritonavir—two tablets once daily	Protein binding is high (about 99%) for all drugs	Ombitasvir and paritaprevir are eliminated in feces	• Fatigue and nausea	• CYP3A4 substrates • Alfuzosin, amiodarone, astemizole, terfenadine, cisapride, ergot derivatives, lovastatin, simvastatin, atorvastatin, orally-administered midazolam, triazolam, quetiapine, quinidine, salmeterol, sildenafil • Enzyme inducers
Dasabuvir	Tablets containing 250 mg of dasabuvir—one tablet twice daily (morning and evening)		Excreted in the bile and eliminated in the feces	• Fatigue and nausea	
Grazoprevir/ elbasvir	Tablets containing 100 mg of grazoprevir and 50 mg of elbasvir—one tablet once daily	Extensively binding to plasma proteins Terminal $t_{1/2}$ approximately 31 and 24 h, respectively	Biliary and faecal with <1% recovered in urine	• Fatigue and headache	• CYP3A and Pgp inducers • Strong CYP3A inhibitors • OATP1B1 inhibitors

with amiodarone is contraindicated because of a serious risk of fatal bradycardia or asystole.

The combination sofosbuvir/ledipasvir can be used with all antiretrovirals. However, in tenofovir-containing regimens, tenofovir concentration can rise and renal function should be carefully monitored, if other therapeutic options are not possible. Even efavirenz-containing regimens require caution as tenofovir levels can increased. This concern has been recently solved with the approval of tenofovir alafenamide (TAF), that considerably reduces the risk of this pharmacokinetic interaction.

Sofosbuvir and Velpatasvir

In vitro, three CYP isoforms (CYP2B6, CYP2C8 and CYP3A4) have been found to be responsible for velpatasvir metabolism, whereas *in vivo* velpatasvir is essentially unmodified. Velpatasvir transport is operated by P-gp and BCRP and, to a limited extent, by organic anion transporting polypeptide (OATP) 1B1.

As for ledipasvir, co-medication of velpatasvir and drugs transported by P-gp and/or BCRP need caution, because of the possible increase of their plasma concentration. Therefore, co-administration with P-gp, BCRP, OATP and CYP substrates having a narrow therapeutic window could potentially have clinical consequences due to increased drug exposure.

In HIV-HCV coinfected patients, sofosbuvir/velpatasvir should not be administered with efavirenz, etravirine and nevirapine due to pharmacokinetic interactions and increased risk of toxicity.

Sofosbuvir, Velpatasvir and Voxilaprevir

Since voxilaprevir AUC and maximum concentration were found to be 112–435%, and 147–680% higher, respectively, in the presence of food, the tablet containing these molecules should be taken during meal [14].

Both velpatasvir and voxilaprevir inhibit P-gp, BCRP, OATP1B1 and OATP1B3. In patients with moderate liver cirrhosis (Child-Pugh B patients) the administration of sofosbuvir/velpatasvir/voxilaprevir is not recommended, and is absolutely contraindicated when liver dysfunction becomes severe (Child-Pugh C patients), due to the significant increase of voxilaprevir AUC in these patients.

Proton pump inhibitors can be given at a dose not exceeding 20 mg omeprazole and, if possible, 4 h after sofosbuvir/velpatasvir/voxilaprevir administration, since velpatasvir solubility decreases as pH increases. In HIV-HCV coinfected patients, the co-administration with efavirenz, etravirine and nevirapine and the protease inhibitor associations atazanavir/ritonavir and lopinavir/ritonavir is not recommended. Efavirenz causes a 50% decrease in velpatasvir exposure, whereas atazanavir causes a fourfold increase in voxilaprevir exposure. Tenofovir-based regimens should be monitored for renal adverse events.

Ritonavir-Boosted Paritaprevir, Ombitasvir and Dasabuvir

Paritaprevir is a HCV protease inhibitor predominantly metabolized by CYP3A4 and primarily excreted into the feces.

Ombitasvir is an nonstructural protein 5A (NS5A) inhibitor that predominantly undergoes hydrolysis and is eliminated with the feces. It can be partially subjected to CYP3A4-mediated metabolism.

Dasabuvir is a non-nucleoside inhibitor of HCV RNA-dependent RNA polymerase, undergoing hepatic CYP2C8- and to a lesser extent CYP3A4-mediated metabolism. Its main metabolite is excreted into the bile and eliminated with the feces. In genotype 1 patients, dasabuvir is given in combination with ritonavir/paritaprevir/ombitasvir. Patients with mild liver cirrhosis (Child-Pugh A) don't require dose adjustment, whereas the combination of ritonavir-boosted paritaprevir and ombitasvir with or without dasabuvir should not be administered in case of decompensated liver cirrhosis (Child-Pugh B and C).

The antiretroviral drug **ritonavir** is a strong inhibitor of CYP3A4 and markedly increases the plasma concentrations of many drugs metabolized by this cytochrome. Because of this characteristic, it is used as a pharmacokinetic enhancer of paritaprevir, but, if co-administered with other CYP3A4 substrates, can lead to serious adverse events. For this reason a wide range of drugs are contraindicated in association with ritonavir (i.e. alfuzosin, amiodarone, astemizole, terfenadine). Since the administration of enzyme inducers (carbamazepine, phenytoin, phenobarbital, rifampicin, St John's wort, enzalutamide) may compromise antiviral efficacy, and enzyme inhibitors (azole antifungals, some macrolide antibiotics) may increase paritaprevir exposure, the co-administration of a ritonavir-boosted regimen with these drugs is not recommended.

Paritaprevir, dasabuvir and ritonavir may inhibit drug transporters. In particular, the drug inhibits OATP1B1/B3, P-gp and BCRP, whereas dasabuvir and ritonavir inhibit P-gp and BCRP, but not OATP. Because of the metabolic profile of these drugs and ritonavir characteristics, drug-drug interactions during these regimens cannot be excluded. Therefore, based on the guidelines of both the European Medicines Agency and the US Food and Drug Administration, a comprehensive program investigating the drug-drug interactions occurring with these drugs has been started. Thus, drug interactions need to be carefully considered and the therapeutic regimen could require dosage adjustment, modifications of the timing of administration or additional monitoring. Additional caution has to be taken in HIV co-infected patients, in which ritonavir should be avoided if they are treated with atazanavir and darunavir. Other drugs used against HIV, such as efavirenz, etravirine, cobicistat and nevirapine are not indicated, whereas rilpivirine should only be used under ECG monitoring, because of the risk of cardiac toxicity.

Grazoprevir and Elbasvir

According to in vitro data, grazoprevir and elbasvir are partially metabolized by CYP3A4, although no metabolites have been detected in plasma [14]. Grazoprevir is transported by P-gp and OATP1B1, while elbasvir is a substrate of P-gp. In patients with moderate or severe hepatic impairment (Child-Pugh B and C) the administration of this combination is not recommended due to pharmacokinetic concerns, whereas renal impairment is not a contraindication and doesn't require any dose adjustment. Drugs metabolized by CYP3A and transported by Pgp need additional monitoring and often dose reduction. Currently, only nucleos(t)ide reverse transcriptase inhibitors can be used as antiretrovirals in combination with grazoprevir and elbasvir (e.g. abacavir, lamivudine, tenofovir).

Glecaprevir and Pibrentasvir

The combination of glecaprevir and pibrentasvir is contraindicated in case of moderate or severe hepatic impairment (Child-Pugh B or C). As with the grazoprevir/elbasvir combination, co-administered drugs whose disposition depends on CYP3A require additional caution or dose reduction. Doses of omeprazole greater than 40 mg may lead to a profound decrease in glecaprevir concentrations, since glecaprevir solubility decreases as pH increases, even though the co-administration has not yet been rigorously studied. Glecaprevir/pibrentasvir is contraindicated with atazanavir-containing regimens in HIV coinfected patients and is not recommended with other HIV protease inhibitors and with inducing non-nucleoside reverse transcriptase inhibitors (efavirenz, etravirine and nevirapine). The other antiretroviral drugs, including cobicistat, can be co-administered in elvitegravir-containing regimens.

In conclusion, because of their efficacy, safety and tolerability, the best options for all both "treatment-naïve" and "treatment-experienced" patients, including those without cirrhosis and those with either compensated (Child-Pugh A) and decompensated (Child-Pugh B and C) cirrhosis, are represented by DAA-based regimens without interferon (IFN) and ribavirin. The therapeutic choice has to be based on the HCV genotype/subtype, the severity of liver disease, and/or prior therapy. In HIV-coinfected patients, treatment or dose adjustments may be required due to drug-drug interactions.

As mentioned before, HCV has six main genotypes (labelled 1–6) with multiple subtypes. The most frequent genotypes worldwide are 1–3. As described in details below, genotyping is fundamental for planning the HCV treatment and personalize HCV therapy. The recommended therapeutic regimens illustrated below are listed in the EASL [14] and American Association for the Study of Liver Diseases (AASLD) and Infectious Diseases Society of America (IDSA) [15] guidelines. AASLD-IDSA also suggest possible alternative regimens (www.hcvguidelines.org).

- **Genotype 1**
  - **Genotype 1a**
    For treatment-naive patients with HCV genotype 1a, characterized by a higher relapse rate than patients with HCV genotype 1b, there are four regimens of similar efficacy, i.e. sofosbuvir/velpatasvir, glecaprevir/pibrentasvir, sofosbuvir/ledipasvir, grazoprevir/elbasvir.
  - **Genotype 1b**
    For treatment-naive patients infected with HCV genotype 1b, five recommended regimens are available: sofosbuvir/velpatasvir, glecaprevir/pibrentasvir, sofosbuvir/ledipasvir, grazoprevir/elbasvir and paritaprevir/ombitasvir/dasabuvir boosted with ritonavir.

    Patients with genotype 1 HCV infections who cannot be subtyped should be treated as genotype 1a patients, since this subtype has a greater risk of relapse when compared with genotype 1b.
- **Genotype 2**
  Sofosbuvir/velpatasvir and glecaprevir/pibrentasvir are the two first line treatment regimens recommended for genotype 2 patients, both treatment-naïve and experienced.
- **Genotype 3**
  The response of genotype 3 to DAAs currently available is less satisfying hat of genotypes 1 and 2. According to AASLD guidelines, the recommended regimens are sofosbuvir/velpatasvir and glecaprevir/pibrentasvir, whereas EASL guidelines also indicate sofosbuvir/velpatasvir/voxilaprevir as a further option.
- **Genotype 4**
  According to the EASL guidelines, patients with HCV genotype 4 have four therapeutic options: glecaprevir/pibrentasvir, grazoprevir/elbasvir and two sofosbuvir-based regimens, namely ledipasvir/sofosbuvir and sofosbuvir/velpatasvir.
- **Genotype 5 or 6**
  Although few data are available for patients infected with HCV genotype 5 or 6, based on emerging data, sofosbuvir/ledipasvir, glecaprevir/pibrentasvir, sofosbuvir/velpatasvir are currently recommended [16].

53.4 Future Perspectives for Hepatitis Treatment

53.4.1 Future Treatment Options for HBV

The main goal of HBV infection treatment is the clearance of HBsAg, with the aim of avoiding the risk of post-treatment virologic relapse and liver disease progression, and decreasing HCC risk. Since HBV DNA is integrated into the host genome, its eradication may not be feasible, but treatment of earlier stages of liver disease would theoretically have a greater impact on reducing the risk of developing HCC. Currently, pre-clinical and early clinical studies are investigating two novel treatment options, i.e. direct antivirals and immunotherapeutic agents. The formers, which have been designed to decrease HBsAg release in serum, include HBV entry inhibitors, drugs silencing or disrupting covalently closed circular DNA (cccDNA), genetic approaches by means of siRNA or anti-sense oligonucleotides targeting viral transcripts, and modulators of nucleocapsid assembly. As immunotherapeutic agents, toll-like receptors 7 (TLR7) agonists and other agents that are able to restore INF responsiveness or affect other antiviral innate pathways are currently under investigation. Moreover, the ability of some new cancer immunotherapies to restore anti-tumor adaptive immunity in chronic HBV patients has been investigated.

In the future, the goal of new antiviral therapies is likely to be represented by a combination therapy, targeting multiple pathways of HBV and restoring immune response against HBV.

As far as the HBV-HDV coinfection is concerned, this is treated with PegIFN-α, nevertheless the success rate is low. Several clinical trials are evaluating new candidates to be used mainly in combination with PegIFN-α and/or NAs. Some of these compounds are HBV/HDV entry inhibitors (Myrcludex-B) [17, 18], nucleic acid polymers that inhibit the release of HBsAg [19] and inhibitors of the prenylation of the large HDV antigen [20]. In order to rescue patients who do not respond to PegIFN-α or to improve the success rate of treatment of naïve patients, the enrolment in these new clinical trials should be considered as a possible choice option.

53.4.2 Future Perspectives for the Treatment of HCV

At present, several studies are investigating new agents for the treatment of HCV, although in recent years several drugs with high successful rate have gained approval. Some issues still remain to be addressed and represent a challenge for future drug development. For example, the successful rates of available agents is very high in most populations that have access to a cure, but not in all patient sub-populations, including cirrhotic genotype 3 patients, individuals with decompensated cirrhosis, and those who fail DAA treatment. Moreover, new techniques for HCV testing and diagnosis, and increasing access to expensive therapies to the whole world population represent future research goals.

Self Study

Questions

1. Which statement is true?
   (a) Ritonavir is approved for treatment of HCV of all genotypes.
   (b) Only sofosbuvir-based regimens are indicated for genotype 2 HCV.
   (c) The antiretroviral drug **ritonavir** is a strong inhibitor of CYP3A4 and is used in association with DAAs as a pharmacokinetic enhancer of paritaprevir.
   (d) Sofosbuvir is transported by P-gp, and metabolized by cytochrome P450 3A4.
2. Which statement is true?
   (a) Interferon is usually administered for the entire life of the patient.
   (b) Nucleos(t)ide analogues (NAs) have all high barrier to HBV resistance.
   (c) Mother-to-child transmission is never occurring for HBV.
   (d) Entecavir and tenofovir are classified as drugs with high barrier to HBV resistance.

Answers

1. Which statement is true?
   (a) Ritonavir is part of a combination therapy indicated for genotype 1b HCV therapy.
   (b) Sofosbuvir/velpatasvir and glecaprevir/pibrentasvir are the two first line treatment regimens recommended for genotype 2 patients.
   (c) **The antiretroviral drug ritonavir is a strong inhibitor of CYP3A4 and markedly increases the plasma concentrations of many drugs metabolized by this cytochrome. Because of this characteristic, it is used as a pharmacokinetic enhancer.**
   (d) Sofosbuvir is transported by P-gp, whereas cytochrome P450 is not involved in its metabolism.
2. Which statement is true?
   (a) Interferon therapy has generally a limited duration.
   (b) Among the five NAs approved for chronic HBV treatment (lamivudine, adefovir, entecavir, telbivudine and tenofovir), three (lamivudine, adefovir, telbivudine) have low barrier and two (entecavir, tenofovir) high barrier to HBV resistance.
   (c) The perinatal or mother-to-child transmission (MTCT) of HBV is one of the major risk factors of chronic HBV infection.

(d) **Differently from the other NAs, entecavir and tenofovir have a high barrier to HBV resistance.**

References

1. Harris RJ, Thomas B, Griffiths J, Costella A, Chapman R, Ramsay M, et al. Increased uptake and new therapies are needed to avert rising hepatitis C-related end stage liver disease in England: modelling the predicted impact of treatment under different scenarios. J Hepatol [Internet]. 2014 [cited 2018 Sep 27];61:530–7. Available from: http://linkinghub.elsevier.com/retrieve/pii/S0168827814003183.
2. WHO. Global hepatitis report, 2017. Geneva: World Health Organization; 2017.
3. Tu T, Bühler S, Bartenschlager R. Chronic viral hepatitis and its association with liver cancer. Biol Chem [Internet]. 2017 [cited 2018 Sep 27];398:817–37. Available from: http://www.degruyter.com/view/j/bchm.2017.398.issue-8/hsz-2017-0118/hsz-2017-0118.xml.
4. Schweitzer A, Horn J, Mikolajczyk RT, Krause G, Ott JJ. Estimations of worldwide prevalence of chronic hepatitis B virus infection: a systematic review of data published between 1965 and 2013. Lancet (London, England) [Internet]. 2015 [cited 2018 Sep 27];386:1546–55. Available from: https://linkinghub.elsevier.com/retrieve/pii/S014067361561412X.
5. Lok ASF, McMahon BJ, Brown RS, Wong JB, Ahmed AT, Farah W, et al. Antiviral therapy for chronic hepatitis B viral infection in adults: a systematic review and meta-analysis. Hepatology [Internet]. 2016 [cited 2018 Sep 27];63:284–306. Available from: http://www.ncbi.nlm.nih.gov/pubmed/26566246.
6. Terrault NA, Bzowej NH, Chang K-M, Hwang JP, Jonas MM, Murad MH, et al. AASLD guidelines for treatment of chronic hepatitis B. Hepatology [Internet]. 2016 [cited 2018 Sep 27];63:261–83. Available from: http://www.ncbi.nlm.nih.gov/pubmed/26566064.
7. Marcellin P, Ahn SH, Chuang W-L, Hui AJ, Tabak F, Mehta R, et al. Predictors of response to tenofovir disoproxil fumarate plus peginterferon alfa-2a combination therapy for chronic hepatitis B. Aliment Pharmacol Ther [Internet]. 2016 [cited 2018 Sep 27];44:957–66. Available from: http://www.ncbi.nlm.nih.gov/pubmed/27629859.
8. Marcellin P, Ahn SH, Ma X, Caruntu FA, Tak WY, Elkashab M, et al. Combination of tenofovir disoproxil fumarate and peginterferon α-2a increases loss of hepatitis B surface antigen in patients with chronic hepatitis B. Gastroenterology [Internet]. 2016 [cited 2018 Sep 27];150:134–44.e10. Available from: http://www.ncbi.nlm.nih.gov/pubmed/26453773.
9. Mazzaro C, Dal Maso L, Urraro T, Mauro E, Castelnovo L, Casarin P, et al. Hepatitis B virus related cryoglobulinemic vasculitis: a multicentre open label study from the Gruppo Italiano di Studio delle Crioglobulinemie - GISC. Dig Liver Dis [Internet]. 2016 [cited 2018 Sep 27];48:780–4. Available from: https://linkinghub.elsevier.com/retrieve/pii/S1590865815303480.
10. Brown RS, McMahon BJ, Lok ASF, Wong JB, Ahmed AT, Mouchli MA, et al. Antiviral therapy in chronic hepatitis B viral infection during pregnancy: a systematic review and meta-analysis. Hepatology [Internet]. 2016 [cited 2018 Sep 27];63:319–33. Available from: http://www.ncbi.nlm.nih.gov/pubmed/26565396.
11. Jonas MM, Lok ASF, McMahon BJ, Brown RS, Wong JB, Ahmed AT, et al. Antiviral therapy in management of chronic hepatitis B viral infection in children: a systematic review and meta-analysis. Hepatology [Internet]. 2016 [cited 2018 Sep 27];63:307–18. Available from: http://www.ncbi.nlm.nih.gov/pubmed/26566163.
12. Polaris Observatory HCV Collaborators, Zeuzem S, Manns M, Altraif I, Duberg A-S, Muljono DH, et al. Global prevalence and genotype distribution of hepatitis C virus infection in 2015: a modelling study. Lancet Gastroenterol Hepatol [Internet]. 2017 [cited 2018 Sep 27];2:161–76. Available from: https://linkinghub.elsevier.com/retrieve/pii/S2468125316301819.
13. European Union HCV Collaborators, Robbins S, Zeuzem S, Negro F, Buti M, Duberg A-S, et al. Hepatitis C virus prevalence and level of intervention required to achieve the WHO targets for elimination in the European Union by 2030: a modelling study. Lancet Gastroenterol Hepatol [Internet]. 2017 [cited 2018 Sep 27];2:325–36. Available from: https://linkinghub.elsevier.com/retrieve/pii/S2468125317300456.
14. Pawlotsky J-M, Negro F, Aghemo A, Berenguer M, Dalgard O, Dusheiko G, et al. EASL recommendations on treatment of hepatitis C 2018. J Hepatol [Internet]. 2018 [cited 2018 Sep 27];69:461–511. Available from: https://www.sciencedirect.com/science/article/pii/S0168827818319688?via%3Dihub.
15. Chung RT, Ghany MG, Kim AY, Marks KM, Naggie S, Vargas HE, et al. Hepatitis C guidance 2018 update: AASLD-IDSA recommendations for testing, managing, and treating hepatitis C virus infection. Clin Infect Dis [Internet]. 2018 [cited 2018 Sep 28]. Available from: https://academic.oup.com/cid/advance-article/doi/10.1093/cid/ciy585/5095352.
16. AASLD/IDSA HCV Guidance Panel. Hepatitis C guidance: AASLD-IDSA recommendations for testing, managing, and treating adults infected with hepatitis C virus. Hepatology [Internet]. 2015 [cited 2018 Sep 27];62:932–54. Available from: http://www.ncbi.nlm.nih.gov/pubmed/26111063.
17. Bogomolov P, Alexandrov A, Voronkova N, Macievich M, Kokina K, Petrachenkova M, et al. Treatment of chronic hepatitis D with the entry inhibitor myrcludex B: first results of a phase Ib/IIa study. J Hepatol [Internet]. 2016 [cited 2018 Sep 27];65:490–8. Available from: https://linkinghub.elsevier.com/retrieve/pii/S0168827816301489.
18. Blank A, Markert C, Hohmann N, Carls A, Mikus G, Lehr T, et al. First-in-human application of the novel hepatitis B and hepatitis D virus entry inhibitor myrcludex B. J Hepatol [Internet]. 2016 [cited 2018 Sep 27];65:483–9. Available from: https://linkinghub.elsevier.com/retrieve/pii/S0168827816301453.
19. Al-Mahtab M, Bazinet M, Vaillant A. Safety and efficacy of nucleic acid polymers in monotherapy and combined with immunotherapy in treatment-naive Bangladeshi patients with HBeAg+ chronic hepatitis B infection. PLoS One [Internet]. 2016 [cited 2018 Sep 27];11:e0156667. Available from: http://dx.plos.org/10.1371/journal.pone.0156667.
20. Durantel D, Zoulim F. New antiviral targets for innovative treatment concepts for hepatitis B virus and hepatitis delta virus. J Hepatol [Internet]. 2016 [cited 2018 Sep 27];64:S117–31. Available from: https://linkinghub.elsevier.com/retrieve/pii/S0168827816001239.

Portal Vein Embolization (PVE) and Partial TIPE ALPPS: Beyond the Limitations of PVE

54

Yutaka Suzuki and Yoshihiro Sakamoto

Key Concepts

- Portal vein embolization (PVE) is an important and indispensable procedure performed to ensure the safety of major hepatectomy.
- About 20% of patients who undergo PVE cannot undergo subsequent hepatectomy, often because of tumor progression during the waiting period, which lasts 3–8 weeks.
- Two-stage hepatectomy (TSH) and associating liver partition and portal vein ligation for staged hepatectomy (ALPPS) have been developed and applied for patients that the planned hepatectomy cannot be performed by PVE. But, original ALPPS is associated with high morbidity and mortality rates.
- Partial TIPE ALPPS can be safely applied in patients to overcome the limitations of conventional PVE.

54.1 Introduction

Major hepatectomy is often necessary for the treatment of advanced biliary cancer, hepatocellular carcinoma (HCC), or colorectal liver metastasis. However, extensive hepatectomy in patients for whom the future liver remnant (FLR) volume will be insufficient and in patients with impaired hepatic functional reserve can result in postoperative liver failure and subsequent death. To prevent such liver failure, portal vein embolization (PVE) aimed at increasing the FLR volume is often performed before major hepatectomy. In this chapter, the history, methods, efficacy, and limitations of PVE performed before major hepatectomy are summarized, and a potential breakthrough in the limitations of PVE is described.

54.2 History

In 1920, Rous et al. showed, in a rabbit model, that ligation of portal branches to a part of the liver leads to atrophy in the region deprived of portal blood but to hypertrophy of the hepatic tissue that receives portal blood in excess [1]. In 1975, Honjo et al., applying portal branch ligation as a new preoperative procedure, documented tumor shrinkage after the ligation in 20 patients with HCC [2].

In 1982, Makuuchi et al. performed PVE 20 days before hepatectomy in a patient with gallbladder cancer and then in 1990 reported the results of PVE performed before major hepatectomy in 14 patients with biliary cancer [3]. In a consecutive series of 84 patients reported by Imamura et al., also in 1990, PVE performed before hepatectomy resulted in a median 30% (0–171%) increase in FLR volume over the original FLR volume, with diabetes mellitus, a high total bilirubin level at the time of PVE, and male sex shown to be factors that limited the organ hypertrophy [4]. In 1996, Nagino et al. described an ipsilateral approach to PVE, with the PVE catheter placed in the right anterior portal branch in patients for whom right portal branch resection was anticipated [5]. Further, Nagino et al. reported a series of left and right trisectional PVEs achieved by means of this ipsilateral approach [6]. Curative major hepatectomy preceded by PVE, in comparison to limited biliary resection without PVE, improve long-term outcomes of patients with cholangiocarcinoma. Sequential arterial embolization and PVE have been performed to decrease tumor viability in patients with HCC, and PVE has been used to aid aggressive tumor resection in patients with bilateral colorectal metastasis [7]. Thus, preoperative

Y. Suzuki · Y. Sakamoto (✉)
Hepato-Biliary-Pancreatic Surgery Division, Kyorin University Hospital, Tokyo, Japan
e-mail: ysuzuki@ks.kyorin-u.ac.jp; yosakamo@ks.kyorin-u.ac.jp

F. Radu-Ionita et al. (eds.), *Liver Diseases*, https://doi.org/10.1007/978-3-030-24432-3_54

PVE has become an indispensable ancillary procedure for resection of biliary cancer, HCC, and metastatic liver tumor.

54.3 Mechanism of PVE-Induced Hypertrophy

The mechanism underlying hepatic hypertrophy after PVE has not been fully clarified, but the resulting increase in portal venous pressure or portal venous flow is thought to induce accelerated hepatocyte turnover in the FLR. Portal vein flow increases in the non-embolized lobe, and shear stress occurs in the sinusoidal endothelium [8]. Nitric oxide, hepatocyte growth factor, and interleukin-6 are then released from sinusoidal endothelium and hepatocytes, promoting liver hypertrophy [9, 10]. Ozawa et al. reported that the liver hypertrophy occurs as a result of enhanced mitochondrial oxidative phosphorylation elicited by the increase in portal vein flow [11, 12]. To the contrary, embolized hepatocytes undergo apoptotic change. Imamura et al. reported that, numerous binuclear hepatocytes and mitotic figures were observed in the nonembolized lobe. In the embolized lobe, hepatocyte atrophy and large sinusoidal areas were evident, especially in the pericentral field. However, there was no inflammatory cell infiltration or necrotic reaction [4].

54.4 Approaches to the Portal Vein for PVE

There are two main PVE techniques: transileocolic portal vein embolization (TIPE) and percutaneous transhepatic portal vein embolization (PTPE). These two techniques represent two different approaches to the portal vein. TIPE is performed via mini-laparotomy under general anesthesia. The catheter is advanced through the ileocolic vein, making antegrade embolization possible. The mini-laparotomy also makes possible the gathering of intraperitoneal information, including whether peritoneal seeding has occurred. PTPE is performed under local anesthesia and ultrasound guidance. In the early days of PVE, TIPE was performed more frequently than PTPE. Since the early 2000s, PTPE has been the preferred method because of improvements in the devices used and improvement of the interventional techniques.

54.4.1 TIPE Technique

When TIPE is performed, the patient is placed under general anesthesia, and a small pararectal incision is made. The abdominal cavity is explored for the presence of peritoneal seeding and/or ascites. If found, samples are submitted for pathological examination.

The end of the ileum-end is pulled out through the small pararectal incision, and the mesenteric serosa was incised to expose the ileocolic vein. A guidewire is inserted into the vein, and a sheath is inserted over the guidewire.

The next steps are best performed by an interventional radiologist. Portography is performed, especially for visualization of the right and left portal branches. The portal venous pressure is measured, and if it is above 30 cm H_2O, the planned PVE is abandoned.

To block blood supply to the right lobe, the right posterior portal branch should be embolized first. P6 and P7 are embolized separately. The anterior section is embolized next. This is because the catheter advances easily into the anterior section, and thus if this section is embolized first, there is a risk that the catheter will dislodge the newly created thrombus. After embolization, portal venous pressure is again measured.

54.4.2 PTPE Technique (Fig. 54.1)

When PTPE is performed, the patient is given a local anesthetic, and the portal branch is punctured under ultrasound guidance. There are two approaches to PTPE: a contralateral approach by which the portal branch in the FLR is punctured and an ipsilateral approach by which the portal branch in the segment of the liver to be resected is punctured. In the case, for example, of right PVE performed via contralateral approach, the umbilical portion of the left branch of the portal vein is punctured, and the right branch of the portal vein is embolized. In the ipsilateral approach, a right portal branch, P5, P6, P7, or P8, is punctured for embolization. The contralateral approach is technically easier than the ipsilateral approach in terms of catheter operation and embolization. However, the contralateral approach poses risks. There is the possibility of a major complication, such as arterial injury, bile duct bleeding, or portal vein thrombosis in the FLR. Thus, the ipsilateral approach should be the first-choice strategy. However, if the tumor is located in the puncture route, the ipsilateral approach should not be considered.

The puncture route should be determined carefully under ultrasound guidance. P5 or P8 is punctured with an 18G needle. After the tip of the needle is positioned in the portal vein, a guidewire is inserted into the portal vein and superior mesenteric vein, and a sheath is inserted over the guidewire. A balloon catheter is advanced into the main portal vein, portography is performed, and portal venous pressure is measured. The balloon catheter is inserted into the posterior branch of the portal vein. Embolization is performed by injection of gelatin sponge particles and coils or absolute ethanol. Thereafter, the anterior branch of the portal vein is embolized. The embolic materials should be injected carefully to avoid their migration into the main portal vein or contralateral portal vein, which can put at risk the opportunity for major hepatectomy.

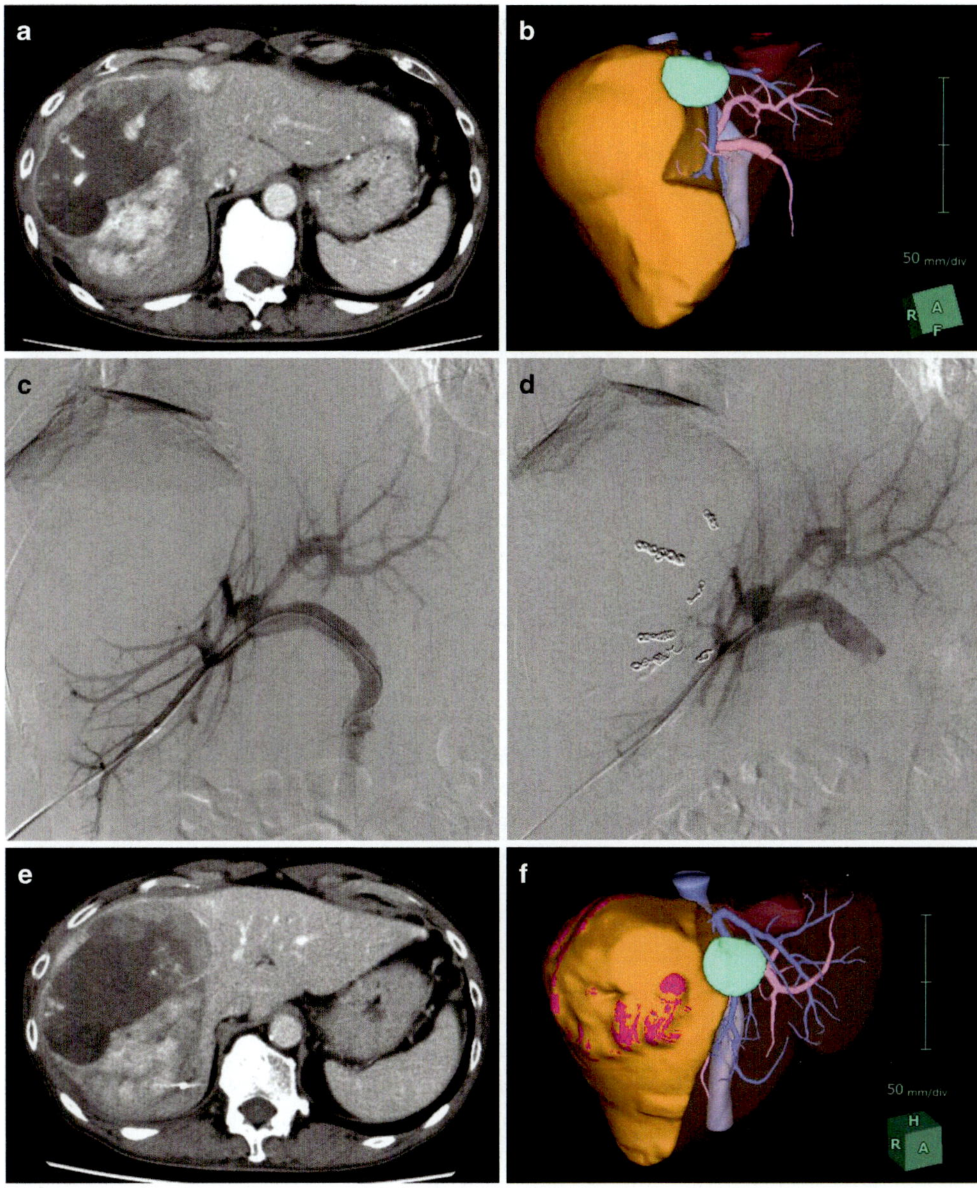

Fig. 54.1 PTPE in a case of hepatocellular carcinoma. (**a**) Portal phase contrast enhanced computed tomography image revealed a 13-cm inhomogeneously enhanced tumor in the right liver lobe. (**b**) Further study revealed intrahepatic metastases of approximately 1 cm in segments 8 and 3. Right hepatectomy and limited hepatectomies (S8 and S3) were planned, but the future remnant liver volume would have been 43%. Therefore, PTPE was performed. P6 was punctured and a 5 Fr sheath was inserted. (**c**) The tumors were not contrasted upon portography, and the branches of right portal vein were compressed. (**d**) The branches of the right portal vein (P5, P6, P7, and P8) were embolized separately with the use of gelatin sponge particles and coils. (**e**, **f**) Four weeks after embolization, the remnant liver volume had increased to 54%. Extended right hepatectomy and resection of segment 2 were then performed

54.5 Embolic Materials

Various embolic materials are used for PVE: gelatin sponge particles [3], gelatin powder combined with thrombin [13], cyanoacrylate combined with ethiodized oil [14], fibrin glue combined with ethiodized oil [15], absolute ethanol [16], and polyvinyl alcohol and coils [17].

Complete embolization is achieved with absolute ethanol and cyanoacrylate through damage done to the sinusoidal cells. However, severe tissue injury and liver dysfunction can also result [18]. Furthermore, the injection of absolute alcohol results in severe pain. When gelatin sponge particles are used for embolization, the sponge is cut to a diameter of 1–2 mm. When gelatin sponge is used alone, recanalization can occur. Recanalization after PVE is a severe problem [19], so coil embolization is added. It is important to push the coil into the distal end of the portal branch. A coil placed in the proximal end of the portal branch is unstable and migrates easily. The coil is made of platinum, so magnetic resonance imaging is possible after coil embolization.

54.6 Potential Complications of PVE

54.6.1 Bleeding

Bleeding can result from accidental puncture of the hepatic artery, hepatic vein, or bile duct. Accidental puncture of the hepatic artery in particular can lead to intra-abdominal bleeding. This is because of the high vascular pressure. Bleeding from the hepatic vein or bile duct is always temporary because of the low vascular pressure.

54.6.2 Portal Thrombosis and Coil Migration

Portal thrombosis and/or coil migration can occur after PVE. Portal thrombosis is the result of excessive or erroneous embolization, and coil migration is usually the result of placement of an inappropriately sized coil.

54.6.3 Bile Leakage

There is an increased risk of bile leakage through the portal vein puncture line in patients with obstructive jaundice. This risk is due to the high pressure and dilatation of the biliary tree. When abdominal pain and/or fever is present after PTPE, imaging should be performed to check for accumulation of intraabdominal fluid. Paracentesis should be considered for patients in whom such ascites develops.

54.7 Outcomes of PVE

Performance of PVE before major hepatectomy for hilar cholangiocarcinoma was first reported in 1990 [3]. Nagino et al. reported the usefulness of PVE in patients undergoing extended hepatectomy for cholangiocarcinoma or gallbladder cancer [19]. Both the volume of the nonembolized lobe and the volumetric ratio of the nonembolized lobe to the whole liver were significantly greater after PVE than before PVE. However, 19.6% of their reported patients did not undergo subsequent hepatectomy because of tumor progression during the waiting period or because peritoneal dissemination, liver metastasis, and/or locally advanced cancer was found upon laparotomy. Overall, resectability and long-term survival were better among patients with cholangiocarcinoma than among patients with gallbladder cancer.

Yamashita et al. reported surgical outcomes after PVE performed in patients with HCC, biliary tract cancer, and colorectal liver metastasis [20]. In each group, the resulting increase in FLR volume was 10%. Major complications occurred in 4.7% of patients with HCC, 11% with biliary tract cancer, and 3.4% with colorectal liver metastasis and did not differ significantly. There was also no significant difference between these groups in hepatic insufficiency (0%, 2.3%, and 3.4%, respectively), 90-day liver-related mortality (0%, 0%, and 0%, respectively), or 90-day overall mortality (0%, 0.8%, and 1.7%, respectively). The planned hepatectomy was not carried out, however, in 5.7% of the HCC patients, 21.5% of the biliary cancer patients, and 22.1% of the patients with colorectal liver metastasis. This was because of tumor progression or poor general status.

Abdalla et al. compared long-term outcomes between patients who did and did not undergo PVE before surgical treatment of their various hepatobiliary malignancies [21]. No significant survival difference was found between the two groups of patients. Similar results were obtained in patients with colorectal liver metastasis.

54.8 Beyond the Limitations of PVE: Associating Liver Partition and Portal Vein Embolization for Staged Hepatectomy

As noted above, the planned hepatectomy cannot be performed in about 20% of patients who have undergone PVE. This is often because of tumor progression during the waiting period. Associating liver partition and portal vein embolization for staged hepatectomy (ALPPS) might reach beyond the limitations of PVE.

ALPPS has been performed enthusiastically mainly in Europe and South America to minimize the waiting period associated with PVE [19]. Originally applied in cases of bilobar colorectal liver metastasis, ALPPS is performed as follows: Tumors in the lateral segment are resected locally. The right branch of the portal vein is then ligated and divided, and the liver parenchyma is transected on the right side of the umbilical portion in segment 4, and the middle hepatic vein is ligated and divided. The right hepatic artery (RHA) and right hepatic vein (RHV) are preserved. These procedures comprise the first-stage surgery, and 7–10 days is allowed to pass between the first and second stages. The second-stage surgery comprises right hemihepatectomy, which is performed by ligation and division of the remnant RHA, right hepatic duct, and RHV. The advantages of ALPPS over conventional PVE are accelerated hypertrophy of the FLR; the volume gain occurs within 7–10 days. The disadvantages of ALPPS are high morbidity and mortality rates [21–24].

In an Italian multicenter study, the reported median increase in FLR volume was 63% of the original volume (60.5% in cases of colorectal liver metastasis, 76.5% in cases of biliary cancer, and 56.5% in cases of HCC) over a median period of 7 days [23]. However, mortality within 90 days was 20%, with 70% of the deaths due to post-hepatectomy liver failure and 80% to septic shock. In a recent randomized controlled study in which ALPPS was compared with conventional two-stage hepatectomy (TSH), the liver volume increase after the first-stage surgery and the rate at which the second-stage surgery was completed were significantly greater after ALPPS than after TSH (68% vs. 36%, respectively, and 92% vs. 57%, respectively) [24]. No significant between-group difference was found in morbidity or 90-day mortality (43% vs. 43%, respectively, and 8.3% vs. 6.1%, respectively). A meta-analysis comparing ALPPS and TSH has been reported [25]. However, 6–8% surgical mortality after hepatectomy is high and not acceptable in Japan, where the nationally reported mortality is 2.7% [26]

To overcome the high morbidity rates associated with ALPPS, several authors have reported modified ALPPS procedures. Robles et al. described use of a tourniquet instead of partitioning the liver [27] and named their procedure "associating liver tourniquet and portal ligation for staged hepatectomy" (ALTPS). In lieu of partitioning the liver, a groove 1 cm deep is made along the partition line, and a tourniquet is tied tightly enough to occlude all vessels that connect the two lobes. Among their 22 patients, the median increase in liver volume 7 days after this first-stage surgery was 61%. There was no tumor progression after this first-stage surgery, but mortality after the second-stage surgery was 9%.

Gall et al. reported use of radiofrequency ablation along the Rex-Cantlie line in lieu of partitioning the liver, and they named this first-stage surgery radiofrequency-assisted liver partition with portal vein ligation (RALPP) [28]. They performed RALPP in five patients with colorectal liver metastasis and compared the outcomes against those of patients who underwent PVE. The median increase in liver volume was significantly greater in the RALPP group than in the PVE group (62.3% vs. 24.6%, respectively). The interval between the first- and second-stage surgeries was significantly shorter in RALPP group than the PVE group (22 days vs. 55 days, respectively). The morbidity rate was 20%, but there was no mortality at 90 days.

Sakamoto et al. reported a modification termed partial TIPE ALPPS [29, 30]. Partial partition of the liver parenchyma along the Rex-Cantlie line is performed instead of complete transection of segment 4, and instead of portal vein ligation, the right branch of the portal vein is embolized by transileocolic approach. The key features of this procedure are the no-touch policy regarding the hepatoduodenal ligament designed to avoid adhesion formation that would affect the second-stage surgery, partial partition of the liver with preservation of the middle hepatic vein and gallbladder, and guidance based on digital subtraction images. Volume gain of the FLR was 65.9% on day 7 and 70.5% on day 14. The interval between the first- and the second-stage surgeries was 17 days. Partial TIPE ALPPS was shown to increase safety, especially that associated with the first-stage surgery. Partial TIPE ALPPS can be safely applied even in patients with perihilar cancer, which is generally considered a contraindication for standard ALPPS [30].

Results to date suggest that partial TIPE ALPPS will provide opportunities for major hepatectomy in patients for whom the problem of an insufficient FLR volume cannot be resolved by means of conventional PVE or TSH.

Self Study

Question

Which of the statements below is true?

(a) Half of patients who undergo PVE cannot receive subsequent hepatectomy due to tumor progression, severe liver dysfunction, and/or insufficient increase in liver volume.
(b) In TIPE, management of the catheter is easier than in PTPE, but it is necessary to perform laparotomy with general anesthesia.
(c) Severe pain occurs during injection of the absolute ethanol used for embolization.
(d) Mortality after application of the original ALPPS procedure is less than 5%, and the procedure is very safe.

Answers

(a) False. Several authors reported that 20% of patients who undergo PVE cannot undergo subsequent hepatectomy.
(b) True. In TIPE, operation of the catheter is easy, but it is necessary to perform laparotomy with general anesthesia.
(c) True. Severe pain occurs after injection due to tissue injury, and liver dysfunction develops after embolization. In most cases, the pain and liver dysfunction resolve within a short time.
(d) False. The surgical mortality rate after application of the original ALPPS procedure is reported to be 5–9% in patients with colorectal liver metastasis.

References

1. Rous P, Larimore LD. Relation of the portal blood to liver maintenance: a demonstration of liver atrophy conditional on compensation. J Exp Med. 1920;31(5):609–32.
2. Honjo I, Suzuki T, Ozawa K, Takasan H, Kitamura O. Ligation of a branch of the portal vein for carcinoma of the liver. Am J Surg. 1975;130(3):296–302.
3. Makuuchi M, Thai BL, Takayasu K, Takayama T, Kosuge T, Gunven P, et al. Preoperative portal embolization to increase safety of major hepatectomy for hilar bile duct carcinoma: a preliminary report. Surgery. 1990;107(5):521–7.
4. Imamura H, Shimada R, Kubota M, Matsuyama Y, Nakayama A, Miyagawa S, et al. Preoperative portal vein embolization: an adult of 84 patients. Hepatology. 1999;29(4):1099–105.
5. Nagino M, Nimura Y, Kamiya J, Kondo S, Kanai M. Selective percutaneous transhepatic embolization of the portal vein in preparation for extensive liver resection: the ipsilateral approach. Radiology. 1996;200(2):559–63.
6. Nagino M, Nimura Y, Kamiya J, Kondo S, Uesaka K, Kin Y, et al. Right or left trisegment portal vein embolization before

hepatic trisegmentectomy for hilar bile duct carcinoma. Surgery. 1995;117(6):677–81.
7. Aoki T, Imamura H, Hasegawa K, Matsukura A, Sano K, Sugawara Y, et al. Sequential preoperative arterial and portal venous embolizations in patients with hepatocellular carcinoma. Arch Surg. 2004;139(7):766–74.
8. Sato Y, Koyama S, Tsukada K, Hatakeyama K. Acute portal hypertension reflecting shear stress as a trigger of liver regeneration following partial hepatectomy. Surg Today. 1997;27(6):518–26.
9. Schoen JM, Wang HH, Minuk GY, Lautt WW. Shear stress-induced nitric oxide release triggers the liver regeneration cascade. Nitric Oxide. 2001;5(5):453–64.
10. Maruhashi S, Sakon M, Nagano H, Gotoh K, Hashimoto K, Kubota M, et al. Effect of portal hemodynamics on liver regeneration studied in a novel portohepatic shunt rat model. Surgery. 2004;136(5):1028–37.
11. Ozawa K, Takasan H, Kitamura O, Mizukami T, Kamano T. Effect of ligation of portal vein on liver mitochondrial metabolism. J Biochem. 1971;70(5):755–64.
12. Ozawa K, Yamada T, Honjo I. Role of insulin as a portal factor in mitochondrial metabolism. Ann Surg. 1974;180(5):716–9.
13. de Baere T, Roche A, Vavasseur D, Therasse E, Indushekar S, Elias D, et al. Portal vein embolization: utility for including left hepatic lobe hypertrophy before surgery. Radiology. 1993;288(1):73–7.
14. Nagino M, Nimura Y, Hayakawa N. Percutaneous transhepatic portal embolization using newly devised catheters: preliminary report. World J Surg. 1993;17(4):520–4.
15. Shimamura T, Nakajima Y, Une Y, Namieno T, Ogasawara K, Yamashita T, et al. Efficacy and safety of preoperative percutaneous transhepatic portal embolization with absolute ethanol; a clinical study. Surgery. 1997;121(2):135–41.
16. Madoff DC, Hicks ME, Abdalla EK, Morris JS, Vauthey JN. Portal vein embolization with polyvinyl alcohol particles and coils in preparation for major liver resection for hepatobiliary malignancy; safety and effectiveness; study in 26 patients. Radiology. 2003;227(1):251–60.
17. de Baere T, Roche A, Elias D, Lasser P, Lagrange C, Bousson V. Preoperative portal vein embolization for extension of hepatectomy indications. Hepatology. 1996;24(6):1386–91.
18. Yokoyama Y, Nagino M, Nishio H, Ebata T, Igami T, Nimura Y. Recent advances in the treatment of hilar cholangiocarcinoma: portal vein embolization. J Hepatobiliary Pancreat Surg. 2007;14(5):447–54.
19. Nagino M, Kamiya J, Nishio H, Ebata T, Nimura Y. Two hundred forty consecutive portal vein embolizations before extended hepatectomy for biliary cancer. Surgical outcome and long-term follow-up. Ann Surg. 2006;243(3):364–72.
20. Yamashita S, Sakamoto Y, Yamamoto S, Takemura N, Omichi K, Shinkawa H, et al. Efficacy of preoperative portal vein embolization among patients with hepatocellular carcinoma, biliary tract cancer, and colorectal liver metastasis: a comparative study based on single-center experience of 319 cases. Ann Surg Oncol. 2017;24(6):1557–67.
21. Abdalla EK, Barnett CC, Doherty D, Curley SA, Vauthey JN. Extended hepatectomy in patients with hepatobiliary malignancies with and without preoperative portal vein embolization. Arch Surg. 2002;137(6):675–81.
22. Schnizbauer AA, Lang SA, Goessmann H, Nadalin S, Baumgart J, Farkas SA, et al. Right portal vein ligation combined with in situ splitting induces rapid left lateral liver lobe hypertrophy enabling 2-staged extended right hepatic resection in small-for-size setting. Ann Surg. 2012;255(3):405–14.
23. Serenari M, Zanello M, Schadde E, Toschi E, Ratti F, Gringeri E, et al. Importance of primary indication and liver function between stages: results of a multicenter Italian audit of ALPPS 2012–2014. HPB. 2016;18(5):419–27.
24. Sandstrom P, Rosok BI, Sparrelid E, Larsen PN, Larsson AL, Lindell G, et al. ALPPS improves resectability compared with conventional two-stage hepatectomy in patients with advanced colorectal liver metastasis. Results from a Scandinavian multicenter randomized control trial (LIGRO trial). Ann Surg. 2018;267(5):833–40.
25. Zhou Z, Mingxing X, Lin N, Pan C, Zhou B, Zhong Y, et al. Associating liver partition and portal vein ligation for staged hepatectomy versus conventional two-stage hepatectomy: a systemic review and meta-analysis. World J Surg Oncol. 2017;15(1):227. https://doi.org/10.1186/s12957-017-1295-0.
26. Othubo T, Kobayashi S, Sano K, Misawa T, Ota T, Katagiri S, et al. Safety-related outcomes of the Japanese Society of Hepato-Biliary-Pancreatic Surgery board certification system for expert surgeons. J Hepatobiliary Pancreat Sci. 2017;24(5):252–61.
27. Robles R, Parrilla P, Lopez-Conesa A, Brusadin R, de la Pena J, Fuster M, et al. Tourniquet modification of the associating liver partition and portal ligation for staged hepatectomy procedure. Br J Surg. 2014;101(9):1129–34.
28. Gall TM, Sodergren MH, Frampton AE, Spalding DR, Habib NA, Pai M. Radio-frequency-assisted liver partition with portal vein ligation (RALPP) for liver regeneration. Ann Surg. 2014;261(2):e45–6.
29. Sakamoto Y, Inagaki F, Omichi K, Ohkura N, Hasegawa K, Kokudo N. Associating liver partial partition and transileocecal portal vein embolization for staged hepatectomy. Ann Surg. 2016;264(6):e21–2.
30. Sakamoto Y, Matsumura M, Yamashita S, Ohkura N, Hasegawa K, Kokudo N. Partial TIPE ALPPS for perihilar cancer. Ann Surg. 2018;267(2):e18–20.

Endoscopic and Pharmacological Treatment of Esophageal Varices

55

Antonio Facciorusso, Rosario Vincenzo Buccino,
and Nicola Muscatiello

Key Concepts

- Bleeding from gastroesophageal varices (GEV) represents a potentially lethal complication of liver cirrhosis. Gastroscopy is the milestone as a screening test for varices; however, non-invasive elastography techniques offer valuable alternatives.
- Non-selective beta-blockers (NSBBs) and terlipressin represent the most commonly used pharmacological agents for prevention and management of acute bleeding, respectively.
- Novel evidence suggest beneficial effects with the use of other molecules such as carvedilol or simvastatin.
- Endoscopic band ligation is the most effective endoscopic treatment in the setting of either acute bleeding and primary/secondary prevention and it has nearly completely replaced sclerotherapy in the clinical practice.

55.1 Introduction

Bleeding from gastroesophageal varices (GEVs) represents a dreadful complication of liver cirrhosis, associated with a mortality that, in spite of recent progress, is still in the order of 10–20% at 6 weeks [1]. At diagnosis, up to 50% patients with compensated cirrhosis and even more with impaired liver function have developed GEV [2]. Among patients without varices at diagnosis, annual incidence of GEV development is about 5–9% [3, 4]; similar is the rate of progression from small to large varices.

Several scores based on predictors of the risk of first variceal bleeding have been proposed in the past, among them the North Italian Endoscopic Club (NIEC) score is the most validated and widely accepted [5, 6]. This score, developed in the late 1980s, is based on three main endoscopic/clinical features, namely impairment of liver function (classified according to Child-Pugh score), size of varices and presence of red colour signs over the varices (red wales, red spots, diffuse redness) [5].

High mortality rates observed in patients with variceal bleeding are not only due to hemorrhage but also to infections, acute kidney injury (AKI) and liver failure [7].

Aim of this chapter is to provide an overview on recent improvements and latest developments concerning the pharmacological and endoscopic treatment of esophageal varices, particularly based on the most robust evidence-based findings.

55.2 Pathophysiology and Endoscopic Characteristics of Esophageal Varices

Portal hypertension is initiated by an increase in outflow resistance from the portal-venous bed, and it is further worsened by splanchnic arterial dilation, which increases portal-venous inflow in cirrhosis.

Intrahepatic vascular bed is physiologically at high-flow and low-resistance. Hepatic parenchyma is deeply altered in cirrhotic patients, thus leading to dramatic increase in vascular resistance from portal-venous bed. As a results, liver releases several vasodilators such as nitric oxide (NO) that determines splanchnic arterial dilation and consequently portal overflow [8].

Once portal hypertension occurs, a collateral circulation develops to return blood to the systemic circulation. This is the underlying mechanisms of GEVs development and bleeding.

Clinically, GEVs are classified by location into esophageal and gastric varices.

Esophageal varices are often graded by size as:

- F1: small, straight varices (Fig. 55.1)
- F2: enlarged, tortuous varices, occupying less than one third of the lumen (Fig. 55.2)

A. Facciorusso (✉) · R. V. Buccino · N. Muscatiello
Gastroenterology Unit, Department of Medical Sciences, University of Foggia, Foggia, Italy

F. Radu-Ionita et al. (eds.), *Liver Diseases*, https://doi.org/10.1007/978-3-030-24432-3_55

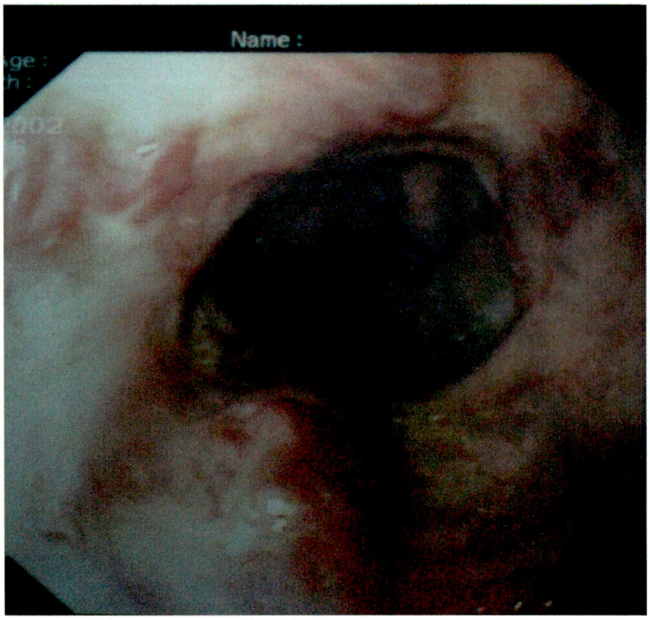

Fig. 55.1 Small varices classified as F1

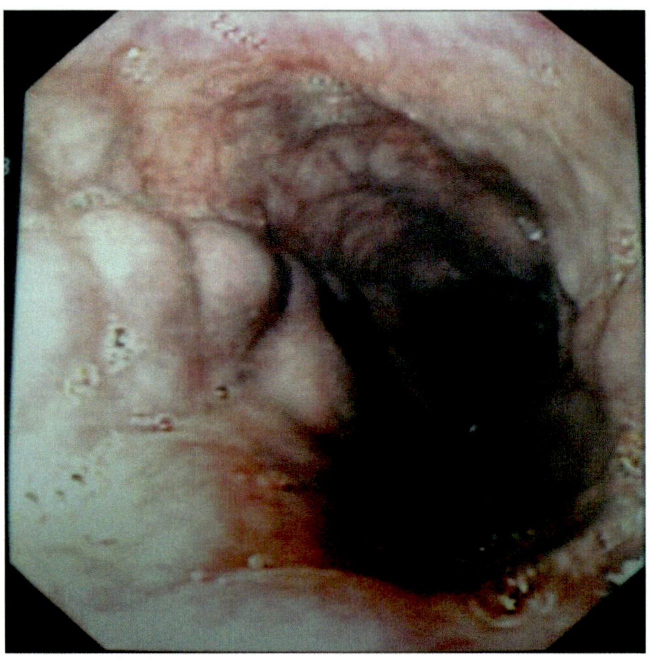

Fig. 55.2 Enlarged, tortuous varices, occupying less than one third of the lumen, classified as F2

- F3: large, coil-shaped varices, occupying more than one third of the lumen (Fig. 55.3)

Gastric varices (which are not object of the current chapter) are classified by location into:

- Gastroesophageal varices (GOVs-gastric varices in continuity with esophageal varices) type 1 (GOV1: along the

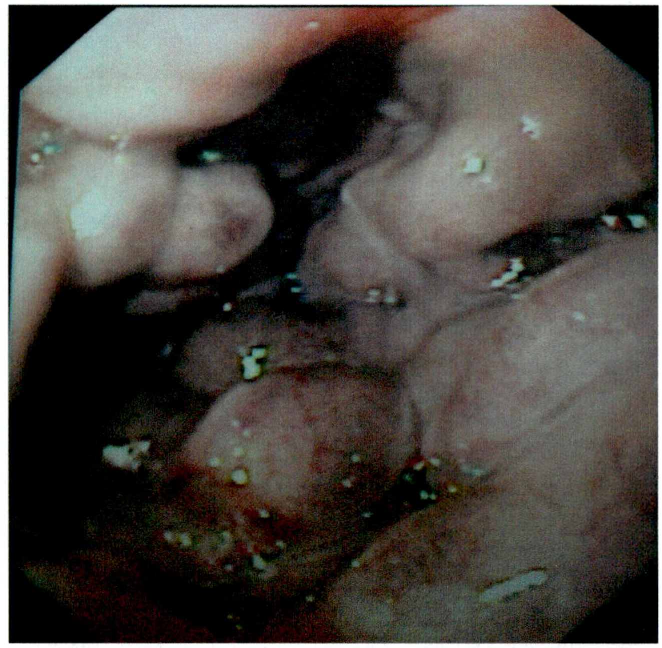

Fig. 55.3 Large, coil-shaped varices, occupying more than one third of the lumen, classified as F3

lesser curve) or type 2 (GOV2: along the greater curve extending towards the fundus of the stomach).
- Isolated gastric varices (IGVs) type 1 (IGV1: isolated cluster of varices in the fundus of the stomach) or type 2 (IGV2: isolated gastric varices in other parts of the stomach).

GOVs (particularly GOV1) are usually associated with large esophageal varices.

As previously described, not only the size of esophageal varices but also some specific endoscopic features may represent predictors of bleeding such as white nipples (Fig. 55.4) or red wale marks. All of these endoscopic features constitute signs of variceal wall weakness, thus claiming for prompt endoscopic prophylactic treatment (see below).

55.3 Screening of EVs in Cirrhotic Patients

The gold standard to assess the presence and severity of portal hypertension remains the hepatic venous pressure gradient (HVPG). However, this invasive procedure is routinely performed only in highly-specialized centers and it is not completely devoid of potential complications such as hemorrhage or infections.

Currently gastroscopy is the milestone as a screening test for varices and it is routinely offered once the diagnosis of cirrhosis is confirmed because of its excellent diagnostic accuracy and potential therapeutic approach [5, 9].

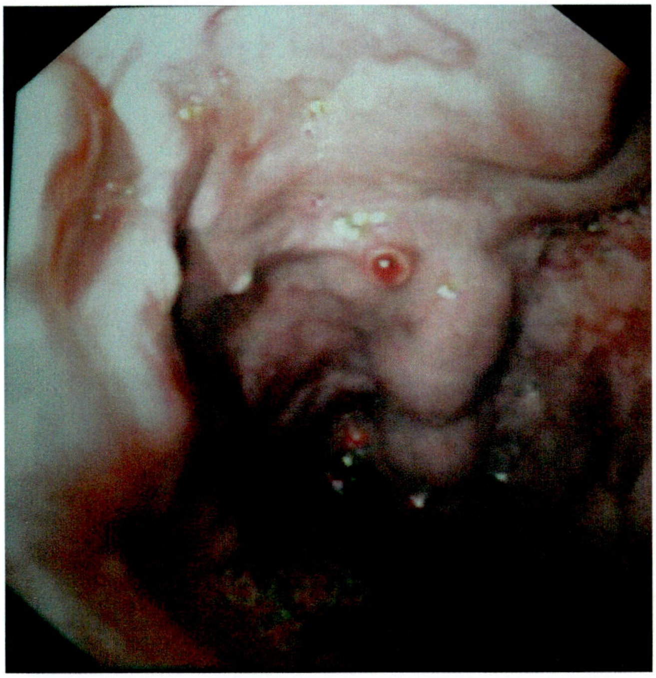

Fig. 55.4 Large esophageal varices with white nipple signs. White nipples constitute signs of variceal wall weakness and represent an important predictor of bleeding

The recent development of non-invasive assessment using elastography techniques offers valuable alternatives. The rationale of using liver stiffness measurement (LSM) in this field is that liver fibrosis is the major trigger of portal hypertension (as previously described) hence measuring non-invasively hepatic fibrosis may help to discriminate patients at high risk of developing GEVs and first episode of bleeding from low-risk subjects [10–12].

As liver disease progresses, the role of extrahepatic factors (vasoactive molecules) in determining portal pressure increase becomes more important. Therefore, as portal hypertension becomes more severe, the correlation between LS and HVPG is attenuated [13], and in such cases the measurement of spleen stiffness (SS) seems to be more reliable. In fact, since the portal vein receives blood from the splenic vein, any increase in portal pressure is theoretically transmitted to the spleen with a subsequent increase in intrasplenic pressure and related increased stiffness [14].

In a recent meta-analysis correlation coefficient between LS and HVPG was 0.783 (95% CI, 0.737–0.823), however this coefficient dropped for high values of HVPG (HVPG > 12 mmHg) probably due to the aforementioned reasons [15]. Summary sensitivity and specificity were 87% (95% CI 76–94%) and 85% (95% CI, 77–91%), respectively, thus indicating good diagnostic performance of LSM, with a cut-off value widely ranging from 8.74 to 25 kPa and an area under receiving operator curve (AUROC) of 0.90 [15].

As a result of these new evidences, recent Baveno VI consensus introduced a new statement on cirrhotic patients who may safely avoid screening gastroscopy [16]:

- Patients with a liver stiffness <20 kPa and with a platelet count >150,000 have a very low risk of having varices requiring treatment, and can avoid screening endoscopy (level of evidence 1b; grade of recommendation A)
- These patients can be followed up by yearly repetition of LSM and platelet count (5;D)
- If liver stiffness increases or platelet count declines, these patients should undergo screening gastroscopy (5;D)

Concerning surveillance gastroscopy, the new statements (changed from Baveno V) are as following [16]:

- In compensated patients with no varices at screening endoscopy and with ongoing liver injury (e.g. active drinking in alcoholics, lack of response in HCV), surveillance endoscopy should be repeated at 2 year intervals (5;D).
- In compensated patients with small varices and with ongoing liver injury (e.g. active drinking in alcoholics, lack of SVR in HCV), surveillance endoscopy should be repeated at 1 year intervals (5;D).
- In compensated patients with no varices at screening endoscopy in whom the etiological factor has been removed and who have no co-factors (e.g. obesity), surveillance endoscopy should be repeated at 3 year intervals (5;D).
- In compensated patients with small varices at screening endoscopy in whom the etiological factor has been removed and who have no co-factors, surveillance endoscopy should be repeated at 2 year intervals (5;D).

This approach has been validated in several series and constitutes the current state of art in the field [17–20].

55.4 Pharmacological Treatment in the Prevention and Management of Variceal Bleeding

55.4.1 Non-selective Beta-Blockers (NSBBs)

Standard NSBBs (propranolol, nadolol and timolol) decrease portal pressure by reducing portal-collateral blood flow through reduction of the cardiac index (via beta1-receptor blockade) and splanchnic vasoconstriction (via beta2-adrenoceptor blockade) [4, 21–23].

Moreover, NSBBs have been shown to exert other beneficial effects in cirrhotics by increasing gut motility and reducing bacterial translocation thus potentially decreasing the rate of infections and their severity, as suggested by some recent reports [24–27].

While the role of NSBBs in cirrhotic patients has been recently questioned in light of the striking results of some retrospective studies which concluded that NSBBs are associated to decrease survival in subjects with refractory ascites (RA) [28] and spontaneous bacterial peritonitis (SBP) [29], these findings have been debunked in more recent series and two meta-analysis [30–33].

The great debate raised about this topic led to an interesting "window hypothesis" for beta-blocker therapy, in which Krag et al. proposed that beta-blockers improve survival within only a narrow window in the natural history of cirrhosis and are either ineffective or harmful outside of this window [34]. According to this theory, in advanced cirrhosis excessive beta-adrenergic activity suppression determines decreased perfusion to vital organs and subsequently increased risk for the HRS [1] and end-organ damage [1, 35]. However, supporting evidences of this theory are quite discordant and exactly when the "window" closes is still up for debate [36]. The recent meta-analysis published by our group and based on 3 randomized controlled trials (RCTs) and 13 observational studies revealed that overall survival was comparable between the two groups (hazard ratio = 0.86, 0.71–1.03, p = 0.11) and no difference in SPB (odds ratio = 0.78, 0.47–1.29, p = 0.33) and HRS incidence (odds ratio = 1.22, 0.48–3.09; p = 0.67) was observed [33]. Therefore, we concluded that NSBBs should not be routinely withheld in cirrhotic patients even in presence of ascites and the decision should be taken individually [33].

Another source of concern when using NSBBs in cirrhotics is the safety. In fact, beta-blockers are well known to determine a number of side effects such as hypotension, bradycardia, rush or fatigue. Interestingly, our meta-analysis showed that pooled rate of treatment interruption was 18.6% (5.2–32.1%) [33], undoubtedly a non-negligible incidence but not that high as previously postulated.

Anyway, a long-term satisfactory hemodynamic response (decrease of HVPG to 12 mmHg or below or at least by 20% of its baseline value) is only obtained in 33–50% of patients. In non-responders, addition of low doses of an NO-donor such as isosorbide-5-mononitrate (ISMN) causes an additional decrease in portal pressure, while increasing side effects [37, 38].

The recommended dosages of NSBBs and most frequent side effects are listed in Table 55.1.

Table 55.1 Pharmacological agents used in the prevention of variceal bleeding

Drug	Mechanism of action; route of administration	Dosage	Side effects
Propranolol	Beta1 and beta2 blocker; oral	Start with 10–20 mg twice daily and increase the dose every 2–3 days up to the maximal tolerated dose Maximal dose: 320 mg/day	Bradycardia, orthostatic hypotension, bronchospasm, erectile dysfunction
Nadolol	Beta1 and beta2 blocker; oral	Start with 20 mg daily and increase the dose every 2–3 days up to the maximal tolerated dose Maximal dose: 160 mg/day	Bradycardia, orthostatic hypotension, bronchospasm, erectile dysfunction
Isosorbide-mononitrate (ISMN)	Nitric Oxide donor; oral	Start with 10 mg daily at night and increase the dose after 2–3 days up to 20 mg twice a day Maximal dose: 40 mg/day	Headache, orthostatic hypotension
Carvedilol	Beta-1 and beta-2 blocker with intrinsic anti-α1 activity; oral	Start with 3.125 mg twice daily and increase the dose every 2–3 days up to 12.5 mg/day Maximal dose: 25 mg/day	Arterial hypotension, sodium retention, ascites
Terlipressin	Long-acting vasopressin analogue Splanchnic vasoconstriction, increase in systemic vascular resistance; intravenous	2 mg injection every 4 h for 24–48 h, then 1 mg/4 h for up to 5 days Maximal dose: 8 mg/day for 24–48 h 4 mg/day thereafter	Abdominal pain, arterial hypertension; less than 3% ischaemia (peripheral, intestinal or myocardial)
Somatostatin	Peptide hormone, inhibits glucagon and facilitates adrenergic vasoconstriction; intravenous	Bolus 250 μg followed by continuous i.v. infusion 250–500 μg/h for up to 5 days Maximal dose: 500 μg/h	Hyperglycaemia, vomiting
Octreotide	Long-acting somatostatin analogue; intravenous	Bolus 50 μg i.v., followed by continuous i.v. infusion 50 μg/h for up to 5 days Maximal dose: 50 μg/h	Hyperglycaemia, vomiting
Simvastatin	Improves endothelial dysfunction and reduces intra-hepatic vascular resistance; oral	20 mg once a day After 2 weeks, increase to 40 mg/day if CPK and ALT do not increase over twice the baseline values Maximal dose: 40 mg/day	Elevated aminotransferases Up to 3% rhabdomyolysis in advanced cirrhosis

55.4.2 Carvedilol

In addition to the aforementioned mechanisms of action of NSBBs, carvedilol has an intrinsic anti-α-adrenergic activity and the potential to release NO. Carvedilol is the sole agent to exert a potential effect on the major driver of portal hypertension by decreasing intrahepatic resistance. This is why it is more effective in lowering portal hypertension than traditional NSBBs [39, 40]; however, therapeutic window is narrower and only low doses are recommended.

Of note, a single primary prophylaxis RCT showed that carvedilol prevented a first GEV bleeding episode more effectively than repeat endoscopic ligation, although this requires confirmation in further studies [41].

In conclusion, despite interesting preliminary results, carvedilol still remains an option only in specialized centers due to the concerns on the safety and the uncertainty on long-term effects.

55.4.3 Terlipressin

Terlipressin is a long-acting synthetic vasopressin analogue and exerts a significant action as splanchnic vasoconstrictor with also systemic circulatory effects, such as increasing arterial pressure and systemic vascular resistance, and decreasing cardiac output. Due to its long biological activity, terlipressin can be administered every 4 h as repeat intravenous injections, although if it is given as a continuous infusion the total dose may be decreased. Due to intravenous administration, this agent is only used for short periods, which in practice is limited to the treatment of acute variceal bleeding (2–5 days) or type-I HRS (1–2 weeks) [42]. Because of potential ischaemic and arrhythmic complications, terlipressin should not be used in patients with a history of coronary, cerebrovascular, peripheral or visceral arterial diseases. Also, it should be used with caution in elderly and/or hypertensive patients.

55.4.4 Somatostatin and Its Analogues

Somatostatin and analogues (octreotide, vapreotide) cause splanchnic vasoconstriction by inhibiting the release of vasodilator glucagon and also by a local mesenteric vasoconstrictive effect [43]. However, the primary mechanism may be through blunting of postprandial splanchnic hyperemia [44].

While continuous infusion of somatostatin has a mild but sustained effect in reduction of portal pressure [45], octreotide does not result in sustained reduction in portal pressure due to rapid desensitization [46].

Unlike other vasoactive drugs, somatostatin and analogues have fewer side effects; therefore their use is recommended in patients at higher risk of ischemia.

55.4.5 Simvastatin

Simvastatin decreases intrahepatic vascular resistance resulting in vasodilation of liver vasculature in cirrhotic liver; this occurs because of upregulation of NO production through an enhancement in endothelial NO synthase activity as shown recently in both animals and humans [47, 48]. In a placebo-controlled double-blind RCT of 59 patients, 1-month simvastatin administration was associated with a significant reduction in HVPG 8%, with 32% of hemodynamic responders. These effects were additive with those of beta-blockers [48].

A recent RCT compared the addition of simvastatin versus placebo in patients receiving standard therapy (ligation and drugs) and, although it showed a lacking effect on recurrent variceal hemorrhage, it showed a beneficial effect on survival [49].

55.5 Endoscopic Treatments of Esophageal Varices

55.5.1 Sclerotherapy

Sclerosants are chemical agents able to induce sclerosis when injected in or around the varices. Several agents have been used for long time in human medicine to induce phlebitis and thrombosis of varices with subsequent obliteration. In many western countries polidocanol is commonly adopted for control of variceal hemorrhage. The type of needle used is usually 23 G or 25 G and injections can be made into (intravariceal injection) or around the varices (paravariceal injection) [50]. For the intravariceal technique, the first injection is usually made just below bleeding site in the varix. Subsequent injections are made at all varices around gastroesophageal junction. Proximal injections are made at 2 cm intervals up to 5–6 cm from gastroesophageal junction.

Usually treatment is repeated at 1–3 week intervals until obliteration and then every 3 months.

Most commonly observed complications are chest pain (about 10%), ulcers (20–60%), strictures (mostly asymptomatic, in up to 40% of cases) [51]. Risk of rebleeding is 15–50% in first 24 h. Other rare complications include perforation, mediastinitis, pericarditis, pneumothorax, spinal cord paralysis and mesenteric vein thrombosis [51].

Therefore, due to the high rate of potentially severe complications, sclerotherapy is generally restricted to the very uncommon situation where variceal ligation is not technically feasible.

55.5.2 Endoscopic Variceal Band Ligation (EVBL)

EVBL is cornerstone for the endoscopic management of esophageal varices, both in the case of acute bleeding and as prophylaxis. Variceal ligation results in ischemic necrosis of banded tissue and thrombosis of varices (24–48 h).

The band ligator is attached to the shaft of endoscope. After advancing the endoscope towards the varix which needs to be banded, suction is applied till "red out" occurs and then the band is fired. It is important at this point not to release suction until after a band has been successfully applied. This is required to minimize the risk of iatrogenic bleeding. The bands are placed in distal 5 cm of esophagus in spiral fashion from the gastro-esophageal junction and moving upwards.

Final results are shown in Fig. 55.5.

Since early 1990s EVBL has been found to be superior and safer to endoscopic injection sclerotherapy for active variceal bleeding [52]. These findings were confirmed in several subsequent series and recent meta-analyses [53, 54].

The incidence of post-banding ulcer bleeding is 2.6–7.3% [55]. Less frequent complications are chest pain, infections, and strictures.

55.5.3 Other Endoscopic Treatments

Sengstaken-Blakemore tube, originally described in the 1950s, represents still an useful device in the case of severe bleeding able to buy time for patients who will need a more definitive treatment such as transjugular intrahepatic portosystemic shunt (TIPS).

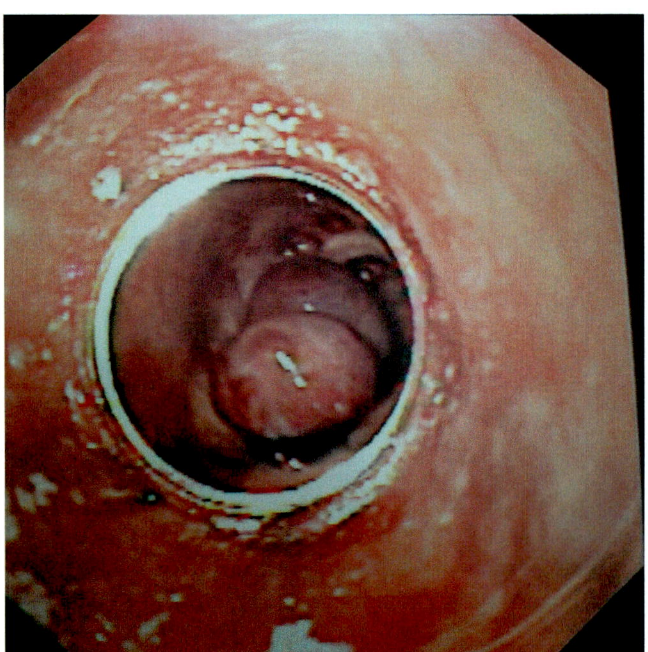

Fig. 55.5 Results of endoscopic band ligation of F3 esophageal varices

Based on the same principle, over the last 5 years several studies have demonstrated the feasibility of controlling active bleeding from esophageal varices with an endoscopically placed stent in the esophagus. Initial bleeding control rates of 80–90% have been reported with minimal side effects [56]. Also, the stent placement can occur at the bedside and can come handy as a rescue therapy. The stent can be easily removed after 7 days.

TC-325 (Hemospray®, Cook Medical, Winston-Salem, North Carolina, USA) is a haemostatic powder which, when put in contact with moisture (e.g., blood or tissue) in the gastrointestinal tract, becomes cohesive and adhesive forming a mechanical barrier that adheres to and covers the bleeding site, achieving very rapid haemostasis [57]. After approximately 24 h, the adherent layer subsequently sloughs off into the lumen from the mucosal wall and is eliminated [57].

Using a delivery system dedicated to endoscopic applications, it has been shown to be effective in peptic ulcer bleeding [57, 58], tumour-related bleeding [59] and patients with lower gastrointestinal bleeding [60]. Hemospray® mainly serves as a bridge towards more definitive endotherapy, with no major adverse events or device-related mortalities. Furthermore, this therapy offers an interesting option for transient haemostasis that does not require specific expertise in therapeutic endoscopy.

Following interesting results of several pilot studies and case reports [61–64], a recent RCT randomized 86 cirrhotic patients with acute variceal bleeding to either immediate endoscopy with haemostatic powder application within 2 h of admission, followed by early elective endoscopy on the next day or to early elective endoscopy only (control group) [65]. Out of 43 patients in the study group, 5 required rescue endoscopy versus 13 in the control group ($p = 0.034$), whereas 6-week survival was significantly improved in the study group (7% vs. 30%, $p = 0.006$) [65].

55.6 Overall Management of Esophageal Varices

55.6.1 Primary Prophylaxis

In patients who do not have gastroesophageal varices, a large multicenter RCT showed no differences between placebo and NSBBs in the prevention of varices [4]. Therefore, no specific treatment for portal hypertension is recommended in this setting.

Patients with varices at screening gastroscopy need to be stratified by the risk of hemorrhage into (1) high-risk patients, i.e., those with medium/large varices or those with small varices that have red wale signs, or in Child C stage; and (2) low risk patients, i.e. those with small varices without red wale signs or occurring in a Child A or B patient [66].

In patients with medium/large varices, quality trials have shown that NSBBs are as effective as EVBL in preventing first variceal hemorrhage [67, 68], and the recommendation is to use therapy based on local resources, expertise and patient preference [16].

In patients with high-risk small varices the mainstay of treatment is NSBB because technically performing EBVL in these varices may be challenging (although there is no clear evidence for this).

In patients with low-risk small varices, there is limited evidence that shows that their growth may be slowed by the use of NSBB [69]. Therefore, the use of NSBB in this setting is considered optional and should be discussed with the patient.

Carvedilol is more effective than traditional NSBB in reducing HVPG but has not been adequately compared head-to-head to traditional NSBB in clinical trials [16].

55.6.2 Acute Bleeding

Acute variceal hemorrhage is a medical emergency requiring intensive care. The basic medical principles of airway, breathing and circulation are followed to achieve hemodynamic stability. Blood transfusion is done conservatively for a target hemoglobin level between 7 and 8 g/dL because excessive blood volume restitution can increase portal pressure [70, 71]. Recommendations regarding management of coagulopathy and thrombocytopenia cannot be made on the basis of currently available data, and management should be individually adopted [16].

Antibiotic prophylaxis is an integral part of therapy for patients with cirrhosis presenting with upper gastrointestinal bleeding and should be instituted from admission [16]. Intravenous ceftriaxone 1 g/24 h or quinolones should be considered as first-line empirical therapy [72].

Safe vasoactive drugs are started as soon as possible, prior to diagnostic endoscopy. Endoscopy is done as soon as possible and not beyond 12 h after presentation. If a variceal source is confirmed, EVBL is the procedure of choice, but sclerotherapy is an option when EVBL is technically difficult [16].

TIPS is recommended in patients who fail standard combination therapy with endoscopic and pharmacological therapy, however salvage TIPS is accompanied by a very high mortality. Predictors of failure are Child class C, HVPG > 20 mmHg and active bleeding at endoscopy [66].

The use of early (pre-emptive) TIPS (within about 48 h of admission) in patients at high risk of failing standard therapy has been shown to reduce mortality [73]. These patients are specifically those who are Child C or are Child B with active hemorrhage at the time of diagnostic endoscopy. In these patients it is recommended to consider early preemptive TIPS, while all others should continue standard therapy with vasoactive drugs continued for 2–5 days depending on control of bleeding and severity of liver disease [16, 66].

Balloon tamponade or novel stents are only used as a temporary measure to control bleeding while a definitive therapy (TIPS or endoscopic therapy) is planned.

55.6.3 Secondary Prophylaxis

Given the high risk of rebleeding in patients who survive an episode of variceal hemorrhage (up to 60%), secondary prophylaxis is an essential part of the management of these patients.

Secondary prophylaxis with NSBBs should be started as soon as the intravenous vasoactive drug is discontinued.

Studies comparing pharmacological therapy (NSBB plus ISMN) vs. EVBL show no differences in recurrent hemorrhage, but there is a suggestion of a beneficial effect on survival with pharmacological therapy in the long term [74, 75]. The combination of pharmacological (NSBB alone or NSBB + ISMN) plus EVBL is associated with lower rebleeding rates than either therapy alone and constitutes the treatment of choice [76].

In patients who experience recurrent variceal hemorrhage despite the combination of pharmacologic and endoscopic treatment, TIPS should be provided [77].

55.7 Conclusions

In the last two decades significant advances in the field of portal hypertension have improved the clinical care and survival of patients with cirrhosis and esophageal varices. In addition to better treatment strategies and improved therapeutic options, the issue of risk stratification has become more important so that, within each clinical stage, different patient subpopulations have been identified that require a different management. Finally, impact of novel effective antiviral treatments are likely to have a significant impact on the natural course of cirrhosis, hence also on the risk of variceal bleeding. Clearly, further research is necessary to explore new pharmacological options that would allow a majority of patients to be hemodynamic responders, thereby foregoing the need for HVPG measurements and even the need for endoscopic therapy.

Self Study

Questions

1. Which statement is true?
   (a) Non-selective beta-blockers (NSBBs) are less effective than endoscopic variceal band ligation (EVBL) as primary prophylaxis of variceal bleeding.
   (b) NSBBs are usually prescribed in monotherapy as secondary prophylaxis of variceal bleeding.

   (c) NSBBs are as effective as EVBL in primary prophylaxis of variceal bleeding.
   (d) a, b.
2. Which statement is true?
   (a) According to Baveno VI criteria, screening gastroscopy is indicated in all cirrhotic patients.
   (b) According to Baveno VI criteria, screening gastroscopy is not indicated in patients with a liver stiffness <20 kPa and with a platelet count >150,000.
   (c) According to Baveno VI criteria, screening gastroscopy is contraindicated in cirrhotic patients.
   (d) None of the above.

Answers

1. Which statement is true?
   (a) NSBBs lead to similar results as EVBL in primary prophylaxis of variceal bleeding. In the case of small varices NSBBs are usually preferred as EVBL may appear challenging in this subset of patients.
   (b) Cornerstone of secondary prophylaxis of variceal bleeding is the association of NSBBs and EVBL.
   (c) Randomized controlled trials and meta-analyses showed that association of NSBBs and EVBL is not superior to NSBBs alone in primary prophylaxis of variceal bleeding-CORRECT.
2. Which statement is true?
   (b) According to Baveno VI criteria gastroscopy is not indicated in patients with a liver stiffness <20 kPa and with a platelet count >150,000-CORRECT.

References

1. Ge PS, Runyon BA. Treatment of patients with cirrhosis. N Engl J Med. 2016;375(8):767–77.
2. Kovalak M, Lake J, Mattek N, et al. Endoscopic screening for varices in cirrhotic patients: data from a national endoscopic database. Gastrointest Endosc. 2007;65:82–8.
3. Merli M, Nicolini G, Angeloni S, et al. Incidence and natural history of small esophageal varices in cirrhotic patients. J Hepatol. 2003;38:266–72.
4. Groszmann RJ, Garcia-Tsao G, Bosch J, et al. Beta-blockers to prevent gastroesophageal varices in patients with cirrhosis. N Engl J Med. 2005;353:2254–61.
5. The North Italian Endoscopic Club for the Study, Treatment of Esophageal Varices. Prediction of the first variceal hemorrhage in patients with cirrhosis of the liver and esophageal varices. A prospective multicenter study. N Engl J Med. 1988;319:983–9.
6. Garcia-Tsao G, Bosch J. Management of varices and variceal hemorrhage in cirrhosis. N Engl J Med. 2010;362:823–32.
7. Hernández-Gea V, Berbel C, Baiges A, García-Pagán JC. Acute variceal bleeding: risk stratification and management (including TIPS). Hepatol Int. 2018;12(Suppl 1):81–90.
8. Schiff ER, Maddrey WC, Reddy KR. Schiff's diseases of the liver. 12th ed. Hoboken, NJ: Wiley-Blackwell; 2017. p. 304–8.
9. Beppu K, Inokuchi K, Koyanagi N, Nakayama S, Sakata H, et al. Prediction of variceal hemorrhage by esophageal endoscopy. Gastrointest Endosc. 1981;27:213–8.
10. Roccarina D, Rosselli M, Genesca J, Tsochatzis EA. Elastography methods for the non-invasive assessment of portal hypertension. Expert Rev Gastroenterol Hepatol. 2018;12(2):155–64.
11. Karatzas A, Konstantakis C, Aggeletopoulou I, Kalogeropoulou C, Thomopoulos K, Triantos C. Non-invasive screening for esophageal varices in patients with liver cirrhosis. Ann Gastroenterol. 2018;31(3):305–14.
12. Gomez-Moreno AZ, Pineda-Tenor D, Jimenez-Sousa MA, Sánchez-Ruano JJ, Artaza-Varasa T, Saura-Montalban J, Ryan P, Resino S. Liver stiffness measurement predicts liver-related events in patients with chronic hepatitis C: a retrospective study. PLoS One. 2017;12(9):e0184404.
13. Vizzutti F, Arena U, Rega L, Pinzani M. Non-invasive diagnosis of portal hypertension in cirrhotic patients. Gastroenterol Clin Biol. 2008;32:80–7.
14. Mazur R, Celmer M, Silicki J, Hołownia D, Pozowski P, Międzybrodzki K. Clinical applications of spleen ultrasound elastography - a review. J Ultrason. 2018;18(72):37–41.
15. Sharma P, Kirnake V, Tyagi P, Bansal N, Singla V, et al. Spleen stiffness in patients with cirrhosis in predicting esophageal varices. Am J Gastroenterol. 2013;108:1101–7.
16. de Franchis R, Baveno VI Faculty. Expanding consensus in portal hypertension: Report of the Baveno VI Consensus Workshop: Stratifying risk and individualizing care for portal hypertension. J Hepatol. 2015;63(3):743–52.
17. Augustin S, Pons M, Maurice JB, Bureau C, Stefanescu H, Ney M, Blasco H, Procopet B, Tsochatzis E, Westbrook RH, Bosch J, Berzigotti A, Abraldes JG, Genescà J. Expanding the Baveno VI criteria for the screening of varices in patients with compensated advanced chronic liver disease. Hepatology. 2017;66(6):1980–8.
18. Jangouk P, Turco L, De Oliveira A, et al. Validating, deconstructing and refining Baveno criteria for ruling out high-risk varices in patients with compensated cirrhosis. Liver Int. 2017;37(8):1177–83.
19. Abraldes JG, Bureau C, Stefanescu H, et al. Noninvasive tools and risk of clinically significant portal hypertension and varices in compensated cirrhosis: the "anticipate" study. Hepatology. 2016;64:2173–84.
20. Garcia-Tsao G, Abraldes JG, Berzigotti A, et al. Portal hypertensive bleeding in cirrhosis: risk stratification, diagnosis, and management: 2016 practice guidance by the American Association for the study of liver diseases. Hepatology. 2017;65(1):310–35.
21. Calés P, Oberti F, Payen JL, et al. Lack of effect of propranolol in the prevention of large oesophageal varices in patients with cirrhosis. Eur J Gastroenterol Hepatol. 1999;11:741–5.
22. Lebrec D, Poynard T, Hillon P, et al. Propranolol for prevention of recurrent gastrointestinal bleeding in patients with cirrhosis. N Engl J Med. 1981;305:1371–4.
23. Poynard T, Calès P, Pasta L, et al. Beta-adrenergic-antagonist drugs in the prevention of gastrointestinal bleeding in patients with cirrhosis and esophageal varices. N Engl J Med. 1991;324:1532–8.
24. Merli M, Lucidi C, Di Gregorio V, Giannelli V, Giusto M, Ceccarelli G, Riggio O, Venditti M. The chronic use of beta-blockers and proton pump inhibitors may affect the rate of bacterial infections in cirrhosis. Liver Int. 2015;35(2):362–9.
25. Reiberger T, Ferlitsch A, Payer BA, et al. Non-selective betablocker therapy decreases intestinal permeability and serum levels of LBP and IL-6 in patients with cirrhosis. J Hepatol. 2013;58:911–21.
26. Mookerjee RP, Pavesi M, Thomsen KL, Mehta G, Macnaughtan J, Bendtsen F, Coenraad M, Sperl J, Gines P, Moreau R, Arroyo V, Jalan R. CANONIC Study Investigators of the EASL-CLIF Consortium. Treatment with non-selective beta blockers is associated with reduced severity of systemic inflammation and improved

survival of patients with acute-on-chronic liver failure. J Hepatol. 2016;64(3):574–82.
27. Senzolo M, Cholongitas E, Burra P, Leandro G, Thalheimer U, Patch D, Burroughs AK. beta-Blockers protect against spontaneous bacterial peritonitis in cirrhotic patients: a meta-analysis. Liver Int. 2009;29(8):1189–93.
28. Sersté T, Francoz C, Durand F, et al. Beta-blockers cause paracentesis-induced circulatory dysfunction in patients with cirrhosis and refractory ascites: a cross-over study. J Hepatol. 2011;55:794–9.
29. Mandorfer M, Bota S, Schwabl P, et al. Nonselective β blockers increase risk for hepatorenal syndrome and death in patients with cirrhosis and spontaneous bacterial peritonitis. Gastroenterology. 2014;146:1680–1690.e1.
30. Bossen L, Krag A, Vilstrup H, et al. Non-selective β-blockers do not affect mortality in cirrhosis patients with ascites: post hoc analysis of three RCTs with 1198 patients. Hepatology. 2015; https://doi.org/10.1002/hep.28352.
31. Bhutta AQ, Garcia-Tsao G, Reddy KR, et al. Beta-blockers in hospitalised patients with cirrhosis and ascites: mortality and factors determining discontinuation and reinitiation. Aliment Pharmacol Ther. 2017;47(1):78–85.
32. Chirapongsathorn S, Valentin N, Alahdab F, et al. Nonselective β-blockers and survival in patients with cirrhosis and ascites: a systematic review and meta-analysis. Clin Gastroenterol Hepatol. 2016;14(8):1096–104.
33. Facciorusso A, Roy S, Livadas S, Fevrier-Paul A, Wekesa C, Kilic ID, Chaurasia AK, Sadeq M, Muscatiello N. Nonselective beta-blockers do not affect survival in cirrhotic patients with ascites. Dig Dis Sci. 2018;63(7):1737–46.
34. Krag A, Wiest R, Albillos A, et al. The window hypothesis: haemodynamic and non-haemodynamic effects of betablockers improve survival of patients with cirrhosis during a window in the disease. Gut. 2012;61:967–9.
35. Ge PS, Runyon BA. The changing role of beta-blocker therapy in patients with cirrhosis. J Hepatol. 2014;60(3):643–53.
36. Ge PS, Runyon BA. When should the β-blocker window in cirrhosis close? Gastroenterology. 2014;146(7):1597–9.
37. Garcia-Pagan JC, Navasa M, Bosch J, et al. Enhancement of portal pressure reduction by the association of isosorbide-5-mononitrate to propranolol administration in patients with cirrhosis. Hepatology. 1990;11:230–8.
38. Bureau C, Péron J-M, Alric JL, et al. 'A La Carte' treatment of portal hypertension: adapting medical therapy to hemodynamic response for the prevention of bleeding. Hepatology. 2002;36:1361–6.
39. Sinagra E, Perricone G, D'Amico M, et al. Systematic review with meta-analysis: the haemodynamic effects of carvedilol compared with propranolol for portal hypertension in cirrhosis. Aliment Pharmacol Ther. 2014;39:557–68.
40. Reiberger T, Ulbrich G, Ferlitsch A, et al. Carvedilol for primary prophylaxis of variceal bleeding in cirrhotic patients with haemodynamic non-response to propranolol. Gut. 2013;62:1634–41.
41. Tripathi D, Ferguson JW, Kochar N, et al. Randomized controlled trial of carvedilol versus variceal band ligation for the prevention of the first variceal bleed. Hepatology. 2009;50:825–33.
42. Facciorusso A, Chandar AK, Murad MH, Prokop LJ, Muscatiello N, Kamath PS, Singh S. Comparative efficacy of pharmacological strategies for management of type 1 hepatorenal syndrome: a systematic review and network meta-analysis. Lancet Gastroenterol Hepatol. 2017;2(2):94–102.
43. Wiest R, Tsai MH, Groszmann RJ. Octreotide potentiates PKC-dependent vasoconstrictors in portal-hypertensive and control rats. Gastroenterology. 2000;120:975–83.
44. Buonamico P, Sabba C, Garcia-Tsao G, et al. Octreotide blunts post-prandial splanchnic hyperemia in cirrhotic patients: a double-blind randomized echo-Doppler study. Hepatology. 1995;21:134–9.
45. Cirera I, Feu F, Luca A, et al. Effects of bolus injections and continuous infusions of somatostatin and placebo in patients with cirrhosis and portal hypertension. A double-blind hemodynamic investigation. Hepatology. 1995;22:106–11.
46. Escorsell A, Bandi JC, Andreu V, et al. Desensitization to the effects of intravenous octreotide in cirrhotic patients with portal hypertension. Gastroenterology. 2001;120:161–9.
47. Abraldes JG, Rodrıguez-Vilarrupla A, Graupera M, et al. Simvastatin treatment improves liver sinusoidal endothelial dysfunction in CCl4 cirrhotic rats. J Hepatol. 2007;46(6):1040–6.
48. Abraldes JG, Albillos A, Banares R, et al. Simvastatin lowers portal pressure in patients with cirrhosis and portal hypertension: a randomized controlled trial. Gastroenterology. 2009;136:1651–8.
49. Abraldes JG, Villanueva C, Aracil C, et al. Addition of simvastatin to standard therapy for the prevention of variceal rebleeding docs not reduce rebleeding but increases survival in patients with cirrhosis. Gastroenterology. 2016;150(5):1160–70.
50. Sarin SK, Nanda R, Sachdev G, Chari S, Anand BS, Broor SL. Intravariceal versus paravariceal sclerotherapy: a prospective, controlled, randomised trial. Gut. 1987;28:657–62.
51. Kapoor A, Dharel N, Sanyal AJ. Endoscopic diagnosis and therapy in gastroesophageal variceal bleeding. Gastrointest Endosc Clin N Am. 2015;25(3):491–507.
52. Stiegmann GV, Goff JS, Michaletz-Onody PA, et al. Endoscopic sclerotherapy as compared with endoscopic ligation for bleeding esophageal varices. N Engl J Med. 1992;326:1527–32.
53. Laine L, Cook D. Endoscopic ligation compared with sclerotherapy for treatment of esophageal variceal bleeding. A meta-analysis. Ann Intern Med. 1995;123:280–7.
54. Singh P, Pooran N, Indaram A, Bank S. Combined ligation and sclerotherapy versus ligation alone for secondary prophylaxis of esophageal variceal bleeding: a meta-analysis. Am J Gastroenterol. 2002;97:623–9.
55. Tierney A, Toriz BE, Mian S, Brown KE. Interventions and outcomes of treatment of postbanding ulcer hemorrhage after endoscopic band ligation: a single-center case series. Gastrointest Endosc. 2013;77:136–40.
56. Cardenas A, Fernandez-Simon A, Escorcell A. Endoscopic band ligation and esophageal stents for acute variceal bleeding. Clin Liver Dis. 2014;18:793–808.
57. Sung JJ, Luo D, Wu JC, et al. Early clinical experience of the safety and effectiveness of Hemospray in achieving hemostasis in patients with acute peptic ulcer bleeding. Endoscopy. 2011;43:291–5.
58. Haddara S, Jacques J, Lecleire S, et al. A novel hemostatic powder for upper gastrointestinal bleeding: a multicenter study (the "GRAPHE" registry). Endoscopy. 2016;48:1084–95.
59. Pittayanon R, Prueksapanich P, Rerknimitr R. The efficacy of Hemospray in patients with upper gastrointestinal bleeding from tumor. Endosc Int Open. 2016;4:E933–6.
60. Holster IL, Brullet E, Kuipers EJ, et al. Hemospray treatment is effective for lower gastrointestinal bleeding. Endoscopy. 2014;46:75–8.
61. Ibrahim M, El-Mikkawy A, Mostafa I, et al. Endoscopic treatment of acute variceal hemorrhage by using hemostatic powder TC-325: a prospective pilot study. Gastrointest Endosc. 2013;78:769–73.
62. Ibrahim M, El-Mikkawy A, Abdalla H, et al. Management of acute variceal bleeding using hemostatic powder. United European Gastroenterol J. 2015;3:277–83.
63. Holster IL, Poley JW, Kuipers EJ, et al. Controlling gastric variceal bleeding with endoscopically applied hemostatic powder (Hemospray™). J Hepatol. 2012;57:1397–8.
64. Stanley AJ, Smith LA, Morris AJ. Use of hemostatic powder (Hemospray) in the management of refractory gastric variceal hemorrhage. Endoscopy. 2013;45(Suppl 2):E86–7.
65. Ibrahim M, El-Mikkawy A, Abdel Hamid M, Abdalla H, Lemmers A, Mostafa I, Devière J. Early application of haemostatic pow-

der added to standard management for oesophagogastric variceal bleeding: a randomised trial. Gut. 2019;68(5):844–53.
66. Bari K, Garcia-Tsao G. Treatment of portal hypertension. World J Gastroenterol. 2012;18(11):1166–75.
67. Gluud LL, Klingenberg S, Nikolova D, Gluud C. Banding ligation versus b-blockers as primary prophylaxis in esophageal varices: systematic review of randomized trials. Am J Gastroenterol. 2007;102:2842–2848; quiz 2841, 2849.
68. Bosch J, Abraldes JG, Berzigotti A, Garcia-Pagan JC. Portal hypertension and gastrointestinal bleeding. Semin Liver Dis. 2008;28:3–25.
69. Merkel C, Marin R, Angeli P, Zanella P, Felder M, Bernardinello E, Cavallarin G, Bolognesi M, Donada C, Bellini B, Torboli P, Gatta A. A placebo-controlled clinical trial of nadolol in the prophylaxis of growth of small esophageal varices in cirrhosis. Gastroenterology. 2004;127:476–84.
70. Kravetz D, Sikuler E, Groszmann RJ. Splanchnic and systemic hemodynamics in portal hypertensive rats during haemorrhage and blood volume restitution. Gastroenterology. 1986;90: 1232–40.
71. Castañeda B, Morales J, Lionetti R, Moitinho E, Andreu V, Pérez-Del-Pulgar S, Pizcueta P, Rodés J, Bosch J. Effects of blood volume restitution following a portal hypertensive related bleeding in anesthetized cirrhotic rats. Hepatology. 2001;33:821–5.
72. Fernández J, Ruiz del Arbol L, Gómez C, Durandez R, Serradilla R, Guarner C, Planas R, Arroyo V, Navasa M. Norfloxacin vs ceftriaxone in the prophylaxis of infections in patients with advanced cirrhosis and hemorrhage. Gastroenterology. 2006;131:1049–56.
73. García-Pagán JC, Caca K, Bureau C, Laleman W, Appenrodt B, Luca A, Abraldes JG, Nevens F, Vinel JP, Mössner J, Bosch J. Early use of TIPS in patients with cirrhosis and variceal bleeding. N Engl J Med. 2010;362:2370–9.
74. Gluud LL, Langholz E, Krag A. Meta-analysis: isosorbide-mononitrate alone or with either b-blockers or endoscopic therapy for the management of oesophageal varices. Aliment Pharmacol Ther. 2010;32:859–71.
75. Lo GH, Chen WC, Lin CK, Tsai WL, Chan HH, Chen TA, Yu HC, Hsu PI, Lai KH. Improved survival in patients receiving medical therapy as compared with banding ligation for the prevention of esophageal variceal rebleeding. Hepatology. 2008;48:580–7.
76. Gonzalez R, Zamora J, Gomez-Camarero J, Molinero LM, Bañares R, Albillos A. Meta-analysis: combination endoscopic and drug therapy to prevent variceal rebleeding in cirrhosis. Ann Intern Med. 2008;149:109–22.
77. Luca A, D'Amico G, La Galla R, Midiri M, Morabito A, Pagliaro L. TIPS for prevention of recurrent bleeding in patients with cirrhosis: meta-analysis of randomized clinical trials. Radiology. 1999;212:411–21.

Procedure for Gastric Variceal Bleeding: From BRTO to PARTO to CARTO, Three Decades of Progress

56

Edward Wolfgang Lee and Damian Hall

Key Concepts

- GV bleeding (GVB) is a significant, life-threatening complication of portal hypertension
- BRTO is a safe and effective treatment option for gastric variceal bleeding
- Modified BRTO includes CARTO and PARTO
- CARTO and PARTO have amended some of the disadvantages of BRTO using a balloon and sclerosing agents to improve the clinical outcomes and safety profiles of BRTO

56.1 Introduction

Balloon-Occluded Transvenous Retrograde Obliteration (BRTO) is a minimally invasive, image-guided procedure in which occlusion of gastric varices and its pathological portosystemic shunt, is achieved with sclerosants, embolic agents, and more recently, combinations of plugs and coils [1–4]. The procedure has been developed in Asia for more than two decades and now emerging globally as an important adjunct to currently available treatment options for gastric varices with spontaneous gastrorenal or gastrocaval shunt. In addition, it may provide additional benefits including treatment of overt hepatic encephalopathy and improvement in hepatic synthetic function [3–6]. Although there is no official guideline, BRTO is currently accepted with several indications. It is primarily performed on patients requiring secondary prevention of recurrent gastric variceal bleeding but has also found a place in primary prophylaxis of gastric variceal hemorrhage (common in Japan and South Korea), and bleeding ectopic varices with gastrorenal or gastrocaval shunt [7, 8].

The current concept of BRTO is much older than most may realize. Thought to have been theorized as far back as the 1970s, it was first documented by Olson et al. at Indiana University in 1984 [9]. That case report described a novel intervention for the treatment of bleeding gastroesophageal varices in patients with spontaneous gastrorenal shunts, utilizing a combination of ethanol sclerosant, coils, and balloon catheter. Two previous attempts to treat that patient's esophageal and gastric varices with coils alone had proven unsuccessful. The major factor preventing complete treatment in those failed two episodes was thought to be the large outflow tract created by the spontaneous gastrorenal shunt, which enabled subsequent enlargement of any remaining varices within the larger shunt [9]. Beyond the work of Olson and his colleagues, BRTO did not gain much favor in North America and Europe for another 25 years. It was not until the work of Kanagawa et al. in Japan in the early 1990s that the procedure began to generate significant interest. It has been hypothesized that one of the main reasons for this disinterest in the West stems from the concurrent development and advancement of the Transjugular Intrahepatic Portosystemic Shunt (TIPS) procedure in those years, with Eastern and Western practices differently focusing on BRTO and TIPS, respectively [6, 8, 10, 11].

The Western approach has consistently favored TIPS, and it has been argued that this focus stems from an overall approach to varices as a symptom of elevated portal pressures, rather than a focus on addressing varices independently from the underlying portal venous hypertension. Specifically, the Western approach tends to prioritize decompression of the portal venous system as the primary means of treating varices, whereas the Eastern approach favors directly intervening as varices arise [6, 11, 12]. Modern BRTO was resurrected by Kanagawa and colleagues in Japan, in August 1990, and culminating in the 1996 publication "*Treatment of*

E. W. Lee, MD, PhD, FSIR (✉)
Interventional Radiology and Liver/Pancreas Transplant Surgery, UCLA Medical Center, Los Angeles, CA, USA
e-mail: EdwardLee@mednet.ucla.edu

D. Hall, MD
Interventional Radiology, UCLA Medical Center, Los Angeles, CA, USA
e-mail: hallx717@umn.edu

F. Radu-Ionita et al. (eds.), *Liver Diseases*, https://doi.org/10.1007/978-3-030-24432-3_56

Gastric Fundal Varices by Balloon-Occluded Retrograde Transvenous Obliteration" [4]. Since that time, it has been widely adopted in Japan and Korea and is progressively becoming accepted in the West as an important addition to current treatment options for patients with portal hypertension and gastric varices [6, 8, 11].

56.2 Techniques and Outcomes of BRTO

56.2.1 Patients

Currently, the primary patient population for BRTO or modified BRTO procedure is cirrhotic patients with portal hypertension, of which alcoholic cirrhosis, hepatitis C, and non-alcoholic steatohepatitis constitute the majority of contributing etiologies [8, 13, 14]. As the liver gets cirrhotic, its ability to perform both synthetic and anabolic functions begin to falter. Portal hypertension in the context of cirrhosis is frequently a chronic, progressive condition, leading to a variety of adverse outcomes [5, 15–18]. In addition to the inherent decline in liver functioning and subsequent adverse outcomes, portal hypertension frequently leads to the development a spontaneous portosystemic shunt (SPSS), connecting with esophageal varices or less commonly, gastric varices [5, 19]. Portal blood seeks the outflow tract of least resistance and can lead to SPSS with gastrorenal, gastrophrenic, or gastrocaval shunt, along with combinations thereof [48]. Both esophageal and gastric varices are prone to hemorrhage. In addition, the gastric varices (GV) are challenging to treat endoscopically due to its location in gastric fundus which is technically more challenging [20]. Also, these shunts frequently form large vascular spaces with multiple inflow and outflow tracts, prompting the development of novel occlusion and obliteration therapies. GV bleeding (GVB) is a significant, life-threatening complication of portal hypertension [16, 21–24]. While GVB occurs less frequently than esophageal varices (EV), they are known to occur at lower portal pressures and are associated with significant mortality. Patients with gastric varices require significant medical resources. They frequently necessitate the involvement of multiple specialties; endoscopic treatment is attempted initially but is often insufficient in these patients [16, 21–24]. In the US, the primary treatment for patients who fail to respond to endoscopic ligation or banding of varices is TIPS. However, TIPS has its own set of inherent risks and limitations, and while it has been found to be an effective treatment for esophageal varices, outcomes for gastric varices have been mixed [11, 25, 26]. The details on TIPS are described in a different chapter.

56.2.2 Outcomes of BRTO

BRTO has proven itself to be a reliable and efficacious therapy for treatment of gastric varices (GV) (Table 56.1). Unlike esophageal varices, which are more common, GVs are known to bleed in the absence of markedly elevated portal pressures and additionally confer high levels of mortality relating to significant blood loss [8, 27–30]. A recent meta-analysis by

Table 56.1 A summary of BRTO for gastric variceal bleeding

Authors	Study design	Treatment received	N	Technical success rate (%)	Obliteration (%)	Sclerosant type	Rebleeding (%)	1-Year mortality (%)
Chu et al. (2018) [43]	Retro	BRTO	142	90–96	95–96	EO or STS	1.3–3.8 (1 year)	–
Kobayakawa et al. (2017) [42]	Pros	BRTO	45	100	93	5% EO	0	–
Chang et al. (2016) [48]	Retro	PARTO	19	95	95	Gelfoam	0	15
Gwon et al. (2015) [44]	Pros	PARTO	73	100	99	Gelfoam	0	
Lee et al. (2014) [3]	Retro	CARTO	20	100	100	Gelfoam	0	5
Gwon et al. (2013) [1]	Retro	PARTO	20	100	100	Gelfoam	0	–
Jang et al. (2012) [57]	Retro	BRTO	183	97	52	5% EO	21	14
Sabri et al. (2011) [50]	Retro	BRTO	22	91	89	3% STS	0	–
Kasuga et al. (2010) [65]	Pros	BRTO	21	95	100	5% EO	0	10
Akahoshi et al. (2008) [37]	Pros	BRTO	68	93	97	5% EO	14	4 (3 years)
Cho et al. (2007) [20]	Pros	BRTO	49	84	80	5% EO	0	17
Hiraga et al. (2007) [66]	Pros	BRTO	34	97	91	5% EO	3	10
Ninoi et al. (2005) [59]	Pros	BRTO	78	87	95	5% EO	2	7
Kitamoto et al. (2002) [67]	Pros	BRTO	24	96	88	5% EO	9	4
Chikamori et al. (2001) [68]	Pros	BRTO	52	–	100	5% EO	0	8
Hirota et al. (1999) [40]	Pros	BRTO	20	100	75	5% EO	–	5 (3 years)
Kanagawa et al. (1996) [4]	Pros	BRTO	32	100	97	5% EO	0	–
Koito et al. (1996) [69]	Pros	BRTO	30	100	100	5% EO	10	–

BRTO balloon-occluded retrograde transvenous obliteration, *CARTO* coil-assisted retrograde transvenous obliteration, *PARTO* plug-assisted retrograde transvenous obliteration, *GV* gastric varices, *Pros* prospective study, *Retro* retrospective study

Park et al. in 2014 reviewed 24 uncontrolled studies, including 23 retrospectives and one prospective study, evaluated the clinical success of the procedure, defined as no recurrence or rebleed of gastric varices [8]. They further expanded this success rate to include complete obliteration of gastric varices observed at any point post-procedure and found that the pooled clinical success rate was nearly 98% [8].

Failure to achieve obliteration of varix, while uncommon, can be characterized based on several specific issues [8]. First, the gastrorenal shunt may not be fully occluded by the balloon-catheter, either due to the size of a shunt, or rapid flow around the balloon. Due to reports of failure based on high flow shunts, some authors have suggested partial embolization of the outflow tract, typically the renal vein, in advance of the BRTO procedure. Secondly, tortuous shunts, comprised of highly complex variceal complexes with multiple in- or outflow tracts, may preclude the possibility of complete obliteration. Lastly, insufficient volume of sclerosant has been thought to be a common cause of incomplete obliteration. These three causes of incomplete obliteration are frequently encountered together and have continued to spur further evolution of the BRTO procedure.

56.2.3 BRTO vs. Endoscopic Treatment

At present, the standard of care for GVB in the US is typically endoscopic banding or injection of N-butyl-2-cyanoacrylate glue [31–36]. A 2009 study by Hong et al. compared the outcomes of GVB treatment with endoscopic treatment vs. BRTO in Korean patients with high risk GV [35]. High-risk was defined as greater than or equal to 5 mm in diameter, GV with red spots, or GV with Child-Pugh liver cirrhosis rating of B or C. They found that endoscopic treatment and BRTO had similar therapeutic efficacies. However, there was an interesting difference in technical success and occurrence of rebreeding. For those patients treated with endoscopic treatment, 100% achieved technical success, while those receiving BRTO only achieved 76.9%. Significant rebleeding occurred in 71.4% of the endoscopy treated patients, but only 15.4% of the BRTO patients [35]. BRTO further proved to be an effective rescue treatment for those previously treated GVB. Park and colleagues found that all patients treated with rescue BRTO due to rebleeding after initial endoscopic treatment achieved technical success and had no rebleeding events during the median follow-up period of 17 months [8]. Park and colleagues concluded that while both therapies have somewhat similar efficacies, BRTO has a unique role as a rescue treatment for those GVB patients experiencing rebleeding events [8]. They note that this results in large part due to the difficulty of repeat endoscopic glue injection due to glue polymerization.

56.2.4 Conventional BRTO: Technique

The first modern description of the procedure, as noted by Kanagawa and colleagues in the early 1990s, involved insertion of a balloon catheter into the outflow tract (e.g., gastro-renal shunt) of the target gastric varix or variceal complex via a transfemoral approach [4, 13, 20, 37–40]. The balloon was then inflated to block outflow. Then, retrograde venography was conducted to assess the shunt and gastric varices and its in- and outflow tracts and collateral vessels. They also used this venography to determine the amount of sclerosant needed to apply, which corresponded to 6–60 mL of ethanolamine oleate (EO). The sclerosant utilized in this first manuscript was a 5% EO and remained behind the occlusion balloon, exerting its effect on the shunt and gastric variceal vascular tissue, for 30 min to hours. After this time, the balloon catheter was removed [4, 13, 20, 37–40]. The procedure described by Olson et al. in 1984 utilized a very similar methodology, with the exception that absolute alcohol instead of EO was used as the sclerosant [9].

It should be noted that EO has the potential to cause hemolysis and renal insufficiency. It is for this reason that balloon occlusion is necessary for the conventional BRTO. Balloon occlusion does not, however, prevent all EO from escaping the variceal complex and circulating systemically. To prevent the leak of EO causing hemolysis, haptoglobin has been prophylactically utilized (haptoglobin is an agent that binds free hemoglobin and functions as an antidote to the rapid hemolysis that may be observed by extravasation of sclerosant). Haptoglobin, while commercially manufactured and clinically available in Japan, was not available to Western clinicians, likely contributing to the weariness with which US clinicians view sclerosant such as EO. Patients were administered 4000 U of haptoglobin peripherally, prior to the BRTO procedure [2, 6, 8, 20].

When a sclerosing agent is used, its ability to remain within the vessel or tissue of interest is paramount. Distribution within the circulatory system or extravasation within adjacent tissues has the potential to cause serious adverse reactions (AE) ranging from incomplete obliteration to anaphylaxis [2, 6, 8, 20]. With respect to BRTO, stasis of the sclerosant within the SPSS and gastric varices is achieved with the help of an occlusion balloon that effectively blocks flow [2, 6, 8, 13, 20, 41]. Despite this, many BRTO patients experience some form of AE, including fever, hematuria, hemolysis somewhat more common than back or abdominal pain [8, 42]. Presently a variety of adjunct tools are implemented, including both plugs and coils, enabling and improving obliteration of more complex variceal systems [2, 5, 43, 44].

56.2.5 The Occlusion-Balloon: Dwell-Time and Rupture

While BRTO does exhibit significant improvement in both technical and clinical success, it does have a number of important complications and limitations [13, 44]. Some of these complications and limitations are due to using an indwelling balloon for shunt occlusion. First, significant balloon dwell-time is required to achieve adequate stagnation of the sclerosant and avoid leakage into the systemic circulation. Studies have found that balloon dwell-time varies widely from several hours to greater than 24 h [2, 45, 46]. Dwell-time is ultimately left to the operator's clinical judgement but has generally been found to correlate with the overall size of the varices [46]. Length of dwell-time can be further determined based on the ability to aspirate blood freely through the balloon catheter along with sclerosant, indicating incomplete thrombus formation. In this scenario, the balloon catheter would remain inflated and additional sclerosant is often added to ensure complete obliteration of the gastrorenal shunt [46].

A 2007 study by Cho et al. investigated clinical and technical outcomes of 49 BRTO patients. The authors found that procedure times ranged from 30 to 120 min and included 5–20 min of fluoroscopy time, which varied with the complexity of the variceal complex [20]. More recent studies examining total balloon dwell-time in US patients have documented subsequent balloon catheter dwell-times ranging from 4 to 24 h [47]. While these methods do vary considerably, the resources required post-procedure are highly variable as well [47]. The dwell time or wait time involves waiting for the formation of a thrombus in the gastric varices and can be done either in the ED or wards from which the patient was referred or with an ICU admission, depending on the institutional policies. In the past, overnight inflation was the standard of care at many Western institutions. More recently, however, US clinicians have engaged to limit this recovery time, not only to reduce costs but also to reduce the risk of complications from indwelling catheters [47].

BRTO Balloon rupture is also a serious concern when attempting BRTO. Although the procedure has been continuously refined over the past three decades, a small number of BRTO patients experienced this complication [43]. In 2018 Chu et al. examined 142 BRTO procedures from January 2002 to June 2015 and found that six patients with a balloon rupture [43]. It should be additionally noted that while rupture has been hypothesized to occur after various insults, ranging from interaction with sclerosant to insufficient physical characteristics, it is a process that is not fully understood [43].

56.2.6 Sclerosants and Transvenous Obliteration

The concept of using sclerosant for the obliteration of varices is neither new nor novel. Beginning in the 1970s, various published reports detail percutaneous transhepatic obliteration (PTO), which is the antegrade counterpart of the retrograde BRTO approach. Early work also pursued obliteration from a variety of approaches, including coils, gelfoam, and sclerosants ranging from dextrose and thrombin to ethanol [5, 6, 13, 48, 49]. Based on ability to cause sclerosis of vasculature, ethanol would be the ideal candidate for interventional procedures requiring transvenous obliteration. It cannot, however, be mixed or satisfactorily bound to a contrast agent that would enable monitoring of its distribution. As such, ETOH was rapidly discarded in favor of more novel compounds that could necessarily function as sclerosants while also facilitating visualization through modern imaging modalities.

When the procedure was revived in the early 1990s, it was done with ethanolamine oleate, a sclerosant most Western clinicians had never encountered. Ethanolamine oleate (EO), typically mixed with lipiodol, has now been used in BRTO for more than two decades [20, 49]. However, EO has several important potential adverse reactions that continue to concern physicians in the West. Major complications range from hemolysis, hemoglobinuria, and kidney injury to anaphylaxis [20, 40, 49]. Therefore, different sclerosing agents were evaluated in the West. Often known by its trade name Sotradecol, sodium tetradecyl sulfate (STS) is also a widely used sclerosant for BRTO, available in liquid and foam forms. Foam types of a sclerosing agent, such as STS, are thought to be more effective as they are likely better able to coat the endothelium of varix better than liquid, which more readily washes away. They are typically prepared in an institution-specific ratio of 3% STS, contrast media, and room air [2, 49, 50]. It has shown to be an effective sclerosant, capable of venous obliteration in conditions as varied as lower extremity varicose veins and varicocele [51, 52]. STS has been shown to obliterate GV and shunts with reduced AE associated with EO [49].

It should be noted that other non-sclerosing agents are also becoming popular adjuncts for the obliteration of spontaneous portosystemic shunts, embodied in so-called modified BRTO procedures [3, 5, 44]. In recent years, gelfoam has established itself as an effective embolizing agent in both PARTO (Vascular Plug-Assisted Retrograde Transvenous Obliteration) [1, 44] and CARTO (Coil-Assisted Retrograde Transvenous Obliteration) [3, 5]. The gelfoam itself functions as a matrix precipitating formation of thrombus, through vascular spasm, platelet agglutination, and ultimately, the formation of an occlusive thrombosis (Fig. 56.1).

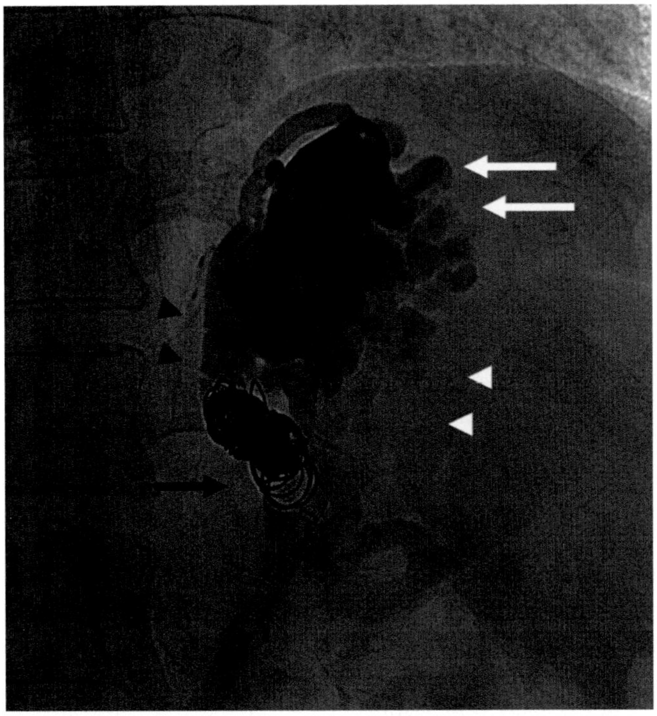

Fig. 56.1 A radiographic illustration of CARTO. Large gastric varices (white arrows) and gastro-renal shunt (black arrowheads) are completely embolized and obliterated with gelfoam. The outflow track of gastro-renal shunt is embolized with multiple coils (black arrow) to replace an indwelling balloon in BRTO to ensure no gelfoam leaks into the systemic circulation. The white arrowheads denote gastric fundus

56.3 Modified BRTO

56.3.1 PARTO

Plug-assisted BRTO or PARTO, as it is commonly known, is a more recent improvement on the decades-old BRTO procedure that employs vascular plugs rather than balloon occlusion to facilitate obliteration of the SPPS, along with the added benefit of faster recovery with no waiting period for balloon dwell-time [1, 44]. Vascular plugs have been employed for the obliteration of vascular malformations for nearly two decades and have been shown to effectively treat a variety of conditions ranging from pulmonary AV malformation to large retroperitoneal shunts, making them ideal for transvenous obliteration of SPPS [51, 53, 54]. Another significant advantage of PARTO is the absence of sclerosants. Ethanolamine oleate and STS, the two most commonly used transvenous sclerosants are known to have significant adverse effect profiles and may induce complications as described above [2, 44, 48, 49]. As such, gelatin, foam, or combination compounds, with dramatically improved safety profiles, may be used. This means that unlike BRTO, clinicians performing PARTO do not need to wait for sclerosis of efferent veins in larger GV or SPPS formations [44, 55]. Finally, the most advantageous aspect of the PARTO procedures is that it can be performed and completely obliterate GV in a single, one-time procedure, avoiding the risks associated with additional interventions [2, 44, 48, 49, 55]. As with BRTO, PARTO does introduce the potential for recurrence or worsening of esophageal varices. However, these are thought to be treated best with close observation and endoscopic ligation as necessary [2, 44, 48, 49].

The first publication describing PARTO and its outcomes, from Gwon and colleagues in 2013, reported successful obliteration via induction of thrombosis in gastrorenal shunt and GV in 20 patients [1]. The study, while only involving 20 patients, demonstrated the technical success of the plug-assisted procedure and did so without the dwell-time required by conventional BRTO [1]. Gwon reported a mean procedure time from vascular plug placement to vascular plug detachment of 22 min with a range of 10–84 min, demonstrating a dramatic reduction in overall procedure time. Gwon employed a gelatin sponge-foam along with vascular plugs and achieved both 100% clinical and technical success rates. In 2015, Gwon and his colleagues reinforced this data with a prospective multicenter study that found a greater than 98% success rate with no recurrent GVB or hepatic encephalopathy [44]. Follow-up CT on these patients found marked shrinkage or total obliteration of GV or SPPS with no cases of variceal bleeding in all patients. Again, showing a progressive refinement of the procedure with improving outcomes [44].

56.3.2 CARTO

In recent years, there has been a need to improve upon the BRTO or PARTO because of several fundamental limitations. First, larger gastrorenal shunts/SPSS have proven to be a challenge for PARTO. Higher rates of blood flow found in these larger vascular spaces make occlusion with the mesh plugs challenging to achieve. Size is also an issue. Plugs are not currently available in diameters larger than 22 mm, which are capable of occluding shunts no larger than 18 mm [2, 3, 5]. Although the use of multiple, overlapping plugs has been considered, they likely would not result in complete occlusion. It has also been noted that the complex course of the IVC-renal vein shunt presents the additional challenge of advancing the relatively larger sheath required to deploy vascular plugs [5]. Because of these limitations, the CARTO procedure has recently come to fill the need for occlusion of more complex SPSSs. CARTO or Coil-Assisted retrograde transvenous obliteration maintains the original BRTO goal of retrograde transvenous occlusion but does so with detachable coils rather than plugs, the initial improvement over the use of an occlusive balloon [2, 3]. In practice, detachable-coils are placed to occlude the efferent shunt (outflow track), and retrograde gel-foam embolization is used to achieve thrombosis. This enables the occlusion of larger shunts with permanent obliteration. CARTO provides the resource savings of PARTO, which includes decreased care related to balloon dwell-time, but with the ability to tackle more extensive and complex gastrorenal shunts with complete and permanent occlusion [3, 5].

CARTO can additionally be separated into two approaches, designated as CARTO I and CARTO II. CARTO I is performed similarly to PARTO, with coils substituting for a vascular plug while CARTO II can be described as hewing to the standard BRTO approach [2]. An occlusion balloon is introduced into the gastrorenal shunt, with multiple coils advanced and deployed through the balloon catheter. The occlusion balloon is removed after complete obliteration has been attained [2]. For the purposes of this chapter, CARTO will indicate CARTO I, the balloon-less procedure.

From a technical perspective, CARTO has demonstrated an ability to effectively treat larger and more complex SPSS. Lee et al. studied 20 patients receiving CARTO from 2012 to 2013 and examined the incidence of post-PARTO variceal bleeding, finding that all 20 patients achieved clinical success without subsequent variceal bleeding, with a mean duration of 2.82 ± 0.56 h [3]. CARTO has the potential to produce outcomes comparable to PARTO and BRTO with the ability to obliterate larger and more complex gastrorenal shunts.

56.4 More Indications for BRTO

56.4.1 BRTO, PARTO, CARTO: Hepatic Encephalopathy and Synthetic Function

BRTO and modified BRTO have additional benefits relating to hepatic reserve that highlight their markedly different approaches relative to TIPS. One of the major limitations to more widespread acceptance of the TIPS procedure is the worsening of hepatic function observed with abrupt drops in portal pressure [13, 46]. While TIPS can be thought of as decompressing the portal circulation, BRTO can be considered as a type of portal re-compression therapy, owing to the increased flow that is now circulating through the portal system in anterograde direction. Therefore, there are also reports of complications of portal hypertension such as splenomegaly and ascites [8, 20, 32, 43, 49, 56, 57]. A further disadvantage of re-compression is the worsening of esophageal varices and portal hypertensive gastropathy after BRTO [8, 37, 58, 59]. In addition, BRTO is known to be additionally useful in those patients that are not candidates for TIPS owing to hepatic encephalopathy [20, 40]. TIPS is not considered first-line treatment for refractory ascites or hepatorenal syndrome because of its unacceptable incidence of portosystemic hepatic encephalopathy [11, 17, 60].

Outcomes relating to liver functioning are generally determined with two major metrics. MELD or The Model for End-Stage Liver Disease produces a score that is based on bilirubin, creatinine, and International Normalized Ratio (INR). Child-Pugh (CP) is based on similar criteria, however also considers the presence or absence of ascites and encephalopathy. Of these two metrics, MELD is typically used as an indicator of a hepatic reserve, or present functionality, providing an objective indication of post-procedural outcomes in cirrhotic patients [61, 62]. In 2013 Saad et al. examined the effects of BRTO in 29 patients without TIPS, and found significant improvement in synthetic function, noted by a significant improvement in MELD score between 1.5 and 3 months post-BRTO [62]. Nearly a third of patients did, however, experience worsening of ascites, with or without hydrothorax, with significant ongoing debate regarding exact pathophysiology relative to *portal re-compression* [62]. With regard to hepatic encephalopathy, a small study by Mukund et al. in 2012 found BRTO to be effective at treating HE, even with only partial obliteration [63]. They reported 86% resolution of HE comprising six of seven patients based on WH scores [63].

PARTO has also shown comparable success for patients with hepatic encephalopathy [1, 44]. Gwon and colleagues' study in on 20 patients, published in 2013, found greater than two in three patients observed improvements in Child-Pugh score within 1 month of PARTO [1]. They additionally found that patients experienced significantly improved INR, a measure of hepatic synthetic functioning [1]. A more recent study of PARTO in 73 patients with GV and hepatic encephalopathy with other portosystemic shunts. Of the 16 patients identified with refractory HE, no cases of HE were found post-PARTO based on West Haven Score (WH) [44].

Beyond the technical success of the CARTO procedure, patients have previously been shown to experience significant improvement in overt hepatic encephalopathy and may also experience increased hepatic synthetic capacity after obliteration of SPSSs [3, 5, 64]. A recent study by Lee and colleagues examined 43 patients undergoing CARTO specifically indicated by overt hepatic encephalopathy and found a 91% clinical success rate constituting an improvement in WH score [5]. Of those 43 patients, nearly two in three were found to have complete resolution of their HE symptoms within the follow-up period lasting a mean of 755 days [5]. This same study additionally found that less than 3% of patients had major complications requiring further treatment, with no procedural deaths reported [5]. This further indicates that CARTO is a safe and effective option for the treatment of refractory overt hepatic encephalopathy.

56.5 Summary

As far back as the 1970s interventionists had conceived endovascular procedures for the treatment of portal hypertension and its complications, including gastric and esophageal varices. Although exact methods have evolved somewhat over the years, BRTO or Balloon-Occluded Retrograde Transvenous Obliteration has hewn to several major concepts. In Western countries, it is an endovascular intervention that functions as an adjunct or alternative treatment to Transjugular Intrahepatic Shunt or TIPS, while in Asia is accomplishes the same task, but is often performed prophylactically, in lieu of TIPS.

From its beginning as a theoretical approach to the treatment of spontaneous portosystemic shunt, BRTO has proven to be an effective means of treating GV bleeding. BRTO and modified BRTO have also recently established themselves as an effective therapy for the obliteration of SPPS complicated by hepatic encephalopathy. All three procedures, BRTO, PARTO, and CARTO, employ varied strategies, with the goal of treating gastric varices that are often difficult to effect with typical endoscopic therapy alone. While all three procedures demonstrate improvement in MELD or WH score, it should be noted that these same studies often document a worsening or smaller improvement in Child-Pugh score, which includes complications such as ascites, likely resulting from the *re-compressive* aspects of the BRTO technique.

Ultimately, BRTO/PARTO/CARTO represents variations on a spectrum of *re-compressive* therapy that has only recently come into playfield in the West. There is great potential to apply these techniques to selective patients with no other options for treating fetal gastric variceal bleeding and medically refractory hepatic encephalopathy. Similar to other high-risk patients, a multi-disciplinary team approach to these patients requiring BRTO/PARTO/CARTO is absolutely critical for optimizing patient care.

Self Study

Questions

1. Which statement is true?
   (a) BRTO and modified BRTO is to treat esophageal varices.
   (b) Gastric variceal bleeding always occurs at the highest portosystemic gradient.
   (c) CARTO requires sclerosing agent such as EO.
   (d) TIPS should not be performed in patients with severe hepatic encephalopathy.
2. Which statement is true?
   (a) BRTO should not be performed in patients with HE as BRTO may worsen HE.
   (b) BRTO creates a shunt between a portal vein and a hepatic vein.
   (c) SPSSs can be often seen in patients with cirrhosis and portal hypertension
   (d) PARTO requires sclerosing agent such as EO

Answers

1. Which statement is true?
   (d) TIPS should not be performed in patients with severe hepatic encephalopathy.
2. Which statement is true?
   (c) SPSSs can be often seen in patients with cirrhosis and portal hypertension

References

1. Gwon DI, Ko GY, Yoon HK, et al. Gastric varices and hepatic encephalopathy: treatment with vascular plug and gelatin sponge-assisted retrograde transvenous obliteration--a primary report. Radiology. 2013;268:281–7.
2. Kim DJ, Darcy MD, Mani NB, et al. Modified balloon-occluded retrograde transvenous obliteration (BRTO) techniques for the treatment of gastric varices: vascular plug-assisted retrograde transvenous obliteration (PARTO)/coil-assisted retrograde transvenous obliteration (CARTO)/balloon-occluded antegrade transvenous obliteration (BATO). Cardiovasc Intervent Radiol. 2018;41:835–47.
3. Lee EW, Saab S, Gomes AS, et al. Coil-assisted retrograde transvenous obliteration (CARTO) for the treatment of portal hypertensive variceal bleeding: preliminary results. Clin Transl Gastroenterol. 2014;5:e61.
4. Kanagawa H, Mima S, Kouyama H, et al. Treatment of gastric fundal varices by balloon-occluded retrograde transvenous obliteration. J Gastroenterol Hepatol. 1996;11:51–8.
5. Lee EW, Saab S, Kaldas F, et al. Coil-assisted retrograde transvenous obliteration (CARTO): an alternative treatment option for refractory hepatic encephalopathy. Am J Gastroenterol. 2018;113:1187.
6. Saad WE. The history and evolution of balloon-occluded retrograde transvenous obliteration (BRTO): from the United States to Japan and back. Semin Intervent Radiol. 2011;28:283–7.
7. Arai H, Abe T, Shimoda R, et al. Emergency balloon-occluded retrograde transvenous obliteration for gastric varices. J Gastroenterol. 2005;40:964–71.
8. Park JK, Saab S, Kee ST, et al. Balloon-occluded retrograde transvenous obliteration (BRTO) for treatment of gastric varices: review and meta-analysis. Dig Dis Sci. 2015;60:1543.
9. Olson E, Yune HY, Klatte EC. Transrenal-vein reflux ethanol sclerosis of gastroesophageal varices. AJR Am J Roentgenol. 1984;143:627–8.
10. Kim SK, Lee KA, Sauk S, et al. Comparison of transjugular intrahepatic portosystemic shunt with covered stent and balloon-occluded retrograde transvenous obliteration in managing isolated gastric varices. Korean J Radiol. 2017;18:345–54.
11. Saad WE, Darcy MD. Transjugular intrahepatic portosystemic shunt (TIPS) versus balloon-occluded retrograde transvenous obliteration (BRTO) for the management of gastric varices. Semin Intervent Radiol. 2011;28:339–49.

12. Ryan BM, Stockbrugger RW, Ryan JM. A pathophysiologic, gastroenterologic, and radiologic approach to the management of gastric varices. Gastroenterology. 2004;126:1175–89.
13. Saad WE. Balloon-occluded retrograde transvenous obliteration of gastric varices: concept, basic techniques, and outcomes. Semin Intervent Radiol. 2012;29:118–28.
14. Saad WE, Simon PO Jr, Rose SC. Balloon-occluded retrograde transvenous obliteration of gastric varices. Cardiovasc Intervent Radiol. 2014;37:299–315.
15. Chao Y, Lin HC, Lee FY, et al. Hepatic hemodynamic features in patients with esophageal or gastric varices. J Hepatol. 1993;19:85–9.
16. de Franchis R, Primignani M. Natural history of portal hypertension in patients with cirrhosis. Clin Liver Dis. 2001;5:645–63.
17. Garcia-Pagan JC, Barrufet M, Cardenas A, et al. Management of gastric varices. Clin Gastroenterol Hepatol. 2014;12:919.
18. Lopera JE. Gastric varices. Radiographics. 2013;33:100–1.
19. Laleman W, Simon-Talero M, Maleux G, et al. Embolization of large spontaneous portosystemic shunts for refractory hepatic encephalopathy: a multicenter survey on safety and efficacy. Hepatology. 2013;57:2448–57.
20. Cho SK, Shin SW, Lee IH, et al. Balloon-occluded retrograde transvenous obliteration of gastric varices: outcomes and complications in 49 patients. AJR Am J Roentgenol. 2007;189:W365–72.
21. Binmoeller KF, Borsatto R. Variceal bleeding and portal hypertension. Endoscopy. 2000;32:189–99.
22. Segawa M, Sakaida I. Diagnosis and treatment of portal hypertension. Hepatol Res. 2009;39:1039–43.
23. Toubia N, Sanyal AJ. Portal hypertension and variceal hemorrhage. Med Clin North Am. 2008;92:551–74, viii.
24. Turon F, Casu S, Hernandez-Gea V, et al. Variceal and other portal hypertension related bleeding. Best Pract Res Clin Gastroenterol. 2013;27:649–64.
25. Kirby JM, Cho KJ, Midia M. Image-guided intervention in management of complications of portal hypertension: more than TIPS for success. Radiographics. 2013;33:1473–96.
26. Ninoi T, Nakamura K, Kaminou T, et al. TIPS versus transcatheter sclerotherapy for gastric varices. AJR Am J Roentgenol. 2004;183:369–76.
27. Maruyama H, Yokosuka O. Current management of gastric varices. JNMA J Nepal Med Assoc. 2007;46:143–50.
28. Sarin SK, Agarwal SR. Gastric varices and portal hypertensive gastropathy. Clin Liver Dis. 2001;5:727–67, x.
29. Sarin SK, Lahoti D, Saxena SP, et al. Prevalence, classification and natural history of gastric varices: a long-term follow-up study in 568 portal hypertension patients. Hepatology. 1992;16:1343–9.
30. Yoshida H, Mamada Y, Taniai N, et al. Treatment modalities for bleeding esophagogastric varices. J Nippon Med Sch. 2012;79:19–30.
31. Ali SM, Wu S, Xu H, et al. A prospective study of endoscopic injection sclerotherapy and endoscopic variceal ligation in the treatment of esophageal varices. J Laparoendosc Adv Surg Tech A. 2017;27:333–41.
32. Emori K, Toyonaga A, Oho K, et al. Balloon-occluded retrograde transvenous obliteration versus endoscopic injection sclerotherapy for isolated gastric varices: a comparative study. Kurume Med J. 2014;60:105–13.
33. Caldwell S. Gastric varices: is there a role for endoscopic cyanoacrylates, or are we entering the BRTO era? Am J Gastroenterol. 2012;107:1784–90.
34. Al-Osaimi AM, Caldwell SH. Medical and endoscopic management of gastric varices. Semin Intervent Radiol. 2011;28:273–82.
35. Hong CH, Kim HJ, Park JH, et al. Treatment of patients with gastric variceal hemorrhage: endoscopic N-butyl-2-cyanoacrylate injection versus balloon-occluded retrograde transvenous obliteration. J Gastroenterol Hepatol. 2009;24:372–8.
36. Huang YH, Yeh HZ, Chen GH, et al. Endoscopic treatment of bleeding gastric varices by N-butyl-2-cyanoacrylate (Histoacryl) injection: long-term efficacy and safety. Gastrointest Endosc. 2000;52:160–7.
37. Akahoshi T, Hashizume M, Tomikawa M, et al. Long-term results of balloon-occluded retrograde transvenous obliteration for gastric variceal bleeding and risky gastric varices: a 10-year experience. J Gastroenterol Hepatol. 2008;23:1702–9.
38. Akahoshi T, Tomikawa M, Kamori M, et al. Impact of balloon-occluded retrograde transvenous obliteration on management of isolated fundal gastric variceal bleeding. Hepatol Res. 2012;42:385–93.
39. Fukuda T, Hirota S, Sugimura K. Long-term results of balloon-occluded retrograde transvenous obliteration for the treatment of gastric varices and hepatic encephalopathy. J Vasc Interv Radiol. 2001;12:327–36.
40. Hirota S, Matsumoto S, Tomita M, et al. Retrograde transvenous obliteration of gastric varices. Radiology. 1999;211:349–56.
41. Sonomura T, Ono W, Sato M, et al. Three benefits of microcatheters for retrograde transvenous obliteration of gastric varices. World J Gastroenterol. 2012;18:1373–8.
42. Kobayakawa M, Kokubu S, Hirota S, et al. Short-term safety and efficacy of balloon-occluded retrograde transvenous obliteration using ethanolamine oleate: results of a prospective, multicenter, single-arm trial. J Vasc Interv Radiol. 2017;28:1108–1115 e2.
43. Chu HH, Kim M, Kim HC, et al. Long-term outcomes of balloon-occluded retrograde transvenous obliteration for the treatment of gastric varices: a comparison of ethanolamine oleate and sodium tetradecyl sulfate. Cardiovasc Intervent Radiol. 2018;41:578–86.
44. Gwon DI, Kim YH, Ko GY, et al. Vascular plug-assisted retrograde transvenous obliteration for the treatment of gastric varices and hepatic encephalopathy: a prospective multicenter study. J Vasc Interv Radiol. 2015;26:1589–95.
45. Saad WE, Kitanosono T, Koizumi J, et al. The conventional balloon-occluded retrograde transvenous obliteration procedure: indications, contraindications, and technical applications. Tech Vasc Interv Radiol. 2013;16:101–51.
46. Saad WE, Sabri SS. Balloon-occluded retrograde transvenous obliteration (BRTO): technical results and outcomes. Semin Intervent Radiol. 2011;28:333–8.
47. Sabri SS, Saad WE. Balloon-occluded retrograde transvenous obliteration (BRTO): technique and intraprocedural imaging. Semin Intervent Radiol. 2011;28:303–13.
48. Chang MY, Kim MD, Kim T, et al. Plug-assisted retrograde transvenous obliteration for the treatment of gastric variceal hemorrhage. Korean J Radiol. 2016;17:230–8.
49. Kim YH, Kim YH, Kim CS, et al. Comparison of balloon-occluded retrograde transvenous obliteration (BRTO) using ethanolamine oleate (EO), BRTO using sodium tetradecyl sulfate (STS) foam and vascular plug-assisted retrograde transvenous obliteration (PARTO). Cardiovasc Intervent Radiol. 2016;39:840–6.
50. Sabri SS, Swee W, Turba UC, et al. Bleeding gastric varices obliteration with balloon-occluded retrograde transvenous obliteration using sodium tetradecyl sulfate foam. J Vasc Interv Radiol. 2011;22:309–16; quiz 316.
51. Gandini R, Chiocchi M, Konda D, et al. Transcatheter foam sclerotherapy of symptomatic female varicocele with sodium-tetradecyl-sulfate foam. Cardiovasc Intervent Radiol. 2008;31:778–84.
52. Yamaki T, Nozaki M, Sakurai H, et al. Prospective randomized efficacy of ultrasound-guided foam sclerotherapy compared with ultrasound-guided liquid sclerotherapy in the treatment of symptomatic venous malformations. J Vasc Surg. 2008;47:578–84.
53. Kessler J, Trerotola SO. Use of the Amplatzer Vascular Plug for embolization of a large retroperitoneal shunt during transjugular intrahepatic portosystemic shunt creation for gastric variceal bleeding. J Vasc Interv Radiol. 2006;17:135–40.

54. Yoo H, Ko GY, Gwon DI, et al. Preoperative portal vein embolization using an amplatzer vascular plug. Eur Radiol. 2009;19:1054–61.
55. Park JK, Cho SK, Kee S, et al. Vascular plug-assisted retrograde transvenous obliteration of portosystemic shunts for refractory hepatic encephalopathy: a case report. Case Rep Radiol. 2014;2014:391420.
56. Itou C, Koizumi J, Hashimoto T, et al. Balloon-occluded retrograde transvenous obliteration for the treatment of gastric varices: polidocanol foam versus liquid ethanolamine oleate. AJR Am J Roentgenol. 2015;205:659–66.
57. Jang SY, Kim GH, Park SY, et al. Clinical outcomes of balloon-occluded retrograde transvenous obliteration for the treatment of gastric variceal hemorrhage in Korean patients with liver cirrhosis: a retrospective multicenter study. Clin Mol Hepatol. 2012;18:368–74.
58. Kiyosue H, Tanoue S, Kondo Y, et al. Balloon-occluded retrograde transvenous obliteration of complex gastric varices assisted by temporary balloon occlusion of the splenic artery. J Vasc Interv Radiol. 2011;22:1045–8.
59. Ninoi T, Nishida N, Kaminou T, et al. Balloon-occluded retrograde transvenous obliteration of gastric varices with gastrorenal shunt: long-term follow-up in 78 patients. AJR Am J Roentgenol. 2005;184:1340–6.
60. Rossle M, Piotraschke J. Transjugular intrahepatic portosystemic shunt and hepatic encephalopathy. Dig Dis. 1996;14(Suppl 1):12–9.
61. Kumamoto M, Toyonaga A, Inoue H, et al. Long-term results of balloon-occluded retrograde transvenous obliteration for gastric fundal varices: hepatic deterioration links to portosystemic shunt syndrome. J Gastroenterol Hepatol. 2010;25:1129–35.
62. Saad WE, Wagner CC, Al-Osaimi A, et al. The effect of balloon-occluded transvenous obliteration of gastric varices and gastrorenal shunts on the hepatic synthetic function: a comparison between Child-Pugh and model for end-stage liver disease scores. Vasc Endovascular Surg. 2013;47:281–7.
63. Mukund A, Rajesh S, Arora A, et al. Efficacy of balloon-occluded retrograde transvenous obliteration of large spontaneous lienorenal shunt in patients with severe recurrent hepatic encephalopathy with foam sclerotherapy: initial experience. J Vasc Interv Radiol. 2012;23:1200–6.
64. Suraweera D, Sundaram V, Saab S. Evaluation and management of hepatic encephalopathy: current status and future directions. Gut Liver. 2016;10:509–19.
65. Kasuga A, Mizumoto H, Matsutani S, et al. Portal hemodynamics and clinical outcomes of patients with gastric varices after balloon-occluded retrograde transvenous obliteration. J Hepatobiliary Pancreat Sci. 2010;17:898–903.
66. Hiraga N, Aikata H, Takaki S, et al. The long-term outcome of patients with bleeding gastric varices after balloon-occluded retrograde transvenous obliteration. J Gastroenterol. 2007;42:663–72.
67. Kitamoto M, Imamura M, Kamada K, et al. Balloon-occluded retrograde transvenous obliteration of gastric fundal varices with hemorrhage. AJR Am J Roentgenol. 2002;178:1167–74.
68. Chikamori F, Kuniyoshi N, Shibuya S, et al. Eight years of experience with transjugular retrograde obliteration for gastric varices with gastrorenal shunts. Surgery. 2001;129:414–20.
69. Koito K, Namieno T, Nagakawa T, et al. Balloon-occluded retrograde transvenous obliteration for gastric varices with gastrorenal or gastrocaval collaterals. AJR Am J Roentgenol. 1996;167:1317–20.

Endoscopy and Endoscopic Ultrasound for the Evaluation and Treatment of Gastric and Ectopic Varices

57

Mihai Rimbaş and Alberto Larghi

Key Concepts

- Acute variceal bleeding from gastric varices is one of the most serious complications of portal hypertension, being associated with an increased mortality;
- Bleeding from ectopic gastrointestinal varices occurs much less frequently than in esophagogastric varices, but the clinical course is usually more severe;
- The endoscopic injection of N-butyl-2-cyanoacrylate has become accepted as the primary intervention for bleeding gastrointestinal varices and is being preferred over other therapies;
- Endoscopic ultrasound can assess directly the variceal blood flow and thus identify the potential for recurrent bleeding of the gastrointestinal varices;
- Endoscopic ultrasound can also guide endoscopic treatment of complex variceal bleeding with direct glue injection and/or coil embolization, and can also direct subsequent endoscopic treatments until complete obliteration of the varices is obtained.

57.1 Introduction

Development of varices of the gastrointestinal (GI) tract is a consequence of an increased pressure in the portal venous system, a condition referred to as portal hypertension (PH). While most of the patients with PH have liver cirrhosis, PH can also develop in the absence of cirrhosis, i.e. "non-cirrhotic PH", which has multiple recognized etiologies, including extrahepatic thrombosis of the portal vein or of its tributary mesenteric vessels, infection (such as schistosomiasis), autoimmunity, drugs, immunodeficiency, or idiopathic causes.

Varices are present in about 50% of patients with PH and, at least in those with liver cirrhosis, they form at a rate of 5–15% per year. Acute variceal bleeding (AVB) is the most serious complication of PH. It occurs in one third of patients with GI varices and it is associated with an increased mortality up to 20% at 6 weeks in patients with already decompensated liver cirrhosis [1]. Noteworthy, bleeding from GI varices is usually better tolerated in patients with non-cirrhotic PH due to their preserved liver function.

Establishing the correct diagnosis in cases of acute GI bleeding is very important. In patients with known liver cirrhosis or PH, any upper GI bleeding needs to be emergently evaluated endoscopically and the source of bleeding should be considered of variceal origin until proven otherwise. On the other hand, variceal bleeding can represent the initial clinical presentation of a previously unknown cirrhotic or non-cirrhotic patient with PH. The outcome of an AVB episode mostly depends on the control of the active bleeding and the avoidance of major complications usually related to the presence of an impaired liver function. Notably, only 50% of these patients stop bleeding spontaneously [2], thus a short time accessibility to a GI endoscopy Unit with experience in variceal management is of utmost importance.

The management of patients with variceal hemorrhage requires a multidisciplinary approach, which includes intensivists, endoscopists, interventional radiologists, hepatologists,

M. Rimbaş (✉)
Gastroenterology Department, Colentina Clinical Hospital, Bucharest, Romania

Internal Medicine Department, Carol Davila University of Medicine, Bucharest, Romania
e-mail: mihai.rimbas@umfcd.ro

A. Larghi
Digestive Endoscopy Unit, Fondazione Policlinico Universitario A. Gemelli, IRCCS, Rome, Italy

F. Radu-Ionita et al. (eds.), *Liver Diseases*, https://doi.org/10.1007/978-3-030-24432-3_57

and surgeons. Standard diagnostic upper GI endoscopy should always be preceded by proper patient resuscitation in order to restore and maintain hemodynamic stability, and by endotracheal intubation in cases of altered consciousness to protect the airways during the endoscopic examination to avoid aspiration. Volume replacement through a venous central line should be given to maintain a systemic blood pressure greater than 100 mmHg, with caution not to overload the patient because this may result in difficulty in achieving bleeding control and in a higher risk of re-bleeding [3]. Hemoglobin level should be maintained between 7 and 8 g/dl through blood transfusion, which is associated with reduction in further bleeding, in complications rates and in mortality [4].

At present there are no absolute contraindications regarding the coagulation parameters that preclude the performance of the endoscopic treatment. However in patients with AVB, efforts to improve the coagulation status before performing the endoscopic procedure should be attempted [5]. Vasoactive drugs, such as somatostatin, vasopressin, and their analogs octreotide and terlipressin, which determine constriction of the mesenteric arterioles and decrease in the portal blood flow, should also be administered as soon as possible before endoscopy, and continued for up to 3–5 days in cases of confirmed AVB [6]. Their early utilization reduces the rate of active bleeding, and in combination with endoscopic therapy improves hemostasis and reduces short-term mortality, transfusion requirement, and duration of hospitalization [7]. In patients with cirrhosis presenting with upper GI bleeding, it is also important to administer broad spectrum antibiotic prophylaxis (such as intravenous ceftriaxone 1 g/24 h) to prevent spontaneous bacterial peritonitis, and lactulose or rifaximin that may avoid the occurrence of hepatic encephalopathy [6].

In these patients upper GI endoscopy is an emergency and should be performed within 12 h from presentation [6]. In the absence of a QT prolongation or other contraindications, i.v. administration of 250 mg of erythromycin 30–120 min before endoscopy should be considered to increase gastric motility and promote emptying of the stomach from blood clots [6]. This results in an improved endoscopic visualization and in a significant decrease in the need for repeat endoscopy [8]. On the contrary, nasogastric aspiration or lavage are not routinely recommended based on the available literature.

The goal of endoscopic treatment is obliteration of the variceal bleeding vessel(s), which must be followed by additional endoscopic re-evaluation to confirm variceal obturation and to assess the need for retreatment. In cases in which endoscopic control of variceal bleeding fails, other rescue procedures, such as transjugular intrahepatic portosystemic shunt (TIPSS), balloon-occluded retrograde transvenous obliteration (BRTO), or creation of a surgical porto-caval shunt must be considered early in the course of the acute event. It should be remembered that Child-Pugh and MELD scores, besides failure to achieve primary hemostasis, predict the 6-week mortality in AVBs occurring in cirrhotic patients [6]. Therapy with non-selective beta-blockers on the long term is considered necessary for all surviving an AVB episode, if not otherwise contraindicated [6].

57.2 Gastric Varices

Gastric varices (GVs) are identified endoscopically in about 20% of patients with PH [9, 10]. Sixty-five percent of these patients present with AVB within 2 years [11], which is usually more severe and associated with a higher mortality rate than bleeding from esophageal varices [12]. Gastric varices appear endoscopically as protruding lesions into the gastric lumen, which sometimes can be confounded with a submucosal lesion. Their appearance as a cluster of varices, or in connection with the esophageal varices helps distinguish them from other types of lesions. Nonetheless, without an active bleeding site, small lesions can be difficult to be localized endoscopically, likewise to what happens with larger lesions when the stomach is filled up with blood clots in cases of AVB.

Similarly to esophageal varices, GVs are located within the submucosa layer, but are anatomically different from the former. In many cases, GVs are composed by multiple variceal veins, interconnected to each other and forming a variceal net spreading over the gastric fundus, which has usually more than one feeding vessel. Therefore, it is understandable why rubber band ligation or clipping are not effective, and sometimes even dangerous [13], in treating such complex vascular structures.

According to Sarin's classification, GVs are divided in four subtypes considering their location and isolation status, as shown in Fig. 57.1—GOV 1: gastroesophageal varices along the lesser curvature of the stomach, the most frequently encountered (75% of GVs); GOV 2: gastric varices in the fundus continuing esophageal varices along the greater curvature of the stomach; IGV 1: isolated gastric varices in the fundus, and IGV 2: isolated gastric varices at other loci in the stomach, which are extremely rare [14]. IGVs result more frequently than GOVs from segmental PH due to splenic vein thrombosis. Noteworthy, IGV 1, although less frequently encountered, bleed much more frequently (about 90%) than other types of GVs, as described in a prospective study on 568 consecutive patients with GVs [9]. What exactly triggers an AVB episode from a gastric varix is unknown. However, a number of risk factors for GVs bleeding have been identified, such as advanced Child-Pugh stage, presence of variceal red spots, and an increase in variceal size [15].

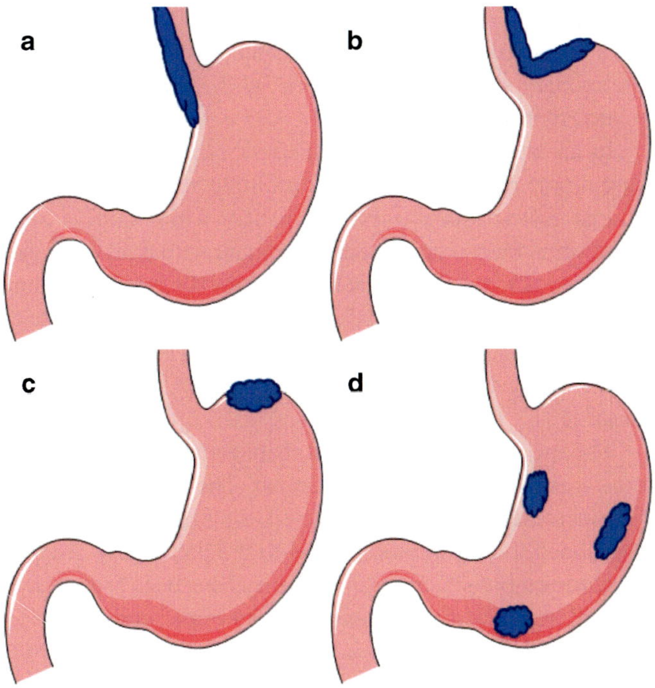

Fig. 57.1 Types of gastric varices according to Sarin's classification: (**a**) Gastroesophageal varices type 1 (GOV 1). (**b**) Gastroesophageal varices type 2 (GOV 2). (**c**) Isolated gastric varices type 1 (IGV 1). (**d**) Isolated gastric varices type 2 (IGV 2)

An upper GI endoscopic procedure in a patient at high risk of GVs acute bleeding starts with the search for the source of bleeding. Careful exploration of the esophagus, the duodenum and the gastric antrum to rule out other causes of bleeding should be performed first. In cases in which the fundus is filled up with blood clots and the examination was started with the patient on the left decubitus, a change to the right decubitus can be helpful to move part of the clots away from the gastric fundus in order to be able to better assess for the presence of GVs. Actively bleeding GVs, those with stigmata of recent bleeding (such as a fibrin plug) or GVs with endoscopic red signs should be targeted first by the endoscopic treatment.

57.2.1 Endoscopic Treatment

The therapeutic role of endoscopy in treating GVs has been described for the first time by Soehendra et al. in 1986, who performed injection of glue directly into a gastric varix [16]. Since then, endoscopic injection of N-butyl-2-cyanoacrylate (NBC), also known as cyanoacrylate glue, has become accepted as the primary intervention for actively bleeding GVs and is being preferred over other therapies [17, 18], according to multiple society guidelines [6]. However, the American Association for the Study of Liver Disease (AASLD) still recommends TIPSS as the first treatment modality for cardio-fundal varices, while NBC injection is recognized as an alternative to TIPSS in case the latter is not technically feasible [14]. N-butyl-2-cyanoacrylate, however, is not FDA approved for this use in the USA due to the fear of systemic embolism. In Canada, a similar compound, 2-octylcyanoacrylate, is presently used in clinical practice [19].

A previous or an active bleeding from GVs are clear-cut indications for GVs treatment, with the therapeutic goal to achieve variceal obliteration and cessation of the hemorrhage. In a study on 77 patients with previous GVs bleeding, after a median follow-up of 26 months, endoscopic treatment with NBC was associated with lower re-bleeding (15% vs. 55%) and mortality rates (3% vs. 25%) compared to beta-blockers [20]. Injection of NBC has been proven to be more effective and safer than endoscopic band ligation (EBL) and injection of sclerosants in this subset of patients with GVs [21]. For patients with GOV 1 varices, EBL can also be used to treat the GVs [6]. In a non-randomized study on 162 patients with GOV 1 varices, successful hemostasis with EBL was similar to that with NBC (85% vs. 89%, $p = 0.7$). However, a higher incidence of re-bleeding from the post-treatment ulcer (16% vs. 5%, $p = 0.04$), and a higher mortality rate (23% vs. 14%, $p < 0.001$) over a follow-up of 42 days was associated with EBL treatment [22]. Moreover, a recent systematic review has suggested that endoscopic NBC injection may be more effective than EBL in terms of preventing re-bleeding from GVs [23]. However, this inference was based on very low quality evidence data and other studies are needed before any conclusion can be drawn.

Injection of NBC is, therefore, considered at present the best endoscopic treatment for GVs to achieve control of bleeding and decrease the re-bleeding rates. The presence of large (>10 mm) GOV 2 or IGV 1 varices without previous bleeding episodes might also constitute an indication for prophylactic endoscopic treatment. In a randomized study [24] on 89 patients followed for a mean of 26 months with large (>10 mm) GOV 2 or IGV 1 GVs and no previous bleeding episodes, bleeding occurred in a significantly smaller proportion of patients prophylactically treated with NBC injection (10%), than in those treated with beta-blockers (38%) or no treatment (53%). In this study, the size of the varix (>20 mm), a MELD score ≥17 and presence of portal hypertensive gastropathy were all associated with an increased risk of GVs bleeding. However, further data are needed to better evaluate the risk/benefit of prophylactic endoscopic treatment of large (>10 mm) GOV 2 or IGV 1 varices with NBC in this patient population [6].

Cyanoacrylate, upon contact with water or blood, undergoes rapid polymerization and transformation into a hard plug, leading to obstruction of the varix. Some centers use for fluoroscopic visualization a mixture of N-butyl-2-cyanoacrylate and Lipiodol typically in a 1:1 ratio, usually delivered through a regular endoscopic needle into the variceal lumen. Each injecting shot should contain no more than 1–2 mL of glue and an equal volume of Lipiodol. Fluoroscopy should be used in real time to trace the opaque mixture within the varix if Lipiodol mixture is being used, and to identify signs of embolization, which should determine prompt cessation of the injection. More recently the use of Lipiodol has been abandoned and undiluted glue has been injected intravariceally into the GVs followed by injection of 2 ml of normal saline to deliver the entire glue from the injector into the varix.

The maximum dose of cyanoacrylate glue to be used has not yet been established [25]. The total dose administered is at the discretion of the endoscopist and is based on the size of the GV and the result of the initial injection. However, a study comparing glue injection in patients with cirrhosis and those with extrahepatic portal venous obstruction (EHPVO) showed that patients with EHPVO required higher volumes of glue and more glue sessions for GVs obliteration [26]. At the end of the injection, the needle should be withdrawn while flushed with saline or sterile water to decrease the risk of needle embedment. Injections can be repeated until GVs appear occluded, which can be judged by probing the lesion with the closed needle catheter. After the injection, the needle is immediately withdrawn and kept outside the endoscope to prevent glue blockage of the endoscope working channel. Once outside the patient, the injector needle is cut and only then extracted from the working channel of the endoscope [26].

After initial hemostasis is achieved, the recommendations are to repeat NBC injection on a 2–4 week basis until variceal obliteration is achieved, and for GVs type GOV 1 and GOV 2 to eradicate esophageal varices as well. The American Society of Gastrointestinal Endoscopy (ASGE) does not have a recommendation for secondary prophylaxis, and there is a lack of consistent evidence for the combination of glue injection and non-selective beta-blockers for the secondary prophylaxis of GVs bleeding. In one randomized trial on 95 patients, there was no difference in re-bleeding rates between those who received a combination therapy (NBC injections until GV obliteration and non-selective beta blockers) and those treated with glue injections alone for up to 3 years (52% versus 47%). Mortality rates were also similar between the two groups [27]. However, combination therapy is still recommended at present [28].

Endoscopic glue therapy for GVs has been reported to achieve hemostasis in more than 90% of cases in most series [28]. There have been, however, a number of adverse events related to the procedure, including further hemorrhage [29], with re-bleeding rates as high as 15–30% after glue injections alone [30], and embolization of glue material, which has been reported in several observational studies [31–35], with also fatal outcomes [36–39]. However, in a series of 753 patients [40], complications of endoscopic glue therapy for GVs included infection (1.4%) and distant embolization (pulmonary or systemic; 0.7%), while the complication-related mortality rate was 0.5%.

In an attempt to decrease the risk of embolization, one case report presented the use of multiple clips positioned on a large gastric fundal varix in a patient with a large gastrorenal shunt before endoscopic treatment with 8 ml of cyanoacrylate, 25 ml lauromacrogol and 10 ml of sodium morrhuate, with good final results and without occurrence of any embolism. However, placement of one of the clips was associated with rupture of the varix and variceal hemorrhage [13].

The use of NBC for variceal management requires, however, a multidisciplinary assessment. The risk of embolization increases with greater injected volumes, and as already mentioned, besides embolization to the pulmonary arteries, systemic embolism and even fatalities have been reported. In a small series of five patients with systemic embolism following endoscopic NBC injection, the mortality rate was 40%, and the overall re-bleeding rate after anticoagulation was 20% [41]. Upon review of imaging studies, three of the five patients had evident portosystemic shunts, while the remaining two cases had no prominent vascular anomaly. In a thorough review of the literature [41], including 27 studies, the authors found that the majority of occurrences were represented by pulmonary embolism (44%) and splenic infarction (33%), while only a few events were attributed to cardiac abnormalities such as patent foramen ovale, with right-to-left shunt, which was however not solidly proven. Therefore, while the known presence of a patent foramen ovale represents an absolute contraindication to variceal NBC injection, the exclusion of the presence of septal defects prior to the endoscopic treatment is not recommended at the present time, especially in patients who are presenting with AVB. The authors emphasized the importance of the technique utilized with injection of only small amounts of NBC mixture each time, which can minimize the risk of embolization [41]. It is also justified to perform BRTO-assisted GV obliteration for patients with large gastrorenal or splenorenal shunts by occlusion of the draining veins using a balloon device, followed by injection of the sclerosing agent directly into the variceal veins, thus preventing the occurrence of systemic NBC embolism.

With regard to EBL, the procedure is used in GOV 1 if technically feasible, and works by capturing all or part of the GV within the ligating device. Thrombosis of the varix is followed within a few days by tissue necrosis sloughing off, which leaves a superficial ulcer that rapidly heals. More than one band can be deployed in a single endoscopic session.

Endoscopic sclerotherapy of GVs using polidocanol, absolute alcohol, ethanolamine oleate and sodium tetradecyl sulfate has also been reported in small uncontrolled series, but appeared less effective in the control of bleeding from GVs than from esophageal varices [23]. Other treatments including loop ligation and endoscopic human thrombin injection have been tested in some centers with good initial results [23], but their use remains experimental.

The endoscopic treatment of acute GVs bleeding may be extremely difficult in patients with severe bleeding due to impaired endoscopic view with impossibility in the visualization of the bleeding vessel(s). In such cases, balloon tamponade could represent a temporary option to attempt bleeding control, while definitive treatment is being arranged. However, it can be associated with serious complications, such as aspiration pneumonia, esophageal necrosis or even perforation. Another way to temporary stop the bleeding is through the use of a hemostatic powder (TC-325 or Hemospray, Cook Medical, Winston-Salem, North Carolina, USA), which forms a cohesive mechanical barrier covering the bleeding site in AVB, resulting in temporary hemostasis in the majority of patients. Its use allows early elective endoscopy to be safely and effectively performed on the next day within 12–24 h [42]. The use of the hemostatic powder should also be considered as a rescue therapy for failure of primary endoscopic therapy or for early relapse of bleeding.

57.2.2 The Role of Endoscopic Ultrasound

The role of standard GI endoscopy is sometimes limited since it visualizes only the gastric mucosa and cannot evaluate deeper structures of the GI wall and beyond it. Differently, endoscopic ultrasound (EUS) is able to visualize the five layers of the GI wall, including intramural varices, as well as, surrounding vascular structures. Indeed, EUS detects GVs almost twice more often as compared with standard upper GI endoscopy (Fig. 57.2) [43, 44]. In a study on 52 patients with liver cirrhosis, GVs were detected in 30.8% of the patients by EUS as compared to 17.3% by standard endoscopy [43]. At EUS examination, GVs are seen as tubular anechoic structures located just beneath the muscularis mucosae layer, into the submucosal layer of the gastric wall (Fig. 57.3). The use of Doppler easily differentiates GVs from other types of submucosal lesions, which is important in order to avoid taking endoscopic biopsies. Gastric varices can also be easily measured by EUS, and their size strongly correlates with their blood flow volume [45]. Moreover, feeding perforating vessels can also be visualized by EUS in roughly 80% of cases, traversing the muscularis propria and connecting the submucosal varices to the esophagogastric collateral veins [46].

Endoscopic ultrasound has been also utilized to evaluate the response to previous endoscopic treatment. Successful obliteration is confirmed by absence of blood flow on color or pulsed Doppler examinations. In a retrospective study enrolling 101 patients who were treated with NBC injection after an episode of GVs hemorrhage, significantly lower rebleeding rates were seen in those in whom EUS was aggressively used during follow-up (biweekly) to assess complete obliteration and guide the subsequent need for repeat endoscopic treatment sessions (19% vs. 45%, $p = 0.005$) [47].

Since the re-bleeding risk in GVs is associated with persistent variceal flow, a possible role of therapeutic EUS for GVs was foreseen. Besides confirming cessation of variceal blood flow, indicative of variceal obliteration [48], EUS allows the endosonographer to very precisely deliver under real time ultrasound control the therapeutic agent into the varix or into its feeding vessel(s) [49, 50] (Fig. 57.4). Table 57.1 presents all the studies evaluating EUS-guided treatments of GVs. In the first such study by Romero-Castro et al. [49], five patients were treated by EUS-guided injection of NBC. The perforating veins feeding the GVs were targeted until no flow was visible on Doppler EUS examination. GVs eradication was confirmed in all five patients after

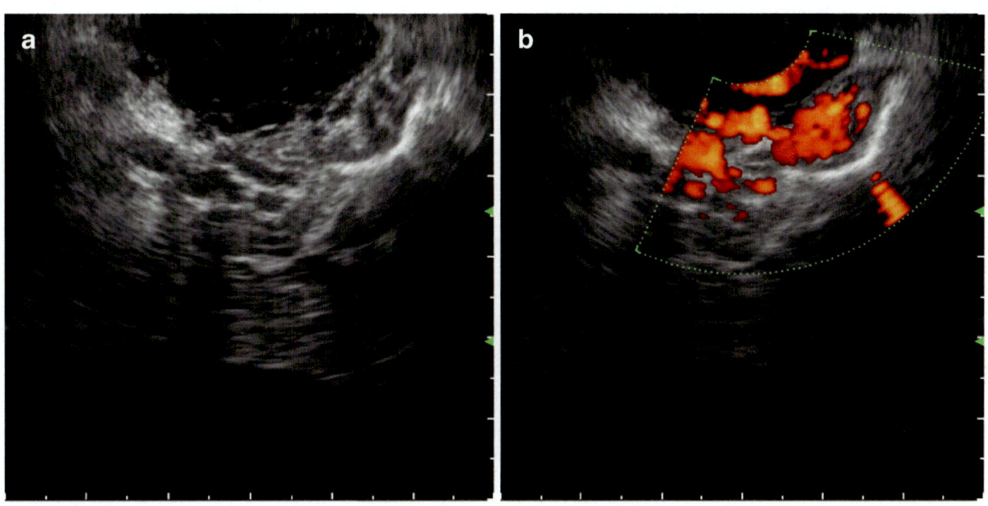

Fig. 57.2 (**a**) EUS view from the gastroesophageal junction with multiple small (<5 mm) gastric varices seen within the submucosal layer, which were not detected by standard endoscopy. (**b**) Doppler confirmation of flow within the variceal vessels

a mean of 1.6 endoscopic sessions, with no procedural-related complications, and no recurrent bleeding over 10 months of follow-up. However, the authors stated that identification of the feeding vessel was extremely difficult and time consuming.

In another single-center study on 40 patients (13 with active bleeding), EUS-guided NBC injection was performed into the perforating veins located within the gastric wall, with subsequent sessions performed until GVs were eradicated [50]. Control of acute bleeding was obtained in all cases, with only two complications (transient bacteriemia in one case and recurrence of bleeding in another one) [50]. The results of this study highly suggested that active bleeding from GVs could be successfully treated endoscopically under EUS guidance, without the need for cleaning up the gastric cavity from blood clots, because with EUS structures are recognized without the need for endoscopic view.

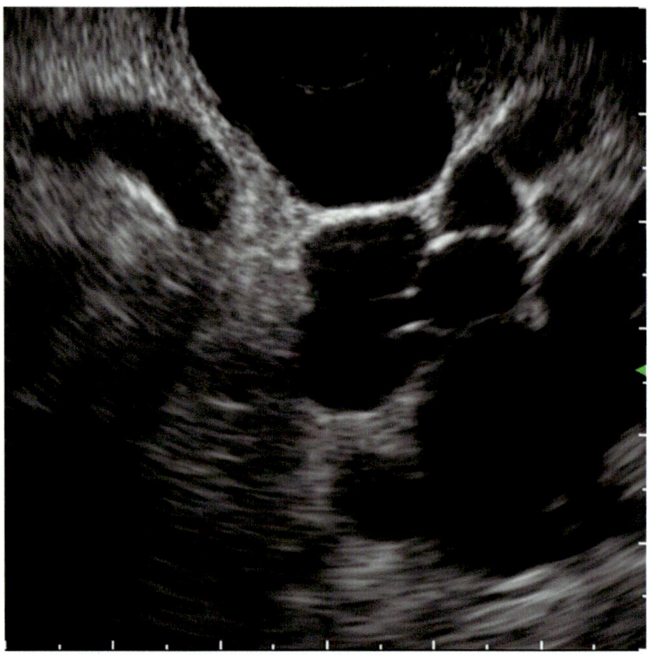

Fig. 57.3 EUS appearance of a large cluster of gastric varices interconnected to each other

In a small case series of eight patients [54], another therapeutic agent (thrombin) was administered under EUS-guidance until variceal flow obliteration or until a maximum dose of 10,000 IU was reached. In two of the three patients with active hemorrhage the treatment was successful. In the third one, variceal obliteration was not achieved despite injection of the maximum dose of thrombin. On the other hand, complete variceal obliteration was achieved in all the five patients electively treated to prevent future bleeding. In one case, however, complete restoration of blood flow within the gastric varices was observed after 8 months of follow-up. There were no procedure-related complications.

Another way to treat GVs is by performing EUS-guided intravascular embolization using metal coils available from interventional radiology, which are covered with synthetic fibers. They can be delivered into the target varix under EUS guidance by using standard fine needle aspiration (FNA) needles [59]. Importantly, their size needs to be tailored based upon the size of the varix in order to achieve the best results [60]. In a first feasibility study on four patients with GVs, two of whom were actively bleeding [57], insertion of stainless steel coils (MReye; IMWCE, Cook Medical, Limerick, Ireland) targeting the feeding perforating collaterals was performed, resulting in complete obliteration of the GVs in three of the four patients, with no recorded complications.

In a subsequent retrospective multicenter study [58], EUS-guided NBC injection was compared with EUS-guided coil embolization in 19 and 11 patients, respectively. GVs obliteration rates were comparable between the two groups (90.9% vs. 94.7%), but complete obliteration was achieved more often in the coil group after a single endoscopic session (52.6% vs. 81.8%). Surprisingly, 47% of the patients in the NBC group had asymptomatic glue embolism detected by CT scan that was performed as per protocol in all patients, occurrence that was not recorded in the coil group.

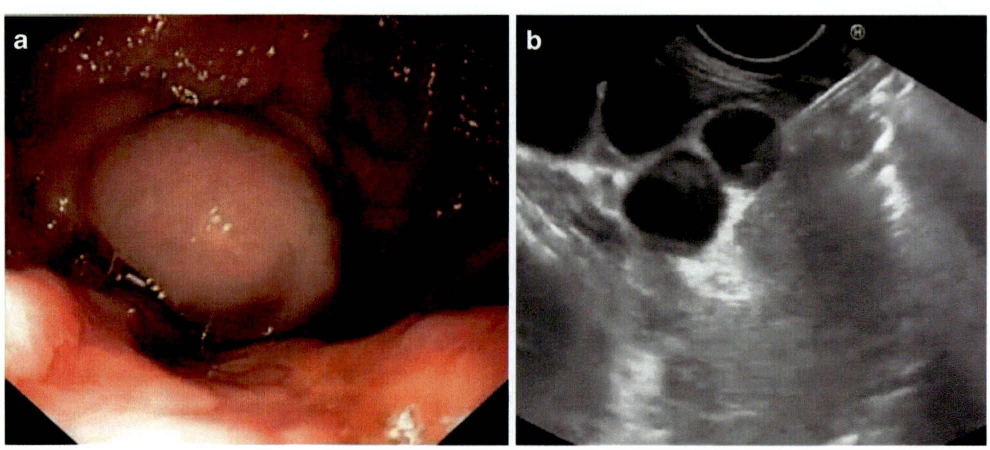

Fig. 57.4 (**a**) Endoscopic view of a large (>10 mm) fundal gastric varix with no stigmata of recent hemorrhage. (**b**) A standard FNA needle is inserted into the variceal lumen for EUS-guided glue injection

Table 57.1 Summary of studies evaluating EUS-guided treatments of gastric varices

Author (year)	Number of patients	Type of treatment	No. of sessions (average)	Confirmed obliteration	Post-treatment bleeding episodes from GV (Follow-up)	Complications
Bhat[R] (2016) [51]	152[a]	CYA and coils	1.1	93%	8%[b] (mean 14.5 mo)	3% mild abdominal pain
						1% pulmonary embolism
						3% minor bleeding from coil extrusion
Binmoeller[R] (2011) [52]	30	CYA and coils	1.0	96%	4% (mean 6.4 mo)	0%
Dedania[CR] (2018) [53]	1	STS and coils	2	Yes	0% (1 week)	None
Frost[R c] (2018) [54]	8	THR	1	87.5%	12.5% (mean 24 mo)	0%
Fujii-Lau[R] (2016) [55]	5	CYA and coils (3)	1.2	60%	0% (mean 24 mo)	0%
		Coils (2)				
Gonzales[R] (2012) [56]	3	PDL or CYA	1.0	100%	0% (mean 9.3 mo)	0%
Gubler[R] (2014) [50]	40[d]	CYA (38)	1.4	NR	15% (mean 60 mo)	2.5% minor bleeding from varix ulcer
		CYA and coils (2)				2.5% transient bacteremia
Romero-Castro[P] (2007) [49]	5	CYA	1.6	100%	0% (mean 10 mo)	0%
Romero-Castro[P] (2010) [57]	4	Coils	1.0	75%	0% (mean 5 mo)	0%
Romero-Castro[R] (2013) [58]	30	Coils (11)	1.3 (coils)	91% (coils)	0% (mean 17.2 mo)	9.1% in coil (1 bleed from EV)
		or CYA (19)	1.5 (CYA)	100% (CYA)		58% in CYA (9 asymptomatic pulmonary embolism; 1 fever; 1 chest pain)

Adapted after: Rimbaş M, et al. Endoscopic Ultrasound for the Hepatologist: A Comprehensive Review. Semin Liver Dis. 2018; 38: 145–159.
CYA cyanoacrylate, *GV* gastric varices, *R* retrospective, *mo* months, *THR* thrombin, *STS* sodium tetradecyl sulfate, *NR* not reported, *P* prospective, *PDL* polidocanol
[a]5% had active bleeding and 26% were treated for primary prophylaxis
[b]3% in the group with confirmed variceal obliteration
[c]Three patients had acute variceal bleeding and five were treated for elective prevention
[d]32.5% had active bleeding and 10% were treated for primary prophylaxis

In another large retrospective study on 152 patients with fundal GVs, seven of whom had active hemorrhage, 105 recent bleeding, and 40 were treated as a primary prophylaxis, combined EUS-guided treatment with coil insertion and NBC injection was performed [51]. The hypothesis behind the study was that the coil promotes clot aggregation, working as a scaffold to retain the glue for achieving maximal varix obliteration (Fig. 57.5). The procedure was technically successful and clinically effective in all but one patient. A mean of 1.4 (range 1–4) coils, and a mean volume of 2 ml (range 0.5–6) of NBC were utilized per patient [51]. After a mean of 1.1 treatment sessions, complete GVs obliteration was confirmed in 93% of the cases by EUS examination, while GVs bleeding occurred in only 3% of these cases after a mean follow-up interval of more than 1 year. Symptomatic pulmonary embolization occurred in only one patient (<1%).

In another report of the combined EUS-guided treatment with coil embolization and cyanoacrylate glue injection, GVs treatment was performed across the diaphragmatic crus, in an anterograde fashion, on 30 patients in one single treatment session, until absence of variceal flow was obtained [52]. With the echoendoscope positioned in the distal esophagus, much of the difficulty resulting from working with the echoendoscope in the retroflexed position was obviated. The procedure was technically successful in all patients. Ninety-six percent of them had persistent complete GVs obliteration after this single treatment session, which lasted for more than 6 months of follow-up. Only one patient had recurrent bleeding within the first month after the initial procedure.

Based on the data available so far, GVs treatment strategy should imply achievement of GVs obliteration whenever possible at the first endoscopic session, with follow-up EUS examination to confirm it, or to guide the need of more endoscopic treatments. Because of the very low risk of coil migration and no risk of embolism, EUS-guided coil insertion is being favored over GVs glue injection by some centers, though not supported by any strong available evidence. Noteworthy, combination therapy of coils and glue appears safe and effective, possibly associated with a reduced risk of embolization, but its costs are significantly higher than of NBC alone. Despite all of the above arguments, at present the only clear indication for EUS-guided treatment is when conventional endoscopic NBC injection fails to control GVs bleeding [61].

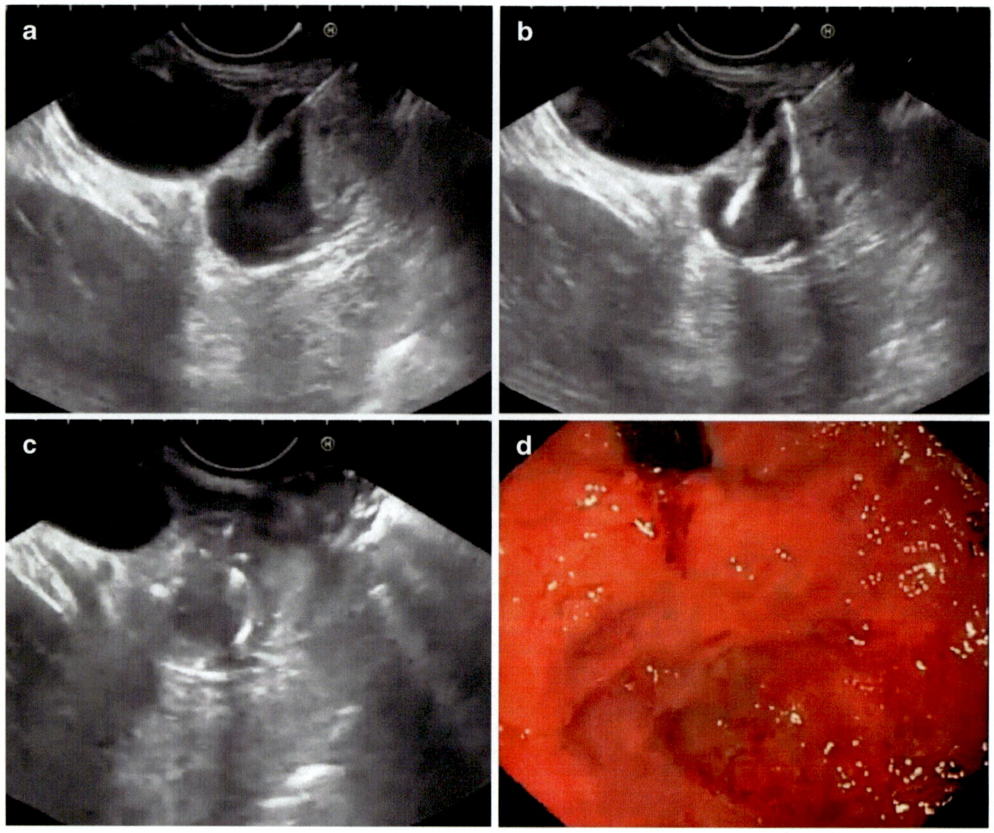

Fig. 57.5 EUS-guided GVs coil embolization. (**a**) Large group of gastric varices seen from the cardia with a standard 19G FNA inserted. (**b**) Initial placement of a coil inside the variceal lumen. (**c**) EUS image of the final result after combined coil insertion and glue injection with complete variceal lumen obliteration. (**d**) Endoscopic view of the gastric fundus after follow-up showing complete disappearance of the gastric varices

Regarding the primary prophylactic treatment of GVs, a subgroup analysis of 40 patients with large GVs and no bleeding history [51] who were treated with a combination of EUS-guided coil and glue application showed that only two bleeding episodes occurred after a mean follow-up of 449 days, supporting the results of a previous study with endoscopic NBC injection [24]. Even though these results are promising, more data are needed before any definitive conclusions can be drawn.

57.3 Ectopic Varices

Ectopic GI varices (i.e. not located in the esophagus or the stomach) are rare, being found in about 1% of patients with PH [10], and are often asymptomatic. They are vascular venous structures protruding into the lumen of the GI tract and similarly to GVs when they bleed, which occurs much less frequently than with esophago-gastric varices, the clinical course is severe [10]. Bleeding from ectopic varices (EVs) is more frequently encountered in patients with prehepatic portal hypertension than in those with liver cirrhosis [62]. Other etiologies independent of PH include familial varices, previous surgery with intra-abdominal adhesions, previous trauma with development of arterio-venous malformations, mesenteric vein thrombosis, or lymphoid hyperplasia [63]. The association of PH, prior abdominal surgery and hematochezia usually characterizes the hemorrhage from small intestinal varices [64]. Their localization and anatomy are, however, very heterogeneous and their rarity makes treatment standardization difficult. In general, the greater the size of the ectopic varices, the greater the chance of their bleeding [63]. The evaluation and treatment should therefore be made on a case-by-case basis and founded on vascular anatomy [14]. The clinical suspicion for the presence of small intestinal varices is very important for the diagnosis, which can be made with a contrast-enhanced thin-slice CT scanning in the portal venous phase, after administration of large-volume of water-soluble diluted oral contrast [14]. Confirmation could be made by endoscopic examination of the small bowel. Most frequently, ectopic varices are located at the level of surgical stomas, in the duodenum, jejunoileum, and rectum.

Management of ectopic variceal bleeding requires a good definition of their vascular supply [14]. The optimal treatment of patients with acute bleeding from ectopic varices is at present still unclear. Management options include, besides endoscopic treatment, TIPSS or BRTO, while traditional treatment has been surgery. The small number of published cases does not allow drawing firm conclusions. A guideline of the AASLD recommends TIPSS as the preferred first approach for prevention of re-bleeding in patients with ectopic GI varices [65]. However, TIPSS is associated with a number of complications and requires close follow-up for many years.

Endoscopic control of bleeding can be achieved, depending on their location and on the expertise of the center where diagnosis is made, by band ligation, injection of sclerosants or endosonographic placement of coils. As with GVs, reducing of the injected volumes of sclerosant is advocated in order to decrease the risk of embolism following the procedure. In the past, their management relied for years on surgical segmental resection of the involved intestinal area, which appears to successfully control the variceal bleeding and should always be taken into account when all the other methods fail. Radiological techniques, which are less invasive, can also be considered in these patients [66].

57.3.1 Duodenal and Jejunal Varices

Of the ectopic varices, those located in the duodenum (and especially the duodenal bulb) are particularly prone to bleed, and when this occurs the mortality can be as high as 40% [67]. Duodenal varices are usually found within the working length of a standard gastroscope and on occasion they can be incidentally discovered in patients with PH. The situation is different in the case of acute variceal bleeding, when endoscopy plays more than a diagnostic role, being the main treatment modality.

The small bowel bleeding from varices distal to the duodenum usually presents with profuse melena or hematochezia of sudden onset, or with intraperitoneal bleeding [63, 68]. In patients who present with GI bleeding and are hemodynamically stable without signs of severe bleeding, the first test that is usually performed after a negative upper GI endoscopy and colonoscopy have excluded other sources of bleeding is videocapsule endoscopy (VCE). Consideration should be given in performing the examination early (less than 3 days after hospital admission) in order to have a better detection rate of the bleeding vascular lesion [69]. The varices appear as bluish distended vascular lesions, but in the case of ongoing bleeding, the only sign could be the presence of fresh or degraded blood within the intestinal lumen. If no source of bleeding is identified after VCE and the bleeding continues, the next logical step is to perform deep small bowel enteroscopy, if available. Several methods of deep enteroscopy have been described such as single balloon, double balloon, and spiral enteroscopy. These procedures are indicated in patients with ongoing bleeding in a good enough health to tolerate the procedure. Push enteroscopy is an option in centers where deep enteroscopy is not available, but is able to evaluate only the proximal jejunum. Another possibility is intraoperative enteroscopy when regular small bowel enteroscopy does not identify the bleeding source, in cases of hemodynamic instability from ongoing bleeding, or if there are contraindications to deep enteroscopy, such as in the case of dense abdominal adhesions.

For duodenal varices, there are a number of case reports of successful endoscopic band ligation. Endoscopic sclerosant and NBC injection were also found to be effective in controlling bleeding from duodenal and jejunal varices. No severe adverse events were reported in the majority of the reported cases [70, 71]. However, cerebral infarction, along with multiple asymptomatic systemic emboli were recognized postprocedurally in a patient with patent foramen ovale [72], and re-bleeding rates of up to 50% have been reported [70].

For jejunal varices, there are only a few case reports describing successful glue treatment performed during push- or deep enteroscopy [73, 74]. However, if this treatment strategy should be generalized is unknown, but in our opinion it should be tried first, if available.

With regard to EUS, in a case report coil embolization and NBC injection emergently pursued at the patient's bedside in ICU was successful in achieving hemostasis from a duodenal varix after failed initial endoscopic injection of ethanolamine [71]. EUS has also been found to be useful in detecting ectopic varices. A case of diagnosis by EUS of bleeding from duodenal varices in a 6-year-old girl, who was transplanted for biliary atresia has been reported [75]. Indeed, the first report of EUS-guided coil embolization of bleeding GI varices was a patient with refractory bleeding secondary to choledocho-jejunal varices [76]. Successful therapeutic EUS-guided coil embolization and NBC injection in two different patients with acute duodenal variceal bleeding have also been described [77, 78]. In one case, however, the glue cast produced compression of the common bile duct resulting in obstructive jaundice. In another small case series of three patients, EUS-guided coil insertion with or without NBC injection was successfully used to treat duodenal varices [55]. No further episodes of bleeding were reported over a median follow-up of 12 months (range 1–104).

57.3.2 Choledochal Varices

Choledochal varices cannot be detected by standard gastrointestinal endoscopy. In a study on 56 patients with portal vein thrombosis, common bile duct (CBD) varices were diagnosed by EUS in 59% patients, a frequency slightly higher than that of transabdominal ultrasound (TUS) [79]. Three types of choledochal varices have been described. (i) paracholedochal, the most common, running parallel to the CBD; (ii) epicholedochal or intramural, the least common; and (iii) submucosal varices, which can protrude into the CBD lumen. Interestingly, in the previously aforementioned study [79] in 19% of the patients EUS revealed a different subtype of varices as compared to TUS. In this study nine patients had obstructive jaundice and proceeded to therapeutic ERCP, which resulted in hemobilia in two. Thus, it has been established that EUS should be performed as a diagnostic test prior to ERCP to search for choledochal varices in cases with portal vein thrombosis and obstructive jaundice [79]. As previously mentioned, successful EUS-guided treatment of bleeding ectopic choledocho-jejunal anastomotic varices was first reported in 2008 [76]. In another study [55], five patients underwent EUS-guided coil injection with or without concomitant NBC injection to treat choledochal varices. During a median follow-up of 12 (range 1–104) months, two patients did not have recurrent bleeding, while in the remaining three, the bleeding decreased significantly.

57.3.3 Rectal and Colonic Varices

Colonic varices are very rarely encountered. Their presence represents a very rare cause of lower GI hemorrhage that could be associated with PH, while other reported cases were idiopathic [80, 81]. They are usually extensive, associated with ileal varices as well and congestive changes of the ileo-colonic mucosa [82]. Decompression of the portal system represents the treatment of choice in cases associated with PH, while ileo-colectomy is reserved for the idiopathic causes.

Rectal varices appear endoscopically as venous dilatations usually located in the inferior rectum in close connection to the hemorrhoidal plexus and can be very easily diagnosed by a regular endoscopic examination (Fig. 57.6). Bleeding from rectal varices is very rare, but can be very severe. Because of the rarity of this event, like in the case of other ectopic varices, the management of bleeding rectal varices is at present not standardized. A number of case reports have shown endoscopic sclerotherapy or EBL to be able to control the bleeding [83]. In a retrospective study of 34 patients who were treated endoscopically for rectal varices, 25 patients underwent sclerotherapy (mean of 2.7 sessions) and nine patients EBL (mean of 2.2 sessions) [84]. There was only one complication (bleeding from post-treatment ulcer), encountered in the EBL group. The rectal varices recurrence rate was also higher in the EBL group (56%) compared to the sclerotherapy group (33%), as was the re-bleeding rate (44% in the EBL group compared to 0% in the sclerotherapy group) ($p < 0.05$). This study, although small and retrospective, is the only evidence suggesting that sclerotherapy might be superior to EBL in the treatment of bleeding rectal varices [84].

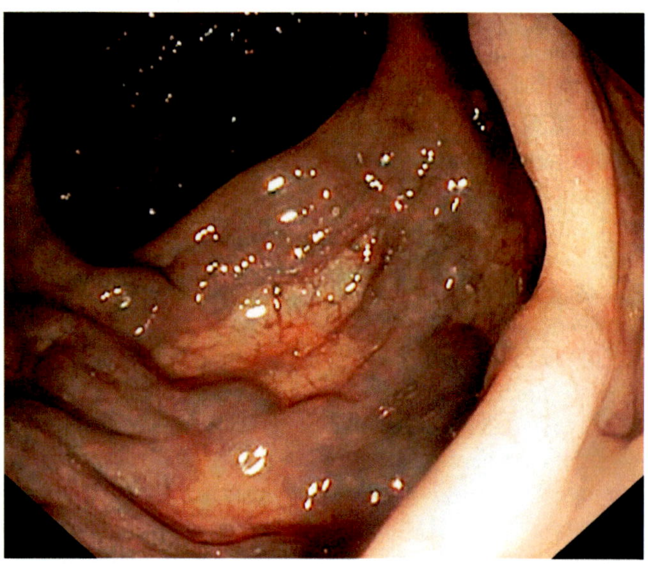

Fig. 57.6 Endoscopic view of multiple tortuous rectal varices interconnected to each other

Similarly to its performances in the upper GI tract, EUS is able to identify varices in the rectum in patients with PH, performing better than standard gastrointestinal endoscopy. Venous dilations of the rectum are rather common in PH, as was proved in a study on 96 patients with cirrhosis, in whom deep rectal varices were detected in 51%, and peri-rectal and para-rectal varices in 40% and 37%, respectively [85]. Of the 83 patients with no rectal varices on standard endoscopy, 39 (47%) had varices at EUS [85]. Although they have a much smaller incidence of bleeding than varices in the upper GI tract, EUS-guided NBC injection alone or in combination with coil placement to treat bleeding rectal varices have been successfully reported [86, 87].

57.4 Conclusions

Bleeding episodes from gastric and ectopic GI varices are less frequent than from esophageal varices but are usually associated with a more severe clinical course. The standard endoscopic management of bleeding GVs or EVs includes N-butyl-2-cyanoacrylate injection to obliterate the variceal lumen. EUS is useful in confirming complete obliteration of the variceal veins and guide subsequent endoscopic treatments until this is achieved. Moreover, EUS-guided treatment of bleeding GVs or EVs using glue and/or coil embolization represent an important therapeutic tool and can control the bleeding in the vast majority of cases. The value of GI endoscopy in treating patients with GVs or EVs with no previous bleeding as primary prophylaxis needs further investigation.

Self Study

Questions

1. **Which statement is true?**
   (a) Endoscopic injection of N-butyl-2-cyanoacrylate in bleeding gastric varices is considered at present the best endoscopic treatment to achieve control of bleeding and decrease the re-bleeding rates.

(b) Isolated gastric varices type 1 are best treated by endoscopic band ligation.
(c) The presence of asymptomatic gastric varices with no episodes of previous bleeding should be endoscopically treated in all cases.
(d) In patients with previous bleeding from gastric varices, endoscopic treatment is not associated with any improvement in re-bleeding or mortality rates compared to beta-blockers alone.

2. **Which statement is true?**
(a) Endoscopic ultrasound (EUS) is not able to perform better than standard gastrointestinal endoscopy in the detection of gastric varices.
(b) Gastric varices are seen by EUS to be located precisely into the mucosal layer of the gastrointestinal wall.
(c) The use of EUS clearly differentiates gastric varices from other types of submucosal lesions of the gastric wall.
(d) Feeding vessels for gastric varices cannot be properly seen by EUS.

Answers

1. **Which statement is true?**
(a) CORRECT ANSWER. Injection of N-butyl-2-cyanoacrylate has been proven to be more effective and safer than endoscopic band ligation and injection of sclerosants in multiple studies in patients with bleeding gastric varices.
(b) Only for patients with GOV 1 gastric varices, endoscopic band ligation can also be used for endoscopic treatment.
(c) According to some studies, the presence of large (>10 mm) gastric varices without previous bleeding episodes might also constitute an indication for prophylactic endoscopic treatment.
(d) In a study on 77 patients with previous gastric variceal bleeding, after a median follow-up of 26 months, endoscopic treatment with N-butyl-2-cyanoacrylate was associated with lower re-bleeding (15% vs. 55%) and mortality rates (3% vs. 25%) compared to beta-blockers alone.

2. **Which statement is true?**
(a) Endoscopic ultrasound detects gastric varices almost twice more often as compared with standard upper gastrointestinal endoscopy.
(b) At EUS examination, gastric varices are seen as tubular anechoic structures located just beneath the muscularis mucosae layer, into the submucosal layer of the gastric wall.
(c) CORRECT ANSWER. The use of Doppler easily differentiates GVs from other types of submucosal lesions, which is important in order to avoid taking endoscopic biopsies.
(d) Feeding perforating vessels can also be visualized by EUS in roughly 80% of cases, traversing the muscularis propria and connecting the submucosal varices to the esophagogastric collateral veins.

References

1. Sarin SK, Kumar A, Angus PW, Baijal SS, Baik SK, Bayraktar Y, et al. Diagnosis and management of acute variceal bleeding: Asian Pacific Association for Study of the Liver recommendations. Hepatol Int. 2011;5(2):607–24.
2. Sanyal AJ. General principles of the management of variceal hemorrhage. In: UpToDate; 2017. online; topic last updated: Feb 21.
3. Cerqueira RM, Andrade L, Correia MR, Fernandes CD, Manso MC. Risk factors for in-hospital mortality in cirrhotic patients with oesophageal variceal bleeding. Eur J Gastroenterol Hepatol. 2012;24(5):551–7.
4. Villanueva C, Colomo A, Bosch A, Concepción M, Hernandez-Gea V, Aracil C, et al. Transfusion strategies for acute upper gastrointestinal bleeding. N Engl J Med. 2013;368(1):11–21.
5. Vieira da Rocha EC, D'Amico EA, Caldwell SH, Flores da Rocha TR, Soares E Silva CS, Dos Santos Bomfim V, et al. A prospective study of conventional and expanded coagulation indices in predicting ulcer bleeding after variceal band ligation. Clin Gastroenterol Hepatol. 2009;7(9):988–93.
6. de Franchis R, Baveno VI. Faculty. Expanding consensus in portal hypertension: report of the Baveno VI Consensus Workshop: stratifying risk and individualizing care for portal hypertension. J Hepatol. 2015;63(3):743–52.
7. Wells M, Chande N, Adams P, Beaton M, Levstik M, Boyce E, et al. Meta-analysis: vasoactive medications for the management of acute variceal bleeds. Aliment Pharmacol Ther. 2012;35(11):1267–78.
8. Barkun AN, Bardou M, Martel M, Gralnek IM, Sung JJ. Prokinetics in acute upper GI bleeding: a meta-analysis. Gastrointest Endosc. 2010;72(6):1138–45.
9. Sarin SK, Lahoti D, Saxena SP, Murthy NS, Makwana UK. Prevalence, classification and natural history of gastric varices: a long-term follow-up study in 568 portal hypertension patients. Hepatology. 1992;16(6):1343–9.
10. Norton ID, Andrews JC, Kamath PS. Management of ectopic varices. Hepatology. 1998;28(4):1154–8.
11. Bosch J, Garcia-Pagan JC. Prevention of variceal rebleeding. Lancet. 2003;361(9361):952–4.
12. Wani ZA, Bhatt RA, Bhadoria AS, Maiwall R, Choudhury A. Gastric varices: classification, endoscopic and ultrasonographic management. J Res Med Sci. 2015;20(12):1200–7.
13. Li H, Ye D, Kong D. Endoscopic clipping prior to N-butyl-2-cyanoacrylate injection for gastric varices with a large gastrorenal shunt. Endoscopy. 2018;50(4):E102–3.
14. Garcia-Tsao G, Abraldes JG, Berzigotti A, Bosch J. Portal hypertensive bleeding in cirrhosis: risk stratification, diagnosis, and management: 2016 practice guidance by the American Association for the study of liver diseases. Hepatology. 2017;65(1):310–35.
15. Kim T, Shijo H, Kokawa H, Tokumitsu H, Kubara K, Ota K, et al. Risk factors for hemorrhage from gastric fundal varices. Hepatology. 1997;25(2):307–12.

16. Soehendra N, Nam VC, Grimm H, Kempeneers I. Endoscopic obliteration of large esophagogastric varices with bucrylate. Endoscopy. 1986;18(1):25–6.
17. Lo GH, Lai KH, Cheng JS, Chen MH, Chiang HT. A prospective, randomized trial of butyl cyanoacrylate injection versus band ligation in the management of bleeding varices. Hepatology. 2001;33(5):1060–4.
18. Garcia-Tsao G, Sanyal AJ, Grace ND, Carey WD. Practice Guidelines Committee of American Association for Study of Liver Diseases; Practice Parameters Committee of American College of Gastroenterology. Prevention and management of gastroesophageal varices and variceal hemorrhage in cirrhosis. Am J Gastroenterol. 2007;102(9):2086–102.
19. Rengstorff DS, Binmoeller KF. A pilot study of 2-octyl cyanoacrylate injection for treatment of gastric fundal varices in humans. Gastrointest Endosc. 2004;59(4):553–8.
20. Mishra SR, Chander Sharma B, Kumar A, Sarin SK. Endoscopic cyanoacrylate injection versus beta-blocker for secondary prophylaxis of gastric variceal bleed: a randomised controlled trial. Gut. 2010;59(6):729–35.
21. Bajaj JS, Sanyal AJ. Methods to achieve hemostasis in patients with acute variceal hemorrhage. In: UpToDate; 2017. online; topic last updated: May 05.
22. Lo GH, Lin CW, Perng DS, Chang CY, Lee CT, Hsu CY, et al. A retrospective comparative study of histoacryl injection and banding ligation in the treatment of acute type 1 gastric variceal hemorrhage. Scand J Gastroenterol. 2013;48(10):1198–204.
23. Ríos Castellanos E, Seron P, Gisbert JP, Bonfill CX. Endoscopic injection of cyanoacrylate glue versus other endoscopic procedures for acute bleeding gastric varices in people with portal hypertension. Cochrane Database Syst Rev. 2015;5:CD010180.
24. Mishra SR, Sharma BC, Kumar A, Sarin SK. Primary prophylaxis of gastric variceal bleeding comparing cyanoacrylate injection and beta-blockers: a randomized controlled trial. J Hepatol. 2011;54(6):1161–7.
25. Hou MC, Lin HC, Lee HS, Liao WC, Lee FY, Lee SD. A randomized trial of endoscopic cyanoacrylate injection for acute gastric variceal bleeding: 0.5 mL versus 1.0 mL. Gastrointest Endosc. 2009;70(4):668–75.
26. Sharma BC, Varakanahalli S, Singh JP, Srivastava S. Gastric varices in cirrhosis vs. extrahepatic portal venous obstruction and response to endoscopic N-butyl-2-cyanoacrylate injection. J Clin Exp Hepatol. 2017;7(2):97–101.
27. Hung HH, Chang CJ, Hou MC, Liao WC, Chan CC, Huang HC, et al. Efficacy of non-selective β-blockers as adjunct to endoscopic prophylactic treatment for gastric variceal bleeding: a randomized controlled trial. J Hepatol. 2012;56(5):1025–32.
28. Garcia-Pagán JC, Barrufet M, Cardenas A, Àngels E. Management of gastric varices. Clin Gastroenterol Hepatol. 2014;12(6):919–28.
29. Kok K, Bond RP, Duncan IC, Fourie PA, Ziady C, van den Bogaerde JB, et al. Distal embolization and local vessel wall ulceration after gastric variceal obliteration with N-butyl-2-cyanoacrylate: a case report and review of the literature. Endoscopy. 2004;36(5):442–6.
30. Sarin SK, Mishra SR. Endoscopic therapy for gastric varices. Clin Liver Dis. 2010;14(2):263–79.
31. Alexander S, Korman MG, Sievert W. Cyanoacrylate in the treatment of gastric varices complicated by multiple pulmonary emboli. Intern Med J. 2006;36(7):462–4.
32. Huang YH, Yeh HZ, Chen GH, Chang CS, Wu CY, Poon SK, et al. Endoscopic treatment of bleeding gastric varices by N-butyl-2-cyanoacrylate (Histoacryl) injection: long term efficacy and safety. Gastrointest Endosc. 2000;52(2):160–7.
33. Rosch W, Rexroth G. Pulmonary, cerebral and coronary emboli during bucrylate injection of bleeding fundic varices. Endoscopy. 1998;30(8):S89–90.
34. Turler A, Wolff M, Dorlars D, Hirner A. Embolic and septic complications after sclerotherapy of fundic varices with cyanoacrylate. Gastrointest Endosc. 2001;53(2):228–30.
35. Upadhyay AP, Ananthasivan R, Radhakrishnan S, Zubaidi G. Cortical blindness and acute myocardial infarction following injection of bleeding gastric varices with cyanoacrylate glue. Endoscopy. 2005;37(10):1034.
36. Saracco G, Giordanino C, Roberto N, Ezio D, Luca T, Caronna S, et al. Fatal multiple systemic embolisms after injection of cyanoacrylate in bleeding gastric varices of a patient who was noncirrhotic but with idiopathic portal hypertension. Gastrointest Endosc. 2007;65(2):345–7.
37. Rickman OB, Utz JP, Aughenbaugh GL, Gostout CJ. Pulmonary embolization of 2-octyl cyanoacrylate after endoscopic injection therapy for gastric variceal bleeding. Mayo Clin Proc. 2004;79(11):1455–8.
38. Tan YM, Goh KL, Kamarulzaman A, Tan PS, Ranjeev P, Salem O, et al. Multiple systemic embolisms with septicemia after gastric variceal obliteration with cyanoacrylate. Gastrointest Endosc. 2002;55(2):276–8.
39. Audibert M, Schoeffler M, Wallet F, Duperret S, Mabrut JY, Bancel B, et al. Acute fatal pulmonary embolism during cyanoacrylate injection in gastric varices. Gastroenterol Clin Biol. 2008;32(11):926–30.
40. Cheng LF, Wang ZQ, Li CZ, Lin W, Yeo AE, Jin B. Low incidence of complications from endoscopic gastric variceal obturation with butyl cyanoacrylate. Clin Gastroenterol Hepatol. 2010;8(9):760–6.
41. Tseng Y, Ma L, Luo T, Zeng X, Wei Y, Li L, et al. Thromboembolic events secondary to endoscopic cyanoacrylate injection: can we foresee any red flags? Can J Gastroenterol Hepatol. 2018:2018:1940592.
42. Ibrahim M, El-Mikkawy A, Abdel Hamid M, Abdalla H, Lemmers A, Mostafa I, et al. Early application of haemostatic powder added to standard management for oesophagogastric variceal bleeding: a randomised trial. Gut. 2019;68:844. https://doi.org/10.1136/gutjnl-2017-314653. pii: gutjnl-2017-314653.
43. Lee YT, Chan FK, Ching JY, Lai CW, Leung VK, Chung SC, et al. Diagnosis of gastroesophageal varices and portal collateral venous abnormalities by endosonography in cirrhotic patients. Endoscopy. 2002;34(5):391–8.
44. Choudhuri G, Dhiman RK, Agarwal DK. Endosonographic evaluation of the venous anatomy around the gastro-esophageal junction in patients with portal hypertension. Hepatogastroenterology. 1996;43(11):1250–5.
45. Imamura H, Irisawa A, Shibukawa G, Takagi T, Hikichi T, Obara K, et al. Echo-endoscopic analysis of variceal hemodynamics in patients with isolated gastric varices. Endosc Ultrasound. 2014;3(4):238–44.
46. Ginès A, Fernández-Esparrach G. Endoscopic ultrasonography for the evaluation of portal hypertension. Clin Liver Dis. 2010;14(2):221–9.
47. Lee YT, Chan FK, Ng EK, Leung VK, Law KB, Yung MY, et al. EUS-guided injection of cyanoacrylate for bleeding gastric varices. Gastrointest Endosc. 2000;52(2):168–74.
48. Iwase H, Suga S, Morise K, Kuroiwa A, Yamaguchi T, Horiuchi Y. Color Doppler endoscopic ultrasonography for the evaluation of gastric varices and endoscopic obliteration with cyanoacrylate glue. Gastointest Endosc. 1995;41(2):150–4.
49. Romero-Castro R, Pellicer-Bautista F, Jimenez-Saenz M, Marcos-Sanchez F, Caunedo-Alvarez A, Ortiz-Moyano C, et al. EUS-guided injection of cyanoacrylate in perforating feeding veins in gastric varices: results in 5 cases. Gastointest Endosc. 2007;66(2):402–7.
50. Gubler C, Bauerfeind P. Safe and successful endoscopic initial treatment and long-term eradication of gastric varices by endoscopic ultrasound-guided histoacryl (N-butyl-2-cyanoacrylate) injection. Scand J Gastroenterol. 2014;49(9):1136–42.

51. Bhat YM, Weilert F, Fredrick RT, Kane SD, Shah JN, Hamerski CM, et al. EUS-guided treatment of gastric fundal varices with combined injection of coils and cyanoacrylate glue: a large U.S. experience over 6 years (with video). Gastrointest Endosc. 2016;83(6):1164–72.
52. Binmoeller KF, Weilert F, Shah JN, Kim J. EUS-guided transesophageal treatment of gastric fundal varices with combined coiling and cyanoacrylate glue injection. Gastrointest Endosc. 2011;74(5):1019–25.
53. Dedania B, Kukreja K, Davee T, Bhutani MS. Endoscopic ultrasound-guided sclerosant injection and coil embolization of bleeding gastric varices. Endoscopy. 2018;50(3):283–5.
54. Frost JW, Hebbar S. EUS-guided thrombin injection for management of gastric fundal varices. Endosc Int Open. 2018;6(6):E664–8.
55. Fujii-Lau L, Law R, Wong Kee Song L, Gostout CJ, Kamath PS, Levy MJ. Endoscopic ultrasound (EUS)-guided coil injection therapy of esophagogastric and ectopic varices. Surg Endosc. 2016;30(4):1396–404.
56. Gonzalez J, Giacino C, Pioche M, Vanbiervliet G, Brardjanian S, Ah-Soune P, et al. Endoscopic ultrasound-guided vascular therapy: is it safe and effective? Endoscopy. 2012;44(5):539–42.
57. Romero-Castro R, Pellicer-Bautista F, Giovannini M, Marcos-Sánchez F, Caparros-Escudero C, Jiménez-Sáenz M, et al. Endoscopic ultrasound (EUS)-guided coil embolization therapy in gastric varices. Endoscopy. 2010;42(Suppl 2):E35–6.
58. Romero-Castro R, Ellrichmann M, Ortiz-Moyano C, Subtil-Inigo JC, Junquera-Florez F, Gornals JB, et al. EUS-guided coil versus cyanoacrylate therapy for the treatment of gastric varices: a multicenter study. Gastrointest Endosc. 2013;78(5):711–21.
59. Rose S. Mechanical devices for arterial occlusion and therapeutic vascular occlusion utilizing steel coil technique: clinical applications. AJR Am J Roentgenol. 2009;192(2):321–4.
60. Hall PS, Teshima C, May GR, Mosko JD. Endoscopic ultrasound-guided vascular therapy: the present and the future. Clin Endosc. 2017;50(2):138–42.
61. Tang RS, Teoh AY, Lau JY. EUS-guided cyanoacrylate injection for treatment of endoscopically obscured bleeding gastric varices. Gastrointest Endosc. 2016;83(5):1032–3.
62. Henry Z, Uppal D, Saad W, Caldwell S. Gastric and ectopic varices. Clin Liver Dis. 2014;18(2):371–88.
63. Helmy A, Al Kahtani K, Al Fadda M. Updates in the pathogenesis, diagnosis and management of ectopic varices. Hepatol Int. 2008;2(3):322–34.
64. Cappell MS, Price JB. Characterization of the syndrome of small and large intestinal variceal bleeding. Dig Dis Sci. 1987;32(4):422–7.
65. Boyer TD, Haskal ZJ. American Association for the Study of Liver Diseases. The role of transjugular intrahepatic portosystemic shunt (TIPS) in the management of portal hypertension: update 2009. Hepatology. 2010;51(1):306.
66. Park CJ, Lee BE, Jeon HK, Kim GH, Song GA, Ko SH, et al. Case of bleeding ileal varices after a colectomy diagnosed by capsule endoscopy. Korean J Gastroenterol. 2018;71(6):349–53.
67. Kakizaki S, Toyoda M, Ichikawa T, Sato K, Takagi H, Arai H, et al. Clinical characteristics and treatment for patients presenting with bleeding duodenal varices. Dig Endosc. 2010;22(4):275–81.
68. Sato T, Akaike J, Toyota J, Karino Y, Ohmura T. Clinicopathological features and treatment of ectopic varices with portal hypertension. Int J Hepatol. 2011;2011:960720.
69. Singh A, Marshall C, Chaudhuri B, Okoli C, Foley A, Person SD, et al. Timing of video capsule endoscopy relative to overt obscure GI bleeding: implications from a retrospective study. Gastrointest Endosc. 2013;77(5):761–6.
70. Park SW, Cho E, Jun CH, Choi SK, Kim HS, Park CH, et al. Upper gastrointestinal ectopic variceal bleeding treated with various endoscopic modalities: case reports and literature review. Medicine (Baltimore). 2017;96(1):e5860.
71. Kinzel J, Pichetshote N, Dredar S, Aslanian H, Nagar A. Bleeding from a duodenal varix: a unique case of variceal hemostasis achieved using EUS-guided placement of an embolization coil and cyanoacrylate. J Clin Gastroenterol. 2014;48(4):362–4.
72. Abbar B, Vimpere D, Khater S, Cellier C, Diehl JL. Cerebral infarction following cyanoacrylate endoscopic therapy of duodenal varices in a patient with a patent foramen ovale. Intern Emerg Med. 2018;13(5):817–9.
73. Getzlaff S, Benz CA, Schilling D, Riemann JF. Enteroscopic cyanoacrylate sclerotherapy of jejunal and gallbladder varices in a patient with portal hypertension. Endoscopy. 2001;33(5):462–4.
74. Hekmat A, Al-toma A, Mallant MPJH, Mulder CJJ, Jacobs MAJM. Histoacryl obliteration of jejunal varices. In: Atlas of double balloon enteroscopy. Munich: Medconnect GmbH; 2007. p. 57–8.
75. Curcio G, Pisa MD, Miraglia R, Catalano P, Barresi L, Tarantino I, et al. Case of obscure-overt gastrointestinal bleeding after pediatric liver transplantation explained by endoscopic ultrasound. World J Gastrointest Endosc. 2012;4(12):571–4.
76. Levy MJ, Wong Kee Song LM, Kendrick ML, Misra S, Gostout CJ. EUS-guided coil embolization for refractory ectopic variceal bleeding. Gastrointest Endosc. 2008;67(3):572–4.
77. Cook DJ, Fuller HD, Guyatt GH, Marshall JC, Leasa D, Hall R, et al. Risk factors for gastrointestinal bleeding in critically ill patients. Canadian Critical Care Trials Group. N Engl J Med. 1994;330(6):377–81.
78. Lakhtakia S, Pericherla B, Bhardwaj K, Ramchandani M, Gupta R, Reddy N. Common bile duct compression caused by cyanoacrylate glue injection into bleeding duodenal varices: a rare adverse event (with videos). Gastrointest Endosc. 2014;79(6):1005–6; discussion 1007.
79. Grgurevic I, Kujundzic M, Banic M, Kusec R, Bokun T, Vukelic-Markovic M, et al. Subtypes and clinical significance of common bile duct varices in portal vein thrombosis: diagnosis and follow-up by Doppler US and EUS. Abdom Radiol (NY). 2016;41(3):476–84.
80. Nikolopoulos N, Xynos E, Datsakis K, Kasapidis P, Vassilakis JS. Varicosis coli totalis: report of a case of idiopathic aetiology. Digestion. 1990;47(4):232–5.
81. Simvoulakis E, Viazis N, Pipis P, Stefanidis G, Avgerinos A. Diffuse idiopathic colonic varices presenting with lower gastrointestinal bleeding in an elderly patient: a case report and review of the literature. Acta Gastroenterol Belg. 2006;69(1):15–9.
82. Al-toma A, Craanen ME, Jacobs MAJM. Idiopathic varicosis coli. In: Atlas of double balloon enteroscopy, vol. 63. Munich: Medconnect GmbH; 2007.
83. Khalloufi KA, Laiyemo AO. Management of rectal varices in portal hypertension. World J Hepatol. 2015;7(30):2992–8.
84. Sato T, Yamazaki K, Akaike J, Toyota J, Karino Y, Ohmura T. Retrospective analysis of endoscopic injection sclerotherapy for rectal varices compared with band ligation. Clin Exp Gastroenterol. 2010;3:159–63.
85. Wiechowska-Kozlowska A, Bialek A, Milkiewicz P. Prevalence of deep rectal varices in patients with cirrhosis: an EUS-based study. Liver Int. 2009;29(8):1202–5.
86. Sharma M, Somasundaram A. Massive lower GI bleed from an endoscopically inevident rectal varices: diagnosis and management by EUS (with videos). Gastrointest Endosc. 2010;72(5):1106–8.
87. Weilert F, Shah JN, Marson FP, Binmoeller KF. EUS-guided coil and glue for bleeding rectal varix. Gastrointest Endosc. 2012;76(4):915–6.

Portacaval Shunting for Portal Hypertension

58

Francis G. Celii, Jayesh M. Soni, and Anil K. Pillai

Key Concepts

- Overview of Portal Hypertension
- Current Treatment Options
  - Surgical Shunts, TIPS Shunt, DIPS Shunt, Transjugular Mesocaval Shunts
  - Description of shunts anatomy, clinical indication/contraindications, technical considerations, and complications
  - Potential complications and long-term outcomes of different portocaval shunt procedures,
  - Future Directions

58.1 Overview of Portal Hypertension

Portal hypertension is a clinical condition characterized by a portosystemic gradient exceeding 5 mmHg. Cirrhosis contributes to the majority of cases with less than 10% arising from noncirrhotic etiology. Pathophysiological mechanisms for the development of portal hypertension are categorized into two broad theories, forward and backward flow theories. In the latter, cirrhosis causes fibrosis and architectural distortion of the liver, leading to increased intrahepatic vascular resistance. Elevated pressure in the portal system eventually leading to reversal of flow within the portal vein, known as hepatofugal flow ensues. In the former, hyperdynamic mesenteric circulation mediated by vasoactive compounds such as Nitrous Oxide (NO), Vascular Endothelial Growth Factor (VEGF), and Tumor Necrosis Factor (TNF) α results in hyper dynamic circulation and increased forward flow [1, 2].

The downstream clinical effects of elevated portal pressure are mainly threefold and include variceal bleeding, ascites and hepatic encephalopathy [3]. When these complications occur, cirrhosis is said to be decompensated with a life expectancy that now plummets to only 2 years from a 12-year life expectancy seen in a compensated cirrhotic patient. Variceal bleeding is a medical emergency with a 7–12% mortality. The onset of ascites portends a poor prognosis with a 1-year and 5-year mortality rate of 15% and 44% respectively. Hepatic encephalopathy is seen in half the patients with portal hypertension.

Other less common clinical manifestations of portal hypertension include hepatorenal syndrome, hepatopulmonary syndrome, hypersplenism, bacterial peritonitis, hepatic hydrothorax, and portal hypertensive biliopathy.

F. G. Celii
University of Texas Health Science Center, Houston, TX, USA
e-mail: Francis.G.Celii@uth.tmc.edu

J. M. Soni · A. K. Pillai (✉)
Diagnostic and Interventional Imaging, University of Texas Health Science Center, Houston, TX, USA
e-mail: Jayesh.Soni@uth.tmc.edu; Anil.K.Pillai@uth.tmc.edu

F. Radu-Ionita et al. (eds.), *Liver Diseases*, https://doi.org/10.1007/978-3-030-24432-3_58

Definition

Portal hypertension condition in which the portosystemic blood pressure gradient is above 5 mmHg.

Hepatofugal or Non-forward portal flow (NFPF) is defined as an abnormal flow pattern where portal venous flow is retrograde from the periphery of the liver towards the porta hepatis.

Hepatic Venous Pressure Gradient (HVPG) is defined as the gradient in pressure between the portal vein and the inferior vena cava (IVC).

- Normal portal pressure is defined as HVPG of ≤5 mmHg.
- Subclinical portal hypertension is defined as HVPG 6–9 mmHg.
- Clinically significant portal hypertension (CSPH) is defined as HVPG of ≥10 mmHg, at which point varices may develop [4].
- Measurement of HVPG provides independent prognostic information on survival.
- HPVG helps assess the risk of decompensation after resection in patients with compensated cirrhosis and hepatocellular cancer

The diagnosis of portal hypertension is made on a clinical basis when a patient with cirrhosis presents with complications of portal hypertension. Direct portal vein measurement via a transhepatic, transjugular or umbilical vein approach is the gold standard but is invasive with a risk of bleeding. The wedged hepatic venous pressure (WHVP) can be measured using a balloon catheter which is wedged in the hepatic vein. Subsequently, the balloon is deflated to measure the free hepatic venous pressure (FHVP). The corrected sinusoidal HVPG is calculated by subtracting the free hepatic venous pressure (FHVP, which reflects intra-abdominal pressure) from the wedged hepatic venous pressure (WHVP, which reflects hepatic sinusoidal portal venous pressure and intra-abdominal pressure). The technique is accurate in the majority of patients with cirrhosis that involves sinusoidal scarring. Other methods to diagnose portal hypertension include ultrasound and elastography; however, ultrasound lacks the sensitivity, and elastography, though it has good correlation with liver fibrosis, is an indirect measure of portal hypertension and is susceptible to confounding factors; additionally, it does not account for extrahepatic causes of portal hypertension [5].

Cirrhosis can remain compensated for many years before the development of a decompensating event. Decompensation includes the development of any of the abovementioned complications of portal hypertension. Managing portal hypertension revolves around preventing or treating its complications. The former (preventing complications) is applicable in patients with compensated cirrhosis (Child-Pugh A) while the later (treating complications) is applicable in decompensated cirrhosis (Child-Pugh B or C). Preventing complications of portal hypertension involves regular screening of patients with Child-Pugh A cirrhosis with endoscopy and managing the portal blood pressure medically. The goal of preventative measures is to avoid the first variceal bleed, which is termed primary prophylaxis. Discussion of preventative measures is beyond the scope of this chapter and discussed elsewhere in this book.

Variceal bleeding is the most dreaded complication of portal hypertension with a 1-year mortality of 50% [6]. Endoscopic therapy (either variceal ligation or sclerotherapy) is the first line treatment for acute variceal hemorrhage. However, when rebleeding occurs, more definite therapy is required. This definitive treatment to reduce portal hypertension, outside of liver transplant, is by creation of a portacaval shunt to decompress the system. Historically, surgical shunts, whereby a connection between the portal vein and vena cava provides a low resistance outlet, and consequently lowers variceal pressures, preventing bleeds. Today, surgical shunts are not commonly used for the treatment of portal hypertension as percutaneous options have largely replaced them, but they should still be understood as they do have potential clinical scenarios of utility (Fig. 58.1).

58.2 Current Treatment Options

58.2.1 Surgical Shunts

Three categories of surgical shunts including total, selective and partial shunts have been described. Portacaval and mesocaval shunts are examples of total Portacaval shunts (TPCS). End-to-side portacaval shunt is created by ligating the portal vein and connecting the proximal stump of the ligated portal vein to the side of the inferior vena cava (Fig. 58.2). Mesocaval shunt are created between the superior mesenteric vein and the inferior vena cava. Although total shunts were remarkably effective in preventing variceal bleeding, operative mortality was high and the incidence of hepatic encephalopathy and liver failure were not acceptable [7–9]. To reduce the risks, selective shunts including the proximal and distal splenorenal shunts were described. Splenorenal shunts maintain forward flow to the liver while decompressing the gastro-esophageal varices (Fig. 58.2).

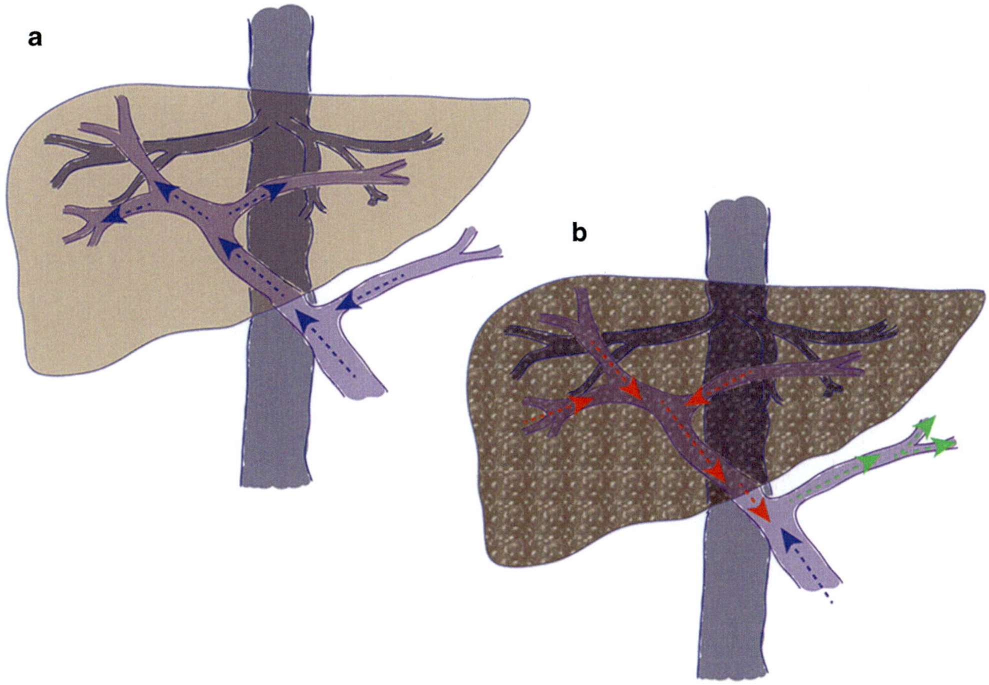

Fig. 58.1 Illustration depicting the normal flow (**a**) and hepatofugal flow seen in portal hypertensive pathology (**b**)

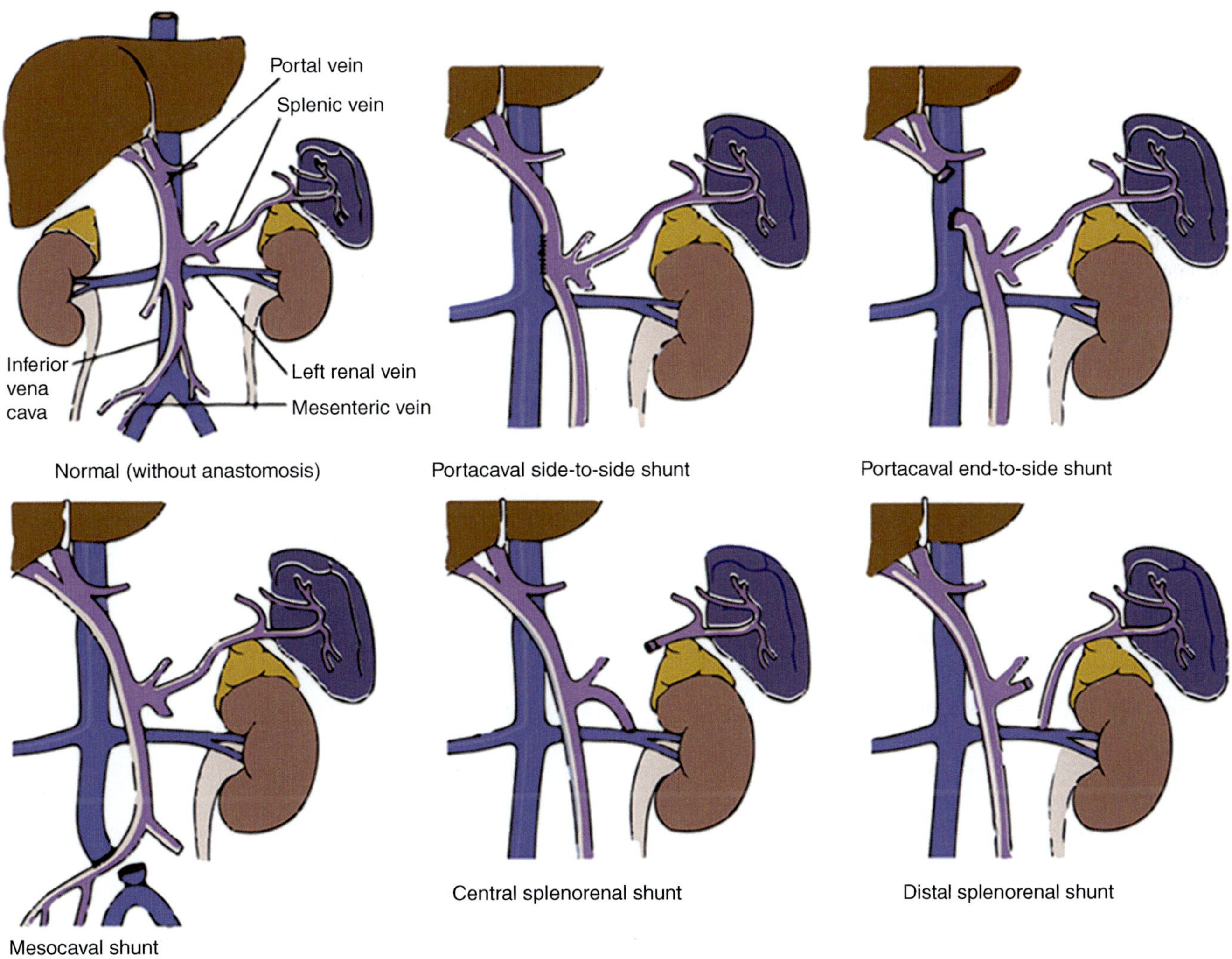

Fig. 58.2 Diagrams of common surgical shunts compared to normal vascular anatomy

Definition
Distal Splenorenal Shunts (DSRS) are created by ligating the distal splenic vein and connecting the proximal arm of the ligated splenic vein to the left renal vein in order to decompress the gastro-esophageal varices.

Definition
Proximal Splenorenal Shunts (PSRS) are created by ligating the proximal splenic vein and the distal arm is connected into the left renal vein, taking portal pressure away from the site of confluence with the superior mesenteric vein.

Clinical trials comparing TPCS to DSRS did not show significant differences in rebleeding, encephalopathy, or mortality. In addition, trials comparing DSRS with sclerotherapy found that patients had worse survival after DSRS even though that arm had better bleeding control [10]. As a result, prophylactic shunt surgery was rapidly abandoned and became only indicated as a salvage therapy.

Partial shunts including calibrated small-diameter portocaval H-graft shunts were eventually designed with the same end goal as DSRS. If the volume of shunted portal blood could be regulated, suppression of variceal bleeding without incurring hepatic encephalopathy or liver dysfunction could be achieved. There have been few RCTs to date evaluating the efficacy of this shunt. Partial shunts were shown to have better encephalopathy-free survival compared to total surgical shunts, and are easier to handle in subsequent transplants, but more data is needed [11, 12].

Ideal surgical shunt candidates in which PCS may be attempted are those who have well-preserved liver function but fail emergent endoscopic therapy or those who are not excellent surgical candidates, but have a contraindication to TIPS placement.

58.2.2 Percutaneous Shunts

58.2.2.1 Transjugular Intrahepatic Portosystemic Shunt (TIPS)

Creation of a transjugular intrahepatic portosystemic shunt (TIPS) is a well-established procedure recommended for patients suffering from sequelae of portal hypertension that is refractory to medical management. An effective end-to-end portacaval shunt between a branch of the portal vein and usually the right hepatic vein, which flows into the inferior vena cava, is created to decompress the portal system (Fig. 58.3). TIPS is performed in the interventional radiology lab with moderate sedation or general anesthesia. Creation of a TIPS shunts is preferred over surgical shunts in patients who are transplant candidates as the extra-hepatic anatomy is not altered.

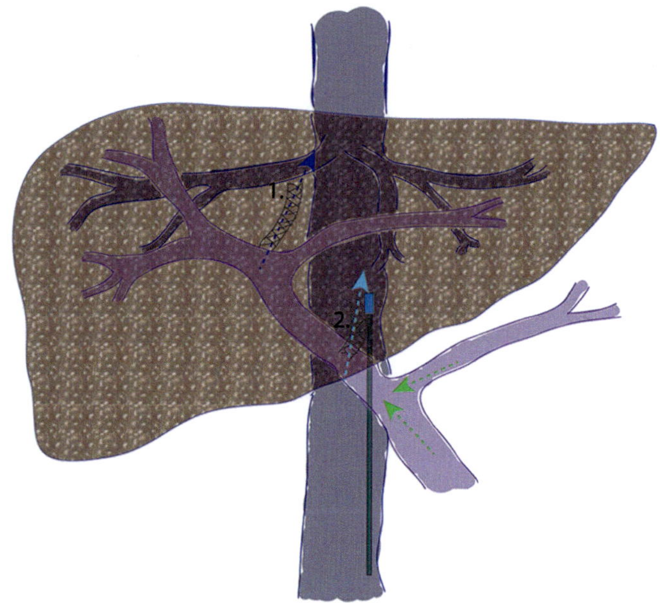

Fig. 58.3 Illustration demonstrating placement and flow of TIPS procedure (1) and DIPS procedure (2) using IVUS and improved portal flow (blue arrows)

The most widely supported indications for TIPS include secondary prevention of variceal bleeding and refractory ascites. Multiple randomized controlled studies and several meta-analyses have proven the utility of TIPS creation in both these conditions. It has been shown to be superior in long-term prevention of rebleeding compared to endoscopic therapy [13]. In the treatment of refractory ascites, TIPS has been shown not only to control ascites in 70% of cases [14], it has also been shown to increase transplant-free survival as compared to large volume paracentesis (LVP) [14–16]. The meta-analysis summarizing five of the six RCTs found a 7.1-fold reduction in the risk of recurrent tense ascites after TIPS [11, 17, 18]. The first line treatment for acute variceal bleeding includes vasoactive pharmacotherapy and endoscopic sclerotherapy or banding. Failure to achieve hemostasis occurs in 20% of patients undergoing the first line treatment [3]. TIPS is considered the second line treatment due to higher incidence of hepatic encephalopathy but achieves hemostasis in 95% of acute variceal bleeding [19].

The utility of TIPS shunt creation in the treatment of Budd-Chiari Syndrome (BCS) is highly dependent on etiology. In primary BCS the patency and long-term survival is promising [20]. It has been postulated that using TIPS to return intravascular volume from the splanchnic circulation to the systemic circulation should improve renal status in cirrhotic patients with hepatorenal syndrome. Currently, there is 2B evidence [21] for using TIPS in the treatment of hepatorenal syndrome. One study even screened patients likely to benefit by verifying response to combination therapy of midodrine, octreotide, and albumin. They then saw further normalization of kidney function with the implementation of TIPS [22, 23]. Portal Hypertensive gastropathy has only level 4 evidence to support the use of TIPS for primary treatment [22, 24]. It has been shown to improve endoscopic endpoints and clinically stop hemorrhage in a case study.

Contraindications to TIPS placement a mostly related to the hemodynamic changes that take place after TIPS placement. Severe congestive heart failure, tricuspid regurgitation, and severe pulmonary hypertension (mean pulmonary pressure >45 mmHg) are all absolute contraindications due to the massive increase in preload that results after blood is shunted from the portal vein to the IVC. If there is evidence that the patient's cardiopulmonary system cannot handle the increased load from the shunt, it should not be placed. Other absolute contraindications are multiple hepatic cysts, bacteremia or sepsis, and unrelieved biliary obstruction. Relative contraindications include portal venous thrombosis, hepatocellular cancer, moderate pulmonary hypertension, obstruction of all hepatic veins, uncorrectable coagulopathy or thrombocytopenia, and existing hepatic encephalopathy [25].

The overall goal is the placement of a stent allowing for portal flow from the portal vein to the Inferior vena cava through the hepatic veins, thus creating a low resistance shunt to relieve elevated portal pressures. This reduction of the portosystemic gradient is successful in over 90% of cases [21]. This is accomplished by obtaining vascular access to the right jugular vein, traversing the superior vena cava through the right atrium, and into the inferior vena cava. From this point, the right or middle hepatic vein is cannulated and hepatic pressures are recorded. Next, a needle assembly is advanced over the wire through a sheath and used to traverse the liver parenchyma and enter the portal vein. After establishing access to the portal vein, portal pressures are obtained. Subsequently, the parenchymal tract is dilated with a balloon catheter and the stent graft is deployed. It is vital to ensure that the appropriate size endograft is selected so that it completely covers the tract, decreasing chances of stent stenosis from fibrous tissue overgrowth at the hepatic venous end. Furthermore, angiographic evidence of reversal of hepatofugal flow and decreased varices, as well as treatment to HVPG of less than 12 mmHg significantly decreases the likelihood of variceal rebleeding (seen in Fig. 58.4).

Complication rates continue to decrease as technique improves. Currently, only 3% of patients experience major complications and the likelihood of minor complications is

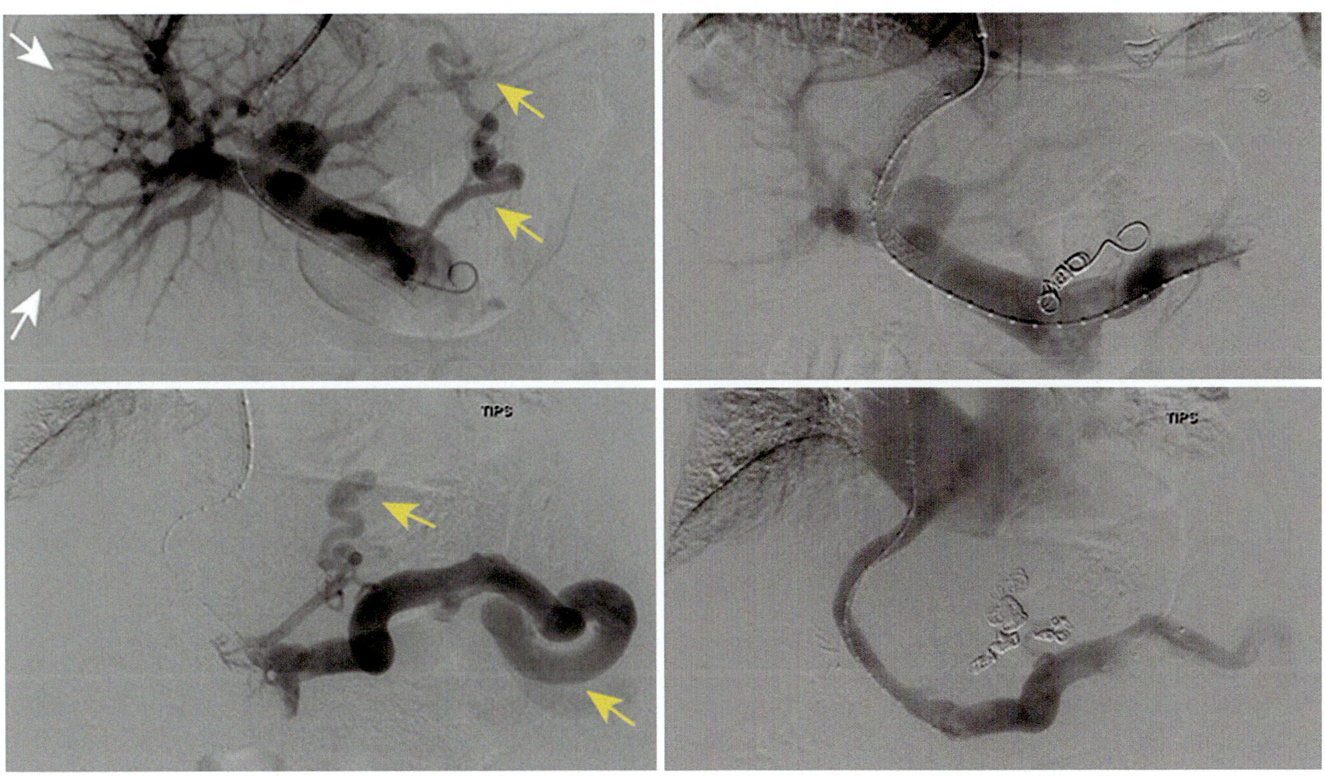

Fig. 58.4 TIPS Procedure showing resolution portal hepatic congestion (white arrow) and gastro-esophageal varices (yellow arrows) before (left) and after (right) shunt placement

reported at 4% [26]. In addition, procedural mortality is only 1.7% [26]. Of the complications that patients may experience, the most commonly encountered are hepatic encephalopathy, variceal hemorrhage, and stent dysfunction. TIPS stent dysfunction can happen due to technical failure (e.g. stent shortening that leads to thrombosis, or biliary stent fistula), parenchymal stenosis due to excessive fibrotic healing response, or late "Pseudo-intimal" hyperplasia of the hepatic vein [27].

In response to the relatively high rates of stent dysfunction, bare metal stents (BMS) were presumed to be more susceptible to the pseudo-intimal hyperplasia and polytetrafluoroethylene (PTFE)-covered stents were introduced to prevent this stenosis. At this point, the evidence is robust enough to deem PTFE-covered stents as superior to bare metal stents [28–30] as a strong meta-analysis that includes four RCTs demonstrated that covered stents are almost 5 times more likely to retain primary patency, two-thirds less likely to have rebleeding as a complication, and survival is superior with an odds ratio of 1.85 [31]. It appears that covered stents are less predisposed to pseudo-intimal hyperplasia and this is thought to be the reason for better patency rates. It has been demonstrated that stent to inferior vena cava distance (SIVCD) has no negative effect on primary patency of TIPS when performed with covered stents as opposed to BMS [27]. In terms of sizing, 10-mm PTFE-covered stent have been shown to better control refractory ascites in patients with cirrhosis, compared with an 8-mm stent, and importantly, without increasing the incidence of hepatic encephalopathy [17]. As a result, the American Association for the Study of Liver Diseases (AASLD) now recommends the use of PTFE covered stents over bare metal stents.

As an important way to manage patients with uncontrollable variceal bleeding and recurrent variceal bleeding, studies on the outcomes of early TIPS placement have shown that risk stratification is vital. Those patients with a persistent HPVG at 20 mmHg or above were at higher risk for recurrent bleeding despite best medical therapy and were shown to benefits from early TIPS intervention. Early TIPS intervention has been shown to have improved 1-year survival of 86% over 76% in the drug + Endoscopic Therapy (ET) group for acute variceal bleeding [32–35].

58.2.2.2 Direct Intrahepatic Portacaval Shunt (DIPS)

The Direct Intrahepatic Portacaval Shunt (DIPS) was first described by Petersen et al. [36] as a response to common failures observed when performing the more established TIPS procedure. The goal was to address parenchymal tract overgrowth at the hepatic venous end and prevent the most common cause of TIPS failure by means of bypassing it completely. In addition, exclusion of the hepatic vein allows for the DIPS procedure to treat those with hepatic veno-occlusive disease (i.e. Budd-Chiari Syndrome). Direct Intrahepatic Portacaval Shunt (DIPS) is a modification to the original TIPS procedure where an artificial communication between the IVC and portal vein is created through the caudate lobe. DIPS also allows for decreased radiation exposure due to real-time image guidance as intravascular ultrasound (IVUS). IVUS is used to navigate from the IVC to the portal vein (See Figs. 58.3 and 58.5). The other described benefit of this modification is that the much shorter liver tract decreases susceptibility to stent stenosis from fibrous tissue overgrowth [37, 38].

Indications for the DIPS procedure are identical to that of the TIPS; however, the evidence backing these indications is not as robust at this point as DIPS is still a relatively new procedure. However, it seems to have good indication for portal hypertension secondary to hepatic veno-occlusive disease, patients with difficult vascular anatomy, those with unsuitable parenchymal tract [39], and DIPS may be considered in patients needing secondary intervention after an occluded TIPS [40].

Contraindications to DIPS mirror those of TIPS, with absolute contraindications being severe congestive heart failure, tricuspid regurgitation, severe pulmonary hypertension, multiple hepatic cysts, bacteremia or sepsis, and unrelieved biliary obstruction. Relative contraindications are fewer without obstruction of hepatic or portal veins being as much a concern. Moderate pulmonary hypertension, uncorrectable coagulopathy or thrombocytopenia, and existing hepatic encephalopathy are still relative contraindications [25].

The DIPS procedure begins with femoral venous access for introduction of the IVUS catheter which is placed in the retrohepatic IVC. Next, an echo tip trocar needle is advanced from a jugular access point to the same level of the IVC. Portal access is then created by advancement of the echo tip trocar needle under real-time ultrasound guidance through the liver and into the portal vein. This can be confirmed with aspiration or contrast-injection. Rest of the procedure is similar to a conventional TIPS procedure.

Complications of DIPS placement are identical to those of TIPS placement and include hepatic encephalopathy, variceal hemorrhage, and stent dysfunction. Although the theoretical risk of stent occlusion by parenchymal tract hypertrophy is reduced, more evidence is needed to substantiate this conclusion. Additionally, in patients with extrahepatic portal vein anatomy, there have been minor complications due to hemoperitoneum.

58.2.2.3 Percutaneous Mesocaval Shunt

One of the main benefits of using a mesenteric vessel as a connection to the systemic vasculature is the preservation of native portal venous anatomy in order for subsequent liver transplantation. This was the concept behind surgical mesocaval shunts, and has now been adapted as a percutaneous procedure. The percutaneous mesocaval shunt also allows

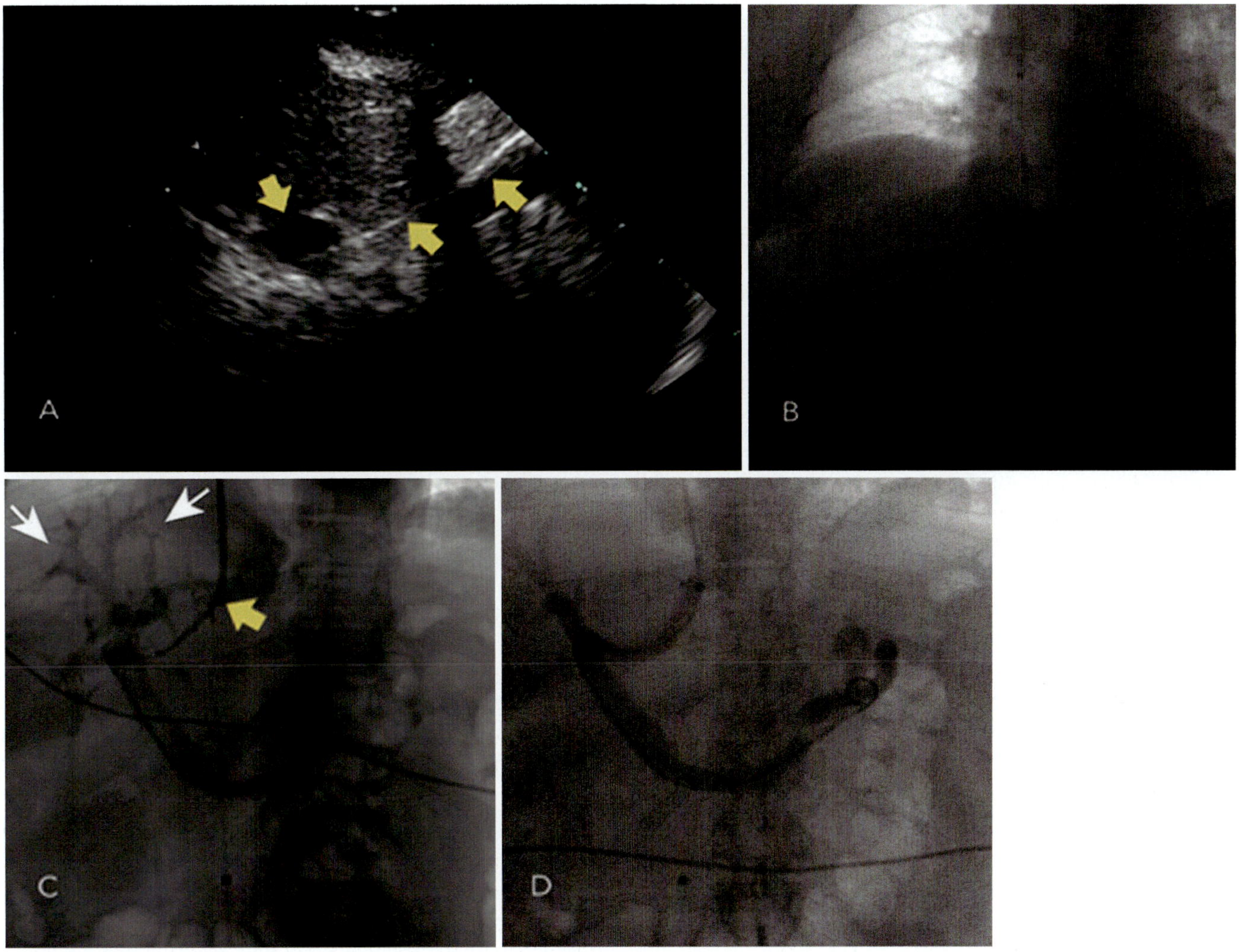

Fig. 58.5 DIPS Procedure showing echogenic needle (yellow arrows) traversing the IVC through the caudate lobe and into the portal vein (**a**), measuring catheter before stent placement (**b**) and after (**c**) demonstrating resolution of portal hepatic congestion (white arrows), (**d**) Completion venography after placement of a DIPS from the IVC to left portal vein

for patients with chronically occluded portal veins, who are not good candidates for TIPS, to have their portal hypertension treated [37].

Indications are again identical to the TIPS procedure; however, percutaneous mesocaval shunts (PMCS) allow for the circumvention of absolute and relative contraindications based on hepatic anatomy that can make TIPS difficult (Hepato-occlusive venous disease, severe hepatic cysts, etc.).

Absolute contraindications are still severe congestive heart failure, tricuspid regurgitation, severe pulmonary hypertension, multiple hepatic cysts, bacteremia or sepsis, and unrelieved biliary obstruction. Moderate pulmonary hypertension, uncorrectable coagulopathy or thrombocytopenia, and existing hepatic encephalopathy are still relative contraindications.

A transjugular or percutaneous mesocaval shunt procedure beings with a retrieval device, usually a snare basket, being placed through the internal jugular vein down to the IVC near the level of the desired shunt. After bowel preparation and prophylactic antibiotics, a 20-gauge Chiba needle is directed through the anterior abdominal wall under CT-guidance. It is advanced through-and-through the SMV and into the IVC. A wire is advanced through the chiba needle and introduced into the previously place snare. The wire is snared and pulled out through the jugular sheath, effectively leaving a wire percutaneously that travels from SMV to IVC and out the jugular sheath. Then a catheter is advanced over the wire, keeping a second wire as the safety wire. Using the working wire, access is obtained further into the SMV. At this point, the percutaneous safety wire is removed, and the stent can be advanced over the working wire. After dilation, pressures and venogram can be taken to confirm appropriate placement and function of the shunt [41] (Fig. 58.6).

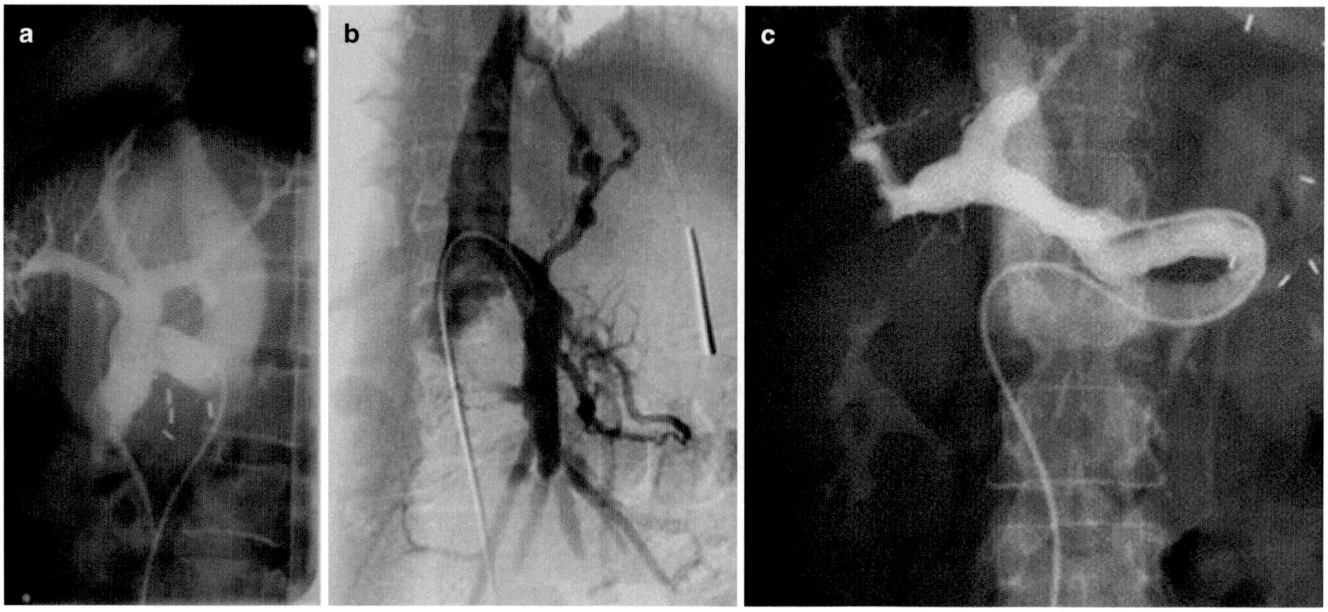

Fig. 58.6 Surgical Shunts visualized via angiography: Portacaval shunt (**a**), Mesocaval shunt (**b**), and Distal splenorenal shunt (**c**)

58.3 Comparison of Available Portocaval Shunting Procedures (Table 58.1)

Table 58.1 Comparison of relative complications across portacaval shunt types

Complications	Surgical shunt	TIPS	DIPS	Mesocaval
Operative mortality	+++	+	+	++
Cont. variceal bleeding	–	+	+	+
Hepatic encephalopathy	+++	+++	+++	?
Stent dysfunction	+	++	–	?
Acute liver failure	+	+	+	–
Hemoperitoneum	–	–	+	++
Bile Leaks	–	+	–	–

58.4 Future Directions

The DIPS procedure appears to be an excellent alternative to the standard TIPS treatment. The main advantages over a TIPS placement are that common failures due to bile leaks, tract hyperplasia, and hepatic vein occlusion are either excluded or much less likely (e.g. tract hyperplasia). Additionally, intravascular US used in DIPS placement allows for visualization portal vein puncture, the most technically challenging and dangerous aspect of TIPS creation. Finally, the widened indications for patients with altered intrahepatic anatomy and portal veno-occlusive disease of the hepatic or portal vein are more easily circumvented [36]. Further studies are currently needed to better quantify the complication rates for DIPS as well as randomized clinical trials to compare TIPS against DIPS on a broader level with stratification based on indication.

Self Study

Questions

1. Which is not an absolute contraindication to TIPS placement?
   (a) Severe Pulmonary Hypertension
   (b) Hepatocellular Carcinoma
   (c) Severe Congestive Heart Failure
   (d) Multiple Hepatic Cysts
2. Which statement is true?
   (a) Early TIPS treatment improves outcome in patients with persistently high HVPG
   (b) DIPS significantly increases patency rates compared to TIPS
   (c) Covered (PTFE) stent grafts have similar patency to Bare metal stents
   (d) TIPS placement for the treatment of refractory ascites is effective is 90% of patients

Answers

1. Which is not an absolute contraindication to TIPS placement?
   (a) Severe pulmonary hypertension is an absolute contraindication TIPS placement as shunt creation will rapidly increase portal venous return to the right side of the heart, leading to exacerbation of pulmonary hypertension, which can lead to right heart failure and circulatory collapse.

(b) CORRECT ANSWER. Hepatocellular carcinoma is a not an absolute contraindication to TIPS. HCC most commonly arises in a background of cirrhosis and as such will likely have sequelae of portal hypertension that may benefit from TIPS. Unless the HCC is directly occluding the majority of the hepatic veins, portal vein, or their is a large degree portal venous thrombosis (PVT), HCC does not present issues with shunt placement.

(c) Severe congestive heart failure is also an absolute contraindication to TIPS, for similar reasons as severe pulmonary hypertension. The rapid increase blood volume returning to the right side of the heart is likely to overload the already failing heart and lead to circulatory collapse and death.

(d) A multitude of hepatic cysts can lead to compression of venous structures, obstruction of parenchymal tracts, and increased risk of hemorrhage.

2. Which statement is true?

(a) CORRECT ANSWER. Studies have shown that patients who fail to respond to Endoscopic therapy and medical management with a decrease in HVPG below 20 mmHg are at significantly increased risk of rebleed and benefit from early intervention with TIPS placement.

(b) Although theoretically performing DIPS increases the patency rates compare to TIPS as the hepatic venous stenosis from TIPS creation is avoided, not enough studies have been conducted to evaluate the potential benefit of increased patency.

(c) Many RCTs have demonstrated improved patency, survival and decreased rates of bleeding with use of PTFE covered stents compared to bare metal stents. In fact, the AASLD now officially recommends the use of PTFE covered stents over bare metal stents.

(d) TIPS placement in the setting of refractory ascites results in 70% resolution of ascites in addition to a significant improvement in transplant free survival

References

1. Benoit JN, Womack WA, Hernandez L, Neil Granger D. "Forward" and "backward" flow mechanisms of portal hypertension: relative contributions in the rat model of portal vein stenosis. Gastroenterology. 1985;89:1092–6.
2. Iwakiri Y. Pathophysiology of portal hypertension. Clin Liver Dis. 2014;18:281–91.
3. Garcia-Tsao G. Current management of the complications of cirrhosis and portal hypertension: variceal hemorrhage, ascites, and spontaneous bacterial peritonitis. Gastroenterology. 2001;120:726–48.
4. Reiberger T, Püspök A, Schoder M, et al. Austrian consensus guidelines on the management and treatment of portal hypertension (Billroth III). Wien Klin Wochenschr. 2017;129:135–58.
5. Roccarina D, Rosselli M, Genesca J, Tsochatzis EA. Elastography methods for the non-invasive assessment of portal hypertension. Expert Rev Gastroenterol Hepatol. 2018;12:155–64.
6. Graham DY, Smith JL. The course of patients after variceal hemorrhage. Gastroenterology. 1981;80:800–9.
7. Jackson FC, Perrin EB, Felix WR, Smith AG. A clinical investigation of the portacaval shunt. V. Survival analysis of the therapeutic operation. Ann Surg. 1971;174:672–701.
8. Rueff B, Prandi D, Degos F, Sicot J, Degos JD, Sicot C, Maillard JN, Fauvert R, Benhamou JP. A controlled study of therapeutic portacaval shunt in alcoholic cirrhosis. Lancet. 1976;1:655–9.
9. Resnick RH, Iber FL, Ishihara AM, Chalmers TC, Zimmerman H. A controlled study of the therapeutic portacaval shunt. Gastroenterology. 1974;67:843–57.
10. Henderson JM, Kutner MH, Millikan WJ Jr, Galambos JT, Riepe SP, Brooks WS, Bryan FC, Warren WD. Endoscopic variceal sclerosis compared with distal splenorenal shunt to prevent recurrent variceal bleeding in cirrhosis. A prospective, randomized trial. Ann Intern Med. 1990;112:262–9.
11. D'amico G, Pagliaro L, Bosch J. The treatment of portal hypertension: a meta-analytic review. Hepatology. 1995;22:332–54.
12. Sarfeh IJ, Rypins EB. Partial versus total portacaval shunt in alcoholic cirrhosis. Results of a prospective, randomized clinical trial. Ann Surg. 1994;219:353–61.
13. Papatheodoridis GV, Goulis J, Leandro G, Patch D, Burroughs AK. Transjugular intrahepatic portosystemic shunt compared with endoscopic treatment for prevention of variceal rebleeding: a meta-analysis. Hepatology. 1999;30:612–22.
14. Salerno F, Cammà C, Enea M, Rössle M, Wong F. Transjugular intrahepatic portosystemic shunt for refractory ascites: a meta-analysis of individual patient data. Gastroenterology. 2007;133:825–34.
15. Bureau C, Thabut D, Oberti F, et al. Transjugular intrahepatic portosystemic shunts with covered stents increase transplant-free survival of patients with cirrhosis and recurrent ascites. Gastroenterology. 2017;152:157–63.
16. Bai M, Qi X-S, Yang Z-P, Yang M, Fan D-M, Han G-H. TIPS improves liver transplantation-free survival in cirrhotic patients with refractory ascites: an updated meta-analysis. World J Gastroenterol. 2014;20:2704–14.
17. Miraglia R, Maruzzelli L, Tuzzolino F, Petridis I, D'Amico M, Luca A. Transjugular intrahepatic portosystemic shunts in patients with cirrhosis with refractory ascites: comparison of clinical outcomes by using 8- and 10-mm PTFE-covered stents. Radiology. 2017;284:281–8.
18. D'Amico G, Luca A. TIPS is a cost effective alternative to surgical shunt as a rescue therapy for prevention of recurrent bleeding from esophageal varices. J Hepatol. 2008;48:387–90.
19. Boyer TD, Haskal ZJ. AASLD practice guidelines the role of transjugular intrahepatic portosystemic shunt (TIPS) in the management of portal hypertension update 2009. Hepatology. 2010;51:306.
20. Hayek G, Ronot M, Plessier A, Sibert A, Abdel-Rehim M, Zappa M, Rautou P-E, Valla D, Vilgrain V. Long-term outcome and analysis of dysfunction of transjugular intrahepatic portosystemic shunt placement in chronic primary Budd-Chiari syndrome. Radiology. 2017;283:280–92.
21. Fidelman N, Kwan SW, LaBerge JM, Gordon RL, Ring EJ, Kerlan RK Jr. The transjugular intrahepatic portosystemic shunt: an update. AJR Am J Roentgenol. 2012;199:746–55.
22. Siramolpiwat S. Transjugular intrahepatic portosystemic shunts and portal hypertension-related complications. World J Gastroenterol. 2014;20:16996–7010.
23. Wong F, Pantea L, Sniderman K. Midodrine, octreotide, albumin, and TIPS in selected patients with cirrhosis and type 1 hepatorenal syndrome. Hepatology. 2004;40:55–64.
24. Mezawa S, Homma H, Ohta H, Masuko E, Doi T, Miyanishi K, Takada K, Kukitsu T, Sato T, Niitsu Y. Effect of transjugular intrahepatic portosystemic shunt formation on portal hyperten-

sive gastropathy and gastric circulation. Am J Gastroenterol. 2001;96:1155–9.
25. Patidar KR, Sanyal AJ. Transjugular intrahepatic portosystemic shunt for refractory ascites in patients with high model for end-stage liver disease scores. Clin Liver Dis. 2016;7:84–7.
26. Franklin VR, Simmons LQ, Baker AL. Transjugular intrahepatic portosystemic shunt: a literature review. J Diagn Med Sonogr. 2018;34:114–22.
27. Andring B, Kalva SP, Sutphin P, Srinivasa R, Anene A, Burrell M, Xi Y, Pillai AK. Effect of technical parameters on transjugular intrahepatic portosystemic shunts utilizing stent grafts. World J Gastroenterol. 2015;21:8110–7.
28. Bureau C, Garcia-Pagan JC, Otal P, et al. Improved clinical outcome using polytetrafluoroethylene-coated stents for TIPS: results of a randomized study. Gastroenterology. 2004;126:469–75.
29. Bureau C, Pagan JCG, Layrargues GP, et al. Patency of stents covered with polytetrafluoroethylene in patients treated by transjugular intrahepatic portosystemic shunts: long-term results of a randomized multicentre study. Liver Int. 2007;27:742–7.
30. Perarnau JM, Le Gouge A, Nicolas C, et al. Covered vs. uncovered stents for transjugular intrahepatic portosystemic shunt: a randomized controlled trial. J Hepatol. 2014;60:962–8.
31. Triantafyllou T, Aggarwal P, Gupta E, Svetanoff WJ, Bhirud DP, Singhal S. Polytetrafluoroethylene-covered stent graft versus bare stent in transjugular intrahepatic portosystemic shunt: systematic review and meta-analysis. J Laparoendosc Adv Surg Tech A. 2018;28:867–79.
32. Garcia-Pagán JC, Di Pascoli M, Caca K, et al. Use of early-TIPS for high-risk variceal bleeding: results of a post-RCT surveillance study. J Hepatol. 2013;58:45–50.
33. Deltenre P, Trépo E, Rudler M, et al. Early transjugular intrahepatic portosystemic shunt in cirrhotic patients with acute variceal bleeding: a systematic review and meta-analysis of controlled trials. Eur J Gastroenterol Hepatol. 2015;27:e1–9.
34. Monescillo A, Martínez-Lagares F, Ruiz-del-Arbol L, et al. Influence of portal hypertension and its early decompression by TIPS placement on the outcome of variceal bleeding. Hepatology. 2004;40:793–801.
35. Garcia-Tsao G, Bosch J. Management of varices and variceal hemorrhage in cirrhosis. N Engl J Med. 2010;362:823–32.
36. Petersen B, Uchida BT, Timmermans H, Keller FS, Rosch J. Intravascular US-guided direct intrahepatic portacaval shunt with a PTFE-covered stent-graft: feasibility study in swine and initial clinical results. J Vasc Interv Radiol. 2001;12:475–86.
37. Casadaban LC, Gaba RC. Percutaneous portosystemic shunts: TIPS and beyond. Semin Intervent Radiol. 2014;31:227–34.
38. Petersen BD, Clark TWI. Direct intrahepatic portocaval shunt. Tech Vasc Interv Radiol. 2008;11:230–4.
39. Kawahara Y, Tanaka Y, Isoi N, et al. Direct intrahepatic portocaval shunt for refractory hepatic hydrothorax: a case report. Acute Med Surg. 2017;4:306–10.
40. Kirby JM, Cho KJ, Midia M. Image-guided intervention in management of complications of portal hypertension: more than TIPS for success. Radiographics. 2013;33:1473–96.
41. Nyman UR, Semba CP, Chang H, Hoffman C, Dake MD. Percutaneous creation of a mesocaval shunt. J Vasc Interv Radiol. 1996;7:769–73.

59 Systemic Therapy of Advanced Liver Cancer

Matthias Ocker

> **Key Concepts**
> - Liver cancer (HCC) still represents a global unmet medical need, ranking among the top ten cancer diseases and causes of cancer related deaths in both men and women [1].
> - Molecular targeted therapy was shown to have only limited efficacy.
> - It is recommended to use chemotherapy only in selected patients with good performance status and preserved liver function, usually without cirrhosis.
> - Immunotherapeutic approaches (checkpoint inhibitors, combinations) are a novel treatment option

59.1 Introduction

Liver cancer (HCC) still represents a global unmet medical need, ranking among the top ten cancer diseases and causes of cancer related deaths in both men and women [1]. While the majority of cases still occurs in Asia and Africa, incidence rates are continuously rising also in Western countries due to the high prevalence of hepatitis C infection and the steep increase in non-alcoholic fatty liver diseases and non-alcoholic steatohepatitis, which is expected to rise further until 2030 [2, 3]. As HCC usually develops on the basis of underlying cirrhosis (due to various pathophysiologic conditions), treatment options, esp. for advanced stages, are still limited. Due to this complex etiology, HCC is considered a disease within a disease and makes the identification of unanimous oncogenic drivers and thus also of potential drug targets very challenging [4].

The only curative treatment options today are surgical resection and liver transplantation, both being applicable only to early stage HCCs. Transplantation is further limited by the availability of donor organs, while resection is often impacted by early relapse. For intermediate stages, several locoregional therapies like radiofrequency or microwave ablation, transarterial chemoembolization (TACE), cryoablation, electroporation or transarterial radioembolization and radiotherapy have been established that could be applied repeatedly (also during transplant waiting time) in an adjuvant setting [5]. For advanced (metastatic or venous invasive) HCC, only little progress has been made since the approval of the multi-kinase inhibitor sorafenib about a decade ago. In this chapter, current and emerging treatment options including cancer immunotherapy approaches for advanced HCC are further discussed.

59.2 Conventional Chemotherapy for Advanced HCC

HCC is considered to be highly resistant to chemotherapeutic agents, probably due to the intrinsically high metabolic capacity of liver parenchymal cells which is e.g. linked to the high expression of efflux pumps as well as to factors associated with altered microenvironment in HCC like fibrosis, chronic inflammation or disturbed blood flow in cancers. Furthermore, high expression of potential drug resistance genes like heat-shock proteins or p53 mutations are commonly observed [6].

Several drugs have been evaluated as single agents or in combination studies, including doxorubicin, 5-fluorouracil, irinotecan, gemcitabine, and others. Most studies showed modest activities with only minimal improvement in overall survival and overall response rates usually below 20% [5, 6]. Combination studies usually showed significant toxicities and it is recommended to use chemotherapy only in selected patients with good performance status and preserved liver function, usually without cirrhosis.

M. Ocker (✉)
Translational Medicine Oncology, Bayer AG, Berlin, Germany

Charité University Medicine Berlin, Berlin, Germany
e-mail: matthias.ocker@bayer.com, matthias.ocker@charite.de

F. Radu-Ionita et al. (eds.), *Liver Diseases*, https://doi.org/10.1007/978-3-030-24432-3_59

59.3 Molecularly Targeted Therapy

The identification of distinct oncogenic drivers has led to the development of highly potent and specific drugs like crizotinib for ALK-translocated lung cancer or imatinib for chronic myeloid leukemia and gastrointestinal stroma tumors. Despite a huge number of clinical trials using targeted agents [7], today only four small molecule kinase inhibitors (sorafenib, regorafenib, lenvatinib, cabozantinib) could show a survival benefit in clinical studies of advanced HCC [8–12].

Sorafenib, an oral multi-kinase inhibitor, achieved overall survival of 10.7 months vs. 7.9 months of controls in advanced HCC [8]. Lenvatinib, another multi-kinase inhibitor with strong anti-angiogenic properties, showed increased overall survival (18.7 months) in a non-controlled phase 2 study of advanced HCC [13] and proved to be non-inferior to sorafenib in a recently published phase 3 study [11].

Regorafenib is a derivative of sorafenib with enhanced potency towards inhibition of antiangiogenic targets like VEGFR1-3, TIE2 and other kinases like PDGFR, FGFR, KIT or BRAF [14]. Regorafenib increased overall survival vs. placebo (10.6 months vs. 7.8 months) in a phase 3 study (RESORCE) of second line setting after sorafenib treatment [10]. Noteworthy, patients intolerant to sorafenib also do not benefit from regorafenib therapy and thus still represent an unmet medical need [15].

Cabozantinib inhibits both MET and VEGFR signaling and showed signs of efficacy in a phase 2 study [12]. Recently, the phase 3 study (CELESTIAL) of cabozantinib in a second line setting after sorafenib progression met its primary endpoint and reached an overall survival of 10.2 months vs. 8.0 months in the placebo arm [16] leading to regulatory submission in 2018.

While sorafenib received approval for first line therapy, regorafenib and cabozantinib are used in a second line setting. Approval of lenvatinib is expected in 2018 for first line therapy. All compounds are recommended for use in patients with Child-Pugh A and selected (low) Child-Pugh B status only.

Several studies investigated combinations of targeted agents, esp. sorafenib, with chemotherapy or other kinase inhibitors. The combination of sorafenib with doxorubicin failed to show a survival benefit in a phase 3 study [17] and a combination trial of sorafenib with the EGFR inhibitor erlotinib even demonstrated a worse outcome [18]. Overall, such combination therapies only provide a modest benefit to the patient but usually show an increase in drug related toxicities.

The combination of targeted agents with locoregional therapies like TACE has also been investigated. Sorafenib was used in intermediate stage multinodular HCC in combination with doxorubicin-eluting beads during TACE in the phase 2 SPACE trial. The procedure proved to be clinically feasible and led to a prolonged time to progression but without improvement in overall survival [19]. In the STORM study, sorafenib was investigated in an adjuvant setting against placebo but was shown not to be effective here [20].

59.4 Immunotherapy

The connection between inflammation and cancer was described by Rudolf Virchow more than 150 years ago and it took more than a century to re-discover the connection of cancer formation and wound healing [21]. As HCC commonly develops on the basis of chronic inflammatory diseases like HBV or HCV infection or (non-) alcoholic steatohepatitis and as so far no unique oncogenic driver has been identified in HCC [22], the concept of using the immune system to tackle HCC is very attractive [23]. Also, locoregional therapies can activate T cells in experimental models and lead to enhanced anti-tumor activity in HCC [24, 25]. The discovery of specific checkpoint inhibitors to overcome T cell inactivation in cancer was key to develop specific drugs which have now become a central pillar for modern oncology therapy in various indications [26]. As the ratio between suppressive (regulatory) and cytotoxic T cells has already been shown to be associated with improved survival in HCC [27], several checkpoint inhibitors have been studied in clinical trials now. Interestingly, also sorafenib has been shown to reduce regulatory T cells [23]. Studies in non-HCC patients already showed a long-lasting anti-tumor response of a combination of pembrolizumab and lenvatinib [15, 28].

As of March 2018, a total of 54 studies investigating the immune checkpoint inhibitors ipilimumab (CTLA-4), tremelimumab (CTLA-4), nivolumab (PD-1), pembrolizumab (PD-1), atezolizumab (PD-L1), durvalumab (PD-L1) or avelumab (PD-L1) in advanced hepatocellular carcinoma are listed on clinicaltrials.gov (Table 59.1).

The CTLA-4 inhibiting antibody tremelimumab showed a favourable safety and efficacy profile in phase 1 with 17.6% partial responses and 76.4% disease control rate. Interestingly, tremelimumab also evoked an anti-viral response in HCV positive patients [29]. In combination with locoregional therapies, tremelimumab confirmed the hypothesis of activating cytotoxic T cells, leading to a median overall survival of 12.3 months [30].

Based on the phase 1/2 (CheckMate-040) data, the anti-PD-1 antibody nivolumab was recently granted accelerated approval by FDA for the treatment of advanced HCC. In this study, 3.2% of patients experienced a complete response. The median overall survival was 28.6% in sorafenib-naïve patients with an overall survival rate of 73% at 12 months and safety seemed slightly better than for the CTLA-4 antibody [31]. The randomized controlled phase 3 trial CheckMate-459 vs. sorafenib did not meet its primary endpoint (OS).

Table 59.1 Studies with immune checkpoint inhibitors listed on clinicaltrials.gov (as of March 19, 2018)

Target	Drug	NCT	Phase	Regimen	Line of therapy	Comment
PD-L1	Avelumab	NCT03389126	2	Mono	After sorafenib	
PD-L1	Avelumab	NCT03289533	1b	+ Axitinib	First line	
PD-L1/ CTLA-4	Durvalumab/ Tremelimumab	NCT03298451	3	Combo	First line	
PD-L1/ CTLA-4	Durvalumab/ Tremelimumab	NCT02519348	2	Combo	After sorafenib	
PD-L1	Durvalumab	NCT03257761	1	+ Guadecitabine	After sorafenib	
PD-L1/ CTLA-4	Durvalumab/ Tremelimumab	NCT02821754	1/2	Combo + locoregional therapy	After sorafenib	RFA, Cryoablation or TACE
PD-L1	Durvalumab	NCT02572687	1	+ Ramucirumab	After sorafenib	
PD-L1	Atezolizumab	NCT03434379	3	+ Bevacizumab	First line	
PD-1	Pembrolizumab	NCT02658019	2	Mono	After sorafenib	
PD-1	Pembrolizumab	NCT03006926	1b	+ Lenvatinib	First line	
PD-1	Pembrolizumab	NCT02702414	2	Mono	After sorafenib	KEYNOTE-224
PD-1	Pembrolizumab	NCT02702401	3	Mono	After sorafenib	KEYNOTE-240
PD-1	Pembrolizumab	NCT03337841	2	Mono	Neoadjuvant	
PD-1	Pembrolizumab	NCT03163992	2	Mono	After sorafenib	
PD-1	Pembrolizumab	NCT03316872	2	+ radiotherapy	After sorafenib	
PD-1	Pembrolizumab	NCT03099564	1	+ Y90 radioembolization	First line	
PD-1	Pembrolizumab	NCT03397654	1/2	+ TACE	First line	TACE followed by Pembrolizumab
PD-1	Pembrolizumab	NCT02940496	1/2	Mono	After sorafenib	
PD-1	Pembrolizumab	NCT03419481	2	Mono	After sorafenib	HBV positive patients
PD-1	Pembrolizumab	NCT03062358	3	Mono	After sorafenib	KEYNOTE-394
PD-1	Pembrolizumab	NCT02509507	1b/2	+ Talimogene Laherparepvec	First line	MASTERKEY-318
PD-1	Pembrolizumab	NCT03347292	1b	+ Regorafenib	First line	
PD-1	Pembrolizumab	NCT03211416	1/2	+ Sorafenib	First line	
PD-1	Pembrolizumab	NCT03095781	1	+ XL888	After sorafenib	
PD-1	Pembrolizumab	NCT02595866	1	Mono	After sorafenib	HIV positive patients
PD-1	Pembrolizumab	NCT02432963	1	+ p53 modified vaccinia virus	After sorafenib	
PD-1	Pembrolizumab	NCT02178722	1/2	+ Epacadostat	After sorafenib	KEYNOTE-037/ECHO-202
PD-1	Pembrolizumab or Nivolumab	NCT03259867	2	+ transarterial tirapazamine	After sorafenib	TATE-PD1
PD-1	Pembrolizumab	NCT01174121	2	+ tumor infiltrating lymphocytes	After sorafenib	
PD-1	Pembrolizumab	NCT03277352	1/2	+ INCAGN01876	After sorafenib	
PD-1	Nivolumab	NCT03382886	1	+ bevacizumab	After sorafenib	NUANCE
PD-1	Nivolumab	NCT03033446	2	+ Y90 radioembolization	All	
PD-1	Nivolumab	NCT03299946	1	+ Cabozantinib	Neoadjuvant	CaboNivo

(continued)

Table 59.1 (continued)

Target	Drug	NCT	Phase	Regimen	Line of therapy	Comment
PD-1	Nivolumab	NCT03071094	1/2	+ Pexa-Vec	First line	
PD-1	Nivolumab	NCT02576509	3	Mono	First line	Study did not meet its primary endpoint (OS)
PD-1/ CTLA-4	Nivolumab/ Ipilimumab	NCT03222076	2	Combo	All	
PD-1	Nivolumab	NCT03380130	2	+ Y90 SIRT		SIRT followed by Nivolumab
PD-1	Nivolumab	NCT03383458	3	Mono	Adjuvant	CheckMate 9DX
PD-1/ CTLA-4	Nivolumab/ Ipilimumab	NCT03203304	1	+ radiotherapy	All	
PD-1/ CTLA-4	Nivolumab/ Ipilimumab	NCT01658878	1/2	Combo	First line	CheckMate040
PD-1	Nivolumab	NCT02423343	1/2	+ Galunisertib	After sorafenib	
PD-1	Nivolumab	NCT03418922	1	+ Lenvatinib	First line	
PD-1	Nivolumab	NCT02828124	1/2	Mono	After sorafenib	
PD-1	Nivolumab	NCT02837029	1	+ Y90 Therasphere	All	
PD-1	Nivolumab	NCT03439891	2	+ Sorafenib	First line	
PD-1	Nivolumab	NCT02859324	1/2	CC-122	After sorafenib	
PD-1	Nivolumab	NCT03143270	1	+ TACE	All	TACE followed by Nivolumab
PD-1	Nivolumab	NCT02705105	1/2	+ Mogamulizumab	After sorafenib	
PD-1	Nivolumab	NCT03071757	1	+ ABBV-368	After sorafenib	
PD-1	Nivolumab or Ipilimumab	NCT03126110	1/2	+ INCAGN01876	After sorafenib	
PD-1	Nivolumab or Ipilimumab	NCT03241173	1/2	+ INCAGN01949	After sorafenib	
PD-1	Nivolumab	NCT02465060	2			NCI-MATCH
CTLA-4	Tremelimumab	NCT01853618	1	+ locoregional therapy	After sorafenib	RFA, Cryoablation or TACE
CTLA-4	Tremelimumab	NCT01008358	2	Mono	After sorafenib	

Combinations of CTLA-4 and PD-1/PD-L1 have shown superior efficacy in patients with malignant melanoma [32, 33] and are currently also investigated in HCC. Preliminary results of a combination of durvalumab and tremelimumab phase 1/2 study presented at ASCO 2017 showed a confirmed overall response rate of 17.5% (30% in non-HBV and non-HCV patients) and a disease control rate 57.5% and 70.0%, respectively [34].

Although immunotherapy trials are still ongoing, the available data already indicate that this approach is feasible in HCC patients and can be an alternative to sorafenib, esp. in addition to locoregional therapies [7].

59.5 Future Perspective and Biomarkers

An important learning from successful trials in HCC is that patient selection is key to translate antitumor efficacy into prolonged survival. Interestingly, the underlying etiology seems less important than the overall patient performance as reflected by Child-Pugh status [35]. Beyond clinical status, the identification of predictive biomarkers would strongly foster the success of new drugs in HCC, not limited to targeted agents but especially also to immunotherapy approaches. The mutational load of a tumor seems to be a better predictor than the expression of PD-1/PD-L1 itself, as it is still unclear where this expression needs to predominantly occur (stroma/tumor) and what would be a useful overall cut-off [36]. Unfortunately, HCC shows rather an intermediate mutational burden and neoantigen load compared to e.g. melanoma or lung cancers [37]. Mutations that are commonly found in HCC samples include TERT, p53 and cell cycle control genes (e.g. TP53, CDKN2A), Wnt/β-catenin signaling, chromatin remodeling and the PI3K pathway [4, 22, 38]. Biomarker studies in HCC have previously been limited by the availability of biopsy material, which was not mandatory for setting the initial diagnosis. More recently, European guidelines recommend taking biopsies from patients in clinical studies [39]. Evolving technologies using liquid biopsies will help to overcome the sampling error of biopsies and help to increase our knowledge on oncogenic drivers in HCC. Enrichment of biomarker-selected patients using novel trial designs (e.g. umbrella or basket studies) seems necessary to further evolve the treatment options for HCC patients.

Self Study

Questions

1. Which statement is true?
   (a) Kinase inhibitors, e.g. sorafenib or regorafenib, are approved for treatment of all HCCs.
   (b) Combination therapies of kinase inhibitors with e.g. chemotherapy usually demonstrate improved efficacy and survival in HCC.
   (c) Combination with locoregional approaches prolongs time to progression.
   (d) Sorafenib is effective in an adjuvant setting.
2. Which statement is true?
   (a) Taking biopsies is not recommended for HCC.
   (b) Immune checkpoint combination therapies are considered feasible and achieve higher response rates in non-viral HCCs.
   (c) Sorafenib increases infiltration of regulatory T cells to HCC.
   (d) HCC shows very high mutational load.

Answers

1. Which statement is true?
   (a) Kinase inhibitors are approved for advanced stages of HCC only (BCLC C) with preserved liver function (Child-Pugh A–low B) good clinical performance score (PS 1–2). Chemotherapy is used in BCLC D while locoregional therapies, transplantation or surgical resection are used in early HCC.
   (b) Combination of different targeted agents are often limited by additive toxicity. Combination of sorafenib with doxorubicin failed to show a survival benefit and combination with erlotinib even demonstrated a worse outcome.
   (c) CORRECT ANSWER. Although overall survival was not improved in the SPACE study (sorafenib in combination with doxorubicin-eluting TACE), time to progression was prolonged.
   (d) In the STORM study, sorafenib did not show efficacy in an adjuvant setting against placebo.
2. Which statement is true?
   (a) European guidelines now recommend taking biopsies from HCC patients in clinical studies to improve biomarker discovery.
   (b) CORRECT ANSWER. Several clinical trials are currently ongoing and preliminary data show a higher response rate and disease control rate in non-viral HCC.
   (c) Sorafenib reduces the number of regulatory T cells and thus potentially improves the immunologic control of HCC.
   (d) HCC has an intermediate mutational load compared to e.g. melanoma or lung cancer. Commonly found mutations include TERT, p53 and cell cycle control as well as WNT/β-catenin signaling and other pathways without having identified a clear oncogenic driver so far.

References

1. Siegel RL, Miller KD, Jemal A. Cancer statistics, 2018. CA Cancer J Clin. 2018;68(1):7–30.
2. Petrick JL, Braunlin M, Laversanne M, Valery PC, Bray F, McGlynn KA. International trends in liver cancer incidence, overall and by histologic subtype, 1978-2007. Int J Cancer. 2016;139(7):1534–45.
3. Petrick JL, Kelly SP, Altekruse SF, McGlynn KA, Rosenberg PS. Future of hepatocellular carcinoma incidence in the United States forecast through 2030. J Clin Oncol. 2016;34(15):1787–94.
4. Khemlina G, Ikeda S, Kurzrock R. The biology of Hepatocellular carcinoma: implications for genomic and immune therapies. Mol Cancer. 2017;16(1):149.
5. Gosalia AJ, Martin P, Jones PD. Advances and future directions in the treatment of hepatocellular carcinoma. Gastroenterol Hepatol (N Y). 2017;13(7):398–410.
6. Eatrides J, Wang E, Kothari N, Kim R. Role of systemic therapy and future directions for hepatocellular carcinoma. Cancer Control. 2017;24(3):1073274817729243.
7. Gerbes A, Zoulim F, Tilg H, Dufour JF, Bruix J, Paradis V, et al. Gut roundtable meeting paper: selected recent advances in hepatocellular carcinoma. Gut. 2018;67(2):380–8.
8. Llovet JM, Ricci S, Mazzaferro V, Hilgard P, Gane E, Blanc JF, et al. Sorafenib in advanced hepatocellular carcinoma. N Engl J Med. 2008;359(4):378–90.
9. Cheng AL, Kang YK, Chen Z, Tsao CJ, Qin S, Kim JS, et al. Efficacy and safety of sorafenib in patients in the Asia-Pacific region with advanced hepatocellular carcinoma: a phase III randomised, double-blind, placebo-controlled trial. Lancet Oncol. 2009;10(1):25–34.
10. Bruix J, Qin S, Merle P, Granito A, Huang YH, Bodoky G, et al. Regorafenib for patients with hepatocellular carcinoma who progressed on sorafenib treatment (RESORCE): a randomised, double-blind, placebo-controlled, phase 3 trial. Lancet. 2017;389(10064):56–66.
11. Kudo M, Finn RS, Qin S, Han KH, Ikeda K, Piscaglia F, et al. Lenvatinib versus sorafenib in first-line treatment of patients with unresectable hepatocellular carcinoma: a randomised phase 3 non-inferiority trial. Lancet. 2018;391:1163.
12. Kelley RK, Verslype C, Cohn AL, Yang TS, Su WC, Burris H, et al. Cabozantinib in hepatocellular carcinoma: results of a phase 2 placebo-controlled randomized discontinuation study. Ann Oncol. 2017;28(3):528–34.
13. Ikeda K, Kudo M, Kawazoe S, Osaki Y, Ikeda M, Okusaka T, et al. Phase 2 study of lenvatinib in patients with advanced hepatocellular carcinoma. J Gastroenterol. 2017;52(4):512–9.
14. Wilhelm SM, Dumas J, Adnane L, Lynch M, Carter CA, Schutz G, et al. Regorafenib (BAY 73-4506): a new oral multikinase inhibitor of angiogenic, stromal and oncogenic receptor tyrosine kinases with potent preclinical antitumor activity. Int J Cancer. 2011;129(1):245–55.
15. Kudo M. Systemic therapy for hepatocellular carcinoma: 2017 update. Oncology. 2017;93(Suppl 1):135–46.

16. Abou-Alfa GK, Meyer T, Cheng AL, El-Khoueiry AB, Rimassa L, Ryoo BY, et al. Cabozantinib (C) versus Placebo (P) in patients (pts) with advanced hepatocellular carcinoma (HCC) who have received prior sorafenib: results from the randomized phase III CELESTIAL trial. J Clin Oncol. 2018;36(Suppl 4S):207.
17. Abou-Alfa GK, Johnson P, Knox JJ, Capanu M, Davidenko I, Lacava J, et al. Doxorubicin plus sorafenib vs doxorubicin alone in patients with advanced hepatocellular carcinoma: a randomized trial. JAMA. 2010;304(19):2154–60.
18. Zhu AX, Rosmorduc O, Evans TR, Ross PJ, Santoro A, Carrilho FJ, et al. SEARCH: a phase III, randomized, double-blind, placebo-controlled trial of sorafenib plus erlotinib in patients with advanced hepatocellular carcinoma. J Clin Oncol. 2015;33(6):559–66.
19. Lencioni R, Llovet JM, Han G, Tak WY, Yang J, Guglielmi A, et al. Sorafenib or placebo plus TACE with doxorubicin-eluting beads for intermediate stage HCC: the SPACE trial. J Hepatol. 2016;64(5):1090–8.
20. Bruix J, Takayama T, Mazzaferro V, Chau GY, Yang J, Kudo M, et al. Adjuvant sorafenib for hepatocellular carcinoma after resection or ablation (STORM): a phase 3, randomised, double-blind, placebo-controlled trial. Lancet Oncol. 2015;16(13):1344–54.
21. Coussens LM, Werb Z. Inflammation and cancer. Nature. 2002;420(6917):860–7.
22. Llovet JM, Villanueva A, Lachenmayer A, Finn RS. Advances in targeted therapies for hepatocellular carcinoma in the genomic era. Nat Rev Clin Oncol. 2015;12(7):408–24.
23. Elsegood CL, Tirnitz-Parker JE, Olynyk JK, Yeoh GC. Immune checkpoint inhibition: prospects for prevention and therapy of hepatocellular carcinoma. Clin Transl Immunol. 2017;6(11):e161.
24. Hansler J, Wissniowski TT, Schuppan D, Witte A, Bernatik T, Hahn EG, et al. Activation and dramatically increased cytolytic activity of tumor specific T lymphocytes after radio-frequency ablation in patients with hepatocellular carcinoma and colorectal liver metastases. World J Gastroenterol. 2006;12(23):3716–21.
25. Behm B, Di Fazio P, Michl P, Neureiter D, Kemmerling R, Hahn EG, et al. Additive antitumour response to the rabbit VX2 hepatoma by combined radio frequency ablation and toll like receptor 9 stimulation. Gut. 2016;65(1):134–43.
26. Pardoll DM. The blockade of immune checkpoints in cancer immunotherapy. Nat Rev Cancer. 2012;12(4):252–64.
27. Gao Q, Qiu SJ, Fan J, Zhou J, Wang XY, Xiao YS, et al. Intratumoral balance of regulatory and cytotoxic T cells is associated with prognosis of hepatocellular carcinoma after resection. J Clin Oncol. 2007;25(18):2586–93.
28. Kudo M. Immuno-oncology in hepatocellular carcinoma: 2017 Update. Oncology. 2017;93(Suppl 1):147–59.
29. Sangro B, Gomez-Martin C, de la Mata M, Inarrairaegui M, Garralda E, Barrera P, et al. A clinical trial of CTLA-4 blockade with tremelimumab in patients with hepatocellular carcinoma and chronic hepatitis C. J Hepatol. 2013;59(1):81–8.
30. Duffy AG, Ulahannan SV, Makorova-Rusher O, Rahma O, Wedemeyer H, Pratt D, et al. Tremelimumab in combination with ablation in patients with advanced hepatocellular carcinoma. J Hepatol. 2017;66(3):545–51.
31. El-Khoueiry AB, Sangro B, Yau T, Crocenzi TS, Kudo M, Hsu C, et al. Nivolumab in patients with advanced hepatocellular carcinoma (CheckMate 040): an open-label, non-comparative, phase 1/2 dose escalation and expansion trial. Lancet. 2017;389(10088):2492–502.
32. Larkin J, Chiarion-Sileni V, Gonzalez R, Grob JJ, Cowey CL, Lao CD, et al. Combined nivolumab and ipilimumab or monotherapy in untreated melanoma. N Engl J Med. 2015;373(1):23–34.
33. Postow MA, Chesney J, Pavlick AC, Robert C, Grossmann K, McDermott D, et al. Nivolumab and ipilimumab versus ipilimumab in untreated melanoma. N Engl J Med. 2015;372(21):2006–17.
34. Kelley RK, Abou-Alfa GK, Bendell JC, Kim TY, Borad MJ, Yong WP. Phase I/II study of durvalumab and tremelimumab in patients with unresectable hepatocellular carcinoma (HCC): phase I safety and efficacy analyses. J Clin Oncol. 2017;35(15 Suppl):4073.
35. Bruix J, Cheng AL, Meinhardt G, Nakajima K, De Sanctis Y, Llovet J. Prognostic factors and predictors of sorafenib benefit in patients with hepatocellular carcinoma: analysis of two phase III studies. J Hepatol. 2017;67(5):999–1008.
36. Morfouace M, Hewitt SM, Salgado R, Hartmann K, Litiere S, Tejpar S, et al. A transatlantic perspective on the integration of immuno-oncology prognostic and predictive biomarkers in innovative clinical trial design. Semin Cancer Biol. 2018;52:158.
37. Schumacher TN, Schreiber RD. Neoantigens in cancer immunotherapy. Science. 2015;348(6230):69–74.
38. Nault JC, Galle PR, Marquardt JU. The role of molecular enrichment on future therapies in hepatocellular carcinoma. J Hepatol. 2018;69:237.
39. EASL-EORTC. clinical practice guidelines: management of hepatocellular carcinoma. J Hepatol. 2012;56(4):908–43.

Embolization Therapy for Liver Cancer

60

Lukas Luerken and Lukas Beyer

Key Concepts

- The concept of TACE is based on minimally invasive induction of tumor necrosis by a high local concentration of a chemotherapeutic agent and an embolic/ischemic effect.
- TACE is the treatment of first choice for patients with intermediate HCC stage BCLC B, but may also be considered in individual cases for patients with early stage A (stage migration) and advanced stage C (segmental PVT).
- Current studies suggest that TACE is also an effective and safe alternative for the treatment of non-resectable liver metastases from colorectal carcinomas and other tumor entities, but there is not yet sufficient evidence as of 2019.
- Currently available methods are cTACE using Lipiodol, DEB-TACE using drug eluting beads and DSM-TACE using dissolvable starch microspheres.
- As of 2019, there is still no agreement on the best TACE technique and different options for patient selection, retreatment schemes, drugs and embolic agents are still in use.

60.1 Introduction

The concept of transarterial chemoembolization (TACE) is based on the minimally invasive induction of tumor necrosis by a high local concentration of a chemotherapeutic agent and an embolic effect. The embolic effect causes ischemia on the one hand and an increased local dwell time of the chemotherapeutic agent in the tumor on the other. Since both HCC and secondary liver tumors receive a large part of their blood supply from the hepatic arteries, but healthy liver tissue is primarily supplied with blood portalvenously, transarterial application is particularly suitable for achieving the highest possible concentration of the chemoembolisate in the tumor.

For the first time TACE was mentioned as an alternative therapy for patients with HCC in 1985 [1], since then it has taken a stable place in the multimodal oncological therapy of primary malignant liver tumors and is also gaining increasing importance in the treatment of secondary malignant liver tumors. In the following, both the general technical procedure for TACE, the indications for TACE as well as the various methods of TACE currently available will be presented.

60.2 Indications

The European Association for the Study of the Liver (EASL) [2] recommends TACE in its guidelines for the treatment of HCC in the version of 2018 for patients with non-resectable HCC in intermediate stage according to the criteria of the Barcelona Clinic Liver Cancer staging system (BCLC B) (Fig. 60.1) [3]. This is defined as multinodular, non-resectable disease with preserved liver function and good clinical status of the patient. There is a high level of evidence for first-line treatment with TACE for this tumor stage.

Also, for patients with tumor stage A, TACE is sometimes considered if, for example, resection and ablation is not possible for technical reasons [4]. This procedure is called stage migration. Similarly, treatment with TACE can keep patients with tumor stage A waiting for a liver transplant longer on the transplant list [5]. A further study from 2013 also shows that TACE reduces the risk of recurrence after liver transplantation [6].

Recent studies suggest that TACE may also be an option for patients with advanced stage C HCC with segmental portal vein invasion. A 2017 study with 238 patients observed

L. Luerken (✉) · L. Beyer
Department of Radiology, University Hospital Regensburg, Regensburg, Germany
e-mail: Lukas.luerken@ukr.de; lukas.beyer@ukr.de

F. Radu-Ionita et al. (eds.), *Liver Diseases*, https://doi.org/10.1007/978-3-030-24432-3_60

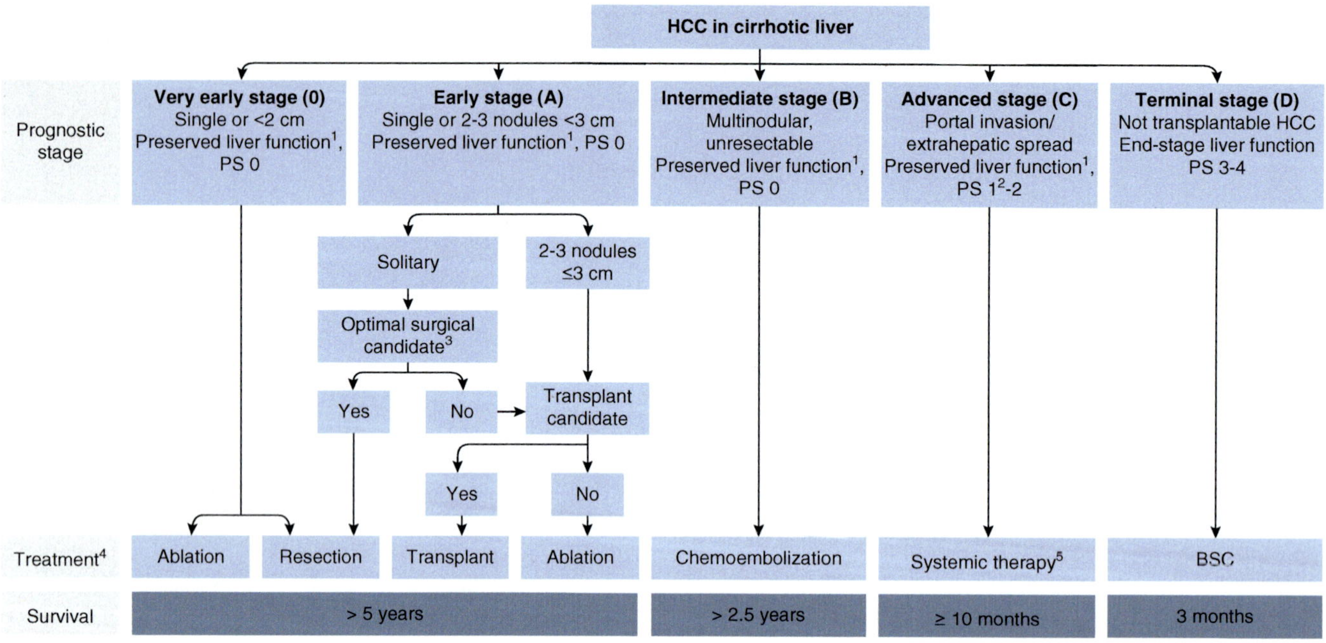

Fig. 60.1 Treatment schema of the European Association for the Study of the Liver (EASL). TACE is recommended for patients with non-resectable HCC in intermediate stage (multinodular, non-resectable disease with preserved liver function and good clinical status)

that patients with central portal vein thrombosis (PVT) survived an average of 6.4 months after TACE, while patients with segmental PVT survived an average of 20.0 months after TACE [7].

Adverse prognostic factors for TACE in HCC are tumor diameter of more than 5 cm, more than four lesions, cirrhosis of the liver with stage Child-Pugh B, and unselective chemoembolization. Poor ECOG status (ECOG PS ≥ 2) and Child-Pugh C are considered absolute contraindications. Although an extrahepatic tumour manifestation is generally also considered a contraindication, selected patient groups may benefit from TACE [18].

If, after two treatments with TACE, there is no response to therapy in the sense of no tumour necrosis or no change in the size of the vital part of the tumour or even tumour progression, no further TACE should be administered and the therapy should be switched to systemic therapy.

The majority of all secondary liver tumors are metastases of colorectal cancer (CRC) and occur in about 25% of all patients with CRC [8]. Even though there is a steadily growing number of studies suggesting that TACE is a safe and effective therapy alternative for patients with non-resectable liver metastases [9], there are still no recommendations for TACE in guidelines due to the not yet sufficient evidence. The same also applies to liver metastases of other tumour entities, for example cholangiocellular carcinoma (CCC) and neuroendocrine tumours (NET).

Since TACE is primarily understood as a palliative rather than a curative treatment approach, repeated treatments of patients are recommended. There is no consensus on the intervals between TACE treatments, the most common being intervals of 4–8 weeks between two treatments. At the latest after the second treatment, imaging should be performed with a contrast-enhanced MRI or CT to monitor the success of the therapy.

Since TACE induces tumor ischemia/infarction but has no direct effect on tumor size, new imaging criteria had to be developed to assess the success of treatment. For the assessment of HCC, the modified RECIST (mRECIST) criterion was developed, which is based on a single measurement of the longitudinal axis of the enhancing part of the tumor tissue. mRECIST is a reliable response marker and independent prognostic factor for survival after TACE and can therefore be used as a guide for potential therapeutic changes [10].

60.3 Technique

Possible access paths for TACE are transfemoral puncture as well as transbrachial and transradial access.

The relatively short access path as well as the normally large diameter of the AFC speak for a femoral access. It is important to puncture the AFC at the level of the femoral head in order to ensure sufficient compressibility of the vessel after the intervention and to reduce the risk of secondary bleeding. Bleeding into the retroperitoneal space after AFC puncture is a feared complication with a mortality rate of 10% and occurs after 0.1–0.7% of all punctures [11].

Both transbrachial and transradial punctures have a significantly lower risk of relevant bleeding than transfemoral punctures. The complication rate for transbrachial access though is not negligible with 12.5% [12] but can be slightly

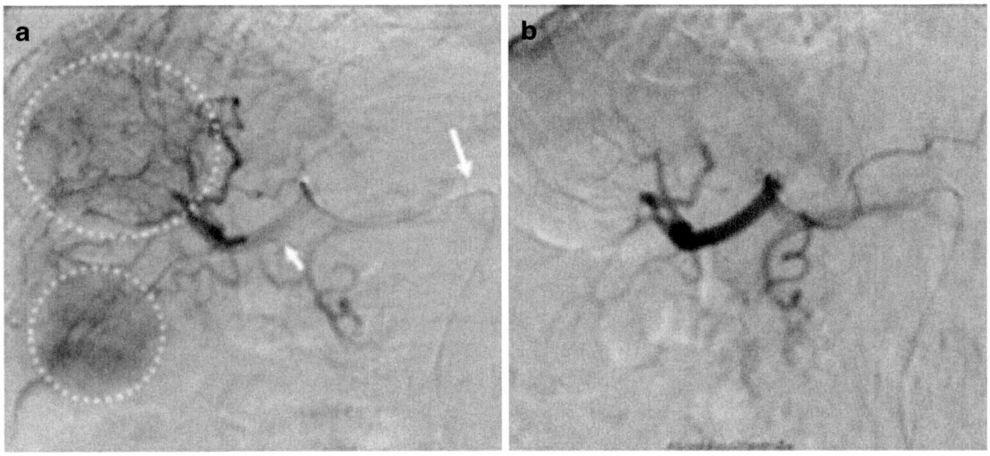

Fig. 60.2 (**a**) Patient with two large HCC in the right lobe of the liver. The truncus coeliacus (long arrow) was probed with a 5F cobra catheter. The tip of the catheter was placed in the hepatica propria (short arrow). After injecting the catheter with a contrast medium, the two HCC show themselves as "tumor blushes" due to their strong arterial vascularization. (**b**) After successful embolization with DSM and Farmorubicin, a contrast-enhanced final check is performed again. No tumor blushes are recognizable as signs of the embolic effect

reduced with vascular occlusion systems such as Angioseal and Exoseal.

Since the transradial access is the access path of choice in guidelines for coronary interventions, various studies exist which confirm an overall lower complication level for the transradial access compared to transfemoral access [13]. Also, stroke risk does not seem to be increased with transradial interventions compared to transfemoral interventions [14].

Disadvantages of transbrachial and transradial puncture are the longer access path and the somewhat more complicated probing of the aorta abdominalis over the aortic arch. Access via the patient's left arm is preferred due to the shorter access route.

Depending on the experience of the interventionalist, the puncture can be performed conventionally or under ultrasound-guidance. For all three access routes, a 4-F or 5-F sheath is suitable for TACE. In most cases, a cobra catheter with a length of 65 cm is used as a probing catheter for the coeliac trunk when performing femoral access. In cases where the coeliac trunc leaves the aorta in a steep angle, a retreat catheter (e.g. SOS-Omni, AngioDynamics, Latham NY, USA) may facilitate access. When probing from a cranial direction via transbrachial and transradial puncture, the angle of the coeliac trunc is usually flatter than 90°, so a less strongly curved catheter is sufficient for stable probing in most cases, but it should have a length of at least 90 cm (transbrachial) or 110 cm (transradial) (e.g. Ultimate 1, Merit medical, Jordan UT, USA).

For first-time TACE treatments, if no thin-layer CT-angiography is available for orientation, the AMS should be probed and visualized to identify possible aberrant hepatic arteries. Subsequently, an overview angiography with catheter position in the coeliac trunc should also be performed. Subsequently, the A. hepatica communis is probed with a microcatheter in coaxial technique, from where a new angiography is obtained (Fig. 60.2).

Identification of A. gastrica dextra and sinistra, gastroduodenalis, cystica and possible vessel variations (e.g. exit of A. gastrica dextra from the left A. hepatica or a pancreaticoduodenal arcade originating from A. hepatica propria, but also from AV fistulas and shunts) is necessary to avoid false embolization.

60.4 Technical Advances

The more superselective the tumour feeders can be probed, the better a tumour embolization can be achieved while protecting the surrounding healthy liver parenchyma. In order to achieve complete and superselective embolization, all tumor feeders must be identified. The simplest and most effective way to visualize the tumor including all tumor supplying vessels is to perform a 3D angiography with a flat panel detector (so called Cone-Beam-CT). Using automated tumor-feeder detection software, even tiny feeder vessels can be detected, visualized three-dimensionally and then embolized ultraselectively [22]. This approach helps to increase local tumor control, preserve the hepatic function and reduce the extent of complications (especially post-embolization syndrome) [15].

60.5 Methods

Essentially, three TACE procedures are available: conventional TACE (cTACE), TACE with drug-eluting beads (DEB-TACE) and TACE with dissolvable-starch-microspheres (DSM-TACE).

60.5.1 cTACE

cTACE is the oldest method for TACE and was first mentioned in 1985. The evidence on cTACE is mainly based on two large meta-analyses in which randomized, controlled studies on the efficacy of cTACE with cisplatin or doxorubicin were evaluated in comparison to Best Supportive Care (BSC) in HCC patients not eligible for surgical therapy [16, 17]. These analyses demonstrated a significant advantage of cTACE over BSC in terms of mean survival time of patients.

In cTACE, Lipiodol (Guerbet, Paris, France) is used as a carrier for a chemotherapeutic agent. Various therapeutics are available, including doxorubicin, epirubicin, idarubicin and cisplatin. A water-in-oil emulsion of Lipiodol and the respective chemotherapeutic agent is produced manually, which is mixed approx. 10–20 times in the "push and pull" process via a 3-way tap, so that droplets with a diameter of 70–100 μm are formed. This mixture is then selectively or superselectively introduced into the tumor supplying arteries via a microcatheter, followed by embolizing particles.

Several options are available as embolizates. Absorbable gelatin (Gelfoam, Pfizer, New York, USA) is most commonly used, alternatives are degradable starch microspheres or permanent materials including polyvinyl alcohols, uncalibrated and calibrated microspheres.

A review from 2016, which analyzed data from 101 clinical studies up to 2013 confirmed the previously known data on the efficacy and safety of cTACE with a median survival of 19.4 months after cTACE [19]. Furthermore, a progression-free-survival of 57.2% was observed 6 months after intervention. The most common adverse events were related to postembolization syndrome, which is characterized by fever (17.2%), pain in the right upper quadrant (11%), and nausea and/or vomiting (6%). The results of a randomized trial published in 2017 suggest that prophylactic intravenous dexamethasone on days 1–3 after TACE may reduce the incidence of postembolization syndrome [20].

60.5.2 DEB-TACE

DEB-TACE was introduced 10 years ago with the aim of improving the results of cTACE and minimising the side effects of the procedure. It is based on the use of microspheres that are capable of binding the cytotoxic drug through an ion exchange mechanism and then slowly release it within the target lesion in a controlled manner over a prolonged period of time. This favourable pharmacokinetic profile increases the exposure of the tumor to the chemotherapeutic agent and minimises associated toxicity due to reduced systemic drug circulation [21].

DEB-TACE has the same clinical applications as cTACE to treat selectively targetable liver lesions in an asymptomatic patient without impaired liver function, metastatic spread or portal vein thrombosis. A study published in 2012 reported unprecedented results in over 100 HCC patients with early and intermediate stage disease: The mean OS was 48.6 months (BCLC A: 54.2 months and BCLC B: 47.7 months) [23].

However, the choice of DEB-TACE over cTACE continues to be debated given the high costs and the controversial results of comparative studies [24, 25]. There is still no agreement on the best TACE technique and different options for patient selection, retreatment schemes, drugs and embolic agents are still in use.

60.5.3 Comparison of DEB-TACE and cTACE

The PRECISION V study published in 2010 was the first to show a lack of superiority of DEB-TACE over cTACE and demonstrated no statistical difference in overall response between these regimens, although the radiological response rate was slightly higher in the DEB-TACE arm [24].

Four years later, the results were confirmed by a randomized controlled trial by Golfieri et al., which found no significant difference in local and overall tumor response rates of cTACE and DEB-TACE [25]. The median time to progression (TTP) was 9 months in both arms ($p = 0.766$) and overall survival after 1 year and 2 years was 86.2% and 56.8%, respectively, after DEB-TACE, and 83.5% and 55.4% after cTACE ($p = 0.949$). The study was terminated prematurely, as the interim analysis showed no significant advantage of DEB-TACE over cTACE.

However, it is important to note, that some of the studies that showed non-superiority of DEB-TACE reported lower rates of adverse events in the DEB-TACE group. The PRECISION V study, for example, indicates that DEB-TACE has a higher tolerability, significantly lower liver toxicity and fewer doxorubicin-associated side effects. Golfieri et al. also conclude that DEB-TACE may lead to a lower incidence of post-embolization syndrome.

To summarize, despite the theoretical advantages of DEB-TACE, in particular with regard to pharmacodynamics, the routine use of DEB-TACE remains the subject of controversial scientific debate due to the lack of evidence of its superiority over cTACE while at the same time is it associated with higher costs.

60.5.4 DSM-TACE

In recent years, DSM-TACE has emerged as an alternative chemoembolization method. Instead of Lipiodol or drug eluting beads, dissolvable starch microspheres are used to obtain a transient occlusion of target vessels. The most common embolization agent is Embocept (PharmaCept GmbH, Berlin, Germany). DSM provide a well-defined, compared to Lipiodol and DEB reasonably shorter and transient vessel occlusion time of 35–50 min, combined with the ability to bind chemotherapeutical agents. Potential advantages of this method may be a reduced vascular epithelial growth factor (VEGF) response, which is discussed to be a predictor for poor response to TACE [26], and a lower risk for adverse events due to embolization of non-target vessels. Partial reperfusion after embolization can be observed after a time of 10–15 min [27], making DSM-TACE a possible alternative for patient scenarios, where selective embolization can't be obtained, for example in bilobar or disseminated disease. First studies describe a good technical efficacy and safety for DSM-TACE [28, 29], but as of 2019 there is still a lack of evidence.

Self Study

Questions

1. Which statement is correct:
   (a) According to the EASL guidelines for HCC, TACE should primarily be performed in patients with advanced HCC stage BCLC C.
   (b) TACE may be considered for patients with early HCC stage BCLC A.
   (c) The evidence for benefits of TACE in patients with intermediate HCC Stage BCLC B compared to system therapy with sorafenib is scarce.
   (d) If, after two treatments with TACE, tumor progression is observed, at least a third treatment session should be performed.
2. Which statement is correct:
   (a) DSM-TACE has a vessel occlusion time of approximately 6 weeks.
   (b) DEB-TACE is more suitable for lesser selective embolizations in disseminated disease than cTACE.
   (c) Transradial approach has a lower risk for adverse events compared to brachial and femoral approach.
   (d) To induce maximum tumor-necrosis, chemoembolization with DSM must be followed by embolizing particles like calibrated microspheres or gelfoam.

Answers

1. Which statement is correct:
   (a) TACE is the treatment of choice for patients with HCC BCLC B. Recent studies suggest, that patients with HCC stage BCLC C and segmental portal vein infiltration may profit from TACE.
   (b) Patients with early HCC stage BCLC A may be treated with TACE if resection or ablation is not possible, this procedure is called stage migration. CORRECT.
   (c) Evidence for TACE as first line treatment in patients with intermediate HCC Stage BCLC B is strong.
   (d) If tumor progression or a non-response to TACE is observed after two treatments, no further TACE should be administered and therapy should be switched to system therapy.
2. Which statement is correct:
   (a) Vessel occlusion time of DSM-TACE is approximately 35–50 min.
   (b) Tumor feeders should be probed as superselective as possible when performing cTACE and DEB-TACE.
   (c) Transradial approach has a significantly lower risk for adverse events compared to brachial and femoral approach. CORRECT.
   (d) Application of embolizing particles like absorbable gelatin, degradable starch microspheres or permanent materials including polyvinyl alcohols, uncalibrated and calibrated microspheres

References

1. Hidaka H, Kobayashi H, Ohyama M, et al. Transarterial chemoembolization therapy of hepatocellular carcinoma using anticancer agents (mitomycin C and/or adriamycin) suspended in lipiodol. Nihon Igaku Hoshasen Gakkai zasshi Nippon acta radiologica. 1985;45(11):1430–40.
2. European Association for the Study of the Liver. Electronic address: easloffice@easloffice.eu; European Association for the Study of the Liver. EASL Clinical Practice Guidelines: Management of hepatocellular carcinoma. J Hepatol. 2018;69(1):182. https://www.sciencedirect.com/science/article/pii/S0168827818302150. Accessed January 31, 2019.
3. Llovet JM, Brú C, Bruix J. Prognosis of hepatocellular carcinoma: the BCLC staging classification. Semin Liver Dis. 1999;19:329–38. https://doi.org/10.1055/s-2007-1007122.
4. Raoul J-L, Sangro B, Forner A, et al. Evolving strategies for the management of intermediate-stage hepatocellular carcinoma: available evidence and expert opinion on the use of transarterial chemoembolization. Cancer Treat Rev. 2011;37:212–20. https://doi.org/10.1016/j.ctrv.2010.07.006.
5. Frangakis C, Geschwind J-F, Kim D, et al. Chemoembolization decreases drop-off risk of hepatocellular carcinoma patients on the liver transplant list. Cardiovasc Intervent Radiol. 2011;34:1254–61. https://doi.org/10.1007/s00270-010-0077-7.
6. Pompili M, Francica G, Ponziani FR, Iezzi R, Avolio AW. Bridging and downstaging treatments for hepatocellular carcinoma in patients on the waiting list for liver transplantation. World J Gastroenterol. 2013;19:7515–30. https://doi.org/10.3748/wjg.v19.i43.7515.
7. Prajapati HJ, Kim HS. Treatment algorithm based on the multivariate survival analyses in patients with advanced hepatocellular carcinoma treated with trans-arterial chemoembolization. PLoS One. 2017;12:e0170750. https://doi.org/10.1371/journal.pone.0170750.
8. Hackl C, Neumann P, Gerken M, Loss M, Klinkhammer-Schalke M, Schlitt HJ. Treatment of colorectal liver metastases in Germany:

a ten-year population-based analysis of 5772 cases of primary colorectal adenocarcinoma. BMC Cancer. 2014;14:810. https://doi.org/10.1186/1471-2407-14-810.
9. Massmann A, Rodt T, Marquardt S, et al. Transarterial chemoembolization (TACE) for colorectal liver metastases--current status and critical review. Langenbecks Arch Surg. 2015;400:641–59. https://doi.org/10.1007/s00423-015-1308-9.
10. Gillmore R, Stuart S, Kirkwood A, et al. EASL and mRECIST responses are independent prognostic factors for survival in hepatocellular cancer patients treated with transarterial embolization. J Hepatol. 2011;55(6):1309–16.
11. Stone PA, Campbell JE. Complications related to femoral artery access for transcatheter procedures. Vasc Endovascular Surg. 2012;46:617–23. https://doi.org/10.1177/1538574412457475.
12. Lupattelli T, Clerissi J, Clerici G, et al. The efficacy and safety of closure of brachial access using the AngioSeal closure device: experience with 161 interventions in diabetic patients with critical limb ischemia. J Vasc Surg. 2008;47:782–8. https://doi.org/10.1016/j.jvs.2007.11.050.
13. Valgimigli M, Gagnor A, Calabró P, et al. Radial versus femoral access in patients with acute coronary syndromes undergoing invasive management: a randomised multicentre trial. Lancet. 2015;385:2465–76. https://doi.org/10.1016/S0140-6736(15)60292-6.
14. Patel VG, Brayton KM, Kumbhani DJ, Banerjee S, Brilakis ES. Meta-analysis of stroke after transradial versus transfemoral artery catheterization. Int J Cardiol. 2013;168:5234–8. https://doi.org/10.1016/j.ijcard.2013.08.026.
15. Miyayama S, Yamashiro M, Ikuno M, Okumura K, Yoshida M. Ultraselective transcatheter arterial chemoembolization for small hepatocellular carcinoma guided by automated tumor- feeders detection software: technical success and short-term tumor response. Abdom Imaging. 2014;39(3):645–56.
16. Cammà C, Schepis F, Orlando A, et al. Transarterial chemoembolization for unresectable hepatocellular carcinoma: meta-analysis of randomized controlled trials. Radiology. 2002;224:47–54. https://doi.org/10.1148/radiol.2241011262.
17. Llovet JM, Bruix J. Systematic review of randomized trials for unresectable hepatocellular carcinoma: chemoembolization improves survival. Hepatology (Baltimore, Md). 2003;37:429–42. https://doi.org/10.1053/jhep.2003.50047.
18. Kirstein MM, Voigtländer T, Schweitzer N, Hinrichs JB, Marquardt J, Wörns MA, Kloeckner R, Fründt TW, Ittrich H, Wacker F, Rodt T, Manns MP, Wege H, Weinmann A, Vogel A. Transarterial chemoembolization versus sorafenib in patients with hepatocellular carcinoma and extrahepatic disease. U Eur Gastroenterol J. 2018;6(2):238–46.
19. Lencioni R, de Baere T, Soulen MC, Rilling WS, Geschwind J-FH. Lipiodol transarterial chemoembolization for hepatocellular carcinoma: a systematic review of efficacy and safety data. Hepatology. 2016;64:106–16.
20. Ogasawara S, Chiba T, Ooka Y, Kanogawa N, Motoyama T, Suzuki E, et al. A randomized placebo-controlled trial of prophylactic dexamethasone for transcatheter arterial chemoembolization. Hepatology. 2017;
21. Varela M, Real MI, Burrel M, Forner A, Sala M, Brunet M, et al. Chemoembolization of hepatocellular carcinoma with drug eluting beads: efficacy and doxorubicin pharmacokinetics. J Hepatol. 2007;46:474–81.
22. Ronot M, Abdel-Rehim M, Hakimé A, Kuoch V, Roux M, Chiaradia M, et al. Cone-beam CT angiography for determination of tumor-feeding vessels during chemoembolization of liver tumors: comparison of conventional and dedicated-software analysis. J Vasc Interv Radiol. 2016;27:32–8.
23. Burrel M, Reig M, Forner A, et al. Survival of patients with hepatocellular carcinoma treated by transarterial chemoembolisation (TACE) using Drug Eluting Beads. Implications for clinical practice and trial design. J Hepatol. 2012;56(6):1330–5.
24. Lammer J, Malagari K, Vogl T, et al. Prospective randomized study of doxorubicin-eluting-bead embolization in the treatment of hepatocellular carcinoma: results of the PRECISION V study. Cardiovasc Intervent Radiol. 2010;33(1):41–52.
25. Golfieri R, Giampalma E, Renzulli M, et al. Randomised controlled trial of doxorubicin-eluting beads vs conventional chemoembolisation for hepatocellular carcinoma. Br J Cancer. 2014;111(2):255–64.
26. Poon RT, Lau C, Yu WC, Fan ST, Wong J. High serum levels of vascular endothelial growth factor predict poor response to transarterial chemoembolization in hepatocellular carcinoma: a prospective study. Oncol Rep. 2004;11:1077–84.
27. Håkansson L, Håkansson A, Morales O, Thorelius L, Warfving T. Spherex (degradable starch microspheres) chemo-occlusion—enhancement of tumor drug concentration and therapeutic efficacy: an overview. Semin Oncol. 1997;24:S6–100–S6-109.
28. Schicho A, Pereira PL, Haimerl M, et al. Transarterial chemoembolization (TACE) with degradable starch microspheres (DSM) in hepatocellular carcinoma (HCC): multi-center results on safety and efficacy. Oncotarget. 2017;8:72613–20.
29. Orlacchio A, Chegai F, Francioso S, et al. Repeated transarterial chemoembolization with degradable starch microspheres (DSMs-TACE) of unresectable hepatocellular carcinoma: a prospective pilot study. Curr Med imag Rev. 2018;14:637–45.

Ablation of Hepatocellular Carcinoma

61

Lukas Beyer and Lukas Luerken

Key Concepts

- Ablation or resection is the treatment of choice for very early stage and early stage HCC according to the criteria of the Barcelona Clinic Liver Cancer staging system
- Most ablation procedures are based on irreversible cell damage caused by heating above 60 °C
- Combination with transarterial chemoembolization improves local tumor control for HCC larger than 3 cm
- Compared to radiofrequency ablation, microwave ablation has theoretical advantages due to the higher possible energy output
- Irreversible electroporation is a novel ablation procedure that is not heat-based and can therefore be used in the vicinity of large bile ducts and vessels

61.1 Introduction

Thermal ablation procedures were developed in the 1980s for minimally invasive and percutaneous use [1]. A distinction has to be made between thermodestructive procedures, which usually allow heat of 60–100 °C to act on the target tissue, and hyperthermia procedures (target temperatures approx. 42–45 °C). While hyperthermia is usually used supportively for radio- or chemotherapy to improve local efficacy, thermodestruction, hereafter referred to as thermoablation, is based on the irreversible complete destruction of biological tissue due to protein denaturation [2]. This complete and irreversible process is achieved within a few seconds after a target temperature of 60 °C has been reached.

Cold based methods (cryotherapy) with target temperatures below −20 °C have also been developed. In contrast to protein denaturation, however, the radicality of cold-based methods is controversial. Even at temperatures below −50 °C, the cell damage induced by the cold, such as membrane ruptures, vascular and capillary thrombosis and apoptosis, can be reversible at least in some tumor cells.

Percutaneous applicators make it technically possible to introduce thermal energy. The diameter of today's applicators is usually between 14 and 18 gauge, which makes them no more traumatic than standard probes for obtaining histological material. Depending on the manufacturer and method, the number of applicators used varies between one and several applicators, whereby the time required for the placement of the applicators increases with the number of applicators and, especially in the case of multi-applicator technology, novel navigation procedures have an added value.

In the 1990s, numerous Phase 1 and Phase 2 studies were conducted, which demonstrated the effectiveness of thermoablative procedures using sonographic, computed tomography or magnetic resonance imaging. Numerous groups used either light (laser-induced thermotherapy) or electric current (radio frequency ablation, RFA) [3, 4] for the energy input of the heat-based procedures.

Although laser light has methodological advantages for the visualization of thermal effects for therapy control, RFA has gained widespread acceptance due to its simpler handling, cheaper materials, better miniaturization and better controllability and is still regarded today as the standard method of thermal ablation. However, microwave ablation (MWA) has evolved considerably in recent years. While the radicality and controllability is comparable to the radio frequency method, many working groups prefer the MWA to the RFA due to the time advantage.

In tumors in the vicinity of blood-flowed vessels from a size of approx. 3 mm, incomplete ablation with residual

L. Beyer (✉) · L. Luerken
Department of Radiology, University Hospital Regensburg, Regensburg, Germany
e-mail: lukas.beyer@ukr.de; lukas.luerken@ukr.de

F. Radu-Ionita et al. (eds.), *Liver Diseases*, https://doi.org/10.1007/978-3-030-24432-3_61

tumor cells along the vessel walls can occur due to heat sink effect [5]. Since in hepatocellular carcinoma a curative result for the patient can only be expected in the case of complete ablation, further procedures, such as irreversible electroporation (IRE), have recently been developed to improve selectivity [6].

In our decade, thermal ablation methods have become established in the healthcare system and, in spite of the expandable evidence, are an integral part of guideline-oriented therapy, especially for HCC, but also for secondary liver tumors. Although the motto "surgery first" still seems to prevail, percutaneous tumor ablation is already on a par with open surgery, at least for hepatocellular carcinoma. Percutaneous ablation procedures enjoy a high level of patient acceptance due to the better tolerability of thermal ablation and the associated lower side effect rates.

61.2 Indications

The European Association for the Study of the Liver (EASL) guidelines for the treatment of HCC in the version 2018 [7] recommend resection and ablation or transplantation for very early stage and early stage HCC according to the criteria of the Barcelona Clinic Liver Cancer staging system (Fig. 61.1).

Very early HCC (BCLC stage 0) is defined in patients with well-preserved liver function (Child-Pugh A) presenting with a single tumor <2 cm in diameter without vascular invasion. Recent studies have shown excellent 5-year survival rates of 80% in patients with very early stage HCC after resection [8]. Given that percutaneous ablation can produce a complete tumor necrosis with an adequate safety margin, resection and RFA are likely to be comparable in their outcome for small HCC less than 2–3 cm. This assumption is supported by a systematic meta-analysis consisting of 17 studies (8420 patients), which concludes that patients with very early HCC treated by RFA have a comparable life expectancy to patients after resection [9].

Early HCC (BCLC stage A) is defined in patients with preserved liver function presenting with a single tumour >2 cm or 2–3 modules <3 cm in diameter. Although data is scarce, studies suggest 5-year median survival rates of 50–70% after resection, liver transplant or local ablation [10].

A 2017 Cochrane Review compared safety and efficacy of different treatment options for very early and early HCC. The review included a total of 18 randomized controlled trials, four of which (593 patients) compared surgical resection with RFA. The authors found no evidence of a difference in all-cause mortality between resection and RFA. The incidence of severe adverse events after resection was significantly higher (23.3% vs. 1.7%) [11]. When weighing between resection and ablation, it is crucial that the prognosis after resection is highly dependent on the progress of the liver dysfunction, whereas prognosis after ablation is determined by the rapid drop of primary efficacy with increasing tumor size.

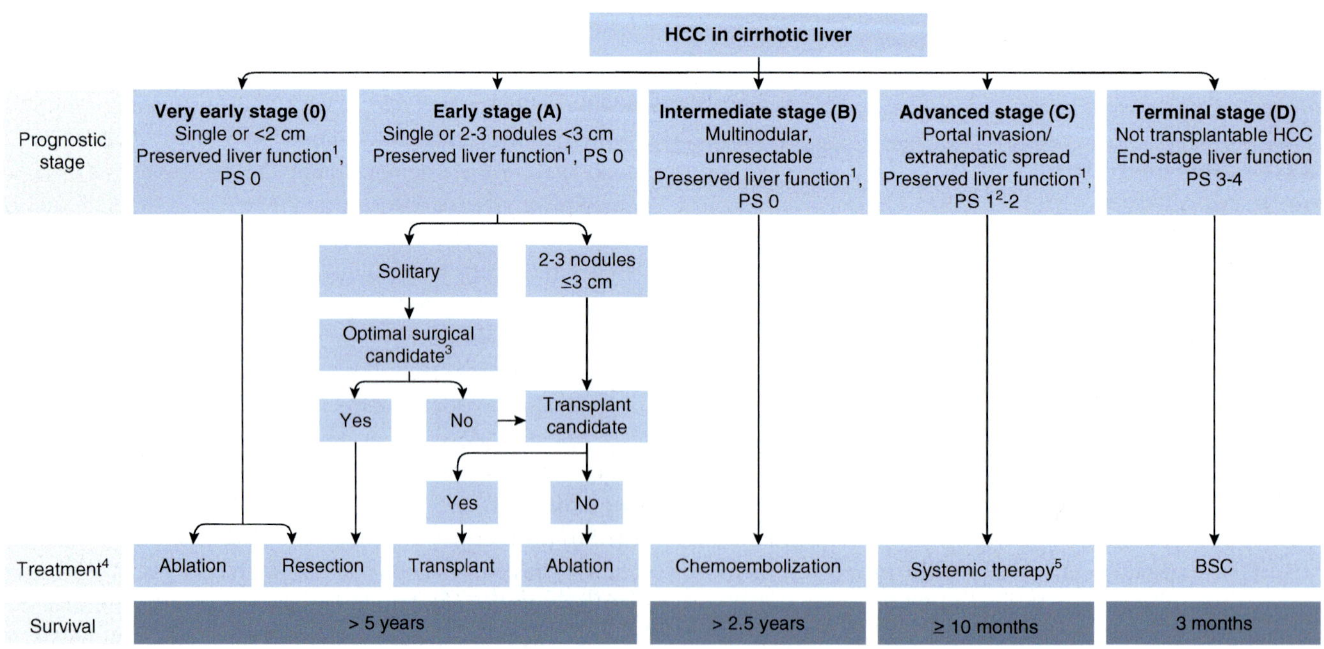

Fig. 61.1 Treatment schema of the European Association for the Study of the Liver (EASL). Ablation is recommended as an alternative to resection or transplantation for very early and early stages (single tumour or 2–3 tumours <4 cm with preserved liver function and good clinical status)

61.2.1 At-Risk Localizations and Adverse Events

Studies have shown that around 30% of patients referred for ablation were drifted to palliative treatment because of an at-risk localization or an at-risk patient profile (Kim et al. 2013). Although certain locations in the liver are associated with risk of complications, special techniques haven been developed in recent years to safely and efficiently treat these patients.

The risk of a diaphragmatic injury or a hollow organ perforation is associated with a location of the tumor near the diaphragm or colon/stomach (Kang et al. 2011). Peritoneal insufflation dextrose solution ("hydrodissection") or CO_2 ("pneumodissection") to separate the liver from the endangered organ nevertheless allows safe treatment of these patients by means of thermal ablation. Alternatively, non-thermal irreversible electroporation can be used for these patients, but at significantly higher time and effort. Studies have shown that the treatment of tumors at these sites does not lead to reduced efficacy compared to other, less vulnerable locations (Teratani et al. 2006).

The risk of a bile duct injury with development of biliomas, cholestasis or bile duct fistulas is significantly increased in centrally located tumors in the vicinity of the primary bile ducts. The use of thermodestructive methods for immediate perihilary HCC is therefore still contraindicated according to current opinion. For these patients, irreversible electroporation is often the only potentially curative therapy option for small, irresectable tumors.

Although a subcapsular situation was long considered an unfavorable prognostic factor, this was proven wrong in a propensity score analysis of 2016 with over 500 patients (Fig. 61.2) [12]. The thermocoagulation of the ablation tract ("tract ablation"), indirect puncture with interposition of non-tumorous liver tissue and the no-touch technique involving several probes placed tangentially to the tumor can reduce the risk of tumor cell seeding in these patients to less than 1% (Nakagomi et al. 2014).

61.2.2 Tumor Size

Selected patients with tumors greater than 3 cm can be reasonably treated with ablation. Although good results can also be achieved for large HCC, primary efficacy and results decrease significantly with increasing size. However, the ablation of large tumors in particular benefits from increasing improvements in percutaneous ablation technology, in particular the use of multi-applicator systems and modern navigation systems [13, 14]. Several mostly retrospective studies report acceptable efficacy rates of more than 80% for ablation of HCC ≥5 cm by multipolar RFA or MWA and 1-year survival rates above 80% with only low morbidity (Lin, Cheng, Chen M, & Lin, 2015; Liu et al. 2013).

Another approach in large HCC is to combine RFA with transarterial chemoembolization. Recent meta-analyzes have shown that the combination of RFA and transarterial chemoembolization (TACE) significantly increases overall and recurrence-free survival, without significant differences in

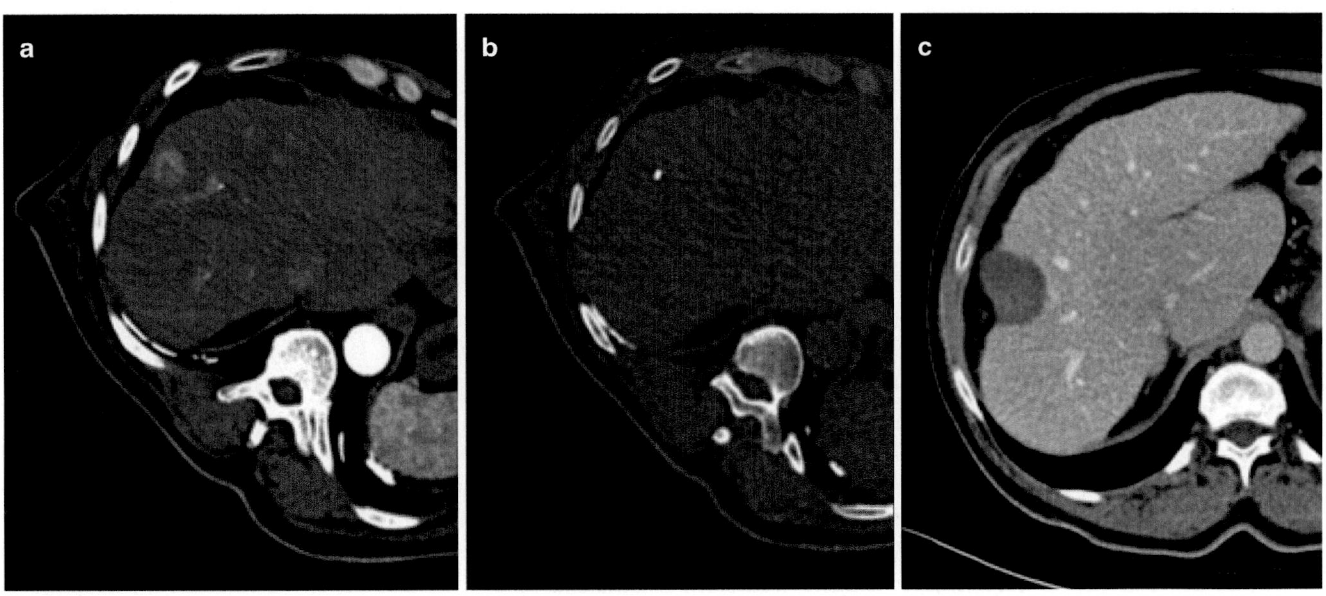

Fig. 61.2 (**a**) Hypervascular, subcapsular HCC in liver segment VIII. (**b**) The microwave antenna was placed cranio-caudally tangentially to the HCC to avoid tumor seeding and too close proximity to the diaphragm. (**c**) CT shows complete response with hypodense coagulation necrosis 6 weeks after ablation

major complications [15]. For small HCC (<3 cm), combination therapy with TACE has no advantages over ablation alone (Shibata et al. 2009).

61.3 Technical Aspects

61.3.1 Radiofrequency-Ablation (RFA)

In radiofrequency-ablation (RFA), an alternating current field with frequencies between 375 and 480 kHz is applied to the tissue to induce an ion movement that leads to the generation of a relevant frictional heat. Temperatures above 60 °C lead to irreversible protein denaturation and thus to cell damage due to coagulation necrosis [16]. Temperatures between 90 and 100 °C are considered optimal target temperatures for RFA. In RFA, the electrical energy is applied by special electrodes. These radiofrequency electrodes essentially consist of an insulated metal shaft with one to six active electrode tips and are also called ablation probes or applicators. An RF generator generates the high-frequency, sinusoidal alternating current, which is emitted into the surrounding tissue via the active electrode tips. Most generators, however, also regulate the power output individually on the basis of the permanently measured parameters resistance (impedance) and/or temperature in the tissue. This control is intended to keep the target temperature in the tissue at a constant level and thus prevent premature carbonisation of the tissue. In the so-called monopolar technique, the current is dissipated via up to four cutaneously attached neutral electrodes. With the bipolar technique, the current is conducted between two tips of the RF electrode. In multipolar systems, the current flows between two to a maximum of six individually inserted bipolar RF probes.

The first monopolar needle-like ablation probes could only generate small necrosis zones. Probe geometries expandable up to 5 cm like umbrellas (Starburst, Angiodynamics, NY, USA and LeVeen, Boston Scientific, MA, USA) were developed to induce larger lesions. Perfused ablation probes (Starburst Talon, Angiodynamics, NY, USA) have an additional lumen through which cooled saline solution is guided to the active electrode tip. This cooling of the electrode tip reduces carbonization effects. The increased local ion concentrations of NaCl additionally reduce tissue resistance, allowing higher energies to be applied, resulting in larger ablation areas [17].

In the case of ablations in the vicinity of larger vessels, the heat-sink-effect (RFA) can lead to a considerable dissipation of the generated heat. As a result, the temperature around the vessel is not sufficient to cause tissue necrosis. The consequence is a zonal lack of ablation, which leads to a local relapse if the tumor is insufficiently covered. At some centers a technically complex modulation of the blood flow is used during ablation in order to reduce the influence of the heat sink effect. This can be done by mechanically closing the "cooling" vessels (e.g. using balloon catheters) in the hepatic vein or portal vein. In the vicinity of large vessels, microwave ablation and irreversible electroporation are advantageous due to the higher energy output respectively the non-thermal mechanism.

61.3.2 Microwave Ablation (MWA)

Microwave ablation (MWA) is based on the emission of electromagnetic waves in the frequency range between 900 and 2500 MHz. The microwaves generate an alternating electromagnetic field whose polarity changes 10^9 times per second. Dipole molecules align their charge at this alternating field. Since the most important dipole for hyperthermal ablation is the water molecule (H_2O), tissues with high water content are particularly susceptible [18]. The water molecules are excited by the periodically changing orientation of their charges in the electromagnetic alternating field. This oscillation increases the kinetic energy of the water molecules and leads to tissue heating due to friction.

In contrast to RFA, which uses high-frequency alternating current, MWA does not require a neutral electrode for a closed circuit. This allows several applicators to be used at the same time. Some systems support the synchronous use of up to three applicators, thus increasing the achievable ablation zone compared to sequential use [13]. If the probes are operated phase-synchronously, the synergistic effect based on constructive interference is exploited, which enables more efficient tissue heating and higher temperatures and leads to a larger continuous ablation area [18].

Since MWA is not dependent on the transmission of an electric current in the tissue, there are some advantages over RFA. Using MWA, a larger ablation area can be achieved in a shorter time compared to RFA [19]. In addition, MWA is less vulnerable to the heat sink effect than RFA, which means that treatment efficiency is less affected by vessels in the vicinity of the tumor. A number of studies comparing RFA with MWA are available. In all available studies, the overall survival between RFA and MWA was not significantly different. There are contradictory results regarding the technical success rate: some studies indicated a lower local recurrence rate for MWA than for RFA [20], while others could not show any difference [21]. The complication rates seem comparable. Similarly, recent meta-analyses indicate similar efficacy between the two percutaneous techniques, with one study showing possible superiority of MWA in larger HCCs [22].

61.3.3 Irreversible Electroporation (IRE)

Electroporation is a technique for the permeabilization of cell membranes by external electric fields [23]. Although the exact molecular mechanisms have not been conclusively clarified, it is assumed that the process of electroporation is associated with the formation of nanopores in the bilipid layer [24]. The transient permeabilization of the cell membrane with restoration of membrane integrity with limited cell injury is referred to as reversible electroporation. Extensive permeabilization of the cell membrane leading to loss of homeostasis and cell death is called irreversible electroporation (IRE). IRE was developed in clinical settings as an ablation technique for the focal destruction of malignant tumors in solid organs.

A special characteristic of IRE is the damage to the cell membrane alone; tissue architecture to be spared [25]. Although histopathological analyses suggest that both necrosis and apoptosis are involved [26], the molecular mechanisms of cell death after IRE remain unclear. Two possible explanations for cell death are the permanent lysis of the cell membrane or the loss of homeostasis.

One of the main advantages of IRE over the established thermodestructive methods MWA and RFA is that it is not influenced by local blood flow and therefore tumors in the immediate vicinity of large blood vessels can be treated. In addition, vessels and bile ducts in the ablation area remain intact while RFA and MWA destroy these structures in the necrosis area [25]. Overall, IRE seems to be a useful therapy option for the treatment of HCC which cannot be treated with thermodestructive methods due to their location.

The decisive limitation of the IRE is the tumor diameter. To achieve complete ablation, the tumor diameter should not exceed 3 cm [27]. Irreversible electroporation can lead to cardiac arrhythmias such as ventricular tachycardia or atrial fibrillation, especially in the treatment of liver tumors below the right half of the diaphragm. Modern devices synchronize the pulse delivery with the patient's ECG so that the pulses are delivered at the time of the absolute refractory time of the cardiomyocytes. The pulses can also cause contractions of the skeletal muscles. Therefore, a deep neuromuscular blockade during general anesthesia is necessary for the duration of the IRE.

Self-Study

Questions

1. Which statement is correct:
   (a) According to the EASL guidelines for HCC, ablation should primarily be performed in patients with intermediate HCC stage BCLC B.
   (b) Subcapsular HCC should not be treated by ablation because of the high risk of tumor seeding.
   (c) HCC immediately adjacent to a central bile duct can be safely treated using microwave ablation, but not radiofrequency ablation.
   (d) Hydrodissection can be used to safely treat HCC adjacent to the colon or stomach.
2. Which statement is correct:
   (a) MWA is independent of the transmission of an electric current in the surrounding tissue.
   (b) IRE is especially suitable for large HCC > 5 cm because multiple electrodes can be placed surrounding the tumor.
   (c) For HCC > 3 cm, ablation should be combined with systemic treatment.
   (d) Resection improves overall survival compared to ablation for HCC < 2 cm.

Answers

1. Which statement is correct:
   (a) Ablation is one of three curative options for patients with HCLC BCLC 0 and A. TACE is the treatment of choice for patients with HCC BCLC B.
   (b) Recent data suggests subcapsular location of HCC is not an unfavourable prognostic factor. Techniques such as indirect puncture and needle tract coagulation or "no-touch" ablation using multiple probes can be used to avoid tumour seeding.
   (c) All thermodestructive ablation techniques such as RFA and MWA are considered contraindicated next to major central bile ducts. Alternatively, irreversible electroporation can be used.
   (d) Hydrodissection uses artificial ascites to protect thermosensitive structures such as the stomach or colon during thermal ablation. Alternatively, CO_2-dissection or irreversible electroporation can be used. CORRECT
2. Which statement is correct:
   (a) MWA is based on the emission of electromagnetic waves and not electric current. CORRECT
   (b) The main limitation of IRE is the tumor diameter with high local recurrence rates for tumors exceeding 3 cm. For large tumors multi-probe RFA or MWA are the technique of choice.
   (c) The STORM trial failed show improved recurrence-free survival for a combination of resection or ablation and sorafenib. However, several meta-analysis showed improved recurrence-free and overall survival for the combination of TACE and ablation in patients with HCC > 3 cm.
   (d) A large systematic meta-analysis (8420 patients) showed that patients with very early HCC treated by RFA have a comparable life expectancy to patients after resection

References

1. Goldberg SN, Gazelle GS, Dawson SL, Rittman WJ, Mueller PR, Rosenthal DI. Tissue ablation with radiofrequency: effect of probe size, gauge, duration, and temperature on lesion volume. Acad Radiol. 1995;2(5):399–404.
2. Lewin JS, Connell CF, Duerk JL, Chung YC, Clampitt ME, Spisak J, Gazelle GS, Haaga JR. Interactive MRI-guided radiofrequency interstitial thermal ablation of abdominal tumors: clinical trial for evaluation of safety and feasibility. J Magn Reson Imaging. 1998;8(1):40–7.
3. Hosten N, Puls R, Kreissig R, Wlodarczyk W, Stroszczynski C, Hentschel M, Felix R. In vivo temperature measurements and MR-thermometry during laser-induced interstitial thermotherapy (LITT) of liver metastasis. Eur Radiol. 2000;10(Suppl 1)
4. Vogl TJ, Mueller PK, Hammerstingl R, Weinhold N, Mack MG, Philipp C, Deimling M, Beuthan J, Pegios W, Riess H, Felix R. Malignant liver tumors treated with MR imaging-guided laser-induced thermotherapy: technique and prospective results. Radiology. 1995;196:257–65.
5. Curley SA, Izzo F. Radiofrequency ablation of primary and metastatic hepatic malignancies. Int J Clin Oncol. 2002;7(2):72–81.
6. Al-Sakere B, Andre F, Bernat C, et al. Tumor ablation with irreversible electroporation. PLoS One. 2007;2(11):e1135.
7. European Association for the Study of the Liver. Electronic address: easloffice@easloffice.eu; European Association for the Study of the Liver. EASL clinical practice guidelines: management of hepatocellular carcinoma. J Hepatol. 2018;69(1):182. https://www.sciencedirect.com/science/article/pii/S0168827818302150. Accessed January 31, 2019.
8. Roayaie S, Obeidat K, Sposito C, Mariani L, Bhoori S, Pellegrinelli A, et al. Resection of hepatocellular cancer ≤2 cm: results from two Western centers. Hepatology. 2013;57:1426–35.
9. Cucchetti A, Piscaglia F, Cescon M, Colecchia A, Ercolani G, Bolondi L, et al. Cost-effectiveness of hepatic resection vs. percutaneous radiofrequency ablation for early hepatocellular carcinoma. J Hepatol. 2013;59:300–7.
10. Forner A, Reig ME, de Lope CR, Bruix J. Current strategy for staging and treatment: the BCLC update and future prospects. Semin Liver Dis. 2010;30:61–74.
11. Majumdar A. Management of people with early- or very early-stage hepatocellular carcinoma: an attempted network meta-analysis. Cochrane Database Syst Rev. 2017;3:CD011650.
12. Kang TW, Lim HK, Lee MW, Kim Y, Rhim H, Lee WJ, et al. Long-term therapeutic outcomes of radiofrequency ablation for subcapsular vs. nonsubcapsular hepatocellular carcinoma: a propensity score matched study. Radiology. 2016;280:300–12.
13. Harari CM, Magagna M, Bedoya M, Lee FT Jr, Lubner MG, Hinshaw JL, et al. Microwave ablation: comparison of simultaneous and sequential activation of multiple antennas in liver model systems. Radiology. 2016;278(1):95–103.
14. Beyer LP, et al. Stereotactically navigated percutaneous microwave ablation (MWA) compared to conventional MWA: a matched pair analysis. Int J Comput Assist Radiol Surg. 2018;13(12):1991.
15. Yang D-J, Luo K-L, Liu H, Cai B, Tao G-Q, Su X-F, et al. Meta-analysis of transcatheter arterial chemoembolization plus radiofrequency ablation versus transcatheter arterial chemoembolization alone for hepatocellular carcinoma. Oncotarget. 2017;8(2):2960–70.
16. Goldberg SN, Gazelle GS, Compton CC, Mueller PR, Tanabe KK. Treatment of intrahepatic malignancy with radiofrequency ablation: radiologic-pathologic correlation. Cancer. 2000;88(11):2452–63.
17. Goldberg SN, Gazelle GS, Solbiati L, Rittman WJ, Mueller PR. Radiofrequency tissue ablation: increased lesion diameter with a perfusion electrode. Acad Radiol. 1996;3(8):636–44.
18. Lubner MG, Brace CL, Hinshaw JL, Lee FT Jr. Microwave tumor ablation: mechanism of action, clinical results, and devices. J Vasc Interv Radiol. 2010;21(8 Suppl):S192–203.
19. Brace CL. Radiofrequency and microwave ablation of the liver, lung, kidney, and bone: what are the differences? Curr Probl Diagn Radiol. 2009;38(3):135–43.
20. Abdelaziz A, Elbaz T, Shousha HI, Mahmoud S, Ibrahim M, Abdelmaksoud A, Nabeel M. Efficacy and survival analysis of percutaneous radiofrequency versus microwave ablation for hepatocellular carcinoma: an Egyptian multidisciplinary clinic experience. Surg Endosc. 2014;28(12):3429.
21. Lu MD, Xu HX, Xie XY, Yin XY, Chen JW, Kuang M, Xu ZF, Liu GJ, Zheng YL. Percutaneous microwave and radiofrequency ablation for hepatocellular carcinoma: a retrospective comparative study. J Gastroenterol. 2005;40(11):1054.
22. Facciorusso A, Di Maso M, Muscatiello N. Microwave ablation vs. radiofrequency ablation for the treatment of hepatocellular carcinoma: a systematic review and meta-analysis. Int J Hyperthermia. 2016;32:339–44.
23. Neumann E, Schaefer-Ridder M, Wang Y, Hofschneider PH. Gene transfer into mouse lyoma cells by electroporation in high electric fields. EMBO J. 1982;1(7):841–5.
24. Weaver JC, Chizmadzhev YA. Theory of electroporation: a review. Bioelectrochem Bioenerg. 1996;41(2):135–60. https://doi.org/10.1016/S0302-4598(96)05062-3.
25. Lee EW, Chen C, Prieto VE, Dry SM, Loh CT, Kee ST. Advanced hepatic ablation technique for creating complete cell death: irreversible electroporation. Radiology. 2010;255(2):426–33. https://doi.org/10.1148/radiol.10090337.
26. Al-Sakere B, André F, Bernat C, et al. Tumor ablation with irreversible electroporation. PLoS One. 2007;2(11):e1135. https://doi.org/10.1371/journal.pone.0001135.
27. Yeung ES, Chung MW, Wong K, Wong CY, So EC, Chan AC. An update on irreversible electroporation of liver tumours. Hong Kong Med J. 2014;20(4):313–6.
28. Kim, Y., Lim, H. K., Rhim, H., Lee, M. W., Choi, D., Lee, W. J., … Yoo, B. C. (2013). Ten-year outcomes of percutaneous radiofrequency ablation as firstline therapy of early hepatocellular carcinoma: Analysis of prognostic factors. Journal of Hepatology, 58(1), 89–97. https://doi.org/10.1016/j.jhep.2012.09.020.
29. Kang, T. W., Rhim, H., Lee, M. W., Kim, Y., Choi, D., Lee, W. J., & Lim, H. K. (2011). Radiofrequency Ablation for Hepatocellular Carcinoma Abutting the Diaphragm: Comparison of Effects of Thermal Protection and Therapeutic Efficacy. American Journal of Roentgenology, 196(4), 907–913. https://doi.org/10.2214/AJR.10.4584.
30. Teratani, T., Yoshida, H., Shiina, S., Obi, S., Sato, S., Tateishi, R., … Omata, M. (2006). Radiofrequency ablation for hepatocellular carcinoma in so-called high-risk locations. Hepatology, 43(5), 1101–1108. https://doi.org/10.1002/hep.21164.
31. Nakagomi, R., Tateishi, R., Shiina, S., Imamura, J., Fujiwara, N., Asaoka, Y., … Koike, K. (2014). Drastically Reduced Neoplastic Seeding Related to Radiofrequency Ablation for Hepatocellular Carcinoma. The American Journal of Gastroenterology, 109(5), 774–776. https://doi.org/10.1038/ajg.2014.42.
32. Lin, C.-C., Cheng, Y.-T., Chen M, W.-T., & Lin, S.-M. (2015). The Effectiveness of Multiple Electrode Radiofrequency Ablation in Patients with Hepatocellular Carcinoma with Lesions More than 3 cm in Size and Barcelona Clinic Liver Cancer Stage A to B2. Liver Cancer, 5(1), 8–20. https://doi.org/10.1159/000367755.
33. Liu, Y., Zheng, Y., Li, S., Li, B., Zhang, Y., & Yuan, Y. (2013). Percutaneous microwave ablation of larger hepatocellular carcinoma, 68(1). https://doi.org/10.1016/j.crad.2012.05.007.
34. Shibata, T., Isoda, H., Hirokawa, Y., Arizono, S., Shimada, K., & Togashi, K. (2009). Small Hepatocellular Carcinoma: Is Radiofrequency Ablation Combined with Transcatheter Arterial Chemoembolization More Effective than Radiofrequency Ablation Alone for Treatment? Radiology, 252(3), 905–913. https://doi.org/10.1148/radiol.2523081676.

62 Laparoscopic Liver Resection

Riccardo Memeo, Guido Fiorentini, and Luca Aldrighetti

Key Concepts

- Laparoscopic liver resections is performed both for benign and malignant disease.
- Potentially, there is no limit embodied by the kind of disease or the number of liver lesions for minimally-invasive approach.
- Lesions invading major vessels' walls (e.g. portal or hepatic vein infiltration) contraindicate laparoscopic approach.
- Laparoscopic hepatic procedures encompass a wide range of difficulty level, which is different for minor or major resections and according to the location in the liver. Indication to laparoscopic approach is therefore conditioned by individual expertise in the field.
- Proper post-operative hepatic function is guaranteed by adequate future remnant liver, which is assessed before major procedures (at least 30% in healthy liver; 50% or more in injured liver).

62.1 Introduction

Laparoscopic liver surgery, since first reports in 1991 by Reich [1], has developed increasing the number of centers began practicing minimally invasive surgery of the liver, even if a slower adoption compared to other laparoscopic procedure, due to the initial high risk of bleeding and inadequate oncological results and necessity of contemporary of high experience in hepatobiliary and minimally invasive advanced surgery. Started as a promising concept, MILS has progressively become a solid practice, reaching more than 10,000 cases described in literature. This spread, probably due to the progress of technology and the increasing experience and indication in expert centers, has generated an increasing interest in minimally invasive surgery. For this reason, in recent years, some consensus conference has indicated which should be the direction for the development of this surgical approach of liver lesions. Louisville consensus conference [2], defined the indication of MILS, identifying some concept that actually are fundamental for MILS:

Currently acceptable indications for laparoscopic liver resection (LLR): solitary lesions 5 cm or less located in liver segments 2–6

LLR approach to left lateral sectionectomy should be considered standard practice.

Although all types of liver resection can be performed laparoscopically, major liver resections (e.g., right or left hepatectomies) should be reserved for experienced surgeons.

Conversion should be considered prudent surgical practice rather than failure.

Indications for surgery for benign hepatic lesions should not be widened simply because the surgery can be done laparoscopically.

Although data presented on colorectal metastases did not reveal an adverse effect of the laparoscopic approach on oncological outcomes in terms of margins or survival, adequacy of margins and ability to detect occult lesions are concerns.

Recently, a second International Consensus Conference was held in Morioka [3], 2014, confirmed that:

MINOR LLRs had become standard practice and that MAJOR liver resections were still innovative procedures in the exploration phase. Continued cautious introduction of MAJORLLRs was recommended.

R. Memeo
General Surgery and Liver Transplantation Unit, Policlinico di Bari, Bari, Italy

G. Fiorentini (✉) · L. Aldrighetti
Hepatobiliary Surgery Division, San Raffaele University Hospital, Milan, Italy
e-mail: fiorentini.guido@hsr.it; aldrighetti.luca@hsr.it

F. Radu-Ionita et al. (eds.), *Liver Diseases*, https://doi.org/10.1007/978-3-030-24432-3_62

Based on this consideration, we can consider the rapid diffusion and evolution of LLS in recent decade, with consolidation of results and development of high volume centers [4]. Literature confirms that no difference were evidenced with open surgery in terms of oncological a short terms results [5], despite MILS guarantees less postoperative pain and shorter postoperative stay.

Even if an increasing interest has been demonstrated in literature with series from all around the world, MILS remains a kind of surgery that could be addressed in expert centers [6].

62.2 Indications

Laparoscopic liver surgery is finding more and more applications since its first introduction almost 25 years ago [7]. The range of indications is wide, encompassing primary and secondary, benign and malignant diseases. Few of the most frequent indications for laparoscopic liver resection are presented, divided as benign, primary malignant and metastatic disease.

62.2.1 Benign Disease

62.2.1.1 Simple Liver Cyst

Simple liver cysts originate from hamartomatous tissue, are benign and do not communicate with the biliary tree; they can arise sporadically or in the context of polycystic liver or polycystic kidney/liver disease.

While usually asymptomatic in most of the cases, in other cases the symptoms they can be responsible of are mainly related to their dimensions, potentially causing compression on the thoracic or abdominal wall and discomfort. Whether a liver cyst is in close vicinity with the hepatic hilum, an intra-hepatic bile ducts obstruction can be observed on imaging, causing segmental intra-hepatic bile ducts dilation. In presence of any of these conditions, a laparoscopic fenestration is indicated, in which the more superficial layer of the cyst is resected allowing its spontaneous drainage into the abdominal cavity. Final aim of such procedure is to relieve the cyst's content rather than completely removing it: actually, major vessels and portal pedicles lie behind posterior walls of the cyst, preventing a complete excision without harvesting liver parenchyma through a formal resection.

Whether malignancy was suspected pre-operatively or the post-operative finding was consistent with a definitive pathology of malignancy (e.g. mucinous cystic adenocarcinoma), a formal resection will be required to radicalize the field. Even in this case, such procedure can be tackled laparoscopically, in accordance to the local expertise of the center [8].

Other common benign indications for laparoscopic liver procedures encompass liver angiomas and focal nodular hyperplasia, whose resection is indicated basing on the risk of traumatic rupture.

62.2.2 Primary Malignant Disease

Hepatocellular carcinoma (HCC) and intra-hepatic cholangiocarcinoma (ICC) accounts for primary malignant liver diseases.

62.2.2.1 Hepatocellular Carcinoma

Hepatocellular carcinoma accounts for more than 50% of the indications of laparoscopic liver procedures for malignant disease [9]. Typically, HCC arises on fibrotic and cirrhotic livers on a background of chronic hepatitis. Despite the presence of cirrhosis, laparoscopic approach is preferred to open as its benefits and advantages have been highlighted in reducing collateral circles brake-down in the abdominal wall with fewer post-operative ascitic decompensation and post-operative morbidities. In fact, since Louisville's consensus in 2008 [2], laparoscopy became the standard of care to perform procedures like left lateral sectionectomy in cirrhotic Child A patients and should represent the approach of first choice in cirrhotic patients requiring minor liver resections [10]. Major liver resections are considered more challenging operations, confined to surgeons who have completed the learning curve on minor procedures. Nevertheless, the oncologic outcomes of laparoscopic resections for HCC have been observed to overlap with open in retrospective series, even for major hepatectomies [11, 12].

Further extension to the application of laparoscopy in the treatment of HCC, other than minor and major resections, has been the introduction of thermal ablation (radiofrequency—RFA and microwave—MWA) for nodules inferior to 3 cm otherwise not achievable percutaneously. It was recently observed laparoscopic thermal ablation is a safe treatment option for early-stage HCC, with inferior local tumor progression rates for MWA (MWA vs. RFA = 8.3% vs. 21.2%, $p = 0.034$), maintaining similar respective overall and disease-free survival rates [13].

62.2.2.2 Intrahepatic Cholangiocarcinoma

Traditionally, since the early development of laparoscopic liver surgery, patients affected by cholangiocarcinoma have been excluded from laparoscopic series. The main reasons for this reside in the needing to perform major resections and the necessity of performing a lymphadenectomy of the hepatic pedicle [14] (Fig. 62.1a, lymphadenectomy of the hepatic pedicle). Actually, laparoscopic lymphadenectomy is itself a technically demanding procedure, requiring a skeletonization of vascular structures like the celiac trunk, the

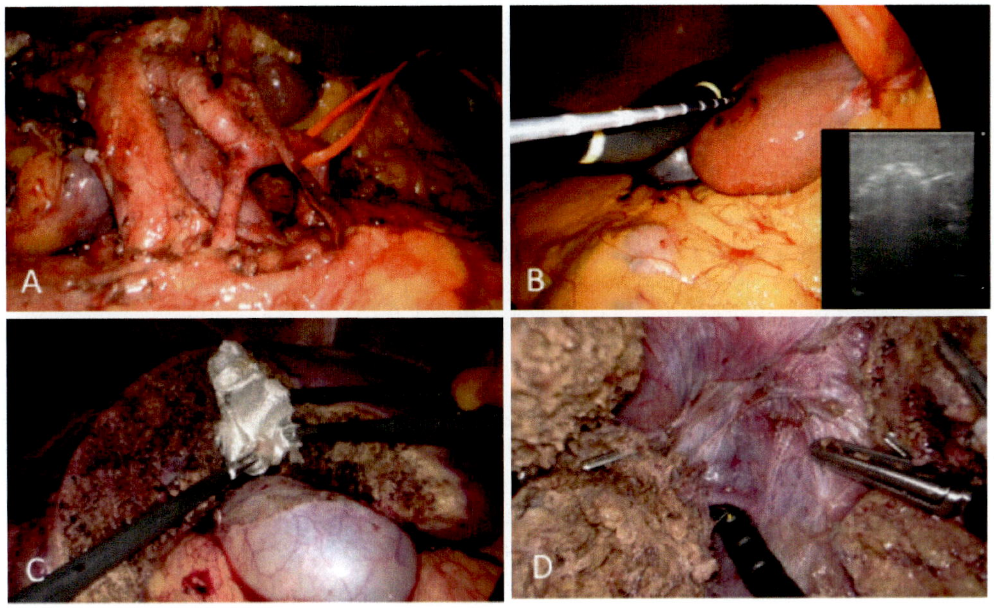

Fig. 62.1 (**a**) Lymphadenectomy of hepatic pedicle with skeletonization of common bile duct, portal vein, hepatic artery (from left to right). (**b**) Intraoperative ultra-sound guided microwave ablation. (**c**) ALPPS stage 1—*in situ* liver partition. (**d**) ALPPS stage 2—completion of right lobectomy after future remnant liver induced hypertrophy

proper hepatic artery, the portal vein and the common bile duct. Nevertheless, recently there are more series describing laparoscopic resections for ICC [15], showing less perioperative morbidity and faster functional recovery, without compromising oncologic outcomes [16].

62.2.3 Metastatic Disease

Colorectal cancer metastasis (CRCM) to the liver account for the most frequent indication to liver resection in laparoscopic liver surgery after HCC. Other metastatic lesions to the liver encompass breast and prostatic cancer and neuroendocrine tumors.

Focusing on CRCM, there are three main topics regarding the synchronicity, the possibility of executing a preoperative neoadjuvant chemotherapy and the numerosity of lesions: of these, the first two are beyond the focus of the present discussion, which is aimed to show the applicability of minimally-invasiveness to resective liver surgery.

The item concerning the number of lesions and the locations of the lesions inside the liver, introduces the topic of parenchymal sparing resections, for the possibility of performing not just formal resections (like segmentectomies, sectionectomies and hepatectomies), but also multiple wedge resections—for more superficial tumours—with associated intra-operative thermal ablation (Fig. 62.1b, intraoperative thermal ablation)—for deeper parenchymal lesions. This scenario increases the amount of metastatic patients who can benefit of laparoscopic liver resections, even in presence of multiple and bilobar disease [17]. Currently, there are no guidelines or recommendations concerning the maximum number of lesions to be harvested or the maximum number of resections recommended for a laparoscopic case, and this limit is therefore individually set by surgeons mainly basing on individual experience.

Other, more complex, procedures whose aim is to increase the future remnant liver, like ALPPS (Associating Liver Partitioning and Portal vein Ligation for Staged Hepatectomy), are technically demanding operations to be performed in laparoscopy, requiring a two-staged major liver resection (Fig. 62.1c, d, ALPPS stage 1 and 2). There are some described reports in literature, even if laparoscopy is far from becoming the standard of care for this procedure [18, 19].

In any case whereas laparoscopy is doable for a minimally-invasive treatment of CRCM, a quicker recovery has been observed, definitely leading to a faster return to chemotherapy [20], other than described benefit from a biological standpoint [21].

62.3 Preparation

Minimally invasive surgery requires an operating room organized to safe perform surgical procedures. First of all, a laparoscopic trolley equipped with light source, laparoscope and camera unit, video monitor and insufflator is necessary. Recently, modern operating theatre has ceiling-mounted trolley with a better ergonomic and occupation of space in the room. Light source, quality of laparoscope and screens are actually extremely important to achieve a correct view during laparoscopic dissection and transection to reduce at minimum the risk of bleeding. Constant pneumoperitoneum insufflator represents today an important help for surgeon in case of necessity of prolonged suction, permitting an easier control of the bleeding. In modern MIS, it is mandatory to have the possibility to perform intraoperative ultrasound, to easily guide the surgeon during the surgical procedure. Increasing quality of video support has introduced recently the possibility to have a 4k view or a 3d view, increasing the quality of intraoperative view. With the progression of technology, the introduction of even more complex devices permits to perform safer surgical procedure, with reduced risk of massive bleeding during liver transection, due to the introduction of energy based sealer and ultrasonic dissector.

Concerning laparoscopic instruments, the ideal concept is that the same set of open surgical instrument should be available in laparoscopy. Extremely important is the use of bipolar forceps, dissectors, vascular clamp, bulldog, needle driver, Goldfinger, precise suction instrument.

In most of cases, surgeon stands between the legs, with assistant on the side, opposite to the scrub nurse. Video monitors are placed at both side of the head of the patient, in order to allow all surgical team to assist the operation.

In selected cases, patient could be positioned in different way, to achieve a better exposition of deep segments. In case of intraoperative bleeding or complication needing rapid conversion, surgeon, assistant and equipment need to be ready for conversion to open procedure.

62.4 Surgical Technique

Minimally invasive liver resection needs to be planned, understanding patient anatomy and relation among arterial, portal, hepatic vein and biliary structure. The analysis of the surgical case should be discussed in multidisciplinary team, with the analysis of CT scan and MRI, better supported by a 3d model that could be extremely important for 3-dimensional orientation of the lesion and to calculate future remnant liver in case of project of major hepatic resection.

In case of MIS, all instrument should be prepared and tested before surgery, as well a conventional operation box of instrument should be in the operating room ready for conversion. It's extremely important to perform laparoscopic liver surgery with at least two expert hepatobiliary surgeon and an adequate nursing staff.

Laparoscope is extremely important, preferring 30° scope (even better if flexible) to explore difficult angle during resection. The introduction of 3d camera and 4k screen facilitate the resection due to the high definition and visualization of structures during the resection.

Collaboration with anesthesiologist is mandatory to reduce the risk of complication during the surgical procedure. Low CVP should be monitored and during surgery, and management of pneumoperitoneum should be performed informing the anesthesiologist.

Patient's and trocar positioning is fundamental for the correct execution of the surgery. Usually patient is positioned in French position (surgeon among the leg's of patient), except for resection in posterior segments of the liver, in which patient is placed on left lateral decubitus. Surgeon stands between legs of the patient with nurse lateral to the surgeon. The assistant usually are placed on left and right side of the patient. All operators and nurse should have easy access to a screen in order to actively participate to the surgical procedure.

Umbilical open access is preferred to Veres, and after the induction of pneumoperitoneum, all ports are placed under view of the surgeon. Ports should be place din function of the localization of lesion, with the possibility to add extra ports in case of need, even transthoracically.

An extremely careful exploration of the abdominal cavity should be performed, and a doppler ultrasound is mandatory at the beginning of the procedure. This is necessary to comprehend if further lesion are present and to better interpretation the anatomy of the liver intraoperatively. Pringle maneuver should be always prepared, after opening the pars flaccida, even if we don't preview to clamp the hepatic pedicle. This is a safe procedure, that allow to be safe in case of unexpected bleeding. Pedicle clamp is possible for 15 min with 5 min of release.

One of the fundamental moments of liver resection is parenchymal transection. Bleeding control can be considered more complicated in laparoscopy compared to open surgery, and so bleeding should be prevented, instead of treatment. Deep transection, close to large vessel, need to be careful and the use of energy devices did cannot avoid the knowledge of liver anatomy and laparoscopic ultrasonography, who can be fundamental to avoid major hepatic bleeding. In dissection of deep vessels, identification and selective control is mandatory, to avoid laceration of pedicles, especially hepatic veins. The use of clips and vascular suture could be useful to control glissonian pedicles or large hepatic veins. Meticulous intrahepatic dissection guarantees the best rate of success to perform even major hepatectomies. Once hepatectomy is completed, specimen must be extract in a plastic bag, via enlargement of trocar incision, Pfannenstiel incision, or previous surgery scar. Drainage is placed via a trocar orifice, depending of surgeon habitude.

62.4.1 Wedge Resection

This kind of resection is usually the first performed by a hepatobiliary surgeon who approaches minimally invasive surgery. This non-anatomical resection, usually don't require liver mobilization. A pringle preparation in recommended, especially in initial experience. Transection could be performed after the determination of correct resection margin with ultrasonography, and use of clip is determined in function on depth of resection

62.4.2 Anatomical Segmentectomy

Segmentectomy is a formal resection whereas the complete area of liver corresponding to the vascularization of a segmental pedicle is removed.

Traditionally, *laparoscopic segments* have always been distinguished from *non-laparoscopic* ones, to highlight differences in the surgical accessibility between anterior segments—3, 4b, 5, 6 and posterior and superior segments—4a, 7, 8, which are technically more difficult. Anatomical segmentectomies have become an important surgical technique capable of minimizing loss of functional liver [22], and can be performed laparoscopically for any segment of the liver, basing on the degree of complexity and the level of expertise of individual surgeons.

62.4.3 Left Lateral Lobectomy

Considered as the gold standard of minimally invasive liver resection [3], it actually represents the standard of care. Falciform ligament and left triangular ligaments are sectioned at the beginning of the procedure. Lesser omentum opening is useful either to perform pringle maneuver or to verify the presence of aberrant left hepatic artery. Transection line should be performed ideally on the left side of the coronary ligament. Opening of parenchymal bridge among segment III and IV should be opened to correct expose the glissonian pedicle of segment III and II. Energy devices could be used in the superficial layer of the liver, in order to easily access to a correct visualization of glissonian pedicle. Once glissonian pedicle of segment III is dissected and taped, Hem o Lock or vascular suture could be used to transect the pedicle and to access to segment II pedicle, who is dissected, encircled and sectioned and sutured. Parenchymal transection continues cranially, up to the visualization of left hepatic vein who is usually stapled with an amount of parenchyma around.

62.4.4 Left Hepatectomy

Left hepatectomy is one of the procedures accounted as advanced according to Ban-Wakabayashi's score and should therefore be tackled once the learning curve on minor procedures is completed.

The procedure is presented in a step-by-step fashion (Fig. 62.2 step-by-step left hepatectomy), following a primary anterior approach (inflow interruption–parenchymal transection–outflow interruption).

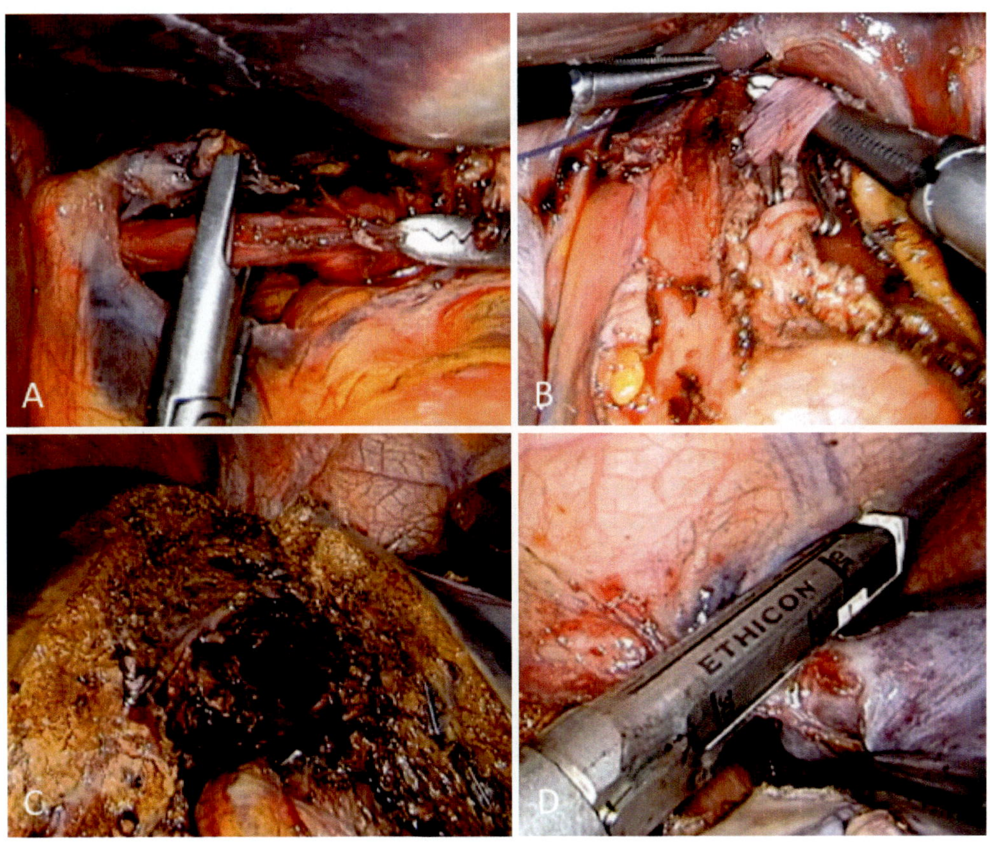

Fig. 62.2 Left hepatectomy step-by-step. (**a**) Left hepatic artery interruption. (**b**) Left portal vein isolation. (**c**) Parenchymal transection. (**d**) Left hepatic vein interruption

A. Interruption of the pars flaccida of the hepatoduodenal ligament gives access to the left lateral aspect of the hepatic pedicle, where the left hepatic artery is interrupted between clips (Fig. 62.2a).
B. The left portal vein is isolated and interrupted between vascular clips (Fig. 62.2b).
C. An intermittent extra-corporeal Pringle maneuver is set up through an umbilical lace and a chest tube, permitting an avascular transection with intermittent pedicle clamping (10 min of ischemia are alternated to 5 min of reperfusion).
D. The parenchymal transection is performed through an ultrasonic dissector and an energy device (Fig. 62.2c). Vascular structures are clipped or sealed with wet bipolar forceps, according to dimensions.
E. The left hepatic vein is isolated intra-parenchymally and stapled (Fig. 62.2d).

At the end of procedure, the specimen is extracted through a Pfannenstiel incision or a small mid-line incision (if a midline scar is present as consequence of a previous open procedure) in a retrieval bag. No drain tubes are left in place if no bile is observed during the procedure itself, in accordance with enhanced recovery after surgery (ERAS) philosophy applied to liver surgery.

62.4.5 Right Hepatectomy

Compared to left hepatectomy, this procedure is more complex compared to left hepatectomy and requires a solid experience in minor liver resection and left hepatectomies. Falciform and round ligament are sectioned and pringle maneuver is prepared after incision of the pars flaccida. Identification and section of cystic duct and cystic artery is done, and gallbladder is partially detached and used as tool to be grasped and give better exposition. Cystic stump is gently retracted in order to lift up the bile duct and identify right branch of hepatic artery and portal vein. Hepatic artery is divided among hem o lock clips, after verification of contralateral arterial signal at ultrasound. Right branch of portal vein is dissected and resected often with vascular stapler, after identification of origin of left branch, in order to avoid stenosis. Once artery and portal vein are sectioned, demarcation appears among left vascularized liver and right nonvascularized part. Parenchymal dissection is performed following the caudal approach, straight on the right border of the vena cava. During the dissection, middle hepatic vein branches to segment V and VIII are clipped and divided, as well as at the level of hilar plate, biliary structure are identified and clipped. Parenchymal dissection continues up to the identification of right hepatic vein who is dissected, encircled and stapled.

62.5 Peri-operative Management

An institutional protocol is presented for the peri-operative management of patients operated for laparoscopic liver resections as part of a local ERAS program [23]. The same protocol is equally applied to patients both undergoing minor and major resections.

- Day −1: an oral carbohydrate loading is administered to patients the night before and 3 h before the procedure.
- Day 0: After surgery, patients are allowed to drink water in the evening. Vital signs are monitored hourly through the first night-time.
- Day 1: blood tests including liver function tests (LFT) are collected; out of bed (at least 2 h in the morning and 2 h in the afternoon). Walking is encouraged. Solid food since morning and light meals are given, if no post-operative nausea is present. Two liters of a balanced i.v. electrolytic solution are administered.
- Day 2: blood tests including LFT are repeated. Walking is recommended. Urine catheter and i.v. infusions are discontinued. Drain tubes are removed if no bile is evident at this time. Patient is started on a full diet.
- Day 3: blood tests including LFT are repeated. Paravertebral analgesia and i.v. pain medications are discontinued. Discharge criteria are evaluated.
- Day 4: discharge is considered if discharge criteria are satisfied (patient is motivated to leave hospital; adequate oral feeding; satisfying pain management through p.o. medications; first flatus occurred; no post-operative complications are encountered).

62.5.1 Pain Management

Before the general anesthesia induction, a right paravertebral catheter is placed at T12 level according to the risk of conversion which is evaluated basing on previous abdominal surgeries, the type of resection (e.g. whether a major hepatectomy is planned) and the estimated degree of complexity of the procedure.

1 g of i.v. paracetamol and 30 mg of ketorolac are given at the end of procedure.

Post-operatively, paracetamol 1 g Q 6 h is administered i.v.; paravertebral infusion with naropine/sufentanil is administered until POD 3–4. Tapentadol 50 mg p.o. Q 12 h is administered since POD 1; i.v. pain medications are discontinued since POD 2–3 and paracetamol 1 g p.o. every 8 h is given since day 2 replacing i.v. administrations.

Ketorolac 30 mg i.v. p.r.n. is administered inpatient as rescue for pain exacerbation.

At the time of discharge, paracetamol 1 g p.o. Q 8 h and tapentadol 50 mg p.o. Q 12 h of are prescribed for 1 week.

62.5.2 NG Tubes, Abdominal Drains

A naso-gastric tube is placed after general anesthesia and is removed before the end of procedure.

Abdominal drains are not routinely placed, for neither minor nor major resections. The following conditions have been identified as the necessity to monitor for bile leakage:

- if the resection is performed in superior/postero-superior areas (which can be difficultly achieved percutaneously in case of a post-operative collection);
- if, during transection, a bile leakage is observed or biliostasis is not satisfying at the end of the procedure.

Post-operatively, drains are removed between POD 2 and 3 if no bile is encountered nor abdominal complications are suspected.

To summarize, ERAS protocol for patients undergoing laparoscopic liver resections contemplate a quick return to preoperative condition within 2 days from the time of surgery, having infusions and lines discontinued and oral feeding resumed as soon as possible.

62.6 Conclusion

Initially applied to *laparoscopic* liver segments, the development of technique and technologies expanded indications to more and more difficult resections, encompassing *non-laparoscopic* liver segments, major resections and extending indications from benign disease to HCC, ICC and multiple metastatic disease. These evolutions make possible an increasing number of patients can take advantages of benefits from minimally-invasive liver surgery without compromising safety profiles and oncologic outcomes.

Self Study

Questions

1. Which statement is true?
   (a) Minor liver resections only are the correct indication for laparoscopic approach.
   (b) Patients with liver cirrhosis should not be tackled with laparoscopy due to risk of liver decompensation.
   (c) Only benign disease can be tackled laparoscopically because of oncological concernings.
   (d) Laparoscopy is associated with reduced intraoperative bleeding, faster postoperative recovery and fewer post-operative complications.
2. Which statement is false?
   (a) CO_2 pneumoperitoneum in laparoscopy significantly increases the risk of air embolism, in comparison to open surgery.
   (b) Careful anaesthesiological intraoperative management is mandatory to perform resections with reduced blood loss by keeping hypovolemic state and low CVP.
   (c) Fast-track protocols in laparoscopic liver surgery lead to a faster resume of chemotherapy in patients affected my metastatic colorectal cancer.
   (d) Bilobar disease is not a contraindication to minimally-invasiveness due to associated intraoperative thermal ablations, parenchymal sparing resections and staged hepatectomies.

Answers

1. Which statement is true?
   (a) False. Both minor and major resections are indications for laparoscopic liver procedures.
   (b) False. Laparoscopy is related to fewer liver decompensation rate in patients with cirrhosis, mainly because of the inferior collateral circles breakdown in the abdominal wall.
   (c) False. Both malignancies and benign disease are approached with laparoscopy.
   (d) **True**.
2. Which statement is false?
   (a) **False**. The risk of CO_2 embolism is unremarkable during laparoscopic procedures, mainly because most of the carbon dioxide is exchanged at lungs during ventilation and then is expelled.
   (b) True.
   (c) True. Patients undergone laparoscopic liver procedures have been shown faster resume of adjuvant therapies.
   (d) True.

References

1. Reich H, McGlynn F, DeCaprio J, Budin R. Laparoscopic excision of benign liver lesions. Obstet Gynecol. 1991;78(5 Pt 2):956–8.
2. Buell JF, Cherqui D, Geller DA, O'Rourke N, Iannitti D, Dagher I, et al. The international position on laparoscopic liver surgery: the Louisville statement, 2008. Ann Surg. 2009;250(5):825–30.
3. Wakabayashi G, Cherqui D, Geller DA, Buell JF, Kaneko H, Han HS, et al. Recommendations for laparoscopic liver resection: a report from the second international consensus conference held in Morioka. Ann Surg [Internet]. 2015;261(4):619–29.
4. Jia C, Li H, Wen N, Chen J, Wei Y, Li B. Laparoscopic liver resection: a review of current indications and surgical techniques. HepatoBiliary Surg Nutr. 2018;7(4):277–88.

5. Morise Z. Status and perspective of laparoscopic repeat liver resection. World J Hepatol. 2018;10(7):479–84.
6. Hallet J, Pessaux P, Beyfuss KA, Jayaraman S, Serrano PE, Martel G, et al. Critical appraisal of predictive tools to assess the difficulty of laparoscopic liver resection: a systematic review. Surg Endosc. 2019;33:366.
7. Morise Z, Wakabayashi G. First quarter century of laparoscopic liver resection. World J Gastroenterol. 2017;23(20):3581–8. https://doi.org/10.3748/wjg.v23.i20.3581. Review. PubMed PMID: 28611511, PubMed Central PMCID: PMC5449415.
8. Smerieri N, Fiorentini G, Ratti F, Cipriani F, Belli A, Aldrighetti L. Laparoscopic left hepatectomy for mucinous cystic neoplasm of the liver. Surg Endosc. 2018;32(2):1068–9. https://doi.org/10.1007/s00464-017-5736-1. PubMed PMID: 28733729.
9. Nguyen KT, Gamblin TC, Geller DA. World review of laparoscopic liver resection-2,804 patients. Ann Surg. 2009;250(5):831–41. https://doi.org/10.1097/SLA.0b013e3181b0c4df. Review. PubMed PMID: 19801936.
10. Fuks D, Aldrighetti L, Jiao LR, Wakabayashi G, Limongelli P. Laparoscopic management of hepatocellular carcinoma: a critical reappraisal. Surg Laparosc Endosc Percutan Tech. 2017;27(4):203–5. https://doi.org/10.1097/SLE.0000000000000415. Review. PubMed PMID: 28520651.
11. Yoon YI, Kim KH, Kang SH, Kim WJ, Shin MH, Lee SK, Jung DH, Park GC, Ahn CS, Moon DB, Ha TY, Song GW, Hwang S, Lee SG. Pure laparoscopic versus open right hepatectomy for hepatocellular carcinoma in patients with cirrhosis: a propensity score matched analysis. Ann Surg. 2017;265(5):856–63. https://doi.org/10.1097/SLA.0000000000002072. PubMed PMID: 27849661.
12. Goh EL, Chidambaram S, Ma S. Laparoscopic vs open hepatectomy for hepatocellular carcinoma in patients with cirrhosis: a meta-analysis of the long-term survival outcomes. Int J Surg. 2018;50:35–42. https://doi.org/10.1016/j.ijsu.2017.12.021. Review. PubMed PMID: 29284151.
13. Santambrogio R, Chiang J, Barabino M, Meloni FM, Bertolini E, Melchiorre F, Opocher E. Comparison of laparoscopic microwave to radiofrequency ablation of small hepatocellular carcinoma (≤3 cm). Ann Surg Oncol. 2017;24(1):257–63. https://doi.org/10.1245/s10434-016-5527-2. PubMed PMID: 27581608; PubMed Central PMCID: PMC5827943.
14. Fiorentini G, Ratti F, Cipriani F, Palombo D, Catena M, Paganelli M, Aldrighetti L. Minimally invasive approach to intrahepatic cholangiocarcinoma: technical notes for a safe hepatectomy and lymphadenectomy. Ann Laparosc Endosc Surg. 2017;2:68.
15. Levi Sandri GB, Spoletini G, Mascianà G, Colasanti M, Lepiane P, Vennarecci G, D'Andrea V, Ettorre GM. The role of minimally invasive surgery in the treatment of cholangiocarcinoma. Eur J Surg Oncol. 2017;43(9):1617–21. https://doi.org/10.1016/j.ejso.2017.02.012. Review. PubMed PMID: 28292628.
16. Lee W, Park JH, Kim JY, Kwag SJ, Park T, Jeong SH, Ju YT, Jung EJ, Lee YJ, Hong SC, Choi SK, Jeong CY. Comparison of perioperative and oncologic outcomes between open and laparoscopic liver resection for intrahepatic cholangiocarcinoma. Surg Endosc. 2016;30(11):4835–40. PubMed PMID: 26902611.
17. Omichi K, Shindoh J, Cloyd JM, Mizuno T, Chun YS, Conrad C, Aloia TA, Tzeng CD, Vauthey JN. Liver resection is justified for patients with bilateral multiple colorectal liver metastases: a propensity-score-matched analysis. Eur J Surg Oncol. 2018;44(1):122–9. https://doi.org/10.1016/j.ejso.2017.11.006. PubMed PMID: 29208318, PubMed Central PMCID: PMC5742306.
18. Machado MA, Surjan RC, Bassères T, Makdissi FF. Totally laparoscopic ALPPS for multiple and bilobar colorectal metastases (with video). J Visc Surg. 2017;154(2):131–2. https://doi.org/10.1016/j.jviscsurg.2016.11.004. PubMed PMID: 28159501.
19. Machado MA, Surjan R, Basseres T, Makdissi F. Total laparoscopic reversal ALPPS. Ann Surg Oncol. 2017;24(4):1048–9. https://doi.org/10.1245/s10434-016-5620-6. PubMed PMID: 27734177.
20. Kawai T, Goumard C, Jeune F, Savier E, Vaillant JC, Scatton O. Laparoscopic liver resection for colorectal liver metastasis patients allows patients to start adjuvant chemotherapy without delay: a propensity score analysis. Surg Endosc. 2018;32(7):3273–81. https://doi.org/10.1007/s00464-018-6046-y. PubMed PMID: 29340819.
21. Fretland AA, Sokolov A, Postriganova N, Kazaryan AM, Pischke SE, Nilsson PH, Rognes IN, Bjornbeth BA, Fagerland MW, Mollnes TE, Edwin B. Inflammatory response after laparoscopic versus open resection of colorectal liver metastases: data from the oslo-CoMet trial. Medicine (Baltimore). 2015;94(42):e1786. https://doi.org/10.1097/MD.0000000000001786. Erratum in: Medicine (Baltimore). 2016;95(10):e367e. PubMed PMID: 26496309; PubMed Central PMCID: PMC4620756.
22. Ishizawa T, Gumbs AA, Kokudo N, Gayet B. Laparoscopic segmentectomy of the liver: from segment I to VIII. Ann Surg. 2012;256(6):959–64. https://doi.org/10.1097/SLA.0b013e31825ffed3. PubMed PMID: 22968066.
23. Ratti F, Cipriani F, Reineke R, Catena M, Comotti L, Beretta L, Aldrighetti LAM. Impact of Enhanced Recovery After Surgery (ERAS) approach and minimally-invasive techniques on outcome of patients undergoing liver surgery for hepatocellular carcinoma. A comparative study from a single institution. Clin Nutr ESPEN. 2016;12:e41. https://doi.org/10.1016/j.clnesp.2016.02.036. PubMed PMID: 28531699.

New Loco Regional Approaches to Treat Liver Cancer

63

Shaikh Afaq, Jayesh M. Soni, and Anil K. Pillai

Key Concepts

Overview of Loco regional treatments for Hepatocellular cancer

Tumor Ablative treatments:

- Radiofrequency Ablation
- Microwave ablation
- Cryoablation
- Irreversible electroporation
- Chemical Ablation
- Stereotactic radiation treatment

Endovascular treatments:

- Trans-arterial Chemoembolization
- Trans-arterial Bland embolization
- Trans-arterial drug eluting bead embolization
- Trans-arterial Radio embolization

Future Direction:

- Immunotherapy

63.1 Introduction

Hepatocellular carcinoma is responsible for 12,000 deaths per year in the United States. The incidence of the disease is approximately 2.5 per 100,000 population. It is third most common malignancy in adults. Incidence is higher in men than women, and in African Americans than Caucasians [4]. Worldwide, over a million deaths per year (about 10% of all deaths in the adult age range) can be attributed to hepatocellular carcinoma. Surgical treatments including hepatic resection and liver transplantation are considered as the most effective treatment of HCC. The vast majority of HCC patients are not suitable for curative treatment. Henceforth, novel minimally invasive interventional radiology techniques have come in existence over the past two decades as the mainstay for managing HCC [2]. We will discuss the basic applicability and designs of these techniques along with their outcomes. The image-guided loco-regional treatment for patients with unresectable Hepatocellular carcinoma can be broadly classified into ablative and endovascular techniques.

63.2 Ablative Techniques

Ablative techniques involve destruction of tumor by thermal, electrical and chemical agents. Thermal ablative techniques involve either heating or freezing tissues to tumoricidal temperatures. Radiofrequency, microwave, laser and high intensity focused ultrasound ablation causes frictional heating in tissues to lethal temperatures of above 60 °C. Cryo-ablation induces ice formation and tissue destruction at temperatures between −20 and −40 °C [5]. Irreversible electroporation (IRE) utilizes electric energy to create nanopores in the cell membrane facilitating osmotic cell death. Percutaneous chemical ablation (PCA) is performed by injecting absolute alcohol or other sclerosant agents directly into the tumor microenvironment. The common theme in all ablative techniques in precise placement of a needle/needles into the tumor. The choice of tumoricidal agent is governed by patient factors, tumor characteristics, local availability, operator preference and expertise. In the following sections we will look into each specific ablative technique.

S. Afaq
University of Texas Health Science Center, Houston, TX, USA
e-mail: Shaikh.afaq@uth.tmc.edu

J. M. Soni · A. K. Pillai (✉)
Diagnostic and Interventional Imaging, University of Texas Health Science Center, Houston, TX, USA
e-mail: Jayesh.Soni@uth.tmc.edu; Anil.K.Pillai@uth.tmc.edu

F. Radu-Ionita et al. (eds.), *Liver Diseases*, https://doi.org/10.1007/978-3-030-24432-3_63

63.2.1 Radiofrequency Ablation

RFA is the most studied ablative technique. An alternating electric current between 200 and 1200 kHz is passed between two electrodes (needle tip and the grounding pads) and the patient in series. Rapid motion of polar water molecules creates frictional heating in the tissues. The heat generated is inversely proportional to the surface area of the electrode. Heating around the needle tip is much higher than at the grounding pad. RFA has many advantages—it is minimally invasive with acceptable morbidity, it enables excellent local tumor control, it has promising long-term survival, and can be combined with other locoregional techniques like chemoembolization. In the guidelines proposed by EASL and AASLD, Radiofrequency ablation is recommended as a non-surgical technique for the treatment of early stage HCC (Child A or B), solitary HCC up to three nodules <3 cm in size. Combined treatment with TACE is a good alternative for the larger tumor measuring more than 3 cm [6]. Limitations of RFA include tumor size >3 cm and heat sink effect. Heat is transmitted in tissue by conduction. As the tumor size extends beyond 3 cm, the conduction of heat to the periphery of the tumor is limited by formation of gas bubbles (charring) near the needle tip (Fig. 63.1). Gas is a poor conductor of heat and decreases the tumoricidal effect. Another well-known phenomenon limiting RFA ablation is "Heat-sink" effect (Fig. 63.2). The convected heat from the adjacent large vessel can decrease the ablation effect by lowering the temperature near the flowing vessel [9]. If the tumor is located close to an organ, collateral thermal injury can develop. Most vulnerable organs are colon, diaphragm, gall bladder and central bile duct. For minimizing thermal injury to the GI tract and diaphragm, tissue separation techniques like hydrodissection (D5W) or CO_2 to separate the organs at risks from the ablation zone is carried out [8].

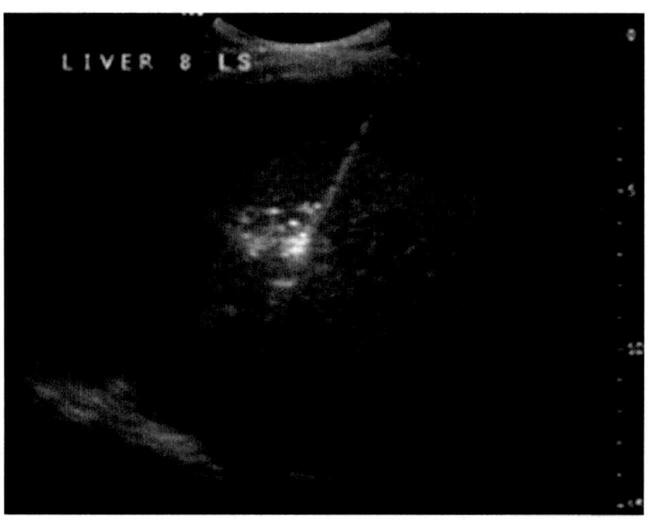

Fig. 63.1 Formation of gas bubbles near the needle tip limits the ability To transfer heat to the periphery of the tumor during RFA ablation

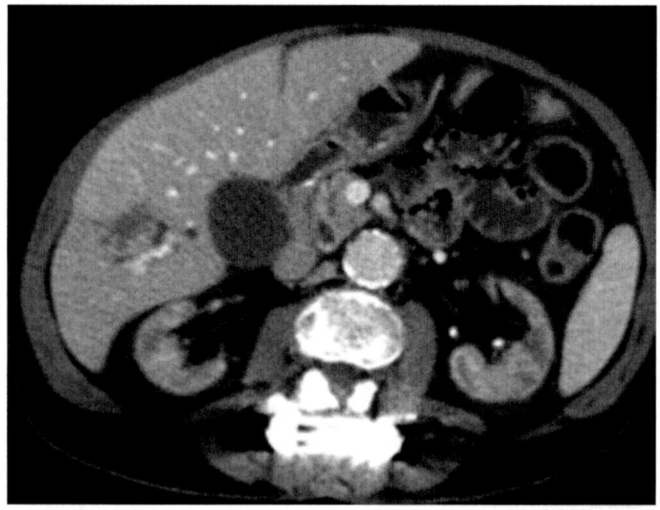

Fig. 63.2 Tumor recurrence (dark arrow) due to heat sink effect from a portal vein branch (white arrow) after RFA

An extensive meta-analysis of 82 independent reports including 3670 patients, reported by Mulier et al. revealed that the overall mortality was 0.5% and major/minor complication rate was 8.9%. These most common complications were abdominal hemorrhage, abdominal infection (abscess), liver failure, biliary tract damage. RFA is associated with much less complication than surgical treatment with the overall survival rates being 60–70% at 5 years [10] (Level 1). Hence, it is the ideal treatments of patients within the Milan criteria.

63.2.2 Microwave Ablation

Image-guided, percutaneous microwave ablation (MWA) is a fairly recent and promising method in the field of thermal ablation. Unlike RFA, microwave ablation utilizes electromagnetic waves oscillating between 900 and 2450 MHz to induce movement of water molecules and create frictional heating. Formation of gas bubbles does not limit the ability of microwaves unlike RFA and thus larger tumors can be treated. Heat sink effect is also less with MWA. Collateral damage to surrounding structures is still a concern especially to bowel, gall bladder and biliary tree. Large scale randomized prospective clinical trials comparing MVA and RFA are needed to determine the future clinical role of MWA [7]. Early MWA equipment was faced with much scrutiny given the technical problems including inadequate power handling to exceeding probe gauge, poor predictability of the field pattern and uncontrolled back heating "Comet effect" (Fig. 63.3). MWA was first used clinically in 2001 in 107 HCCs ranging from 0.8 to 6.4 cm using either a single antenna (in 46 nodules) or multiple antennae (61 nodules).

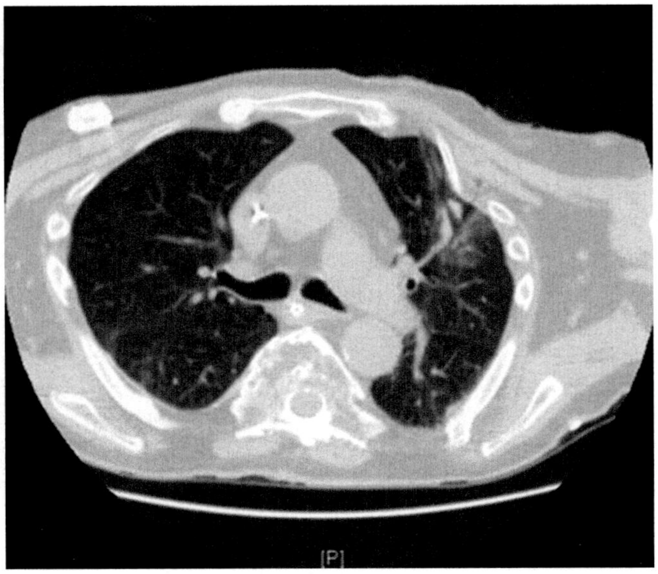

Fig. 63.3 Tail burn in the soft tissue (arrow) after MWA

Technical success was achieved in 98% of tumors <2 cm and 92% of nodules >2 cm, while local recurrence was found in 2% of nodules <2 cm and in 8% of nodules >2 cm [11]. In 2005, Lu et al. [12] reported the results of a retrospective study comparing percutaneous MWA with RFA. The mean diameter of HCC nodules was 2.5 ± 1.2 cm in MWA group and 2.6 ± 1.2 cm in RFA group. A single insertion was applied for tumors <2.0 cm while multiple insertions were used for tumors >2 cm. RFA was performed by using a 290 kHz-RF generator with a maximum power output of 200 W. Complete ablation rates were 98.6% in <3.0 cm tumors and 83.3% in >3.0 cm tumors in the MWA group. The numbers comparatively in the RFA group were 98% and 81% respectively. The differences between the two groups were not statistically significant. Complications and long term survivals were also equivalent in the two groups.

However, with the upgrade of MWA devices there have been early clinical trials showing promising results in treating hepatic tumors >3 cm. Yin et al. [13] treated with percutaneous RFA or MVA 109 patients with HCC measuring between 3 and 7 cm. They reported a complete ablation of 92.6%, a local recurrence in 22% of patients and a 3 year survival rate of 31%. Still no statistical difference between the complete ablation rate between RFA and MVA. Though recent improvement of ablation microwave technology has significantly improved clinical efficacy, its superiority or inferiority over RFA is yet to be determined.

63.2.3 Cryoablation

Cryoablation (CA) is a less prevalent percutaneous ablative therapy for HCC, and current evidence about its usefulness is limited. Cryoablation destroys tissue by the application of alternating freezing and thawing leading to apoptotic cell death by osmotic damage. The currently available cryosystems use argon and helium gas based on the Joule Thomson effect [14]. There is direct cellular injury (which relies on ice crystal formation in extracellular and intracellular spaces) and vascular related injury (which occurs as a result of vasoconstriction and a decrease in the flow of blood). Comparisons of Cryoablation to other modalities for HCC are limited [14]. A multicenter randomized controlled trial [15] of Cryoablation versus RFA was published in 2015 which included a total of 260 patients with Child Pugh Class A or B cirrhosis and onc or two HCC lesions <4 cm, treatment naïve, without metastasis. Patients were randomly assigned to Cryoablation (m = 180) and RFA (n = 180). The primary endpoints were local tumor progression at 3 years after treatment and safety. Local tumor progression rates at 1, 2 and 3 years were 3%, 7% and 7% for Cryoablation and 9%, 11% and 11% for RFA (P = 0.043). For lesions >3 cm in diameter, the local tumor progression rate was significantly lower in the Cryoablation group versus the RFA group. The 1 year, 3 year and 5 year survival rates were 97%, 67%, and 40% for Cryoablation and 97%, 66%, and 38% for RFA, respectively [15]. According to Wang et al. the recurrence free survival rate and overall survival rate were not significantly different between two groups. In terms of complication, the major complication rate between percutaneous Cryoablation and RFA was also comparable. Although the safety profile of Cryoablation overall is comparable, and there is less chance of damage to blood vessels and gall bladder, it is important to discuss the clinical relevance of "Cryo-Shock". Cryo-shock is a rare, but fatal Cryoablation-related complication leading to multi organ failure experienced by few patients after hepatic cryotherapy. Patients suffer from severe coagulopathy and DIC, similar to septic shock but without evidence of systemic sepsis. Severe DIC necessitating repeated transfusions of fresh frozen plasma, cryoprecipitate, platelets, and tranexamic acid has been observed in some patients. According to a survey study, Cryo-Shock occurred in about 1% of patients who underwent hepatic cryosurgery, but the exact rate of Cryo-Shock in percutaneous Cryoablation remains unknown [15]. The incidence of bleeding complication after CA is slightly more compared to coagulative techniques like MWA and RFA.

63.2.4 Irreversible Electroporation (IRE)

Irreversible electroporation (IRE) is a new non-chemical, non-thermal ablation treatment during which alteration of trans-membrane potential disrupts the integrity of the membrane resulting in cellular death [16]. The technique is currently undergoing clinical evaluation for small sized HCC. In the early experience, IRE was hampered by cardiac toxicity

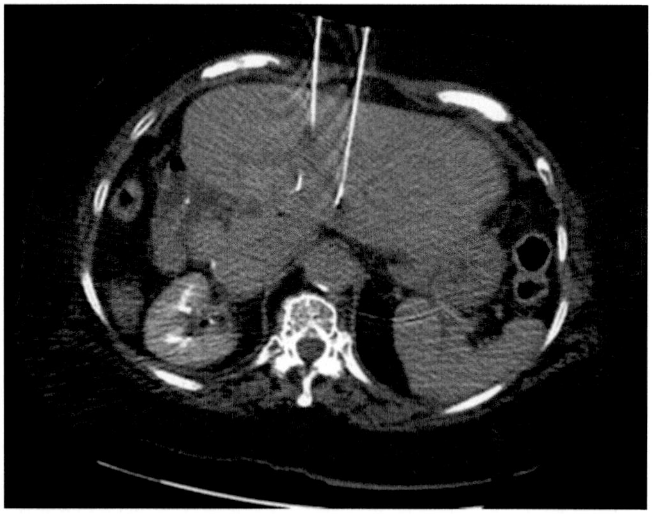

Fig. 63.4 Lesion near the portal vein treated with IRE to avoid heat sink

and arrhythmias. Since the introduction of cardiac synchronization with IRE treatment delivery, the safety of IRE for liver ablation has been established in several case series and a systematic review. Like thermal ablation, the best results with IRE are seen after treating tumors <3 cm [16]. Since IRE does not induce thermal coagulative necrosis it becomes the ablative tool of choice is patients with tumors close to vital structures like portal vein and biliary system. IRE does not suffer from the effects of heat sink unlike thermal techniques (Fig. 63.4).

63.2.5 Chemical Ablation

Introduced more than 30 years ago for local treatment of Hepatocellular cancer, this technique is not very prevalent in the western world. Absolute alcohol is injected directly into the tumor after percutaneous access using a special type of needle with tines to induce coagulative necrosis by protein denaturation and vascular occlusion. Alcohol ablation is cheap, does not cause collateral damage, and is not affected by heat sink. The penetration of alcohol into the tumor is variable. Multi-septate tumor limits diffusion of alcohol to all parts of the tumor leading to local recurrence. With introduction of thermal ablation techniques, alcohol ablation has fallen out of favor. Several Randomized studies have shown superiority of RFA over alcohol ablation.

63.3 Endovascular Techniques

63.3.1 TACE

For patients who are not candidates for surgical treatments and ablation either due to tumor size or distribution, trans catheter embolization is the mainstay treatment option with proven survival benefits [17]. The normal liver receives a dual blood supply from the hepatic artery (25%) and the portal vein (75%). As HCC grows, it increasingly depends on the hepatic artery for blood supply and once a tumor nodule reaches a diameter of 2 cm or more, most of the blood supply derives from the hepatic artery. This unique property of HCC provides the rationale for the use of trans arterial therapies. Trans arterial chemoembolization consists of the selective angiographic occlusion of the tumor arterial blood supply with a variety of embolizing agents with the precedence of local chemotherapy infusion.

Conventional Trans arterial chemoembolization (TACE) uses a mixture of chemotherapeutic agent (e.g. doxorubicin or cisplatin) and lipiodol which is the recommended standard of care for the treatment of intermediate stage HCC [18]. Drug-eluting beads (DEBs) is a novel system consistent of embolic microspheres preloaded with doxorubicin, that ensure the controlled release over time of chemotherapy and thus provide a combined local ischemic and cytotoxic effect. This results in lower systemic doxorubicin concentrations than conventional TACE and higher intra-tumor retention [18]. Patients with more advanced liver disease might benefit from DEB-TACE due to lower systemic chemotherapy concentrations. Lencioni R et al. published in May of 2016 SPACE trial aimed at comparing DEB-TACE with doxorubicin-eluting beads on Sorafenib versus just Deb-TACE alone. Patients with intermediate stage (BCLC B) multinodular HCC without macrovascular invasion or extrahepatic spread were randomized 1:1 to DEB-TACE (150 mg doxorubicin) plus sorafenib 400 mg twice daily or just DEB-TACE with placebo (Table 63.1). The primary end point was time to tumor progression (TTP) [19]. No unexpected adverse events related to Sorafenib were observed. The overall response rate for patients in the sorafenib and placebo groups with post-baseline scans were 55.9% and 41.3% respectively and the disease control rate was 89.2% and 76.1% respectively. However, median TTP for subjects receiving sorafenib plus DEB-TACE or placebo plus DEB-TACE was similar (169 days versus 166 days) proving that while TACE alone may not provide all beneficial effects combining it with systemic chemotherapy is both safe and technically feasible [19]. Contraindications include encephalopathy and large burden metastatic disease outside the liver. TACE is also contra-indicated in patients with portal vein thrombosis due to concern that further decrease to the blood supply of the liver can prove to be deleterious. Therefore, it is best to exercise extreme precaution and/or avoid TACE in patients with advanced cirrhosis. Other complications include post-embolization syndrome (fever, nausea, elevated liver function tests); Gastrointestinal ulceration (3–5%), rare pancreatitis or cholecystitis (<1%), due to embolization of other vessels. The survival rates of TACE are approximately 60–80% at 1 year and 30–60% at 2 years. Studies have even shown that TACE combined with Radiofrequency ablation

Table 63.1 BCLC classification

BCLC stage	Performance status	Tumor features	Liver functions	Treatment options	Survival data
0	0	Single < 2 cm	No PH Nor T bili	Surgery or ablation	OS >60 months 5 years—75%
A	0	Single < 5 cm Three <3 cm	Child A	Transplant Ablation	OS >60 months 5 years—75%
B	0	Multinodular	CP A-B	Transarterial treatments	OS 20 months SD 14–45 months
C	1–2	Vascular invasion Metastatic	CP A-B	Sorafenib	OS 11 months SD 6–14 months
D	3–4	Any	CP C	Supportive care	OS <3 months

improves the overall survival compared with that of TACE Alone. Anti-VEGF antibodies in combination with TACE and p53 gene therapy in combination with TACE are under study. Ultra-selective catheterization of tumor feeding arteries is also under consideration.

63.3.2 Bland Embolization

Bland embolization aims to increase tumor ischemia by peripheral vessel occlusion with the use of a permanent embolic agent without combining chemotherapeutic agents or iodized oil [20].

A study published in July 2008 by Keigo et al. shows that bland embolization using super absorbed polymer (SAP) microspheres as an initial therapeutic option for previously untreated hepatocellular carcinoma ineligible for resection or ablation is a safe and very promising option. Fifty-nine patients were allocated to this study and a total of 121 sessions of SAP trans-arterial embolization were performed. The mean period of repeated SAP-TAE was 15.6 months and it exceeded 1 year and 2 years in 32 (54%) and 15 (25%) patients, respectively. Thirteen (22%) patients underwent repeated SAP-TAE alone, and the remaining 46 (78%) patients underwent subsequent chemoembolization [21].

No major complication was observed and post embolization syndrome was minimal after SAP-TAE. Overall survival rates were 100% and 83% at 1 years and 2 years, respectively, and median survival time was 30 months. In conclusion, SAP-TAE was a safe and repeatable option as the induction therapy for HCC unamenable to surgery or ablation [21].

63.3.3 Y-90

Yttrium-90 radio embolization is a catheter based therapy that delivers internal radiation to hepatic tumors in the form of microspheres. It can be delivered to the hepatic tumor as either a constituent of a glass microsphere (Thera sphere), or a biocompatible resin-based microsphere (Sirsphere). Once embedded within the tumor microcirculation, these microspheres emit Beta radiation at therapeutic levels [22]. Y-90 unlike other modalities discussed above such as TACE and RFA is less often associated with toxicities such as abdominal pain, fever, nausea, and vomiting. In fact, there is a significant body of evidence supporting its safety and efficacy. The selection process for patients undergoing radio-embolization and their subsequent pretreatment evaluation is similar. Patients' eligibility for repeat radio embolization should be evaluated following every treatment. A study by Carr in 2004 reports on the safety and efficacy of Thera sphere for inoperable HCC [23]. Sixty-five patients with biopsy-proven HCC received a median radiation dose of 134 Gy. Median survival was 649 days and 302 days for Okuda Stage I and Okuda II patients respectively compared with 244 days and 64 days respectively for historical controls. These findings were supported by Geschwind et al. in 2004 [24] who reported on 80 patients from a relatively large database of 121 who were treated with Thera sphere.

Although further clinical investigation is warranted and should be directed towards a more rigorous approach to investigating patient selection criteria, as well as optimal dosimetry to obtain the desired therapeutic effect, there is no question about the inevitable application of radio embolization in patients with advanced HCC. A study by Chow et al. published in 2018 March compared Radio embolization to Sorafenib for Advanced HCC. Significantly fewer patients in the Radio embolization group had grade >3 Adverse effects (36 of 130 [27.7%] versus 82 of 162 [50.6%]), $p < 0.01$ [25], while overall survival did not differ between radio-embolization and Sorafenib. The improved toxicity profile of Radio embolization may inform treatment choice in selection patients.

63.3.4 Stereotactic Body Radiotherapy (SBRT)

SBRT refers to the use of a few fractions, generally fewer than 10, of potent doses of highly conformal radiation therapy with high geometric precision and accuracy to ablate the tumor. The main advantage of SBRT is that it is noninvasive. Radiation liver damage has been the concern with external beam radiation. In carefully selected patients with good liver functions, SBRT has been shown to be comparable to TACE and RFA. In patients with decompensated liver disease, the use of SBRT is limited.

63.4 Immunotherapy

There are four major immunotherapeutic approaches for HCC. These include Adoptive Cell therapy, HCC vaccines, oncolytic viruses and immune checkpoint inhibitors [26]. Adoptive cell therapy is an immunotherapeutic approach that kills cancer cells using patients' own lymphocytes. It functions by stimulating or loading autologous lymphocytes with cytokines or tumor antigens, cultivating them ex vivo and then reinfusing them into the patient. Adoptive immunotherapy includes cytokine-induced killer cells, tumor infiltrating lymphocytes, natural killer cells, and chimeric antigen receptor cells [26].

Cancer vaccination is performed using antigenic substances to activate tumor specific immune responses that can reduce tumor load and prevent tumor relapse. HCC vaccines include cancer cells, antigen peptides, and DNA-based vaccines, and some of these effectively inhibit tumor recurrence and metastasis. Oncolytic virotherapy includes engineering of wild-type viruses that selectively replicate in tumor cells and cause lysis without harming normal tissues. The mechanism underlying the antitumor activity of oncolytic viruses involves direct killing of cancer cells by expanding in them and causing cell lysis [26].

Immune checkpoint inhibitors reactivate tumor specific T cells and develop an antitumor effect by suppressing checkpoint-mediated signaling. Common immune checkpoint proteins include cytotoxic T lymphocyte-associated antigen-4 (CTLA-4), programmed cell death protein-1, programmed cell death ligand 1, VISTA, TIM-3, LAG-3 and OX40. CTLA-4 and PD-1 inhibitors have been well characterized and have been approved by FDA for treating melanomas, with some progress in their application in treating Hepatocellular carcinomas [26].

63.5 Conclusion

While there is still more research as our techniques continue to evolve there have been some major achievements made with non-surgical treatments. BCLC stage A patients can be treated with RFA with RFA and microwave ablation achieving similar outcomes and with less complications (with microwave ablation avoiding the heat-sink effect) compared to surgical treatments. Trans arterial embolization can be used for BCLC stage B patients and can be applied with chemotherapy or Yttrium-90 radio-embolization or even RFA. For extensive disease Yttrium-90 is a great option as it offers a better toxicity profile compared to the chemoembolization. With so many different trans-arterial options, a meta-analysis to find the optimal trans-catheter embolization was inevitable. Katsanos et al. [27] performed a meta-analysis which included the network of evidence of 55 randomized controlled trials (12 direct comparisons) with 5763 patients with preserved liver function and unresectable HCC (intermediate to advanced stage). All embolization strategies achieved a significant survival gain over control treatment. However, TACE, DEB-TACE, Trans-arterial Radio embolization and adjuvant systemic agents did not confer any survival benefit over Bland embolization lone. Estimated median survival was 13.9 months in control, 18.1 months in TACE, 20.6 months with DEB-TACE, 20.8 months with bland TAE, 30.1 months in TACE plus external radiotherapy, and 33.3 months in TACE plus liver ablation. Trans arterial RE was the safest treatment. And while the quality of evidence remained mostly low to moderate because of clinical diversity, chemoembolization combined with external radiotherapy or local liver ablation showed to significantly improve tumor response and patient survival rates over embolization (See Fig. 63.3). For BCLC stage C HCC there has been an equivalent survival demonstrated along with lower toxicity for trans arterial therapy compared to systemic therapy alone.

Self Study

Questions

1. Which is the following is a tumor ablative modality that can be use in tumors located in the hepatic hilum?
   (a) Microwave ablation
   (b) Radiofrequency ablation
   (c) Irreversible electroporation
   (d) Cryoablation
2. Heat sink effect is a major limitation in which of the following ablative modalities?
   (a) Chemical ablation
   (b) Irreversible electroporation
   (c) Laser ablation
   (d) Radiofrequency ablation
3. The recommended ideal tumor size for ablative modalities currently in practice is?
   (a) 2–3 cm
   (b) 1–2 cm
   (c) 3–5 cm
   (d) 5–9 cm

4. Which endovascular treatment has shown a superior survival benefit for BCLC B HCC within the Milan criteria?
   (a) TACE
   (b) Y-90 Radio-embolization
   (c) Bland Embolization
   (d) No difference in outcomes
5. Abscopal effect of ablation refers to
   (a) Complete tumor ablation from thermal techniques
   (b) Augmented response to immunotherapy after ablation
   (c) Undesirable effects of immunotherapy
   (d) Side effect of microwave ablation causing tumor progression

Answers

1. Which is the following is a tumor ablative modality that can be use in tumors located in the hepatic hilum?

   Correct Answer C. Tumors at the hepatic hilum are risky to treat with thermal ablation techniques due to the proximity to the main bile ducts. Thermal injury can lead to biliary strictures. Irreversible electroporation does not cause coagulative necrosis. Collateral damage to biliary system does not occur with this modality.
2. Heat sink effect is a major limitation in which of the following ablative modalities?

   Correct Answer: D. Heat sink effect is due to presence of a blood vessel in the vicinity of a tumor that is being thermally ablated. As the temperature cannot be maintained in the tumoricidal range due to flowing blood in the vicinity of the tumor, local recurrence can occur. This is a major issue with RFA. It also occurs in MWA and Cryoablation to a lesser extend.
3. The recommended ideal tumor size for ablative modalities currently in practice is?

   Correct Answer: A. The AASLD and EASL recommendation for thermal ablation are tumors below 3 cm. Multiple studies have shown that as the tumor becomes larger, the local recurrence rate increases. With MWA larger tumors could be targeted, but there is limited data.
4. Which endovascular treatment has shown a superior survival benefit for BCLC B HCC within the Milan criteria?

   Correct Answer: D. There is no survival benefit among all the endovascular treatment options. DEB-TACE and Y-90 has a better safety profile.
5. Abscopal effect of ablation refers to

   Correct Answer: B. Immune modulators like Tremelimumab in combination with ablation in patients with advanced hepatocellular carcinoma causes an augmented immune response referred to as Abscopal effect. J Hepatol. 2017 Mar; 66(3): 545–551

References

1. Golabi P, Fazel S, Otgonsuren M, et al. Mortality assessment of patients with hepatocellular carcinoma according to underlying disease and treatment modalities. Medicine. 2017;96(9):e5904.
2. Ramesh H. Resection for Hepatocellular carcinoma. J Clin Exp Hepatol. 2014;4(3):S90–6.
3. Raza A, Sood GK. Hepatocellular carcinoma review: current treatment, and evidence-based medicine. World J Gastroenterol. 2014;20(15):4115–27.
4. Mazzanti R, Arena U, Tassi R. Hepatocellular carcinoma: where are we? World J Exp Med. 2016;6(1):21–36.
5. Goldberg SN, Gazelle GS, Mueller PR. Thermal ablation therapy for focal malignancy. a unified approach to underlying principles, techniques, and diagnostic imaging guidance. Am J Rentgenol Diagn Imag Relat Sci. 2000;174(2):323.
6. Rhim H, Lim HK. Radiofrequency ablation of hepatocellular carcinoma: pros and cons. Gut Liver. 2010;4(1):S113–8.
7. Poggi G, Tosoratti N, Montagna B, et al. Microwave ablation of hepatocellular carcinoma. World J Hepatol. 2015;7(25):2578–89.
8. Liu CH, Yu CY, Chang WC, et al. Computed tomographic-guided percutaneous radiofrequency ablation with hydro dissection of hepatic malignancies in the Subcapsular location: evaluation of safety and technical efficacy. J Chin Med Assoc. 2016;79(2):93–100.
9. Pillai K, Akhter J, Chua TC, et al. Heat sink effect on tumor ablation characteristics as observed in monopolar radiofrequency, bipolar radiofrequency, and microwave, using ex vivo calf liver model. Medicine. 2015;94(9):e580.
10. Rhim H, Lim HK, Choi D. Current status of radiofrequency ablation of hepatocellular carcinoma. World J Gastrointest Surg. 2010;2(4):128–36.
11. Lu MD, Chen JW, Xie XY, et al. Hepatocellular carcinoma: US guided percutaneous microwave coagulation therapy. Radiology. 2001;221(1):167–72.
12. Lu MD, Xu HX, Xie XY, et al. Percutaneous microwave and radiofrequency ablation for Hepatocellular carcinoma: a retrospective comparative study. J Gastroenterol. 2005;40(11):1054–60.
13. Yin XY, Xie XY, Lu MD, et al. Percutaneous thermal ablation of medium and large hepatocellular carcinoma: long-term outcome and prognostic factors. Cancer. 2009;115(9):1914–23.
14. Doo Song K. Percutaneous cryoablation for hepatocellular carcinoma. Clin Mol Hepatol. 2016;22(4):509–15.
15. Wang C, Wang H, Yang W, et al. Multicenter randomized controlled trial of percutaneous Cryoablation versus radiofrequency ablation in hepatocellular carcinoma. Hepatology. 2015;61(5):1579–90.
16. Zimmerman A, Grand D, Charpentier KP. Irreversible electroporation of HCC: patient selection and perspectives. J Hepatocell Carcinoma. 2017;4:49–58.
17. Song MJ, Bae SH, Lee JS, et al. Combination trans arterial chemoembolization and radiofrequency ablation therapy for early HCC. Korean J Intern Med. 2016;31(2):242–52.
18. Song JE, Kim DY. Conventional versus drug-eluting beads TACE for HCC. World J Hepatol. 2017;9(18):808–14.

19. Lencioni R, Llovet JM, Han G, et al. Sorafenib or placebo plus TACE with Doxorubicin-eluting beads for Intermediate stage HCC: the SPACE trial. J Hepatol. 2016;64(5):1090–8.
20. Tzochatzis EA, Fatourou E, O'Birne J, et al. TACE and bland embolization for HCC. World J Gastroenterol. 2014;20(12):3069–77.
21. Osuga K, Hori S, Hirasishi K, et al. Bland embolization of HCC using superabsorbent polymer microspheres. Cardiovasc Intervent Radiol. 2008;31(6):1108–16.
22. Kallini JR, Gabr A, Salem R, et al. Trans arterial radio embolization with yttrium-90 for the treatment of HCC. Adv Ther. 2016;33:669–714.
23. Carr BI. Hepatic arterial 90Yttrium glass microspheres (Therasphere) for unresectable HCC: interim safety and survival data on 65 patients. Liver Transpl. 2004;10(2):S107–10.
24. Geschwind JF, Salem R, Carr BI, et al. Yttrium 90 microspheres for the treatment of HCC. Gastroenterology. 2004;127(5):S194–205.
25. Chow PKH, Gandhi M, Tan SB, et al. SIRveNIB: selective internal radiation therapy versus Sorafenib in Asia-Pacific Patients with HCC. J Clin Oncol. 2018;36(19):1913–21.
26. Pardee AD, Butterfield LH. Immunotherapy of HCC. Oncoimmunology. 2012;1(1):48–55.
27. Katsanos K, Kitrou P, Spiliopoulos S, et al. Comparative effectiveness of different trans-arterial embolization therapies alone or in combination with local ablative or adjuvant systemic treatments for unresectable HCC: a network meta-analysis of randomized controlled trials. PLoS One. 2017;12(9):e0184597.

Hepatic Encephalopathy

64

Stephen M. Riordan

Key Concepts

- With the exception of the rare patient with hepatic encephalopathy (HE) due to a congenital urea cycle enzyme defect, HE occurs either as a consequence of severe acute, chronic or acute-on-chronic liver disease or in the setting of porto-systemic venous shunting.
- Evolving evidence points to key roles for both ammonia and inflammation in the pathogenesis of HE.
- The more rapidly progressive clinical course of HE arising in acute liver failure (ALF) and acute-on-chronic liver failure (ACLF), compared to that of HE complicating cirrhosis and chronic porto-systemic shunting, is best explained by differences in the rapidity of ammonia-generated glutamine accumulation within astrocytes and the extent to which this can be effectively counter-balanced by regulatory osmotic processes.
- Contrasting effects of acute and chronic increases in ammonia and glutamate concentrations on astrocyte function and neuronal transmission, along with differences in the potential for inflammation to complicate these various clinical scenarios, are also important.
- Treatments aimed at reversing ammonia accumulation and preventing or suppressing systemic and neural inflammation form the bases of current therapeutic strategies.
- Consideration for emergency liver transplantation based on prognostic criteria and careful assessment for, and effective management of, cerebral oedema are of paramount importance in the management of HE in patients with ALF.
- The new concept that disturbances in the intestinal microbiome are associated with systemic inflammation in cirrhotic patients with HE offers the potential for various gut-flora altering therapies to be beneficial in this group not only as a consequence of their conventional role in modulating the intestinal metabolism of ammonia but also via anti-inflammatory effects.

S. M. Riordan (✉)
Gastrointestinal and Liver Unit, Prince of Wales Hospital, Prince of Wales Clinical School, University of New South Wales, Sydney, NSW, Australia
e-mail: Stephen.Riordan@health.nsw.gov.au

Hepatic encephalopathy (HE) encompasses a spectrum of neuropsychiatric manifestations, ranging from covert disturbances such as deficits in memory and learning evident only by psychometric testing (referred to as minimal HE) through to clinically overt disturbances reflected by changes in personality, inversion of the sleep cycle, confusion and, in its most extreme form, coma [1] (Table 64.1). HE, in either of its covert or overt forms, occurs either as a consequence of severe acute, chronic or acute-on-chronic liver disease or in the setting of porto-systemic venous shunting. The exception is the rare patient with HE due to a congenital urea cycle enzyme defect.

The occurrence of HE defines the often rapidly progressive entity of acute liver failure (ALF), in which severe liver damage occurs in a patient without underlying chronic liver disease. In the chronic liver disease setting, HE is highly prevalent, occurring in up to 80% of patients with cirrhosis when both MHE and overt forms are taken in to account [2] and not only adversely impacts both quality of life and daily functioning but also is independently predictive of an increased mortality rate [3]. HE is also commonly encountered in the syndrome of acute on chronic liver failure (ACLF), in which an acute decompensation of hepatic

F. Radu-Ionita et al. (eds.), *Liver Diseases*, https://doi.org/10.1007/978-3-030-24432-3_64

Table 64.1 The West Haven criteria for grading the severity of overt hepatic encephalopathy (HE) [1]

Grade	Manifestations
1	Trivial lack of awareness; euphoria; anxiety; shortened attention span; impaired performance in basic arithmetic.
2	Lethargy; apathy; minimal disorientation in time and space; subtle changes in personality; inappropriate behaviour; asterixis.
3	Somnolence but responsive to verbal stimuli; gross disorientation; bizarre behaviour.
4	Coma.

Table 64.2 Differential diagnoses of hepatic encephalopathy

Category	Examples
Intracranial pathology	Haemorrhage Infarction Tumour Abscess Meningitis Encephalitis Epilepsy/post-seizure encephalopathy
Neuropsychiatric disorders	Organic brain syndromes
Toxic encephalopathies	Alcohol intoxication Alcohol withdrawal Wernicke-Korsakoff syndrome Psychoactive drugs Salicylate intoxication Heavy metal intoxication
Metabolic encephalopathies	Electrolyte imbalance Hypoxia Carbon dioxide narcosis Hypoglycaemia Uraemia Ketoacidosis

function in a patient with pre-existing, but clinically stable chronic liver disease follows a precipitating insult, often infective or hepatotoxin-related [4].

Importantly, none of the clinical manifestations of HE are specific for an hepatic aetiology of encephalopathy, such that it is imperative to exclude alternative neuropsychiatric diagnoses by appropriate clinical assessment and further investigations, including various laboratory markers, cerebral imaging and electroencephalography (Table 64.2). Unlike in the ALF setting, the blood ammonia level is of relatively little clinical value for establishing the diagnosis of HE in the more chronic scenarios of cirrhosis and chronic porto-systemic shunting, as levels in these clinical contexts do not reliably correlate with HE grades [5]. Practical bedside tests such as trail-making tests are easily administered and generally provide useful information in patients with low grade HE who are able to co-operate, although educational status and familiarity consequent to repeated testing can confound interpretation of results, and various computerised psychometric and neurophysiological tests are more widely used these days for this purpose [6].

64.1 Developments in Pathophysiologic Understanding

Accumulation of unmetabolised ammonia plays a fundamental role in the pathogenesis of HE. Evolving evidence points to an additional and important mechanistic role for inflammation, with complex interactions between ammonia metabolism and inflammation promoting dysfunction of astrocytes, neuronal transmission, blood-brain barrier permeability, cerebral blood flow and cerebral energy production. The more rapidly progressive clinical course of HE arising in ALF and ACLF, compared to that of HE complicating cirrhosis and chronic porto-systemic shunting, is best explained by differences in the rapidity of ammonia-generated glutamine accumulation within astrocytes and the extent to which these metabolic abnormalities can be effectively counter-balanced by regulatory osmotic processes. Contrasting effects of acute and chronic increases in ammonia and glutamate concentrations on astrocyte function and neuronal transmission, along with differences in the potential for inflammation to complicate these various clinical scenarios, are also important. Treatments aimed at reversing ammonia accumulation and preventing or suppressing systemic and neural inflammation form the bases of current therapeutic strategies.

64.1.1 The Role of Ammonia in the Pathogenesis of HE Occurring in ALF, Cirrhosis and Chronic Porto-Systemic Shunting

64.1.1.1 In ALF

HE in ALF is often rapidly progressive and frequently associated with the development of cerebral oedema and intracranial hypertension, especially at more advanced HE grades (grades 3 and 4). Cerebral oedema in ALF is predominantly intracellular in aetiology, due to a combination of osmotic, oxidative and nitrosative stresses, largely the consequence of increased metabolism of ammonia to glutamine in astrocytes. Osmotic stress related to ammonia in this circumstance is related to the rapidity with which high levels of glutamine are generated, overwhelming the capacity of astrocytes to compensate by losing osmolytes such as myoinositol and up-regulating water channels such as aquaporin-4. These compensatory mechanisms attempting to counter-regulate ammonia-induced oxidative stress on astrocytes contribute to the potential for extracellular cerebral oedema to occur, although the extent to which extracellular factors account for cerebral oedema is only modest when compared to intracellular processes. Markedly reduced cerebral energy production consequent to a toxic effect of ammonia on cellular metabolism also occurs [7].

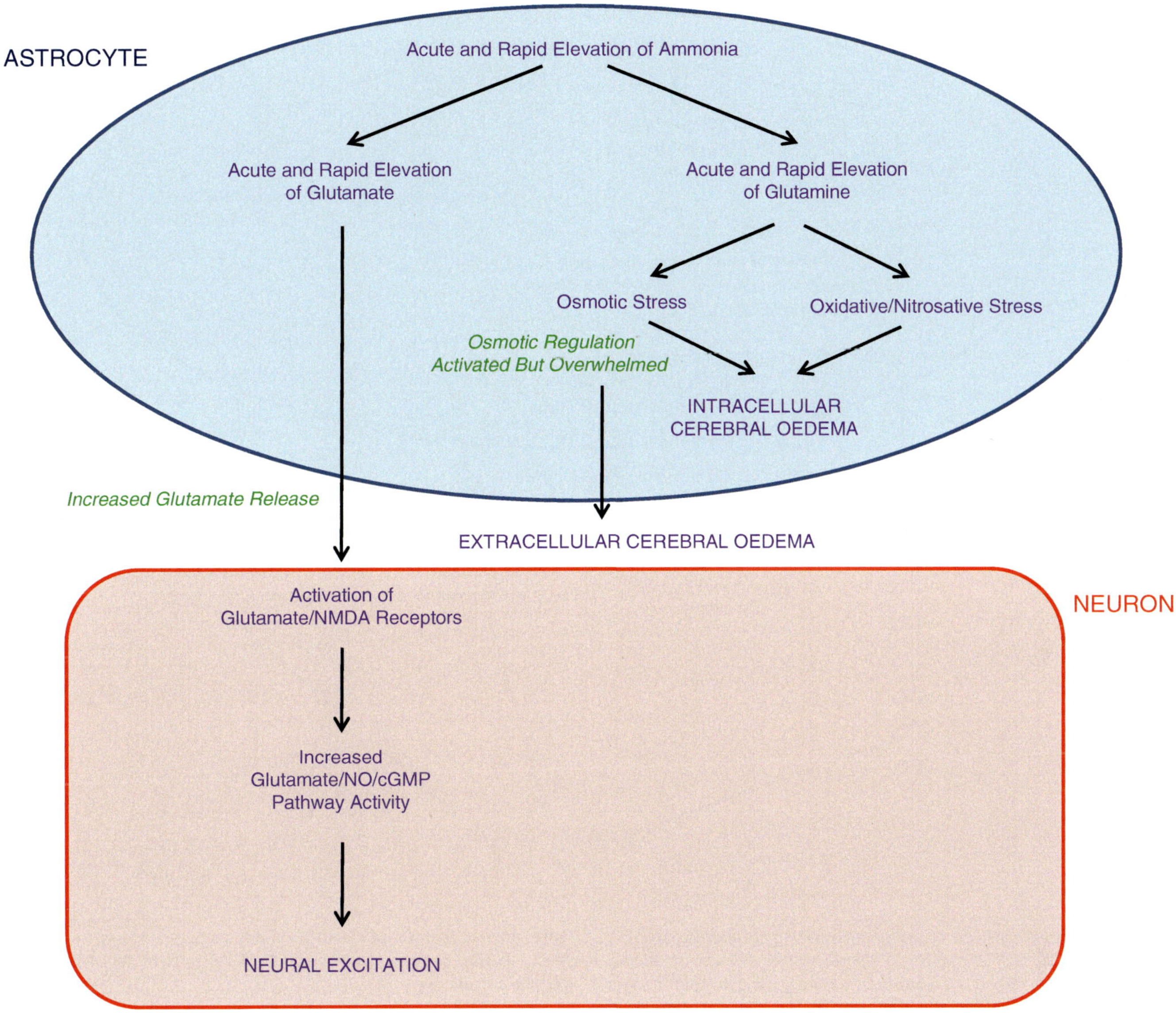

Fig. 64.1 Current concepts of the pathophysiology of hepatic encephalopathy (HE) in acute liver failure (ALF), demonstrating the key effects of ammonia on the astrocyte and neuron. *cGMP* cyclic guanosine monophosphate, *NMDA* N-methyl-D-aspartate, *NO* nitric oxide

In addition to cerebral oedema related to disturbed ammonia metabolism, excitatory neurotransmission, stemming from the excessive generation within astrocytes and subsequent release of glutamate from ammonia, leading to neuronal activation triggered via glutamate/N-methyl-D-aspartate (NMDA) receptors and the glutamate-nitric oxide (NO)-cyclic guanosine monophosphate (cGMP) pathway and reflected clinically by manifestations such as agitation and seizure activity, often subclinical, is a key pathophysiological process responsible for HE in ALF [6, 8, 9] (Fig. 64.1).

64.1.1.2 In Cirrhosis and Chronic Porto-Systemic Shunting

The effects on the astrocyte of the more gradual, chronic elevation in intracellular ammonia that occurs in cirrhosis and chronic porto-systemic shunting, in which circumstances patients' capacities for ammonia detoxification in alternative sites to the damaged or bypassed liver are often severely limited by factors such as associated skeletal muscle wasting and zinc deficiency, differ in several important respects from those that occur acutely in ALF. Most importantly, the slower rates of glutamine accumulation in astrocytes in the former settings allow for more effective osmotic regulation that prevents or at least greatly limits osmotic stress of astrocytes and, hence, intracellular cerebral oedema [10, 11]. Indeed, cerebral oedema of sufficient extent to be detectable by computerised tomography is generally not apparent in cirrhotic patients with HE, even at high grade [12], although more sensitive imaging modalities, such as magnetic resonance imaging, demonstrate that

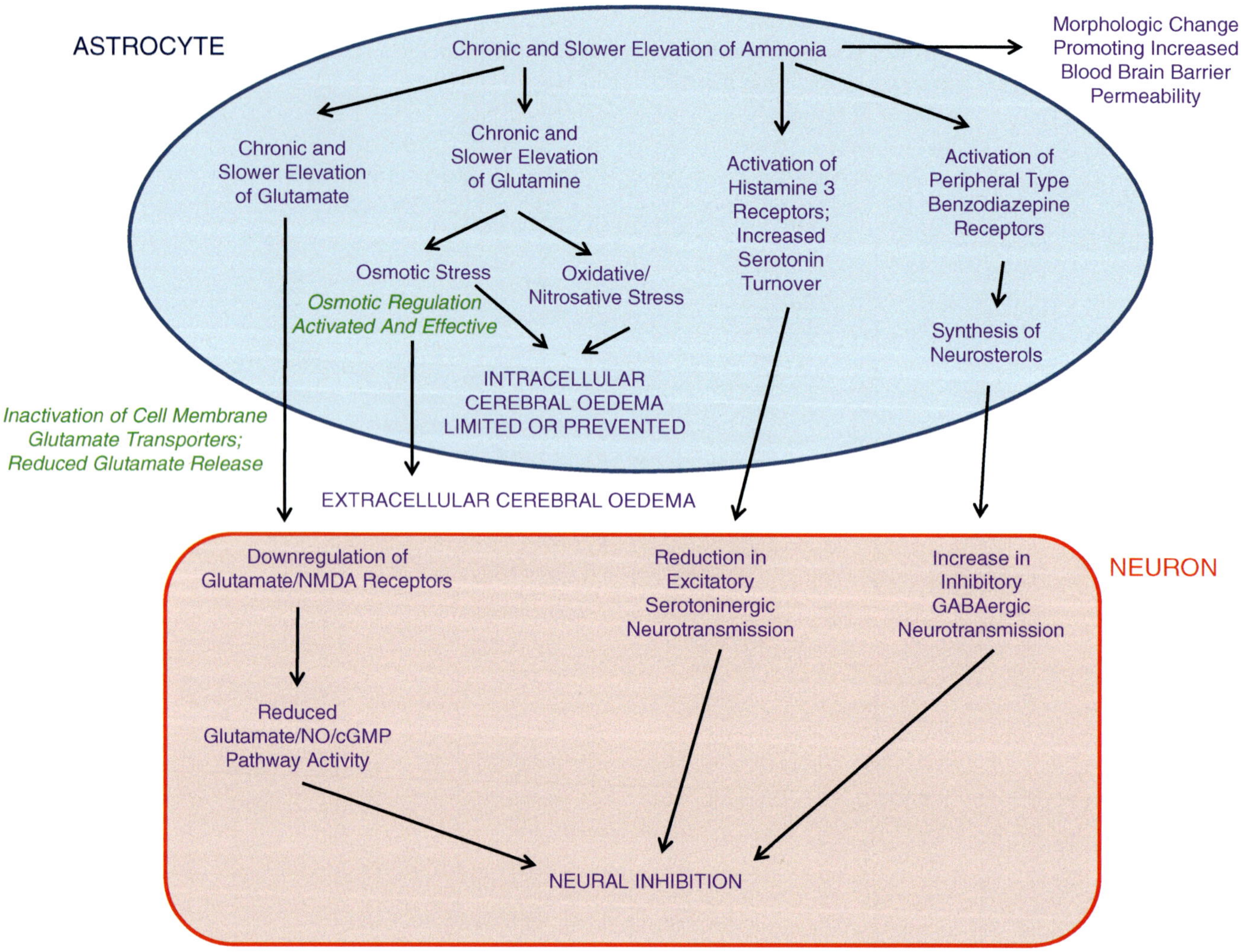

Fig. 64.2 Current concepts of the pathophysiology of hepatic encephalopathy (HE) in cirrhosis and chronic porto-systemic shunting, demonstrating the key effects of ammonia on the astrocyte and neuron, highlighting some important differences in end-effects compared to those in acute liver failure (ALF). *cGMP* cyclic guanosine monophosphate, *GABA* γ-amino-butyric acid, *NMDA* N-methyl-D-aspartate, *NO* nitric oxide

cerebral oedema, predominantly extracellular and only low-grade, does occur, even in those patients with only MHE [13]. As in the ALF setting, the counter-regulatory mechanisms that limit osmotic stress on astrocytes likely contribute to the development of this extracellular cerebral oedema [14] (Fig. 64.2). Nonetheless, low-grade cerebral oedema is unlikely the predominant mechanism for HE in cirrhosis and chronic port-systemic shunting [15].

This seems more related to disturbed neurotransmission resulting in neuro-inhibition, a phenomenon in marked contrast to the neuro-excitatory state occurring in encephalopathic ALF patients. This occurs largely as a result of prolonged exposure of astrocytes to increased ammonia levels, resulting in effects on three key neurotransmitter pathways, namely the glutamate-NO-cGMP pathway [16], the serotonergic pathway [17] and the gamma-aminobutyric acid (GABA)ergic pathway [6, 18] (Fig. 64.2).

Other deleterious effects of chronically elevated ammonia levels, potentially contributing to HE, have been demonstrated. A disturbance in blood brain barrier permeability related to the development of a type II Alzheimer phenotype by astrocytes in the setting of chronic exposure to increased ammonia has been proposed [15], given that astrocytes contribute importantly to the blood brain barrier. In addition, CBF is substantially reduced in cirrhotic patients with clinically overt HE [19], due to reduced cerebral energy production, with both phenomena significantly correlated with increased blood ammonia levels [20] (Fig. 64.2).

64.1.2 The Role of Inflammation in the Pathogenesis of HE Occurring in ALF, Cirrhosis and Chronic Porto-Systemic Shunting

Increasing evidence points to an important role of pro-inflammatory mediators, produced either systemically or within the brain as a result of either the severe underlying liver injury, accumulation of ammonia and lactate or complicating bacterial or fungal infection, in promoting HE in ALF [21, 22], in which an often marked systemic inflammatory response frequently occurs [23]. Important interactions between ammonia and inflammation in promoting HE have also been demonstrated in cirrhosis and chronic porto-systemic shunting, especially in the setting of inflammation resulting from super-imposed bacterial or fungal infection. Cirrhotic patients display significant deteriorations in psychometric test scores following hyperammonaemia induced in the setting of inflammation due to super-imposed infection, but not when hyperammonaemia is induced in the non-inflammatory state, suggesting that pro-inflammatory mediators are important in modulating the cerebral effects of ammonia in cirrhosis [24].

Increased circulating pro-inflammatory cytokines are also produced by a disturbed gut microbiome in cirrhotic patients, resulting in a systemic inflammatory state even in the absence of overt infection [25]. Disturbances in the colonic mucosal microbiome have been demonstrated in cirrhotic patients with an history of HE compared to cirrhotic patients with no prior history of HE. In those with a history of HE, significantly lower levels of *Roseburia* species and increased abundance of *Enterococcus*, *Veillonella*, *Megasphaera* and *Burkholderia* are evident. Genera over-expressed in the colonic mucosa in the HE group were found on network analysis to be significantly associated with both poor cognition and systemic inflammation, as reflected by serum levels of pro-inflammatory cytokines [26]. Taken together, the findings suggest that a disturbed gut microbiome in cirrhotic patients with an history of HE, detected at the colonic mucosal level, may contribute significantly to systemic inflammation, which, in turn, adversely affects cognition. Another study has demonstrated that dysbiosis is associated with systemic inflammation in cirrhotic patients with HE and that specific gut microbial families, namely autochthonous taxa negatively and *Enterobacteriaceae* positively, correlate with hyperammonaemia-associated astrocytic changes in glutamine and glutamate [27]. These findings provide rationale to investigate the use of gut flora-altering therapies in the treatment of cirrhotic patients with HE as potential modulators of systemic inflammation, beyond their conventional role in reducing the intestinal production of ammonia.

Systemic and neural inflammation have the potential to promote HE via various mechanisms, ultimately leading to increased oxidative and nitrosative stress in astrocytes, increased blood brain barrier permeability, increased cerebral blood flow, cerebral oedema and an exacerbation of ammonia-mediated deleterious effects, as outlined in Fig. 64.3 [21, 22, 28–36].

64.1.3 The Two-Phase Roles of Ammonia and Inflammation in the Pathogenesis of HE Occurring in ACLF

HE in ACLF is often rapidly progressive. A two-phase explanation for the occurrence of cerebral oedema in ACFL patients with HE has been proposed, in which an initial intracellular component due to a sudden and rapid accumulation of ammonia-derived glutamine, analogous to that occurring in the ALF setting, is followed by increased blood-brain barrier permeability mediated by pro-inflammatory cytokines that promotes increased extracellular water accumulation [14]. Nonetheless, cerebral oedema generally develops to a lesser extent in ACLF than in ALF [37] and is generally predominantly extracellular [38]. As in cirrhosis and chronic porto-systemic shunting, cerebral oedema sufficient to be detectable by computerised tomography occurs in only a small minority of ACLF patients, even when the HE grade is high (grade 3 or 4) [12].

64.2 Management

Fundamentally, treatment of HE is aimed at correcting hyperammonaemia and inflammation and their consequences, including cerebral oedema when present, while adopting measures to at least limit the degree of underlying liver damage and, in the settings of cirrhosis and ACLF, identifying and correcting precipitating factors. Given the differing clinical course of HE in ALF and ACLF as compared to that arising in cirrhosis and porto-systemic shunting, as well as the potentials for more rapid progression of the underlying liver injury and development of multi-organ failure in the former contexts, the management of HE complicating ALF and ACLF must be considered separately from that occurring in other settings. In all circumstances, careful assessment for and correction of a systemic inflammatory response syndrome, defined by abnormalities in body temperature, heart rate, respiratory rate, PaCO2 level and white blood cell count [23], and an high index of suspicion for complicating bacterial or fungal infection must be maintained. In the latter

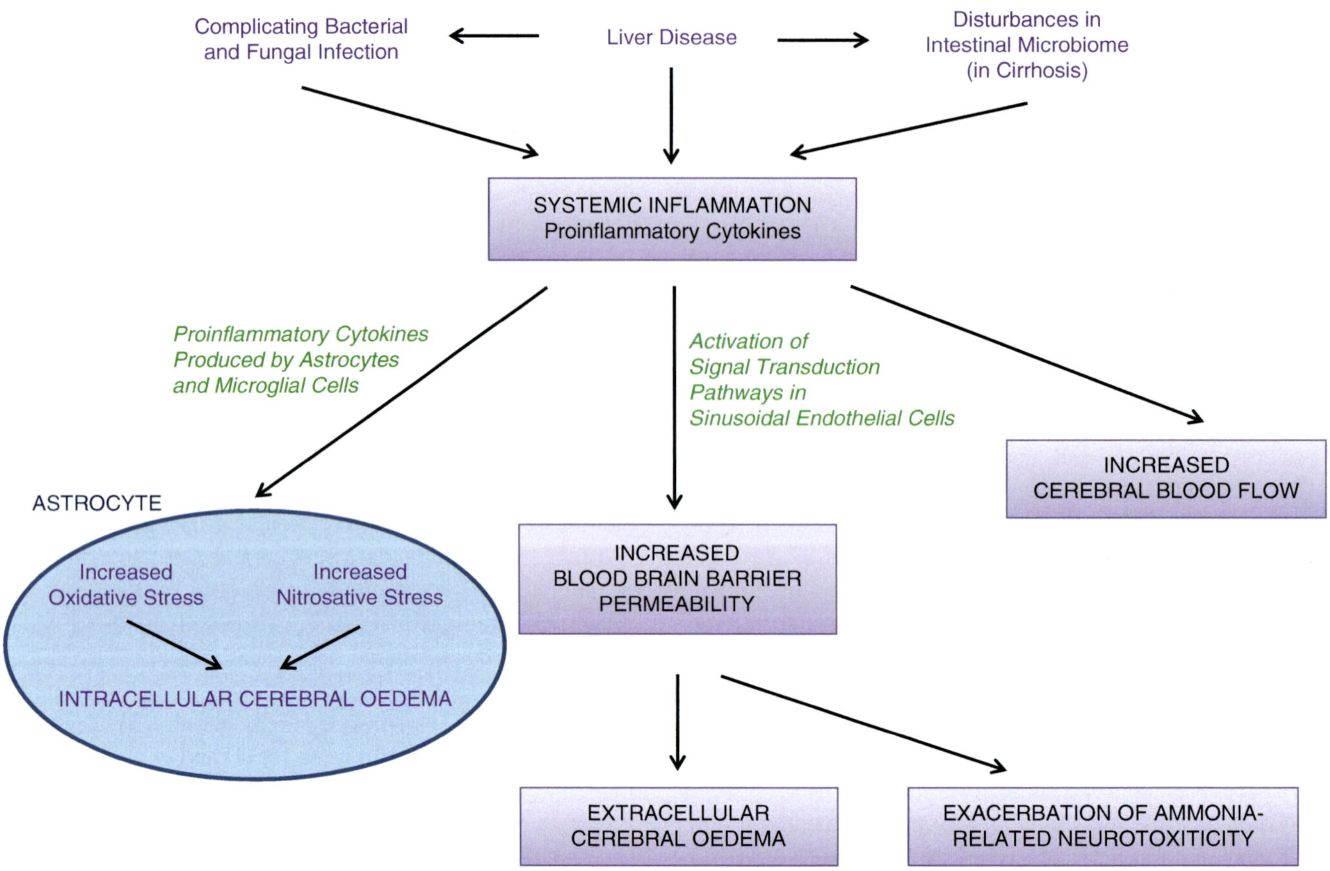

Fig. 64.3 Mechanisms by which inflammation contributes to the pathogenesis of hepatic encephalopathy (HE)

regard, some centres favour the commencement of prophylactic broad-spectrum antibiotics while awaiting results of a septic screen, especially in patients with more advanced grades of HE (grade 3 or grade 4). Enteral nutrition is generally preferable to the parenteral route in order to limit the likelihood of septic complications. A potential role for N-acetylcysteine in limiting or reversing oxidative stress in astrocytes and attenuating neuroinflammation has also recently been proposed, given both its anti-oxidant and anti-inflammatory properties and since it has been shown to cross the blood-brain barrier [31].

64.2.1 Treatment of HE in ALF (Table 64.3)

Along with the institution of specific therapies to limit the extent of liver damage in those with treatable aetiologies, consideration for emergency liver transplantation based on prognostic criteria and careful assessment for, and effective management of, cerebral oedema are of paramount importance in ALF patients. Selection criteria for liver transplantation in ALF are based on indices identifying the most severely affected group, having a poor prognosis with medical management alone and are not currently standardised.

Table 64.3 Approach to the management of hepatic encephalopathy (HE) in acute liver failure (ALF)

Intervention	
Consideration of emergency liver transplantation according to prognostic criteria, such as the King's College criteria [39]	
Commence specific therapies for treatable causes	
Aetiology	Treatment
Paracetamol	N-acetylcysteine
Hepatitis B virus	Entecavir or tenofovir
Herpes simplex virus	Acyclovir
Autoimmune	Corticosteroids
Budd-Chiari syndrome	Thrombolysis, decompressive shunt
Lymphoma	Chemotherapy
Pregnancy-associated	Delivery
Intracranial pressure monitoring in patients with advanced HE grades	
Strategies to reverse cerebral oedema (see text)	
Strategies to reverse neuroinflammation High index of suspicion for and aggressive treatment of complicating bacterial or fungal infection Possible role for prophylactic, broad-spectrum antibiotic use in advanced HE grades Possible role for N-acetylcysteine	

Nonetheless, those formulated at King's College Hospital are the most widely applied [39]. In the original analyses, positive predictive values for death (the proportions of those patients fulfilling criteria who died) in patients with paracetamol and non-paracetamol aetiologies of ALF were 84% and 98%, respectively, while negative predictive values (the proportions of those patients not fulfilling criteria who survived) were 86% and 82%, respectively. The findings suggest that ALF patients fulfilling the King's College criteria should be considered for urgent liver transplantation, even with HE grade is not advanced, with the exception of non-acidotic paracetamol-related ALF patients, in whom advanced HE grade is a prognostic factor. Conversely, lack of fulfilment of prognostic criteria in current use do not reliably predict spontaneous survival, especially in cases unrelated to paracetamol, and emergency liver transplantation should still be considered for this group.

Potential transplant candidates should be urgently transferred to a liver transplant unit at an early HE stage, ideally before cerebral oedema has developed. Various strategies are available to prevent or treat cerebral oedema and optimise cerebral perfusion in those with grade 3 or 4 HE. Elective mechanical ventilation, along with positioning of the patient 20–30° head-up and minimising endotracheal suctioning, patient turning and other tactile stimulation are all important measures to prevent surges in intracranial pressure that can provoke or exacerbate cerebral oedema. Intracranial pressure monitoring, with sufficient clotting factor support to achieve an international normalised ratio ≤ 2 and platelet transfusions to achieve a count $\geq 50 \times 10^9$/L at the time of insertion of the transducer, remains controversial on account of risks of haemorrhagic and infective complications, but can be of considerable value in determining intracerebral pressure and cerebral perfusion pressure (the difference between mean arterial pressure and intracranial pressure) and thereby guiding further therapy in ALF patients with grade 3 or 4 HE [40]. In particular, a cerebral perfusion pressure <50 mmHg due to arterial hypotension in ALF is an indication for use of vasopressor agents, provided that intravascular volume status is adequate. Conversely, when cerebral perfusion pressure is reduced to <50 mmHg due to an increase in intracranial pressure, or when the latter exceeds 25 mmHg irrespective of cerebral perfusion pressure, bolus intravenous injection of mannitol (0.5 g/kg body weight) is considered first-line treatment [41]. Continuous veno-veno haemodiafiltration, rather than intermittent haemodialysis in order to reduce the likelihood of systemic arterial hypotension that might result in a fall in cerebral perfusion pressure [42] and with the aim of removing two to three times the volume of mannitol given, is required to properly manage intracranial hypertension in ALF patients in oliguric renal failure. Induction of moderate hypothermia (32–33 °C) can be beneficial for otherwise uncontrolled increases in intracranial pressure [43], while reduction in cerebral blood flow by means of hyperventilation is appropriate in the subgroup with cerebral hyperaemia, as reflected by an increased reverse jugular venous oxygen saturation of at least 75%. Artificial liver support using modalities such as plasmapheresis and extracorporeal albumin dialysis may also have a role in reducing cerebral oedema in the ALF setting [44, 45]. Thiopentone may be helpful in cases of otherwise intractable cerebral oedema, but has the potential to promote or exacerbate haemodynamic instability. Prophylactic anti-epileptic therapy reduces the incidence of subclinical epilepsy which can exacerbate cerebral oedema [9].

Importantly, earlier disease recognition likely accounts for the significantly reduced prevalence of intracranial hypertension complicating ALF demonstrated at admission to a large, dedicated liver intensive care unit over recent decades (from 76% during the period from 1984 to 1988 to 20% during the period from 2004 to 2008), while improvements in modern liver intensive care based on a better understanding of pathogenesis and availability of emergency liver transplantation in a timely manner, before patients become untransplantable, presumably are responsible for the significantly reduced mortality rate in those with intracranial hypertension from 95% to 55% during this time [46].

64.2.2 Treatment of HE in Cirrhosis (Table 64.4)

Most episodes of HE complicating cirrhosis are secondary to a clinically apparent precipitating event that requires appropriate additional treatment. Several precipitating factors may be operative in a given patient at the same time. Most manifestations of overt HE complicating cirrhosis improve with medical treatment, although refractory syndromes such as dementia, spastic paraparesis, cerebellar degeneration and extrapyramidal movement disorders are well-recognised. The latter may gradually improve following successful liver transplantation. MHE commonly persists in cirrhotic patients after resolution of overt HE and requires on-going medical therapy [47]. Medical therapy for HE complicating cirrhosis is aimed at reducing the intestinal production and systemic absorption of ammonia and/or promoting increased systemic metabolism of absorbed ammonia. Several recent studies have investigated whether systemic inflammation in cirrhosis can be modulated by gut flora-altering treatments, given data that a disturbed intestinal microbiome may contribute to systemic inflammation in this group.

64.2.2.1 Reducing the Intestinal Production and Systemic Absorption of Ammonia

While intestinal production of ammonia can be effectively reduced by dietary protein restriction, patients with cirrhosis require daily protein intakes of 1.2–1.5 g/kg body weight to maintain nitrogen balance and long-term restriction to below this range must be avoided in order to avoid protein energy malnutrition. In patients whose total daily dietary protein tol-

Table 64.4 Management of hepatic encephalopathy (HE) complicating cirrhosis

Intervention	Examples
Correction of precipitating factors	Gastrointestinal haemorrhage Infection Constipation Uraemia Hypokalaemia Hyponatraemia Systemic alkalosis Use of benzodiazepines Porto-systemic shunting Progressive liver damage Development of hepatocellular carcinoma
Ammonia-lowering treatments	Prevent excessive dietary protein intake Non-absorbable disaccharides (lactulose, lactitol) Rifaximin Probiotics, synbiotics, faecal microbial transplantation L-ornithine-L-aspartate Sodium benzoate Zinc Glycerol phenylbutyrate Possible role for Sodium phenylbutyrate
Strategies to reverse neuroinflammation	High index of suspicion for and aggressive treatment of complicating bacterial or fungal infection Possible role for prophylactic, broad-spectrum antibiotic use in advanced HE grades Possible role for N-acetylcysteine Reduction in systemic inflammation due to disturbed intestinal microbiome (lactulose, rifaximin, probiotics, possible role for synbiotics, possible role for faecal microbial transplantation)
Liver transplantation	Failed medical therapies, especially for HE occurring in association with other manifestations of severe hepatic functional decompensation

erance is below this level, supplementation with vegetable, rather than animal, protein can result in significant improvements in nitrogen balance without precipitating or worsening HE, possibly due to the increased fibre content of vegetable protein [48]. Non-absorbable disaccharides are considered first line pharmacological therapy for reducing the intestinal production and systemic absorption of ammonia in cirrhotic patients with overt HE. The lowered colonic pH resulting from their fermentation by gut flora to acetic and lactic acids is both hostile to the survival of urease-producing intestinal bacteria and reduces ammonia absorption by non-ionic diffusion. Lactulose (galactosidofructose) is the most commonly used of these [5]. The daily dose of lactulose should be titrated to result in two to four soft, acidic stools ($pH < 6$) daily. Meta-analyses suggest that oral lactitol (galactosidosorbitol) is as effective as lactulose for treating overt HE in cirrhosis and is more palatable, aiding compliance [49]. Disaccharide enemas have a role in those patients in whom oral or nasogastric administration is impossible [50]. Compared to placebo or no treatment, oral lactulose or lactitol therapy significantly reduces the likelihood of no improvement in overt HE in patients with cirrhosis (relative risk 0.62; 95% confidence interval 0.46–0.84) [51, 52]. Lactulose is also considered first line therapy for MHE complicating cirrhosis [53], with the likelihood of no improvement in psychometric test scores significantly reduced by lactulose therapy compared to placebo or no treatment [54, 55].

Antibiotics such as neomycin, metronidazole, vancomycin and rifaximin also reduce intestinal ammonia production and are beneficial in the treatment of overt HE complicating cirrhosis [5]. However, the potential for adverse effects (ototoxicity and renal toxicity with neomycin; peripheral neuropathy with metronidazole and development of resistant *Enterococcus* strains with vancomycin) limits their use. Rifaximin is a well-tolerated, broad spectrum antibiotic with low risk of inducing bacterial resistance. Meta-analyses indicate that the efficacy of rifaximin for treating overt HE in cirrhosis is comparable to that of the non-absorbable disaccharides [56, 57]. The combination of rifaximin and lactulose may be more effective than lactulose alone for treating overt HE in patients with cirrhosis [58]. Rifaximin is also of proven value for the management of MHE in this group [59–61], apparently without significantly altering the composition of the faecal microbiome, although the relative abundances of genus *Veillonella* and *Streptococcus* were lowered [61].

The promotion of urease-negative bacteria within the intestine by use of probiotic and synbiotic (probiotic plus fermentable fibre) preparations, as an alternative strategy to antibiotic or disaccharide therapies for reducing the intestinal production of ammonia, has been shown to significantly improve MHE complicating cirrhosis and reduce the likelihood of development of overt HE [62–65]. Notably, probiotic and synbiotic treatments were found to be better tolerated than lactulose, a factor favouring improved compliance [62]. Recent data suggest that faecal microbial transplantation of microbiota shown to be deficient in HE, resulting in increased faecal microbial diversity and beneficial taxa, may reduce the likelihood of recurrent HE in cirrhosis [66].

64.2.2.2 Increasing the Systemic Metabolism of Ammonia

Ornithine and aspartate are important substrates involved in the systemic metabolism of ammonia to urea and glutamine, respectively. L-ornithine-L-aspartate thus provides substrates for each of these ammonia detoxification pathways. Recent analyses have confirmed significant beneficial effects of treatment compared to placebo or no intervention in cirrhotic patients with both overt HE and MHE [67, 68]. The efficacy of L-ornithine-L-aspartate therapy was comparable to that of lactulose [67]. Treatment with sodium benzoate, which reduces systemic ammonia levels by the formation of hippurate, is also of proven value [69]. Whether there is benefit in combining these strategies to increase the systemic metabolism of ammonia with therapies that reduce ammonia production, such as non-absorbable disaccharides and/or rifaximin, remains to be properly assessed. A controlled trial of oral zinc supplementation in addition to other therapies, including lactulose, found significant improvement in psychometric test scores in the group receiving zinc [70]. A randomized, double-blind, placebo-controlled study of glycerol phenylbutyrate, which acts by promoting ammonia removal via the kidney in the form of urinary phenylacetylglutamine, has demonstrated a significantly beneficial effect in preventing recurrent episodes of overt HE in patients with cirrhosis [71]. A beneficial effect of sodium phenylbutyrate has also been suggested recently in a preliminary analysis [72], although randomized, controlled trial data are currently lacking.

64.2.2.3 Reducing Systemic Inflammation by Modulation of the Intestinal Microbiome

To date, assessment of this evolving therapeutic concept has been conducted only in cirrhotic patients with MHE, using treatment with lactulose [73], rifaximin [59] and probiotics [74]. Modulation of systemic levels of pro-inflammatory and anti-inflammatory cytokines has been demonstrated, associated with clinical improvement (Table 64.5). Whether a change in intestinal microbial function rather than its composition is predominantly responsible [25] remains to be fully determined. Further delineation of the possible anti-systemic inflammatory effects of these and other gut flora-altering therapies, including synbiotics and intestinal microbial transplantation, along with stratification of the relative benefit of this potential mechanism of action on HE management as opposed to their anti-ammonia effects in various clinical contexts, are awaited.

Table 64.5 Studies investigating whether systemic inflammation can be reduced by gut flora altering therapies in cirrhotic patients with minimal hepatic encephalopathy (MHE)

Treatment	Trends in systemic levels of parameters measured	Clinical correlates
Lactulose [73]	Significant reductions in TNF-α, IL-6 and IL-18	Improvement in psychometric test scores
Rifaximin [59]	Significant reduction in IL-10	Improvement in driving simulator performance
Probiotics [74]	Significant reduction in IL-6	Reduced need for hospitalisation for HE

TNF tumour necrosis factor, *IL* interleukin

64.2.3 HE in Chronic Portal-Systemic Shunting

HE complicating spontaneous or surgically-created portal-systemic anastomoses or radiologically-placed transjugular intrahepatic portal-systemic shunt procedures is usually successfully managed as in cirrhosis, as discussed above. Transhepatic or percutaneous transparaumbilical embolization or surgical ligation of portal-systemic shunts is occasionally of benefit in such patients when HE is refractory to other modalities [75, 76]. Similarly, refractory HE complicating TIPSS may be successfully managed by the implantation of a reducing stent, especially in patients in whom hepatic function is well maintained and porto-systemic shunting is taken to be the major factor responsible for the HE [77].

64.2.4 HE in Acute on Chronic Liver Failure (ACLF)

Reversal of the precipitating factor and support of all other failing organ systems are crucial to the management of patients with HE complicating ACLF, which is often complicated by associated multi-organ failure. The use of emergency liver transplantation as a rescue procedure is hampered by the high frequency of concomitant conditions that contraindicate the procedure, such as unresolved infection and circulatory failure. Given the low incidence of intracranial hypertension demonstrated in patients with even advanced HE grades in this syndrome [12], invasive intracranial pressure monitoring is generally not required. The medical management of HE in ACLF currently relies on those measures outlined above for patients with overt HE complicating cirrhosis, such as non-absorbed disaccharides and rifaximin, although little data are currently available regarding efficacies in this particular syndrome.

The possible role of artificial liver support using extracorporeal albumin dialysis to improve HE refractory to medical treatments in ACLF has been assessed in two multi-centre, randomised, controlled trials [78, 79]. In the first of these, conducted in 70 cirrhotic patients in grade 3 or 4 HE, most with ACLF, significantly more frequent improvement and faster reduction in HE grade were apparent in patients managed with extracorporeal albumin dialysis in combination with standard medical treatment compared to patients managed with standard medical treatment alone [78]. Conversely, a significant difference in rates of HE improvement associated with extracorporeal albumin dialysis and standard medical treatment compared with standard treatment alone was not demonstrated in a subsequent, larger analysis of 189 patients with ACLF [79].

Self Study

Question

1. Which of the following statements is/are true?
   (a) Cerebral oedema rarely occurs in hepatic encephalopathy (HE) complicating acute liver failure (ALF), even at advanced HE grades (grade 3 or grade 4).
   (b) Excitatory neurotransmission via neuronal activation of glutamate/N-methyl-D-aspartate (NMDA) receptors and the glutamate-nitric oxide (NO)-cyclic guanosine monophosphate (cGMP) pathway is a key pathophysiological process responsible for HE in ALF.
   (c) A cerebral perfusion pressure (the difference between mean arterial pressure and intracranial pressure) <50 mmHg is always an indication for bolus intravenous injection of mannitol (0.5 g/kg body weight).
2. Which of the following statements is/are true?
   (a) As in ALF, cerebral oedema is a key clinical feature in cirrhotic patients with high grade HE (grades 3 and 4).
   (b) Disturbed neurotransmission resulting in neuro-inhibition is an important feature of the pathogenesis of HE in cirrhosis.
   (c) A disturbed intestinal microbiome contributes to the pathogenesis of HE via pro-inflammatory mechanisms.

Answers

1. Which of the following statements is/are true?
   (a) This is false. Cerebral oedema often complicates advanced grades of HE (grades 3 or 4) in ALF. This is predominantly intracellular in aetiology, due to a combination of osmotic, oxidative and nitrosative stresses, largely the consequence of increased metabolism of ammonia to glutamine in astrocytes. Osmotic stress related to ammonia in this circumstance is related to the rapidity with which high levels of glutamine are generated, overwhelming the capacity of astrocytes to compensate by losing osmolytes such as myoinositol and up-regulating water channels such as aquaporin-4.
   (b) This is true and reflected clinically by features such as agitation and seizure activity.
   (c) This is false. A cerebral perfusion pressure <50 mmHg due to arterial hypotension in ALF is an indication for use of vasopressor agents, provided that intravascular volume status is adequate. Conversely, when cerebral perfusion pressure is reduced to <50 mmHg due to an increase in intracranial pressure, or when the latter exceeds 25 mmHg irrespective of cerebral perfusion pressure, bolus intravenous injection of mannitol (0.5 g/kg body weight) is considered first-line treatment.
2. Which of the following statements is/are true?
   (a) This is false. Unlike in the ALF setting, the slower rate of glutamine accumulation in astrocytes in cirrhosis allows for more effective osmotic regulation that prevents or at least greatly limits osmotic stress of astrocytes and, hence, cerebral oedema. Indeed, cerebral oedema of sufficient extent to be detectable by computerised tomography is generally not apparent in cirrhotic patients with HE, even at high grade.
   (b) This is true, in marked contrast to the neuro-excitatory state occurring in encephalopathic ALF patients. This neuro-inhibition in cirrhotic patients with HE arises largely as a result of prolonged exposure of astrocytes to increased ammonia levels, resulting in effects on three key neurotransmitter pathways, namely a reduction in excitatory glutamate-NO-cGMP neurotransmission, a reduction in excitatory serotonergic neurotransmission and an increase in inhibitory gamma-aminobutyric acid (GABA)ergic neurotransmission.
   (c) This is true, providing rationale to further investigate the use of gut flora-altering therapies in the treatment of cirrhotic patients with HE as potential modulators of systemic inflammation, beyond their conventional role in reducing the intestinal production of ammonia.

References

1. Conn HO, Leevy CM, Vlahcevic ZR, et al. Comparison of lactulose and neomycin in the treatment of chronic portal-systemic encephalopathy. A double blind controlled trial. Gastroenterology. 1977;72:573–83.
2. Groeneweg M, Quero J, De Bruijn I, et al. Subclinical hepatic encephalopathy impairs daily functioning. Hepatology. 1998;28:45–9.
3. Gadiparthi C, Cholankeril G, Yoo ER, Hu M, Wong RJ, Ahmen A. Waitlist outcomes in liver transplant candidates with high MELD and severe hepatic encephalopathy. Dig Dis Sci. 2018;63:1647–53.
4. Moreau R, Jalan R, Gines P, et al. Acute-on-chronic liver failure is a distinct syndrome that develops in patients with acute decompensation of cirrhosis. Gastroenterology. 2013;144:1426–77.
5. Riordan SM, Williams R. Treatment of hepatic encephalopathy. N Engl J Med. 1997;337:473–9.
6. Prakash R, Mullen KD. Mechanisms, diagnosis and management of hepatic encephalopathy. Nat Rev Gastroenterol Hepatol. 2010;7:515–25.
7. Ott P, Clemmensen O, Larsen FS. Cerebral metabolic disturbance in the brain during acute liver failure: from hyperammonaemia to energy failure and proteolysis. Neurochem Int. 2005;47:13–8.
8. Rose C. Effect of ammonia on astrocytic glutamate release/uptake mechanisms. J Neurochem. 2006;97(Suppl 1):11–5.

9. Ellis AJ, Wendon JA, Williams R. Subclinical seizure activity and prophylactic phenytoin infusion in acute liver failure; a controlled clinical trial. Hepatology. 2000;32:666–9.
10. Bernal W, Hall C, Karvellas C, et al. Arterial ammonia and clinical risk factors for encephalopathy and intracranial hypertension in acute liver failure. Hepatology. 2007;46:1844–52.
11. Wright G, Soper R, Brooks HF, et al. Role of aquaporin-4 in the development of brain oedema in liver failure. J Hepatol. 2010;53:91–7.
12. Joshi D, O'Grady J, Patel A, et al. Cerebral oedema is rare in acute-on-chronic liver failure patients with high grade hepatic encephalopathy. Liver Int. 2014;34:362–6.
13. Kale RA, Gupta RK, Saraswat VA, et al. Demonstration of interstitial cerebral edema with diffusion tensor MR imaging in type C hepatic encephalopathy. Hepatology. 2006;43:698–706.
14. Chavarria L, Oria M, Romero-Gimenez J, et al. Brain magnetic resonance in experimental acute-on-chronic liver failure. Liver Int. 2013;33:294–300.
15. Cauli O, Llansola M, Agusti A, et al. Cerebral oedema is not responsible for motor or cognitive deficits in rats with hepatic encephalopathy. Liver Int. 2014;34:379–87.
16. Butterworth RF. Pathophysiology of hepatic encephalopathy: the concept of synergism. Hepatol Res. 2008;38:S116–21.
17. Palomero-Gallagher N, Zilles K. Neurotransmitter receptor alterations in hepatic encephalopathy: a review. Arch Biochem Biophys. 2013;536:109–21.
18. Ahboucha S, Butterworth RF. The neurosteroid system: an emerging therapeutic target for hepatic encephalopathy. Metab Brain Dis. 2007;22:291–308.
19. Keiding S, Pavese N. Brain metabolism in patients with hepatic encephalopathy studied by PET and MR. Arch Biochem Biophys. 2013;536:131–42.
20. Iversen P, Sorenson M, Bak L, et al. Low cerebral oxygen consumption and blood flow in patients with cirrhosis and an acute episode of hepatic encephalopathy. Gastroenterology. 2009;136:863–71.
21. Odeh M. Pathogenesis of hepatic encephalopathy: the tumour necrosis factor-alpha theory. Eur J Clin Invest. 2007;37:291–304.
22. Bernal W, Donaldson P, Underhill J, Wendon J, Williams R. Tumour necrosis factor genomic polymorphism and outcome of acetaminophen (paracetamol)-induced acute liver failure. J Hepatol. 1998;29:53–9.
23. Members of the American College of Chest Physicians/Society of Critical Care Medicine Consensus Conference Committee. American College of Chest Physicians/Society of Critical Care Medicine Consensus Conference: Definitions for sepsis and organ failure and guidelines for the use of innovative therapies in sepsis. Crit Care Med. 1992;20:864–74.
24. Shawcross DL, Davies NA, Williams R, Jalan R. Systemic inflammatory response exacerbates the neuropsychological effects of induced hyperammonemia in cirrhosis. J Hepatol. 2004;40:247–54.
25. Bajaj JS, Ridlon JM, Hylemon PB, et al. Linkage of gut microbiome with cognition in hepatic encephalopathy. Am J Physiol Gastrointest Liver Physiol. 2012;302:G168–75.
26. Bajaj JS, Hylemon PB, Ridlon JM, et al. Colonic mucosal microbiome differs from stool microbiome in cirrhosis and hepatic encephalopathy and is linked to cognition and inflammation. Am J Physiol Gastrointest Liver Physiol. 2012;303:G675–85.
27. Ahluwalia V, Betrapally NS, Hylemon PB, et al. Impaired gut-liver–brain axis in patients with cirrhosis. Sci Rep. 2016;6:26800.
28. Moldawer LL, Marano MA, Wei H, et al. Cachectin/tumor necrosis factor-α alters red blood cell kinetics and induces anemia in vivo. FASEB J. 1989;3:1637–43.
29. Blei AT. Brain edema and portal-systemic encephalopathy. Liver Transpl. 2000;6(Suppl 1):S14–20.
30. Anderson AK, Ronnback L, Hansson E. Lactate induces tumour necrosis factor-alpha, interleukin-6 and interleukin-1 beta release in microglial- and astroglial-enriched primary cultures. J Neurochem. 2005;93:1327–33.
31. Bemeur C, Butterworth RF. Liver-brain proinflammatory signalling in acute liver failure: role in the pathogenesis of hepatic encephalopathy and brain edema. Metab Brain Dis. 2013;28:145–50.
32. Coltart I, Tranah TH, Shawcross DL. Inflammation and hepatic encephalopathy. Arch Biochem Biophys. 2013;536:189–96.
33. Jalan R, Olde Damink SW, Hayes PC, Deutz NE, Lee A. Pathogenesis of intracranial hypertension in acute liver failure: inflammation, ammonia and cerebral blood flow. J Hepatol. 2004;41:613–20.
34. Strauss G, Adel-Hansen B, Kirkegaard P, et al. Liver function, cerebral blood flow autoregulation, and hepatic encephalopathy in fulminant hepatic failure. Hepatology. 1997;25:837–9.
35. Didier N, Romero IA, Creminon C, et al. Secretion of interleukin-1β by astrocytes mediates endothelin-1 and tumour necrosis factor-α effects on human brain microvascular endothelial cell permeability. J Neurochem. 2003;86:246–54.
36. Duchini A. Effects of tumour necrosis factor-α and interleukin-6 on fluid-phase permeability and ammonia diffusion in CNS-derived endothelial cells. J Invest Med. 1996;44:474–82.
37. Garcia-Martinez R, Cordoba J. Acute-on-chronic-liver failure: the brain. Curr Opin Crit Care. 2011;17:177–83.
38. Nath K, Saraswat VA, Krishna YR, et al. Quantification of cerebral edema on diffusion tensor imaging in acute-on-chronic liver failure. NMR Biomed. 2008;21:713–22.
39. O'Grady JG, Alexander GJ, Hayllar KM, et al. Early indicators of prognosis in fulminant hepatic failure. Gastroenterology. 1989;97:439–45.
40. Rajajee V, Fontana RJ, Courey AJ, Patil PG. Protocol based invasive intracranial pressure monitoring in acute liver failure: feasibility, safety and impact on management. Crit Care. 2017;21:178.
41. Wendon JA, Harrison PM, Keays R, et al. Cerebral blood flow and metabolism in fulminant hepatic failure. Hepatology. 1994;19:1407–13.
42. Davenport A, Will EJ, Davidson AM. Improved cardiovascular stability during continuous modes of renal replacement therapy in critically ill patients with acute hepatic and renal failure. Crit Care Med. 1993;21:328–38.
43. Jalan R, Olde Damink SW, Deutz NE, et al. Moderate hypothermia in patients with acute liver failure and uncontrolled intracranial hypertension. Gastroenterology. 2004;127:1338–46.
44. Stenbog P, Busk T, Larsen FS. Efficacy of liver assisting in patients with hepatic encephalopathy with special focus on plasma exchange. Metab Brain Dis. 2013;28:333–5.
45. Pugliese F, Ruberto F, Perrella SM, et al. Modifications of intracranial pressure after molecular adsorbent recirculating system treatment in patients with acute liver failure: case reports. Transplant Proc. 2007;39:2042–4.
46. Bernal W, Hyyrylainen A, Gera A, et al. Lessons from look-back in acute liver failure? A single centre experience of 3300 patients. J Hepatol. 2013;59:74–80.
47. Bajaj JS, Schubert CM, Heuman DM, et al. Persistence of cognitive impairment after resolution of overt hepatic encephalopathy. Gastroenterology. 2010;138:2332–40.
48. Bianchi GP, Marchesini G, Fabbri A, et al. Vegetable versus animal protein diet in cirrhotic patients with chronic encephalopathy: a randomized cross-over comparison. J Intern Med. 1993;233:385–92.
49. Camma FF, Tine F, et al. Lactitol in treatment of chronic hepatic encephalopathy. A meta-analysis. Dig Dis Sci. 1993;38:916–22.
50. Uribe M, Campollo O, Vargas F, et al. Acidifying enemas (lactitol and lactose) vs. nonacidifying enemas (tap water) to treat acute portal-systemic encephalopathy: a double-blind, randomized clinical trial. Hepatology. 1987;7:639–43.

51. Als-Nielsen B, Gluud LL, Gluud C. Non-absorbable disaccharides for hepatic encephalopathy: systematic review of randomised trials. BMJ. 2004;328:1046.
52. Sharma P, Sharma BC, Sarin SK. Predictors of non-response to lactulose in patients with cirrhosis and hepatic encephalopathy. Eur J Gastroenterol Hepatol. 2010;22:526–31.
53. Dhiman RK, Saraswat VA, Sharma BK, et al. Minimal hepatic encephalopathy: consensus statement of a working party of the Indian National Association for Study of the Liver. J Gastroenterol Hepatol. 2010;25:1029–41.
54. Luo M, Li L, Lu CZ, et al. Clinical efficacy and safety of lactulose for minimal hepatic encephalopathy: a meta-analysis. Eur J Gastroenterol Hepatol. 2011;23:1250–7.
55. Sharma P, Sharma BC, Sarin SK. Predictors of nonresponse to lactulose for minimal hepatic encephalopathy in patients with cirrhosis. Liver Int. 2009;29:1365–71.
56. Jiang Q, Jiang XH, Zheng MH, et al. Rifaximin versus nonabsorbable disaccharides in the management of hepatic encephalopathy: a meta-analysis. Eur J Gastroenterol Hepatol. 2008;20:1064–70.
57. Eltawil KM, Laryea M, Peltekian K, Molinari M. Rifaximin vs conventional oral therapy for hepatic encephalopathy: a meta-analysis. World J Gastroenterol. 2012;18:767–77.
58. Sharma BC, Sharma P, Lunia MK, et al. A randomized, double-blind, controlled trial comparing rifaximin plus lactulose with lactulose alone in treatment of overt hepatic encephalopathy. Am J Gastoenterol. 2013;108:1458–63.
59. Bajaj JS, Heuman DM, Wade JB, et al. Rifaximin improves driving simulator performance in a randomized trial of patients with minimal hepatic encephalopathy. Gastroenterology. 2011;140: 478–87.
60. Sidhu SS, Goyal O, Mishra BP, et al. Rifaximin improves psychometric performance and health-related quality of life in patients with minimal hepatic encephalopathy (the RIME trial). Am J Gastroenterol. 2011;106:307–16.
61. Kaji K, Takaya H, Saikawa S, et al. Rifaximin ameliorates hepatic encephalopathy and endotoxaemia without affecting the gut microbiome diversity. World J Gastroenterol. 2017;23:8355–66.
62. Shukla S, Shukla A, Mehboob S, Guha S. Meta-analysis: the effects of gut flora modulation using prebiotics, probiotics and synbiotics on minimal hepatic encephalopathy. Alim Pharmacol Ther. 2011;33:662–71.
63. Viramontes Horner D, Avery A, Stow R. The effects of probiotics and symbiotics on risk factors for hepatic encephalopathy: a systematic review. J Clin Gastroenterol. 2017;51:312–23.
64. Cao Q, Yu CB, Yang SG, et al. Effect of probiotic treatment on cirrhotic patients with minimal hepatic encephalopathy: a meta-analysis. Hepatobiliary Pancreat Dis Int. 2018;17:9–16.
65. Liu Q, Duan ZP, Ha DK, Bengmark S, Kurtovic J, Riordan SM. Synbiotic modulation of gut flora: effect on minimal hepatic encephalopathy in patients with liver cirrhosis. Hepatology. 2004;39:1441–9.
66. Bajaj JS, Kassam Z, Fagan A, et al. Fecal microbiota transplant from a rational stool donor improves hepatic encephalopathy: a randomized clinical trial. Hepatology. 2017;66:1727–38.
67. Mai M, Yang Z, Qi X, Fan D, Han G. l-ornithine-l-aspartate for hepatic encephalopathy in patients with cirrhosis: a meta-analysis of randomised controlled trials. J Gastroenterol Hepatol. 2013;28:783–92.
68. Varakanahalli S, Sharma BC, Srivastava S, Sachdeva S, Dahale AS. Secondary prophylaxis of hepatic encephalopathy in cirrhosis of liver: a double-blind randomized controlled trial of L-ornithine L-aspartate versus placebo. Eur J Gastroenterol Hepatol. 2018;30:951–8.
69. Sushma S, Dasarathy S, Tandon RK, et al. Sodium benzoate in the treatment of acute hepatic encephalopathy: a double-blind randomized trial. Hepatology. 1992;16:138–44.
70. Takuma Y, Nouso K, Makino Y, Hayashi M, Takahashi H. Clinical trial: oral zinc in hepatic encephalopathy. Alim Pharmacol Ther. 2010;32:1080–90.
71. Rockey DC, Vierling JM, Mantry P, et al. Randomized, double-blind, controlled study of glycerol phenylbutyrate in hepatic encephalopathy. Hepatology. 2014;59:1073–83.
72. Weiss N, Tripon S, Lodey M, et al. Treating hepatic encephalopathy in cirrhotic patients admitted to ICU with sodium phenylbutyrate: a preliminary study. Fundam Clin Pharmacol. 2018;32:209–15.
73. Jain L, Sharma BC, Srivastava S, Puri SK, Sharma P, Sarin S. Serum endotoxin, inflammatory mediators, and magnetic resonance spectroscopy before and after treatment in patients with minimal hepatic encephalopathy. J Gastroenterol Hepatol. 2013;28:1187–93.
74. Dhiman RK, Rana B, Garg A, et al. Efficacy and safety of a probiotic preparation in the secondary prophylaxis of hepatic encephalopathy in cirrhotic patients: interim results of a double blind, randomized, placebo controlled study. Hepatology. 2012;56:255A.
75. Laleman W, Simon-Talero M, Maleux G, et al. Embolization of large spontaneous portosystemic shunts for refractory hepatic encephalopathy: a multicentre survey on safety and efficacy. Hepatology. 2013;57:2448–57.
76. Park HY, Tsauo J, Shin JH, Kim PH. Percutaneous transparaumbilical embolization of spontaneous portosystemic shunts for the treatment of hepatic encephalopathy. J Vasc Interv Radiol. 2017;28:1563–8.
77. Hauenstein KH, Haag K, Ochs A, Langer M, Rossle M. The reducing stent: treatment for transjugular intrahepatic portosystemic shunt-induced refractory hepatic encephalopathy and liver failure. Radiology. 1995;194:175–9.
78. Hassanein TI, Tofteng F, Brown RS, et al. Randomized controlled study of extracorporeal albumin dialysis for hepatic encephalopathy in advanced cirrhosis. Hepatology. 2007;46:1853–62.
79. Banares R, Nevens F, Larsen FS, et al. Extracorporeal albumin dialysis with the molecular adsorbent recirculating system in acute-on-chronic liver failure: the RELIEF trial. Hepatology. 2013;57:1153–62.

Management of Ascites

65

Michela Triolo and Vincenzo La Mura

Key Concepts

- Ascites is the most common complication of cirrhosis. It is associated with a high risk of further complications such as dilutional hyponatremia, spontaneous bacterial peritonitis (SBP), refractory ascites and hepatorenal syndrome (HRS)
- Diuretics are the mainstay of treatment for uncomplicated ascites. However, the development of any complication requires a specific approach which can consist of drug implementation (e.g. antibiotics for SBP, terlipressin and albumin for acute and rapidly progressive HRS) and, in patients with refractory ascites, can consider transjugular intrahepatic porto-systemic shunt (TIPS) allocation.
- Liver transplantation represents the best treatment of patients with complicated ascites which is a clinical hallmark of poor survival. In several countries refractory ascites is considered an exception to the MELD score in the allocation of priority in patients with cirrhosis on the waiting list

M. Triolo
Medicina Interna, Istituto di Ricovero e Cura a carattere Scientifico (IRCCS) San Donato, Università degli Studi di Milano, San Donato Milanese, MI, Italy

V. La Mura (✉)
Fondazione IRCCS Cà Granda, Ospedale Maggiore Policlinico, U.O.C. Medicina Generale Emostasi e Trombosi, Dipartimento di Scienze Biomediche per la Salute, Università degli studi di Milano, Milan, Italy

CRC "A.M. and A. Migliavacca" Center for liver disease, Division of Gastroenterology and Hepatology, Fondazione IRCCS Cà Granda Ospedale Maggiore Policlinico, Università degli studi di Milano, Milan, Italy
e-mail: vincenzo.lamura@unimi.it

65.1 Introduction

Ascites is the most common of the three major complications related with cirrhosis, being the others hepatic encephalopathy and variceal hemorrhage [1]. Ascites is associated with a high incidence of further complications of cirrhosis. In fact, patients with ascites have a high risk of developing dilutional hyponatremia, bacterial infections, in particular spontaneous bacterial peritonitis (SBP), and a specific type of acute kidney injury (AKI), namely hepatorenal syndrome (HRS) [1].

65.2 Classification and Management of Ascites

Ascites can be classified into complicated and uncomplicated ascites. Complicated ascites is defined in association with at least one among hyponatremia, refractoriness to diuretic treatment, acute kidney injury and SBP [1]. In addition, ascites can be quantified in three grades according to its amount in the peritoneal cavity: (1) mild ascites only detectable by ultrasound; (2) moderate ascites with symmetrical distension of the abdomen; (3) large ascites. The first step in the management of ascites is to collect a detailed medical history and to perform liver and renal blood tests and an abdominal ultrasound. A paracentesis should be performed in all patients with first onset of grade 2/3 ascites and/or acutely decompensated. Peritoneal fluid analysis can provide relevant information such as the confirmation of ascites as a consequence of portal hypertension [serum albumin ascites gradient (SAAG) $\geq$1.1 g/dl], the presence/absence of an SBP (neutrophil cell count [250 cells/μl]) and the risk of developing SBP during follow-up (total protein content <1.5 g/dl) [1]. Before discussing the specific treatment of ascites, it should be highlighted that an important issue in the management of patients with cirrhosis is the treatment of the underlying cause of liver disease. In fact, several data suggest that the antiviral treatment of HBV and HCV and/or alcohol abstinence may lead

F. Radu-Ionita et al. (eds.), *Liver Diseases*, https://doi.org/10.1007/978-3-030-24432-3_65

to a progressive improvement of liver function with the potential prevention of the first episode of ascites in patients with compensated cirrhosis and the potential improvement of the response to diuretics in already decompensated patients.

65.2.1 Uncomplicated Ascites

The treatment of uncomplicated ascites should be adapted to the ascites grade. The clinical impact of grade 1 ascites have not been extensively investigated and no specific treatment has been suggested. The aim of treatment of moderate ascites is to induce a negative sodium balance with a moderate restriction in salt intake and diuretic use to increase renal sodium excretion.

65.2.1.1 Sodium Intake Restriction

Although there is no clear evidence of the efficacy of low sodium intake in the management of ascites in cirrhosis, the current guidelines suggest a moderate restriction of dietary salt (80–120 mmol of sodium/day, equivalent to approximately 4.6–6.9 g of salt/day) [1]. A lower sodium intake is often intolerable to patients, and also might worsen the malnutrition frequently observed in these patients [2].

65.2.1.2 Diuretics

Renal sodium retention in patients with ascites due to cirrhosis is mainly due to increased proximal as well as distal tubular sodium reabsorption [3]. The mediators of the enhanced proximal tubular reabsorption of sodium have not been elucidated completely, while aldosterone stimulates renal sodium reabsorption along the distal tubule by increasing both the permeability of the luminal membrane of principal cells to sodium and the activity of the Na/K ATPase pump in the basolateral membrane, therefore, aldosterone antagonists, such as spironolactone are used for first-line diuretics to treat ascites [3]. Aldosterone antagonists should be administered starting from 100 to 200 mg/day. A stepwise increase of aldosterone antagonist doses (up to 400 mg/day) may be effective in mobilizing ascites in 60–80% of nonazotemic cirrhotic patients with a first episode of ascites [1]. A long-standing debate in the management of ascites is whether aldosterone antagonists should be given alone or in combination with a loop diuretic (i.e., furosemide). Since the effect of aldosterone is slow, as it involves interaction with a cytosolic receptor and then a nuclear receptor, a sequential increase of antialdosteronic drugs requires a long time to find the effective dose, especially for patients with recurrent ascites [3]. A combined diuretic treatment has been proposed with the administration of a low dose of furosemide (up to 160 mg/day) and 100–400 mg/day of an antialdosteronic drug [3].

Amiloride can be substituted for spironolactone in patients with tender gynecomastia. However, amiloride is more expensive and has been shown to be less effective than an active metabolite of spironolactone [1]. Triamterene, metolazone, and hydrochlorothiazide have also been used for ascites [1]. Hydrochlorothiazide can also cause rapid development of hyponatremia when added to the combination of spironolactone and furosemide; it should be used with extreme caution or avoided [1]. In all patients, diuretic dosage should be adjusted to achieve a rate of weight loss of no greater than 0.5 kg/day in patients without peripheral edema and 1 kg/day in those with peripheral edema to prevent diuretic-induced renal failure and/or hyponatremia [1]. Following mobilization of ascites, diuretics should be reduced to maintain patients with minimal or no ascites to avoid diuretic-induced complications.

65.2.1.3 Complications of Diuretic Therapy

The use of diuretics may be associated with several complications such as renal failure, hepatic encephalopathy, electrolyte disorders, gynecomastia, and muscle cramps [1, 4]. Diuretic-induced renal failure is most frequently due to intravascular volume depletion that usually occurs as a result of an excessive diuretic therapy [1, 4]. Diuretic therapy has been classically considered a precipitating factor of hepatic encephalopathy. Hypokalemia may occur if patients are treated with loop diuretics alone. Hyperkalemia may develop as a result of treatment with aldosterone antagonists or other potassium-sparing diuretics, particularly in patients with renal impairment. Hyponatremia is another frequent complication of diuretic therapy, most experts agree that diuretics should be stopped temporarily in patients whose serum sodium decreases to less than 120–125 mmol/L. Gynecomastia is common with the use of aldosterone antagonists, but it does not usually require discontinuation of treatment. Finally, diuretics may cause muscle cramps [1, 4]. If cramps are severe, diuretic dose should be decreased or stopped and albumin infusion may relieve symptoms [1, 4].

65.2.2 Large Ascites

In patients with large ascites the first-line treatment should be the combination of large volume paracentesis (LVP) and infusion of albumin because is more effective than diuretics and significantly shortens the duration of hospital stay [1, 3]. In addition, the frequency of hyponatremia, renal impairment, and hepatic encephalopathy is significantly lower with paracentesis than with diuretic treatment. Hemorrhagic complications after LVP are infrequent even in patients with INR >1.5 and platelet count <50,000/μl [5]. Thus, there are no data to support a systematic use of fresh frozen plasma or pooled platelets before LVP.

The mobilization of ascites can be completed in one single tap. The removal of large volumes of ascitic fluid is associated with circulatory dysfunction characterized by a ≥50% increase of plasma renin activity 1 week after the procedure [6], a reduction of effective blood volume, an acute increase of cardiac output and a reduction in the systemic vascular resistance and arterial blood pressure, a condition known as post-paracentesis circulatory dysfunction (PPCD) [6]. PPCD is a relevant complication, being associated with a rapid recurrence of ascites, a high incidence of HRS, dilutional hyponatremia and death [6]. The most effective method to prevent circulatory dysfunction after LVP is plasma volume expansion. Albumin, at the dose of 8 g/l of ascites removed, is more effective than other plasma expanders for the prevention of PPCD [7] and to reduce the mortality rate in patients with ascites [7]. When less than 5 L of ascites are removed, dextran-70 (8 g/L of ascites removed) or polygeline (150 ml/L of ascites removed) show efficacy similar to that of albumin. However, albumin should be preferred because it is more effective [8]. Patients treated with LVP should immediately receive diuretic treatment after the removal of ascitic fluid to prevent the re-accumulation of ascites [4].

65.2.3 Refractory Ascites

Refractory ascites is defined as "ascites that cannot be mobilized or the early recurrence of which (i.e. after paracentesis) cannot be satisfactorily prevented by sodium restriction and diuretic treatment" [3]. Two different types of RA have been described: diuretic-resistant ascites [that do not respond to dietary sodium restriction and maximal diuretic dose (furosemide 160 mg/day and aldosterone antagonists 400 mg/day)] and diuretic-intractable ascites (caused by the development of diuretic-related complications) [3]. The latter accounts for more than 90% of patients with refractory ascites [3]. Refractory ascites occurs in 5–10% of patients with cirrhosis and ascites and is associated with a low probability of survival, about 50% at 6 months [3]. The treatment includes LVP with albumin, liver transplantation (LT), vasoconstrictors or insertion of a transjugular intrahepatic portosystemic shunt (TIPS). The use of therapies under investigation will also be discussed briefly.

65.2.3.1 Liver Transplantation (LT)

LT represents the best treatment of patients with refractory ascites who have a poor survival, even worse than that predicted by the MELD score. Thus, in several countries refractory ascites is considered an exception to the MELD score and indicates priority for transplantation in waiting list patients [8]. However, many patients with refractory ascites have contraindications to LT. These patients need some other therapeutic options. The same happens for the management of patients with large ascites while on waiting list.

65.2.3.2 Vasoconstrictors

Vasoconstrictors, such as the α1-adrenergic agonist midodrine or the vasopressin-1 (V1) receptor agonist terlipressin may decrease the splanchnic arterial vasodilatation and thereby improve the renal perfusion and filtration [9, 10]. In patients with ascites, a single oral dose of midodrine increases the arterial blood pressure, renal perfusion, glomerular filtration rate (GFR) and sodium excretion but this drug is not recommended as standard of therapy [9]. The administration of terlipressin has been shown to be effective in the treatment of refractory ascites in a small pilot study [10]. However, considering the lack of large prospective studies, and the high risk of adverse events, outpatient administration of terlipressin cannot be recommended.

65.2.3.3 Other Treatments

Radiologists and surgeons have collaborated to develop a device, named alpha pump, that drains ascitic fluid into the urinary bladder [11]. The alpha pump has been recently tested in comparison with therapeutic paracentesis in a randomized clinical trial [11] confirming that it significantly reduces the need for paracentesis with an impact on quality of life, however, alpha pump was associated with a significant higher number of adverse events, among them, AKI after the intervention and the need of re-intervention. Finally, no survival advantages were observed [11].

Vaptans are vasopressin receptor antagonists and have been studied predominantly in heart failure but also in the setting of cirrhosis [12]. Their utility is treating hyponatremia and reducing fluid overload. These drugs appear to correct mild hyponatremia. Unfortunately, a recent meta-analysis showed no beneficial effect of vaptans in the control of ascites, moreover the treatment could be associated with an increased morbidity and mortality [12] therefore the use of this class of drug is not recommendable in clinical practice.

65.2.3.4 Transjugular Intrahepatic Portosystemic Shunts (TIPS)

TIPS decompresses the portal system like a side-to-side portocaval shunt inserted between the portal vein, at high pressure, and the inferior cava vein, at low pressure [13]. In the short-term, TIPS induces an increase of cardiac output, right atrial pressure, and pulmonary artery pressure leading to a secondary reduction in systemic vascular resistance and effective arterial blood volume [13].

International clinical guidelines recommends TIPS as a treatment of medically refractory ascites for patients who do not tolerate repeated LVP [1]. Indeed, LVP has a negative effect on systemic hemodynamics and renal function which often limits its use as a long-term treatment [6]. In contrast, TIPS offers a treatment option which even improves renal function and systemic hemodynamics as well. Within 4 weeks after TIPS, urinary sodium excretion and serum creatinine improve significantly and can normalize within 6–12 months. This is associated with an increase in serum sodium concentration, urinary volume, and glomerular filtration rate together with a normalization of plasma renin activity, aldosterone, and noradrenaline concentrations at 4–6 months of follow-up [13]. These findings strongly suggest that TIPS ameliorates central underfilling.

A recent analysis of the literature showed that TIPS was associated with better control of ascites and a higher incidence of hepatic encephalopathy (HE) than LVP, however results on survival were conflicting. This discrepancy, at least in part, could be explained by distinct selection criteria of the patients and the difference in the technical success rate of the procedures among different studies.

In the most recent randomized control trial, which included also patients with recurrent ascites, not just refractory, TIPS with covered stents improved survival when compared to LVP [14]. Furthermore, patients treated with TIPS had a lower rate of portal hypertension-related bleeding and fewer days of hospitalization than those treated with LVP [14].

Bercu et al. published a single center retrospective series of 92 patients with refractory ascites who underwent covered TIPS. Stents were initially dilated to 6 mm in an attempt to target a PSG of 7–12 mmHg [15]. If the porto-systemic gradient (PSG) response was not adequate (over the threshold of 12 mmHg indicating high risk of variceal bleeding/rebleeding), serial dilation up to the maximum stent diameter was performed. Of the 61 patients with documented follow-up, 90% had a partial or complete ascites response. The TIPS revision rate was 13%. Overall survival was 79% at 365-day follow-up and transplantation-free survival was 75%. Fifty-nine percent of patients had HE, of which 19.7% were severe. These recent investigations suggest TIPS as the primary therapy for the treatment of refractory ascites. Careful selection of patients with preserved liver function and the use of covered stents may further improve both survival and ascites control [13].

Unfortunately, the main limitation to the extensive use of TIPS for the treatment of refractory ascites is the presence of contraindications to TIPS placement, making TIPS use available for less than 40% of patients [13]. An important drawback is the risk of HE which remains frequent and constitutes an invalidating complication after TIPS allocation. This notwithstanding, recently Schepis et al. [16] showed, in a non-randomized study of 42 unselected patients with cirrhosis who received under-dilated TIPS and 53 patients who received TIPS dilated to its nominal diameter, that HE developed in a significantly lower proportion of patients with under-dilated TIPS (27%) than controls (54%) during the first year after the procedure (P = .015) without significant difference in the recurrence of ascites between groups. Hence, under-dilation of stent during TIPS placement may be feasible, associated with lower rates of HE, and effective in the ascites control. However these data need to be validated in adequately sized randomized controlled trials before an under-dilatation of TIPS can be routinely recommended in patients with ascites even more if we think that the lowest the PSG the lowest the risk of variceal bleeding which is lifethreatening.

65.3 Hyponatremia

Hypervolemic hyponatremia is common in patients with decompensated cirrhosis and is related to impaired solute-free water excretion secondary to non-osmotic hypersecretion of vasopressin (the antidiuretic hormone), a decrease in the delivery of pre-urine to the ascending limb of the loop of Henle (the diluting segment of the nephron), and the reduced production of prostaglandins, which results in a disproportionate retention of water relative to sodium retention [17]. Hyponatremia in cirrhosis is arbitrarily defined when serum sodium concentration decreases below 130 mmol/L [17]. Serum sodium concentration is an important marker of prognosis in cirrhosis and the presence of hyponatremia is associated with an impaired survival [17]. Moreover, hyponatremia may also be associated with an increased morbidity, particularly neurological complications, and reduced survival after transplantation [17].

65.3.1 Management of Hyponatremia

The aim of treatment of hypervolemic hyponatremia is to improve the free water excretion with the urine. The administration of hypertonic sodium chloride cannot be recommended since it would further increase ascites and edema. The current available treatments for hypervolemic hyponatremia in cirrhosis include: (1) fluid restriction, (2) albumin and (3) antagonists of AVP V2 receptors (vaptans). Fluid restriction to about 1 L per day has been suggested for these patients but its efficacy is poor [4]. Some reports suggest that albumin may increase the serum sodium concentration in patients with cirrhosis and ascites by increasing the effective circulating volume [18]. A number of evidences show that a short-therapy with vaptans (1 week to 1 month) ameliorates solute-free water excretion and leads to the increase in serum sodium levels in 45–82% of patients without particular side effects on renal function, urine sodium and circulatory function. Satavaptan and tolvaptan were investigated in the treatment of hypervolemic hyponatremia in cirrhotic patients [12]. Satavaptan was more effective than placebo in increasing the serum sodium concentration, but control of ascites was not improved even with an increased morbidity and mortality for unknown reasons [12]. Hence, satavaptan was abandoned. Tolvaptan was more effective than placebo in treating hyponatremia in patients with cirrhosis and ascites, however robust long-term data are still lacking [12]. Thus, nowadays the role of vaptans in the management of hyponatremia in cirrhosis is still uncertain.

65.4 Spontaneous Bacterial Peritonitis (SBP)

SBP is defined as bacterial infection of ascitic fluid without any intra-abdominal, surgically treatable source of infection [19]. The prevalence of SBP is about 20% in hospitalized patients with cirrhosis and ascites [20]. SBP is diagnosed when neutrophil count in ascitic fluid is ≥250 cells/μl [19]. The pathogenesis of SBP includes both a pathological bacterial translocation from the gut to the systemic circulation and an impaired ability of the local and systemic immunity to control the spread of these bacteria [19]. Bacterial translocation occurs because of an intestinal bacterial overgrowth, an increased intestinal permeability, a change in the quality of bacteria and the ineffective activity of the intestinal immune system [19]. SBP is associated with a high risk of AKI and poor short-term survival [20].

65.4.1 Management of SBP: Antibiotic Treatment

Empirical antibiotic therapy must be initiated immediately after the diagnosis of SBP, without the results of ascitic fluid culture [1, 4]. Cefotaxime, a third-generation cephalosporin, has been extensively investigated in patients with SBP because it covers most causative organisms and because of its high ascitic fluid concentrations during therapy [1, 4]. A dose of 4 g/day is as effective as a dose of 8 g/day [1, 4]. A 5-day therapy is as effective as a 10-day treatment [1, 4]. Alternatively, amoxicillin/clavulanic acid, first given intravenously then orally, has similar results with respect to SBP resolution and mortality, compared with cefotaxime [1, 4] and with a much lower cost. Ciprofloxacin, given either for 7 days intravenously or for 2 days intravenously followed by 5 days orally, results in a similar SBP resolution rate and hospital survival compared with cefotaxime, but with a significantly higher cost [1, 4]. Oral ofloxacin has given similar results as intravenous cefotaxime in uncomplicated SBP, without renal failure, hepatic encephalopathy, gastrointestinal bleeding, ileus, or shock [1, 4]. Cefotaxime or amoxicillin/clavulanic acid are effective in patients who develop SBP while on norfloxacin prophylaxis [1, 4]. In hospital acquired episodes of SBP, the efficacy of the above-mentioned antibiotics is poor, because those episodes are frequently sustained by multi-drug-resistant (MDR) bacteria; in this case a broader spectrum empirical antibiotic treatment should be used according to local epidemiology [3]. If ascitic fluid neutrophil count fails to decrease to less than 25% of the pretreatment value after 2 days of antibiotic treatment, there is a high likelihood of failure to respond to therapy [3]. This should indicate modification of antibiotic treatment according to antibiogram or empiric choice or the presence of 'secondary peritonitis'. Hepato-renal syndrome (HRS) occurs in approximately 30% of patients with SBP treated with antibiotics alone, and is associated with a poor survival [20]. The administration of albumin (1.5 g/kg at diagnosis and 1 g/kg on day 3) decreases the frequency of HRS and improves survival. It is unclear whether albumin is useful in the subgroup of patients with baseline serum bilirubin <4 mg/dL and creatinine <1 mg/dL [20]. Until further trials are completed, albumin infusion appears a valuable adjunction to the treatment of SBP.

65.4.2 Prophylaxis of SBP

The probability of SBP recurrence is about 70% at 1 year [1, 4]. In these patients, secondary prophylaxis with norfloxacin was shown to be effective in preventing the recurrence of SBP [1, 4]. Currently, primary prophylaxis of SBP is recommended in two conditions: (1) after episodes of gastrointestinal bleeding and (2) in patients with a protein concentration in ascitic fluid below 1.5 g/dl and advanced liver disease (Child-Pugh C9 and bilirubin ≥3 mg/dl or serum creatinine ≥1.2 mg/dl or serum sodium ≤130 mmol/l) [1, 4]. In patients with gastrointestinal bleeding and severe liver disease (at least two of the following: ascites, severe malnutrition, encephalopathy or bilirubin >3 mg/dl) ceftriaxone is the prophylactic antibiotic of choice [1, 4], while patients with less severe liver disease may be given oral norfloxacin or an alternative oral quinolone to prevent the development of SBP [1, 4]. In patients with a protein concentration in ascitic fluid below 1.5 g/dl, advanced liver disease and without prior SBP norfloxacin (400 mg/day) reduced the risk of SBP and improved survival [1, 4]. Therefore, these patients should be considered for long-term prophylaxis with norfloxacin.

Patients who recover from an episode of SBP have a high risk of developing recurrent SBP. In these patients, the administration of prophylactic antibiotics reduces the risk of recurrent SBP. Norfloxacin (400 mg/day, orally) is the treatment of choice [1, 4]. Nevertheless, this efficacy is counterbalanced by the risk of MDR infection, therefore the indication is for selected patients who cannot be addressed to alternative therapies. Alternative antibiotics include ciprofloxacin (750 mg once weekly, orally) or co-trimoxazole (800 mg sulfamethoxazole and 160 mg trimethoprim daily, orally), but evidence is not as strong as that with norfloxacin [1, 4]. Patients who recover from SBP have a poor long-term survival and should be considered for liver transplantation [1, 4].

65.5 Hepatorenal Syndrome (HRS)

Renal dysfunction is a severe complication of advanced stages of cirrhosis. Traditionally renal dysfunction in patients with liver disease has been defined as a serum creatinine >1.5 mg/dl [19] while AKI has been defined by an absolute increase of serum creatinine more than or equal to 0.3 mg/dl up to 48 h of clinical observation, or by a percentage increase of serum creatinine more or equal to 50% in less than seven days [19]. HRS has been defined as a syndrome that occurs in patients with advanced liver disease, characterized by impaired renal function and marked abnormalities in the arterial circulation and over-activity of the endogenous vasoactive systems. In the kidney, there is marked renal vasoconstriction that results in a low GFR. In the extrarenal circulation there is a predominance of arterial vasodilation that results in the reduction of systemic vascular resistance and arterial hypotension [20]. HRS has been traditionally classified into two different clinical types: type-1 HRS, characterised by a rapidly progressive reduction of renal function, defined by a doubling of the serum creatinine to a level >2.5 mg/dl in less than 2 weeks, and type-II HRS, in which the renal failure does not have a rapidly progressive course [20]. Recently this schematic classification has been questioned and partially modified as the reader can see in the guidelines of the European Association for the Study of the Liver published in 2018 for further details.

65.5.1 Management of HRS

The first measure is to minimize or to stop any potential nephrotoxic drug (i.e., diuretics, antibiotics, NSAIDs, angiotensin-converting enzyme inhibitors, etc.). Then, it is important to verify the presence of hypovolemia and, if present, to correct it. In patients with AKI stage ≥2 (increase of serum creatinine ≥2-fold from baseline) diuretics should be withdrawn and plasma expansion with albumin (1 g/kg of body weight) should be administered [1, 4, 20]. In patients without response of creatinine to albumin expansion HRS diagnosis should be considered whether there has been no recent use of nephrotoxic drugs, no hematuria, no significant proteinuria, no shock and no alterations of renal ultrasonography [1, 4, 20]. Liver transplantation (LT) is the best treatment both for type-1 and type-2 HRS [1, 4, 20]. Unfortunately, not all patients are eligible for LT. Thus, medical treatments have been developed, the most effective being the combination of vasoconstrictors plus albumin. The rationale behind the use of vasoconstrictors is to counteract splanchnic arterial vasodilation. Albumin improves the effective circulating volume [19]. Among vasoconstrictors, terlipressin (i.v. boluses starting from 1 mg/4–6 h to 2 mg/4–6 h or continuous i.v. infusion starting from 2 mg/24 h to 12 mg/24 h, increasing dosage in a stepwise fashion any 48–72 h in case of no response) is the most widely used, while alpha-adrenergic drugs have been claimed to be a potential alternative. Among alpha-adrenergic drugs, midodrine given orally (2.5 up to 12.5 qid) together with octreotide given subcutaneously (125 up to 250 μg bid) [20] or norepinephrine (continuous i.v. infusion starting from 0.5 to 3 mg/h) [20] has been used. Recently, terlipressin was shown to be superior to midodrine plus octreotide in the treatment of type-1 HRS [19]. Norepinephrine is as effective as terlipressin in terms of reversal of type-1 HRS and 1-month survival [20]. Albumin should be administered at a dose of 1 g/kg of body weight for 1 day followed by 20–40 g/day and it should be withdrawn or reduced if signs of pulmonary edema appear [20]. The treatment with vasoconstrictors plus albumin should be continued until serum creatinine reaches a value below 1.5 mg/dl. About 20% of patients may present a recurrence of HRS after treatment withdrawal, and retreatment is usually effective. Some patients may show a continuous recurrence of HRS at any attempt to discontinue terlipressin. For these patients, a high priority on the LT waiting list and/or outpatient infusion has been suggested [20]. The use of TIPS is a potential treatment because it reduces portal hypertension and increases cardiac output. TIPS improves renal perfusion, sodium and water excretion and has been reported to reduce serum creatinine in selected patients with HRS [20]. However, data available on the use of TIPS in patients with type-1 HRS are mainly based on case series and randomized clinical trials are needed to evaluate the use of TIPS in these patients. Both hemodialysis or continuous venous hemofiltration, have been used to treat patients with type 1 HRS [20]. However, published information is very scant and in most studies patients with type 1 HRS have not been differentiated from patients with other causes of renal failure.

65.6 Conclusions/Summary

Ascites is the most frequent complication of patients with portal hypertension. The first line of treatment is represented by diuretic therapy. Albumin, antibiotic therapy, TIPS constitutes a second line of treatment in highly selected patients with complicated ascites.

Self-Study

Questions

1. Which statement/s is/are true?
   - (a) Aldosterone antagonists, such as spironolactone, are used as first-line diuretics drugs to treat patients with portal hypertension related ascites
   - (b) The removal of large volumes of ascitic fluid (over 4 L) does not need plasma volume expansion
   - (c) The most frequent type of "Refractory Ascites" is the diuretic-intractable ascites
2. Which statement/s is/are true?
   - (a) Spontaneous bacterial peritonitis is diagnosed when lymphocytic count in ascitic fluid is ≥250 cells/μl
   - (b) International guidelines recommends TIPS as an efficacious treatment of refractory ascites
   - (c) The combination of vasoconstrictors plus albumin is the most effective medical treatment in the management of hepato-renal syndrome

Answers

1. Which statement/s is/are true?
   - (a) CORRECT—Renal sodium retention in ascites due to cirrhosis is mainly due to increased proximal reabsorption, whose mediators have not been elucidated completely, and distal tubular sodium reabsorption. Aldosterone stimulates renal sodium reabsorption along the distal tubule by increasing both the permeability of the luminal membrane of principal cells to sodium and the activity of the Na/K ATPase pump in the basolateral membrane.
   - (b) INCORRECT—The removal of large volumes of ascitic fluid is associated with post-paracentesis circulatory dysfunction (PPCD), characterized by a ≥50% increase of plasma renin activity 1 week after the procedure, a reduction of effective blood volume, an acute increase of cardiac output and a reduction in the systemic vascular resistance and arterial blood pressure. The most effective method to prevent PPCD is plasma volume expansion, in particular with albumin, at the dose of 8 g/l of ascites removed.
   - (c) CORRECT—Refractory ascites is defined as "ascites that cannot be mobilized or the early recurrence of which cannot be satisfactorily prevented by sodium restriction and diuretic treatment". Two different types of refractory ascites have been described: diuretic-resistant ascites (not responder to dietary sodium restriction and maximal diuretic dose) and diuretic-intractable ascites (caused by the development of diuretic-related complications). The latter accounts for more than 90% of patients with refractory ascites.
2. Which statement/statements is/are true?
   - (a) INCORRECT—Spontaneous bacterial peritonitis is diagnosed when neutrophil count in ascitic fluid is ≥250 cells/μl
   - (b) CORRECT—TIPS can improves survival when compared to large volume paracentesis. Unfortunately, the main limitation to the extensive use of TIPS for the treatment of refractory ascites is the presence of contraindications to TIPS placement, especially HE Under-dilation of stent during TIPS placement may be associated with lower rates of HE, and effective in the ascites control.
   - (c) CORRECT—Hepato-renal syndrome in cirrhosis is mainly due to marked renal vasoconstriction that results in a low GFR as well as predominance of arterial vasodilation in the extrarenal circulation that results in the reduction of systemic vascular resistance and arterial hypotension. The rationale behind the use of vasoconstrictors is to counteract splanchnic arterial vasodilation while albumin improves the effective circulating volume.

References

1. Pericleous M, Sarnowski A, Moore A, Fijten R, Zaman M. The clinical management of abdominal ascites, spontaneous bacterial peritonitis and hepatorenal syndrome: a review of current guidelines and recommendations. Eur J Gastroenterol Hepatol. 2016;28(3):e10–8.
2. Morando F, Rosi S, Gola E, Nardi M, Piano S, Fasolato S, Stanco M, Cavallin M, Romano A, Sticca A, Caregaro L, Gatta A, Angeli P. Adherence to a moderate sodium restriction diet in outpatients with cirrhosis and ascites: a real-life cross-sectional study. Liver Int. 2015;35:1508–15.
3. Piano S, Tonon M, Angeli P. Management of ascites and hepatorenal syndrome. Hepatol Int. 2018;12(Suppl 1):122–34.
4. European Association for the Study of the Liver. EASL Clinical Practice Guidelines for the management of patients with decompensated cirrhosis. J Hepatol. 2018;69:406.

5. Lin S, Wang M, Zhu Y, Dong J, Weng Z, Shao L, Chen J, Jiang J. Hemorrhagic complications following abdominal paracentesis in acute on chronic liver failure: a propensity score analysis. Medicine (Baltimore). 2015;94(49):e2225.
6. Elsabaawy MM, Abdelhamid SR, Alsebaey A, Abdelsamee E, Obada MA, Salman TA, Rewisha E. The impact of paracentesis flow rate in patients with liver cirrhosis on the development of paracentesis induced circulatory dysfunction. Clin Mol Hepatol. 2015;21:365–71.
7. Bernardi M, Caraceni P, Navickis RJ. Does the evidence support a survival benefit of albumin infusion in patients with cirrhosis undergoing large-volume paracentesis? Expert Rev Gastroenterol Hepatol. 2017;11:191–2.
8. Cillo U, Burra P, Mazzaferro V, Belli L, Pinna AD, Spada M, Nanni Costa A, Toniutto P, I-BELT (Italian Board of Experts in the Field of Liver Transplantation). A multistep, consensus-based approach to organ allocation in liver transplantation: toward a "Blended Principle Model". Am J Transplant. 2015;15:2552–61.
9. Ali A, Farid S, Amin M, Kassem M, Al-Garem N. Clinical study on the therapeutic role of midodrine in non azotemic cirrhotic patients with tense ascites: a double-blind, placebo-controlled, randomized trial. Hepatogastroenterology. 2014;61:1915–24.
10. Gow PJ, Ardalan ZS, Vasudevan A, Testro AG, Ye B, Angus PW. Outpatient terlipressin infusion for the treatment of refractory ascites. Am J Gastroenterol. 2016;111:1041–2.
11. Bureau C, Adebayo D, Chalret de Rieu M, Elkrief L, Valla D, Peck-Radosavljevic M, McCune A, Vargas V, Simon-Talero M, Cordoba J, Angeli P, Rosi S, MacDonald S, Malago M, Stepanova M, Younossi ZM, Trepte C, Watson R, Borisenko O, Sun S, Inhaber N, Jalan R. Alfapump® system vs. large volume paracentesis for refractory ascites: a multicenter randomized controlled study. J Hepatol. 2017;67:940–9.
12. Facciorusso A, Amoruso A, Neve V, Antonino M, Prete VD, Barone M. Role of vaptans in the management of hydroelectrolytic imbalance in liver cirrhosis. World J Hepatol. 2014;6:793–9.
13. Rössle M. TIPS: 25 years later. J Hepatol. 2013;59:1081–93.
14. Bureau C, Thabut D, Oberti F, Dharancy S, Carbonell N, Bouvier A, Mathurin P, Otal P, Cabarrou P, Péron JM, Vinel JP. Transjugular intrahepatic portosystemic shunts with covered stents increase transplant free survival of patients with cirrhosis and recurrent ascites. Gastroenterology. 2017;152:157–63.
15. Bercu ZL, Fischman AM, Kim E, Nowakowski FS, Patel RS, Schiano TD, Chang CY, Lookstein RA. TIPS for refractory ascites: a 6-year single-center experience with expanded polytetrafluoroethylene-covered stent-grafts. AJR Am J Roentgenol. 2015;204:654–61.
16. Schepis F, Vizzutti F, Garcia-Tsao G, Marzocchi G, Rega L, De Maria N, Di Maira T, Gitto S, Caporali C, et al. Under-dilated TIPS associate with efficacy and reduced encephalopathy in a prospective, non-randomized study of patients with cirrhosis. Clin Gastroenterol Hepatol. 2018;16:1153–62.
17. Møller S, Krag A, Bendtsen F. Kidney injury in cirrhosis: pathophysiological and therapeutic aspects of hepatorenal syndromes. Liver Int. 2014;34:1153–63.
18. Minhtri K, Nguyen MK, Ornekian V, Kao L, Butch AW, Kurtz I. Defining the role of albumin infusion in cirrhosis-associated hyponatremia. Am J Physiol. 2014;307:G229–32.
19. Ekser B, Mangus RS. Spontaneous bacterial peritonitis. Lancet. 2017;389:735.
20. Angeli P, Gines P, Wong F, Bernardi M, Boyer TD, Gerbes A, Moreau R, Jalan R, Sarin SK, Piano S, Moore K, Lee SS, Durand F, Salerno F, Caraceni P, Kim WR, Arroyo V, Garcia-Tsao G, International Club of Ascites. Diagnosis and management of acute kidney injury in patients with cirrhosis: revised consensus recommendations of the International Club of Ascites. Gut. 2015;64:531–7.

Extracorporeal Non cellular Liver Assisted Devices

66

Mehul Shah and Nikolaos T. Pyrsopoulos

Key Concepts

- Mortality in patients with liver failure remains high.
- Liver assisted devices may assist in bridging patients who are waiting for liver transplantation
- More randomized controlled trials are needed to establish the effective use of liver assisted devices.

66.1 Introduction

Liver is a very complex organ that performs some of the most vital functions such as blood detoxification and purification, synthesis and storage that is crucial in maintaining function of other organs [1]. Even though the liver has the capacity to regenerate there are occasions whereas the insult to the liver is extreme in a such a way that recovery and regeneration is suboptimal and the patient develops cerebral edema, infections and multi-organ failure among others.

Liver diseases are responsible for more than one million deaths worldwide and the number continues to rise as per the study published by Naghavi and colleagues [2]. Some of the deaths are related to acute liver failure while others are due to acute on chronic liver failure. In acute liver failure, the adult mortality is approximately 50% despite the increase in the number of patients receiving liver transplants. In acute on chronic liver failure, the mortality is increasing with repeated hospitalizations due to acute decompensation.

Liver transplantation is a life saving procedure, though mortality while on the least is substantial. In order to decrease the mortality rate there is a high demand for modalities that can bridge the gap until a graft is available. Extracorporeal liver support devices have therefore been developed in order to clinically stabilize the decompensated patient and either act as a bridge to liver transplantation or allow the liver to recover from injury [3].

The ultimate liver assist device would eliminate the need for liver transplantation and may offer a chronic replacement for patient with end stage liver disease, as, potentially in renal dialysis. Liver assist devices are far from ready to be routinely used as renal dialysis but with research in this field we are making remarkable strides towards achieving the goal.

66.2 Types of Extracorporeal Liver Assisted Devices

Effective liver assisted devices would be expected to perform three key functions in patients with liver failure 1) detoxification, 2) synthesis of clinically important proteins and 3) facilitated regeneration of native hepatocytes [4].

Liver assisted devices can be divided into two types:

- Extracorporeal Non Cellular Liver Assisted Devices
- Extracorporeal Cellular Liver Assisted Devices

In this chapter, we will be focusing on the Extracorporeal Non Cellular Liver Assisted Devices (Table 66.1) such as Molecular Adsorbent Recirculating System (MARS™), Fractionated Plasma Separation and Adsorption System—FSPA (Prometheus™), Single Pass Albumin Dialysis System (SPAD), and Selective plasma filtration therapy (SEPET).

Table 66.1 Artificial liver support devices (non-cell based liver support devices)

Molecular Adsorbents Recirculating System (MARS)
Fractionated plasma separation and adsorption (Prometheus)
Single pass albumin dialysis (SPAD)
Selective Plasma Filtration therapy (SPFT)

M. Shah · N. T. Pyrsopoulos (✉)
Division of Gastroenterology and Hepatology, Rutgers—New Jersey Medical School, Newark, NJ, USA
e-mail: ms2828@njms.rutgers.edu; pyrsopni@njms.rutgers.edu

F. Radu-Ionita et al. (eds.), *Liver Diseases*, https://doi.org/10.1007/978-3-030-24432-3_66

These systems are based on the concept of albumin dialysis (removal of albumin bound toxins). These toxins have been associated with Hepatic Encephalopathy (HE), renal failure due to hepatorenal syndrome (HRS) and cardiovascular failure. These devices can also remove water-soluble substances such as creatinine or urea, ammonia, and smaller proteins such as some cytokines, by standard dialysis. Non cellular assisted devices are based on the principles of adsorption and filtration and are aimed at removing circulating toxins by using membranes with different pore sizes and adsorbent columns [5].

66.3 Molecular Adsorbent Recirculating Systems (MARS)

MARS was originally developed by Strange and colleagues [6] in 1993. The system provided a combination of conventional dialysis with hemodialysis against an Albumin dialysate solution over an Albumin impermeable membrane.

MARS consists of an albumin hemodialyzer, a standard hemodialyzer, an activated carbon adsorber and an anion exchanger (Fig. 66.1). This circuit is filled with 600 ml of 20% human albumin solution. The albumin acts as a dialysate and is pumped through a hollow-fibre membrane hemodialyzer (High Flux Dialysis Filter) countercurrent to the blood flow. Protein-bound toxins and water-soluble substances diffuse into the albumin solution. The albumin is then passed through another dialyzer countercurrent to a standard buffered dialysis solution where diffusive clearance of water-soluble substances occurs. The albumin solution is then cleaned of its albumin-bound toxins by passage through an activated carbon adsorber and an anion exchanger [7].

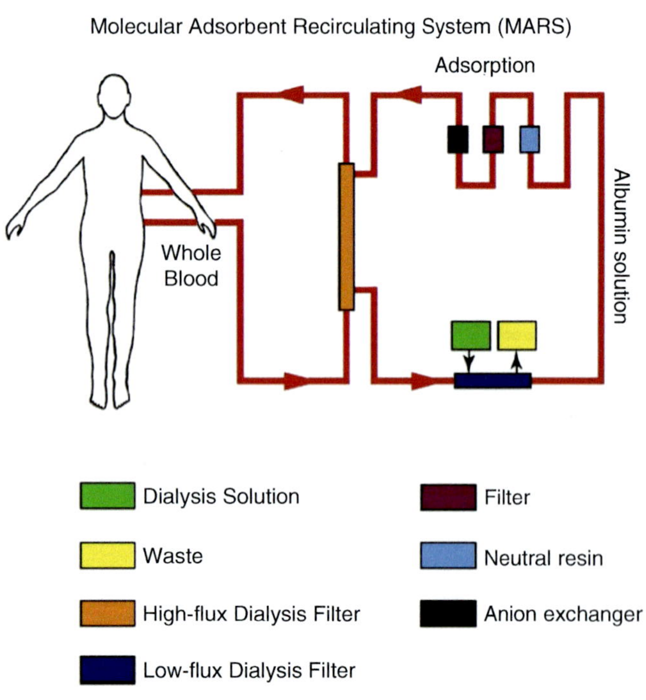

Fig. 66.1 Molecular adsorbent recirculating system

The MARS High Flux dialyzer has a surface area of 2.1 m^2, a membrane thickness of 100 nm and a molecular cut-off of about 50 kDa. The irregularities in the membrane surface provide deep crypts, which act as binding sites for albumin when the circuit is primed with albumin solution. The albumin molecules on the dialysis side of the membrane are in very close proximity to the surface of the membrane in contact with patient's blood. Albumin-bound toxins move by physicochemical interactions between the plasma, albumin molecules bound to the dialysis side of the membrane and the circulating albumin solution. A concentration gradient is maintained by circulation of the albumin solution and disposal of the albumin-bound toxins by passage through the activated charcoal and anion-exchange columns [8, 9].

In the first randomized controlled trial [10], 13 patients with cirrhosis were divided into two groups: A control group (n = 5) receiving standard medical treatment and hemodiafiltration, and a group (n = 8) additionally being treated with MARS. The MARS treatment was applied 1–10 times for 6–8 h. A significant decrease in creatinine and bilirubin levels as well as increase in serum sodium level and prothrombin activity was detected in the MARS group. Mortality of control group was 100% after 7 days, where it was 62.5% in the MARS group.

A prospective, controlled study was performed to test whether hyperbilirubinemia, 30-day survival, and encephalopathy would be improved by extracorporeal albumin dialysis (ECAD) [11]. Twenty-four patients were studied; 23 patients had cirrhosis; one had a prolonged cholestatic drug reaction and was excluded from per protocol (PP) analysis. Patients had a plasma bilirubin greater than 20 mg/dL and had not responded to prior standard medical therapy (SMT). Patients were randomized to receive SMT with ECAD or without (control). ECAD was performed with an extracorporeal device that dialyzes blood in a hollow fiber dialyzer against 15% albumin. Albumin-bound molecules transfer to dialysate albumin that is regenerated continuously by passage through a charcoal and anion exchange column and a conventional dialyzer. ECAD was associated with improved 30-day survival (PP, 11 of 12 ECAD, 6 of 11 controls). Plasma bile acids and bilirubin decreased on average by 43% and 29%, respectively, in the ECAD group after 1 week of treatment, but not in the control group. Renal dysfunction and hepatic encephalopathy improved in the ECAD group, but worsened significantly in the control group. ECAD was safe, with adverse events being rare and identical in both groups. In conclusion, ECAD appeared to be effective and safe for the short-term treatment of patients with cirrhosis and superimposed acute injury associated with progressive hyperbilirubinemia and may be useful for increasing survival in such patients awaiting liver transplantation [11].

A prospective randomized controlled multi-center trial was performed in 19 tertiary hospitals in Europe known as Relief Trial. One hundred eighty-nine patients with acute on chronic liver failure were randomized either to MARS (n = 95) or to standard therapy (SMT) (n = 94). Ten patients (five per group) were excluded due to protocol violations. In addition, 23 patients (MARS: 19; SMT: 4) were excluded from per-protocol (PP) analysis (PP population n = 156). Up to ten 6–8-h MARS sessions were scheduled. The main endpoint was 28-day intention to treat (ITT) and PP survival. There were no significant differences at inclusion, although the proportion of patients with Model for End stage Liver Disease (MELD) score over 20 points and with spontaneous bacterial peritonitis (SBP) as a precipitating event was almost significantly greater in the MARS group. The 28-day survival was similar in the two groups in the ITT and PP populations (60.7% versus 58.9%; 60% versus 59.2% respectively). After adjusting for confounders, a significant beneficial effect of MARS on survival was not observed. MELD score and HE at admission and the increase in serum bilirubin at day 4 were independent predictors of death. At day 4, a greater decrease in serum creatinine (P = 0.02) and bilirubin (P = 0.001) and a more frequent improvement in HE (from grade II–IV to grade 0–I; 62.5% versus 38.2%; P = 0.07) was observed in the MARS group. Severe adverse events were similar. So in conclusion at scheduled doses, a beneficial effect on survival of MARS therapy in patients with acute on chronic liver failure could not be demonstrated. However, MARS has an acceptable safety profile, has significant dialysis effect, and non-significantly improves severe HE [12].

An additional randomized controlled trial of MARS that included 102 patients (n = 53 MARS vs. 49 SMT) in 16 French transplant centers to determine whether MARS improves survival in acute liver failure was contacted. The main end point was to evaluate the 6 month survival. one hundred two patients (mean age, 40.4 years [SD, 13]) were in the modified intention-to-treat (mITT) population. The per-protocol analysis (49 conventional, 39 MARS) included patients with at least 1 session of MARS of 5 h or more. This study showed no survival benefit of MARS at 6 months (84.9% vs. 74.4% SMT, p = 0.28). A significant criticism of this study was the short time from randomization to liver transplantation (median 16.2 h), which may have limited any demonstrable effect from albumin dialysis. This randomized trial of MARS in patients with acute liver failure was unable to provide definitive efficacy or safety conclusions because many patients had transplantation before administration of the intervention. Acute liver failure not caused by paracetamol was associated with greater 6-month patient survival [13].

66.4 Prometheus System

The Prometheus system is based on fractional plasma separation and adsorption (FPSA) and hemodialysis. It uses a membrane with a cut-off of 250 kDa, being permeable for albumin. The toxin-loaded patient albumin crosses the membrane and passes a neutral resin adsorber and an anion exchanger, where the toxins bind to the adsorbers and free albumin is brought back to the patient. The method is combined with additional hemodialysis, therefore being able to remove water-soluble toxins as well as albumin-bound toxins.

A small clinical study was performed including nine patients with acute on chronic liver failure and documented cirrhosis due to alcohol or chronic viral infection, to confirm the efficacy of the system, to outline the effect of the single components and to evaluate the saturation effect of the adsorber columns [14]. It was shown that water-soluble toxins were almost exclusively cleared by the dialyzer, whereas bilirubin was cleared by the adsorber column, as expected. However, the clearance of bilirubin and bile acids strongly decreased in time, suggesting a saturation of the adsorbers. In general, the Prometheus system was shown to be effective in the removal of various toxins and to trigger no adverse events [15–18].

The first Prometheus trial was published in 2003 and included 11 patients with acute on chronic liver failure and accompanying renal failure [19]. While on treatment there was a significant improvement in serum levels of conjugated bilirubin, bile acids, ammonia, cholinesterase, creatinine, urea, and blood pH. Major complication of the procedure included hypotension in two patients due to infection and one patient developed uncontrolled bleeding.

Over the last few years, only a limited number of studies have used clinical endpoints. The most important was the HELIOS study, which was published in 2012 by Kribben et al. [20]. This was a multi-centric randomized controlled trial comparing Prometheus with SMT in 145 patients with acute on chronic liver failure, and the primary endpoint was the probabilities of survival at 28 and 90 days (irrespective of liver transplantation). This RCT scored 3 on the Oxford quality scoring system. This trial failed to prove a survival benefit with Prometheus in the overall patient population, and the patient recruitment was interrupted after the interim analysis (90 patients) due to futility (204 patients were initially planned for inclusion in the study). It is important to note that in the overall population the probability of survival was slightly higher in the Prometheus group compared to the SMT group (90-day survival probability: 47% vs. 38%) but without statistical significance.

66.5 Single Pass Albumin Dialysis (SPAD)

Single Pass Albumin Dialysis (SPAD) applies similar principles. The patient's blood also passes a high flux dialysis membrane. Albumin solution streams along the other side of the membrane counter-directionally, accepting toxins from the plasma. However, in SPAD the albumin solution is discarded after a single passage of the membrane without being recycled. The concept enables CVVHDF using the same dialysis filter [21].

With respect to clinical data on SPAD, only a few case reports were published in the early years, and there are currently no published studies that focus on demonstrating the clinical benefits of SPAD versus standard medical therapy (SMT) in acute liver failure or acute on chronic liver failure. Two retrospective uncontrolled studies reviewing data from patients with liver failure treated with SPAD as rescue therapy were identified. One included pediatric patients with ALF of different etiologies [22], and the other included adults patients with severe liver dysfunction in a context of alcoholic liver disease who were treated with SPAD or Prometheus [23]. Neither of these studies allow us to draw conclusions about the clinical usefulness of SPAD, and they only show us its relative ease of use and the absence of unexpected complications from its use.

The only randomized study using SPAD was recently published by Sponholz et al. [24]. This is a randomized, controlled crossover study comparing the detoxification capacity and influence on clinical and para-clinical parameters of SPAD (4% albumin dialysate solution; 700 mL/h dialysis flow rate) and MARS (20% albumin flow rate equal to the blood flow rate, 2000 mL/h dialysis flow rate). The authors found similar reductions in the total plasma bilirubin levels, without significant differences between the two devices. The reductions in the total bile acids and γ-glutamyl transferase levels in the SPAD arm were non-significant. The creatinine and urea levels were not significantly reduced with SPAD compared to those of MARS. In contrast to other studies, neither MARS nor SPAD induced a reduction in the systemic cytokine levels. Moreover, the patients treated with SPAD presented some metabolic derangements such as increasing lactate levels or decreasing calcium levels, which are probably explained by the preferential use of citrate anti-coagulation with a low dialysis flow rate. The effects of MARS and SPAD on the clinical parameters (HE and hemodynamic status) were small and equivalent. Currently, SPAD may be an easy-to-use alternative to MARS, but the optimal albumin dialysate concentration, dialysate flow rate and treatment regimen are not yet fully established.

66.6 Selective Plasma Filtration Therapy (SEPET)

In Selective Plasma Filtration Therapy (SEPET) the patient's blood is lead through a single-use cartridge containing hollow fibers with a molecular weight cut-off at 100 kDa. A plasma fraction containing several of the accumulated toxins in the blood is discarded after passing the membrane. This fraction contains toxins of small molecular weight and free pro-inflammatory cytokines but not for example immunoglobulins. Molecules with a molecular weight close to 100 kDa pass the membrane in only limited amounts so that large portions of for example albumin, HGF, as well as several clotting factors, are retained. The fluid loss is replaced by electrolyte solution, human albumin solution, fresh frozen plasma or a combination thereof. The system is designed for use with any commercially available kidney dialysis unit and/or plasmapheresis system utilizing hollow-fiber cartridges.

66.7 Discussion

There continues to be great interest and potential for extracorporeal non cellular liver assist devices. At present it is difficult to make an evidence-based recommendation supporting artificial liver assisted devices. Of this group, MARS is the best-studied albumin dialysis technology in acute liver failure and acute on chronic liver failure. Although studies have consistently demonstrated biochemical improvement and improvement in HE with MARS [11], recent large randomized studies in acute on chronic liver failure (RELIEF) [12] and acute liver failure (FULMAR) [13] showed no survival benefit. The HELIOS study examining Prometheus in acute on chronic liver failure was also disappointing [20]. These studies shared some common methodological limitations in study design. Within studies in acute liver failure and acute on chronic liver failure, heterogeneous groups of patients with varying causes with different natural histories were often lumped together. Several studies did not stratify patients based on severity of illness (e.g., MELD, CLIF-SOFA); hence, it is difficult to assess patient matching and, furthermore, the impact of underlying disease on patient mortality with or without treatment. Furthermore due to co-interventions, such as liver transplantation, not all patients received pre-specified durations of extracorporeal non cellular liver assist device therapy. When examining RELIEF AND HELIOS, it may have been more parsimonious to examine only acute on chronic liver failure patients who were candidates for liver transplantation because acute on chronic liver failure patients with multi-organ failure portends poor outcomes. Successfully bridging patients to liver transplantation may warrant further consideration because the primary endpoint over a 30-day to 90-day survival.

66.8 Conclusion

Severe liver failure is associated with high mortality, as patients succumb despite undergoing optimal medical treatment. Liver transplantation can be a life saving procedure though approximately a quarter of patients will succumb while waiting for a liver transplant. Consequently, there is a clear need for liver support systems to provide a "bridge" to a final treatment. Over the last two decades, several artificial liver support systems with promised advances were introduced. However, whether such devices that can lead into survival benefit are still in need.

Self Study

Questions

1. Which of the following is not an Extracorporeal Non Cellular Assisted Device?
   (a) Molecular Adsorbent Recirculating System (MARS™)
   (b) Extracorporeal Liver Assist Device (ELAD®)
   (c) Fractionated Plasma Separation and Adsorption System—FSPA (Prometheus™)
   (d) Single Pass Albumin Dialysis System (SPAD)
   (e) Selective plasma filtration therapy (SEPET)
2. Which of the following non cellular liver assisted devices have survival benefit?
   (a) Molecular Adsorbent Recirculating System (MARS™)
   (b) Fractionated Plasma Separation and Adsorption System—FSPA (Prometheus™)
   (c) Single Pass Albumin Dialysis System (SPAD)
   (d) Selective plasma filtration therapy (SEPET)
   (e) None of the above

Answers

1. Which of the following is not an Extracorporeal Non Cellular Assisted Device?
   (a) Molecular Adsorbent Recirculating System (MARS™). This is a non cellular liver assisted device.
   (b) CORRECT ANSWER. Extracorporeal Liver Assist Device (ELAD®). It is a bioartificial liver assist device.
   (c) Fractionated Plasma Separation and Adsorption System—FSPA (Prometheus™). This is a non cellular liver assisted device.
   (d) Single Pass Albumin Dialysis System (SPAD). This is a non cellular liver assisted device.
   (e) Selective plasma filtration therapy (SEPET). This is a non cellular liver assisted device.
2. Which of the following non cellular liver assisted devices have survival benefit?
   (a) Molecular Adsorbent Recirculating System (MARS™)
   (b) Fractionated Plasma Separation and Adsorption System—FSPA (Prometheus™)
   (c) Single Pass Albumin Dialysis System (SPAD)
   (d) Selective plasma filtration therapy (SEPET)
   (e) CORRECT ANSWER. None of the above

References

1. Sleisenger MH, Feldman M, Friedman LS, et al. Sleisenger and Fordtran's gastrointestinal and liver disease: pathophysiology, diagnosis, management. 9th ed. Philadelphia, PA: Saunders/Elsevier; 2010.
2. Naghavi M, Abajobir AA, Abbafati C, Abbas KM, Abd-Allah F, Abera SF, et al. Global, regional, and national age-sex specific mortality for 264 causes of death, 1980–2016: a systematic analysis for the Global Burden of Disease Study 2016. Lancet. 2017;390(10100):1151–210.
3. Puri P, Anand AC. Liver support devices. Med Update. 2012;22:489–93.
4. O'Grady J. Personal view: current role of artificial liver support devices. Aliment Pharmacol Ther. 2006;23:1549–57.
5. Karvellas CJ, et al. Current evidence for extracorporeal liver support systems in acute liver failure and acute-on-chronic liver failure. Crit Care Clin. 2016;32(3):439–51.
6. Strange J, Mitzner S, et al. Dialysis against a recycled albumin solution enables the removal of albumin-bound toxins. Artif Organs. 1993;17:809–13.
7. Steiner C, Majacher-Peszynska J, Peszynski P, Teasdale D. MARS® liver support therapy. Therapy information for doctors and nurses. Teraklin AG. 2002;1:2.
8. Stange J, Mitzner S. A carrier-mediated transport of toxins in a hybrid membrane. Safety barrier between a patients blood and a bioartificial liver. Int J Artif Organs. 1996;19:677–91.
9. Stange J, Mitzner SR, Risler T, Erley CM, Lauchart W, Goehl H, Klammt S, Peszynski P, Freytag J, Hickstein H, Lohr M, Liebe S, Schareck WP, Hopt UT, Schmidt R. Molecular adsorbent recycling system (MARS): clinical results of a new membrane-based blood purification system for bioartificial liver support. Artif Organs. 1999;23:319–30. https://doi.org/10.1046/j.1525-1594.1999.06122.x.
10. Mitzner SR, Stange J, Klammt S, Risler T, Erley CM, Bader BD, Berger ED, Lauchart W, Peszynksi P, Freytag J, Hickstein H, Loock J, Lohr JM, Liebe S, Emmrich J, Korten G, Schmidt R. Improvement of hepatorenal syndrome with extracorporeal albumin dialysis MARS: results of a prospective, randomized, controlled clinical trial. Liver Transpl. 2000;6:277–86.
11. Heeman U, Treichel U, Loock J, et al. Albumin dialysis in cirrhosis with superimposed acute liver injury: a prospective, controlled study. Hepatology. 2002;36:949–58.
12. Banares R, Nevens F, Larsen FS, Jalan R, Albillos A, Dollinger M, et al. Extracorporeal albumin dialysis with the molecular adsorbent recirculating system in acute-on-chronic liver failure: the RELIEF trial. Hepatology. 2013;57:1153–62.

13. Saliba F, Camus C, Durand F, Mathurin P, Letierce A, Delafosse B, et al. Albumin dialysis with a noncell artificial liver support device in patients with acute liver failure: a randomized, controlled trial. Ann Intern Med. 2013;159:522–31.
14. Evenepoel P, Laleman W, Wilmer A, Claes K, Maes B, Kuypers D, Bammens B, Nevens F, Vanrenterghem Y. Detoxifying capacity and kinetics of prometheus-a new extracorporeal system for the treatment of liver failure. Blood Purif. 2005;23:349–58.
15. Rifai K, Ernst T, Kretschmer U, Bahr MJ, Schneider A, Hafer C, Haller H, Manns MP, Fliser D. Prometheus-a new extracorporeal system for the treatment of liver failure. J Hepatol. 2003;39:984–90.
16. Rifai K, Manns MP. Review article: clinical experience with Prometheus. Ther Apher Dial. 2006;10:132–7.
17. Rifai K, Ernst T, Kretschmer U, Haller H, Manns MP, Fliser D. Removal selectivity of Prometheus: a new extracorporeal liver support device. World J Gastroenterol. 2006;12:940–4.
18. Rifai K, Ernst T, Kretschmer U, Hafer C, Haller H, Manns MP, Fliser D. The Prometheus device for extracorporeal support of combined liver and renal failure. Blood Purif. 2005;23:298–302.
19. Rifai K, Ernst T, Kretschmer U, et al. Prometheus - a new extracorporeal system for the treatment of liver failure. J Hepatol. 2003;39:984–90.
20. Kribben A, Gerken G, Haag S, Herget-Rosenthal S, Treichel U, Betz C, et al. Effects of fractionated plasma separation and adsorption on survival in patients with acute-on-chronic liver failure. Gastroenterology. 2012;142(4):782–9.
21. Chawla LS, Georgescu F, Abell B, Seneff MG, Kimmel PL. Modification of continuous venovenous hemodiafiltration with single-pass albumin dialysate allows for removal of serum bilirubin. Am J Kidney Dis. 2005;45:e51–6.
22. Ringe H, Varnholt V, Zimmering M, Luck W, Gratopp A, Konig K, et al. Continuous veno-venous single-pass albumin hemodiafiltration in children with acute liver failure. Pediatr Crit Care Med. 2011;12(3):257–64.
23. Piechota M, Piechota A. An evaluation of the usefulness of extracorporeal liver support techniques in patients hospitalized in the ICU for severe liver dysfunction secondary to alcoholic liver disease. Hepat Mon. 2016;16(7):e34127.
24. Sponholz C, Matthes K, Rupp D, Backaus W, Klammt S, Karailieva D, et al. Molecular adsorbent recirculating system and single-pass albumin dialysis in liver failure–a prospective, randomised crossover study. Crit Care. 2016;20:2.

Extracorporeal Cellular Liver Assisted Devices

67

Pavan Patel and Nikolaos T. Pyrsopoulos

Key Concepts

- Currently available hepatic assist devices have limited studies in acute liver failure
- Complex physiologic liver functions cannot be emulated despite advances in technology
- Extracorporeal devices may be of benefit in the subset of patients with acute liver failure
- Better randomized-controlled trials with strict inclusion and exclusion criteria as well as high power will need to be undertaken to fully understand the utility of these devices.

67.1 Introduction

Patients with acute liver failure (ALF) require liver transplant for definitive therapy unless the liver is able to regenerate. Many patients however may not survive until a suitable liver is available or may not be candidates for transplant. In addition, patients with long-standing liver disease may undergo sudden onset of decline and acute liver failure which is termed acute on chronic liver failure (ACLF) which may not be amenable to standard medical therapy [1].

Therefore, other treatment modalities that may reduce morbidity and mortality and perhaps serve as a bridge to transplantation may be an additional option. One particular avenue that has been investigated are the hepatic assist devices. Such devices aim to temporarily assume metabolic and excretory functions of the liver and thereby allow stabilization of patients who await transplant. This chapter will focus on the bioartificial devices that incorporate liver cells to accomplish this task [2–6].

P. Patel · N. T. Pyrsopoulos (✉)
Division of Gastroenterology and Hepatology, Rutgers—New Jersey Medical School, Newark, NJ, USA
e-mail: patel338@njms.rutgers.edu; pyrsopni@njms.rutgers.edu

67.2 Bioartificial Liver Support (BALS)

The BALS are based on the concept of dialysis with cell-based techniques that utilize animal or human liver cells to replace all of the intricate detoxification, synthetic (proteins and clotting factors) regulatory (hormones) and immunologic functions of the liver. This is accomplished by incorporating a bioreactor into the extracorporeal circuit that consists of hepatocytes. These cells are cultured in a 3-D matrix and surrounded by fibers that allow capillary perfusion. Oxygen and carbon dioxide are exchanged and glucose is supplied to mimic human physiology [7].

However, the limitations of producing such devices lies in the complexity of the liver functions themselves. The main issues that arise in the development of these devices is the selection of the source of liver cells and the stabilization of normal physiologic function with the artificial bioreactors [8].

The ideal bioartificial liver assist device would use human hepatocytes to closely mimic human physiology. However, a good-quality source of a large number of these cells is not currently available to accomplish this task. Most human hepatocytes would come from unused cadavers or from partial hepatectomy specimens which are uncommon. The quality of these specimens is inadequate as the better-quality ones are usually used for liver transplantation.

Currently the two cell sources that have been used in human clinical trials for bioartificial liver support systems are the human hepatoblastoma cell line, HepG2/C3A and primary hepatocytes from healthy pig livers [9].

C3A cells have numerous proteins that produce anti-inflammatory effects. They express anti-apoptotic and

F. Radu-Ionita et al. (eds.), *Liver Diseases*, https://doi.org/10.1007/978-3-030-24432-3_67

anti-oxidative mechanisms that decrease hepatocellular injury. They also express growth factors that are involved in regeneration of hepatocytes following acute phase response to injury [10].

67.3 Extracorporeal Liver Assist Device

The Extracorporeal Liver Assist Device (ELAD®) is a bioartificial liver assist device. Cartridges containing hollow fibers filled with human hepatoblastoma cell lines, HepG2/C3A, are employed in this device. These cells have hepatocyte properties, such as a functional CYP450 enzyme system and the ability to produce liver-specific proteins. They have shown a higher level of albumin secretion as well. It employs the use of whole blood for perfusion and can be continued for long periods of time [11]. These cell lines are originally from human liver tumor and therefore there is a theoretical risk that tumor dissemination can occur. However, there have been no reports of transmission of cancer thus far in the patients treated with these cells [12].

67.3.1 Extracorporeal Circuit

The system is connected in a closed circuit via venous access gained by placement of a double-lumen dialysis catheter in either the internal jugular or femoral vein. Four ELAD cartridges are used in this circuit to give a hepatocyte mass of 400 g. These cartridges are composed of thousands of hollow fibers that are semipermeable. The C3A cells are grown in the extracapillary space around these hollow fibers. Patient's blood is ultra-filtrated to isolated plasma ultra-filtrate. This plasma is then pumped through these cartridges via a standard dialysis pump at a rate of 150–200 mL/min. Anticoagulation is achieved using heparin with an initial bolus and then continuous infusion to achieve an activated clotting time of 200–250 s. An oxygenator is used to ensure adequate oxygen supply to the cells. Negative pressure is applied across the membranes to achieve an ultra-filtrate before being returned to the patient [13, 14]. A schematic representation can be seen in Fig. 67.1.

67.3.2 Studies

A phase 1 trial was performed in 11 patients most of which had acute liver failure. Improvement in mental status occurred in 8 of the 11 patients. Of the group, 4 were successfully bridged to OLT and six patients died before OLT while 1 survived without OLT [15].

The pilot ELAD study enrolled 24 patients with acute liver failure, 17 of whom had been considered to have potentially recoverable disease (Group 1) and 7 that had been listed for transplant (Group 2). Each of these subsets were then randomly assigned to ELAD vs. control (standard medical therapy). The median period of treatment was 72 h. There were no issues with biocompatibility and patients remained hemodynamically stable on the device. Six patients in Group 1 deteriorated and were placed on the waiting list for OLT. In patients treated with ELAD, ammonia, bilirubin and hepatic encephalopathy improved when compared to standard medical treatment. There was no survival benefit in either group (survival rates were 78% and 75% in Group 1 and 33% and 25% in Group 2) for patients treated with and without ELAD, respectively [14].

In a follow-up study in which ultra-filtrate was used instead of whole blood, Millis et al., studied [5] patients with ALF who were bridged to transplant using ELAD. The patients tolerated the treatment well and the clinical course for the treated patients appeared to be stabilized. The 30-day survival rate was 75%. Other parameters that showed

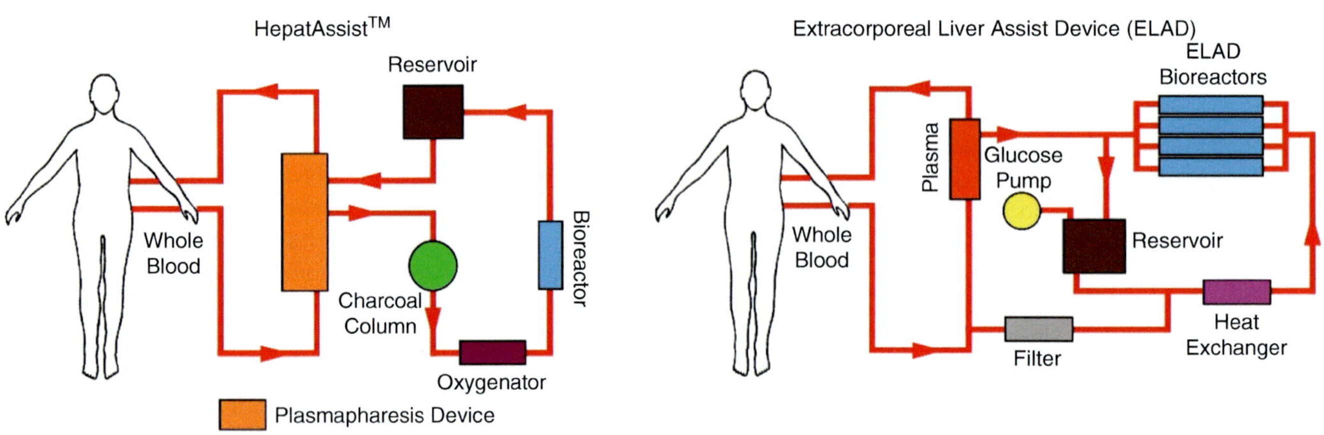

Fig. 67.1 Schematic extracorporeal circuit for HepatAssist and ELAD devices

improvement included mean arterial pressures, cerebral perfusion pressures, and reduction in cardiovascular and ventilator support [13].

An open-label randomized controlled trial was conducted in two Chinese Centers to evaluate ELAD in patients with chronic hepatitis B and C infection. A total of 49 patients were enrolled of which 32 were treated with ELAD. The 28-day transplant-free survival was 47% in the control group vs. 81% in the ELAD group ($p = 0.022$). Total bilirubin level decreased by 25% in the ELAD group vs. 37% increase in the control group ($p < 0.001$). Thrombocytopenia occurred in a majority of patients however with a mean drop in counts of 28% from baseline. However, the counts recovered within 5 days of ELAD discontinuation [16].

More recently, a randomized multi-center clinical trial using ELAD for patients with severe alcoholic hepatitis was published (VTI-208 [Assess Safety and Efficacy of ELAD (Extracorporeal Liver Assist System) in Subjects with Alcohol-Induced Liver Failure]). The study population was defined as adults ≥18 years of age with last drink within 6 weeks of rapid onset of jaundice (serum bilirubin ≥8 mg/dL) and coagulopathy (Maddrey's DF ≥ 32) and Model for End-Stage Liver Disease (MELD) score ≤35. Patients were randomized to ELAD for 3–5 days plus standard of care vs. standard of care alone. Unfortunately, after a minimum follow-up of 91 days, there was no significant difference in overall survival between groups. However, in a pre-specified analysis in patients with MELD < 28 there was a trend toward higher survival at 91 days (68.6% vs. 53.6%; $p = 0.08$). Using regression analysis, high creatinine and INR were associated with negative outcomes. Therefore a new trial investigating the potential benefit of ELAD in younger patients with sufficient renal function and less severe coagulopathy was done in 2018 [10]. Unfortunately, the study failed to meet the primary endpoint of overall survival through 91 days using the Kaplan Meier statistical method. The secondary endpoint of proportion of survivors at study day 91 was also not statistically different between study groups. There were no differences between groups regarding safety and tolerability of the treatment. Therefore, at this time, ELAD cannot be approved for management of either ALF or ACLF until further studies are completed.

Smaller studies have been presented regarding the anti-inflammatory effects of the C3A cells based on data from VTL-208. Plasma from cohorts with severe alcoholic hepatitis that met inclusion criteria were assayed for a variety of inflammatory markers. When compared to controls, levels of procalcitonin and ferritin were significantly reduced in ELAD patients. Levels of Interleukin-1 receptor antagonist (IL-1Ra) which reduces inflammation was higher in the ELAD arm as well. This may suggest that HepG2/C3A cells release products that dampen the inflammatory response [17].

67.4 HepatAssist™

HepatAssist (Alliqua Inc., Langhorne, PA, USA) is made from porcine hepatocytes that are contained within a hollow fiber bioreactor [18]. It uses plasma that is obtained from the patient's blood that is separated via plasmapheresis and then passed through the circuit containing porcine hepatocytes.

67.4.1 Extracorporeal Circuit

The system includes a perfusion pump, a charcoal column, an oxygenator, and custom tubing that connects the various components to a plasmapheresis machine [19]. During its use, plasmapheresis is performed via a double-lumen catheter. The plasma is pumped into the HepatAssist device and continuously circulates the plasma through the hollow fiber reactor. The charcoal provides detoxification and diminishes the toxin load applied to the hepatocytes. The membrane oxygenator ensures adequate oxygen supply. The plasma flows through the hollow fibers that are surrounded by the porcine hepatocytes. There are $5–7 \times 10^9$ cryopreserved porcine hepatocytes attached to beads which are inoculated into the extrafiber compartment. The pore size is small enough to prevent cell debris from passing into the patient [18]. This can be seen in Fig. 67.1. An improved version, HepatAssist-2 was created with an increased cell mass of 15×10^9 hepatocytes.

67.4.2 Studies

The largest, randomized, multicenter trial involving HepatAssist involved 171 patients with ALF or primary nonfunction after liver transplantation. The patients in the HepatAssist group underwent 6 h of treatment with the number of treatments ranging from 1 to 9 (mean 2.9) per patient. The 30-day survival was 71% versus 62% ($P = 0.26$) for the HepatAssist group compared to standard medical therapy, respectively. The study was stopped prematurely due to futility in the safety interim analysis. Though there was no survival benefit in the overall cohort, survival in the subgroup of patients with fulminant or sub-fulminant hepatic failure was significantly higher in the HepatAssist group compared with control with a 44% reduction in mortality ($P = 0.048$). Serum bilirubin had a statistically significant reduction in patients receiving HepatAssist, however there were no changes in encephalopathy, hemodynamics, or other lab values. In the subgroup of patients with acute liver failure, there was a significant difference in the time to death within the first 30 days compared to the control group ($p = 0.009$). No zoonosis or immune reactions were reported though this still remains a concern [18]. Despite the survival benefit identified in a post hoc subgroup analysis, the FDA did not approve the HepatAssist device.

67.5 Modular Extracorporeal Liver Support System (MELS)

MELS was Initially developed by Gerlach et al. in Berlin, Germany using a unique multi-compartment bioreactor unit (CellModule) and detoxification unit (DetoxModule) using the concept of single-pass albumin dialysis for removing albumin-bound toxins [20].

67.5.1 Extracorporeal Circuit

The bioreactor contains three interwoven hollow-fiber membranes aimed at reproducing the liver vascular network [21]. Up to 600 g of porcine hepatocytes or human hepatocytes are inoculated into the extracapillary space. The patient's plasma is separated from the blood via plasma filter and recirculated through the hollow fibers at 200–250 cm^3/min. The device can combine different extracorporeal units that can be personalized to patient needs using either single pass albumin dialysis (SPAD) or continuous veno-venous hemodialysis (CVVHD) [22]. The first system used primary porcine cells from pigs. Later MELS became the only system that used primary human hepatocytes isolated from donor livers as well as porcine hepatocytes.

67.5.2 Studies

In a phase 1 clinical study published in 2003 by Sauer et al., eight patients with acute liver failure were treated with MELS continuously for 8–46 h. All patients were successfully bridged to OLT with 100% 3-year survival. More importantly, the therapy was well tolerated [20].

Due to rising concern for xenogenic infections using porcine cells, primary human cells were isolated from discarded donor organs as an alternative source. Cells from 54 human livers were isolated from grafts that were not suitable for transplant due to a variety of reasons (steatosis, cirrhosis, and fibrosis) [23]. Prepared bioreactors using these cells were then used to treat 8 patients with liver failure for 7–144 h. Once again, no adverse events were observed. Six of these patients were bridged successfully to transplant and the other two were not due to active alcohol consumption. In all patients, neurological and coagulation status improved during the treatment [20].

67.6 Bioartificial Liver Support System (BLSS)

The BLSS system was first developed at the University of Pittsburgh and employed the use of semipermeable cellulose acetate hollow fibers containing porcine hepatocytes. It uses whole blood perfusion instead of plasma [24].

67.6.1 Extracorporeal Circuit

The BLSS consists of a blood pump, heat exchanger to control the temperature of the blood being exchanged, oxygenator, and a bioreactor. The bioreactor contains hollow fibers with cellulose acetate membranes with a 100 kDa size cutoff. About 70–100 g of primary porcine hepatocytes are harvested and infused into the extraluminal space of the bioreactor. After loading these hepatocytes, the bioreactor is kept under physiologic conditions in an incubator prior to use with the patient. Oxygenation and pH control is maintained with the use of mass flow controllers [25].

67.6.2 Studies

The first clinical use of BLSS was in a 41-year old patient with acute liver failure. After treatment with BLSS the patient's ammonia, total bilirubin and lactate all improved. In addition, the coagulation function and clinical symptoms also improved and the patient was removed from the treatment [25].

A phase 1 clinical trial was then done on 4 patients with different etiologies of acute liver failure including acetaminophen toxicity, Wilson's disease, acute alcoholic hepatitis and chemotherapy. The mean ammonia and total bilirubin levels decreased after treatment (33% and 6% respectively). Renal and neurologic function did not improve however and survival data was not mentioned. All patients tolerated the system well [26].

67.7 Conclusions

Though orthotopic liver transplantation is the gold standard therapy for treating acute liver failure, there have been dramatic advances in liver support strategies to cope with the shortage in available donor organs. As outlined above and in Table 67.1, bio-artificial extracorporeal cellular assist devices have shown some promise. However, due to difficulty in creating a well-structured randomized-controlled trial with adequate power is difficult in this diverse population. In addition, standard medical therapy varies from institution to institution and therefore broad applicability is

Table 67.1 Bioartificial liver assist devices study outcomes

Study	N	Device	Cell type	Outcome
VTI-208, 2015 [10]	203	ELAD	Human (cultured C3A)	No survival benefit at 90 days
VTL-308, 2018	151	ELAD	Human (cultured C3A)	No survival benefit at 90 days
Ellis et al. [14]	24	ELAD	Human (cultured C3A)	No survival benefit
Demetriou et al. [18]	171	HepatAssist	Porcine	No survival benefit at 30 days
Sauer et al. [20, 22]	8	MELS	Porcine	100% Survival benefit as bridge to transplant
Mazariegos et al. [26]	4	BLSS	Porcine	No survival data

difficult. Treatment with these devices is usually followed by urgent OLT and therefore the 30-day survival is largely influenced by the outcomes of the OLT. The published results point towards the need for new trials with improvements in the system. The obvious limitations of these support systems are the membranes used for appropriate exchange and the lack of complete physiologic function. The government has yet to approve any of these bioartificial systems for this reason.

In addition, new approaches not using extracorporeal devices such as hepatocyte transplantation, repopulation of decellularized livers, organogenesis and stem cell transplant appear to be appealing. Further research is in need in order to improve survival of this difficult to manage population.

Self Study

Question

1. Which statement is true?
   (a) ELAD employs the use of porcine hepatocytes
   (b) MELS employs the use of only porcine hepatocytes
   (c) HepatAssist employs the use of porcine hepatocytes
   (d) BLSS uses plasma for exchange

Answer

1. Which statement is true?
   (a) ELAD uses human hepatoblastoma cells not porcine hepatocytes
   (b) MELS uses both porcine and human hepatocytes
   (c) CORRECT ANSWER. HepatAssist uses porcine hepatocytes
   (d) BLSS uses whole blood for exchange not plasma

References

1. Jepsen P, Ott P, Andersen PK, Sørensen HT, Vilstrup H. Clinical course of alcoholic liver cirrhosis: a Danish population-based cohort study. Hepatology. 2010;51:1675. https://doi.org/10.1002/hep.23500.
2. Rahman H. Review article: liver support systems in acute hepatic failure. Aliment Pharmacol Ther. 1999;13(10):1255–72. https://doi.org/10.1046/j.1365-2036.1999.00597.x.
3. Riordan SM, Williams R. Extracorporeal support and hepatocyte transplantation in acute liver failure and cirrhosis. J Gastroenterol Hepatol. 1999;14(8):757–70. https://doi.org/10.1046/j.1440-1746.1999.01945.x.
4. Allen JW, Hassanein T, Bhatia SN. Advances in bioartificial liver devices. Hepatology. 2001;34(3):447–55. https://doi.org/10.1053/jhep.2001.26753.
5. Keeffe EB. Liver transplantation: current status and novel approaches to liver replacement. Gastroenterology. 2001;120(3):749–62. https://doi.org/10.1053/gast.2001.22583.
6. Pless G. Artificial and bioartificial liver support. Organogenesis. 2007;3:20. https://doi.org/10.4161/org.3.1.3635.
7. van Wenum M, Chamuleau RA, van Gulik TM, Siliakus A, Seppen J, Hoekstra R. Bioartificial livers *in vitro* and *in vivo* : tailoring biocomponents to the expanding variety of applications. Expert Opin Biol Ther. 2014;14:1745. https://doi.org/10.1517/14712598.2014.950651.
8. Leckie P, Davenport A, Jalan R. Extracorporeal liver support. Blood Purif. 2012;34(2):158–63. https://doi.org/10.1159/000342065.
9. Chen HS, Nyberg SL. Acute liver failure and bioartificial liver support. 8th ed. Amsterdam: Elsevier Inc.; 2018. https://doi.org/10.1016/B978-0-323-40232-3.00128-X.
10. Thompson J, Jones N, Al-Khafaji A, et al. Extracorporeal cellular therapy (ELAD) in severe alcoholic hepatitis: a multinational, prospective, controlled, randomized trial. Liver Transpl. 2018;24:380. https://doi.org/10.1002/lt.24986.
11. Gislason GT, Lobdell DD, Kelly JH, Sussman NL. A treatment system for implementing an extracorporeal liver assist device. Artif Organs. 1994;18(5):385–9. https://doi.org/10.1111/j.1525-1594.1994.tb02220.x.
12. Tritto G, Davies N, Jalan R. Liver replacement therapy. Semin Respir Crit Care Med. 2012;33:70. https://doi.org/10.1055/s-0032-1301736.
13. Millis JM, Cronin DC, Johnson R, et al. Initial experience with the modified extracorporeal liver-assist device for patients with fulminant hepatic failure: system modifications and clinical impact. Transplantation. 2002;74(12):1735–46. https://doi.org/10.1097/01.TP.0000038483.93833.21.
14. Ellis AJ, Hughes RD, Wendon JA, et al. Pilot-controlled trial of the extracorporeal liver assist device in acute liver failure. Hepatology. 1996;24(6):1446–51. https://doi.org/10.1053/jhep.1996.v24.pm0008938179.
15. Sussman NL, Kelly JH. Improved liver function following treatment with an extracorporeal liver assist device. Artif Organs. 1993;17:27. https://doi.org/10.1111/j.1525-1594.1993.tb00381.x.
16. Duan Z, Xin S, Zhang J, et al. Comparison of extracorporeal cellular therapy (ELAD) vs standard of care in a randomized controlled clinical trial in treating Chinese subjects with acute-on-chronic liver failure. Hepatic Med Evid Res. 2018;10:139–52. https://doi.org/10.2147/HMER.S180246.

17. Landeen LK, Lapetoda J, Bedard PW, et al. Sa1449 - inflammation biomarkers decrease during ELAD treatment in alcoholic hepatitis subjects. Gastroenterology. 2018;154(6):S–1117. https://doi.org/10.1016/S0016-5085(18)33716-8.
18. Demetriou AA, Brown RS, Busuttil RW, et al. Prospective, randomized, multicenter, controlled trial of a bioartificial liver in treating acute liver failure. Ann Surg. 2004;239(5):660–70. https://doi.org/10.1097/01.sla.0000124298.74199.e5.
19. Watanabe FD, Mullon CJ, Hewitt WR, et al. Clinical experience with a bioartificial liver in the treatment of severe liver failure. A phase I clinical trial. Ann Surg. 1997;225(5):484–91-4. https://doi.org/10.1097/00000658-199705000-00005.
20. Sauer IM, Kardassis D, Zeillinger K, et al. Clinical extracorporeal hybrid liver support--phase I study with primary porcine liver cells. Xenotransplantation. 2003;10:460–9. https://doi.org/10.1034/j.1399-3089.2003.00062.x.
21. Gerlach JC, Encke J, Hole O, Müller C, Ryan CJ, Neuhaus P. Bioreactor for a larger scale hepatocyte in vitro perfusion. Transplantation. 1994;58:984. https://doi.org/10.1097/00007890-199411150-00002.
22. Sauer IM, Zeilinger K, Pless G, et al. Extracorporeal liver support based on primary human liver cells and albumin dialysis - treatment of a patient with primary graft non-function. J Hepatol. 2003;39:649. https://doi.org/10.1016/S0168-8278(03)00348-9.
23. Sauer IM, Zeilinger K, Obermayer N, et al. Primary human liver cells as source for modular extracorporeal liver support--a preliminary report. Int J Artif Organs. 2002;25:1001.
24. Patzer JF, Mazariegos GV, Lopez R, et al. Novel bioartificial liver support system: preclinical evaluation. Ann N Y Acad Sci. 1999;875:340–52. https://doi.org/10.1111/j.1749-6632.1999.tb08516.x.
25. Mazariegos GV, Patzer JF, Lopez RC, et al. First clinical use of a novel Bioartificial Liver Support System (BLSS). Am J Transplant. 2002;2(3):260–6. https://doi.org/10.1034/j.1600-6143.2002.20311.x.
26. Mazariegos GV, Kramer DJ, Lopez RC, et al. Safety observations in Phase I clinical evaluation of the excorp medical bioartificial liver support system after the first four patients. ASAIO J. 2001;47(5):471–5. https://doi.org/10.1097/00002480-200109000-00015.

Liver Transplantation for Acute and Chronic Liver Failure

68

Tehilla Apfel and Nikolaos T. Pyrsopoulos

Key Concepts
- Liver transplantation is a life-saving procedure for patients with acute and chronic liver diseases.
- Allocation of organs and indications for organ transplantation is an ever developing process, with refinements continuously being implemented in the hopes of developing an equitable way to allocate grafts but some ethical dilemmas have been formulated.
- As the population ages, new considerations for evaluation for cardiovascular risk factors in the pre-listing are required
- New developments in surgical techniques for "splitting" organs and for criteria for graft acceptance such as "extended criteria livers" has increased the graft supply

68.1 Introduction

The American Association for the Study of Liver Diseases (AASLD) and the American Society of Transplantation (AST) issued updated guidelines in 2013 for evaluation of liver transplantation (LT) in adults in acknowledgement of the changing landscape of transplant medicine that has occurred with the development of treatments for viral hepatitis, the increasing longevity of the population, and the impact of the increasing number of patients with metabolic syndrome leading to the development of Non-alcoholic fatty liver disease (NAFLD) [4]. NAFLD has become an increasingly prominent cause of cirrhosis and hepatocellular carcinoma requiring LT [5]. As such the makeup of the individuals eligible for liver transplantation has slowly shifted.

Access to LT has profoundly altered the management of advanced liver disease. Management of decompensated cirrhosis and acute liver failure before the introduction of LT was limited to attempts to treat complications, but without the ability to extend life. Without liver transplantation the 1-year survival rate for patients with decompensated cirrhosis is less than 10%, but increases to 85–90% at 1 year and 75% at 5 years after LT [6]. When liver transplantation is successful it increases life expectancy and enhances quality of life [7].

68.2 Liver Allocation

Prior to 2002, liver allocation was based on the Child-Turcotte-Pugh (CPT) score, which took into account clinical parameters (encephalopathy and ascites) and laboratory values (bilirubin, albumin, and prothrombin time). In the past, a CPT score of 7 or greater was considered the minimum listing criteria for liver transplantation [8]. The Model for End-stage Liver Disease (MELD) score replaced the CPT score as it was found to be a better predictor of mortality for listed patients [9]. The MELD score was initially designed to evaluate 3-month prognosis in patients with cirrhosis undergoing a transjugular intrahepatic portosystemic shunt [10]. It is a mathematical model that is calculated from laboratory values (creatinine, bilirubin, the international normalized ratio of prothrombin time) and does not take into account clinical presentation [11]. In an important paper by Merion et al., transplant survival was observed in patients with a MELD score of at least 18, and increased with higher MELD scores [12]. However, recipients who underwent liver transplantation (LT) with a MELD score less than 15 had higher 1-year mortality rates compared to individuals with comparable MELD scores who remained on the waitlist [7]. This highlights another complexity to organ allocation, the need to

T. Apfel · N. T. Pyrsopoulos (✉)
Division of Gastroenterology and Hepatology, Rutgers—New Jersey Medical School, Newark, NJ, USA
e-mail: ta431@njms.rutgers.edu; pyrsopni@njms.rutgers.edu

F. Radu-Ionita et al. (eds.), *Liver Diseases*, https://doi.org/10.1007/978-3-030-24432-3_68

both offer transplantation to the patients with the greatest need, but also to avoid liver transplantation in patients who could potentially improve without liver transplantation and would therefore be placed at unnecessary risk.

Refining the process to determine the best prognostication score for organ allocation is a dynamic process. Recently, studies showed that incorporating sodium into the MELD score increases its accuracy at predicting survival. A pivotal study showed that by calculating the MELD with sodium (MELD-Na), 7% of waiting-list deaths could be prevented [13]. Hyponatremia was also found to be a marker for increased neurologic dysfunction post-liver transplantation [8]. Therefore, in 2016 the MELD-Na became the predictive model used to facilitate liver allocation by The United Network for Organ Sharing (UNOS) [14]. The MELD-Na score does have some disadvantages as described in Table 68.1 and therefore other predictive models have been proposed, such as a MELD-X calculation which excludes INR, but it has not yet been validated [15].

Additionally, the MELD score does not take into account that many liver conditions have a high risk of morbidity and mortality without significantly affecting the laboratory values incorporated in the MELD-Na score. For this reason, MELD exception points are granted to individuals with hepatocellular carcinoma, hepatopulmonary syndrome, porto-pulmonary hypertension, cholangiocarcinoma, and familial amyloidosis to decrease their waitlist time (Table 68.2) [16].

Deterioration in a patient's quality of life is not reflected adequately in predictive models, including the MELD score. For instance, many patient suffer from life-interfering symptoms such as sever pruritus, fatigue, and in the case of Primary Sclerosing Cholangitis, recurrent bacterial cholangitis [17]. Therefore, in extreme situation MELD exception points can be requested from UNOS on a case by case basis. Studies have shown that patients with a MELD score of less than 15 appear to have better survival without transplantation than with transplantation [18]. That is why patients with a MELD score of less than 10 are not eligible for active listing with UNOS unless they have received exception points [18].

Table 68.1 Limitations of the MELD score

Male gender bias
PT/INR not developed for measuring abnormalities in the setting of cirrhosis
Disadvantageous for candidates with low MELD-Na and complications of cirrhosis
Serum creatinine is not reliable marker of renal function in cirrhosis
Interlaboratory variability of serum creatinine, bilirubin, and INR
Weak predictor of posttransplant mortality as it does not take into account donor characteristics
Bilirubin levels can be influenced by extrahepatic factors

MELD model for end-stage liver disease

Patients with certain clinical presentations including fulminant hepatic failure, primary graft nonfunction, and acute hepatic artery thrombosis are given the highest priority and a status 1A designation and listed first regardless of MELD score [19]. For patients with cirrhosis, the highest MELD score within a specific location and blood group determines the order on the waiting list for liver transplantation. If multiple patients have the same MELD score, priority for liver transplantation is then based on the amount of time spent at the current MELD score. In 2013 "Share-35" was implemented which changed the allocation algorithm, so that liver offers were made within the local organ procurement organization, then regionally. According to the AASLD, Share-35 led to a 6.6% increase in the number of transplants performed for patients with MELD score of 35, with follow-up data showing that this change had not impact on overall waiting-list mortality, post-transplant survival, or liver discard rate [15]. In 2018, a new policy was implemented which changes how livers are allocated in the United States of America. Previously, livers were allocated to recipients based which geographical region the donor was in. The new policy has discarded the idea of regions, and instead livers are offered to recipients based on a radius determined by nautical miles. This policy change was made in hopes of reducing geographic disparity and making the process of liver allocation more equitable [15].

68.3 Orthotopic Liver Transplantation

Orthotopic liver transplantation (OLT) refers to the placement of a new organ in the same location as the ex-planted liver. Although most LT recipients receive a whole organ from a deceased donor, we now are able to split a liver with, most commonly, a pediatric recipient receiving a left lateral segment and an adult recipient the larger right lobe. The method of splitting livers has also allowed for the development of live donor liver transplantations (LDLT) with a part of the liver removed from the donor and given to the recipient. Adult LDLT reduces waiting time for the recipient. In Europe and United States, the graft supply is predominantly deceased donor, with living donor transplant comprises only 4% of all liver transplants [20]. LDLT might raise some concerns due to potential risks to the donor including perioperative morbidity and mortality, economic losses, issues with obtaining life insurance in the future, a lack of data on possible downstream effects after liver surgery which may cause biliary abnormalities and potential medical complications later in life [17, 21]. Additionally, "extended-criteria grafts" are now being employed to increase the donor liver supply. "Extended criteria grafts" are livers that are not normally considered "optimum" such as organs from older donors (age > 55) and from non–heart-beating donors, which often leads to longer cold

Table 68.2 Standardized MELD exceptions per UNOS guidelines

Disease	Diagnostic criteria	Listed MELD SCORE	Adjustments
Cholangiocarcinoma (CCA)	The candidate must meet a specific hospital approved protocol and have documented hilar CCA.	22	10% increase in score every 3 months while on the wait list
Cystic Fibrosis	Reduced pulmonary function and FEV1 < 40%	22	10% increase in score every 3 months while on the wait list
Familial Amyloid Polyneuropathy (FAP)	The candidate has all of the following: 1. Clear diagnosis of FAP. 2. Echocardiogram showing the candidate has an EF > 40% 3. Ambulatory status. 4. Identification of transthyretin (TTR gene) mutation (Val30Met vs. non-Val30Met). 5. Biopsy-proven amyloid in the involved organ.	22	10% increase in score every 3 months while on the wait list
Hepatic Artery Thrombosis (HAT)	The candidate has HAT within 14 days of transplant but does not meet criteria for status 1A	40	NA
Hepatocellular Carcinoma (HCC)	The candidate must meet specific HCC criteria for listing which is based on the number and size of lesions identified.	Calculated MELD score	Every 90 days an additional extension request can be submitted and if approved the MELD score will be adjusted The maximum score is capped at 34 after 5 requests.
Hepatopulmonary Syndrome (HPS)	All of the following: 1. Clinical evidence of portal hypertension. 2. Evidence of a shunt. 3. PaO2 less than 60 mmHg on room air. 4. No significant clinical evidence of underlying primary pulmonary disease	22	10% increase in score every 3 months as long as the PaO2 remains under 60 mmHg
Portopulmonary Hypertension (PHT)	The candidate meets criteria for PHT and shows documentation of post-vasodilator treatment MAP < 35 mmHg and PVR < 400 dynes/s/cm^{-5}	22	10% increase in score every 3 months as long as MPAP remains <35 mmHg
Primary Hyperoxaluria	The candidate has all of the following: 1. Is registered for a combined liver-kidney transplant. 2. Alanine glyoxylate aminotransferase (AGT) deficiency proven by liver biopsy using sample analysis or genetic analysis. 3. GFR ≤ 25 mL/min for 42 or more days	28	10% increase in score every 3 months while on the wait list

MELD model for end-stage liver disease, *FEV1* Forced expiratory volume at 1 s, *EF* ejection fraction, *MPAP* mean pulmonary arterial pressure, *PVR* pulmonary vascular resistance, *GFR* glomerular filtration rate

ischemia time (>10 h) or warm ischemia time (>40 min). Using "extended-criteria graft", however, increases the frequency of biliary complications such as the development of biliary stricture post-transplantation, as well as abdominal hernias, and post-traumatic stress disorder [22].

68.4 Indications for Liver Transplantation

According to the AASLD, evaluation for LT should be considered once a patient with cirrhosis has experienced a complication from his condition such as ascites, hepatic encephalopathy, variceal hemorrhage (Table 68.3) or if her MELD-Na Score is 15 or greater reflecting hepatocellular dysfunction [4]. Referral to a transplant center for evaluation should occur early as to not delay the patient's work-up as decompensation can occur rapidly. Individuals with well-compensated cirrhosis do not require liver transplant evaluation. It is important to always weigh the risk of surgery against an assessment of the potential recipient's prognosis without LT. A not so common, but important indication is acute liver failure (ALF), which accounts for 8% of all transplant cases [23]. ALF is a life threatening presentation of hepatic encephalopathy and liver test abnormalities, especially INR, in patients without previous documented liver disease [24]. Without, transplantation

Table 68.3 Indications for liver transplantation

Acute liver failure
Complications of cirrhosis
Ascites
Chronic gastrointestinal blood loss due to portal hypertensive gastropathy
Hepatic Encephalopathy
Liver cancer
Refractory variceal hemorrhage
Synthetic dysfunction
Liver-based metabolic conditions with systemic manifestations
a1-Antitrypsin deficiency
Familial amyloidosis
Glycogen storage disease
Hemochromatosis
Primary oxaluria
Wilson disease
Systemic complications of chronic liver disease
Hepatopulmonary syndrome
Portopulmonary hypertension

mortality rates have been recorded as high as 50–83% [24]. With LT, survival rates are drastically improved with documented 1-year survival rates are 79% in Europe and 84% in the United States [25].

68.5 Transplantation Evaluation and Listing

Individuals referred to a transplant center are required to undergo rigorous testing and evaluation by a multi-specialty team to determine his or her suitability for listing. As delineated in Table 68.4, the process involves not only medical investigations, but also in-depth examination of the social, psychological, and financial circumstances of the patient to ascertain their ability to successfully navigate the difficulties presented after transplantation. Candidates who meet all the listing criteria should be placed on the waiting list.

Table 68.4 Steps prior to listing

Financial screening	Secure approval for the evaluation
Medical and Hepatology evaluation	Identify interventions such as prophylaxis of variceal hemorrhage or vaccination against hepatitis A and B that are appropriate in any patient with advanced liver disease
Laboratory testing	Assess hepatic synthetic function, serum electrolytes, renal function, viral serologies, markers of other causes of liver disease, tumor markers, ABO-Rh blood typing; 24-h urine for creatinine clearance; urinalysis and urine drug screen
Cardiac evaluation	Electrocardiography and 2-dimensional echocardiography; stress testing and potential cardiac catheterization, cardiology consult if risk factors are present and/or the patient is ≥40 years old
Imaging	Ultrasound with Doppler to document portal vein patency, multi-phase dynamic imaging such as triple-phase CT, MRI, or gadolinium MRI for tumor screening
Cancer Screening	Chest film, prostate-specific antigen level (men), Pap smear and mammogram (women), colonoscopy if the patient is ≥50 years or has PSC
Surgery evaluation	Assessment of technical issues and discuss the risks of the procedure
Anesthesia evaluation	Required if operative risk is unusually high
Dietitian/ Nutritionist	Many patients with cirrhosis have protein-calorie malnutrition
Psychiatry and psychology evaluation	Necessary if there is a history of substance abuse, psychiatric illness, or adjustment difficulties

68.6 Important Medical Concerns for Listing

68.6.1 Age

With an aging population, increased life expectancy, and increasing prevalence of NAFLD, older individual are requiring liver transplant evaluations. The AASLD, recommends evaluating patients based on their physiologic age and not their chronological age to determine whether an older patient can be accepted for LT [4]. Careful attention must still be made to the patient's comorbidities and functional status. Transplantation has been successful in recipients over age 70. However, outcomes have still been reported as inferior to younger individuals, with a reported 73.3% survival at 1 year for individuals >70 years in one single center prospective study compared to reported survival rates of >90% at 1 year patients of all ages combined [26]. Therefore, in a healthy individual older recipient age is not a contraindication.

68.6.2 Obesity

Obesity in liver transplant candidates is on the rise in proportion with the increasing prevalence of NAFLD and obesity in the general population [27]. Obesity and metabolic syndrome are associated with increased risk of complications and poorer outcomes following LT [27]. Therefore, AASLD recommends obese patients with BMI of 30 or more undergo dietary counseling prior to listing. Additionally, BMI of 40 or more is considered a relative contraindication for listing [4].

68.6.3 Coronary Artery Disease

Cardiac evaluation pre-LT is necessary to assess perioperative risk and to evaluate for cardiopulmonary disorders that would lead to poor outcome post-LT [28]. Coronary artery disease (CAD) is equally prevalent in patients with advanced liver disease as it is in the general population [29]. Before listing, cardiac evaluation with stress testing is required if a patient is 40 years or older or shows any signs or symptoms concerning for CAD. Often due to decompensation, patients will require pharmacologic stress testing or cardiac catheterization as they are unable to achieve the targeted heart rate required in standard exercise testing. Special consideration must be taken with cardiac catheterization as patients with advanced liver disease often have abnormal renal function putting them at risk for contrast induced nephropathy. Additionally, cirrhotic patients with coagulopathy or thrombocytopenia are at higher risk for bleeding complications from cardiac catheterization [4]. If significant CAD is found with stenosis >70%, revascularization will be required before listing. Angioplasty with bare metal stent placement is preferred in cirrhotic patients with advanced liver disease as to mitigate the need for dual antiplatelet therapy in patients at high risk for bleeding [30]. Evaluation of valvular heart disease may also be required pre-LT.

68.6.4 Porto-Pulmonary Hypertension

Porto-pulmonary hypertension (POPH) is the presence of elevated mean pulmonary artery pressure (MPAP) over 25 mmHg occurring in the presence of portal hypertension [31]. Approximately, 4–8% of LT candidates are reported to have POPH [32]. Moderate and severe POPH, with MPAP of >35 and >45 respectively are predictors of increased mortality after transplantation [4]. "In a report from the Mayo Clinic, mortality was 50% with MPAP >35 mmHg and 100% with MPAP >50 mmHg" [4]. Therefore, screening for POPH with routine echocardiography is required for pre-LT evaluation. If increased right ventricular systolic pressure is noted, then the patient will require right heart catheterization [4]. This is necessary to confirm the diagnosis, evaluate for elevated pulmonary vascular resistance (PVR) 240-dynes s cm and to assess if a patient's POPH is responsive to vasodilator therapy [4]. If the MPAP can be reduced by vasodilator therapy to less than 35 mmHg and PVR to less than 400 dynes s cm then a LT is still possible with good outcomes [4].

68.6.5 Hepatopulmonary Syndrome

In the setting of chronic liver disease and/or portal hypertension, hepatopulmonary syndrome (HPS) can develop. It is caused by intrapulmonary microvascular dilation that leads to arterial deoxygenation [33]. "Intrapulmonary shunting can be demonstrated by contrast echocardiography or by 99mTC macro aggregated albumin (MAA) lung-brain perfusion scanning" [4]. HPS was reported in 5–32% of adult liver transplant candidates [4]. At Mayo Clinic it was shown that LT offered a large survival benefit, with a 5-year survival rate of 76% in LT recipients vs. 26% of matched controls that were not transplanted [34]. In most cases, LT leads to reversal of HPS, although perioperative mortality is reportedly high in those with severe HPS [4]. "UNOS policy assigns a MELD exception score of 22 for patients with evidence of hepatopulmonary syndrome as evidenced by portal hypertension, intrapulmonary shunting, and a room air PaO2 < 60 mmHg, with a 10% mortality equivalent increase in points every 3 months if the PaO2 remains <60 mmHg" [4]. Therefore, the AASSLD recommends screening LT candidates with pulse oximetry and follow-up arterial blood gas as indicated to detect HPS [35].

68.6.6 Renal Dysfunction

Renal insufficiency in patients with advanced liver disease can be due to many things including hepatorenal syndrome which is potentially reversible. Hepatorenal syndrome, is a type of progressive kidney disease due to underlying changes in the way fluid and electrolytes are moved and stored in patient's with advanced liver disease. It is often difficult to distinguish HRS from primary kidney disease in cirrhotic patients. Regardless of the cause, renal insufficiency is associated with poorer outcomes and decreased survival in cirrhotic patients [17].

Candidates who develop renal failure are eligible for a simultaneous liver-kidney transplantation (SLK) where the candidate receives both a liver and kidney from the same deceased donor (ref). The candidate must be listed for both organs and meet the criteria outlined in Table 68.5.

68.6.7 Tobacco Use

Tobacco use is associated with many adverse outcomes in LT recipients, including cardiovascular events, cancer development and an increased incidence of hepatic artery

Table 68.5 Listing criteria for simultaneous liver-kidney transplantation

Diagnosis	Criteria for listing
CKD as defined as a GFR < 60 mL/min for greater than 90 consecutive days	The candidate must meet one of the following criteria: 1. The candidate has begun regularly administered dialysis as an end-stage renal disease (ESRD) patient 2. At the time of registration on the kidney waiting list or in a date after registration the candidate's most recent measured CrCl or GFR ≤ 30 mL/min
Sustained kidney injury	The candidate must meet one of the following criteria for at least 6 weeks: 1. That the candidate has been on dialysis at least once every 7 days. 2. That the candidate has a measured or calculated CrCl or GFR ≤ 25 mL/min at least once every 7 days.
Metabolic disease	A diagnosis of at least one of the following: Hyperoxaluria, Atypical hemolytic uremic syndrome (HUS) from mutations in factor H or factor I, Familial non-neuropathic systemic amyloidosis, Methylmalonic aciduria

CKD chronic kidney disease, *GFR* glomerular filtration rate, *CrCl* calculated creatinine clearance

Table 68.6 Absolute contraindications to liver transplantation

Brain death
Extrahepatic malignancy
History of malignancy with a disease-free period <2 years
Uncontrolled Sepsis
Active substance or alcohol use abuse
AIDS
Severe cardiopulmonary disease
Inability to comply with medical regimen

AIDS acquired immune deficiency syndrome

thrombosis [36]. The AASLD, recommends that tobacco cessation be required of all patients prior to listing [4].

68.6.8 Absolute Contraindications to Transplantation

Absolute contraindications to liver transplantation have been reduced over the last decade. For example, transplantation in HIV positive individuals without active AIDS is now possible. Additionally, the presence of non-tumoral thrombosis of the portal and splanchnic venous systems, which was previously considered a major contraindication to transplantation, can now be done in selected cases. Table 68.6 lists the current absolute contraindications to LT. However, at this time the indication for pre-transplantation abstinence from alcohol is being heavily debated amongst transplant hepatologists as newer research has shown success with liver transplantation for alcoholic hepatitis with good post-LT rates of alcohol abstinence [37]. Therefore, some transplant centers are allowing LT in patients with active alcohol use who do not have a long history of alcohol dependence.

68.7 Early Post-Liver Transplant Complications

Early post-LT complications are usually related to graft dysfunction, surgical issues, and infection [38]. Primary nonfunction (PNF) is a rare, but life-threatening complication in the immediate post-operative period and has been reported to occur in occurring in 2–6% of transplanted patient [39]. According to the strict criteria established by the United Network for Organ Sharing (UNOS; American transplantation regulatory body), PNF is defined as serum AST levels $\geq$3000 associated with at least one of the following: NR ≥ 2.5, acidosis corresponding to arterial pH ≤ 7.30 or venous pH ≤ 7.25 and/or serum lactate levels $\geq$4 mmol. Recipients develop acute liver failure, encephalopathy, coagulopathy, and renal failure [16]. Risk factors for PNF include older-age donors, DCD donors, prolonged ischemic times and high-risk recipients, however the underlying etiology has not been fully elucidated [40]. Patients with PNF require urgent transplantation and therefore are listed as Status 1A within 7 days of the initial transplantation [16]. A similar entity, primary graft dysfunction also called delayed graft function can be seen in up to 39% of recipients [40]. There is no consensus definition or accepted criteria for this entity though it is associated with elevated aminotransferase levels, bile production and prothrombin time within the first 72 h after transplant [41]. It is due to multiple causes including most prominently severe ischaemic-reperfusion injuries, acute rejection episodes, vascular complications, though in some cases no of these factors are present [41]. Patients with delayed function often require elongated hospital stays and are at risks for secondary complications such as infections, or renal dysfunction. However ultimately the majority of patients have good graft recovery by day 28 [41].

Another life threatening complication is hepatic artery thrombosis (HAT) which occurs in 2–12% of patients. It is a catastrophic event which requires relisting within 7 days for a liver as a status 1A at a MELD score of 40 [16]. Another possible vascular complication is hepatic venous outflow obstruction which is due to stenosis of the anastomosis at the inferior vena cava, and is associated with the presence of ascites and occurs in 1–2% of the cases [17]. Biliary complications occur in 8–15% of the patients and include biliary leaks and strictures [42]. Leaks occur within the first month, while strictures occur later often requiring ERCP for treatment. Diffuse biliary strictures are difficult to treat and transplantation may be required [42]. Overall, the most common post-op complication is postoperative hemorrhage which occurs in ~20% of the patients, and about half will require re-operation. Infectious complications in the early setting are linked to the level of immunosuppression required, the presence of surgical complications, and length of stay in the intensive care unit [17]. The most common infections within the first month are bacterial and originate from the surgical wound site, biliary tree, abdominal cavity, urinary tract, or lungs [17]. Patients with fulminant hepatic failure or immunosuppression prior to transplant are at additional risk for invasive fungal infections immediately after transplant. Infections due to cytomegalovirus and Epstein-Barr virus are also common after the first month of transplantation [17].

68.8 Immunosuppression

Induction and maintenance of immunosuppression have led to an overall decrease in the incidence of both acute and chronic rejection in liver transplant recipients. Induction immunosuppression, given at the time of transplantation, is used by approximately 25% of liver transplant centers and includes antibody therapy with antithymocyte globulin and IL-2 receptor antibodies (basiliximab and daclizumab) [43].

Maintenance immunosuppressive agents are usually given in combinations. There are 4 general classes: corticosteroids, calcineurin inhibitors (CNIs) such as tacrolimus and cyclosporine; antimetabolites (mycophenolate mofetil, azathioprine), and mammalian target of rapamycin (mTOR) inhibitors (sirolimus, everolimus). Induction immunosuppression is tapered in the months following LT to avoid toxicity and lessen the risk of recurrent disease, often by discontinuing maintenance glucocorticoids. As described in Table 68.7, there are many well established side-effects to immunosuppressive agents such as renal toxicity, arterial hypertension, osteopenia, hyperlipidemia, diabetes mellitus, and obesity. Renal insufficiency secondary to cyclosporine or tacrolimus nephrotoxicity affects most of these patients. Hypertension and diabetes are additional cofactors that contribute to renal insufficiency. Preliminary studies show the possibility of reducing CNI doses by adding mycophenolate mofetil or sirolimus, to reduce renal dysfunction. Drug interactions between immunosuppressive agents and other commonly prescribed drugs are well described. Possible interactions should be considered when transplant recipients are using additional medications, including antibiotics, antifungal and antiviral agents, and seizure medications. After the first 90 days following LT, immunosuppression is reduced, as the graft becomes somewhat tolerant to the recipient's immune system. While most liver recipients require lifelong immunosuppressive therapy, there are some recipients in which a phenomenon called operational tolerance may occur, and graft rejection does not occur despite immunosuppression withdrawal [44]. This is specific to liver transplantation as it is not seen with other types of transplants and the frequency of this event is unknown though is estimated at occurring in 20–60% of LT recipients. However, since there is no way at this time to predict which patients will develop tolerance, complete withdrawal of immunosuppression is a rare occurrence [44].

Table 68.7 Common immunosuppressive agents

Agents	Mechanism of action	Major side effects
Prednisone	Cytokine inhibitor (IL-1, IL-2, IL-6, TNF, and IFN-γ)	Hypertension, diabetes mellitus, obesity, osteoporosis, infection, depression, psychosis
Cyclosporine	Calcineurin inhibitor: suppresses IL-2–dependent T-cell proliferation	Renal, neurologic, hyperlipidemia, hypertension, hirsutism
Tacrolimus	Calcineurin inhibitor: suppresses IL-2–dependent T-cell proliferation	Renal, neurologic, diabetes mellitus
Azathioprine	Inhibition of T- and B-cell proliferation by interfering with purine synthesis	Bone marrow suppression, hepatotoxicity
Mycophenolate mofetil	Selective inhibition of T- and B-cell proliferation by interfering with purine synthesis	Diarrhea, bone marrow suppression
Sirolimus/ Everolimus	Inhibition of late T-cell functions	Neutropenia, thrombocytopenia, hyperlipidemia
OKT3 (Muromonab-CD3)	Blocking of T-cell CD3 receptor, preventing stimulation by antigen	Cytokine release syndrome, pulmonary edema, increased risk of infections
Basiliximab/ Daclizumab	Competitive inhibition of IL-2 receptor on activated lymphocytes	Hypersensitivity reactions

IFN interferon, *IL* interleukin

68.9 Acute and Chronic Rejection

Acute cellular rejection (ACR) occurs in 15–30% of transplant recipients [45]. This form of rejection typically occurs within 90 days after liver transplantation, but can occur later on as well. The hallmark morphologic features of ACR are: mixed portal inflammation in the portal triad which is predominantly lymphocytic; nonsuppurative cholangitis involving interlobular bile duct epithelium, bile duct inflammation and damage; and endothelialitis. These three features comprise the "diagnostic triad" of ACR [46]. Liver biopsy with evidence of these pathologic changes and subtherapeutic levels of immunosuppressive medications indicates the presence of acute cellular rejection. However, differentiation between acute rejection and hepatitis from viral disease, drugs, and autoimmunity can be difficult given the overlap of clinical and histologic features [47]. First-line treatment is with high-dose corticosteroids, which 80–90% of patients respond well to, and augmentation of maintenance immunosuppression [17]. A proposed algorithm for treating ACR is depicted in Fig. 68.1.

According to one study, 15.7% of transplant recipients had at least one episode of acute rejection and this was associated with an increased risk of graft failure and death, especially if the episode occurs more than 1 year after transplantation [45].

Chronic rejection occurs in 5–10% of LT recipients and usually occurs between 6 weeks and 6 months after the procedure. Liver biopsy typically shows obliterative arteriopathy with bile duct injury and loss affecting more than 50% of

Fig. 68.1 Algorithm for treating acute cellular rejection

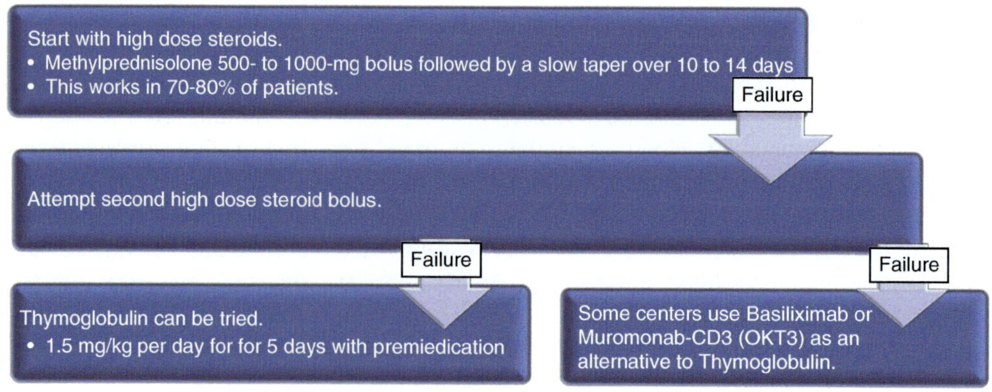

Fig. 68.2 Patient survival among adult deceased donor liver transplant recipients, 2009-2011, by diagnosis [52]. Graft survival estimated using unadjusted Kaplan-Meier methods. *HCV* hepatitis C virus, *ALD* alcoholic liver disease, *Chol. disease* cholestatic disease

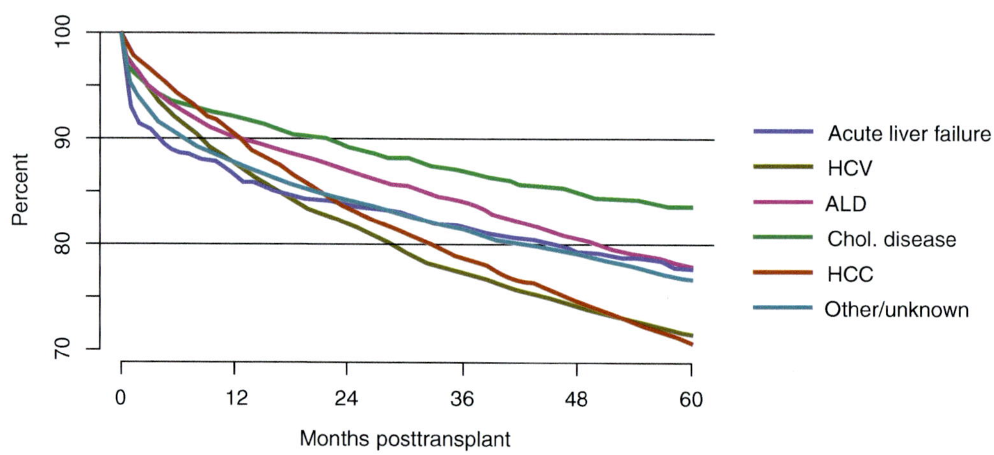

the portal tracts [48]. Recipients with viral hepatitis or autoimmune liver diseases have a 4 times greater risk for developing chronic rejection compared with other recipients [49]. Treatment of chronic rejection requires ramping up the immunosuppressive regimen. This is not always successful and ultimately re-transplantation is required.

68.9.1 Long-Term Outcomes and Reoccurrence of Disease

Outcomes after liver transplantation have continued to improve, with the most recent data analysis as of 2016 with estimated patient and graft survival rates of 93% at 6 months, 90% at 1 year, 75% at 5 years, and 55% at 10 years for all etiologies of liver disease combined [50]. Many factors influence survival rates including baseline characteristics of the donor and recipient, and factors associated with perioperative and post-operative period. Donor parameters that have been shown to be associated with poorer outcomes include advanced age, higher BMI, increased length of hospitalization, use of vasopressors, and the presence of infection [44]. Recipient parameters include urgent indication, the presence of renal dysfunction, older age, mechanical ventilation requirement, poor nutritional status, and the presence of infection [44]. Perioperative factors include cold and warm ischemia time, increased blood product requirements, and complex surgery required for liver placement [44].

Based on data collected from the National Institute of Diabetes and Digestive and Kidney Diseases Liver Transplantation Database, the most common overall causes of death were hepatic (recurrent disease or liver failure) causes (23.9%), malignancy (18.7%), infection (15.9%), cardiovascular disease (12.2%), and renal failure (4.3%) [51].

Survival rates have been shown to differ based on the primary indication for LT as depicted in Fig. 68.2. Notably, patients with HCV and HCC having poorer outcomes at 5 years post-LT. HCV survival rates are expected to increase as more patients with HCV are being treated with direct acting anti-viral medications after LT preventing recurrence of HCV cirrhosis in the new liver though this has not yet been reflected in an increase in long term outcomes.

Generally, patients with cholestatic disease and autoimmune cirrhosis have better survival rates though both diseases have been noted to be associated with reoccurrence. Autoimmune liver diseases have documented survival rates of approximately 90% at 1 year and 70%, at 5 years [53]. However, recurrent disease is common and the prevalence increases with time following LT ranging from 17% to 42% in patients with autoimmune hepatitis, 12–30% in those with primary biliary cirrhosis, and 12–60% in subjects with primary sclerosing cholangitis [54]. One large center reported that 6% of patients with autoimmune hepatitis had progression of disease requiring re-transplantation [55].

Hepatitis B infection after transplantation is increased in patients with high hepatitis B virus DNA levels, hepatitis B e antigen positivity, prior resistance to antiviral therapy, and in patients who are hepatitis B surface antigen negative and receive a liver from a hepatitis B core antibody–positive donor [56]. With implementation of prophylactic regimens using hepatitis B immunoglobulin and nucleoside or nucleotide analogues, patients are able to live disease free, they must be maintained lifelong on antiviral therapy.

Almost all patients with hepatitis C viremia before transplantation will have reinfection of the new liver graft and can have accelerated progression to cirrhosis and therefore treatment is required. The best time for treatment is in the perioperative period since hepatitis C virus RNA levels are at its lowest during the "anhepatic phase" with viral replication starting within hours of transplantation [57].

Nonalcoholic fatty liver disease (NAFLD) reoccurrence is common after transplantation. Risk factors include obesity, diabetes, hyperlipidemia, hypertension, tacrolimus-based immunosuppression, alcoholic cirrhosis as primary indication for transplantation, and steatosis in the liver graft [43]. Rates of reoccurrence range widely, with steatosis reported in 25–100% of livers and nonalcoholic steatohepatitis (NASH) reported in 10–37.5% of livers after transplantation [43]. It has been noted that progression to fibrosis may be more rapid in transplant recipients compared to the original livers [43].

The 5-year patient and graft survivals in adults transplanted for alcoholic liver disease (ALD) are similar to patients transplanted for other indications [50]. However, ALD survival decreases after the 5 year point due to non-liver related morbidity and mortality from cardiorespiratory disease, cerebrovascular events, and de novo malignancy [58]. Interestingly, the incidence rate of de novo malignancies is higher in patients with ALD compared to other LT recipients, especially cancers of the oropharyngeal and lung, which is thought to be related to substance abuse and smoking history [17]. Recidivism in patients after LT is always a concern. In one metanalysis, relapse rates were reported at 2.5 cases per 100 patients per year with heavy alcohol use and 5.6 cases per 100 patients per year with any alcohol use [59]. Additionally, recidivism has not been shown to increase patient or graft mortality [59].

68.9.2 Long-Term Concerns After Liver Transplantation

Recipients after LT are at higher risk of developing metabolic syndrome compared to the general public and increased aggressive management is indicated. This is due to the side-effects of many immunosuppressive agents and the reversal of the pre-transplant catabolic state [60]. The risk of a cardiovascular event, such as acute coronary syndrome, cerebrovascular accident, arrhythmia, congestive heart failure, peripheral artery disease, within 10 years of liver transplantation is over 13%, which correlates with a 64% increased risk compared with the general population [61]. Therefore, aggressive management of risk factors including hyperlipidemia, diabetes mellitus, and obesity must be emphasized in the post-LT population.

68.10 Hypertension

Systemic hypertension is a frequent complication of LT and is related to calcineurin inhibitors inducing renal vasoconstriction, as well as to the effects of other drugs such as glucocorticoids. Unfortunately, a reduction in immunosuppression is generally ineffective in treating hypertension. Medication management is also complicated by the many interactions most anti-hypertensive medications have with immunosuppressive agents. Therefore, dihydropyridine calcium channel blockers (amlodipine, felodipine, nifedipine) are often used first in treating hypertension due to their vasodilatory effects and minimal interaction with the commonly used immunosuppressants [62]. Non-dihydropyridine calcium channel blockers (diltiazem, verapamil) should be avoided as they can cause increased levels of calcineurin inhibitors [43]. Angiotensin-converting enzyme inhibitors and angiotensin receptor blockers are may be less effective early after transplantation, when renin levels are relatively low and may be contraindicated in patients with renal dysfunctions from calcineurin inhibitors [43]. Beta-blockers can also be used effectively in patients with coronary artery disease or patients who are unresponsive to calcium channel blockers [43].

68.11 Obesity

Obesity (body mass index ≥30 kg/m^2) is seen in one-third of patients within the first year after transplantation [17]. Risk factors include elevated body mass index before transplantation, presence of NASH, presence of diabetes after transplantation, glucocorticoid use, increased caloric intake, and decreased physical activity during recuperation from surgery [19]. Pharmacotherapies for weight loss have limited data in liver transplant recipients. Bariatric surgery is an effective means of achieving weight loss and improving obesity-related comorbidities, but there are no clear guidelines for performing bariatric surgery in liver transplant recipients [43]. Immunosuppression with tacrolimus has been reported to result in less weight gain than occurs with cyclosporine, though this may be due to the lower glucocorticoid doses used with tacrolimus [17].

68.12 Diabetes Mellitus

Diabetes mellitus (DM) is common in liver transplant recipients and new-onset diabetes mellitus is estimated to occur in 25–33% of liver transplant recipients [17, 43]. The presence of diabetes is an independent risk factor for mortality [63].

Immunosuppressant medications contribute to diabetes by various mechanisms, including increased insulin resistance, increased gluconeogenesis, and decreased peripheral insulin use [43]. The use of cyclosporine is associated with a lower rate of new-onset diabetes after transplantation when compared with tacrolimus [43]. Other risk factor for DM include: age greater than 50 year old, African American race, body mass index greater than 25 kg/m^2, hepatitis C infection, donor age >60 years old, and a cadaveric donor [43]. Management of liver transplant recipients with diabetes, mirrors that of the general population and often requires treatment with insulin. Monitoring for long-term complications including nephropathy, neuropathy, retinopathy, and cardiovascular disease is essential.

68.13 Dyslipidemia

Hyperlipidemia occurs in up to 50% of patients after transplantation, reflecting a number of factors including diabetes mellitus, obesity, renal dysfunction, and immunosuppressive agents, especially mTOR inhibitors and glucocorticoids [64]. Pharmacologic therapy is indicated if hypercholesterolemia fails to improve with weight reduction and glycemic control. Treatment with statins must be done carefully because they inhibit the cytochrome p450 CYP3A4 pathway leading to increased levels of both the statins and calcineurin inhibitors when used concomitantly [43]. Therefore, statins should be used at the lowest possible doses and the patient must be monitored for development of myalgias. Pravastatin and fluvastatin are the only available statins on the US market that are not metabolized by the CYP3A4 pathway and may be safer to use in LT recipients [43].

68.14 Kidney Disease

Patients after LT are at higher risk for renal dysfunction compared to the general population. Risk factors include the use of calcineurin inhibitors, hypertension, diabetes mellitus, HCV infection [43]. One study showed that chronic renal failure is at high rates in LT recipients with prevalence at 8.0% at 1 year, 13.9% at 3 years, 18.1% at 5 years, and 25.0% at 10 years [65]. Modifications in standard immunosuppressive regimens may be helpful in preventing renal dysfunction. In the perioperative period, antibody induction may be used to allow for delayed introduction of calcineurin inhibitors. A lower dose of calcineurin inhibitors may also be used with adjunctive therapy with mTOR inhibitors or mycophenolate, but some studies have shown that this benefit is not as significant after the first year post-transplantation [43]. Control of baseline risk factors is also important, including glucose and blood pressure control.

68.15 Osteopenia

Osteopenia is frequently seen in liver transplant recipients [17]. Risk factors include poor nutritional status, immobility, glucocorticoid use, increased age, female gender, and the post-menopausal state. In the initial several months after LT, osteopenia is accelerated by high-dose glucocorticoid therapy as well as the use of other immunosuppressive agents. Even prednisone doses as low as 7.5 mg daily have been shown to cause bone loss despite the absence of other risk factors [43].

Increased bone loss leads to a higher incidence of atraumatic fractures, especially in patients with low bone mineral density before transplantation [43]. Treatment with supplemental calcium and vitamin D is required in all post-LT patients, and bisphosphonates should be considered in patients with osteoporosis or recent fractures [17].

68.16 Malignancy

The overall incidence of malignancy in adult liver transplant recipients is nearly 12 times greater than the general population due to the required immunosuppressive agents used. The most common malignancies seen are skin (30.5%), solid organ (38.3%), hematologic (11.3%), and recurrent (19.5%) malignancies [66]. Liver transplant recipients need ongoing age-appropriate surveillance for common tumors such as breast, cervical, and colon cancer [17]. The incidence rates of squamous cell carcinoma and malignant melanoma are respectively 35.7 and 2.8 times higher than the general population [67]. Therefore patients should be educated to always use sun protection with SPF 15 or above, limit sun exposure, and receive annual skin examinations [17]. Posttransplant lymphoproliferative disorder (PTLD) is a common malignancy in liver transplant recipients with an estimated incidence of 2–4% in post-LT recipients and leads to death in 50% of cases [55]. It is seen at increased rates in recipients over the age of 50, with hepatitis C or alcoholic cirrhosis, or recipients of antilymphocyte antibodies [55]. The majority of cases are associated with Epstein–Barr virus infection leading to B-cell proliferation in the setting of decreased T-cell function from immunosuppression [55]. Treatment requires a reduction in immunosuppression. Anti-CD20 antibodies, radiation therapy, or surgery may be necessary in patients who do not improve with decreased immunosuppression or patients with more aggressive disease at initial presentation [55].

68.17 Conclusion

The field of liver transplantation is a dynamic and changing area with new break-throughs and advances allowing for increased accessibility to organ transplantation for those in need. With an aging population, the makeup of transplant recipients is changing and it is expected that NALFD will be the most common indication for transplantation in the near future, as hepatitis C is slowly eradicated. As such, advancements in organ procurement and the methods for allocation will need constant updating as time goes on. At this time, there are not enough organs available, and candidates die while on the waiting list. Alternative avenues to allow for extended life are currently being developed but have not shown the same efficacy as liver transplantation yet.

Self Study

Questions

1. Which statement is true?
   (a) All patients diagnosed with HCC are automatically assigned the status 1A designation.
   (b) Patients with hepatopulmonary syndrome are diagnosed with right heart catheterization and if the pulmonary vascular resistance is responsive to vasodilators the patient can be listed for liver transplantation.
   (c) Post-transplant lymphoproliferative disorder (PTLD) is a common malignancy in liver transplant recipients leads to death in 50% of cases
   (d) Liver transplantation is contraindicated in recipients who are over the age of 70.
2. A 55-year-old man with a PMH significant for well-compensated NASH cirrhosis presents to clinic for follow-up. She complains of dyspnea on exertion. She denies a history of smoking. On examination, she has finger clubbing, but a normal cardiac and respiratory exam. Vitals: T 37.2 °C HR 87 BP 112/60 SpO2 86% on room air. Labs reveal a PaO2 on ABG is 59 mmHg. Chest X-ray is significant for an enlarged mediastinum. Doppler of the lower extremities is negative for deep vein thrombosis.
   What is the next best test to evaluate the patient?
   (a) VQ scan
   (b) CT chest
   (c) Right heart catheterization.
   (d) Contrast echocardiogram
3. A 64 year old man received an orthotopic liver transplant 7 years ago for NASH cirrhosis. He is on tacrolimus for immunosuppression and takes medications for hypertension. On routine labs his creatinine is found to be 2.3 mg/dL and has been rising progressively over the last year. All his other labs values are normal and he has no other complaints.
   What do you consider doing next?
   (a) Plan for dialysis
   (b) Stop tacrolimus and start Basiliximab.
   (c) Stop tacrolimus and start sirolimus
   (d) Stop tacrolimus and start cyclosporine.
   (e) Start prednisone 20 mg.

Answers

1. Which statement is true?
   (a) All patients diagnosed with HCC are automatically assigned the status 1A designation
   (b) Patients with hepatopulmonary syndrome are diagnosed with right heart catheterization and if the pulmonary vascular resistance is responsive to vasodilators the patient can be listed for liver transplantation.
   (c) Posttransplant lymphoproliferative disorder (PTLD) is a common malignancy in liver transplant recipients leads to death in 50% of cases—**CORRECT**
   (d) Liver transplantation is contraindicated in recipients who are over the age of 70.
2. A 55-year-old man with a PMH significant for well-compensated NASH cirrhosis presents to clinic for follow-up. She complains of dyspnea on exertion. She denies a history of smoking. On examination, she has finger clubbing, but a normal cardiac and respiratory exam. Vitals: T 37.2 °C HR 87 BP 112/60 SpO2 86% on room air. Labs reveal a PaO2 on ABG is 59 mmHg. Chest X-ray is significant for an enlarged mediastinum. Doppler of the lower extremities is negative for deep vein thrombosis.
   What is the next best test to evaluate the patient?
   (a) VQ scan
   (b) CT chest
   (c) Right heart catheterization.
   (d) Contrast echocardiogram—**CORRECT**
3. A 64 year old man received an orthotopic liver transplant 7 years ago for NASH cirrhosis. He is on tacrolimus for immunosuppression and takes medications for hypertension. On routine labs his creatinine is found to be 2.3 mg/dL

and has been rising progressively over the last year. All his other labs values are normal and he has no other complaints.

What do you consider doing next?

(a) Plan for dialysis
(b) Stop tacrolimus and start Basiliximab.
(c) Stop tacrolimus and start sirolimus—**CORRECT**
(d) Stop tacrolimus and start cyclosporine.
(e) Start prednisone 20 mg.

References

1. O'Leary JG, Lepe R, Davis GL. Indications for liver transplantation. Gastroenterology. 2008;134(6):1764–76. https://doi.org/10.1053/j.gastro.2008.02.028. Review. PubMed PMID: 18471553.
2. United Network for Organ Sharing (UNOS). Transplants by organ type—2017. Data: Transplant trends. Richmond, VA: UNOS.
3. https://optn.transplant.hrsa.gov/data/view-data-reports/national-data/. Accessed 15 Dec 2018.
4. Martin P, DiMartini A, Feng S, Brown R Jr, Fallon M. Evaluation for liver transplantation in adults: 2013 practice guideline by the American Association for the Study of Liver Diseases and the American Society of Transplantation. Hepatology. 2014;59:1144–65.
5. Charlton MR, Burns JM, Pedersen RA, Watt KD, Heimbach JK, Dierkhising RA. Frequency and outcomes of liver transplantation for nonalcoholic steatohepatitis in the United States. Gastroenterology. 2011;141:1249–53.
6. Lopez P, Martin P. Update on liver transplantation: indications, organ allocation, and long-term care. Mt Sinai J Med. 2006;73:1056–66.
7. Duffy JP, Kao K, Ko CY, Farmer DG, McDiarmid SV, Hong JC, et al. Long-term patient outcome and quality of life after liver transplantation: analysis of 20-year survivors. Ann Surg. 2010;252:652–61.
8. Lucey MR, Brown KA, Everson GT, et al. Minimal criteria for placement of adults on the liver transplant waiting list: a report of a national conference organized by the American Society of Transplant Physicians and the American Association for the Study of Liver Diseases. Liver Transpl Surg. 1997;3:628–37.
9. Bernardi M, Gitto S, Biselli M. The MELD score in patients awaiting liver transplant: strengths and weaknesses. J Hepatol. 2011;54:1297–306.
10. Fede G, D'Amico G, Arvaniti V, Tsochatzis E, Germani G, Georgiadis D, et al. Renal failure and cirrhosis: a systematic review of mortality and prognosis. J Hepatol. 2012;56:810–8.
11. https://optn.transplant.hrsa.gov/resources/allocation-calculators/meld-calculator. Accessed 15 Dec 2018.
12. Merion RM, Schaubel DE, et al. The survival benefit of liver transplantation. Am J Transplant. 2005;5:307–13.
13. Kim WR, Biggins SW, et al. Hyponatremia and mortality among patients on the liver-transplant waiting list. N Engl J Med. 2008;359:1018–26.
14. https://optn.transplant.hrsa.gov/media/1200/optn_policies.pdf. Accessed 15 Dec 2018.
15. https://aasldpubs.onlinelibrary.wiley.com/doi/pdf/10.1002/cld.464. Accessed 15 Dec 2018.
16. https://optn.transplant.hrsa.gov/media/1200/optn_policies.pdf#nameddest=Policy_09. Accessed 10 Jan 2019.
17. Feldman M. Sleisenger and Fordtran's gastrointestinal and liver disease. Philadelphia, PA: Saunders, Elsevier; 2016.
18. Siciliano M, Parlati L, Maldarelli F, Rossi M, Ginanni Corradini S. Liver transplantation in adults: choosing the appropriate timing. World J Gastrointest Pharmacol Ther. 2012;3(4):49–61.
19. Schilsky ML, Moini M. Advances in liver transplantation allocation systems. World J Gastroenterol. 2016;22(10):2922–30.
20. Kato T, Nery JR, Morcos JJ, et al. Successful living related liver transplantation in an adult with fulminant hepatic failure. Transplantation. 1997;64:415–7.
21. Muzaale AD, Dagher NN, Montgomery RA, et al. Estimates of early death, acute liver failure, and long-term mortality among live liver donors. Gastroenterology. 2012;142:273–80.
22. Tector A, Mangus R, Chestovich P, et al. Use of extended criteria livers decreases wait time for liver transplantation without adversely impacting posttransplant survival. Ann Surg. 2006;244:439–50.
23. O'Grady JG, Alexander GJ, Hayllar KM, et al. Early indicators of prognosis in fulminant hepatic failure. Gastroenterology. 1989;97:439–45.
24. Bernal W, Hyyrylainen A, Gera A, et al. Lessons from look-back in acute liver failure? A single centre experience of 3300 patients. J Hepatol. 2013;59:74–80.
25. Freeman RB, Steffick DE, Guidinger MK, et al. Liver and intestine transplantation in the United States, 1997-2006. Am J Transplant. 2008;8:958–76.
26. Lipshutz GS, Hiatt J, Ghobrial RM, Farmer DG, Martinez MM, Yersiz H, et al. Outcome of liver transplantation in septuagenarians: a single-center experience. Arch Surg. 2007;142:775–81; discussion 81–84.
27. Watt KD. Reducing the load: the evolution and management of obesity and nonalcoholic steatohepatitis before liver transplantation. Liver Transpl. 2012;18(Suppl 2):S52–8.
28. McCaughan GW. Trekking new ground: overcoming medical and social impediments for extended criteria liver transplant recipients. Liver Transpl. 2012;18(Suppl 2):S39–46.
29. McAvoy NC, Kochar N, McKillop G, Newby DE, Hayes PC. Prevalence of coronary artery calcification in patients undergoing assessment for orthotopic liver transplantation. Liver Transpl. 2008;14:1725–31.
30. Azarbal B, Poommipanit P, Arbit B, Hage A, Patel J, Kittleson M, et al. Feasibility and safety of percutaneous coronary intervention in patients with end-stage liver disease referred for liver transplantation. Liver Transpl. 2011;17:809–13.
31. Safdar Z, Bartolome S, Sussman N. Portopulmonary hypertension: an update. Liver Transpl. 2012;18:881–91.
32. Kochar R, Nevah Rubin MI, Fallon MB. Pulmonary complications of cirrhosis. Curr Gastroenterol Rep. 2011;13:34–9.
33. Rodriguez-Roisin R, Krowka MJ. Hepatopulmonary syndrome—a liver-induced lung vascular disorder. N Engl J Med. 2008;358:2378–87.
34. Swanson KL, Wiesner RH, Krowka MJ. Natural history of hepatopulmonary syndrome: impact of liver transplantation. Hepatology. 2005;41:1122–9.
35. Arguedas MR, Singh H, Faulk DK, Fallon MB. Utility of pulse oximetry screening for hepatopulmonary syndrome. Clin Gastroenterol Hepatol. 2007;5:749–54.
36. Pungpapong S, Manzarbeitia C, Ortiz J, Reich DJ, Araya V, Rothstein KD, et al. Cigarette smoking is associated with an increased HEPATOLOGY, Vol. 59, No. 3, 2014 MARTIN ET AL. 1161 incidence of vascular complications after liver transplantation. Liver Transpl. 2002;8:582–7.
37. Mathurin P, et al. Early liver transplantation for severe alcoholic hepatitis. N Engl J Med. 2011;365(19):1790–800.
38. Duffy JP, Hong JC, Farmer DG, Ghobrial RM, Yersiz H, Hiatt JR, Busuttil RW. Vascular complications of orthotopic liver transplantation: experience in more than 4,200 patients. J Am Coll Surg. 2009;208(5):896–903.
39. Tannuri U, Tannuri AC. Postoperative care in pediatric liver transplantation. Clinics (Sao Paulo). 2014;69(Suppl 1):42–6.
40. Chen XB, Xu MQ. Primary graft dysfunction after liver transplantation. Hepatobiliary Pancreat Dis Int. 2014;13(2):125–37.

41. Neves DB, Rusi MB, Diaz LG, Salvalaggio P. Primary graft dysfunction of the liver: definitions, diagnostic criteria and risk factors. Einstein (Sao Paulo). 2016;14(4):567–72.
42. Pascher A, Neuhaus P. Bile duct complications after liver transplantation. Transpl Int. 2005;18(6):627–42.
43. Cheung A, Levitsky J. Follow-up of the post-liver transplantation patient. Clin Liver Dis. 2017;21(4):793–813.
44. Song AT, Avelino-Silva VI, Pecora RA, Pugliese V, D'Albuquerque LA, Abdala E. Liver transplantation: fifty years of experience. World J Gastroenterol. 2014;20(18):5363–74.
45. Levitsky J, Goldberg D, et al. Acute rejection increases risk of graft failure and death in recent liver transplant recipients. Clin Gastroenterol Hepatol. 2017;15(4):584–93.
46. Demetris AJ, Batts KP, Dhillon AP, et al. Banff Schema for grading liver allograft rejection: an international consensus document. Hepatology. 1997;25:658–63.
47. Demetris AJ, Adeyi O, Bellamy CO, et al. Liver biopsy interpretation for causes of late liver allograft dysfunction. Hepatology. 2006;44:489–501.
48. Demetris AJ, Murase N, Lee RG, et al. Chronic rejection. A general overview of histopathology and pathophysiology with emphasis on liver, heart and intestinal allografts. Ann Transplant. 1997;2(2):27–44.
49. Jain A, Demetris AJ, Kashyap R, et al. Does tacrolimus offer virtual freedom from chronic rejection after primary liver transplantation? Risk and prognostic factors in 1,048 liver transplantations with a mean follow-up of 6 years. Liver Transpl. 2001;7:623–30.
50. Kim WR, Lake JR, Smith JM, et al. OPTN/SRTR 2015 annual data report: liver. Am J Transplant. 2017;17:174–251.
51. Watt KD, Pedersen RA, Kremers WK, et al. Evolution of causes and risk factors for mortality post-liver transplant: results of the NIDDK long-term follow-up study. Am J Transplant. 2010;10:1420–7.
52. Kim WR, et al. OPTN/SRTR 2016 annual data report: liver. Am J Transplant. 2018;18(S1):172–253.
53. Ilyas JA, O'Mahony CA, Vierling JM. Liver transplantation in autoimmune liver diseases. Best Pract Res Clin Gastroenterol. 2011;25:765–82.
54. Montano-Loza AJ, Bhanji RA, et al. Systematic review: recurrent autoimmune liver diseases after liver transplantation. Aliment Pharmacol Ther. 2017;45(4):485–500.
55. Rowe IA, Webb K, Gunson BK, et al. The impact of disease recurrence on graft survival following liver transplantation: a single centre experience. Transpl Int. 2008;21:459–65.
56. Adil B, Fatih O, Volkan I, et al. Hepatitis B virus and Hepatitis D virus recurrence in patients undergoing liver transplantation for hepatitis B virus and hepatitis B virus plus hepatitis D virus. Transplant Proc. 2016;48:2119–23.
57. Garcia-Retortillo M, Forns X, Feliu A, et al. Hepatitis C virus kinetics during and immediately after liver transplantation. Hepatology. 2002;35:680–7.
58. Jain A, DiMartini A, Kashyap R, et al. Long-term follow-up after liver transplantation for alcoholic liver disease under tacrolimus. Transplantation. 2000;70:1335–42.
59. Dew MA, DiMartini AF, Steel J, et al. Meta-analysis of risk for relapse to substance use after transplantation of the liver or other solid organs. Liver Transpl. 2008;14:159–72.
60. Watt KD, Charlton MR. Metabolic syndrome and liver transplantation: a review and guide to management. J Hepatol. 2010;53:199–206.
61. Madhwal S, Atreja A, Albeldawi M, et al. Is liver transplantation a risk factor for cardiovascular disease? A meta-analysis of observational studies. Liver Transpl. 2012;18:1140–6.
62. Textor SC. De novo hypertension after liver transplantation. Hypertension. 1993;22:257–67.
63. Younossi ZM, Stepanova M, Saab S, et al. The impact of type 2 diabetes and obesity on the long-term outcomes of more than 85 000 liver transplant recipients in the US. Aliment Pharmacol Ther. 2014;40:686–94.
64. Desai S, Hong JC, Saab S. Cardiovascular risk factors following orthotopic liver transplantation: predisposing factors, incidence and management. Liver Int. 2010;30:948–57.
65. Ojo AO, Held PJ, Port FK, et al. Chronic renal failure after transplantation of a nonrenal organ. N Engl J Med. 2003;349:931–40.
66. Zhou J, Hu Z, Zhang Q, et al. Spectrum of de novo cancers and predictors in liver transplantation: analysis of the scientific registry of transplant recipients database. PLoS One. 2016;11:e0155179.
67. Garrett GL, Blanc PD, Boscardin J, et al. Incidence of and risk factors for skin cancer in organ transplant recipients in the United States. JAMA Dermatol. 2017;153:296–303.

69 Surgical Complications Following Liver Transplant and Their Management

Rahul S. Koti, Helen Tzerbinis, and Brian R. Davidson

Key Concepts

- Liver transplantation is now an established treatment for end stage liver disease, resulting in excellent long term survival.
- With advances in anaesthesia and surgical techniques, intraoperative mortality is rare. However postoperative complications are common and have a significant impact on graft and patient survival, and resource utilization.
- Symptoms and signs of complications are masked in the immunosuppressed patient and a high degree of clinical suspicion is crucial.
- Most surgical complications occur within the first few weeks of transplantation.
- The general condition of the transplant recipient, the quality of the donor liver and complexity of the operative procedure are key determinants of outcome.

69.1 Introduction

Liver transplantation is the treatment of choice for end stage liver disease, resulting in 1 year survival reaching 96% and 10 year survival of 75% [1, 2]. With advances in anaesthesia and surgical techniques, intraoperative death is nowadays a rare occurrence. However, liver transplantation surgery remains a complex operation and nearly two thirds of patients develop surgical complications in the postoperative period. Recipients are often debilitated by their end stage liver disease (ESLD) at the time of major transplant surgery which predisposes to postoperative complications. Common surgical complications include postoperative haemorrhage, vascular and biliary complications and wound complications (Table 69.1). They have a significant impact on graft and patient survival. Failed or delayed management of major complications may lead to the need for re-transplantation, a major undertaking with less favourable outcomes than a first liver transplant. Retransplantation also deprives another patient of a transplant organ. Early and effective diagnosis and treatment of postoperative surgical complications is crucial in optimizing transplant outcomes and ensuring best use of the scarce donor organ pool.

69.2 Surgical Complications

69.2.1 Haemorrhage

Postoperative haemorrhage is a common complication of liver transplant. It is also the most common reason for reoperation after liver transplantation either for control of the bleeding or evacuation of the haematoma. Reoperation for postoperative haemorrhage is required in 8–27% of OLT recipients [3] and is associated with significant resource utilization and increased postoperative mortality [4].

The cause of bleeding post transplant is multifactorial but key factors include the presence of portal hypertension and varices in the recipient, the development of coagulopathy during and after transplant and poor function of the transplanted graft.

69.2.1.1 Methods of Ensuring Haemostasis During Transplant

Management of intraoperative coagulopathy is vital to prevent postoperative bleeding.

R. S. Koti · H. Tzerbinis · B. R. Davidson (✉)
HPB and Liver Transplant Unit, Royal Free London NHS Foundation Trust, London, UK

Centre for Surgical Innovation, Organ Repair and Transplantation, Division of Surgery, Hampstead Campus, University College London (UCL), London, UK
e-mail: b.davidson@ucl.ac.uk

F. Radu-Ionita et al. (eds.), *Liver Diseases*, https://doi.org/10.1007/978-3-030-24432-3_69

Table 69.1 Common surgical complications after orthotopic liver transplantation and their incidence

Complications	Incidence	Reference
Postoperative haemorrhage	Common	
Vascular complications	6.8%	[8]
Hepatic artery thrombosis	1–9%	[9]
Hepatic artery stenosis	2–15%	[15]
Hepatic artery pseudoaneurysms	1–3%	[14, 22]
Portal vein thrombosis	2%	[8]
Portal vein stenosis	1%	[28]
Concurrent hepatic artery and portal vein thrombosis	Rare	
Inferior vena cava stenosis or thrombosis	<2%	[30, 31]
Biliary complications	23%	[33]
Bile leaks	8.2%	[33]
Biliary strictures	12.8%	[33]
Anastomotic biliary strictures	12%	[33]
Non anastomotic biliary strictures	10%	[48]
Intra-abdominal infections		
Intra-abdominal abscesses	29%	[54]
Infected bilomas	11.5%	[58, 59]
Liver abscesses	2.6%	[60]
Peritonitis	43%	[54]
Wound complications		
Haematomas	Common	
Superficial and deep wound infections	6–43%	[51, 62, 63]
Wound dehiscence (superficial and deep)	27%	[61]
Incisional hernias	1.7–34.3%	[66]

Bleeding can occur from the extensive raw surfaces created by mobilization of the cirrhotic liver, from the various vascular anastomoses or from the abdominal wound and drain sites. Iatrogenic liver lacerations, usually at organ retrieval and from the gallbladder bed following cholecystectomy on the donor graft are other potential sites for bleeding. Haemostasis during surgery is achieved by suturing of bleeding points, electro-cautery or argon beam coagulation and administration of clotting factors and platelets (see Chap. 71: Surgery in Liver Disease).

69.2.1.2 Post transplant Monitoring of Clotting and Administration of Clotting Factors

Coagulation abnormalities, thrombocytopenia and fibrinolysis which may be related to poor preoperative general condition of the recipient or occur on reperfusion of the transplanted liver are important considerations in the pathogenesis of post liver transplant bleeding. If graft function is good, coagulations factors synthesized by the new liver stop the oozing from raw areas.

In the early postoperative period, the causes of haemorrhage include bleeding from the vascular anastomoses due to technical failure, primary nonfunction or early dysfunction of the graft, iatrogenic injury to the liver and use of anticoagulants such as heparin. In the late postoperative period, percutaneous liver biopsy and endoscopic or percutaneous interventions of the biliary tract may also cause bleeding.

69.2.1.3 Detection, Quantifying and Treating Post op Haemorrhage

Postoperative haemorrhage commonly manifests as fresh blood loss in the abdominal drains or as haemodynamic instability. Coagulopathy is diagnosed and managed as outlined in Chap. 70: Anaesthesia for Liver Transplantation.

If bleeding persists despite correction of coagulopathy or if the patient is losing sufficient blood to become haemodynamically unstable an urgent exploratory laparotomy is required.

At laparotomy, the vascular anastomoses, raw areas on the liver, diaphragm and behind the liver are carefully inspected. Bleeding from the hepatic artery, portal vein and inferior vena cava anastomoses is usually controlled by extra sutures to achieve haemostasis but occasionally the entire anastomosis may have to be refashioned. Bleeding from the peritoneal and retroperitoneal raw areas can be controlled by diathermy, argon beam coagulation or suture ligation. Diaphragmatic collateral vessel near the bare of the liver are associated with the inferior phrenic artery and bleeding from these usually requires suture ligation. Bleeding from the abdominal wound or abdominal drain sites may arise from the abdominal wall due to injury of the superior or inferior epigastric arteries, or superficial circumflex iliac arteries, and is controlled by suture ligation of the bleeding vessel. Often at exploratory laparotomy, an active bleeding source is not to be found but the laparotomy, lavage and evacuation of the blood clot achieves haemostasis.

In a haemodynamically stable patient Ultrasound and CT are useful in establishing whether there is a significant abdominal haematoma and if this warrants evacuation. Re-laparotomy may be required if the haematoma is large and loculated to prevent abdominal compartment syndrome, difficulty in ventilation and possible development of secondary infection.

Diffuse liver parenchymal bleeding causing subcapsular haematoma is rare but occurs from minor injuries during mobilization and handling of the liver and is precipitated by underlying coagulopathy (Fig. 69.1). Selective arterial embolization is recommended for controlling expanding subcapsular haematomas which can compress the underlying liver parenchyma and compromise graft function [5]. Once the bleeding is controlled a subcapsular pigtail catheter can be inserted under ultrasound guidance to drain the haematoma [5]. If expanding subcapsular haematoma is discovered at relaparotomy for bleeding, perihepatic packing or opening of the liver capsule with haemostasis of the underlying raw bleeding surface may be required. Percutaneous endoluminal selective arterial embolization performed under local anaesthesia and sedation is also the best treatment option for bleeding from pancreaticoduodenal and jejunal branches of the superior mesenteric artery, pseudoaneurysms of the

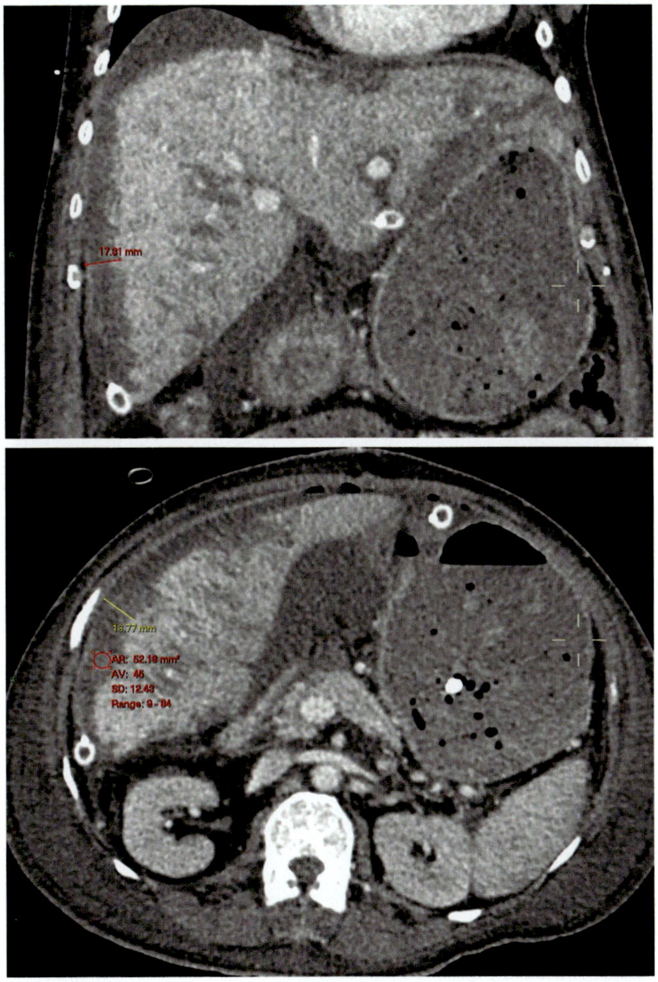

Fig. 69.1 Coronal (top image) and Axial (bottom image) CT scan from a patient post liver transplantation. A large crescent shaped subcapsular haematoma is seen (measured at approximately 18 mm in depth). This fluid is of high attenuation on CT (Hounsfield units measured at 45) consistent with haematoma. The compressive effect of the subcapsular haematoma gives the donor graft an irregular contour

hepatic and splenic artery and bleeding from percutaneous liver biopsy track [6, 7].

In the setting of postoperative bleeding related to poor initial graft function, it is prudent to maintain the clotting with clotting factors until the graft has had an opportunity to function with synthesis of clotting factors. If the graft function remains poor then consideration should be given to re-transplantation.

69.2.2 Vascular Complications

Several vascular anastomoses (hepatic artery, portal vein and vena cava) are carried out during the transplant procedure. Thrombosis or stenosis at these anastomoses are specific vascular complications related to liver transplantation. A large review of 4200 OLT's had a 6.8% incidence of postoperative vascular complications [8]. Hepatic artery thrombosis and portal vein thrombosis occurred in 5% (203 patients) and 2% (84 patients), respectively. For patients with HAT, initial treatment was surgical anastomotic revision or thrombectomy in 71% of patients and catheter based thrombolysis in 11.2%. Retransplantation was required in 75% of patients with HAT. Initial treatment for PVT was thrombolysis in 10 patients, surgical revision or thrombectomy in 22 patients and retransplantation in 20 patients [8]. Although uncommon, vascular complications are a major source of morbidity and mortality. By interrupting blood supply to the liver, they can cause early graft failure, long term graft dysfunction or patient death [8]. Thus all vascular complications are feared and considered life threatening. Hepatic artery thrombosis (HAT) and portal vein thrombosis (PVT) are more common than IVC complications.

69.2.2.1 Hepatic Artery Thrombosis (HAT)

Incidence and Presentation

Hepatic artery thrombosis (HAT) is the most common vascular complication of liver transplantation. The incidence of HAT is between 1% and 9% [9]. Factors increasing the risk of HAT are outlined in Table 69.2. It leads to graft loss or mortality in 56% and 33% of cases, respectively [10].

The majority of publications define early HAT as occurring within 1 month of transplantation [10, 11]. The UK liver advisory group has arbitrarily defined early HAT as an event which occurs between 0 and 21 days after transplantation [12].

Hepatic artery thrombosis results in liver parenchymal ischaemia and biliary tree necrosis leading to graft failure, sepsis, and ultimately multiorgan failure and death. Late HAT may be asymptomatic and found following investigation of graft dysfunction and the finding of diffuse biliary strictures typical of an ischaemic cholangiopathy (Fig. 69.2). The development of arterial collaterals may occur secondary to a slow and progressive reduction in hepatic arterial flow resulting in the milder clinical course in late HAT. Fulminant hepatic failure, however, may occur in both early and late HAT [9].

Diagnosis and Treatment of Early HAT

The mean incidence of early HAT is 3.9% [10]. Early HAT, is usually detected on either routine Doppler ultrasound or following elevation in liver function tests (principally transaminases). Regular postoperative monitoring of the liver vasculature with Doppler ultrasound is common practice, although there are no randomized controlled trials of early Doppler US after OLT showing improved outcome. The hepatic artery supplies high oxygen level arterial blood to the liver and is the main blood supply to

Table 69.2 Causes of early hepatic artery thrombosis (HAT) [8, 11]

Surgical causes (technical complications)
Retrieval injuries (intimal tears and dissection)
Kinking of the artery
Discrepancy in size between donor and recipient arteries
Anastomotic stenosis
Aberrant and accessory arteries requiring complex back-table arterial reconstruction
Small donor or recipient arteries
Poor quality donor or recipient arteries (e.g. atheromatous)
Use of aortohepatic arterial grafts (conduits)
Pretransplant transarterial chemoembolisation for liver cancers
Retransplantation
Paediatric transplants
Non surgical causes
Cigarette smoking
ABO incompatibility
Long cold ischaemia time
Procoagulant states (Janus kinase 2, factor V Leiden deficiency, anticardiolipin antibodies, high haematocrit)
Procoagulant liver diseases (primary sclerosing cholangitis, human immunodeficiency virus)
Fragile arteries (familial amyloid polyneuropathy, alpha-1-antitrypsin deficiency)
Drugs (aprotinin, tranexamic acid)
Massive ascites
Cytomegalovirus

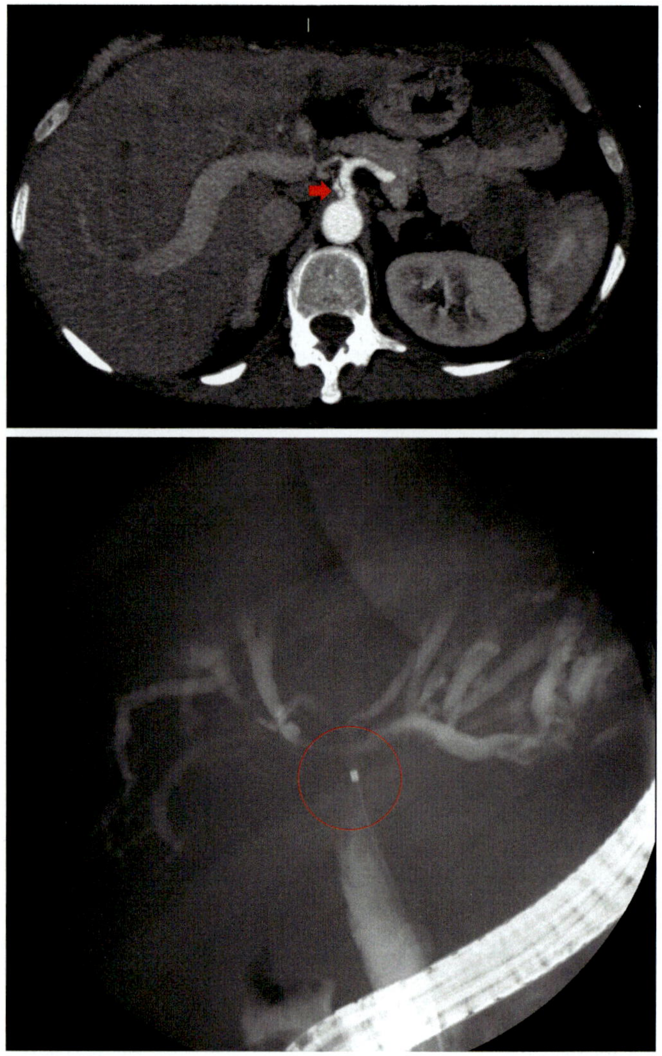

Fig. 69.2 Top image—CT in the late arterial phase demonstrates normal filling of the coeliac trunk and splenic artery but abrupt truncation at the origin of the hepatic artery. A small flap is seen in the artery consistent with a dissection. Bottom image—ERCP performed 3 months later demonstrating an extensive stenosis at the liver hilum with dilated intrahepatic ducts—this is consistent with ischaemic cholangiopathy secondary to loss of hepatic artery

the extra-hepatic biliary tree. Early HAT often presents with biliary tract complications and should be suspected if the patient develops fever, transaminitis or a gram negative sepsis in the early postoperative period. Profound transaminitis is indicative of severe graft dysfunction from development of parenchymal necrosis and cholestasis. Biliary ischaemia leads to development of pathognomonic non-anastomotic biliary strictures, intrahepatic biliary abscesses, cholestasis and cholangitis. The duration and severity of biliary tract ischaemia which can recover if hepatic artery occlusion or stenosis is diagnosed and treated is unknown. Biliary necrosis can also present as a bile leak and sepsis. Untreated early HAT usually leads to graft loss and patient death without urgent intervention [11].

Causes of early HAT have been outlined in Table 69.2.

Diagnosis of HAT

Doppler ultrasound is typically the initial examination for monitoring of vascular integrity in the immediate postoperative period. It is noninvasive and is available by the patient's bedside. The reported sensitivity and specificity of Doppler sonography for HAT range from 54% to 92% and from 64% to 88%, respectively [13]. Visualization of the vessel together with demonstration of flow on Doppler US indicates a patent hepatic artery. However, there may be false positive findings in situations of hypotension, slow flow in the artery, or small caliber artery. Technical factors such as patient position, abdominal dressings, ascites and bowel gas also can limit US examination. Further, US is an indirect test. Doppler US is used as a screening test for HAT. Patients in whom US does not visualize the hepatic artery or does not show a normal arterial waveform require CT angiography or conventional coeliac angiography.

Treatment of Early HAT

The treatment options for early HAT are urgent retransplantation, surgical revascularization, endovascular intervention or observation. Surgical revascularization techniques include thrombectomy, revision of hepatic artery anastomosis or creating an interposition conduit from recipient aorta to donor hepatic artery using a donor iliac artery graft. Endovascular interventions include intra-arterial thrombolysis, percutaneous transluminal angioplasty and stent placement. The best treatment option has not been established and there are no guidelines or randomized controlled trials to guide treatment of HAT. Endovascular treatments are controversial due to potential risks of haemorrhage, dissection and thrombosis, and their efficacy is not proven [14]. The safety and efficacy of thrombolytic treatment has been shown with different dosing regimens, but the best protocol in terms of dose and duration of treatment is not known and there are no specific guidelines for their use [14]. Retransplantation is ultimately required in most patients with HAT. In 133 cases of early HAT, surgical thrombectomy or anastomotic revision was performed in 86 patients of which graft salvage was achieved in only 9 patients (10.5%), retransplantation was required in 71 patients. Six patients died while waiting for retransplantation. Catheter based thrombolysis was performed in 3 patients of which only 1 had graft salvage [8]. In a systematic review of early HAT, revascularisation was attempted in 75% of adults and 64% of children with overall success rate of 56%. In 30% retransplantation was necessary after attempted revascularisation. Retransplantation was the treatment of choice in 53% of cases of early HAT. The overall mortality of retransplantation was 55% [10]. At our institution, experience with thrombolysis for early HAT has not been encouraging. In patients with a patent coeliac trunk and no CT evidence of parenchymal ischaemia a surgical approach with thrombectomy would be considered or formation of an arterial conduit to the infrarenal aorta. Patients with established graft damage at the time of HAT diagnosis would be considered for re-transplant.

Treatment of Late HAT

Late HAT may be treated conservatively if there is evidence of arterial collateralisation with good hepatic perfusion. If late HAT is associated with graft impairment or ischaemic cholangiopathy then retransplantation is required. In a retrospective review of 71 episodes of late HAT conservative management was successful in 13% of patients. The incidence of retransplantation was 41%. In 32%, patients were too ill for retransplantation and died within a month of diagnosis [9]. Endovascular treatment has not generally been successful for late HAT.

69.2.2.2 Hepatic Artery Stenosis

The clinical significance of hepatic artery stenosis (HAS) has not been well defined. This is likely related to whether it is a radiological appearance or producing a true reduction in arterial flow. It is considered a risk factor for development of HAT, for graft ischaemia and for biliary complications. The reported incidence of HAS is between 2% and 15% [15]. Untreated HAS progresses to HAT in 65% of cases [14].

Hepatic artery stenosis most commonly occurs at the site of anastomosis [16]. It can also occur due to kinks in redundant hepatic artery or due to intimal damage from vascular clamp injury [16]. Atheromatous donor or recipient vessels can also cause HAS.

Diagnosis

Severe HAS is defined as resistive index <0.5, peak systolic velocity >400 cm/s and presence of tardus parvus waveform on Doppler ultrasound [17]. More than 50% narrowing of the transverse diameter on angiogram in the presence of clinical suspicion (elevated liver function tests) also suggests significant HAS [14]. Technical factors such as poor surgical technique, redundant length with kink, clamp injury, intimal dissection and acute rejection are considered risk factors for development of HAS.

Clinical presentation can be with abnormal liver function tests alone, biliary complications and cholangitis, or deteriorating graft function. The incidence of biliary complications in patients with HAS is between 22% and 54% [15]. Initial investigation is Doppler US followed by CT angiography or conventional angiography for confirmation of diagnosis.

Treatment

Treatment options for HAS are endovascular intervention, surgical revision of vascular anastomosis and retransplantation. Surgical revision methods include resection of the stenotic segment with primary reanastomosis, interposition artery or vein grafts and vein patch angioplasty [18]. Endovascular intervention consists of percutaneous transluminal balloon angioplasty with or without stent placement. There are no randomized trials comparing efficacy and outcomes of surgery versus endovascular treatment of HAS. In 35 cases of HAS treated by open surgical revision, actuarial patient and graft survival at 4 years were 65% and 56%, respectively [18]. Endovascular treatment is a less invasive alternative to surgery and can be performed with high technical success rate and low morbidity. In a retrospective review [17] of 99 cases of HAS, technical success of endovascular treatment defined as <30% residual stenosis after treatment was accomplished in 91% of cases. Major complications occurred in 7.5%. In another review [15] transluminal intervention and endovascular stent placement, was associated with 5 year graft and patient survival rates of 82.3% and 87.7% respectively.

Patients with HAS who develop deranged liver function tests or biliary complications within 6–12 months of transplantation appear to benefit from endovascular treatment

[19, 20], but whether asymptomatic patients with HAS also benefit is not clear [20, 21].

69.2.2.3 Hepatic Artery Pseudoaneurysms

An arterial pseudoaneurysm is formed following injury to the vascular wall, with resultant leakage of blood which is contained by the tunica adventitia of the vessel or its surrounding tissues.

Hepatic artery pseudoaneurysm (HAP) is a rare but well documented complication following liver transplantation, with a reported incidence between 1% and 3% [14, 22]. The location of the pseudoaneurysm can be either extrahepatic, or less frequently intrahepatic [14].

HAP's most commonly present within the first month following transplantation, but a more delayed appearance has also been described. Common presentations are massive intra-abdominal haemorrhage and shock following rupture or intermittent gastrointestinal bleeding and haemobilia. Obstructive jaundice and deranged liver function tests can also be found in the presence of a pseudoaneurysm that extrinsically compresses the biliary tree. In rare occasions, they may remain quiescent and are found on radiological investigations for non-specific symptoms, including abdominal pain, fever and falling haemoglobin [23–25].

The aetiology varies and it may include infection, instrumentation and biliary leak [22–24]. In a review of 16 OLT's complicated by HAP, the majority of the patients had culture proven bacterial or fungal intra-abdominal infections. A strong association with bile leak and bilioenteric anastomosis was also demonstrated [23]. A technically difficult arterial anastomosis is also considered a risk factor for HAP formation [22, 23]. In a review of 13 OLT's complicated by HAP, intrahepatic pseudoaneurysms were associated with interventional procedures, such as liver biopsy, percutaneous transhepatic cholangiography (PTC) and placement of percutaneous transhepatic biliary drainage catheters (PTBD) [22].

Preoperative diagnosis can be difficult, and frequently pseudoaneurysms are detected during emergency laparotomy for intra-abdominal haemorrhage or infected collections. Multimodality imaging can assist in diagnosis and the methods include Doppler ultrasound scan, contrast-enhanced CT scan, magnetic resonance angiography and formal angiography [22–25].

Treatment may be surgical or by the interventional radiologist. Presentation and location may determine the optimal treatment [14, 22]. Intrahepatic pseudoaneurysms are often treated by selective embolisation with good results in the absence of infection [22]. Pseudoaneurysms involving the main hepatic artery or the anastomosis (Fig. 69.3) frequently require surgical intervention but embolisation of the artery or placement of arterial stent to exclude the pseudoaneurysm may be effective [22, 23, 26]. Surgical approaches include hepatic artery ligation with or without revascularization of the graft [22–26]. Hepatic artery ligation without revascularization is considered a salvage procedure and should only be considered as a lifesaving procedure in the setting of a ruptured HAP [24]. Another surgical approach involves excision of the HAP and immediate revascularization by direct arterial re-anastomosis or by use of an arterial conduit [22–26].

Despite optimal surgical and/or radiological treatment, HAP following liver transplantation is associated with increased mortality and morbidity [14]. Complications include loss or poor graft function requiring retransplantation, sepsis and multiorgan failure, ischaemic cholangiopathy with biliary strictures leading to recurrent cholangitis and bleeding [22–26].

HAP is a rare but serious complication of liver transplantation. It is frequently seen in the setting of intra-abdominal sepsis and biliary leak. High clinical suspicion and vigilance should prompt early investigation and treatment. Management should be achieved in a multimodality approach including surgical and radiological interventional procedures. Unfortunately, a high mortality and morbidity remain high even following successful initial treatment.

69.2.2.4 Portal Vein Thrombosis (PVT)

Portal vein thrombosis after liver transplantation occurred in 2% of cases in a large single centre review of 4200 OLT's [8]. It is commonly a result of technical issues such as small portal vein size, discrepancy in caliber of donor and recipient vessels, redundancy, misalignment, stretching of the anastomosis and use of venous conduits for portal vein reconstruction. Other risk factors include previous portal vein thrombosis, previous splenectomy and hypercoagulable states. Similar to HAT, portal vein thrombosis disrupts blood supply to the liver graft and can lead to graft failure and patient death.

PVT can present acutely with graft failure or with portal hypertension and ascites, gastrointestinal bleeding and elevated transaminases. Diagnosis can be made on Doppler ultrasound and confirmed by contrast enhanced CT scan. Non opacification of the portal vein on contrast CT is indicative of portal vein thrombosis.

Acute portal vein thrombosis is treated by exploratory laparotomy and portal vein thrombectomy. Revision of the portal vein anastomosis or construction of a mesenteric venous jump graft (venous conduit) may be required. Urgent retransplantation is required for patients presenting with acute graft failure and graft necrosis. Chronic portal vein thrombosis presenting with complications of portal hypertension can be treated by creation of a surgical portosystemic shunts if the superior mesenteric or splenic vein remains patent. Asymptomatic patients can be treated with

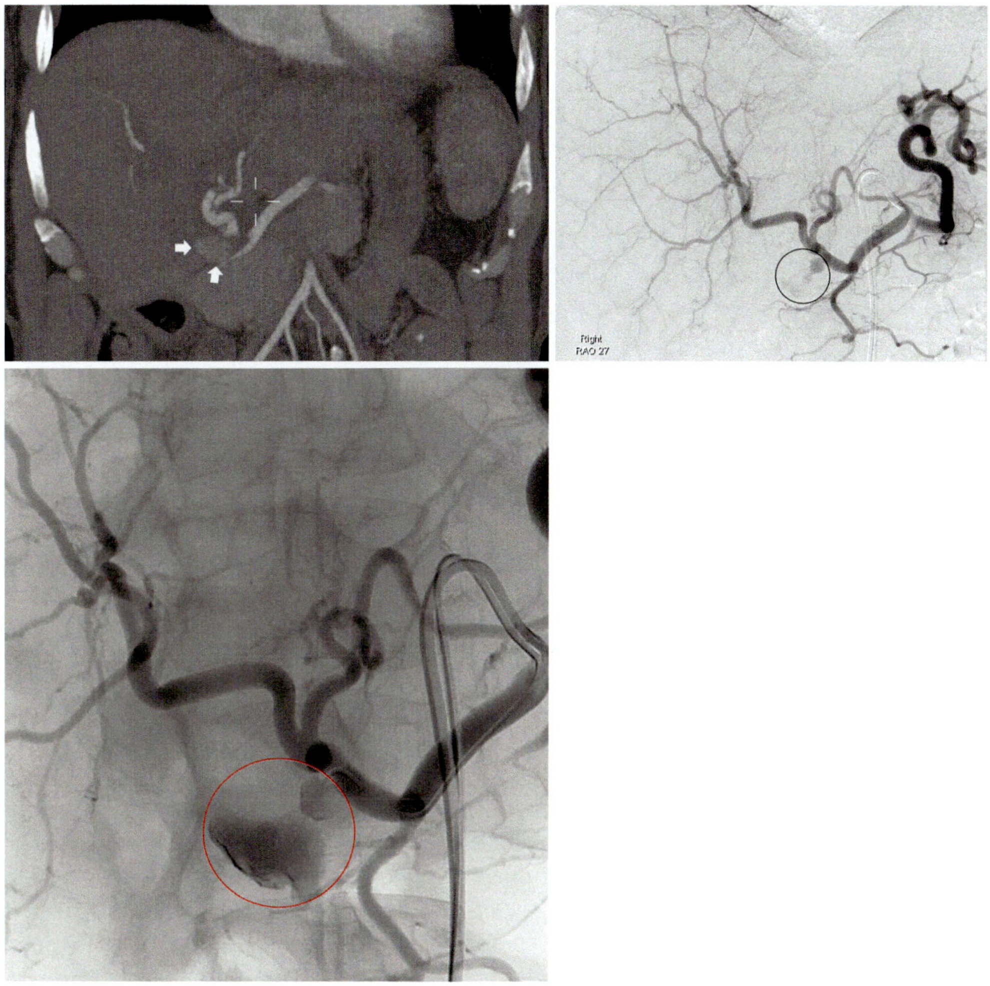

Fig. 69.3 Top left image—CT coronal maximal intensity projection demonstrating a pseudoaneurysm at the hepatic arterial anastomosis (white arrows). Top right image—Angiogram from the coeliac trunk confirms finding on CT (black circle). Bottom left image—Further subselective angiogram via a microcatheter in the neck of the pseudoaneurysm demonstrates its extent (red circle)

anticoagulation without surgical therapy. In 84 patients with post transplant PVT, 48 patients received anticoagulation without surgical therapy, 22 underwent reoperation and thrombectomy, 20 underwent retransplantation, ten had catheter directed therapy and six had portosystemic shunt surgery [8].

Portal vein thrombosis can be more detrimental to graft and patient survival than HAT [8]. This may be due to technical considerations precluding retransplantation. During retransplantation for HAT, arterial reconstruction may be performed by anastomosing the donor artery to recipient common hepatic artery, coeliac trunk or via an arterial conduit to the aorta. However in patients with extensive portal vein thrombosis extending into the mesenteric veins it may not be technically possible to construct alternative portal inflow to the new graft even with construction of a venous conduit. Therefore many patients with portal vein thrombosis may not be candidates for retransplantation [8].

With advances in interventional radiology, minimally invasive treatments have been tried and there are small case series of percutaneous transhepatic thrombolysis, balloon angioplasty and stent placement [27].

69.2.2.5 Portal Vein Stenosis

Portal vein stenosis occurs in less than 1% of patients after liver transplantation. It occurs at the site of the portal vein anastomosis. It can lead to portal vein thrombosis or can present with portal hypertension with gastrointestinal bleeding and ascites. Diagnosis is made on Doppler US and CT angiography and confirmed by percutaneous transhepatic portal venography. The recommended treatment is percutaneous transhepatic balloon angioplasty performed by an interventional radiologist [28] (Fig. 69.4).

69.2.2.6 Concurrent Hepatic Artery and Portal Vein Thrombosis

This is extremely rare and there are only a handful of case reports published in the English literature. Not much is known about its causation. Trauma from vascular intervention such as embolization of hepatic artery pseudoaneurysm and generalized hypercoagulable states are some of the factors reported to precipitate this event. When concurrent HAT and PVT occur in the first few days post transplant complete graft necrosis is inevitable and urgent retransplantation is required. However when the event

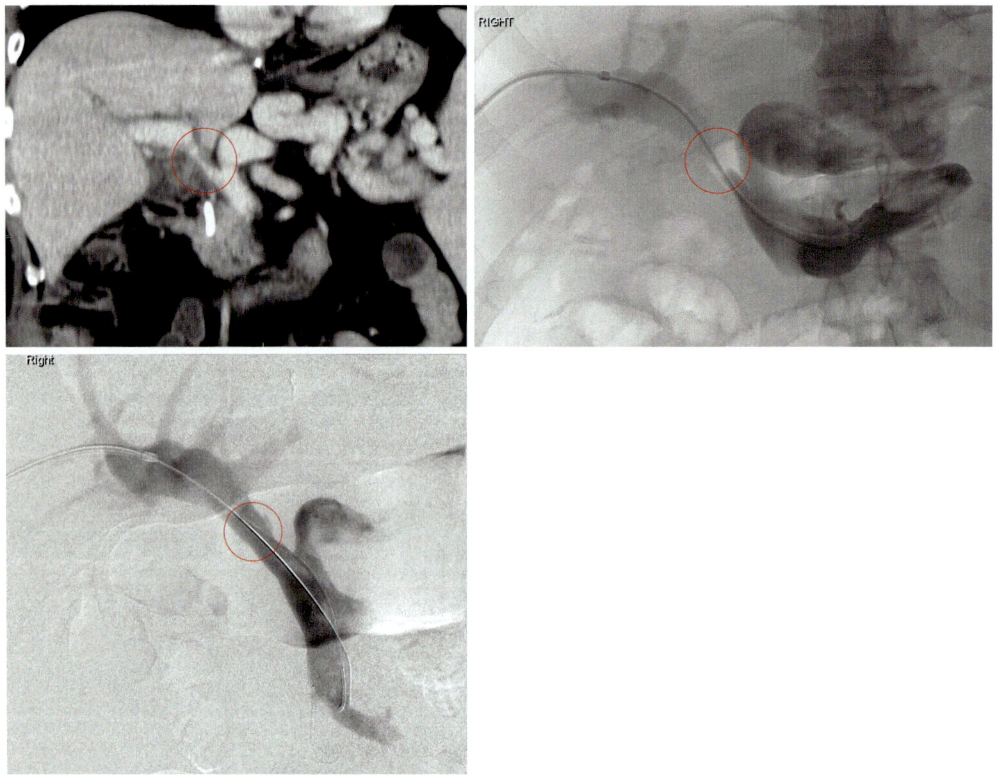

Fig. 69.4 Top left image—CT scan in the portal venous phase showing a relative caliber change in the portal vein at the anastomosis. Top right image—Transhepatic portogram confirming the stricture (red circle). Bottom left image is after balloon angioplasty of the portal anastomosis

occurs late, graft survival has been reported due to development of collateral circulation reconstituting intrahepatic blood flow. These patients have high risk of developing biliary necrosis and ischaemic cholangiopathy and therefore require close surveillance [29].

69.2.2.7 Vena Cava Complications

Stenosis or thrombosis of the inferior vena cava after liver transplantation is rare with an overall incidence of less than 2% [30, 31]. The stenosis or thrombosis occurs at the site of the surgical inferior vena cava anastomosis and can lead to hepatic outflow obstruction. The likely cause depends on the length of time elapsed since the liver transplant operation. When the event occurs acutely, it is due to technical issues such as a tight anastomosis, twisting or misalignment of the IVC, donor recipient size mismatch, or an intimal flap. Late anastomotic stenosis is usually due to perivascular fibrosis or intimal hyperplasia. Extrinsic compression of the IVC can also occur due to an oedematous or hypertrophic liver graft causing outflow obstruction.

The clinical features of hepatic outflow obstruction can include abdominal pain, enlargement and engorgement of the liver, ascites, increased abdominal girth, peripheral oedema and laboratory findings of deteriorating liver function. The liver is enlarged and firm on palpation.

Diagnosis can be made on US and contrast enhanced CT or MRI. Venography and measurement of pressure gradient across the stenosis will confirm the diagnosis of hepatic outflow obstruction [30, 32]. However, it is often not possible to do a gradient measurement if there is outflow occlusion.

Initial treatment is medical with diuretics. When this fails percutaneous balloon angioplasty with or without stent can be considered. IVC stenosis are resistant to angioplasty and have high risk of restenosis with angioplasty alone. IVC stents have good short term success rates but have risk of thrombosis, migration and can interfere with retransplantation. Surgical repair of the IVC anastomosis is technically difficult because of the short length of suprahepatic IVC [30–32]. Ultimately retransplantation is required for many patients.

69.2.3 Biliary Complications

Biliary complications are the most common major post transplant complication and a major source of morbidity after OLT. They increase hospital stay and often require invasive procedures such as Endoscopic Retrograde Cholangio Pancreatography (ERCP), percutaneous transhepatic cholangiography (PTC), surgical reconstruction of the bile duct and even re-transplantation. Biliary complications manifest as bile leaks which occur in the early postoperative period or as biliary obstruction due to anastomotic or non-anastomotic strictures which occur late. In a systematic review [33] of more than 14,000 transplanted patients the mean overall incidence of biliary strictures and bile leaks was 12.8% and 8.2%, respectively. Mortality was 1% for each.

69.2.3.1 Biliary Reconstruction Techniques

The preferred surgical technique for biliary reconstruction during OLT in most centres is a choledochocholedochostomy (duct to duct reconstruction) where the donor bile duct is anastomosed to the recipient bile duct using interrupted or continuous sutures. This is done most commonly as an end to end anastomosis but a side to side anastomosis is equally effective and both techniques have similar risk of biliary complications [34]. A duct to duct anastomosis is physiological, preserves sphincter of Oddi function and maintains endoscopic access to the bile duct.

A Roux en Y choledochojejunostomy, where the donor bile duct is anastomosed to a Roux loop of recipient jejunum, is performed in specific situations such as primary sclerosing cholangitis with involvement of the extrahepatic bile duct, significant discrepancy between donor and recipient ducts, retransplantation, and revision surgery for biliary stricture.

A choledochoduodenostomy, where the donor bile duct is anastomosed directly to recipient duodenum has been described as a safe alternative to choledochojejunostomy by some centres. However the benefits of this technique have not been demonstrated in a randomized trial [35].

Traditionally a T-tube was used for duct to duct reconstruction during OLT to provide radiological access to the bile duct and to monitor bile output postoperatively, a marker of satisfactory graft function. However T-tubes are associated with a risk of ascending cholangitis and bile leak at the time of tube removal in up to 15% of patients. Some studies have, however, reported lower incidence of biliary strictures with use of T-tube [36]. There is no strong evidence to support the routine use of T-Tube for biliary reconstruction during OLT [36, 37] and nowadays most transplant centres only use them when difficulties in reconstruction are encountered.

69.2.3.2 Diagnosis of Biliary Complications

Most biliary complications occur within the first 3 months after OLT. Early diagnosis and prompt intervention has decreased the morbidity and mortality associated with biliary complications after OLT. The coexistence of hepatic artery thrombosis with biliary complications must always be considered and investigation of biliary complications must include careful assessment of the hepatic artery patency and blood flow.

Initial evaluation is with US examination of the liver and Doppler evaluation of the hepatic artery. US is useful in detecting fluid collections and bile duct dilatation but has low sensitivity in diagnosing biliary complications. If Doppler US is suspicious for hepatic artery stenosis or thrombosis, CT angiography or conventional coeliac angiography should be performed to confirm the diagnosis.

Cholangiography either by the endoscopic route (endoscopic retrograde cholangiopancreatography, ERCP) or percutaneous route (percutaneous transhepatic cholangiography, PTC) are the gold standard for diagnosis of biliary complications. However MRCP (Magnetic resonance cholangiopancreatography), which is noninvasive, has sensitivity of 96% and specificity of 94% for diagnosing biliary obstruction in OLT patients [38]. MRCP is therefore an appropriate diagnostic procedure before undertaking invasive procedures such as ERCP and PTC.

69.2.3.3 Bile Leaks

The majority of bile leaks occur at the surgical anastomosis site. Other sites of bile leaks are the liver cut surface when partial grafts are used and after T-tube removal. Occasionally bile leaks can occur after percutaneous liver biopsy. The mean incidence of bile leak after cadaveric OLT was 7.8% [33].

Anastomotic bile leak is considered a technical failure and can occur due to improper surgical technique causing ischaemic necrosis of the anastomosis due to tension at the anastomosis, traction on the stitches, taking large bites or placing too many stitches. Stripping of the extrahepatic bile duct of all surrounding tissues during the retrieval or back table preparation procedures can also lead to ischaemic necrosis of the duct by injuring its blood supply which arises via small branches from the hepatic artery. Hepatic artery thrombosis occurring in the early postoperative period causes necrosis of the entire bile duct with complete disruption of the anastomosis.

Bile leaks can be asymptomatic with elevation in laboratory values of liver function or present with fever, abdominal pain and peritonitis. For suspected duct to duct anastomotic leaks, if a T-tube is in place, a T-tube cholangiogram should be performed to detect the bile leak. In those without a T-tube an ERCP is the investigation of choice for diagnosing the bile leak. Sphincterotomy with placement of a plastic biliary stent at ERCP is successful in resolving 94% of bile leaks [39]. Fluid collections and bilomas are drained by percutaneous methods under US or CT guidance to prevent secondary infection and abscess formation. The bile duct stent is left in situ for at least 2–3 months to allow sufficient time for the leak to heal in the immunosuppressed patient.

There is limited experience in the use of covered self expanding metal stents (cSEMS) for post liver transplant bile leaks. cSEMS are effective in controlling the bile leak (Fig. 69.5) but may be associated with a high risk of stricture at site of previous bile leak. In a review of 17 cases of post liver transplant bile leaks treated by cSEMS placement, 8 cases developed biliary strictures after removal of cSEMS [40]. Prospective studies comparing cSEMS versus plastic

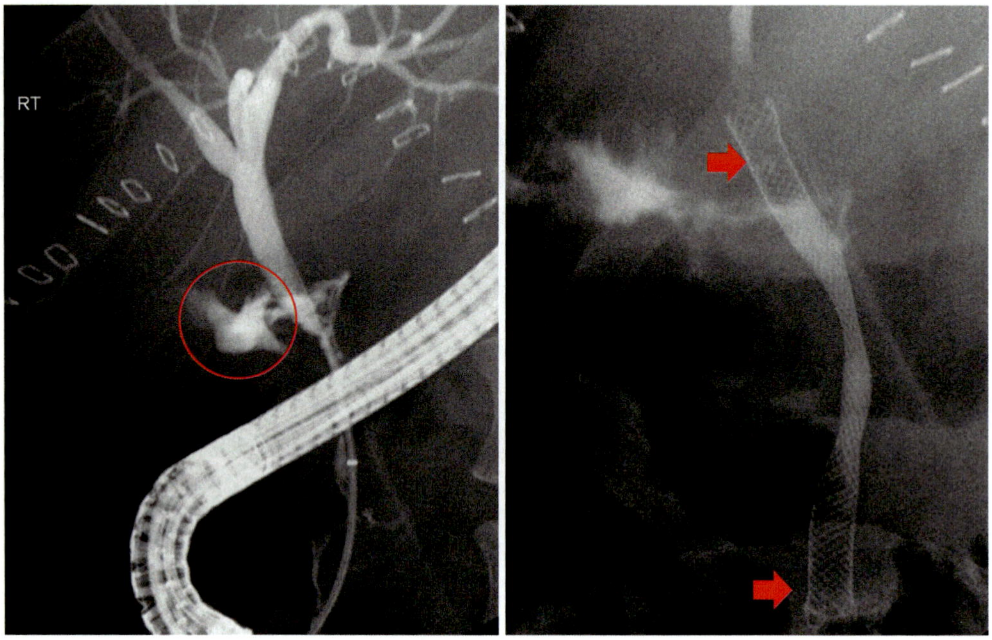

Fig. 69.5 Left hand image—ERCP demonstrating extravasation of contrast at biliary duct to duct anastomosis (red circle). Right hand image—ERCP image, showing placement of a covered metal biliary stent across the anastomosis (red arrows)

stents are required to ascertain the benefits and risks of cSEMS use for bile leaks in OLT patients.

In patients with a choledochojejunostomy anastomotic leak, ERCP is not possible. A PTC with insertion of internal external biliary drain is the preferred initial management. Relaparotomy for revision of the choledochojejunostomy is often required.

69.2.3.4 Biliary Strictures

Biliary strictures can be anastomotic or non anastomotic. Anastomotic strictures are more common. Anastomotic strictures are extrahepatic and occur at the site of surgical biliary anastomosis, whereas nonanastomotic strictures occur at any other site in the biliary tree and can be extrahepatic as well as intrahepatic.

Anastomotic Strictures

The mean incidence of anastomotic strictures is 12% after cadaveric OLT [33] and the majority of them occur within the first year after OLT. They occur as a result of technical issues causing ischemia and scarring of the anastomosis. A previous bile leak is an important risk factor for developing a biliary stricture [41].

Clinical presentation is variable and the diagnosis of biliary obstruction requires a high degree of clinical suspicion. Many patients present with abnormal liver function tests and no symptoms. Others will present with acute cholangitis (fever, rigors, abdominal pain and jaundice). Other presentations are symptoms of jaundice with or without pruritus, or as repeated episodes of fever and abnormal liver function tests. Ultrasound with Doppler is the initial investigation to assess the liver parenchyma, bile ducts and hepatic vasculature. However US has low sensitivity to detect biliary obstruction because many OLT patients do not develop biliary dilatation despite a tight biliary stricture [42]. Therefore if biliary obstruction is suspected, MRCP followed by ERCP or PTC should be performed (Fig. 69.6).

Most transplant centres nowadays use ERCP with balloon dilatation and placement of plastic stent for treatment of anastomotic strictures. Reported long term success rate varies from 64% to 100% [43]. However treatment of the biliary stricture is not usually possible in a single endoscopic intervention and most patients require several ERCP's, usually once every 2–3 months, for repeated balloon dilatation and stent changes. Following endoscopic treatment, patients require long term surveillance since the recurrence rate is high. One study reported recurrence of anastomotic strictures in 25.5% of patients after initial successful course of stent treatment [43]. However recurrences can be treated with further course of endoscopic plastic stents achieving long term stricture resolution in 67% of patients [43]. Although ERCP is an invasive procedure, it is generally well tolerated by patients with one prospective study showing a complication rate of 6.6% per procedure and 20.7% per treated patient [44]. In this study the cumulative rate was higher because most patients require multiple endoscopic interventions for treatment of anastomotic strictures following OLT.

There is limited data on the value of covered self expanding metal stents (cSEMS) in the management of anastomotic biliary strictures after liver transplant. Spontaneous cSEMS migration is known to occur [45, 46]. In a randomized clinical trial [45] comparing cSEMS versus multiple plastic stents in 64 patients, stricture recurrence rates were higher in cSEMS group (32% versus 0%), complications rates

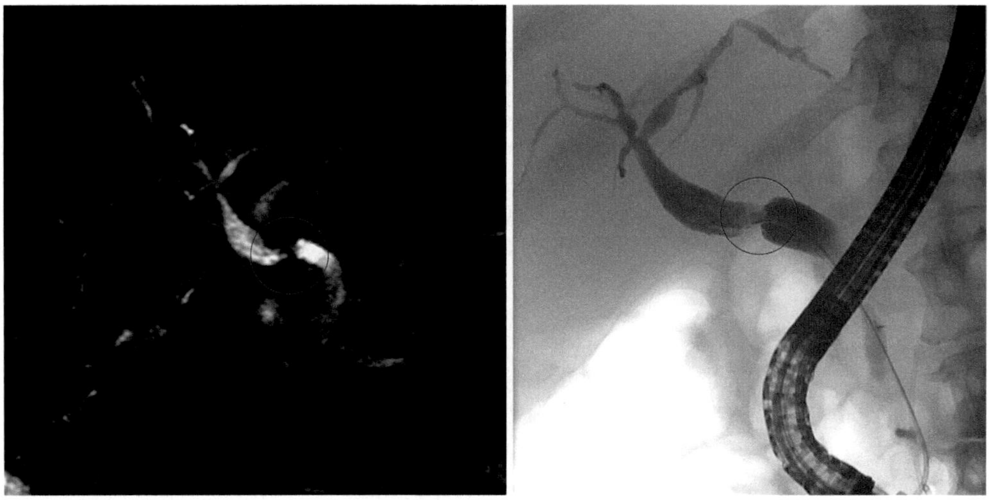

Fig. 69.6 Left hand image—MRCP coronal image showing caliber change at the biliary anastomosis. Right hand image—ERCP image, Cholangiogram confirming the finding on MRCP with tight stricture at the biliary anastomosis

including acute pancreatitis were higher in cSEMS group (23.3% versus 6.4%). Stricture resolution rates were not statistically different (83.3% versus 96.5%) between the two groups. cSEMS migration occurred in 3 cases [45]. cSEMS however may require fewer endoscopic interventions and stent changes. In another randomized clinical trial [46] of 48 patients, cSEMS required a median of 2 endoscopic interventions and a median of 1 stent whereas the plastic stent group required a median of 4 endoscopic interventions and a median of 8 stents until stricture resolution. cSEMS migration occurred in 8 cases [46]. At present, cSEMS may be reserved for use in biliary strictures refractory to treatment with plastic stents, however stent migration will continue to be a problem in these cases too. Further prospective studies are required to investigate duration and cost effectiveness of cSEMS therapy. Trial of newer stents with flared ends or anchoring flaps which may prevent stent migration may also be beneficial.

PTC for balloon dilatation and stent placement is performed in patients in whom ERCP is not successful due to failure to gain access to the bile duct or to cross a tight stricture. Patients with Roux en Y choledochojejunostomy require PTC as endoscopic access is rarely possible. PTC is required in 16–44% of cases [47]. It is more invasive than ERCP but has a high technical success rate. Complications include haemorrhage and bile leak from the liver puncture site. Also, PTC can be difficult and challenging if the intrahepatic bile ducts are not dilated.

Surgery is required for the treatment of bile duct strictures when ERCP and PTC have failed. Surgical biliary reconstruction most commonly consists of conversion to Roux en Y choledochojejunostomy or hepaticojejunostomy when the original procedure was a duct to duct anastomosis. In patients in whom the initial procedure was a Roux en Y choledochojejunostomy, the anastomosis is reconstructed above the previous anastomosis to healthy and well vascularized bile duct and jejunum.

Nonanastomotic Biliary Strictures

Non anastomotic biliary strictures occur secondary to hepatic artery thrombosis, chronic rejection, recurrence of primary sclerosing cholangitis, prolonged warm ischaemia time and use of ABO incompatible grafts. The incidence of non anastomotic biliary stricture after cadaveric OLT is around 10% [48]. Strictures can occur at single or multiple sites and can involve the extrahepatic bile ducts, hilum and intrahepatic bile ducts. The strictures are difficult to treat. The reported success rate of endoscopic therapy is 50–75% [49]. As the obstruction progresses biliary sludge, casts and stones form in the obstructed bile ducts further compounding the obstruction and predisposing to recurrent episodes of cholangitis. Graft loss rate is up to 46% by the end of the second postoperative year [48]. Progression of the anatomical extent of the biliary strictures occurred in 68% of patients with a significant number of patients developing sludge and casts [50]. Cholangitis occurred in 48% of patients and biliary cirrhosis, the end result of long standing biliary obstruction from nonanastomotic strictures, occurred in 28% of patients [50]. Overall, up to 50% of patients with non anastomotic biliary strictures die from complications or require re-transplantation [49].

69.2.4 Intra-abdominal Infections

Intra-abdominal infections present as intra-abdominal abscesses, infected bilomas, liver abscesses or peritonitis. Abdominal infections are a major source of bacterial infections and account for 27–47% of bacterial infections in the early postoperative period after OLT [51]. Risk factors associated with development of intra-abdominal infections after OLT include high pre transplant MELD score, prolonged duration of surgery, retransplantation, Roux en Y biliary anastomosis, and renal replacement therapy after liver transplant [52]. Abdominal infections prolong hospital stay, increase medical costs and graft loss [53].

Peritonitis occurs as a result of technical complications such as biliary or bowel anastomotic leak, or due to bowel perforation. Peritonitis accounted for 43% of intra-abdominal infections in a review of 169 adult OLT's [54]. In a retrospective review of 950 cadaveric OLT's studying peritonitis after liver transplant, bile leak and bowel anastomotic leak or perforation were associated with 28.7% and 18.5% of episodes of peritonitis respectively [52]. Bowel leaks which occur at enteric anastomosis sites are often due to a technical failure. Gastrointestinal perforations after adult OLT are rare and there are only anecdotal reports in the literature. Perforations can occur in the small and large bowel or stomach and duodenum and could be due to iatrogenic injury related to adhesiolysis and diathermy use. Post transplant lymphoproliferative disease (PTLD) is a rare cause of intestinal perforations after OLT and in a review of 5677 adult OLT's, 6 patients with PTLD presented with perforation [55]. Plain X-rays and contrast CT are diagnostic and exploratory laparotomy is required. In the immunosuppressed transplanted patient, clinical features of perforation may be absent or non specific and the interval from clinical onset to surgery can be 2–8 days [56].

Intra-abdominal abscesses after OLT can occur as a result of secondary infection of fluid collections or haematomas. The source may be external contamination such as drains or via haematogenous route or translocation from gut. Small ascitic fluid collections are common after OLT and usually resolve spontaneously in a few days. Small haematomas are also common and usually resolve without complications although complete resolution of some haematomas can take several months. Large haematomas can get infected leading to abscess formation. The gallbladder fossa, hepatorenal pouch and subphrenic spaces are common sites for haematoma and abscess formation. In a retrospective review of 169 OLT patients, intraabdominal infections occurred in 40% of patients in the first 2 months after OLT, with intra-abdominal abscesses comprising 29% of infections [54]. In the presence of immunosuppression, fever and leukocytosis do not correlate well with abdominal sepsis and a low threshold should be maintained to investigate for abdominal infection in OLT recipients with minimum signs and symptoms [54]. US and contrast CT are the investigations of choice and a complex fluid collection with an air fluid level is diagnostic of an abscess. Treatment consists of US or CT guided drainage of abscess and antimicrobial therapy. Intra-abdominal abscesses are significantly associated with patient death and graft loss [57].

Bilomas are localised intra or extrahepatic collections of bile typically associated with bile leaks or strictures. They have a high rate of retransplantation and decreased patient and graft survival. Bilomas may be associated with biliary anastomotic leaks or occur secondary to ischaemic bile duct injury from hepatic artery thrombosis or stenosis. Choledochojejunostomy is also strongly associated with biloma formation [58]. Although initially sterile, superimposed infection can occur. In a review of 492 OLT's 11.5% patients developed one or more bilomas [58, 59]. Clinical presentation was with fever and abdominal pain in 44% and 40% of patients respectively. Thirty-five percent were asymptomatic and were identified only because of abnormal liver enzymes [59]. Common infecting organisms were enterococci, staphylococci and candida species. Contrast enhanced CT and cholangiography are the mainstay of diagnosis. In the absence of graft failure, initial treatment is with percutaneous aspiration or drainage of the biloma, endoscopic stenting and antimicrobial therapy. Retransplantation is required if there is worsening graft function or no clinical improvement with nonsurgical therapy [59].

Pyogenic liver abscesses after OLT are uncommon. In a review of 2715 recipients of organ transplants 12 patients with 14 episode of liver abscesses were identified, all in liver transplant recipients (n = 459) [60]. Fever, chills and abdominal pain were common presenting symptoms. US and contrast enhanced CT were the mainstay of diagnosis. Predisposing factors for liver abscess formation were HAT, cholangitis, choledochojejunostomy, liver biopsy and prior episodes of bacteremia. CT guided drainage was successful in 70% of cases, five patients required retransplantation and five patients died [60].

69.2.5 Wound Complications

Surgical wound complications are the most common surgical problem following liver transplantation [61]. They include wound haematomas, superficial and deep wound infections, wound dehiscence and incisional hernias. Their incidence is related to various factors, including the complexity and duration of the transplant procedure, immunosuppressive treatment and the recipient BMI. Although not usually associated with mortality, their presence can increase morbidity due to increased hospital stay, readmissions and reoperations. They also increase medical costs and affect the patient's quality of life.

Wound haematomas are common after OLT. Portal hypertension and coagulopathy are risk factors for development of wound haematomas. They can delay wound healing or get secondarily infected. Removal of a few skin sutures to allow evacuation of the haematoma is advisable.

Wound infections may be superficial involving the skin and subcutaneous tissue or deep involving the fascia and muscle layers. Superficial and deep wound infections usually occur within the first month after transplantation and commonly present with wound erythema, tenderness and purulent discharge. The incidence of wound and organ/space infections considered together ranges between 6% and 43%. They are associated with prolonged hospitalization and readmission, and higher costs. Risk factors include diabetes, obesity, prolonged surgical procedure, large number of red blood cell transfusions and immunosuppression [51, 62, 63]. Gram positive organisms including *Staphylococcus* and *Enterococcus* species are the most common pathogens, but gram negative bacteria and *Candida* species can also cause wound infections [64, 65]. Multiple pathogens are also common [65]. Removal of skin sutures to release the wound collections and pus, and wound debridement is often required, following which wounds are allowed to heal by secondary intention. Antimicrobial treatment protocols including perioperative prophylaxis and postoperative empirical treatment (until wound culture and antimicrobial sensitivities are available) should be specifically tailored, rather than generalized, to each transplant centre's requirements and always take into consideration that more than one pathogens may be involved.

Superficial wound dehiscence involves the skin and the subcutaneous tissue whereas full-thickness or deep wound dehiscence denotes the involvement of the underlying fascia and muscle, and can lead to evisceration. Wound dehiscence (superficial and deep) occurs in 27% of liver transplant patients. Superficial wound dehiscence can be managed conservatively and healing by secondary intent can be achieved or the wound can be debrided and primarily closed. Another emerging technique is the application of vacuum dressings that promote wound healing by suction approximation of the skin edges and promoting granulation tissue and healing by secondary intention. Full-thickness wound dehiscences are considered a surgical emergency and require reoperation for primary or mesh closure of the abdomen [61].

An abdominal incisional hernia is a defect in the abdominal wall at the site of a previous incision. Incisional hernias following liver transplantation are late complications and their incidence can range between 1.7% and 34.3% [66]. Not all incisional hernias are symptomatic, however they can lead to several complications, including abdominal discomfort and pain, incarceration and strangulation, bowel obstruction, necrosis and perforation of the bowel and cosmesis issues [61, 66]. Risk factors for the formation of an incisional hernia after liver transplantation include surgical site infection, prolonged ICU stay, high BMI, older age (>55 years) and immunosuppression [61, 66–68]. Surgical site infections are strongly associated with the formation of incisional hernias and the underlying mechanism involves impaired wound healing [67]. The association between prolonged ICU stay and incisional hernia has been hypothesised to be related to malnutrition and impaired immune function [66]. A link between obesity and incisional hernia development has been suggested by several studies and this is attributed to the higher intra-abdominal pressures exerted on the abdominal muscles during wound healing, the higher incidence of wound infections as well as the higher occurrence of diabetes mellitus in obese patients [66–68]. Older patients are also more likely to form an incisional hernia after liver transplant due to alterations in their immune system that can lead to a higher rate of wound infections as suggested by one study, although the mechanism behind this is not clear [66]. More than a few studies have shown a relationship between incisional hernia formation and immunosuppression. Several agents have been implicated in the pathogenesis and include mycophenolate mofetil (MMF), steroids and mammalian target of rapamycin (mTOR) inhibitors, such as sirolimus [61, 67]. The type of incision is also important and a J shaped subcostal incision is associated with reduced incidence of wound infection, dehiscence and hernias as compared to the classic Mercedes Benz incision [69]. Clinical follow-up and examination of the patient is important in the identification of incisional hernias, as they can be often missed and thus their management delayed [66]. Treatment of symptomatic incisional hernias is surgical and the preferred method is bridging of the defect with the use of a mesh, either synthetic or biological, as it has been found that direct closure of the abdominal wall with sutures leads to high recurrence rates [66, 70].

69.3 Conclusion

Postoperative surgical complications are a common and important cause of morbidity and mortality after liver transplantation. The results of OLT have improved with advances and improvements in anaesthesia and surgical techniques. In the current era, intraoperative deaths are rare but postoperative complications are a frequent occurrence and prevention of these complications is crucial to the success of OLT. Early diagnosis and treatment of postoperative surgical complications improves graft and patient survival rates but when there is significant graft dysfunction or failure, early retransplantation can save the patients life.

Self Study

Questions

1. Which of the following statements is correct?
   (a) Hepatic artery thrombosis is the most common reason for reoperation following liver transplantation.
   (b) Hepatic artery thrombosis is the most common vascular complication in liver transplantation.
   (c) Hepatic artery thrombosis can have greater impact on graft and patient survival than portal vein thrombosis.
   (d) Laparotomy is indicated for all patients with early bleeding following liver transplantation.

2. Which of the following statements is correct?
   (a) Wound infections in transplant patients are more commonly caused by single organisms and gram negative bacteria are the most frequently isolated bacterial microorganisms
   (b) Incisional hernias are a frequent complication following liver transplantation and should be treated surgically with mesh placement.
   (c) ERCP and/or PTC are the gold standard for biliary leak diagnosis, but MRCP should be the initial investigation when a biliary complication is suspected.
   (d) Covered self-expanding stents are associated with fewer complications and higher success rates when compared to plastic stents in the management of biliary complication and should be the treatment of choice.

Answers

1. Which of the following statements is correct?
   (a) Postoperative haemorrhage is the most common reason for reoperation following liver transplantation. Reoperation is required in 8–27% of OLT recipients
   (b) CORRECT. Hepatic artery thrombosis is the most common vascular complication in liver transplantation occurring in 1–9% of OLT recipients and can leads to graft loss in 56% of the patients and is associated with a 33% mortality.
   (c) Portal vein thrombosis has overall a more detrimental effect on patient and graft survival than hepatic artery thrombosis, as it may involve extension into the mesenteric vessels and thus preclude retransplantation.
   (d) Patients with haemodynamic instability, persisting despite clotting correction, require emergency relaparotomy. However haemodynamically stable patients can have a diagnostic US or CT scan prior to deciding on whether a laparotomy is necessary.
2. Which of the following statements is correct?
   (a) Most common pathogens causing wound infections are gram positive cocci including Staphylococcus and Enterococcus *species* and multiple microorganisms can be isolated. Antimicrobial treatment should be tailored according to each transplant centre's microbiology policy.
   (b) Only patients with symptomatic incisional hernias should be treated surgically. The preferred method of treatment is reconstruction of the abdominal wall with a mesh, as primary closure has high recurrence rates.
   (c) CORRECT. ERCP and/or PTC are the gold standard investigations for diagnosis of biliary complications but should be preceded by MRCP which is a non-invasive investigation and has a high sensitivity and specificity (96% and 94% respectively).
   (d) Currently covered self-expanding stents are reserved for patients with strictures refractory to plastic stent treatment, as there are associated with spontaneous stent migration and higher stricture recurrence rate.

References

1. Kim WR, Lake JR, Smith JM, Schladt DP, Skeans MA, Harper AM, et al. OPTN/SRTR 2016 Annual data report: liver. Am J Transplant. 2018;18(Suppl 1):172–253.
2. NHSBT. NHSBT-liver-transplantation-annual-report-2017-2018. Watford: NHSBT; 2018. https://nhsbtdbe.blob.core.windows.net/umbraco-assets-corp/12250/nhsbt-liver-transplantation-annual-report-2017-2018.pdf.
3. Ertel AE, Wima K, Chang AL, Hoehn RS, Hohmann SF, Edwards MJ, et al. Risk of reoperation within 90 days of liver transplantation: a necessary evil? J Am Coll Surg. 2016;222(4):419–28.
4. Thompson MA, Redden DT, Glueckert L, Smith AB, Crawford JH, Jones KA, et al. Risk factors associated with reoperation for bleeding following liver transplantation. HPB Surg. 2014;2014:816246.
5. Kim DS, Lee SG, Sung GB, Ko GY, Park KM, Kim KH, et al. Management of subcapsular hematoma of the graft after living donor liver transplantation. Liver Transpl. 2006;12(7):1124–8.
6. Jung SW, Hwang S, Namgoong JM, Yoon SY, Park CS, Park YH, et al. Incidence and management of postoperative abdominal bleeding after liver transplantation. Transplant Proc. 2012;44(3):765–8.
7. Hong SS, Kim AY. Early postoperative bleeding after living donor liver transplantation. Abdom Imaging. 2009;34(3):365–70.
8. Duffy JP, Hong JC, Farmer DG, Ghobrial RM, Yersiz H, Hiatt JR, et al. Vascular complications of orthotopic liver transplantation: experience in more than 4,200 patients. J Am Coll Surg. 2009;208(5):896–903; discussion –5.
9. Mourad MM, Liossis C, Gunson BK, Mergental H, Isaac J, Muiesan P, et al. Etiology and management of hepatic artery thrombosis after adult liver transplantation. Liver Transpl. 2014;20(6):713–23.
10. Bekker J, Ploem S, de Jong KP. Early hepatic artery thrombosis after liver transplantation: a systematic review of the incidence, outcome and risk factors. Am J Transplant. 2009;9(4):746–57.
11. Heaton ND. Hepatic artery thrombosis: conservative management or retransplantation? Liver Transpl. 2013;19(Suppl 2):S14–6.
12. Zalewska K. Liver selection policy - ODT Clinical. Watford: NHSBT; 2017. http://www.odt.nhs.uk/pdf/non_compliance_with_selection_and_allocation_policies.pdf.
13. Horrow MM, Blumenthal BM, Reich DJ, Manzarbeitia C. Sonographic diagnosis and outcome of hepatic artery thrombosis after orthotopic liver transplantation in adults. AJR Am J Roentgenol. 2007;189(2):346–51.
14. Piardi T, Lhuaire M, Bruno O, Memeo R, Pessaux P, Kianmanesh R, et al. Vascular complications following liver transplantation: a literature review of advances in 2015. World J Hepatol. 2016;8(1):36–57.
15. Sommacale D, Aoyagi T, Dondero F, Sibert A, Bruno O, Fteriche S, et al. Repeat endovascular treatment of recurring hepatic artery stenoses in orthotopic liver transplantation. Transpl Int. 2013;26(6):608–15.
16. Jain A, Costa G, Marsh W, Fontes P, Devera M, Mazariegos G, et al. Thrombotic and nonthrombotic hepatic artery complications in adults and children following primary liver transplantation with long-term follow-up in 1000 consecutive patients. Transpl Int. 2006;19(1):27–37.

17. Goldsmith LE, Wiebke K, Seal J, Brinster C, Smith TA, Bazan HA, et al. Complications after endovascular treatment of hepatic artery stenosis after liver transplantation. J Vasc Surg. 2017;66(5):1488–96.
18. Abbasoglu O, Levy MF, Vodapally MS, Goldstein RM, Husberg BS, Gonwa TA, et al. Hepatic artery stenosis after liver transplantation--incidence, presentation, treatment, and long term outcome. Transplantation. 1997;63(2):250–5.
19. Rajakannu M, Awad S, Ciacio O, Pittau G, Adam R, Cunha AS, et al. Intention-to-treat analysis of percutaneous endovascular treatment of hepatic artery stenosis after orthotopic liver transplantation. Liver Transpl. 2016;22(7):923–33.
20. Pulitano C, Joseph D, Sandroussi C, Verran D, Strasser SI, Shackel NA, et al. Hepatic artery stenosis after liver transplantation: is endovascular treatment always necessary? Liver Transpl. 2015;21(2):162–8.
21. Taner T, Heimbach J. To stent or not to stent: endovascular treatment of hepatic artery stenosis. Liver Transpl. 2016;22(7):884–5.
22. Marshall MM, Muiesan P, Srinivasan P, Kane PA, Rela M, Heaton ND, et al. Hepatic artery pseudoaneurysms following liver transplantation: incidence, presenting features and management. Clin Radiol. 2001;56(7):579–87.
23. Volpin E, Pessaux P, Sauvanet A, Sibert A, Kianmanesh R, Durand F, et al. Preservation of the arterial vascularisation after hepatic artery pseudoaneurysm following orthotopic liver transplantation: long-term results. Ann Transplant. 2014;19:346–52.
24. Boleslawski E, Bouras AF, Truant S, Liddo G, Herrero A, Badic B, et al. Hepatic artery ligation for arterial rupture following liver transplantation: a reasonable option. Am J Transplant. 2013;13(4):1055–62.
25. Leelaudomlipi S, Bramhall SR, Gunson BK, Candinas D, Buckels JA, McMaster P, et al. Hepatic-artery aneurysm in adult liver transplantation. Transpl Int. 2003;16(4):257–61.
26. Fistouris J, Herlenius G, Backman L, Olausson M, Rizell M, Mjornstedt L, et al. Pseudoaneurysm of the hepatic artery following liver transplantation. Transplant Proc. 2006;38(8):2679–82.
27. Unger LW, Berlakovich GA, Trauner M, Reiberger T. Management of portal hypertension before and after liver transplantation. Liver Transpl. 2018;24(1):112–21.
28. Saad WE. Portal interventions in liver transplant recipients. Semin Intervent Radiol. 2012;29(2):99–104.
29. Khan A, Park P, Oberholzer J, Tzvetanov I, Garcia Roca R, Gaba RC, et al. Concurrent hepatic artery and portal vein thrombosis after orthotopic liver transplantation with preserved allografts. Case Rep Transpl. 2014;2014:384295.
30. Khorsandi SE, Athale A, Vilca-Melendez H, Jassem W, Prachalias A, Srinivasan P, et al. Presentation, diagnosis, and management of early hepatic venous outflow complications in whole cadaveric liver transplant. Liver Transpl. 2015;21(7):914–21.
31. Settmacher U, Nussler NC, Glanemann M, Haase R, Heise M, Bechstein WO, et al. Venous complications after orthotopic liver transplantation. Clin Transplant. 2000;14(3):235–41.
32. Darcy MD. Management of venous outflow complications after liver transplantation. Tech Vasc Interv Radiol. 2007;10(3):240–5.
33. Akamatsu N, Sugawara Y, Hashimoto D. Biliary reconstruction, its complications and management of biliary complications after adult liver transplantation: a systematic review of the incidence, risk factors and outcome. Transpl Int. 2011;24(4):379–92.
34. Davidson BR, Rai R, Kurzawinski TR, Selves L, Farouk M, Dooley JS, et al. Prospective randomized trial of end-to-end versus side-to-side biliary reconstruction after orthotopic liver transplantation. Br J Surg. 1999;86(4):447–52.
35. Bennet W, Zimmerman MA, Campsen J, Mandell MS, Bak T, Wachs M, et al. Choledochoduodenostomy is a safe alternative to Roux-en-Y choledochojejunostomy for biliary reconstruction in liver transplantation. World J Surg. 2009;33(5):1022–5.
36. Riediger C, Muller MW, Michalski CW, Huser N, Schuster T, Kleeff J, et al. T-Tube or no T-tube in the reconstruction of the biliary tract during orthotopic liver transplantation: systematic review and meta-analysis. Liver Transpl. 2010;16(6):705–17.
37. Sotiropoulos GC, Sgourakis G, Radtke A, Molmenti EP, Goumas K, Mylona S, et al. Orthotopic liver transplantation: T-tube or not T-tube? Systematic review and meta-analysis of results. Transplantation. 2009;87(11):1672–80.
38. Jorgensen JE, Waljee AK, Volk ML, Sonnenday CJ, Elta GH, Al-Hawary MM, et al. Is MRCP equivalent to ERCP for diagnosing biliary obstruction in orthotopic liver transplant recipients? A meta-analysis. Gastrointest Endosc. 2011;73(5):955–62.
39. Sendino O, Fernandez-Simon A, Law R, Abu Dayyeh B, Leise M, Chavez-Rivera K, et al. Endoscopic management of bile leaks after liver transplantation: an analysis of two high-volume transplant centers. U Eur Gastroenterol J. 2018;6(1):89–96.
40. Phillips MS, Bonatti H, Sauer BG, Smith L, Javaid M, Kahaleh M, et al. Elevated stricture rate following the use of fully covered self-expandable metal biliary stents for biliary leaks following liver transplantation. Endoscopy. 2011;43(6):512–7.
41. Sundaram V, Jones DT, Shah NH, de Vera ME, Fontes P, Marsh JW, et al. Posttransplant biliary complications in the pre- and post-model for end-stage liver disease era. Liver Transpl. 2011;17(4):428–35.
42. St Peter S, Rodriquez-Davalos MI, Rodriguez-Luna HM, Harrison EM, Moss AA, Mulligan DC. Significance of proximal biliary dilatation in patients with anastomotic strictures after liver transplantation. Dig Dis Sci. 2004;49(7-8):1207–11.
43. Dai SC, Goldberg D, Agarwal A, Ma GK, Yam C, Ahmad NA, et al. Endoscopic therapy is effective for recurrent anastomotic biliary strictures after orthotopic liver transplantation. Ann Hepatol. 2017;16(6):924–31.
44. Holt AP, Thorburn D, Mirza D, Gunson B, Wong T, Haydon G. A prospective study of standardized nonsurgical therapy in the management of biliary anastomotic strictures complicating liver transplantation. Transplantation. 2007;84(7):857–63.
45. Martins FP, De Paulo GA, Contini MLC, Ferrari AP. Metal versus plastic stents for anastomotic biliary strictures after liver transplantation: a randomized controlled trial. Gastrointest Endosc. 2018;87(1):131.e1–e13.
46. Tal AO, Finkelmeier F, Filmann N, Kylanpaa L, Udd M, Parzanese I, et al. Multiple plastic stents versus covered metal stent for treatment of anastomotic biliary strictures after liver transplantation: a prospective, randomized, multicenter trial. Gastrointest Endosc. 2017;86(6):1038–45.
47. Koksal AS, Eminler AT, Parlak E, Gurakar A. Management of biliary anastomotic strictures after liver transplantation. Transplant Rev (Orlando). 2017;31(3):207–17.
48. Guichelaar MM, Benson JT, Malinchoc M, Krom RA, Wiesner RH, Charlton MR. Risk factors for and clinical course of non-anastomotic biliary strictures after liver transplantation. Am J Transplant. 2003;3(7):885–90.
49. Sharma S, Gurakar A, Jabbour N. Biliary strictures following liver transplantation: past, present and preventive strategies. Liver Transpl. 2008;14(6):759–69.
50. Verdonk RC, Buis CI, van der Jagt EJ, Gouw AS, Limburg AJ, Slooff MJ, et al. Nonanastomotic biliary strictures after liver transplantation, part 2: management, outcome, and risk factors for disease progression. Liver Transpl. 2007;13(5):725–32.
51. Romero FA, Razonable RR. Infections in liver transplant recipients. World J Hepatol. 2011;3(4):83–92.
52. Pungpapong S, Alvarez S, Hellinger WC, Kramer DJ, Willingham DL, Mendez JC, et al. Peritonitis after liver transplantation: incidence, risk factors, microbiology profiles, and outcome. Liver Transpl. 2006;12(8):1244–52.
53. Hollenbeak CS, Alfrey EJ, Souba WW. The effect of surgical site infections on outcomes and resource utilization after liver transplantation. Surgery. 2001;130(2):388–95.

54. Reid GE, Grim SA, Sankary H, Benedetti E, Oberholzer J, Clark NM. Early intra-abdominal infections associated with orthotopic liver transplantation. Transplantation. 2009;87(11):1706–11.
55. Cruz RJ Jr, Ramachandra S, Sasatomi E, DiMartini A, de Vera M, Fontes P, et al. Surgical management of gastrointestinal posttransplant lymphoproliferative disorders in liver transplant recipients. Transplantation. 2012;94(4):417–23.
56. de'Angelis N, Esposito F, Memeo R, Lizzi V, Martinez-Perez A, Landi F, et al. Emergency abdominal surgery after solid organ transplantation: a systematic review. World J Emerg Surg. 2016;11(1):43.
57. Hellinger WC, Crook JE, Heckman MG, Diehl NN, Shalev JA, Zubair AC, et al. Surgical site infection after liver transplantation: risk factors and association with graft loss or death. Transplantation. 2009;87(9):1387–93.
58. Said A, Safdar N, Lucey MR, Knechtle SJ, D'Alessandro A, Musat A, et al. Infected bilomas in liver transplant recipients, incidence, risk factors and implications for prevention. Am J Transplant. 2004;4(4):574–82.
59. Safdar N, Said A, Lucey MR, Knechtle SJ, D'Alessandro A, Musat A, et al. Infected bilomas in liver transplant recipients: clinical features, optimal management, and risk factors for mortality. Clin Infect Dis. 2004;39(4):517–25.
60. Tachopoulou OA, Vogt DP, Henderson JM, Baker M, Keys TF. Hepatic abscess after liver transplantation: 1990-2000. Transplantation. 2003;75(1):79–83.
61. Kahn J, Muller H, Iberer F, Kniepeiss D, Duller D, Rehak P, et al. Incisional hernia following liver transplantation: incidence and predisposing factors. Clin Transplant. 2007;21(3):423–6.
62. Natori Y, Kassar R, Iaboni A, Hosseini-Moghaddam SM, Vu J, Husain S, et al. Surgical site infections after liver transplantation: prospective surveillance and evaluation of 250 transplant recipients in Canada. Infect Control Hosp Epidemiol. 2017;38(9):1084–90.
63. Freire MP, Soares Oshiro IC, Bonazzi PR, Guimaraes T, Ramos Figueira ER, Bacchella T, et al. Surgical site infections in liver transplant recipients in the model for end-stage liver disease era: an analysis of the epidemiology, risk factors, and outcomes. Liver Transpl. 2013;19(9):1011–9.
64. Patel G, Huprikar S. Infectious complications after orthotopic liver transplantation. Semin Respir Crit Care Med. 2012;33(1):111–24.
65. Viehman JA, Clancy CJ, Clarke L, Shields RK, Silveira FP, Kwak EJ, et al. Surgical site infections after liver transplantation: emergence of multidrug-resistant bacteria and implications for prophylaxis and treatment strategies. Transplantation. 2016;100(10):2107–14.
66. de Goede B, Eker HH, Klitsie PJ, van Kempen BJ, Polak WG, Hop WC, et al. Incisional hernia after liver transplantation: risk factors and health-related quality of life. Clin Transplant. 2014;28(7):829–36.
67. Smith CT, Katz MG, Foley D, Welch B, Leverson GE, Funk LM, et al. Incidence and risk factors of incisional hernia formation following abdominal organ transplantation. Surg Endosc. 2015;29(2):398–404.
68. Lee JS, Kim JM, Kim KS, Choi GS, Joh JW, Lee SK. Predictors of incisional hernia in adult liver transplant recipients. Hernia. 2019;23:61.
69. Heisterkamp J, Marsman HA, Eker H, Metselaar HJ, Tilanus HW, Kazemier G. A J-shaped subcostal incision reduces the incidence of abdominal wall complications in liver transplantation. Liver Transpl. 2008;14(11):1655–8.
70. den Hartog D, Dur AH, Tuinebreijer WE, Kreis RW. Open surgical procedures for incisional hernias. Cochrane Database Syst Rev. 2008;(3):CD006438.

Anaesthesia for Liver Transplantation

70

Donald M. Milliken, Brian R. Davidson, and Michael D. Spiro

Key Concepts

- Sarcopenia, frailty and poor exercise capacity are prevalent among patients undergoing liver transplantation, and contribute substantially to perioperative risk
- Liver transplantation presents extreme physiological challenges relating to anhepatic physiology and donor graft reperfusion, and these demand proactive management
- Robust management strategies for detecting and treating coagulopathy must be adopted and policies must be in place for managing major blood loss.
- Living donor liver transplantation produces good outcomes for recipients but requires an appreciation of additional technical, logistical and ethical considerations, as well as anaesthetic complexity.

70.1 Introduction

Liver transplantation offers the possibility of long term survival for eligible patients with end-stage liver disease (ESLD) and has overall excellent outcomes with a UK 5-year elective survival rate of over 80% [1]. Most liver transplants are isolated liver grafts from donors who have fulfilled criteria for brainstem death: donation after brain death (DBD). Transplantation of organs recovered by donation after cardiac death (DCD) is increasingly common, and now represents around 20% of the volume in the UK. Transplantations of split liver grafts, reduced size grafts and living donor transplants represent only a small fraction of the liver transplant volume in Western healthcare systems.

The majority of recipients undergoing elective transplantation suffer from chronic liver disease of variable aetiology, most commonly associated with cirrhosis. Approximately 10% of organs go to recipients with acute liver failure—'super-urgent' transplantation—and survival in this group is only slightly inferior to the elective cohort [1].

Evidence is emerging of good results of transplantation in patients with acute on chronic liver failure, with centres reporting 5-year survival in the range of 73–90% [2, 3].

70.2 Preoperative Considerations

Owing to the complex, multi-system nature of ESLD and the risks associated with surgery, candidates for liver transplantation undergo rigorous, multidisciplinary assessment prior to listing for transplant. This assessment includes input from, at minimum, a hepatologist, surgeon, anaesthetist and transplant coordinator, but should also include input from radiologist, dietician, substance misuse counsellor, psychologist and physiotherapist as appropriate.

Liver disease severity is central to the prioritisation of candidates for liver transplant. The most commonly used scoring system is the Model for End-Stage Liver Disease

D. M. Milliken (✉)
Royal Free Perioperative Research, London, UK

Liver Transplant and HPB Anaesthesia, The Royal Free London NHS Foundation Trust, London, UK

B. R. Davidson
Department of Hepato-pancreatico-biliary Surgery, Royal Free Hospital, London, UK
e-mail: b.davidson@ucl.ac.uk

M. D. Spiro
Royal Free Perioperative Research, London, UK

Liver Transplant and HPB Anaesthesia, Royal Free London NHS Foundation Trust, London, UK

The Royal Free London NHS Foundation Trust, University College London, London, UK
e-mail: michaelspiro@nhs.net

F. Radu-Ionita et al. (eds.), *Liver Diseases*, https://doi.org/10.1007/978-3-030-24432-3_70

(MELD), based on an algorithm derived from the biochemical function of the liver [4]. Poorer function results in a higher score and prioritisation on the transplant waiting list. The MELD score correlates with perioperative risk. The risk of adverse perioperative outcomes is also increased by the high and overlapping incidence of frailty, sarcopenia, poor functional capacity and cardiorespiratory pathology in this cohort. Diabetes mellitus, chronic kidney disease and haematological disorders are also frequently identified in the preoperative period and affect perioperative management and outcomes.

70.2.1 Frailty, Sarcopenia and Poor Functional Capacity

Frailty is the age-related syndrome of increased vulnerability to stressors and decreased physiological reserve that results from the accumulation of biological deficits. Though more commonly associated with older patients, the prevalence of frailty is around 15–20% in patients awaiting liver transplantation, and the diagnosis is associated with waiting list and perioperative mortality [5]. Frailty may be measured using one of the validated scales of general frailty in current use and a liver disease-specific frailty measure has recently been developed [4, 6, 7].

Sarcopenia is a syndrome of older age characterised by the loss of skeletal muscle mass and function. It is increasingly recognised in younger patients, particularly those with obesity. It affects around 40% of patients awaiting liver transplantation and is associated with increased waiting list and surgical mortality, complications and length of hospital stay [8, 9]. Sarcopenia may be diagnosed by the presence of low muscle mass (e.g. by cross-sectional imaging), low muscle force (e.g. by handgrip dynamometer) and poor physical function (e.g. by short physical performance battery) [10].

Poor performance on measures of global physical function is associated with a host of adverse outcomes. A reduced six-minute walking distance (6MWD) predicts death on the waiting list for liver transplant candidates [11]. Cardiopulmonary exercise testing (CPET) is the gold standard test of global cardiorespiratory function, and is used routinely in some centres in the assessment of liver transplant candidates. Poor CPET performance is associated with adverse perioperative outcomes, with an anaerobic threshold below 9 ml/min/kg predicting increased surgical mortality in retrospective series, although prospective validation is awaited [12].

The identification of frailty, sarcopenia and poor functional capacity is an essential part of the preoperative assessment of liver transplant candidates. An appreciation of their contribution to increased surgical risk supports listing decisions, patient counselling and tailoring of perioperative care. Crucially, these are all dynamic and reversible conditions that may improve with nutritional and exercise interventions in the preoperative period.

The science and practice of prehabilitation aims to improve preoperative fitness through programmes of physical exercise, nutritional support and psychological interventions. There are clear challenges in applying fitness and exercise regimes in people debilitated by chronic liver disease. However evidence supporting its role in improving preoperative function and perioperative outcomes is emerging. Applied to patients with ESLD, prehabilitation could in theory allow deconditioned, marginal transplant candidates to be placed on the waiting list, prevent death and de-listing while on the waiting list, and improve post-transplant outcomes. Though the benefits of prehabilitation to liver transplant candidates would intuitively seem to be substantial, supporting evidence is awaited.

70.2.2 Cardiorespiratory Pathology

Patients with portal hypertension may develop a significant intrapulmonary shunt as a consequence of abnormal pulmonary haemodynamics and neovascularisation. This condition, the hepatopulmonary syndrome, affects 10% of liver transplant candidates, presenting clinically with reduced resting oxygen saturation, exercise intolerance, and orthodeoxia: improved oxygenation in the supine position [13]. Diagnosis requires the presence of liver disease, a positive contrast-enhanced transthoracic echocardiogram, and an alveolar-arterial oxygen gradient greater than or equal to 15 mmHg (≥20 mmHg if age > 64) [14]. Cases associated with severe hypoxaemia ($PaO2 < 7$ kPa) are associated with increased perioperative mortality and complications [13]. These patients may require ambulatory oxygen therapy and suffer from significant functional impairment. Maintaining adequate intraoperative and postoperative oxygenation is usually possible in mild to moderate disease and is aided by the supine position during surgery.

Pulmonary hypertension in association with portal hypertension, the syndrome of portopulmonary hypertension, is found in approximately 6% of patients considered for liver transplantation [7]. Raised pulmonary artery systolic pressure on preoperative transthoracic echocardiogram should prompt further investigation by right heart catheterisation. Diagnosis requires the presence of portal hypertension, a mean pulmonary artery pressure (mPAP) >25 mmHg, PVR >240 dynes/s per cm^{-5}, pulmonary artery wedge pressure <15 mmHg and the exclusion of other causes of pulmonary hypertension [14]. In mild disease, with mPAP between 25 and 35 mmHg, perioperative risk is only slightly increased. Moderate disease (mPAP 35–45 mmHg) increases both short- and long-term postoperative mortality and severe disease (mPAP > 45 mmHg) is generally considered a contraindication to transplantation [8]. Unexpected increased breathlessness in patients awaiting transplantation, or in patients presenting on the day of planned transplantation, should prompt consideration of repeat echocardiography. Good transplant outcomes have been demonstrated in a series of patients with moderate and severe portopulmonary hypertension who were responsive to vasodilators in the preoperative period [15]. At present transplantation in such patients remains controversial and should be considered on a case-by-case basis.

The characteristic systemic vasodilatation of severe liver disease results in a compensatory increase in the cardiac output and work. It is thought that this, along with direct myocardial toxicity from abnormal metabolites, results in the constellation of features known collectively as cirrhotic cardiomyopathy. Cirrhotic cardiomyopathy typically is characterised by diastolic dysfunction and impaired contractile response to stress. Clinical suspicion may be raised by evidence of abnormal repolarisation including a prolonged QT interval [16]. Intraoperatively this may increase the likelihood of arrhythmia and reduce tolerance of hypo- or hypervolaemia.

70.2.3 Diabetes Mellitus

Diabetes mellitus is common among patients awaiting liver transplantation and is especially prevalent among those with non-alcoholic steatohepatitis (NASH). NASH cirrhosis is an increasingly common indication for transplantation, rising commensurate with population obesity levels. NASH is frequently responsive to lifestyle intervention, which may at the same time improve blood glucose control. Medical management of diabetes in the liver transplant candidate should be according to local guidelines and adjusted according to serial measurement of glycosylated haemoglobin. Where control is poor, patients benefit from early involvement of a diabetes specialist. A diagnosis of diabetes increases the risk of a range of perioperative complications, including acute kidney injury, wound infection, and sepsis [17]. Careful attention to blood glucose control in the perioperative period is essential.

70.2.4 Chronic Kidney Disease

Patients with chronic liver disease may have concomitant chronic kidney disease (CKD) as a direct consequence of their liver disease, as in the hepatorenal syndrome, or due to common causes such as pre-existing diabetes or hypertension. The risk of postoperative acute kidney injury is substantially higher in patients with CKD and should be anticipated. In some centres selected patients with severe CKD may be established on haemofiltration in the pre- and intraoperative periods to optimise electrolytes and acid-base balance.

70.2.5 Coagulopathy and Anaemia

Coagulopathy is a hallmark of severe liver disease and its management is a major intraoperative challenge for the liver transplant anaesthetist. The cell-based model of coagulation explains that coagulation in patients with ESLD is 'rebalanced' with preserved thrombin generation, and that even in the presence of abnormal laboratory coagulation tests they may not exhibit a bleeding tendency. They are however more vulnerable to stressors, including surgical stress, that may increase their risk of haemorrhage, thrombosis, or both [18]. Abnormal coagulation tests in the absence of clinical haemorrhage are not routinely corrected in the preoperative period.

Thrombocytopenia frequently occurs due to bone marrow suppression, splenic sequestration associated with splenomegaly and preoperative bleeding episodes. Preoperative platelet transfusion is uncommon and must be weighed against the risks, including that of transfusion-related acute lung injury.

Anaemia in the liver transplant candidate is common, multifactorial and increases the risk of perioperative transfusion. Preoperative identification and treatment of anaemia as part of a patient blood management strategy may help to reduce transfusion requirements. Patients with iron deficiency may benefit from treatment with intravenous iron (Fig. 70.1).

70.3 Intraoperative Care

Anaesthetic management for liver transplantation is complex, aiming to mitigate against the high risk of major haemorrhage and to maintain stability through the physiological challenges presented by the anhepatic phase and donor organ reperfusion. Intraoperative management may be standardised at each liver transplant center, but it varies considerably between centers. Factors influencing management include the surgical approach (caval replacement or piggyback, with or without a temporary porto-caval shunt or venovenous bypass [VVBP]), the experience of surgeons and anesthetists, case volume, and patient factors. Intraoperative resource and personnel utilisation also varies widely between liver transplant centers and is influenced by the same factors. In general, two experienced anaesthetists are required to deliver safe care.

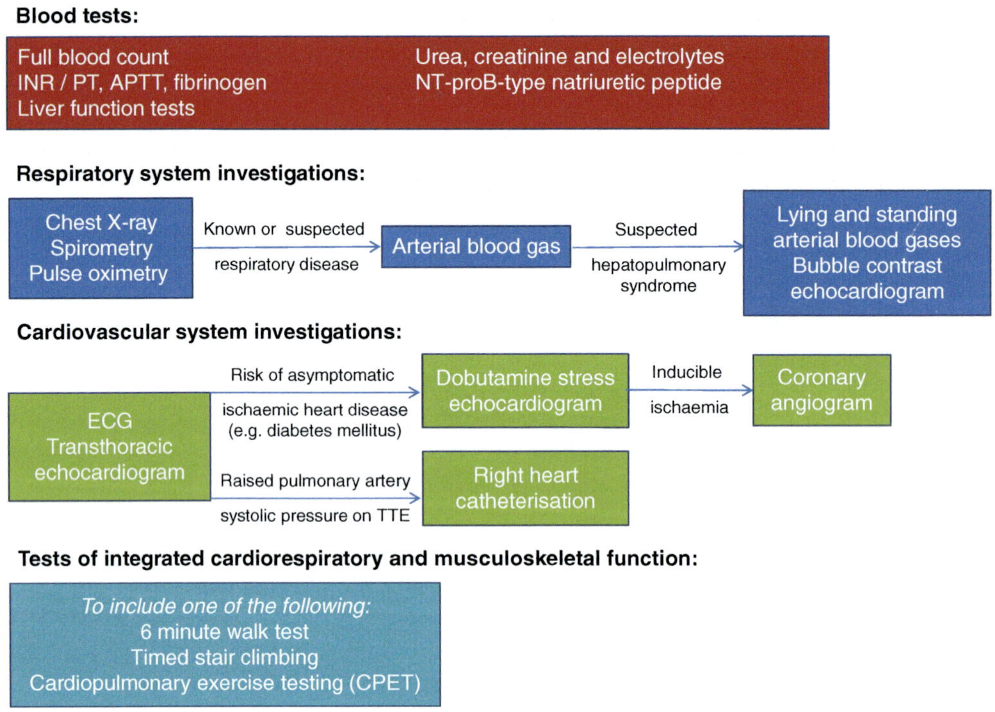

Fig. 70.1 Example of preoperative investigations for liver transplant recipients

70.3.1 Anaesthetic Choice

Anaesthetic techniques vary due to the lack of evidence supporting any one approach over others, but all involve balanced general anaesthesia with invasive monitoring. With the exception of halothane, all volatile anaesthetics are suitable for liver transplantation. Nitrous oxide should not be used to avoid intestinal distension. Intravenous techniques have been used successfully. The use of epidural catheters is discouraged due to the risk of severe and persistent perioperative coagulopathy.

70.3.2 Vascular Access

Line placement should include an arterial line for invasive blood pressure monitoring and some form of multi-lumen central venous access to allow pressure transduction and infusion of multiple drugs. The risk of severe bleeding makes some form of large bore venous access essential. The choices for large-bore venous access are highly variable between institutions, with some centres siting them in central veins, and others preferring to place multiple wide gauge peripheral cannulae.

It is routine practice in some centres to monitor venous pressure both in the SVC and the infrahepatic IVC, in order to estimate the trans-caval pressure gradient during the anhepatic phase. During surgery using the piggyback technique, this gradient indicates the degree of IVC obstruction, and during full caval cross-clamp it indicates the extent of transhepatic venous collateral flow. This traditionally requires access via both the femoral and internal jugular or subclavian approach, but some centres have reported good results measuring infrahepatic pressure at the saphenous vein.

Similarly, practices for arterial access differ widely between transplant centers with some placing a single femoral or radial arterial line, and others routinely placing two arterial lines to allow simultaneous sampling and pressure monitoring.

70.3.3 Haemodynamic Monitoring

Invasive monitoring of at minimum arterial and central venous pressure is standard. In addition to haemodynamic status, arterial and central venous lines allow serial measurement of blood gases, blood glucose, electrolytes and haemoglobin, which is considered routine in most transplant centers.

Pulmonary artery catheters were historically placed for the majority of patients but practice at many centres has evolved over time toward their targeted use for the minority of patients where concerns about newly developed or worsening pulmonary hypertension persist at the time of surgery.

Trans-oesophageal echocardiography is now frequently used for fluid management, monitoring of cardiac function, and identification of intraoperative complications (e.g. pulmonary embolus) [19]. Despite its widespread use, most practitioners are not formally certified, and joint guidelines from the American Society of Echocardiography (ASE) and the Society of Cardiovascular Anesthesiologists

(SCA) state that it is sufficient for anaesthetists to familiarise themselves with a limited number of views that allow a focused assessment of cardiac function and detection of complications [20].

Newer monitors using pulse contour analysis to estimate cardiac output are also used in some centres. While they are easy to use and associated with fewer complications than pulmonary artery catheters, concerns persist about their accuracy in a variety of contexts, including liver transplantation [21].

70.3.4 Point of Care Testing

Frequent intraoperative blood samples allow rapid diagnosis of acid-base, electrolyte and metabolic disturbances, and assessment of coagulopathy and adequacy of transfusion. Aside from guiding transfusion and interventions to correct other derangements, post-reperfusion monitoring of metabolic status and serum lactate can be used to assess initial graft function. With a healthy graft there is often correction of acidaemia and a reduction in serum lactate within hours of graft reperfusion.

Approaches to the assessment and management of intraoperative coagulopathy vary considerably. There is evidence that point of care viscoelastic testing (viscoelastography or viscoelastometry) is beneficial, although use of the technology is at present far from universal [22]. Results of viscoelastic test results are available more quickly than laboratory coagulation tests and they permit targeted correction of specific coagulation abnormalities using blood products and factor concentrates. Use of viscoelastic tests is supported by the European Society of Anaesthesiology guidelines for the management of severe bleeding during major surgery, and there is evidence that their use may reduce bleeding during liver transplantation [23].

70.3.5 Induction and Maintenance

Patients selected for liver transplantation usually have preserved cardiac function, although the cardiovascular physiology in ESLD is significantly altered with often severe peripheral vasodilation and increased cardiac output. However, it is usually not necessary to place an arterial line or a central line/pulmonary artery catheter for invasive monitoring before induction. Cricoid pressure and rapid sequence intubation should be considered in cases of large-volume ascites, encephalopathy, or uraemia. Induction can be accomplished with any IV anaesthetic such as propofol or etomidate, with or without opioids. A short- or intermediate-acting neuromuscular blocking agent should be used to facilitate endotracheal intubation.

Hypotension after induction is common and may persist throughout surgery due to the peripheral vasodilatation of ESLD. It is treated with small boluses of vasoconstrictors (e.g. metaraminol) and, if persistent, by infusion of noradrenaline or other vasopressor.

The pharmacokinetics and pharmacodynamics of any given drug are unpredictable in the setting of liver transplantation due to the effects of ESLD and because of acute changes as the dysfunctional native liver is removed and replaced by a new graft. Initial graft function is unpredictable and difficult to measure, with only secondary indicators such as a reduction in serum lactate providing an index of function.

An orogastric or nasogastric tube should be placed to decompress the stomach and improve surgical access, and temperature monitoring and active warming measures should be instituted as soon as practicable.

70.3.6 Fluid Management and Transfusion

Large volume fluid replacement during liver transplantation is common because of bleeding, ascitic and other fluid losses and fluid shifts. Most centres use a combination of crystalloids and colloids for fluid replacement, with normal saline and albumin the most frequently used in their respective classes [24]. We would advocate for the use of balanced salt solutions where possible, to reduce the risk of hyperchloraemic acidosis associated with infusions of large volumes of normal saline [25]. A rapid transfusion device is typically set up and connected to a large-bore IV line. These devices include efficient warming systems that help to maintain normothermia even during large volume fluid replacement.

Close communication with the blood bank before and during surgery is crucial, with initial provision of blood products guided by a standard protocol. While local practices vary, a typical setup may include 10 units of packed red blood cells (PRC) and 10 units of fresh frozen plasma (FFP) to be brought to the operating room, with four units of single-donor platelets available on request. The use of intraoperative cell salvage is common and may reduce the requirement for allogeneic blood products.

70.4 Key Intraoperative Priorities

Specific haemodynamic targets and management goals vary according to the phase of surgery: dissection, anhepatic, and reperfusion. The surgical approach (bicaval clamp, piggyback, or VVBP) also has a major impact on fluid and hemodynamic management.

70.4.1 Dissection Phase

At incision, acute decompression of ascites and resulting fluid redistribution frequently unmasks intravascular volume depletion and may result in significant hypotension. Adequate volume replacement is essential at this time, and in the absence of anaemia or coagulopathy, colloids may be the fluid of choice.

Depending on the underlying cause of the liver disease and the degree of portal hypertension, bleeding during dissection is highly variable. Patients with extensive varices may bleed briskly and require significant blood product transfusion. Coagulopathy during liver transplantation is very common and may result from dilution/consumption of clotting factors, platelet entrapment, endogenous heparinoid-like substances, and hyperfibrinolysis. Viscoelastic testing may indicate the predominant cause of coagulopathy and allow targeted treatment, for instance with tranexamic acid where there is evidence of hyperfibrinolysis. There is evidence that use of viscoelastic testing may reduce bleeding complications and mortality in high-risk liver transplant patients [26].

Where point of care viscoelastic testing is not used, a combination of empirical administration of blood products and treatment guided by laboratory coagulation tests may be employed. The value of laboratory coagulation tests in guiding the immediate management of haemorrhage is limited due to their turnaround time of over an hour, and by data showing that they do not predict blood loss during transplantation [27, 28]. In the absence of clinical bleeding, moderate abnormalities of coagulation are not normally treated.

Some data indicate that aiming to limit the CVP to less than 5 mmHg, as is well established practice in liver resection surgery, may reduce blood loss during the dissection phase of liver transplantation [29]. A low CVP strategy is facilitated by use of the piggyback technique, where venous return is relatively maintained on vascular exclusion of the recipient liver. Where a caval replacement technique is used, a low initial CVP may result in severe haemodynamic instability on caval cross-clamping. Overall a low CVP strategy is controversial, with many anaesthetists preferring to maintain normovolaemia throughout dissection. When significant blood loss is encountered, viscoelastic testing may allow targeted use of blood products and avoid significant dilutional coagulopathy.

Immediately prior to the anhepatic phase, especially when complete caval occlusion is planned, haemodynamic stability will be better maintained if a normovolaemic state is achieved. The surgeons should perform a test clamp so that the haemodynamic impact can be better anticipated and the fluid and vasoconstrictor therapy can be optimised before the anhepatic phase.

70.4.2 Anhepatic Phase

The dissection phase ends and the anhepatic phase begins with clamping of the native portal vein, hepatic artery and IVC or hepatic vein. The native liver is excised and meticulous haemostasis is achieved. The cooled donor graft is placed into the surgical field after being flushed to remove the organ preservation solution. The suprahepatic and infrahepatic caval and portal vein anastomoses are then completed in that order. In the piggyback approach, only one caval anastomosis needs to be completed. The hepatic artery anastomosis is often performed after restoration of venous blood flow.

The degree of reduction in venous return on vascular exclusion is dependent on the extent of venous collateral flow in the case of a caval replacement and, in the piggyback technique, on the degree of caval obstruction on clamping. Reduced venous return during this phase often requires an increase in vasopressor administration and judicious fluid administration. Aggressive fluid administration should be avoided during this phase because it may lead to fluid overload following reperfusion, with consequent risks of right heart failure and liver engorgement contributing to delayed graft function.

The use of veno-venous bypass (VVBP) has declined significantly over the years, and is subject to centre- and surgeon-specific preferences [30]. While it may improve haemodynamic stability during the anhepatic phase, there is no clear evidence that it improves outcome and it is associated with a significant rate of serious complications [31]. In most centres its role is limited to specific circumstances such as re-transplant, Budd-Chiari syndrome or gross hepatomegaly secondary to polycystic disease. If VVBP is used to blunt the hemodynamic consequences of vascular exclusion, bypass is usually accomplished by cannulation of the femoral and portal veins with diversion to the suprahepatic vena cava through the axillary, subclavian, or jugular vein.

There is some evidence that temporary intraoperative porto-caval shunts may improve short- and long-term graft function [32]. Their use is controversial, however, and many centres reserve them for use only as a temporising measure in cases where a prolonged anhepatic phase is anticipated, for instance due to difficult anastomoses or extensive porto-mesenteric thrombosis.

Coagulopathy during the anhepatic phase is common and multifactorial, and it is not uncommon to encounter significant haemorrhage. Lack of hepatic clearance of endothelial tissue plasminogen activator (tPA) leads to fibrinolysis and this, combined with progressive acidosis due to impaired lactate and citrate metabolism, and hypothermia due to introduction of the cooled graft into the surgical field, are all contributory. Point of care viscoelastic testing is useful in diagnosis and initial management of this coagulopathy, although moderate abnormalities in the absence of surgical bleeding are usually not actively corrected.

Correction of coagulopathy in the setting of clinical bleeding varies according to institutional preferences, although it does appear that administration of packed red blood cells, FFP, platelets and cryoprecipitate remain the preferred method of treating blood loss and coagulopathy during liver transplantation [7]. Some centres have moved toward greater use of fibrinogen concentrate, prothrombin concentrate and specific factor concentrates for haemostatic treatment. Recombinant factor VIIa is usually reserved for cases of very severe bleeding, as current evidence does not support its haemostatic effectiveness and concerns persist regarding thrombotic risk.

Meticulous optimisation of electrolytes and acid-base balance is essential prior to donor organ reperfusion. Reducing serum potassium to the low end of the physiological range with insulin/dextrose or furosemide may prevent severe hyperkalaemia at reperfusion and administration of 5–10 mmol of calcium chloride provides a degree of myocardial, protection. Where acidosis develops during the anhepatic phase, correction with sodium bicarbonate, along with optimal ventilation, will improve tolerance of reperfusion.

70.4.3 Reperfusion Phase

The donor graft is flushed to clear the preservation fluid and the IVC is then unclamped, restoring caval blood flow, venous return and overall haemodynamics. The onset of reperfusion is marked by unclamping of the portal vein anastomosis. Blood from the splanchnic circulation perfuses the new liver, and this is often the most critically unstable period for the anaesthetist to manage. The sudden influx of cold, hyperkalaemic, acidotic fluid from the donor liver, despite flushing the graft, frequently causes a post-reperfusion syndrome of hypotension, bradycardia, vasoplegia and coagulopathy. In severe cases there may be profound haemodynamic instability. The incidence of cardiac arrest requiring cardiac massage within minutes of reperfusion is around 3% [33].

Immediate treatment of haemodynamic instability may require bolus doses of adrenaline, atropine, calcium or sodium bicarbonate. We prefer to treat any evidence of bradycardia immediately with small increments of adrenaline (e.g. 10–20 μg initial dose) and further doses titrated according to effect. In some centres, preoperative placement of defibrillator pads is standard practice to allow rapid treatment of ventricular tachycardia or fibrillation. In cases of cardiac arrest, effective coordination with the surgical team is essential to allow safe CPR. Hypotension and instability may persist beyond immediate reperfusion and may require significant up-titration of vasopressor and inotrope therapy. Extreme cases of post-reperfusion syndrome may respond to administration of methylene blue in addition to conventional therapy [34].

Coagulopathy at reperfusion may be severe and produces characteristic findings on viscoelastic tests, including hyperfibrinolysis and a 'heparin-like effect' due to endogenous heparinoids from the donor liver. In the presence of good graft function, this coagulopathy normally self-corrects within a matter of hours. However with poor initial graft function it may be associated with ongoing severe bleeding and require active management. Care must be taken to avoid over-correction of coagulation abnormalities and induction of a hypercoagulable state which predisposes to hepatic artery thrombosis, a complication which is usually fatal without re-transplant. Surgery concludes with suturing of the biliary anastomoses and wound closure.

70.5 Immediate Postoperative Care

Initial postoperative care takes place in an intensive care setting. Extubation in the operating room at the conclusion of surgery is feasible in a substantial proportion of patients, although practice varies substantially between centres. A further group of patients may be appropriate for extubation within a few hours of admission to the intensive care unit, and a proactive approach to extubation may have substantial benefits for resource utilisation and cost of care without increasing the risk of complications [35].

Postoperative anaemia is common and objective criteria for transfusion including haemoglobin/haematocrit thresholds and clinical triggers should be set to minimise the risk of inappropriate transfusion. The risk of postoperative venous thromboembolism and hepatic artery thrombosis is significant, and prophylactic antiplatelet and anticoagulant therapy should be considered although the evidence for effectiveness is limited.

70.6 Discussion of Adjuvant Drugs

Massive haemorrhage during liver transplantation surgery is associated with decreased graft and patient survival [36]. Octreotide reduces portal venous blood flow, and there is evidence of a trend toward a reduction in intraoperative blood transfusion requirements when it is administered as a continuous intraoperative infusion [37]. There is evidence that tranexamic acid is effective in reducing the requirement for RBC transfusion without any increase in thrombotic risk, and the European Society of Anaesthesiologists recommend that its use is considered for liver transplant [23, 38].

Acute kidney injury after liver transplantation affects 40–70% of patients, with 8–17% requiring renal replacement therapy [39]. While no specific therapy is accepted as providing renal protection, there is some evidence that octreotide infusion may improve intraoperative urine output [40]. While diuretics do not offer renal protection, significant diuresis may in some cases make volume management easier, especially where coagulopathy is treated by the transfusion of large volumes of blood products.

Ionized calcium levels can be significantly decreased during liver transplantation, especially when large volumes of RBC and/or FFP need to be transfused. The citrate load from these products can significantly reduce calcium levels, in particular during the anhepatic phase when capacity to metabolise citrate is further reduced. Administration of calcium chloride or calcium gluconate as infusion or bolus is often required, and calcium levels should be closely monitored.

In addition, the glucose-insulin pathway is frequently impaired in patients with ESLD, and close monitoring of blood glucose levels is required. Administration of steroids for immunosuppression, enhanced glycogenolysis, and insulin resistance of the graft may all contribute to hyperglycemia requiring insulin treatment.

Immunosuppressive therapy is crucial for the success of transplantation. Protocols vary between medical centers, and clear communication is important to ensure delivery of the appropriate immunosuppressant.

70.7 Living Donor Liver Transplantation in Adults

Living donor liver transplantation (LDLT) comprises a small proportion of overall liver transplantation activity in Western healthcare systems [1, 41]. The situation is very different in Asia, where cultural factors lead to very low rates of cadaveric donation, and in this region transplants from living donors form the vast majority of the caseload [42]. LDLT requires two operations: the donor undergoes either a left or right hepatectomy and the recipient undergoes native hepatectomy and orthotopic transplantation of the donor graft. The vast majority of live donations are directed donations from individuals who are related genetically or emotionally to the recipient, although undirected, altruistic donations are possible.

70.7.1 LDLT Recipients

The indications for LDLT are broadly similar to those for deceased donor transplantation, but there are some important differences. Because the choice of recipient in LDLT is usually made by the donor and does not require the equitable allocation of a scarce, shared resource, there is the potential for patients to undergo transplantation who do not qualify for deceased donor transplantation. This includes patients with hepatocellular carcinoma (HCC) falling outside of standard criteria for transplant such as the Milan criteria. Centres have reported acceptable outcomes in patients with more than three lesions, providing that no lesion exceeds 5 cm in diameter [43]. Some studies have reported higher HCC recurrence rates after LDLT than after deceased donor transplantation, although other data contradict this, and there is an absence of prospective studies [44]. In the absence of definitive evidence it is reasonable to assume that recurrence rates are similar.

Patients with less advanced liver disease of any aetiology may be transplanted when the severity of their disease may not yet prioritise them for deceased donor transplantation but where their clinical condition may optimise their outcomes.

70.7.2 Donor Preoperative Assessment

Living donors volunteer to undergo major surgery associated with substantial morbidity and mortality, from which they derive no direct benefit. Accurate assessment and effective communication of risk are therefore crucial to donor preoperative assessment, and strict donor selection criteria are required.

Exclusion criteria vary between centres, but many exclude donors over the age of 55, those with BMI over 30 kg/m^2, significant comorbid disease or hepatosteatosis and those with a post-donation residual liver volume predicted to be less than 30–35% [45, 46]. Preoperative screening aims to uncover occult disease and to assess the severity of known comorbidities.

Assessment of the donor liver aims to quantify the risk of a small-for-size syndrome in recipients, a syndrome of hyperbilirubinaemia, ascites and poor liver function resulting from insufficient postoperative functioning hepatocyte mass. Graft weight to recipient weight (GWRW) ratio and the quality of the donor liver both affect this risk, and are carefully assessed by preoperative imaging and liver biopsy, respectively. Selection of a right or left lobe graft aims to reduce the risk of small-for-size syndrome in the recipient while ensuring adequate residual liver volume in the donor. Right lobe grafts are by far the most common in adults, although some centres have reported good results with dual left lobe grafts [47].

Donors should undergo thorough preoperative psychological assessment to explore their motivation for transplantation and their understanding of the likely short- and long-term consequences of donation [48]. Any concerns that donors are being in any way coerced or unduly influenced by family pressures should be explored in detail, and may preclude donation.

70.7.3 Intraoperative Care of the Living Donor

The considerations for anaesthetic management of the donor are similar to those of patients undergoing hepatectomies. Preoperative placement of a thoracic epidural catheter for postoperative pain control is performed in some transplant centers. There is some evidence that postoperative pain control is better with an epidural technique compared with PCA and that concerns about safety based on possible coagulopathy may not be justified [49, 50]. Other centres have reported good pain control with intrathecal opioids in conjunction with PCA, or with the oblique subcostal approach to transversus abdominis plane block [51, 52].

Induction of anaesthesia can be performed using any intravenous anaesthetic and neuromuscular blocker of choice. Wide-bore intravenous access and invasive arterial blood pressure monitoring are commonly used, and a central venous catheter is used in many centres. An orogastric or nasogastric tube should be placed to improve surgical exposure through decompression of the stomach.

General anaesthesia is standard and may consist of a balanced technique or be combined with intraoperative supplementation of epidural analgesia. Paralysis is maintained throughout the operation. Mobilisation of the liver may lead to brief periods of hypotension due to temporary obstruction of venous return to the heart. These episodes do not usually require active treatment in view of their brevity and donor fitness.

Intravenous fluid is administered cautiously until the graft has been isolated, aiming to minimise blood loss during transection. Many anaesthetists aim to maintain the CVP below 5 mmHg and there is some evidence that this strategy, or an alternative strategy of maintaining the stroke volume variation between 10% and 20%, are associated with reduced blood loss [53]. Although average blood loss at most centers is usually well below 1000 ml, the nature of the procedure warrants vigilance and preparation. A patient blood management strategy incorporating preoperative autologous blood donation, iron supplementation and intraoperative cell salvage may reduce the risk of allogeneic blood transfusion.

In most cases, the patient can be extubated immediately following surgery. Choice of postoperative location is influenced by institutional practices and patient factors, but the intensive care unit, high dependency unit or dedicated postoperative care unit may be appropriate.

70.7.4 Recipient and Donor Outcomes

Recipient post-transplant liver function is critically dependent on graft size, graft quality, portal inflow and venous outflow [40]. Postoperative biliary strictures are common with right lobe grafts, with reported overall rates of biliary complications in the range of 20–30% [54, 55]. Multidisciplinary management of these strictures with involvement of expert interventional radiologists and endoscopists is essential to preserving graft function and quality of life. Survival rates for live donor grafts are similar to those of deceased donor grafts, with rates of 80% at 1 year and 69% at 5 years reported by European registry data [41].

The main cause of donor mortality or need for transplantation is liver insufficiency due to resection of an excessively large volume of liver. The right lobe hepatectomy used in most LDLT carries a mortality risk of approximately 0.5%, and deaths may be attributable to suboptimal donor selection or inappropriately large resection volume [40, 41].

The rate of serious donor complications is around 30%, with biliary anastomotic leaks and infection the most common [40, 41]. Donor comorbidities fail to predict postoperative complications but this is likely due to the low severity of comorbidities among qualifying donors. Donors may take approximately 3–6 months to return to full social and occupational functioning, although the majority, more than 80%, say they would choose to donate again [56].

Self Study

Questions

1. Which of the following statements is true?
   (a) Candidates are prioritised for liver transplant based primarily on an assessment of their frailty.
   (b) Any degree of portopulmonary hypertension is generally considered a contraindication to liver transplantation.
   (c) At the time of transplant, patients may be at increased risk of haemorrhage, thrombosis, or both.
   (d) Preoperative correction of laboratory coagulation tests is important to reduce the risk of intraoperative haemorrhage.
2. Which of the following statements is true?
   (a) European Society of Anaesthesiology guidelines recommend against the use of point-of-care viscoelastic testing in liver transplantation.
   (b) Intraoperative cardiac arrest during orthotopic liver transplantation is very rare.
   (c) The severity of bleeding during surgery does not predict transplant outcomes.
   (d) Living donation may allow candidates to undergo transplantation who would not qualify to receive a deceased donor liver.

Answers

1. Which of the following statements is true?
   (a) Prioritisation is usually based on liver disease severity, and the most commonly used measure is the MELD score.
   (b) Mild portopulmonary hypertension increases perioperative risk only slightly and is not generally considered a contraindication to transplant. Severe portopulmonary hypertension is generally considered a contraindication.
   (c) CORRECT ANSWER. The cell-based model of coagulation explains that while coagulation in chronic liver disease is 'rebalanced', there is an increased vulnerability to stressors that may increase the tendency to thrombosis, haemorrhage, or both.
   (d) Laboratory coagulation tests are poor predictors of surgical bleeding and are not normally corrected preoperatively.
2. Which of the following statements is true?
   (a) ESA guidelines support the use of an algorithmic approach with predefined viscoelastic triggers for the treatment of perioperative bleeding. They also state that there is some evidence to suggest that viscoelastic testing reduces bleeding during liver transplantation.
   (b) The rate of cardiac arrest within minutes of donor organ reperfusion is around 3% in some series.
   (c) Massive haemorrhage during liver transplant surgery predicts worse graft and patient survival.
   (d) CORRECT ANSWER. Candidates with hepatocellular carcinoma falling outside of standard transplantation criteria, and those with liver disease of insufficient severity to prioritise them for deceased donor transplant, may undergo living donor transplant.

References

1. NHS Blood and Transplant. Annual report on liver transplantation 2016/2017. Watford: NHS Blood and Transplant; 2017. Available from: https://nhsbtdbe.blob.core.windows.net/umbraco-assets-corp/5007/annual_liver_transplantation_report_2017.pdf.
2. Chan AC, Fan ST, Lo CM, et al. Liver transplantation for acute-on-chronic liver failure. Hepatol Int. 2009;3(4):571–81. https://doi.org/10.1007/s12072-009-9148-8.
3. Choudhary NS, Saraf N, Saigal S, Soin AS. Liver transplantation for acute on chronic liver failure. J Clin Exp Hepatol. 2017;7(3):247–52. https://doi.org/10.1016/j.jceh.2017.08.001.
4. Malinchoc M, Kamath PS, Gordon FD, Peine CJ, Rank J, Borg PC. A model to predict poor survival in patients undergoing transjugular intrahepatic portosystemic shunts. Hepatology. 2000;31:864–71.
5. Lai JC, Feng S, Terrault NA, Lizaola B, Hayssen H, Covinsky K. Frailty predicts waitlist mortality in liver transplant candidates. Am J Transplant. 2014;14(8):1870–9. https://doi.org/10.1111/ajt.12762.
6. Rolfson DB, Majumdar SR, Tsuyuki RT, Tahir A, Rockwood K. Validity and reliability of the Edmonton Frail Scale. Age Ageing. 2006;35(5):526–9. https://doi.org/10.1093/ageing/afl041.
7. Fried LP, Tangen CM, Walston J, Newman AB, Hirsch C, Gottdiener J, et al. Frailty in older adults: evidence for a phenotype. J Gerontol A Biol Sci Med Sci. 2001;56(3):M146–56.
8. Tandon P, Ney M, Irwin I, Ma MM, Gramlich L, Bain VG, et al. Severe muscle depletion in patients on the liver transplant wait list: its prevalence and independent prognostic value. Liver Transpl. 2012;18(10):1209–16. https://doi.org/10.1002/lt.23495.
9. Kaido T, Ogawa K, Fujimoto Y, Ogura Y, Hata K, Ito T, et al. Impact of sarcopenia on survival in patients undergoing living donor liver transplantation. Am J Transplant. 2013;13(6):1549–56. https://doi.org/10.1111/ajt.12221.
10. Cruz-Jentoft AJ, Baeyens JP, Bauer JM, et al. Sarcopenia: European consensus on definition and diagnosis: report of the European Working Group on sarcopenia in older people. Age Ageing. 2010;39(4):412–23. https://doi.org/10.1093/ageing/afq034.
11. Carey EJ, Steidley DE, Aqel BA, Byrne TJ, Mekeel KL, Rakela J, et al. Six-minute walk distance predicts mortality in liver transplant candidates. Liver Transpl. 2010;16(12):1373–8. https://doi.org/10.1002/lt.22167.
12. Prentis JM, Manas DM, Trenell MI, Hudson M, Jones DJ, Snowden CP. Submaximal cardiopulmonary exercise testing predicts 90-day survival after liver transplantation. Liver Transpl. 2012;18(2):152–9. https://doi.org/10.1002/lt.22426.
13. Aldenkortt F, Aldenkortt M, Caviezel L, Waeber JL, Weber A, Schiffer E. Portopulmonary hypertension and hepatopulmonary syndrome. World J Gastroenterol. 2014;20(25):8072–81. https://doi.org/10.3748/wjg.v20.i25.8072.
14. Krowka MJ, Fallon MB, Kawut SM, Fuhrmann V, Heimbach JK, Ramsay MA, et al. International liver transplant society practice guidelines: diagnosis and management of hepatopulmonary syndrome and portopulmonary hypertension. Transplantation. 2016;100(7):1440–52. https://doi.org/10.1097/TP.0000000000001229.
15. Khaderi S, Khan R, Safdar Z, Stribling R, Vierling JM, Goss JA, et al. Long-term follow-up of portopulmonary hypertension patients after liver transplantation. Liver Transpl. 2014;20(6):724–7. https://doi.org/10.1002/lt.23870.
16. Liu H, Jayakumar S, Traboulsi M, Lee SS. Cirrhotic cardiomyopathy: implications for liver transplantation. Liver Transpl. 2017;23(6):826–35. https://doi.org/10.1002/lt.24768.
17. Serio S, Clements JM, Grauf D, Merchant AM. Outcomes of diabetic and nondiabetic patients undergoing general and vascular surgery. ISRN Surg. 2013;2013:963930. https://doi.org/10.1155/2013/963930.
18. Tripodi A, Mannucci PM. The coagulopathy of chronic liver disease. N Engl J Med. 2011;365(2):147–56. https://doi.org/10.1056/NEJMra1011170.
19. Wax DB, Torres A, Scher C, Leibowitz AB. Transesophageal echocardiography utilization in high-volume liver transplantation centers in the United States. J Cardiothorac Vasc Anesth. 2008;22(6):811–3. https://doi.org/10.1053/j.jvca.2008.07.007.
20. Reeves ST, Finley AC, Skubas NJ, Swaminathan M, Whitley WS, Glas KE, Hahn RT, Shanewise JS, Adams MS, Shernan SK. Basic perioperative transesophageal echocardiography examination: a consensus statement of the American Society of Echocardiography and the Society of Cardiovascular Anesthesiologists. J Am Soc Echocardiogr. 2013;26:443–56.
21. Feltracco P, Biancofiore G, Ori C, Saner FH, Della Rocca G. Limits and pitfalls of haemodynamic monitoring systems in liver transplantation surgery. Minerva Anestesiol. 2012;78(12):1372–84.
22. Mallett SV. Clinical utility of viscoelastic tests of coagulation (TEG/ROTEM) in patients with liver disease and during liver transplantation. Semin Thromb Hemost. 2015;41(5):527–37. https://doi.org/10.1055/s-0035-1550434.

23. Kozek-Langenecker SA, Ahmed AB, Afshari A, Albaladejo P, Aldecoa C, Barauskas G, et al. Management of severe perioperative bleeding: guidelines from the European Society of Anaesthesiology: first update 2016. Eur J Anaesthesiol. 2017;34(6):332–95. https://doi.org/10.1097/EJA.0000000000000630.
24. Schumann R, Mandell S, Michaels MD, et al. Intraoperative fluid and pharmacologic management and the anesthesiologist's supervisory role for nontraditional technologies during liver transplantation: a survey of US Academic Centers. Transplant Proc. 2013;45(6):2258–62.
25. Yunos NM, Kim IB, Bellomo R, et al. The biochemical effects of restricting chloride-rich fluids in intensive care. Crit Care Med. 2011;39(pg):2419–24.
26. Alamo JM, León A, Mellado P, Bernal C, Marín LM, Cepeda C, Suárez G, Serrano J, Padillo J, Gómez MÁ. Is "intra-operating room" thromboelastometry useful in liver transplantation? A case-control study in 303 patients. Transplant Proc. 2013;45:3637–9.
27. Rana A, Petrowsky H, Hong JC, Agopian VG, Kaldas FM, Farmer D, et al. Blood transfusion requirement during liver transplantation is an important risk factor for mortality. J Am Coll Surg. 2013;216(5):902–7. https://doi.org/10.1016/j.jamcollsurg.2012.12.047.
28. Massicotte L, Beaulieu D, Thibeault L, Roy JD, Marleau D, Lapointe R, et al. Coagulation defects do not predict blood product requirements during liver transplantation. Transplantation. 2008;85(7):956–62. https://doi.org/10.1097/TP.0b013e318168fcd4.
29. Massicotte L, Lenis S, Thibeault L, Sassine MP, Seal RF, Roy A. Effect of low central venous pressure and phlebotomy on blood product transfusion requirements during liver transplantations. Liver Transpl. 2006;12:117–23.
30. Barbas AS, Levy J, Mulvihill MS, et al. Liver transplantation without venovenous bypass: does surgical approach matter? Transplant Direct. 2018;4(5):e348. https://doi.org/10.1097/TXD.0000000000000776.
31. Fonouni H, Mehrabi A, Soleimani M, Müller SA, Büchler MW, Schmidt J. The need for venovenous bypass in liver transplantation. HPB. 2008;10(3):196–203. https://doi.org/10.1080/13651820801953031.
32. Pratschke S, Meimarakis G, Bruns CJ, Kaspar M, Prix N, Zachoval R, et al. Temporary intraoperative porto-caval shunt: useless or beneficial in piggy back liver transplantation? Transpl Int. 2013;26(1):90–8. https://doi.org/10.1111/tri.12007.
33. Matsusaki T, Hilmi IA, Planinsic RM, Humar A, Sakai T. Cardiac arrest during adult liver transplantation: a single institution's experience with 1238 deceased donor transplants. Liver Transpl. 2013;19(11):1262–71. https://doi.org/10.1002/lt.23723.
34. Koelzow H, Gedney JA, Baumann J, et al. The effect of methylene blue on the hemodynamic changes during ischemia reperfusion injury in orthotopic liver transplantation. Anesth Analg. 2002;94(4):824–9. Table of contents.
35. Mandell MS, Stoner TJ, Barnett R, Shaked A, Bellamy M, Biancofiore G, et al. A multicenter evaluation of safety of early extubation in liver transplant recipients. Liver Transpl. 2007;13(11):1557–63.
36. Cleland S, Corredor C, Ye JJ, Srinivas C, McCluskey SA. Massive haemorrhage in liver transplantation: consequences, prediction and management. World J Transplant. 2016;6(2):291–305. https://doi.org/10.5500/wjt.v6.i2.291.
37. Byram SW, Gupta RA, Ander M, Edelstein S, Andreatta B. Effects of continuous octreotide infusion on intraoperative transfusion requirements during orthotopic liver transplantation. Transplant Proc. 2015;47(9):2712–4. https://doi.org/10.1016/j.transproceed.2015.07.036.
38. Badenoch A, Sharma A, Gower S, Selzner M, Srinivas C, Wąsowicz M, et al. The effectiveness and safety of tranexamic acid in orthotopic liver transplantation clinical practice: a propensity score matched cohort study. Transplantation. 2017;101(7):1658–65. https://doi.org/10.1097/TP.0000000000001682.
39. Lewandowska L, Matuszkiewicz-Rowinska J. Acute kidney injury after procedures of orthotopic liver transplantation. Ann Transplant. 2011;16(2):103–8.
40. Sahmeddini MA, Amini A, Naderi N. The effect of octreotide on urine output during orthotopic liver transplantation and early postoperative renal function; a randomized, double-blind, placebo-controlled trial. Hepat Mon. 2013;13(9):e12787. https://doi.org/10.5812/hepatmon.12787.
41. Kim WR, Lake JR, Smith JM, Schladt DP, Skeans MA, Harper AM, et al. OPTN/SRTR 2016 Annual data report: liver. Am J Transplant. 2018;18(Suppl 1):172–253. https://doi.org/10.1111/ajt.14559.
42. de Villa VH, Lo CM, Chen CL. Ethics and rationale of living-donor liver transplantation in Asia. Transplantation. 2003;75(3 Suppl):S2–5.
43. Lee SG, Hwang S, Moon DB, Ahn CS, Kim KH, Sung KB. Expanded indication criteria of living donor liver transplantation for hepatocellular carcinoma at one large-volume center. Liver Transpl. 2008;14(7):935–45. https://doi.org/10.1002/lt.21445.
44. Akamatsu N, Sugawara Y, Kokudo N. Living-donor vs deceased-donor liver transplantation for patients with hepatocellular carcinoma. World J Hepatol. 2014;6(9):626–31. https://doi.org/10.4254/wjh.v6.i9.626.
45. Lee SG. A complete treatment of adult living donor liver transplantation: a review of surgical technique and current challenges to expand indication of patients. Am J Transplant. 2015;15(1):17–38. https://doi.org/10.1111/ajt.12907.
46. Walter J, Burdelski M, Bröring DC. Chances and risks in living donor liver transplantation. Dtsch Arztebl Int. 2008;105(6):101–7. https://doi.org/10.3238/arztebl.2008.0101.
47. Lu Q, Wu H, Yan L-N, Chen Z-Y, Fan Y-T, Luo Y. Living donor liver transplantation using dual grafts: ultrasonographic evaluation. World J Gastroenterol. 2010;16(31):3979–83. https://doi.org/10.3748/wjg.v16.i31.3979.
48. British Transplantation Society. BTS UK guidelines: living donor liver transplantation. Macclesfield: BTS; 2015. Available from: https://bts.org.uk/wp-content/uploads/2016/09/03_BTS_LivingDonorLiver-1.pdf.
49. Clarke H, Chandy T, Srinivas C, et al. Epidural analgesia provides better pain management after live liver donation: a retrospective study. Liver Transpl. 2011;17(3):315–23.
50. Choi SJ, Gwak MS, Ko JS, et al. The changes in coagulation profile and epidural catheter safety for living liver donors: a report on 6 years of our experience. Liver Transpl. 2007;13(1):62–70.
51. Ko JS, Choi SJ, Gwak MS, Kim GS, Ahn HJ, Kim JA, et al. Intrathecal morphine combined with intravenous patient-controlled analgesia is an effective and safe method for immediate postoperative pain control in live liver donors. Liver Transpl. 2009;15(4):381–9. https://doi.org/10.1002/lt.21625.
52. Maeda A, Shibata SC, Wada H, Marubashi S, Kamibayashi T, Eguchi H, et al. The efficacy of continuous subcostal transversus abdominis plane block for analgesia after living liver donation: a retrospective study. J Anesth. 2016;30(1):39–46. https://doi.org/10.1007/s00540-015-2085-x.
53. Choi S-S, Kim S-H, Kim Y-K. Fluid management in living donor hepatectomy: recent issues and perspectives. World J Gastroenterol. 2015;21(45):12757–66. https://doi.org/10.3748/wjg.v21.i45.12757.
54. Yaprak O, Dayangac M, Akyildiz M, et al. Biliary complications after right lobe living donor liver transplantation: a single-centre experience. HPB (Oxford). 2012;14(1):49–53. https://doi.org/10.1111/j.1477-2574.2011.00401.x.
55. Soejima Y, Taketomi A, Yoshizumi T, Uchiyama H, Harada N, Ijichi H, et al. Biliary strictures in living donor liver transplantation: incidence, management, and technical evolution. Liver Transpl. 2006;12(6):979–86.
56. Lee SH, Jeong JS, Ha HS, No MJ, Hong JJ, Kwon JS, et al. Decision-related factors and attitudes toward donation in living related liver transplantation: ten-year experience. Transplant Proc. 2005;37(2):1081–4.

71 Surgery in Liver Disease

Saied Froghi, Farid Froghi, and Brian R. Davidson

Key Concepts

- Liver disease affects a wide range of physiological parameters (e.g. clotting, electrolyte disturbance, hyperdynamic circulation)
- Chronic liver disease increases the risk of morbidity and mortality from surgery. Key factors are the severity of liver disease and the extent of the proposed surgical procedure.
- It is important to assess risk preoperatively and meticulously assess individual patient's pre-operative physiological status in a multi-disciplinary manner.
- Scoring systems Child-Turcotte Pugh (CTP) or Model for End-Stage Liver Disease (MELD) can be used to assess risk but should be used as an adjunct to other means of assessing risk (i.e. ASA grading, cardiac risk factors)
- Pre-operative optimisation can improve postoperative outcomes.
- Any major surgical procedure in cirrhotic patients should be carried out by experienced surgeons and anaesthetists in a Liver Unit with the support of hepatologists and HPB surgeons.

71.1 Introduction

People with chronic liver disease may require surgery for their liver condition or may require surgery for an unrelated disorder. The management and outcome of the surgery are dependent on the severity of the underlying liver disease. The incidence of liver disease is on the rise and survival for many liver diseases is improving with new treatments. In Europe alone, around 29 million people are estimated to suffer from chronic liver disease [1]. Recent data suggests that about 0.1% of the European population is affected by cirrhosis, corresponding to 14–26 new cases per 100,000 inhabitants per year or an estimated 170,000 deaths per year [2]. Both cirrhosis and primary liver cancer (incidence of 1–13 new cases) are representative of end-stage liver disease. With almost 10% of cirrhotic patients undergoing surgery during their last year of life [3], this translates into an ever-increasing cohort of patients with complex medical needs undergoing operative management.

Liver surgery was historically a risky procedure as it was associated with much blood loss and high patient morbidity and mortality. Over the past two decades, this field of surgery has expanded vastly due to an improved understanding of the pathophysiology of cirrhosis, improved diagnosis and severity grading, surgical technologies and new surgical techniques. A better understanding of liver anatomy and physiology was incorporated into specific training programmes for surgeons in the rapidly developing speciality of HPB and liver transplant surgery. This combination of developments has resulted in safe surgery being available for highly complex patients.

Patients with chronic liver disease who require surgery need particular attention to a number of factors in the pre-operative and intra-operative period to optimise their care. Such considerations are based on the extent of liver disease and the type of surgery required. Non-hepatic operations tend to be more common than hepatic resection in this group of patients. Irrespective of the nature of surgical procedure common factors are addressed pre-operative and post-operatively to achieve better outcomes.

71.2 Surgical Anatomy of the Liver

Couinaud's description of the eight anatomic segments of the liver is now the most widely accepted nomenclature for liver anatomy. His description of segments was based on portal

S. Froghi · F. Froghi · B. R. Davidson (✉)
University College London (UCL), London, UK
e-mail: s.froghi@nhs.net; farid.froghi@nhs.net; b.davidson@ucl.ac.uk

F. Radu-Ionita et al. (eds.), *Liver Diseases*, https://doi.org/10.1007/978-3-030-24432-3_71

venous inflow which resulted in a safer surgical approach for liver resection surgery. Thorough knowledge of liver anatomy is essential. The liver receives dual blood supply from the portal vein and the hepatic artery, which together with the bile duct form the portal triad. The triad branches to each liver segment within the liver where it is covered by the Glisson's sheath, a continuation of the visceral peritoneal capsule of the liver.

71.2.1 Avoiding Blood Loss During Liver Surgery

Understanding the vascular supply of the liver allows for development and performing vascular exclusion techniques during the division of the liver parenchyma in liver resection surgery. Such techniques can decrease intraoperative bleeding and transfusion by controlling the inflow and outflow of blood to the liver [4]. The concept of hepatic vascular control is based on the known tolerance of liver to ischemia and on the strong evidence that liver tolerates ischemia better than bleeding [5, 6]. This has resulted in the development of ischemic preconditioning and total vascular exclusion techniques (through selective inflow or outflow vascular occlusion) as strategies of blood control during liver surgery (Fig. 71.1) [4]. There is variability of the use of these methods in different centres with variability in the time of occlusion [4, 7]. These methods must be applied with an understanding of its combined effect on the overall physiology of the patient.

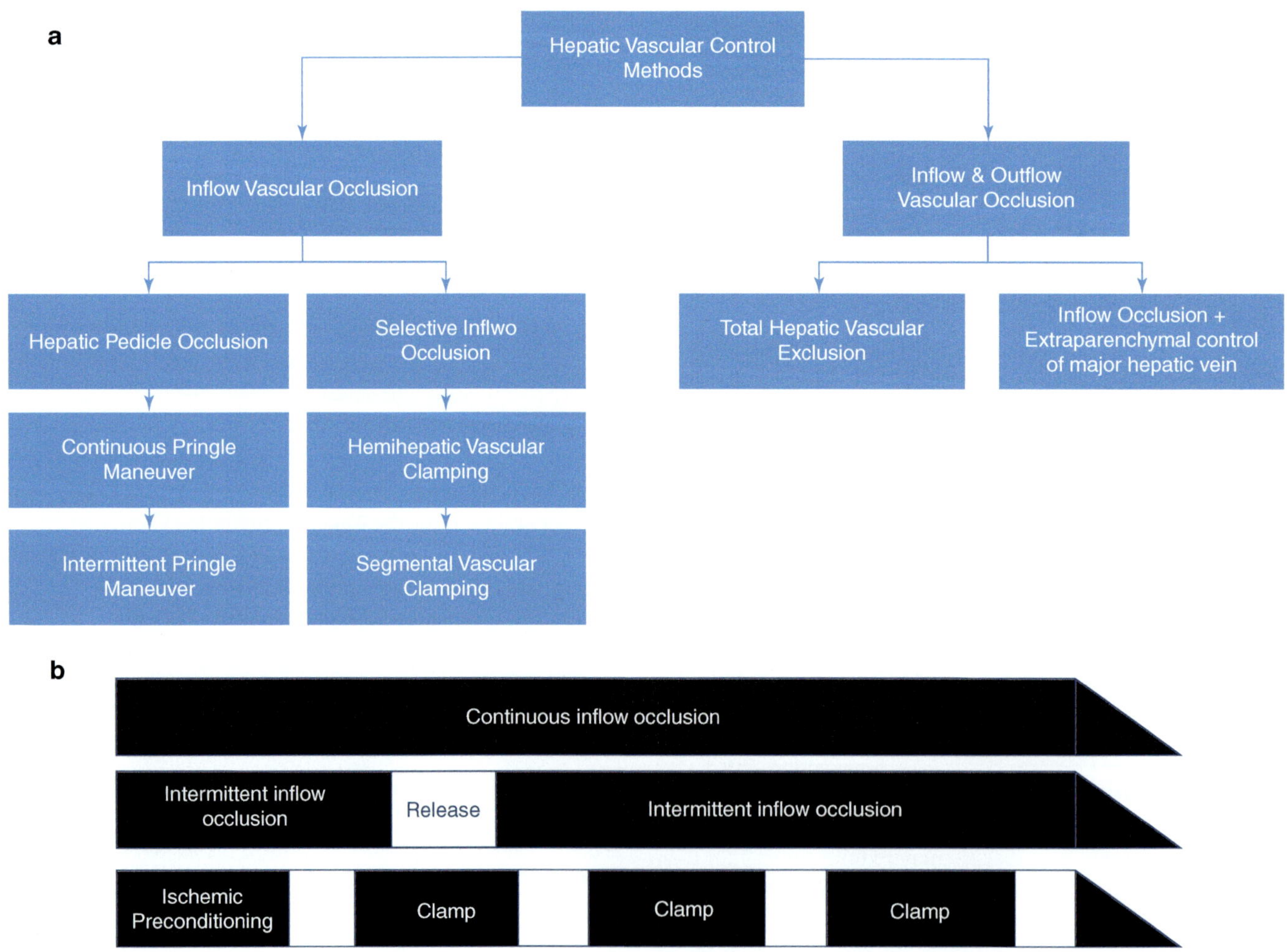

Fig. 71.1 (**a**) Different methods of inflow and outflow techniques. Occlusion can be only inflow or inflow and outflow combined. Depending on the type of surgery different inflow occlusion strategies can be achieved. (**b**) Occlusion can be continuous, intermittent or regular intervals of ischemia and reperfusion to precondition hepatocytes function and reduce the risk of hepatocyte dysfunction. Knowledge of the techniques can aid pre-operative and intra-operative fluid management. For example, a low CVP (<5 mmHg) can be achieved by fluid restriction which can be a useful technique in inflow occlusion as a mean of reducing further blood loss. Equally, techniques such as total vascular occlusion rely on both inflow and outflow occlusion, which in turn can increase the preload on the heart and to counter the physiological imbalance may require volume loading pre- or intra-operatively

71.3 Physiological Changes of Liver Disease and Implications for Surgery

The liver has many physiological roles—synthesis of most serum proteins, metabolism of nutrients and drugs, excretion and detoxification of toxins to name a few. In cirrhosis, these processes are altered, and they can impact on the success of surgery (Fig. 71.2).

71.3.1 Altered Circulation

Cirrhosis creates a hyperdynamic circulation. There is an increase in cardiac output with decreased vascular resistance due to impairment of the autoregulatory mechanism. Consequently, blood flow to the liver is reduced. Portal hypertension develops as a result of poor portal flow. The cirrhotic liver is therefore at risk of hypoxic injury during surgery. Hence, special consideration should be given to the choice of anaesthesia, pre-operative volume status and the choice of surgical procedure for any given pathology (e.g. liver resection vs. transplant for hepatocellular carcinoma, HCC). It is known that inhalational anaesthetic agents have a profound effect on hepatic blood flow. More stable agents such as propofol can reduce hepatic blood flow and hence predispose the liver to hypoxia. Blood flow reduction has a subsequent effect on the pharmacokinetics of the liver, e.g. reduced clearance of endogenous substances. Intra-operative factors such as the volume of blood loss, periods of hypotension, use of vasoactive drugs, and pneumoperitoneum during laparoscopy all can exacerbate susceptibility of the liver to hypoxia [8].

71.3.2 Drug Clearance and Hepatic Encephalopathy

Reduced metabolic capacity of the liver leads to accumulation of endogenous toxins and altered drug metabolism. Cautious use of sedatives and narcotics is advised under such circumstance as they can exacerbate hepatic encephalopathy and would prolong periods of unconsciousness. Hyperammonaemia can further contribute to cerebral dysfunction and therefore careful pre-operative assessment to identify mild hyperammonaemia is necessary to differentiate between hepatic and non-hepatic (e.g. GI bleed, urinary diversion, urea-splitting gram-negative bacteria) causes of raised ammonia. Therefore, a high index of suspicion is used when dealing with the patient who present with neurological symptoms on the background of normal liver function. Delay in diagnosis can have potentially life-threatening consequences such as seizure and coma. If encephalopathy

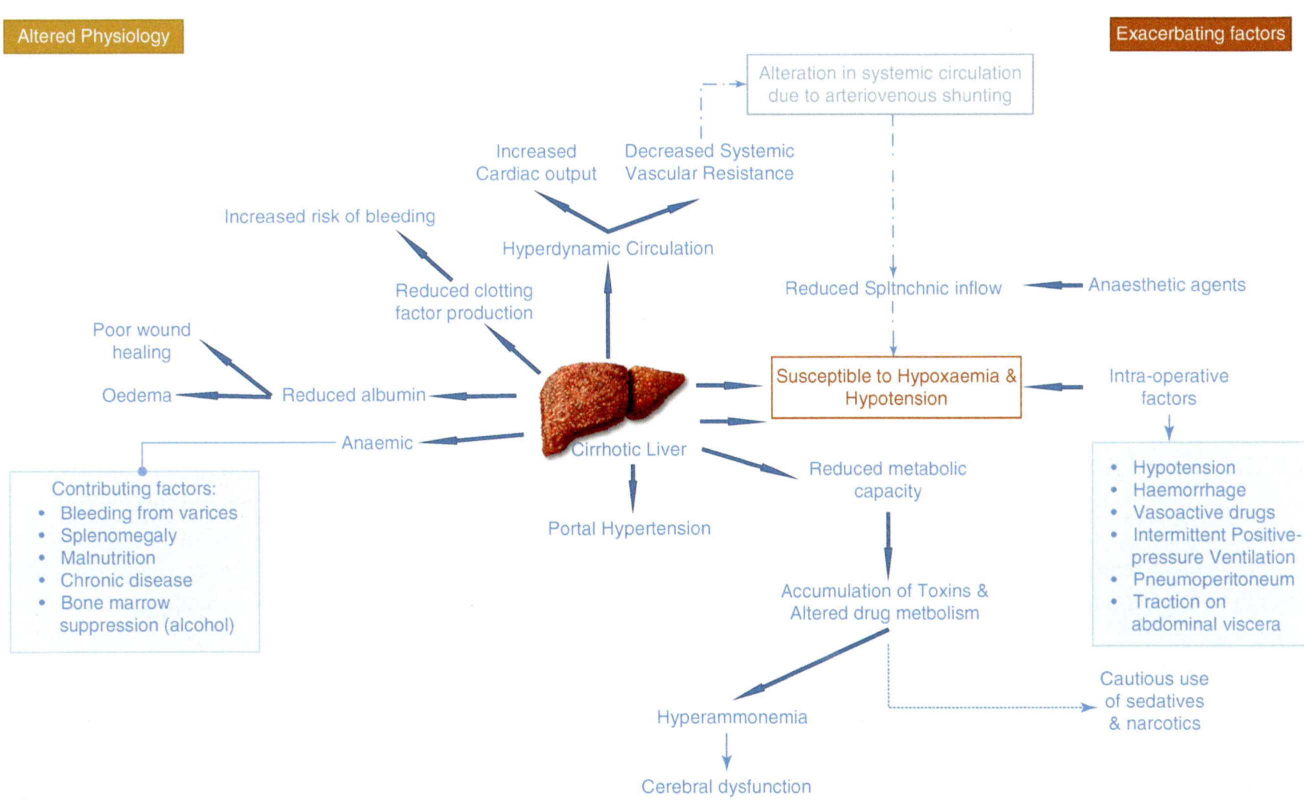

Fig. 71.2 Altered physiology in cirrhotic liver and consequential effects to be considered in patients undergoing surgery

is identified, treatment should be focused on treating the underlying cause of encephalopathy, i.e. correction of electrolyte imbalance, treatment of sepsis or hypoxia [9].

71.3.3 Clotting and Blood Loss

Cirrhotic patients have impaired hepatic synthesis of clotting factors II, VII, IX and X resulting in a risk of bleeding intra- and post-operatively. Bleeding can range from small petechial bleeds to massive gastrointestinal bleeding. Hence, careful planning with detection and correction of coagulopathies should be combined with surgical planning to minimise blood loss. For patients with coagulopathy, administration of fresh frozen plasma (FFP) and vitamin K to correct a prothrombin time (PT) to within 3 s of normal is recommended [10]. If coagulopathy is not corrected with FFP, cryoprecipitate or desmopressin can be used. When available, the aid of thromboelastography (TEG) would limit the use of FFP and reduce side effect by limiting inappropriate administration of blood products. TEG is a novel technique that analyses the interaction between platelets, fibrinogen and clotting factors. It provides an insight into clot development and aids in measuring the strength of fibrin-platelet bonds in whole blood. This kind of qualitative analysis can facilitate the administration of the right blood products at the right time.

As a general rule, a coagulopathy should be corrected in the peri-operative period. If FFP is being used attention should be given to the half-life of the products and the timing of its use (i.e. half-life of vWB factor: 2–5 h; factor VII: 5–7 h and factor VIII 8–12 h [10]). Additionally, cirrhotic patients are often anaemic which requires investigation and treatment before consideration of any surgery. Preoperative correction of low Hb and coagulopathy can limit intra-operative transfusion rate. Intraoperative transfusion is an independent risk factor of increased mortality. Therefore, patients with cirrhosis with a haemoglobin level lower than 10 g/dL should receive a corrective blood transfusion before abdominal surgery [11].

71.3.4 Nutrition, Obesity and Sarcopenia

A low serum albumin level is common in patients with chronic liver disease. It is a sign of impaired hepatocellular protein synthesis and is often associated with the malnourished state seen in advanced cirrhosis. Multiple mechanisms including poor nutritional intake, poor absorption and increased losses lead to sever macro- and micronutrient deficiencies in cirrhotic patients. This and the overall catabolic state in cirrhosis leads to poor wound healing, sepsis, delay in recovery, impaired mobility and respiratory muscle dysfunction from muscle wasting. Hypoalbuminaemia is a predictor of mortality in patients with cirrhosis undergoing surgery. The lower the albumin level, the higher the risk of mortality from surgery in cirrhotic patients. Evidence supports preoperative nutritional assessment and supplementation [10, 12]. In a recent study, Merli et al. [12] concluded that pre-transplant nutritional optimisation leads to a reduced number of infection during hospital stay and malnutrition was an independent risk factor associated with ICU length of stay. More so, preoperative nutritional support leads to better outcomes and may reduce short-term complications [13, 14]. Therefore, correcting the nutrient deficit of the affected patients is mandatory prior to surgery. Avoidance of alcohol and excess fat plus ingestion of 4–6 meals/day containing carbohydrates and protein are the most common recommendations [15]. Close collaboration with a dietician preoperatively helps with optimal timing of surgery. For those cirrhotic patients with obesity (sarcopenic obesity[1]), in addition to medical therapy, close collaboration with bariatric services is recommended, particularly for those patients being considered for liver transplantation. Malnutrition is not the only challenge in sarcopenic obesity; the risk of surgery is increased in obese patients due to a number of added technical challenges (e.g. anaesthetic risks, challenging laparoscopic surgery). Indeed, sarcopenic obesity is associated with increased mortality, sepsis complications, hyperammonaemia, risk of overt hepatic encephalopathy and it's associated with increased length of hospital stay after liver transplantation [14].

71.3.5 Hepato-Renal Syndrome (HRS)

Patient with cirrhosis, particularly those on the transplant waiting list, are at risk of rapid deterioration of their renal function. This is attributed to renal vasoconstriction secondary to the activation of the renin-angiotensin-aldosterone system that comes about as a result of the circulatory changes associated with portal hypertension. HRS is often fatal unless timely liver transplantation is performed. Treatments such as dialysis can prevent advancement of the disease and can be used as a bridging therapy until a patient get a liver transplant. Additionally, any form of elective surgery is avoided in patients with acute renal failure with pre-existing cirrhosis. If patients are being considered for transplantation, terlipressin and albumin along with liver and kidney support systems are considered preoperatively to avoid or reduce the incidence of postoperative complications: prolonged ITU and hospital stay, need for postoperative dialysis, infectious complications, acute rejection, and increased mortality [16, 17].

[1] Sarcopenic obesity: a condition in cirrhotic patients with obesity marked by loss of skeletal muscles and gain of adipose tissue.

71.3.6 Sepsis in Cirrhotic Patients, Particularly SBP

Patients with cirrhosis have impaired immunity and are therefore predisposed to infections with a higher incidence of multi-drug resistance organisms [10]. Sepsis in this group of patients can rapidly worsen liver function and lead to an acute on chronic liver failure state with poor short term prognosis. Therefore, pre-operative assessment should focus on identifying undiagnosed infections and treating pre-existing infections. In patients with cirrhosis and spontaneous bacterial peritonitis (SBP), early use of antibiotics and intravenous albumin administration decreases the risk of developing renal failure and improves survival [18]. Prophylactic antibiotic therapy is recommended for those with low-protein ascites (<1.5 g/dL) and advanced cirrhosis (primary prophylaxis), prior history of SBP (secondary prophylaxis) and gastrointestinal haemorrhage [10, 19].

71.4 Pre-operative Management for Cirrhotic Patients

Multiple factors should be taken into consideration when planning surgery in patients with liver disease (Fig. 71.3). Even in medically fit cirrhotic patients, liver disease poses multiple challenges that make the decision to operate a difficult one. The necessity of the proposed procedure and the magnitude of intervention are key factors. Other vital considerations are non-hepatic comorbidities and the severity of their liver disease. Therefore, appreciation of the risk of surgery is essential for optimal preoperative evaluation of the patients.

Preoperative multi-disciplinary assessment should include an assessment by a hepatologist, gastroenterologist, anaesthetist, intensivist and surgeon experienced in dealing with the liver disease in addition to dietetics and physiotherapy. Ideally, patients with chronic liver disease should be managed and worked up in a Liver unit where facilities exist to deal with episodes of liver failure postoperatively. Hence, high-risk patients should be transferred to or managed along with a tertiary liver unit.

Liaison with the critical care team in the preoperative period is necessary as most patients post-surgery require HDU/ITU bed. This is important particularly for those at high risk (co-morbidity of the severity of liver disease) and emergency operations. Any patient with chronic liver disease should undergo a rapid and detailed nutritional assessment by the dietician team. Particularly those with Child-Pugh class C and those with BMI of <18 as they are at increased risk of decompensation and mortality. Assessment should include determination of BMI, the severity of malnutrition, and consideration of CT and a DEXA scan to assess for sarcopenia.

Biochemical derangements should be identified early and corrected in the perioperative period. This includes early identification and correction of anaemia, clotting abnormalities, renal impairment and electrolyte disturbances. Blood bank should be informed if operating on patients with a high risk of bleeding and those who are coagulopathic to ensure ready availability of matched blood and blood products. Appropriate blood products (FFP, platelets, cryoprecipitate) should be anticipated before surgery and be ready to be utilised immediately if necessary (blood products may be frozen requiring careful rewarming in a water bath prior to clinical use). Theatre staff should be informed of high-risk patients so they can also help in better planning (i.e. utilisation of equipment such as cell saver, different haemostatic products and increased in the number of theatre personnel if anticipating major bleed or any complications).

71.4.1 Auto-Transfusion and Cell Salvage

Cell salvage offers a relatively inexpensive and safe method of avoiding allogenic red cell transfusion during

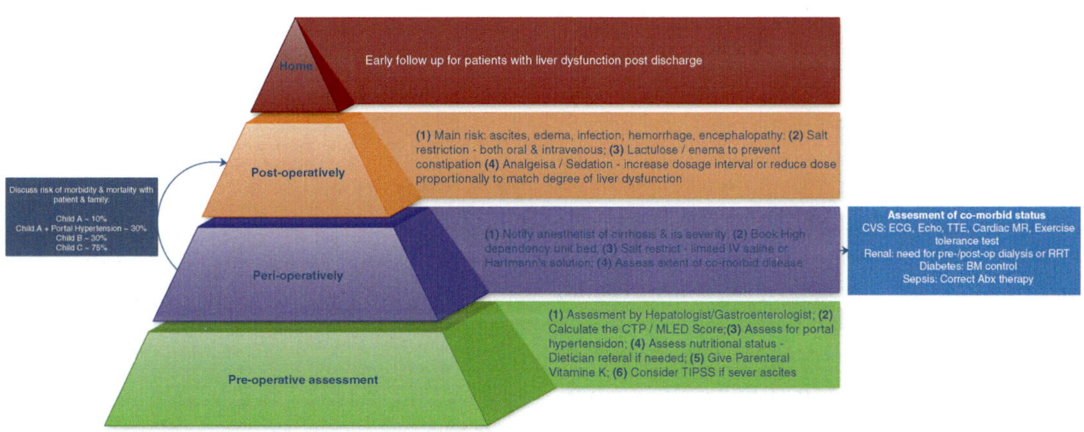

Fig. 71.3 Pre- and peri-operative assessment pyramid for patients with liver disease. Factors to consider at different stages of surgery to optimize care [22]

the intra-operative period. Autologous means of transfusion have gained acceptance in a major surgical procedure where homologous blood transfusion has proven challenging and pose a risk. Therefore, its use is recommended particularly in high-risk surgical patients. There are a number of relative contra-indications that would limit its use such as the presence of infection/sepsis, suspicion of malignancy, haematological disorders such as sickle cell disease, contamination with urine, fat or bowel content.

71.4.2 Pre-operative TIPPS

For the majority of the patient with cirrhosis, the high morbidity and mortality after surgery are due to portal hypertension and liver failure in the postoperative period [9]. Transjugular Intra-hepatic Portosystemic Shunting (TIPS) allows connection of the portal vein to the hepatic veins by allowing the return of the blood to heart while avoiding the liver and therefore reducing the risk of internal bleeding. Hence, it's a meaningful strategy to consider TIPS in cirrhotic patients who are considered for elective surgery to reduce post-operative complications related to portal hypertension [20]. Although more robust evidence regarding utilisation of TIPS in the per-operative period is needed, the general trend is a reduction in morbidity and mortality reported with neoadjuvant TIPS placement. Further, the optimal timing of its placement is subject to debate. Planning for this should take place several weeks prior to elective surgery since it takes a few weeks for the ascitic volume to respond to the intervention. Although TIPS has the added benefit of reducing the risk of internal bleeding, equally by diverting blood from liver parenchyma, it can predispose it to poor hepatic flow and increases the risk of hepatic encephalopathy.

Steps in the pre-operative period should be focused on: optimising patient for surgery and therefore reducing overall risk; taking actions to better plan for surgery as well as steps to ensure adequate treatment post-surgery. Prior to any surgical intervention imaging studies can aid in better planning of the operation. Hence, it's important to have imaging studies to confirm anatomy, the extent of pathology and most importantly to check for degree of venous dilations/varices in the presence of portal hypertension. All of which can help in the assessment of risk pre-operatively.

Assessment of the specific risk in this group of patients is somewhat difficult mostly due to lack of robust studies. The available data tend to be from retrospective studies mostly focused on abdominal surgery [21]. Hence, a more individualised assessment of risk performed by a physician experienced in dealing with liver disease is more favoured.

71.5 Classifying Severity of Liver Disease

The Child-Turcotte-Pugh (CTP) score or model for end-stage liver disease (MELD) score may be used to determine the severity of liver disease and the operative risk for an individual patient. More generic assessment of surgical risk such as the American Society of Anaesthesiologist (ASA) classification is less helpful for this patient group as it is not specific to the liver disease. More useful are the new models for risk estimation in the context of liver disease.

71.5.1 CTP Score

The CTP score is easy to calculate and correlates well with severity of disease and survival. It was originally developed to predict operative risk in patients undergoing portosystemic shunt surgery for variceal bleeds. It has been found to be a useful indicator of operative risk for other surgical procedures in patients with chronic liver disease. CTP score is obtained by adding the score for five parameters: encephalopathy, ascites, bilirubin and albumin level and the degree of coagulopathy. The score ranges from 5 to 15 with a further classification of CTP scores into three classes: Class A (CTP score 5–6), Class B (CTP score 7–9) and Class C (CTP score 10–15), the higher scores reflecting a more severe liver disease and hence higher operative risks. Overall general surgical risk of mortality is considered to be 10% for CTP classes A, 30% for class B and 82% for class C [23]. This means while patients with mild chronic liver disease are able to tolerate surgery, those with higher scores should have a realistic discussion about the associated risk of mortality and non-surgical options. They tend to fall in CTP class C, presenting as an emergency, their risk of mortality is several fold and surgery may have a detrimental effect. Risk of morbidity from surgical procedure also increases with higher classes of CTP classification and can have an impact on the quality of life of the patient. Hence, any intervention should be offered not only with mortality in mind but also with morbidity associated with the intervention and its short and long term impact on the quality of life of the patient.

71.5.2 MELD Score

The MELD score was originally developed to predict mortality after TIPS and now is implemented in risk assessment of patients awaiting liver transplantation, as well as, to predict perioperative mortality risk in abdominal surgery [24]. It has been validated for the prediction of both short- and long-term survival of cirrhotic patients to allow anticipated survival without any interventions to be considered. When applied to the risk assessment of cirrhotic patients undergoing surgery a MELD score of 0–11 correlates with 5–10% 90-day mortality, a score of 12–25 with 25–54% mortality rate, and a score greater than 26 with a 90% postoperative mortality rate [9]. In the non-transplant surgical group, there was approximately a 1% increase in mortality risk per MELD point below a score of 20, whereas there was a 2% increase in mortality risk per MELD point over 20 [25]. A MELD score of greater than 8 in patients undergoing hepatic resection is associated with decreased long-term survival and correlates well with peri-operative mortality [26]. Generally, a MELD score of 14 or greater should be considered as a replacement for CTP class C and as a predictor of being very high risk for abdominal surgery [11].

The above models provide an estimation of operative and post risk as well as an indicator for both short and long term survival. However, there are other factors that need to be considered for risk stratification and prediction in cirrhotic patients undergoing major surgery. For patients with cirrhosis undergoing either elective or emergency surgery, CTP and MELD scores provide a good measure of global liver function and patient's overall risk. Any patient with CTP class B/C or a MELD score of >8 should be carefully assessed for surgery where possible the above risk stratification models should be accompanied with other methods of functional liver assessment. More so, when considering the risk of surgery patient's other comorbid conditions should be taken into account such as their age, BMI, the presence of diabetes, cardiovascular status, renal function and presence of sepsis. This will reveal more about the patient's physiological reserve and ability to cope with the insult of surgery.

71.6 Emergency Surgery in Cirrhotic Patients

When compared to elective, emergency surgery in cirrhotic patients is associated with a sevenfold increased risk of mortality [27]. Morbidity and mortality depend on the severity of cirrhosis (see above), the presence of complications related to liver cirrhosis, e.g. varices, and the nature of the surgical emergency. As a general rule aim should be to optimise patients prior to any operation. However, there is a balance between the time required to investigate and optimise the patient with liver disease and the reduction in the patient's condition secondary to the surgical emergency. For example, patients with a demonstrated radiological evidence of a strangulated hernia with rising lactate are likely to benefit from early intervention rather than a period of pre-operative optimisation. Patients risk of emergency surgery must be weighed against non-intervention, and the discussion needs to be clearly communicated with the patient, their family and the rest of the clinical team. Patients with Child C score who present in an emergency setting are more likely to be considered for a non-operative or palliative measure because surgery may be futile.

71.7 Elective Surgery in Patients with Abnormal Liver Function

For patients requiring elective surgery who are found to have asymptomatic biochemical abnormalities (LFT derangement), these should further be investigated prior to surgery irrespective of level and duration of abnormality. In adults, this normally includes an ultrasound scan and a serology screen looking for chronic liver disease (hepatitis screen [HCV, HBV], anti-mitochondrial Ab, anti-nuclear Ab, anti-smooth muscle Ab, serum immunoglobulins, simultaneous serum ferritin and transferrin saturation).

Patients with a history of alcohol dependence should be referred to alcohol services for clinical assessment including a Fibroscan/ARFI elastography. This allows planning for post-operative management including alcohol withdrawal and commencing treatment. Those presenting with evidence of NAFLD on their ultrasound scan should have an assessment of the risk of advanced fibrosis. Patients at high risk with advanced fibrosis (Fibroscan of >8 kPa) should be referred to a specialist hepatology clinic for further assessment and management plus screening and treatment of portal hypertension and HCC.

If investigations reveal acute hepatitis, then elective surgery should be deferred until the stabilisation of the patient. Further consideration of the type of surgery should be given as mortality differs in non-hepatic operation to hepatic resection in the context of liver disease/cirrhosis (Table 71.1).

71.8 Hepatic Resection in Cirrhotic Patients

71.8.1 Selection of Surgical Procedure

Liver cirrhosis is not only a major risk factor for the development of hepatocellular carcinoma (HCC) but also other extrahepatic malignancies [29]. HCC is the most common primary liver cancer and the second most common cause of cancer-related mortality with its incidence on the rise globally. It is the most common indication for hepatic resection in cirrhotic patients. The severity of liver disease, the extent of the required liver resection and the volume of the anticipated future liver remnant (FLR) should define the operative strategy. Liver transplantation is an ideal treatment for early-stage HCC meeting the Milan criteria (BCLC staging) but is restricted to young patients with limited co-morbidities. Hepatic resection is considered mainly for patients with soli-

Table 71.1 Mortality rates associated with specific types of surgery in patients with cirrhosis—adapted from [28]

	Mortality				
		Child class			
Type of surgery	Overall	A	B	C	MELD score
Appendectomy	9%	NA	NA	NA	NA
Cardiac	16–17%	0–3%	42–50%	100%	NA
Cholecystectomy	1–3%	0.50%	3%	NA	<8 = 0%, ≥8 = 6%
Colorectal cancer surgery	12.50%	6%	13%	27%	NA
Esophagectomy	17%	NA	NA	NA	NA
Hepatic resection	9%	9%	NA	NA	<9 = 0%, ≥9 = 29%
Major abdominal surgery	26–30%	10%	30–31%	76–82%	NA
Total knee arthroplasty	0%	0%	NA	NA	NA
Treatment of hepatic hydrothorax with talc	39%	NA	NA	NA	NA

tary tumours and very well-preserved liver function (CTP class A) [30]. This decision making necessitates a careful patient selection and detailed evaluation of liver function. Unlike other malignancies, the prognosis of HCC in cirrhosis is not only determined by the burden of cancer but also the degree of cirrhosis and its complications (e.g. ascites, portal hypertension, encephalopathy) significantly determine overall mortality [31].

71.8.2 Evaluation of Liver Function and Functional Reserve

Both CTP and MELD score, in addition to BCLC stating system, have led to better risk stratification in patients with HCC leading to a more appropriate patient selection. Patient with early HCC stage and a low CTP score (class A) are generally the most suitable candidates for surgical treatment [32, 33]. On the other hand, more advanced disease and CTP class C patients are considered for non-surgical treatments (i.e. TACE, Radiofrequency ablation, PEIT and HAIC). The MELD score has been shown to be a strong predictor of perioperative mortality. A MELD score of 9 or greater, as well as, tumour size of >5 cm, high tumour grade and absence of tumour capsule are independent predictors of decreased long-term survival [32, 33]. Both CTP classification and ASA grade can also provide useful information about the risks associated with elective hepatic resection [34]. However, they lack quantitative information about the functional reserve of the liver thus lacking accuracy in predictive risk associated with liver surgery in cirrhosis.

71.8.3 Other Methods of Predicting Postoperative Liver Failure

Since CTP provides a rough estimation, current guidelines recommend additional studies to assess liver functional reserve. Indocyanine green retention rate at 15 min (ICGR15) or assessment of severity of portal hypertension provide useful information. Resections are reportedly safe in patients with an ICGR15 less than 20%, while others have suggested a cut-off point of 14% to achieve zero operative mortality [35, 36]. A hepatic venous pressure gradient of >10 mmHg has been shown to be a predictor of unresolved hepatic decompensation after surgery [37]. Presence of portal hypertension is a poor prognostic indicator; its 5-year survival rates are less than 50% [38]. Hence, the presence of portal hypertension is now widely considered a relative contraindication for liver resection. Current western guidelines recommend resection in patients with well-preserved liver function, defined as normal serum bilirubin with either hepatic venous pressure <10 mmHg or platelet count $>100 \times 10^9$/L [29].

Once HCC is suspected detailed imaging is required for staging and surgical planning. Arterial phase CT and/or MRI of the liver are standard. Biopsy tends to be preserved for lesions greater than 2 cm with low alpha-fetoprotein (AFP) where ablative therapy or transplant is contraindicated. Patients should also be screened for extra-hepatic metastasis. These findings should be discussed in the local MDT prior to any plan for resection.

71.8.4 Importance of AFP Levels in Patients with Suspected HCC

AFP is an important biomarker used in diagnosis and monitoring treatment regimen in HCC. It also serves as an indicator of HCC risk mostly in patients with cirrhosis and HCV/HBV infection [39]. Although, it's a cheap screening option, it is only 40–64% sensitive. Only the regenerating hepatocytes or tumours at a very advanced stage produce AFP. More so, levels can be elevated in chronic active hepatitis leading misinterpretation of results. AFP levels also transiently rise post liver resection or following recovery from a toxic injury. Hence, when interpreting AFP levels, it must be interpreted in the clinical context with support from imaging studies.

Preoperative serum AFP level has predictive value for malignant feature and prognosis of HCC. HCC patients with no contraindication of operation and serum AFP < 20 ng/mL can benefit from primary treatment of hepatectomy. While HCC patients with serum AFP higher than 20 ng/mL need comprehensive therapy beside surgical resection and close follow up [40].

Resection of HCC in cirrhotic patients requires expert selection of the candidates—meaning adequate knowledge of the stage of the disease, the risk factors for postoperative morbidity and mortality, recurrence, and survival—and the surgical skills necessary for the planned procedure [41].

Further, the severity of cirrhosis and characteristics of tumour more depicts long-term survival than the type of resection in HCC. The safety and feasibility of surgical resection in selected cirrhotic cases is now well established. The success of an intervention depends on the careful selection of patients with meticulous pre-operative work-up and risk stratification.

71.9 Non-hepatic Surgery in Cirrhotic Patients

71.9.1 Umbilical Hernia Repair (UHR)

An umbilical hernia occurs in about 20% of cirrhotic patients [42], caused mainly by ascites, poor nutritional status and muscle wasting. Ascites should be controlled medically prior to hernia repair. If the ascites is refractory to diuretics, the patient should be considered for a liver transplant with hernia repair during the transplant surgery. If they are not a candidate for transplant, a TIPPS stent may be considered to control ascites prior to hernia repair.

Historically, UHR was associated with high morbidity and mortality in cirrhotic patients. Therefore, the general consensus was to manage uncomplicated umbilical hernias conservatively. However, recent evidence would suggest elective UHR can be performed safely and effectively with improved surgical technique supported by specialist perioperative medical management [43].

71.9.1.1 Emergency UHR

Emergency hernia repair is becoming less common as elective repair is becoming safer and hence more often performed in cirrhotic patients. Morbidity and mortality are higher in the emergency setting and with the severity of the underlying liver disease [43]. There are more wound-related complications following emergency repair. To decrease the risk of emergency hernia repair, elective repair should be carried out whenever possible. If the need for emergency repair arises, this should be done at experienced centres following control of ascites with diuretic therapy and/or percutaneous paracentesis [44]. Preoperative anaemia and electrolyte abnormalities should be aggressively treated. Early referral to the local HPB/transplant unit should be made particularly for those with higher CTP score or evidence of strangulation or decompensation.

71.9.1.2 Elective

Elective UHR is considered a safe approach and is preferred to conservative measures. Eker et al. [45], reports on elective UHR in 30 patients with different CTP scores: six were CTP class A, 19 CTP class B and five were CTP class C. The patient's median MELD score was 12. None of the patients required ITU admission following operation. Only one postoperative complication was reported which was due to pneumonia and decompensated cirrhosis. More so, after a median follow-up period of 25-month only two patients suffered recurrence. Although this was a small study, it supports earlier reports on the safety and effectiveness of elective UHR [46]. Marsman et al. [46] in a retrospective database analysis, compared elective repair (17 patients) versus a conservative approach (13 patients) to umbilical hernia in cirrhotic patients. As would be expected there was a higher rate of incarceration requiring emergency repair in the conservative group. Elective repair, on the other hand, was performed with less morbidity and therefore advocated. Elective repair has been associated with poor outcomes in those >65 years, MELD score >15, and albumin level <3.0 g/dl [47].

Whether nylon or polypropylene mesh should be used for hernia repair in cirrhotic patients has been a matter of debate. In a prospective comparative study, use of mesh in non-complicated UHR in ascitic patients with liver cirrhosis is reported to be associated with less ascitic fluid leakage (15% vs. 30%) and hernia recurrence (10% vs. 35%) compared to primary suture repair [48]. However, higher rates of wound infection (25% vs. 15%) are reported in the mesh group. In a recent randomised control trial [49], the use of mesh in complicated umbilical hernias in cirrhotic patients was considered safe with minimal wound-related morbidity and significantly lower rates of recurrence than conventional fascial repair.

In brief, elective UHR is advised in patients with cirrhosis, and it seems to be well tolerated. However, this group of patients require pre-operative workup to ensure they are well compensated and ascites is under control. This means those medically fit patients with Child A score and no evidence of decompensation can be managed locally and those with higher CTP score or evidence of decompensation should be referred and managed in an HPB unit.

71.9.2 Cholecystectomy

Gallstones are a common finding in patients with cirrhosis with an increased incidence of 9.5–29.4% compared to those without cirrhosis (5.2–12.8%) [50]. Haemolysis and a reduction in gallbladder emptying in cirrhotic patients are contributing factors to the high incidence [51]. The majority are asymptomatic, the minority presenting with biliary pain, cholecystitis or obstructive jaundice [51].

Until recently, cirrhosis was considered to be an absolute or relative contraindication to laparoscopic cholecystectomy (LC). However, LC has been reported to be safe in CTP class A and selected class B [52]. The laparoscopic approach offers the advantage of less blood loss, shorter operative time, and shorter length of hospitalisation in patients with cirrhosis.

CTP class C usually represents the end stage of liver disease and surgery would generally not be indicated for elective procedures [53]. In patients with CTP class C, cholecystostomy is recommended over cholecystectomy. However, if surgery is required, open rather than laparoscopic is recommended [8]. Complication rates are high for CTP class C patients regardless of an open or laparoscopic approach.

Pre-operatively, any patient undergoing LC should have an attempt at control of ascites, correction of coagulopathy with Vit K and FFP (aim for INR < 1.3) and correction of platelet count to >50,000/dL. Patients should have pre-operative imaging (arterial and venous phase CT scan) to help identify abdominal wall varices, re-canalised umbilical vein with choledochal varices and to rule out HCC [54].

71.9.2.1 Emergency

Emergency cholecystectomy in cirrhotic patients is a challenging operation particularly with those who have advanced liver disease. A recent meta-analysis demonstrated patient with cirrhosis who undergo emergency cholecystectomy have a higher morbidity (20.9% vs. 7.99%; p-value: <0.001) and no difference in mortality (0.59% vs. 0.13%; p-value: 0.133) compared to the patients undergoing LC in non-cirrhotic group [55]. Surprisingly, In the 400 patients with liver cirrhosis that were reviewed in the study, only six patients had advanced stage liver disease (PTC class C). The laparoscopic approach to cholecystectomy was associated with less blood loss (113 mL vs. 425 mL; p = 0.015), shorter operative time (123.3 min vs. 150 min, p < 0.042) and shorter length of stay (6 days vs. 12 days, p < 0.001) when compared to open technique in cirrhotic patients [56]. In comparison to non-cirrhotic patients who undergo LC, cirrhotic patients have a higher conversion rate, more bleeding complications and higher overall morbidity [55]. Given the challenges of LC in cirrhotic patients, attempts should be made to refer patients early to HPB centres with the capacity to deal with surgical complications and the episodes of liver decompensation. Even elective cases are suggested to be considered for referral to an HPB Unit.

71.9.2.2 Elective

LC in cirrhosis is associated with better outcomes in the elective as compared to the emergency setting. Reported mortality rates from LC in CTP class A and B is low (0.12% and 0.97% respectively) [57]. The rate for CTP class C, however, have been reported as high as 50–83% and even higher in the emergency settings [57].

MELD score may also be used to predict both mortality and morbidity and may be more accurate than CTP in assessing morbidity [50]. A MELD score of >13 was associated with an increased rate of conversion to open and a high incidence of postoperative complications [50]. A conservative or minimally invasive treatment (antibiotics, percutaneous gallbladder drainage) should be considered in patients with MELD score of >13.

Post-operative complications can be reduced via modifications to a surgical technique such as hepatic pedicle occlusion (Pringle manoeuvre) to reduce bleeding, provide a clear surgical field and avoid damage to vital structures during LC [58]. The Pringle manoeuvre offers a feasible and safe approach to lower the conversion rate in difficult cases. In high-risk patients an alternative surgical strategy is to perform a subtotal LC [59] leaving the patient with a risk of future biliary complications. The need for conversion to open cholecystectomy should not be considered a failure but as a safe strategy to avoid intra- or post-operative complications [59]. Puggioni et al. [55] reviewed 400 patients with cirrhosis undergoing LC; their meta-analyses reported a 7% conversion rate for LC in cirrhotic patients (47% presented with acute cholecystitis). Recently, Machado et al. [57] reported on LC in 1310 cirrhotic patients. The overall conversation rate was 4.5% but was 35% in CTP class C patients. Interestingly, a low platelet count <50,000/dL was associated with a higher rate of conversion in cirrhotic patients undergoing LC [50], presumably related to the severity of portal hypertension and hypersplenism.

In summary, LC is considered a safe approach to CTP class A patients and in a selected number of patients with CTP class B (those without evidence of portal hypertension). Conservative measures should be first line considerations in the management of CTP class C with surgery being considered only in those failing conservative treatment. In patients with cirrhosis, LC should be performed by surgeons with advanced laparoscopic and HPB surgical experience.

71.9.3 Colorectal Surgery

Cirrhosis poses a major challenge in patients requiring major colorectal surgery. Morbidity and mortality rates at 30 days range from 48% to 77% and 21.5–26%, respectively [60]. Patients with cirrhosis have a 6.5-fold increased risk of mortality following bowel surgery [61]. Mortality is higher in emergency surgery and in the presence of portal hypertension. A review of data from the American College of Surgeons National Surgical Quality Improvement Project [62] revealed MELD score of >15 in chronic liver disease patients undergoing colorectal surgery was significantly associated with higher rates of complications, failure to rescue (proportion of death following major complication) and mortality. Subsequent studies confirmed the MELD score as an independent predictor of mortality in cirrhotic patients undergoing bowel surgery regardless of the underlying disease [63]. The higher the MELD score, the higher the risk of death and major morbidity in the 30-days after elective colorectal resection [64]. This re-enforces the importance of risk stratification and pre-operative optimisation to improve the outcome of elective bowel surgery in cirrhotic patients.

Postoperative complications, particularly, infective complications, significantly contribute to mortality following colorectal surgery in cirrhotic patients [65]. Other independent predictors of mortality include age, functional status, ASA classification, ascites, oesophageal varices, disseminated cancer, chronic steroid use, cardiac disease, renal failure, sepsis, ventilatory dependence and emergency operation [63]. These factors should also be considered in conjunction with the MELD or CTP score for a more realistic approach to risk assessment.

A recent review [66] of the Danish database looking at patients with the colorectal disease who underwent surgery between 1996 and 2009, the 30-day mortality after surgery was 8.7% in a patient without liver disease, 13.3% in patients with non-cirrhotic liver disease and 24% in those with cirrhosis. Mortality was greater in patients undergoing colon cancer surgery compared to rectal cancer surgery [66]. Similar, high 30-day mortality rates (13%) were found in patients with colorectal adenocarcinoma by Gervaz et al. [67] in their retrospective study. They reported 1-, 3-and 5-year survival rates of 69%, 49%, and 35%. Significantly better survival rates are described for CTP class A than CTP class B and C. Interestingly, TNM staging of the adenocarcinoma provided no prognostic information in patients with cirrhosis [67]. However, low albumin and prolonged prothrombin time are identified as risk factors for mortality.

Although there is limited data on methods to reduce the risk of colorectal surgery in liver disease recommendations have been made on the importance of perioperative risk assessment and optimisation of physiological markers such as albumin and haematocrit [60]. Laparoscopic rather than open surgery may offer benefit. Martinez et al. [68] reported reduced blood loss, 29% morbidity and no mortality in a small cohort of patients (n = 17) with compensated cirrhosis (CTP A = 12 and CTP B = 5) undergoing laparoscopic bowel resection. Laparoscopic surgery may have favourable outcomes in patients with cirrhosis, but careful patient selection is crucial to reduce associated morbidity and mortality [69]. This depends on a number of factors and a meticulous preoperative assessment of the patient (i.e. identifying and addressing the correctable). Not only the degree of liver disease is a determinant of patients' suitability for laparoscopic surgery, but the nature of the colonic tumour (position and local stage) along with other comorbid conditions (e.g. previous surgery, the presence of cardio-respiratory disease) would be a determining factor. Patients should have their surgery at centres with experienced laparoscopic surgeons and availability of hepatology and HPB surgeons that can assist in all stages of the patient management.

71.9.4 Cardiac Surgery

Cardiac surgery and other surgical procedures that require cardiopulmonary bypass (CPB) have increased rates of mortality in patients with cirrhosis (Table 71.1) [8]. Cardiovascular risk factors are more common in cirrhotic patients than the general population [70], and they are therefore more likely to require cardiac surgery. Identification of those with underlying liver disease is essential to facilitate preoperative planning. As with the other surgeries being performed in cirrhotic patients mentioned above, the mortality following cardiac surgery increases with the severity of liver disease [71]. MELD score has again been shown to reliably identify cirrhotic patients who are at high risk for open heart surgery [72]. Thielmann et al. [71], showed both MELD score and CTP class differed significantly between survivors and nonsurvivors following cardiac surgery both for in-hospital and long-term mortality.

Interestingly, in a study of 55 patients with cirrhosis undergoing cardiac surgery, Lin et al. [73] revealed preoperative serum bilirubin, the EuroSCORE[2], and CABG are major predictors of early and late mortality. In this study, CTP and MELD scores were not strongly predictive of early or late mortality. There were 30 patients in PTC A, 20 in PTC class B and five in PTC C with an overall hospital mortality rate of 16.4%. The actuarial survival rates were 70%, 64%, 56%, and 44% at 1 year, 2 years, 3 years, and 5 years after surgery, respectively. The mortality of

[2]EuroSCORE (European System for Cardiac Operative Risk Evaluation): is a risk model which allows the calculation of risk of death after heart surgery.

patients with liver cirrhosis undergoing open heart surgery increases with the severity of liver disease.

Filsoufi et al. [74], reported on patients with livers disease and a mean MELD score of 14 who had undergone cardiac surgery between 1998 and 2004. Stratified mortality according to CTP class were 11%, 18%, and 67% for class A, B, and C, respectively. The 1-year survival was 80%, 45%, and 16% for CTP class A, B, and C, respectively. Results are suggestive that cardiac surgery can be performed safely in CTP class A patients and a selected number of CTP class B patients. Operative mortality is very high in CTP class C patients, surgery is hazardous, and alternative conservative treatments must be considered [72]. Overall mortality is high in all classes of liver cirrhosis [75]. Short-term, peri-operative mortality is particularly high in class B and C patients [75]. Therefore, when considering surgery in Class B, apart from the severity of liver disease other comorbidities play an important part in decision making (i.e. renal failure, respiratory disease) and overall long-term survival.

Other factors determining the outcome in cirrhotic patients undergoing cardiac surgery have been platelet count, serum cholinesterase level, and Cardio-pulmonary bypass (CPB) time. Low platelet count and serum cholinesterase levels along with longer CPB time were associated with increased mortality [76]. Mortality is even higher in the presence of such factors along with a MELD score >13 [77]. Therefore, when assessing liver disease patients for cardiac surgery, in addition to MELD score other factors (e.g. co-morbidity, platelet count and anticipated bypass period) need to be taken into account to assess the true extent of risk [78].

Modifications to techniques such as off-pump coronary artery bypass in patients with liver cirrhosis have been shown to reduce bleeding and transfusion time [79]. Although off-pump surgery has the aforementioned added advantages, the presence of cirrhosis did not affect morbidity or mortality unless there was severe liver dysfunction [80]. The impact of cirrhosis on preoperative outcomes and health care costs are significant. Therefore, CABG should be performed in carefully selected patients and, whenever possible, without the use of CPB [75]. However, CPB is safe in those compensated cirrhotic patients with a CTP score of <8 and no other significant comorbidity.

71.10 Avoiding Futile Operations

Any surgical treatment in patients with cirrhosis should be undertaken with careful consideration of the severity of liver disease, the likely operative morbidity and mortality and the anticipated length and quality of life for those who survive.

Consideration must also be given to the technical abilities of the surgeon as well as the availability of resources to deal effectively with decompensated cirrhosis in a patient following major surgery [81]. If no HPB medical and surgical expertise is available cirrhotic patients requiring any form of major surgical intervention should be referred to a specialist unit. This allows pre-assessment to be done in conjunction with a hepatology team for optimisation of the background liver disease, the availability of liver surgery expertise if required and a multi-disciplinary team available to treat decompensated cirrhosis. The patient will be assessed by an anaesthetist who is experienced with portal hypertension and the hemodynamic challenges of a cirrhotic patient. Additionally, input from haemophilia team with clotting management can be coordinated and the requirement identified for specialist intensive care monitoring postoperatively.

There are a number of liver-related contraindications to elective surgery (Table 71.2). Acute liver failure [82] defined by the presence of neurologic dysfunction, INR >1.5, with no prior evidence of liver disease and a disease course of fewer than 26 weeks, is considered an absolute contraindication to any form of surgery unless transplantation is being considered. Acute hepatitis and alcoholic hepatitis are also considered contraindications to elective surgery due to increased risk of morbidity and mortality. Surgery should be delayed until the patient's condition is stable both clinically and biochemically.

It is important to identify high-risk patients pre-operatively. Those with high pre-operative serum creatinine (>125 μmol/L) are at increased risk of blood loss, higher postoperative morbidity and have a higher incidence of cardiorespiratory complications [83]. Elective surgery should be postponed until renal function has been stabilised. In those requiring liver resection, the presence of pre-existing renal failure can have fatal consequences if other comorbidities exist and the patient undergoes an extended resection [84].

Futile operations can be avoided by appropriate risk assessment, adequate preoperative optimisation, better operative planning and appropriate level of care postoperatively. Every patient must be discussed individually and assessed on their merits in the context of the severity of background liver disease.

Table 71.2 Contraindication to elective surgery in patients with liver disease [28]

Acute or fulminant liver failure
Acute renal failure
Alcoholic hepatitis
Hypoxaemia
Cardiomyopathy
Severe coagulopathy (despite treatment; prolongation of PT >3 s despite vitamin K; Platelet count of <50,000/mm^3)
Child Class C cirrhosis
Severe chronic hepatitis

71.11 Summary

Liver disease, irrespective of its severity, poses a challenge to surgery. Any degree of liver disease must be investigated and discussed with appropriate members of the MDT team before any planned operations. Preoperative risk assessment and optimisation of the liver function are essential as the liver disease severity score (CTP or MELD) correlates with perioperative mortality. Referral to a specialist HPB centre is necessary for all major surgical procedures in cirrhotic patients as the multi-disciplinary team is essential for preoperative optimisation, determining whether surgery is appropriate, determining the optimal surgical approach and for maximising the chance of survival with anaesthetists and intensivists familiar with the physiology of cirrhotic patients and the availability of hepatology review for those decompensating following surgery.

Risk assessment of patients should not be based solely on CTP or MELD score and a more individualised approach including patients' age, co-morbid status and extent of planned surgery should determine the patient risk and suitability for surgery. In general, patients with CTP class C should be considered as having end-stage liver disease and should not be considered candidates for major surgery unless intensive management can improve the function of chronic liver disease.

Self Study

Questions

1. In patients with cirrhosis undergoing surgery:
   (a) The liver is at increased risk of hypoxia due to arterio-venous shunting
   (b) Sarcopenic obesity can increase the risk of hepatic encephalopathy
   (c) Cardiac output is decreased and systemic vascular resistance increased
   (d) Coagulopathy can only be corrected with FFP
   (e) Sedatives and narcotics should be used judiciously
2. When assessing patients in the pre-operative period:
   (a) Type and extent of surgery does not determine risk
   (b) Biochemical derangements should be investigated and corrected prior to surgery
   (c) Preoperative TIPS is safe in emergency surgery
   (d) Patients with BMI of <18 are at increased risk of decompensation
   (e) Imaging is mandatory prior to surgery
3. Regarding risk classification of liver disease:
   (a) Higher CTP class tolerate invasive procedures well
   (b) A MELD score of 8 or greater should be considered the same as CTP Class C
   (c) Either MELD or CTP is sufficient in determining risk alone
   (d) The risk is higher in the emergency setting for any of CTP classes
   (e) ASA classification is useful in determining risk in cirrhotic patients
4. In hepatic resections in cirrhotic patients
   (a) CTP or MELD score provide sufficient information regarding risk
   (b) ICGR15 of less than 20% is considered safe
   (c) The severity of cirrhosis and tumour characteristic are predictive of long term survival
   (d) Resection is considered safe in hepatic venous pressures >10 mmHg
   (e) A MELD score of 9 or greater is associated with good outcome

Answers

1. In patients with cirrhosis undergoing surgery:
   TTFFT
2. When assessing patients in the pre-operative period:
   FTFTT
3. Regarding risk classification of liver disease:
   FFFTF
4. In hepatic resections in cirrhotic patients
   FTTFF

References

1. Martin Blachier HL, Peck-Radosavljevic M, Valla D-C, Roudot-Thoraval F. The burden of liver disease in Europe: a review of available epidemiological data. Geneva: EASL; 2013.
2. Zatonski WA, et al. Liver cirrhosis mortality in Europe, with special attention to Central and Eastern Europe. Eur Addict Res. 2010;16(4):193–201.
3. Peck-Radosavljevic M, et al. Managing complications in cirrhotic patients. U Eur Gastroenterol J. 2015;3(1):80–94.
4. Chouillard EK, Gumbs AA, Cherqui D. Vascular clamping in liver surgery: physiology, indications and techniques. Ann Surg Innov Res. 2010;4:2.
5. Smyrniotis V, et al. Vascular control during hepatectomy: review of methods and results. World J Surg. 2005;29(11):1384–96.
6. Dixon E, et al. Vascular occlusion to decrease blood loss during hepatic resection. Am J Surg. 2005;190(1):75–86.
7. Lau WY, Lai E, SHY L. Methods of vascular control technique during liver resection: a comprehensive review. Hepatobiliary Pancreat Dis Int. 2010;9(5):473–81.
8. Friedman LS. Surgery in the patient with liver disease. Trans Am Clin Climatol Assoc. 2010;121:192–204; discussion 205.
9. Bhangui P, et al. Assessment of risk for non-hepatic surgery in cirrhotic patients. J Hepatol. 2012;57(4):874–84.

10. Abbas N, et al. Perioperative care of patients with liver cirrhosis: a review. Health Serv Insights. 2017;10:1178632917691270.
11. Befeler AS, et al. The safety of intra-abdominal surgery in patients with cirrhosis: model for end-stage liver disease score is superior to Child-Turcotte-Pugh classification in predicting outcome. Arch Surg. 2005;140(7):650–4.
12. Merli M, et al. Nutritional status: its influence on the outcome of patients undergoing liver transplantation. Liver Int. 2010;30(2):208–14.
13. Harimoto N, et al. Prognostic significance of preoperative controlling nutritional status (CONUT) score in patients undergoing hepatic resection for hepatocellular carcinoma: a multi-institutional study. Ann Surg Oncol. 2018;25(11):3316–23.
14. Schiavo L, et al. Nutritional issues in patients with obesity and cirrhosis. World J Gastroenterol. 2018;24(30):3330–46.
15. Tsiaousi ET, et al. Malnutrition in end stage liver disease: recommendations and nutritional support. J Gastroenterol Hepatol. 2008;23(4):527–33.
16. Guerrero-Dominguez R, et al. Perioperative renal protection strategies in liver transplantation. Nefrologia. 2014;34(3):276–84.
17. Biancofiore G, Davis CL. Renal dysfunction in the perioperative liver transplant period. Curr Opin Organ Transplant. 2008;13(3):291–7.
18. Gustot T, et al. Severe sepsis in cirrhosis. Hepatology. 2009;50(6):2022–33.
19. Jalan R, et al. Bacterial infections in cirrhosis: a position statement based on the EASL Special Conference 2013. J Hepatol. 2014;60(6):1310–24.
20. Jain D, et al. Preoperative elective transjugular intrahepatic portosystemic shunt for cirrhotic patients undergoing abdominal surgery. Ann Gastroenterol. 2018;31(3):330–7.
21. Patel T. Surgery in the patient with liver disease. Mayo Clin Proc. 1999;74(6):593–9.
22. Nicoll A. Surgical risk in patients with cirrhosis. J Gastroenterol Hepatol. 2012;27(10):1569–75.
23. Mansour A, et al. Abdominal operations in patients with cirrhosis: still a major surgical challenge. Surgery. 1997;122(4):730–5; discussion 735–6.
24. Kamath PS, et al. A model to predict survival in patients with end-stage liver disease. Hepatology. 2001;33(2):464–70.
25. Northup PG, et al. Model for end-stage liver disease (MELD) predicts nontransplant surgical mortality in patients with cirrhosis. Ann Surg. 2005;242(2):244–51.
26. Rahbari NN, et al. The predictive value of postoperative clinical risk scores for outcome after hepatic resection: a validation analysis in 807 patients. Ann Surg Oncol. 2011;18(13):3640–9.
27. Carbonell AM, Wolfe LG, DeMaria EJ. Poor outcomes in cirrhosis-associated hernia repair: a nationwide cohort study of 32,033 patients. Hernia. 2005;9(4):353–7.
28. Friedman LS. The risk of surgery in patients with liver disease. Hepatology. 1999;29(6):1617–23.
29. Pinter M, et al. Cancer and liver cirrhosis: implications on prognosis and management. ESMO Open. 2016;1(2):e000042.
30. Zhu Z. Milan criteria and its expansions in liver transplantation for hepatocellular carcinoma. Hepatobiliary Surg Nutr. 2016;5(6):498–502.
31. Cabibbo G, et al. A meta-analysis of survival rates of untreated patients in randomized clinical trials of hepatocellular carcinoma. Hepatology. 2010;51(4):1274–83.
32. Teh SH, et al. Hepatic resection of hepatocellular carcinoma in patients with cirrhosis: model of end-stage liver disease (MELD) score predicts perioperative mortality. J Gastrointest Surg. 2005;9(9):1207–15; discussion 1215.
33. Ercolani G, et al. Liver resection for hepatocellular carcinoma on cirrhosis: univariate and multivariate analysis of risk factors for intrahepatic recurrence. Ann Surg. 2003;237(4):536–43.
34. Schroeder RA, et al. Predictive indices of morbidity and mortality after liver resection. Ann Surg. 2006;243(3):373–9.
35. Llovet JM, Schwartz M, Mazzaferro V. Resection and liver transplantation for hepatocellular carcinoma. Semin Liver Dis. 2005;25(2):181–200.
36. Poon RT, Fan ST. Hepatectomy for hepatocellular carcinoma: patient selection and postoperative outcome. Liver Transpl. 2004;10(2 Suppl 1):S39–45.
37. Bruix J, et al. Surgical resection of hepatocellular carcinoma in cirrhotic patients: prognostic value of preoperative portal pressure. Gastroenterology. 1996;111(4):1018–22.
38. Bruix J, Sherman M. Management of hepatocellular carcinoma: an update. Hepatology. 2011;53(3):1020–2.
39. Baig JA, et al. Hepatocellular carcinoma (HCC) and diagnostic significance of A-fetoprotein (AFP). J Ayub Med Coll. 2009;21(1):72–5.
40. Ma W-j, Wang H-y, Teng L-s. Correlation analysis of preoperative serum alpha-fetoprotein (AFP) level and prognosis of hepatocellular carcinoma (HCC) after hepatectomy. World J Surg Oncol. 2013;11(1):212.
41. Cucchetti A, et al. Current concepts in hepatic resection for hepatocellular carcinoma in cirrhotic patients. World J Gastroenterol. 2012;18(44):6398–408.
42. Coelho JC, et al. Umbilical hernia in patients with liver cirrhosis: a surgical challenge. World J Gastrointest Surg. 2016;8(7):476–82.
43. Hew S, et al. Safety and effectiveness of umbilical hernia repair in patients with cirrhosis. Hernia. 2018;22(5):759–65.
44. Odom SR, et al. Emergency hernia repair in cirrhotic patients with ascites. J Trauma Acute Care Surg. 2013;75(3):404–9.
45. Eker HH, et al. A prospective study on elective umbilical hernia repair in patients with liver cirrhosis and ascites. Surgery. 2011;150(3):542–6.
46. Marsman HA, et al. Management in patients with liver cirrhosis and an umbilical hernia. Surgery. 2007;142(3):372–5.
47. Cho SW, et al. Umbilical hernia repair in patients with signs of portal hypertension: surgical outcome and predictors of mortality. Arch Surg. 2012;147(9):864–9.
48. Youssef YF, El Ghannam M. Mesh repair of non-complicated umbilical hernia in ascitic patients with liver cirrhosis. J Egypt Soc Parasitol. 2007;37(3 Suppl):1189–97.
49. Ammar SA. Management of complicated umbilical hernias in cirrhotic patients using permanent mesh: randomized clinical trial. Hernia. 2010;14(1):35–8.
50. Delis S, et al. Laparoscopic cholecystectomy in cirrhotic patients: the value of MELD score and Child–Pugh classification in predicting outcome. Surg Endosc. 2010;24(2):407–12.
51. Perini MV, Fink MA. Cholecystectomy in cirrhosis. In: Cox MR, Eslick GD, Padbury R, editors. The management of gallstone disease: a practical and evidence-based approach. Cham: Springer International Publishing; 2018. p. 279–89.
52. Pinheiro RS, et al. Laparoscopic cholecystectomy and cirrhosis: patient selection and technical considerations. Ann Laparosc Endosc Surg. 2017;2(3):35.
53. Toro A, Di Carlo I. Caution in the indication for cholecystectomy in patients with modified Child C cirrhosis. HPB. 2011;13(8):592.
54. Nguyen KT, et al. Cirrhosis is not a contraindication to laparoscopic cholecystectomy: results and practical recommendations. HPB (Oxford). 2011;13(3):192–7.
55. Puggioni A, Wong LL. A metaanalysis of laparoscopic cholecystectomy in patients with cirrhosis. J Am Coll Surg. 2003;197(6):921–6.
56. Laurence JM, et al. Laparoscopic or open cholecystectomy in cirrhosis: a systematic review of outcomes and meta-analysis of randomized trials. HPB. 2012;14(3):153–61.

57. Machado NO. Laparoscopic cholecystectomy in cirrhotics. JSLS. 2012;16(3):392–400.
58. Zhao R, et al. Hepatic pedicle occlusion with the pringle maneuver during difficult laparoscopic cholecystectomy reduces the conversion rate. World J Surg. 2019;43:207.
59. Griniatsos J. Factors predisposing to conversion from laparoscopic to open cholecystectomy. Ann Laparosc Endosc Surg. 2018;3(2):12.
60. Paolino J, Steinhagen RM. Colorectal surgery in cirrhotic patients. ScientificWorldJournal. 2014;2014:239293.
61. Masoomi H, et al. Predictive factors of in-hospital mortality in colon and rectal surgery. J Am Coll Surg. 2012;215(2):255–61.
62. Ghaferi AA, et al. Adverse outcomes in patients with chronic liver disease undergoing colorectal surgery. Ann Surg. 2010;252(2):345–50.
63. Hedrick TL, Swenson BR, Friel CM. Model for end-stage liver disease (MELD) in predicting postoperative mortality of patients undergoing colorectal surgery. Am Surg. 2013;79(4):347–52.
64. Lange EO, et al. Relationship between model for end-stage liver disease score and 30-day outcomes for patients undergoing elective colorectal resections: an American college of surgeons-national surgical quality improvement program study. Dis Colon Rectum. 2015;58(5):494–501.
65. Meunier K, et al. Colorectal surgery in cirrhotic patients: assessment of operative morbidity and mortality. Dis Colon Rectum. 2008;51(8):1225–31.
66. Montomoli J, et al. Liver disease and 30-day mortality after colorectal cancer surgery: a Danish population-based cohort study. BMC Gastroenterol. 2013;13:66.
67. Gervaz P, et al. Colorectal adenocarcinoma in cirrhotic patients. J Am Coll Surg. 2003;196(6):874–9.
68. Martínez JL, et al. Laparoscopic-assisted colectomy in patients with liver cirrhosis. Surg Endosc Other Interv Tech. 2004;18(7):1071–4.
69. Adani GL. Colorectal surgery in cirrhotic patients: the role of laparoscopy. Ann Surg. 2014;259(4):e57.
70. Hessheimer AJ, et al. Metabolic risk factors are a major comorbidity in patients with cirrhosis independent of the presence of hepatocellular carcinoma. Eur J Gastroenterol Hepatol. 2010;22(10):1239–44.
71. Thielmann M, et al. Risk prediction and outcomes in patients with liver cirrhosis undergoing open-heart surgery. Eur J Cardiothorac Surg. 2010;38(5):592–9.
72. Vanhuyse F, et al. Cardiac surgery in cirrhotic patients: results and evaluation of risk factors. Eur J Cardiothorac Surg. 2012;42(2):293–9.
73. Lin C-H, Hsu R-B. Cardiac surgery in patients with liver cirrhosis: risk factors for predicting mortality. World J Gastroenterol. 2014;20(35):12608–14.
74. Filsoufi F, et al. Early and late outcome of cardiac surgery in patients with liver cirrhosis. Liver Transpl. 2007;13(7):990–5.
75. Jacob KA, et al. Mortality after cardiac surgery in patients with liver cirrhosis classified by the Child-Pugh score. Interact Cardiovasc Thorac Surg. 2015;20(4):520–30.
76. An Y, Xiao YB, Zhong QJ. Open-heart surgery in patients with liver cirrhosis: indications, risk factors, and clinical outcomes. Eur Surg Res. 2007;39(2):67–74.
77. Morisaki A, et al. Risk factor analysis in patients with liver cirrhosis undergoing cardiovascular operations. Ann Thorac Surg. 2010;89(3):811–7.
78. Murashita T, et al. Preoperative evaluation of patients with liver cirrhosis undergoing open heart surgery. Gen Thorac Cardiovasc Surg. 2009;57(6):293–7.
79. Carr C, Desai J. OPCAB surgery in a cirrhotic hepatocellular carcinoma patient awaiting liver transplant. Ann Thorac Surg. 2004;78(4):1460–2.
80. Gopaldas RR, et al. Cirrhosis as a moderator of outcomes in coronary artery bypass grafting and off-pump coronary artery bypass operations: a 12-year population-based study. Ann Thorac Surg. 2013;96(4):1310–5.
81. Alsina AE, et al. Outcomes of abdominal surgeries in cirrhotic patients performed by liver transplant surgeons: are these safe? Am J Surg. 2018;216(3):518–23.
82. Montrief T, Koyfman A, Long B. Acute liver failure: a review for emergency physicians. Am J Emerg Med. 2019;37:329.
83. Armstrong T, et al. The impact of pre-operative serum creatinine on short-term outcomes after liver resection. HPB. 2009;11(8):622–8.
84. Truant S, et al. Factors associated with fatal liver failure after extended hepatectomy. HPB. 2017;19(8):682–7.

Robotic Liver Resection

72

Amr I. Al Abbas, Jae Pil Jung, and Melissa E. Hogg

Key Concepts
- Robotic liver resection offers certain advantages to and circumvents many of the difficulties encountered in laparoscopic surgery
- Robotic liver resection has the same indications and contraindications as laparoscopic liver resection
- Short and long-term outcomes of robotic liver resection have been non-inferior to the open and laparoscopic approaches
- The learning curve and financial constraints limit wide-spread use of the robotic platform

72.1 Introduction

Minimally invasive approaches have revolutionized the face of surgical practice. These techniques have provided for improved perioperative morbidity and mortality in a variety of surgical specialties [1–4]. Hepato-pancreato-biliary (HPB) surgery, however, is low-volume, technically challenging and morbid rendering the implementation of minimally invasive techniques difficult and this is particularly evident in liver surgery [5–7].

Liver resection is becoming more routine surgery in experienced hands. Laparoscopic techniques are increasingly used with multiple studies showing improved short-term outcomes and oncologic non-inferiority compared to the open approach [8–11]. However, there are a number of limitations to the laparoscopic approach including limited depth perception, restricted movement by rigid instruments and fixed fulcrum at the ports, unnatural ergonomics and difficult suturing [12–16]. These limitations largely persist despite advances in instruments and utilization of single port surgery.

The robotic platform has seen some success in gastrointestinal surgery and circumvents many of the short-comings of laparoscopic surgery. These features included improved three-dimensional imaging, 540-degree movement of instruments, improved dexterity and precision in vascular dissection and intracorporeal suturing [14, 17–19]. This work will cover the operative technique in detail and review some of the published short and long-term outcomes on robotic liver resection (RLR).

A. I. Al Abbas · J. P. Jung
University of Pittsburgh, Pittsburgh, PA, USA
e-mail: alabbasa@upmc.edu

M. E. Hogg (✉)
University of Pittsburgh, Pittsburgh, PA, USA

Northshore University HealthSystem, Evanston, IL, USA
e-mail: MHogg@Northshore.org

72.2 Indications

Table 72.1 shows some of the indications for RLR. The indications for robotic hepatectomy are the same as those for laparoscopic hepatectomy. Although malignancy is the most common indication for robotic liver resection, both benign and malignant tumors can be resected with the robot. Contraindications to use of the robot include invasion of major hepatic vessels, extension into the diaphragm and patient inability to tolerate pneumoperitoneum.

72.3 Operative Technique

72.3.1 Patient Positioning and Port Placement

Patient positioning is contingent upon the patient's body habitus and procedure being performed with the goal of avoiding arm collisions and offering optimal exposure. The patient is typically positioned in supine position, legs parted, in about 30-degree reverse Trendelenburg. However, for right posterior-section liver resection, the patient is positioned in 45–90° left lateral decubitus position without legs parted, in 30-degree reverse Trendelenburg. The assistant

F. Radu-Ionita et al. (eds.), *Liver Diseases*, https://doi.org/10.1007/978-3-030-24432-3_72

Table 72.1 Indications and contraindications of robotic liver resection

Indications	Contraindications
Malignant disease	*General*
Primary hepatocellular carcinoma (HCC)	Any contraindication to open liver resection
Hepatoblastoma	Pneumoperitoneum intolerance
Cholangiocarcinoma	Major vessel invasion or need for vascular reconstruction
Gallbladder carcinoma	*Specific*
Recurrent hepatocellular carcinoma	Dense adhesions
Colorectal liver metastasis	Significant lesion proximity to major vasculature
Other hepatic metastasis[a]	Lesion size prohibits laparoscopic manipulation
Benign disease	
Adenoma	
Benign biliary disease	
Hemangioma/hamartoma	
Recurrent cholangitis	

[a]Metastasis from breast, neuroendocrine carcinoma, pheochromocytoma, endometrial carcinoma, melanoma, clear cell renal metastasis, ovarian carcinoma, and small bowel cancer

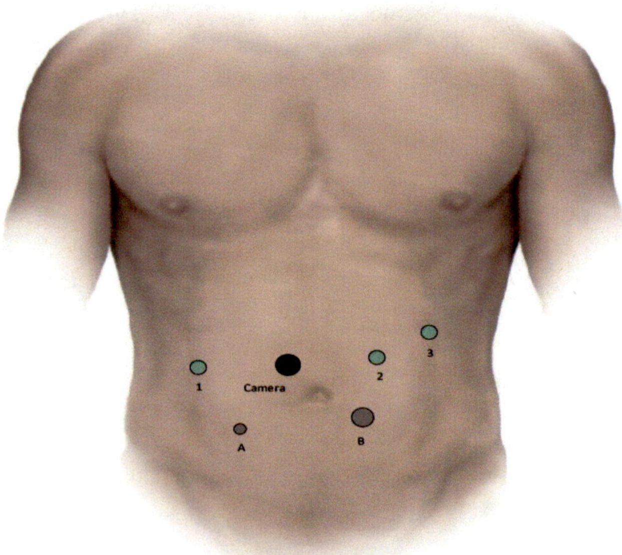

Fig. 72.1 Port-placement for right anterior hepatectomy

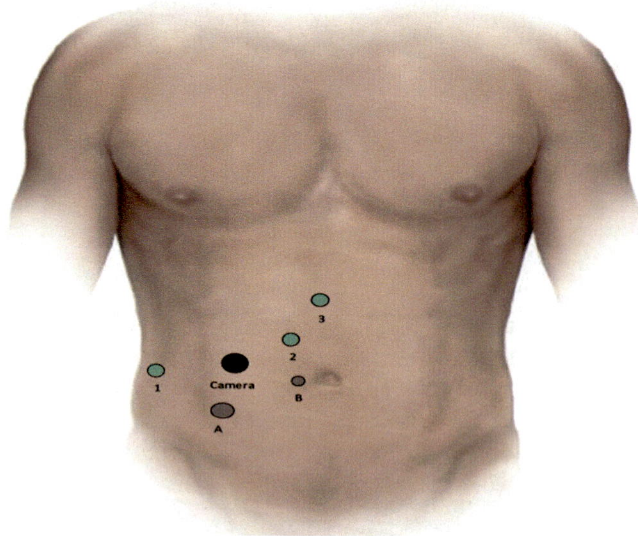

Fig. 72.2 Port-placement for right posterior hepatectomy

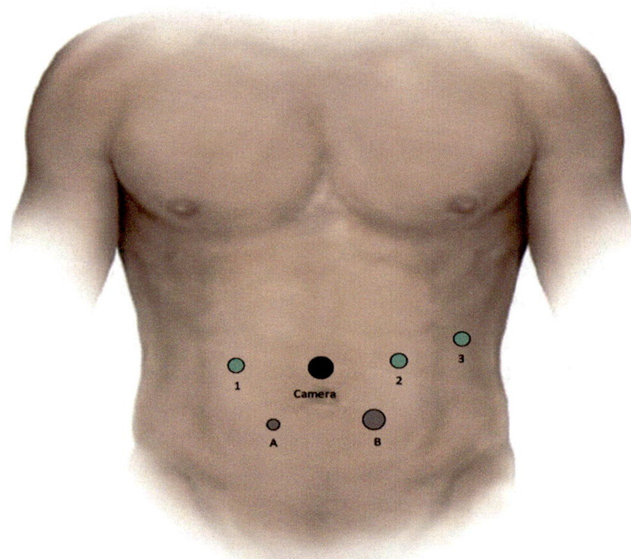

Fig. 72.3 Port-placement for left hepatectomy

surgeon then stands to the left of the patient and pneumoperitoneum is achieved with a 5 mm trocar in the left upper quadrant; however, entry technique will vary by surgeon. Port-placement may vary depending on the location of the lesion. Trocar port-placements for different hepatectomies are shown in Figs. 72.1, 72.2, and 72.3. Trocars are generally placed closer to the transverse umbilical line, shifting towards the left or right depending on lesion location. Laparoscopy is typically performed to exclude the presence of metastasis prior to the procedure and the robot is brought in from the patient's head and the arms are docked. If an Intuitive Surgical (Sunnyvale, CA) Si Robot is used. However, if an Xi is used, docking can occur anywhere, but is usually on the side of the lesion.

72.3.2 Lobectomy (Right and Left Hepatectomy)

Three steps are clearly defined: dissection of the hepatic hilum, ligament and connective tissue dissection around the hepatic plane, and hepatic transection. Surgeons preferences will vary for using the Pringle Maneuver. However, having

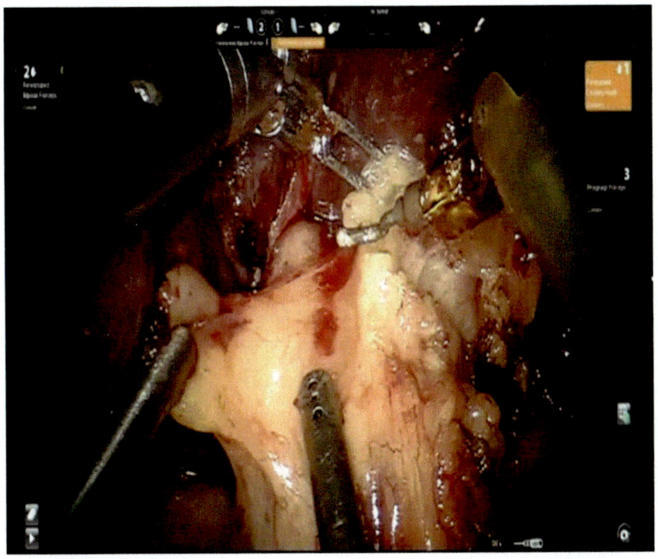

Fig. 72.4 Hepatoduodenal Ligament Isolation

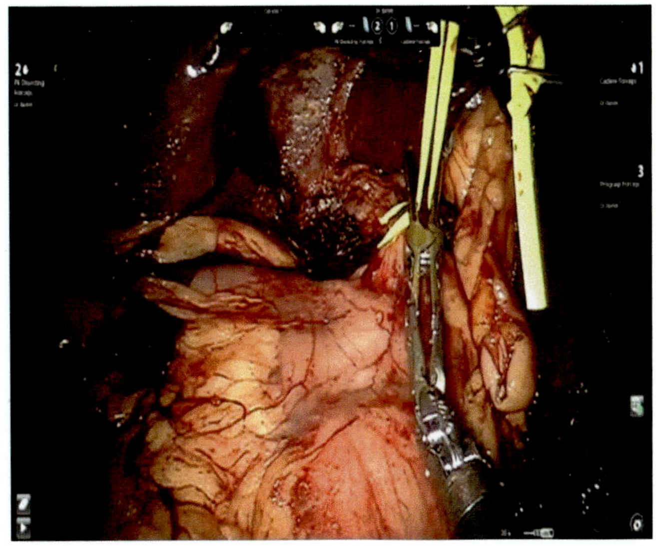

Fig. 72.6 Preparation of bulldog clamp

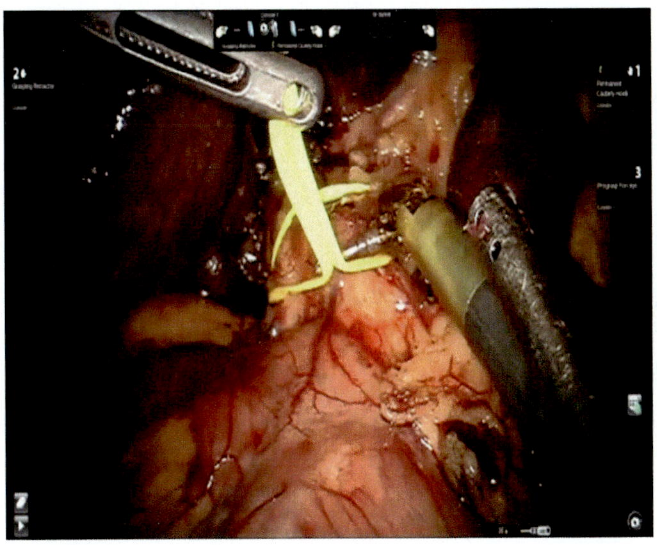

Fig. 72.5 Vessel loop placement around hepatoduodenal ligament

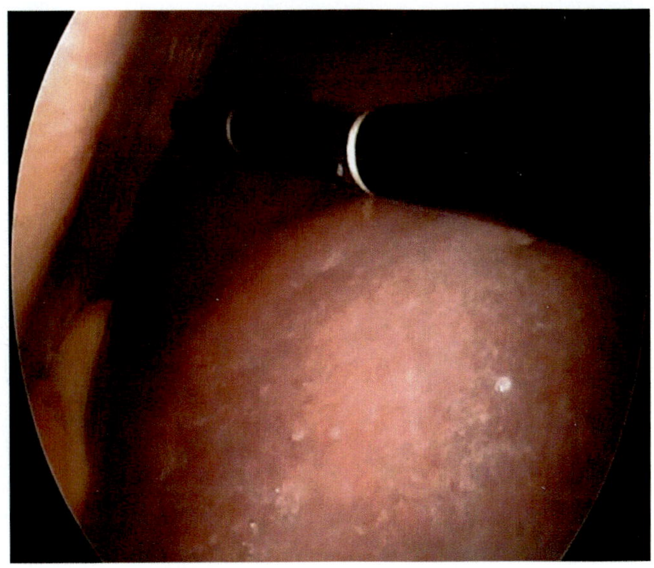

Fig. 72.7 Use of endoscopic ultrasound to identify the lesion

the porta identified and being set up to employ a Pringle at a moment's notice can be a safety step since you can't quickly pinch off the entire porta like in open surgery. The following intra-operative pictures will be used to convey the steps.

I. Pringle Maneuver Set-up
   1. Isolate the hepatoduodenal ligament (Fig. 72.4).
   2. Prepare vessel loop around the hepatoduodenal ligament (Fig. 72.5).
   3. Prepare general-use bulldog clamp (Fig. 72.6).

II. Dissection of the Hepatic Hilum
   1. Identify the location of the liver lesion using laparoscopic ultrasound (Fig. 72.7).
   2. Perform a standard retrograde cholecystectomy (Fig. 72.8).
   3. Dissect the hepatic pedicle with an Intuitive Surgical permanent cautery hook (Sunnyvale, CA).
   4. Portal vein (PV) and hepatic artery dissection.
      a. The right hepatic artery is usually located superior to the PV whereas the left hepatic artery is usually located anterior lateral to the PV.
      b. Isolate and ligate these branches with an Intuitive Weck hem-o-lock large clip applier (Intuitive Surgical, Sunnyvale, CA) (Fig. 72.9).
      c. Alternatively, suture and tie using 3-0 black silk and 5-0 prolene or ligate using laparoscopic clips (Fig. 72.10).

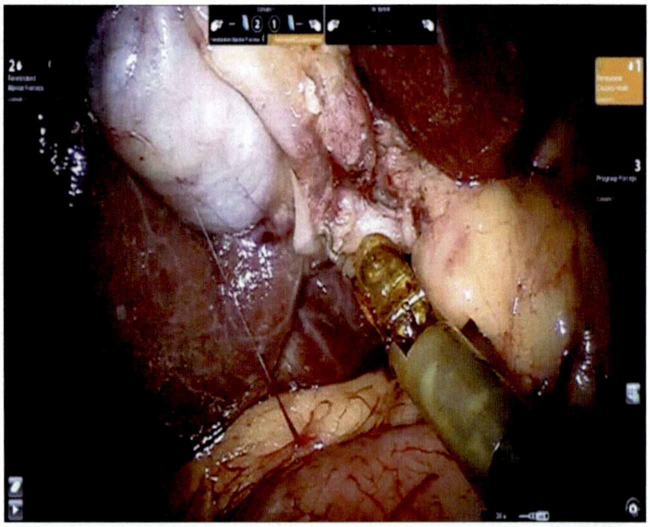

Fig. 72.8 Retrograde cholecystectomy

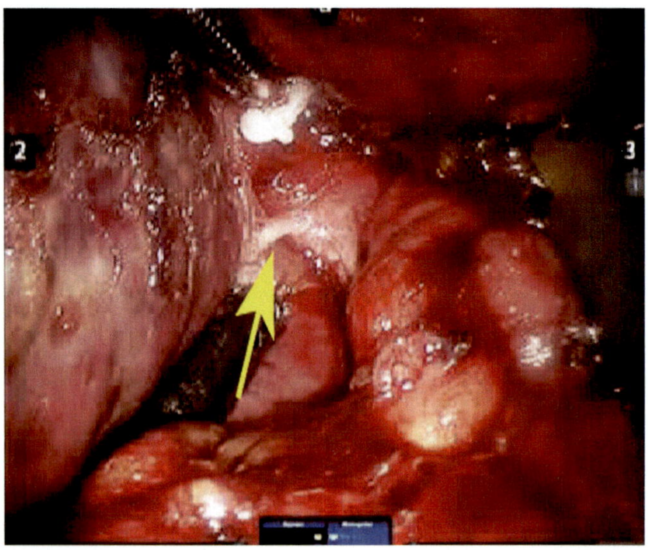

Fig. 72.9 Use of hem-o-lock to isolate and ligate portal vein or hepatic artery branches

   d. Attention should be paid to the small posterior branches of the portal vein to segment I.
   e. Ligate these branches with laparoscopic clips or suture them using 5-0 prolene
   f. Alternatively, the Ligasure (Medtronic, Minneapolis, MN) can be used.
   g. After ligation of these small branches, proceed to isolate the right or left portal vein. It can be sutured using 3-0 black silk or 5-0 prolene. It may also be ligated using a Covidien laparoscopic stapler (Medtronic, Minneapolis, MN) or an Intuitive weck hem-o-lock large clip applier (Figs. 72.11 and 72.12).
5. An optional step when the anatomy is clear and the portal confluence is low, is extrahepatic bile duct dissection.

III. Hepatic Transection

1. Hepatic ligament and connective tissue isolation before resection:
   a. Isolate and section the coronary and falciform ligaments (Fig. 72.13).
   b. The right triangular ligament is dissected along the lateral peritoneal reflection and the along the hepatocaval plane in the case of right lobe resection (Fig. 72.14).
   c. Transect the left triangular ligament in the case of left lobe resections (Fig. 72.15).
   d. In the case of right hepatectomy:
      i. Use the third arm to lift the inferior surface of the right lobe, exposing the inferior vena cava (IVC).
      ii. Ligate minor accessory veins from the IVC with laparoscopic clips or suture using 5-0 Prolene or ligate using the Ligasure.
      iii. If they are large, resection and ligation is performed using the laparoscopic stapler.
      iv. Dissect along the right side of the IVC up to the inferior aspect of the right hepatic vein for right lobar resections.

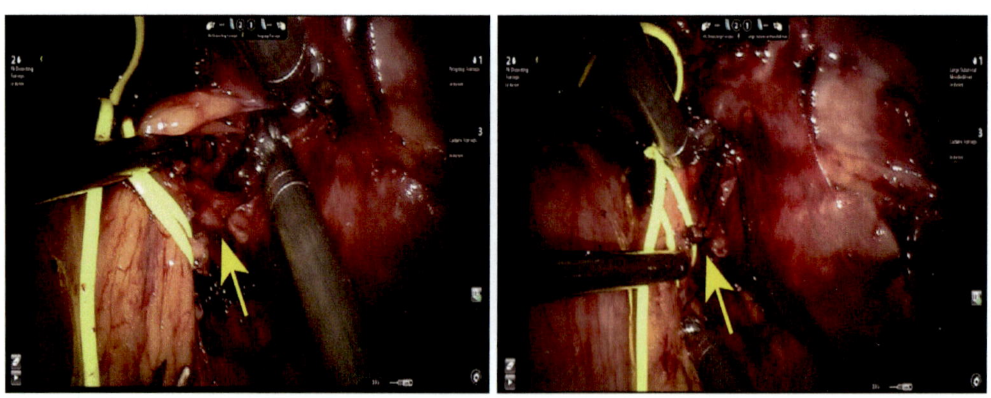

Fig. 72.10 Ligating portal vein and hepatic artery branches using suture

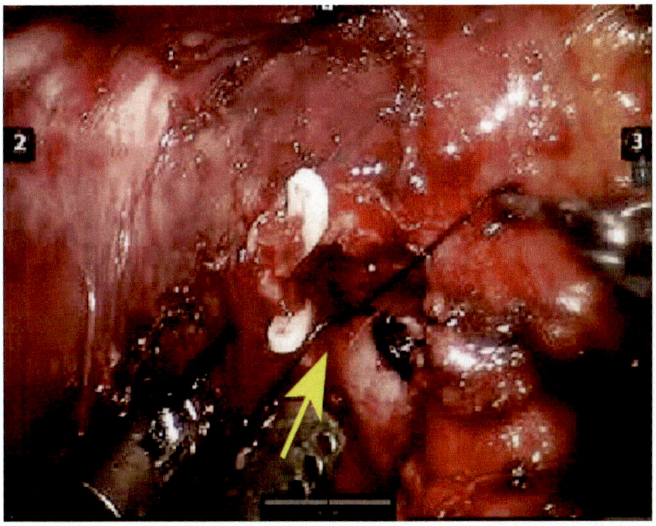

Fig. 72.11 Portal vein isolation and ligation using suture

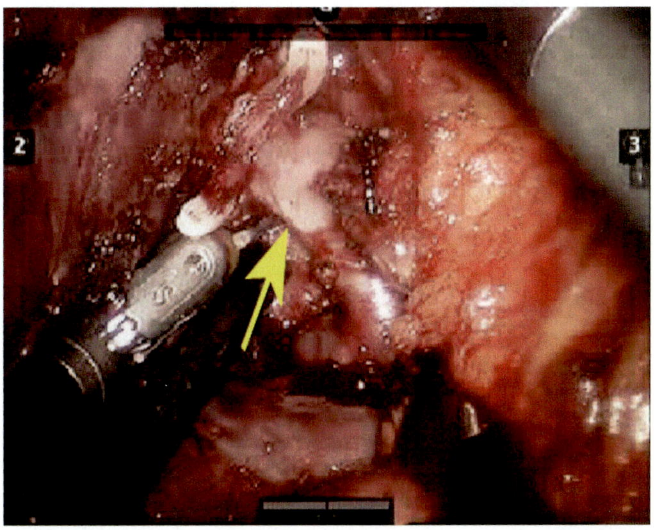

Fig. 72.12 Portal vein isolation and ligation using the weck hem-o-lock large clip applier

2. Liver Transection:
   a. Burn the liver surface to mark along the ischemic demarcation line using an Intuitive permanent cautery hook (Fig. 72.16).
   b. Apply stay sutures using 0-O Vicryl or chromic along the liver border to retract the left or right hepatic lobes and expose the resection line (Fig. 72.17).
   c. Perform the Pringle maneuver by lifting the vessel loops up and clamping them using the bulldog clamp as mentioned above (Fig. 72.6).
   d. Communicate with anesthesia before the case to keep the central venous pressure (CVP) lower than 5 mmHg.

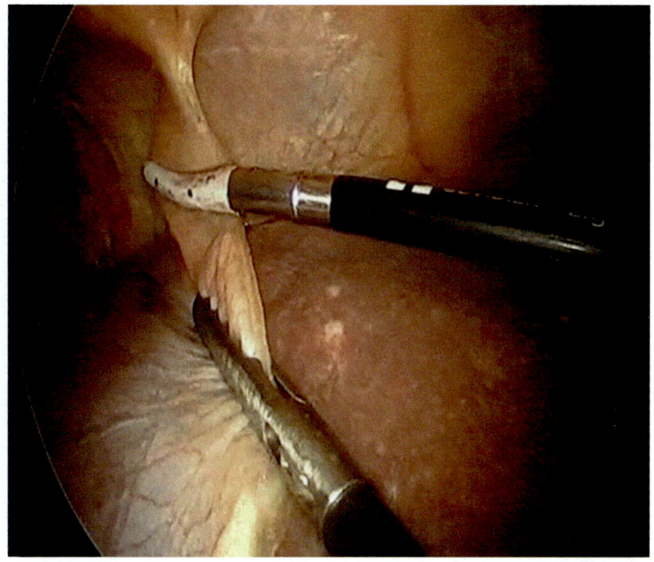

Fig. 72.13 Coronary and falciform ligament isolation and resection

   e. Transection of the liver layer by layer:
      i. Start at the cortical aspect along the burned markings.
      ii. This illustration uses the Intuitive PK dissecting forceps (Intuitive Surgical, Sunnyvale, CA) and Maryland bipolar forceps (Intuitive Surgical, Sunnyvale, CA) for liver resection and control minor bleeding (Fig. 72.18).
      iii. Alternatively, an Intuitive Harmonic ACE or Endowrist Vessel Sealer (Intuitive Surgical, Sunnyvale, CA) can be used in addition to laparoscopic instruments like the Aquamantys bipolar sealers (Medtronic, Minneapolis, MN), the Argon beam coagulator (Medtronic, Minneapolis, MN), and Habib 4X laparoscopic bipolar resection device (AngioDynamics, Queensbury, NY).
      iv. Larger vessels should be resected with a Covidien laparoscopic stapler or ligated/sutured using 3-0 black silk and 5-0 prolene suture (Fig. 72.19).
3. Once done with the subcortical aspect, proceed to resection of the core of the liver parenchyma.
   a. Care must be taken with the bigger venous branches directed to the middle hepatic vein and the Glisson pedicle containing bile ducts.
   b. One option is to use Covidien laparoscopic staplers for transection and ligation of venous branches and the Glisson pedicle during parenchymal liver resection (Fig. 72.20).
   c. Isolate the right or left hepatic vein and ligate it with a Covidien laparoscopic stapler (Fig. 72.21).

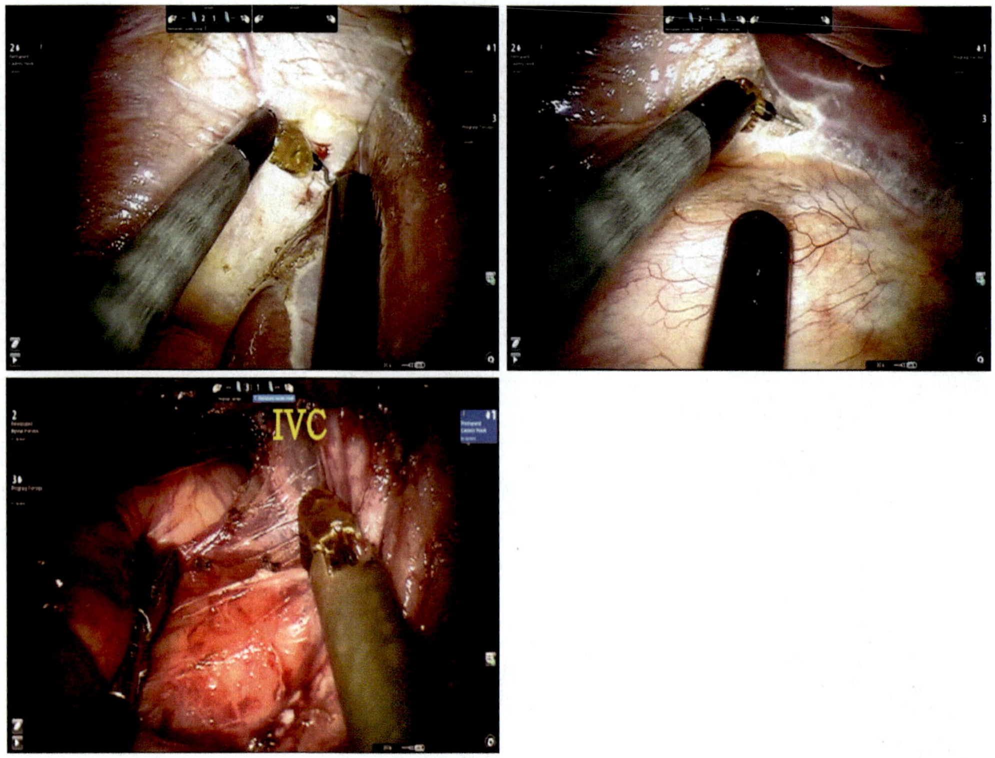

Fig. 72.14 Right triangular ligament dissection

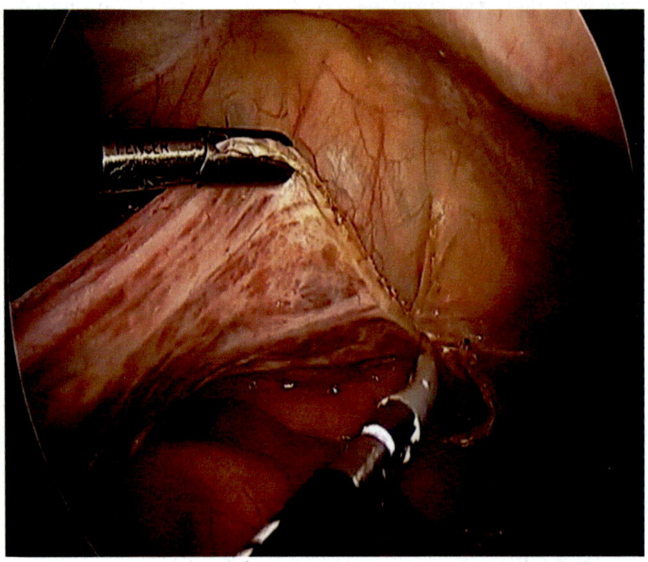

Fig. 72.15 Left triangular ligament transection

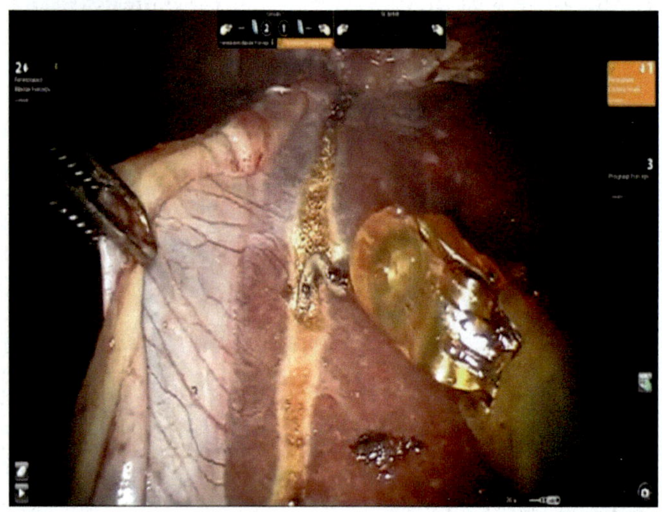

Fig. 72.16 Use of cautery hook to mark along ischemic demarcation line

4. Examine the liver parenchyma for bleeding or bile leak
   a. Bleeding is controlled using the Intuitive permanent cautery hook and surgicel (Johnson and Johnson, New Brunswick, NJ) or using 5-0 prolene sutures (Fig. 72.22).
   b. Suture using 3-0 black silk (Fig. 72.23).
   c. After bleeding control, place dry gauze on the liver surface and de-clamp the bulldog (Fig. 72.24).
   d. Decrease intra-abdominal pressure up to less than 5 mmHg for 5–15 min and recheck for bleeding or bile leak.
   e. Drain placement is at the discretion of the surgeon.
5. Remove the specimen in the endocatch bag and extract it through the lower 12 mm Trocar site after extension of the incision line.
6. After the specimen is removed:

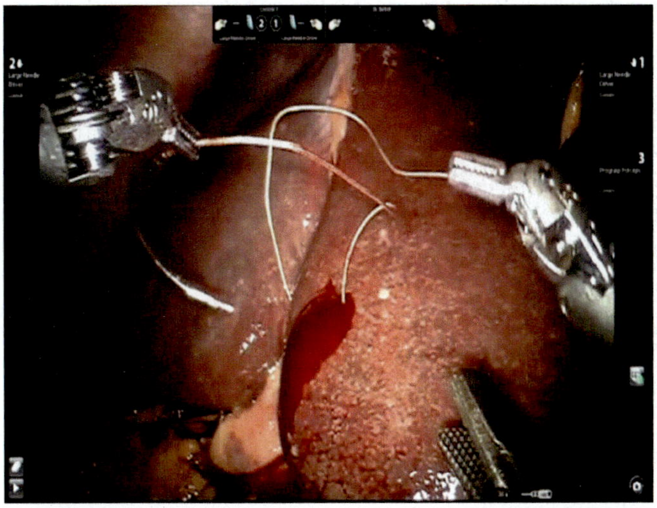

Fig. 72.17 Applying sutures for traction along liver

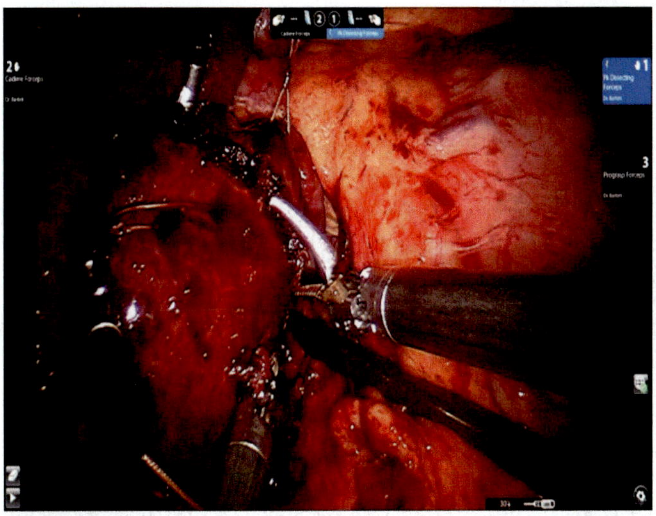

Fig. 72.18 Liver resection and bleeding control using the PK dissecting forceps and Maryland bipolar forceps

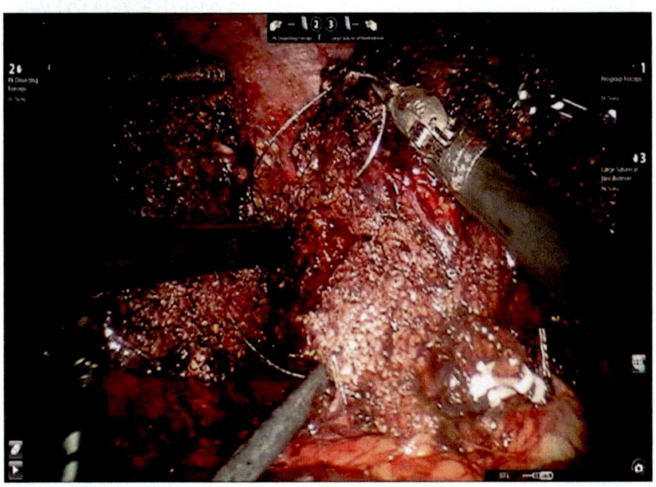

Fig. 72.19 Ligation of larger vessels using suture during liver resection

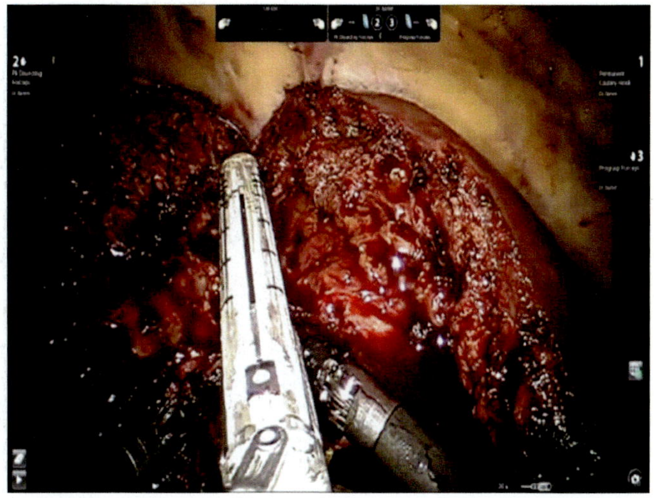

Fig. 72.20 Ligation of venous branches and the Glisson pedicle during parenchymal liver resection

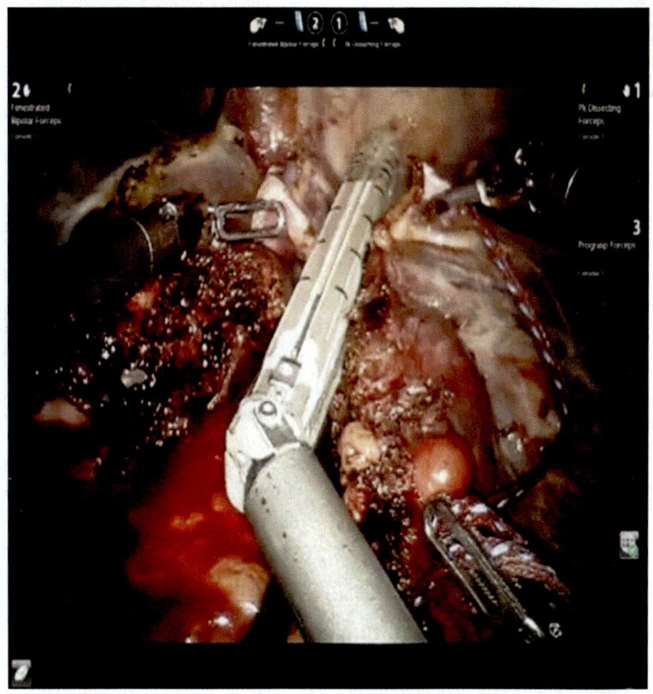

Fig. 72.21 Isolation and ligation of the hepatic vein

a. Undock the robot.
b. Stop pneumoperitoneum.
c. Extract trocars under direct vision.
d. Close port sites.

72.3.3 Segmentectomy (Follow Segmental Anatomy)

I. The ultrasound is used to find the location of the liver lesion.

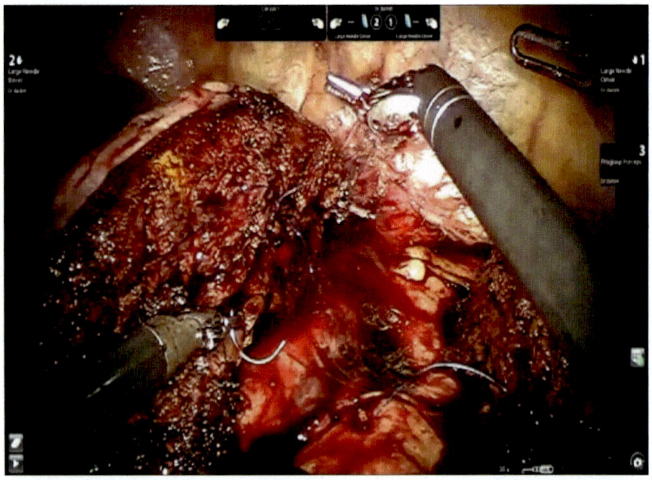

Fig. 72.22 Bleeding controlled using suture

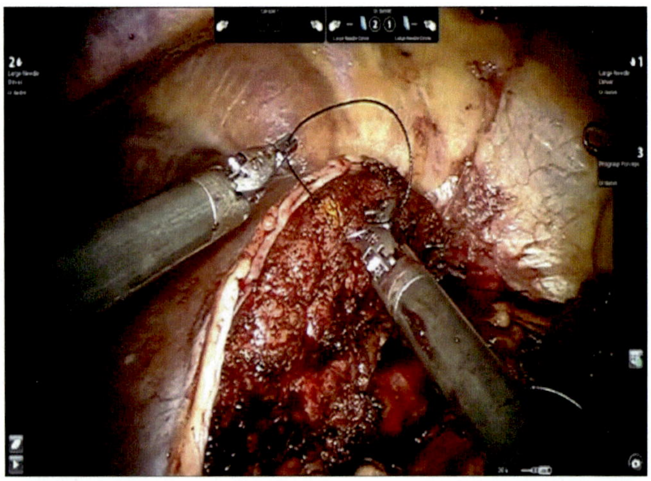

Fig. 72.23 Suturing liver parenchyma

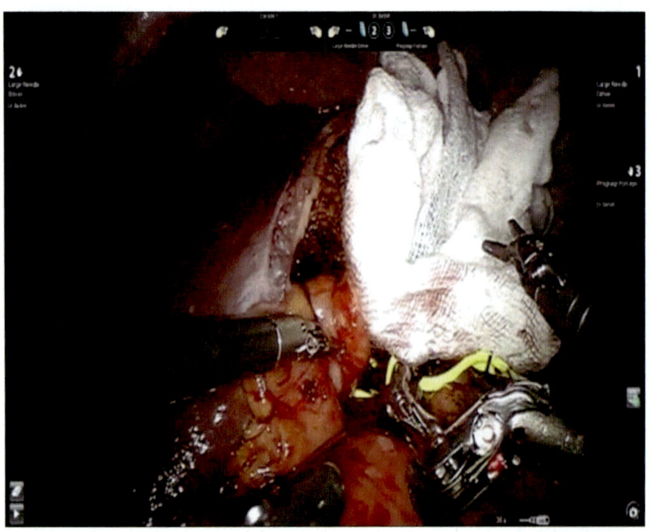

Fig. 72.24 Placing dry gauze on liver surface and de-clamping the bulldog

II. Burn around the liver lesion using the Intuitive permanent cautery hook.
III. Place anchoring 0-Vicryl along the virtual line of the liver segment based on the lesion's location and retract gently.
IV. Perform the Pringle maneuver according to preference as stated previously in the section on lobectomy to achieve hepatic inflow control.
V. Transect layer by layer starting from the surface and proceeding to the core.
VI. Use Intuitive PK dissecting forceps and maryland bipolar forceps for liver transection.
VII. Control minor bleeding with the Intuitive permanent cautery hook, maryland bipolar forceps or the Ligasure.
VIII. Inspect the liver remnant as before and proceed with specimen retrieval and port-closure as stated previously.

72.3.4 Wedge Resection

I. Follows a similar technique to segmentectomy but does not respect segmental anatomy.
II. Typically used for metastatic liver lesions originating from another tumor (e.g. colorectal cancer, pancreatic cancer neuroendocrine tumors, etc).
III. Most resection is performed apart from the liver lesion around 1–2 cm.
   a. An early study showed higher rates of positive margin with wedge resection compared to segmental resection [20]. More recent studies have challenged this and suggest that there is no difference [21–23].
IV. The robotic Aloka drop-in probe (Hitachi, Tokyo, Japan) can be used to determine the location of the liver lesion (Fig. 72.25).
V. Use the Intuitive permanent cautery hook to burn around the liver lesion with a radius of about 2 cm (Fig. 72.26).
VI. Anchoring sutures using 0-O vicryl are placed around the liver lesion and the lesion is retracted gently to avoid rupture (Fig. 72.27).
VII. The Pringle maneuver is applied to achieve hepatic inflow control using the same technique as in lobectomy.
VIII. Intuitive PK dissecting forceps and maryland bipolar forceps are used for liver lesion removal.
IX. Hemostasis is achieved with the Intuitive permanent cautery hook, the maryland bipolar forceps or the Ligasure.
X. Alternative techniques to the PK described above can also be used according to surgeon preference.

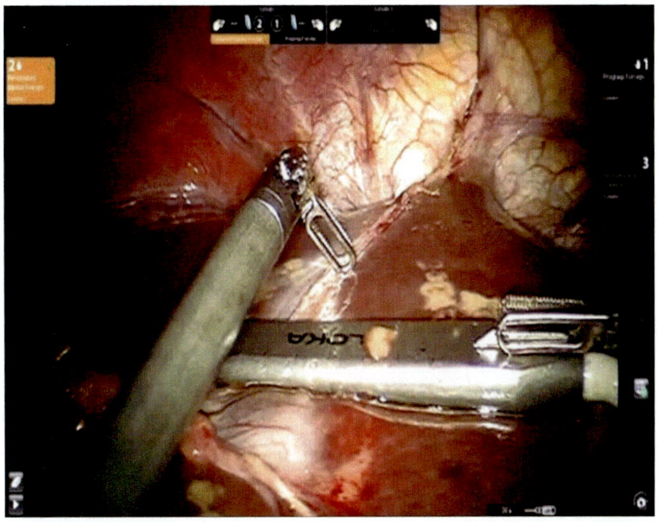

Fig. 72.25 Use of Aloka drop-in probe to locate lesion during wedge resection

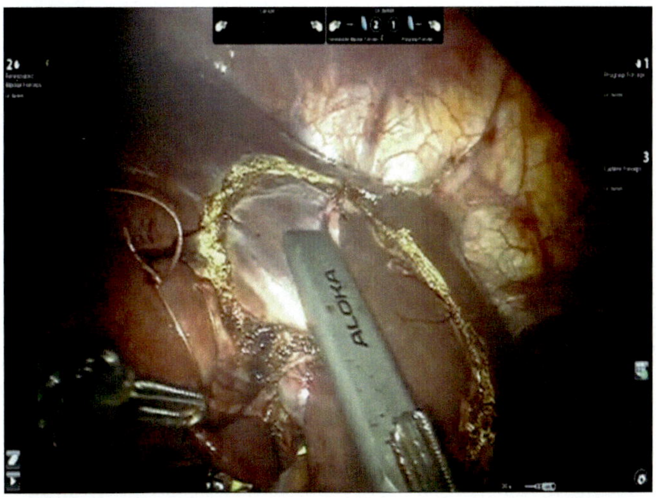

Fig. 72.26 Use of permanent cautery hook to mark around lesion

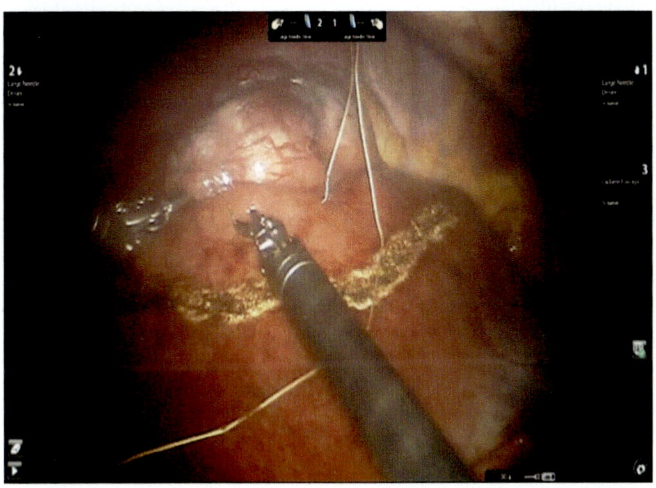

Fig. 72.27 Anchoring suture placement around liver lesion

XI. After examining for liver parenchymal bleeding or bile leak, the wound is closed as stated previously.

72.3.5 Near-Infrared Fluorescence Imaging

One of the unique advantages afforded by the robotic platform includes near-infrared fluorescence imaging. Firefly fluorescence imaging (Intuitive Surgical, Sunnyvale, CA) provides real-time, image-guided identification of key anatomical landmarks using near-infrared technology. This allows for assessing anatomy better than the naked eye. This involves the use of Indocyanine green (ICG) which is a non-toxic fluorophore that appears green upon stimulation with near-infrared light. This has been approved by the Food and Drug Administration (FDA) and been in use for over four decades. Upon injection, arteries and veins are visualized for just under a minute and then it accumulates in the liver. It is secreted in bile about an hour later, allowing for visualization of the biliary tree. This technique allows for differentiating hepatic lesions based on their vascular pattern. Well differentiated HCCs are hyperfluorescent while poorly differentiated HCCs and colorectal metastasis are hypofluorescent [24, 25]. The utility of this technology is endless with future avenues for antibody-conjugated fluorophores for fluorescence guided surgery, real-time microscopy for resection margin evaluation and differentiating between normal versus malignant lymph nodes.

72.4 Outcomes of Robotic Liver Resection

72.4.1 Post-operative Outcomes

Table 72.2 lists some selected major studies on RLR. The most recent systematic review and meta-analysis [26] revealed that most RLRs were wedge or segmental resections (28.67%), followed by right hepatectomy (17.88%) and left lateral segmentectomy (13.22%). Operative time ranged from 200 to 275 min. As expected, series with major hepatectomies tended to have longer operative times. The total rate of conversion was 5.59%, varying from 0% to 55%. The most common indication for conversion was bleeding (46.67%) followed by tumor margin (33.33%). Intraoperative blood loss ranged from 50 to 1800 mL with one series reporting that cirrhotic patients had a median estimated blood loss (EBL) of 400 mL more than non-cirrhotics. The hospital length of stay varied from 4 to 15 days. Interestingly, a study by Tsung et al. had shown that operative time, blood loss and hospital length of stay significantly decreased when comparing surgeries performed early on in the group's experience to surgeries performed later [16]. This highlights the role of a learning curve for robotic liver surgery that ought to be considered when comparing approaches. A recent ACS NSQIP analysis by Zureikat et al. on predictors of conversion for robotic hepatectomy revealed no significant differences between the robotic and laparoscopic approaches to hepatectomy in terms of pure MIS completion rates [27]. Finally, in a relatively large multicenter study on 61 patients undergoing RLR for malignancy, median hospital stay was 5 days and Grade III–IV complications occurred in seven patients with no perioperative mortality recorded [28].

72.4.2 Long-Term Oncologic Outcomes

Studies on long-term oncologic outcomes of RLR are limited. According to the most recent meta-analysis, most of these studies do not differentiate between the different pathologies and reports on oncologic margins showed that they ranged from 8 to 18.7 mm [26]. Recurrence rate in patients with hepatocellular carcinoma (HCC) was 13.5% at 14 month follow-up [26]. A report by Beber et al. showed that there were no significant differences in survival between robotic and laparoscopic liver resection on 14 month follow-up [29]. Wang et al. reported the long-term outcomes of HCC in patients undergoing robotic and open hepatectomy [30]. There were no significant differences between the two groups: similar margin negative resection rates, and similar rates of overall survival and disease free-survival at 1, 2 and 3 years. This was reproduced in another recent study [31]. A recent multicenter study by Khan et al. included 61 patients, 56% who had RLR for HCC, 26% for Cholangiocarcinoma and 18% for gallbladder carcinoma [28]. Most of the resections were non-anatomical (39.3%). At a median follow-up of 75 months, 5-year OS and DFS were 56% and 38%, respectively.

Table 72.2 Selection of recent major studies on robotic liver resection

Study	Year	Center	Sample size (n)	Malignancy (%)
Khan et al. [28]	2018	Multiple	61	61 (100)
Wang et al. [30]	2018	Kaohsiung, Taiwan	63	63 (100)
Chen et al. [31]	2017	Taipei, Taiwan	81	81 (100)
Kingham et al. [32]	2016	New York, NY	64	57 (88)
Sham et al. [40]	2016	Seattle, WA	71	60 (85)
Tsung et al. [16]	2014	Pittsburgh, PA	57	40 (70)

72.4.3 Comparative Outcomes: Robotic vs. Open

Chen et al. showed comparable percentages of major liver resection and cirrhotic patients between the two procedures [31]. However, patients undergoing RLR had a longer operative time, but shorter hospital stay and lower patient controlled anesthesia (PCA) dosages. Multiple studies have shown similar findings [30, 32, 33]. A list of selected comparative case series on RLR and OLR are shown in Table 72.3.

72.4.4 Comparative Outcomes: Robotic vs. Laparoscopic

Differences between the robotic and laparoscopic approaches are less starkly delineated. Yu et al. showed no significant differences in operative time, intra-operative blood loss, post-operative liver function tests, complication rates and hospital stay [34]. Multiple other studies have shown similar findings [16, 26, 35, 36]. However, while Tsung et al. did show longer operative times in the robotic approach, the robotic approach appeared to allow greater rates of completion of major hepatectomy without utilizing hybrid approaches [16]. A systematic review and metanalysis comparing the two approaches showed significant reduction in blood loss and operative times in the robotic approach, but no differences in conversion rates, hospital length of stay (LOS) and morbidity [26]. Details on some large comparative studies are shown in Table 72.4.

Table 72.3 Comparative case series of robotic vs. open liver resection

		Sample size		OR time		Hospital stay		EBL		pRBC transfusion	
Study	Year	RLR	OLR	RLR	OLR	RLR	OLR	RLR	OLR	RLR	OLR
Wang et al. [30]	2018	63	177	296	182	6.21	8.18	NA	NA	NA	NA
Chen et al. [31]	2017	81	81	402	285	8.9	12.3	182	322	0	3
Kingham et al. [32]	2016	64	64	163	210	4	7	100	300	1	9
Sham et al. [40]	2016	71	88	284	269	3.9	7	495	1132	NA	NA
Morel et al. [33]	2015	16	16	352	235	10	16.6	NA	NA	NA	NA

RLR robotic liver resection, *OLR* open liver resection, *OR* operating room, *EBL* estimated blood loss, *pRBC* packed red blood cells, *NA* not applicable

Table 72.4 Comparative case series of robotic vs. laparoscopic liver resection

		Sample size		OR time		Hospital stay		EBL		pRBC transfusion	
Study	Year	RLR	LLR	RLR	LLR	RLR	LLR	RLR	LLR	RLR	LLR
Montalti et al. [36]	2016	36	72	306	295	6	4.9	415	437	NA	NA
Tranchart et al. [35]	2014	28	28	210	176	6	5.5	125	200	2.5	5
Yu et al. [34]	2014	13	17	240.9	291.5	8.9	12.3	342.6	388.5	0	0
Tsung et al. [16]	2014	57	114	253	198.5	4	4	200	100	NA	NA
Packiam et al. [15]	2012	11	18	175	188	4	3	30	30	NA	NA

RLR robotic liver resection, *LLR* laparoscopic liver resection, *OR* operating room, *EBL* estimated blood loss, *pRBC* packed red blood cells, *NA* not applicable

72.4.5 Learning-Curve

The learning curve of RLR is not particularly well investigated. One study by Chen et al. included a series of 183 RLR performed at a single center from 2012 to 2015 [37]. Using the cumulative sum model, they showed that the procedural learning curve was characterized by three main phases: initial (15 patients), intermediate (25 patients), and mature (52 patients). The initial phase was characterized by shorter operation time and hospital stay, whereas the second phase was characterized by less blood loss. In an earlier study by Tsung et al., surgeries performed earlier in the group's experience were compared to those performed later and there was a significant difference in terms of the operative time, blood loss and hospital length of stay: with those performed earlier having longer operative time, more blood loss and longer hospital stay [16]. A recent study included both RLR (40) and LLR (91) to evaluate the learning curve in both approaches. Groups were divided into early and late and the primary end-point was to determine the number of procedures before the difficulty index increased significantly. The difficulty index of RLR was found to be significantly higher when comparing the late group to the early group 7.3 (4.3–10.2) vs. 5.0 (3.0–7.7) ($p < 0.001$). However, the difficulty index did not increase significantly for LLR when comparing the late and early periods [38]. There were no significant differences in post-operative outcomes between RLR and LLR as well as between the subgroups of early and late experience for both types of resection despite the increase in difficulty index. The authors concluded that it was necessary to perform 8–10 robotic procedures of low and intermediate level of difficulty before proceeding to high difficulty resections. A non-exhaustive list of major studies on the learning curve is provided in Table 72.5.

Table 72.5 Selected studies on the learning curve of robotic liver resection

Study	Year	Center	Sample size (n)
Chen et al. [31]	2017	Taipei, Taiwan	183
Efanov et al. [38]	2017	Moscow, Russia	40
Tsung et al. [16]	2014	Pittsburgh, PA	57

72.4.6 Financial Impact

The financial impact of the robotic approach is poorly studied despite the fact that financial constraints are one of the main hindrances for institutions to overcome. One of the first studies to include cost comparing 13 RLRs to matched OLRs and LLRs showed that cost was higher in the RLR group compared to the OLR and the LLR groups ($12,046 versus $10,548 and $7618, respectively) [39]. An early study from the University of Pittsburgh comparing outcomes between robotic and laparoscopic left lateral sectionectomy showed that cost was not significantly different between two approaches when considering direct costs ($5130 versus $4408, $p = 0.401$) [15]. Robotic costs were significantly higher, however, when factoring in indirect costs which were estimated to be 1423$ per-case (total $6553 versus $4408, $p = 0.021$). Another study comparing cost between RLR and LLR revealed that direct costs associated with post-operative care were actually lower in the RLR group ($8570 versus $13,425, $p < 0.001$) [40]. Overall average adjusted direct costs were shown to be $4244 lower in RLR ($14,754 versus $18,998, $p = 0.001$). Daskalaki et al. compared costs between the robotic and open approaches and showed that anesthesiology, operating and recovery room and readmission costs were higher for the robotic group [41]. On the other hand, intensive care unit (ICU) admission, inpatient nursing and pharmacy costs were higher for the open group. Average total costs, including readmissions were $37,518 for the robotic group and $41,948 for the open group. A more recent study has compared costs between the robotic and laparoscopic approaches and showed that total medical costs were significantly higher in the robotic group compared to the laparoscopic group ($11,475 for the robot vs. $6762 for the laparoscopic group, $p = 0.001$) [34]. Further details on cost are shown in Table 72.6.

Table 72.6 Selected comparative case series with cost of robotic liver resection

			Sample size			Average total cost (USD)		
Study	Year	Center	RLR	OLR	LLR	RLR	OLR	LLR
Daskalaki et al. [41]	2017	Chicago, Illinois	68	44	NA	37,518	41,948	NA
Sham et al. [40]	2016	Seattle, WA	71	88	NA	14,754	18,998	NA
Yu et al. [34]	2014	Seoul, South Korea	13	NA	17	11,475	NA	6762
Packiam et al. [15]	2012	Pittsburgh, PA	11	NA	18	6553	NA	4403
Wen-bin et al. [39]	2011	Beijing, China	13	13	13	12,046	10,548	7618

RLR robotic liver resection, *OLR* open liver resection, *LLR* laparoscopic liver resection, *NA* not applicable

72.5 Conclusion

RLR is a safe and feasible approach. While more high-powered studies are necessary to delineate the benefits and risks compared to other approaches, most current studies show promise. Financial constraints may limit wide-spread use of this approach, however further centralization of HPB surgery within referral centers may make this issue moot. An important avenue for future research would be work focused on characterizing the learning curve of RLR in order to ensure safer and more efficient implementation at a system wide-scale.

Self Study

Questions

1. Which of the following statements is true?
   (a) Well differentiated HCCs are hypofluorescent on Firefly fluorescence imaging.
   (b) Segmental resections pose a lower risk of margin positive resections when compared to wedge resection.
   (c) The robotic approach affords greater degree of movement, improved dexterity and precision in vascular dissection and intracorporeal suturing.
   (d) The robotic approach is less useful for more complex hepatic resections when compared to laparoscopy.
2. Which of the following statements is true?
   (a) The robotic approach may contribute to longer operative times, but affords shorter length of stay and less use of patient-controlled anesthesia when compared to the open approach.
   (b) The right hepatic artery is usually located anterolateral to the PV whereas the left hepatic artery is usually located superior to the PV.
   (c) The robotic approach has a higher likelihood of conversion when compared to the laparoscopic approach in liver resection
   (d) Long-term oncologic outcomes with the robotic approach are inferior to those of the laparoscopic approach.

Answers

1. Which of the following statements is true?
   C
2. Which of the following statements is true?
   A

References

1. Aquina CT, Probst CP, Becerra AZ, Iannuzzi JC, Hensley BJ, Noyes K, et al. Missed opportunity: laparoscopic colorectal resection is associated with lower incidence of small bowel obstruction compared to an open approach. Ann Surg. 2016;264(1):127–34.
2. Gietelink L, Wouters MW, Bemelman WA, Dekker JW, Tollenaar RA, Tanis PJ, et al. Reduced 30-day mortality after laparoscopic colorectal cancer surgery: a population based study from the Dutch surgical colorectal audit (DSCA). Ann Surg. 2016;264(1):135–40.
3. McCormack K, Scott NW, Go PM, Ross S, Grant AM, Collaboration EUHT. Laparoscopic techniques versus open techniques for inguinal hernia repair. Cochrane Database Syst Rev. 2003;(1):CD001785.
4. Shaligram A, Unnirevi J, Simorov A, Kothari VM, Oleynikov D. How does the robot affect outcomes? A retrospective review of open, laparoscopic, and robotic Heller myotomy for achalasia. Surg Endosc. 2012;26(4):1047–50.
5. Han HS, Cho JY, Yoon YS, Hwang DW, Kim YK, Shin HK, et al. Total laparoscopic living donor right hepatectomy. Surg Endosc. 2015;29(1):184.
6. Jarnagin WR, Gonen M, Fong Y, DeMatteo RP, Ben-Porat L, Little S, et al. Improvement in perioperative outcome after hepatic resection: analysis of 1,803 consecutive cases over the past decade. Ann Surg. 2002;236(4):397–406; discussion –7.
7. Kim H, Suh KS, Lee KW, Yi NJ, Hong G, Suh SW, et al. Long-term outcome of laparoscopic versus open liver resection for hepatocellular carcinoma: a case-controlled study with propensity score matching. Surg Endosc. 2014;28(3):950–60.
8. Han HS, Shehta A, Ahn S, Yoon YS, Cho JY, Choi Y. Laparoscopic versus open liver resection for hepatocellular carcinoma: case-matched study with propensity score matching. J Hepatol. 2015;63(3):643–50.
9. Nguyen KT, Geller DA. Outcomes of laparoscopic hepatic resection for colorectal cancer metastases. J Surg Oncol. 2010;102(8):975–7.
10. Tranchart H, Di Giuro G, Lainas P, Roudie J, Agostini H, Franco D, et al. Laparoscopic resection for hepatocellular carcinoma: a matched-pair comparative study. Surg Endosc. 2010;24(5):1170–6.
11. Vanounou T, Steel JL, Nguyen KT, Tsung A, Marsh JW, Geller DA, et al. Comparing the clinical and economic impact of laparoscopic versus open liver resection. Ann Surg Oncol. 2010;17(4):998–1009.

12. Ballantyne GH. The pitfalls of laparoscopic surgery: challenges for robotics and telerobotic surgery. Surg Laparosc Endosc Percutan Tech. 2002;12(1):1–5.
13. Berguer R, Rab GT, Abu-Ghaida H, Alarcon A, Chung J. A comparison of surgeons' posture during laparoscopic and open surgical procedures. Surg Endosc. 1997;11(2):139–42.
14. Milone L, Daskalaki D, Fernandes E, Damoli I, Giulianotti PC. State of the art in robotic hepatobiliary surgery. World J Surg. 2013;37(12):2747–55.
15. Packiam V, Bartlett DL, Tohme S, Reddy S, Marsh JW, Geller DA, et al. Minimally invasive liver resection: robotic versus laparoscopic left lateral sectionectomy. J Gastrointest Surg. 2012;16(12):2233–8.
16. Tsung A, Geller DA, Sukato DC, Sabbaghian S, Tohme S, Steel J, et al. Robotic versus laparoscopic hepatectomy: a matched comparison. Ann Surg. 2014;259(3):549–55.
17. Giulianotti PC, Bianco FM, Daskalaki D, Gonzalez-Ciccarelli LF, Kim J, Benedetti E. Robotic liver surgery: technical aspects and review of the literature. Hepatobiliary Surg Nutr. 2016;5(4):311–21.
18. Giulianotti PC, Coratti A, Sbrana F, Addeo P, Bianco FM, Buchs NC, et al. Robotic liver surgery: results for 70 resections. Surgery. 2011;149(1):29–39.
19. Zeh HJ III, Bartlett DL, Moser AJ. Robotic-assisted major pancreatic resection. Adv Surg. 2011;45:323–40.
20. DeMatteo RP, Palese C, Jarnagin WR, Sun RL, Blumgart LH, Fong Y. Anatomic segmental hepatic resection is superior to wedge resection as an oncologic operation for colorectal liver metastases. J Gastrointest Surg. 2000;4(2):178–84.
21. Poultsides GA, Schulick RD, Pawlik TM. Hepatic resection for colorectal metastases: the impact of surgical margin status on outcome. HPB (Oxford). 2010;12(1):43–9.
22. Tang H, Li B, Zhang H, Dong J, Lu W. Comparison of anatomical and nonanatomical hepatectomy for colorectal liver metastasis: a meta-analysis of 5207 patients. Sci Rep. 2016;6:32304.
23. Zorzi D, Mullen JT, Abdalla EK, Pawlik TM, Andres A, Muratore A, et al. Comparison between hepatic wedge resection and anatomic resection for colorectal liver metastases. J Gastrointest Surg. 2006;10(1):86–94.
24. Chung JJ, Kim MJ, Kim KW. Mangafodipir trisodium-enhanced MRI for the detection and characterization of focal hepatic lesions: is delayed imaging useful? J Magn Reson Imaging. 2006;23(5):706–11.
25. Hoekstra LT, de Graaf W, Nibourg GA, Heger M, Bennink RJ, Stieger B, et al. Physiological and biochemical basis of clinical liver function tests: a review. Ann Surg. 2013;257(1):27–36.
26. Qiu J, Chen S, Chengyou D. A systematic review of robotic-assisted liver resection and meta-analysis of robotic versus laparoscopic hepatectomy for hepatic neoplasms. Surg Endosc. 2016;30(3):862–75.
27. Zureikat AH, Borrebach J, Pitt HA, McGill D, Hogg ME, Thompson V, et al. Minimally invasive hepatopancreatobiliary surgery in North America: an ACS-NSQIP analysis of predictors of conversion for laparoscopic and robotic pancreatectomy and hepatectomy. HPB (Oxford). 2017;19(7):595–602.
28. Khan S, Beard RE, Kingham PT, Fong Y, Boerner T, Martinie JB, et al. Long-term oncologic outcomes following robotic liver resections for primary hepatobiliary malignancies: a multicenter study. Ann Surg Oncol. 2018;25:2652.
29. Berber E, Akyildiz HY, Aucejo F, Gunasekaran G, Chalikonda S, Fung J. Robotic versus laparoscopic resection of liver tumours. HPB (Oxford). 2010;12(8):583–6.
30. Wang WH, Kuo KK, Wang SN, Lee KT. Oncological and surgical result of hepatoma after robot surgery. Surg Endosc. 2018;32:3918.
31. Chen PD, Wu CY, Hu RH, Chou WH, Lai HS, Liang JT, et al. Robotic versus open hepatectomy for hepatocellular carcinoma: a matched comparison. Ann Surg Oncol. 2017;24(4):1021–8.
32. Kingham TP, Leung U, Kuk D, Gonen M, D'Angelica MI, Allen PJ, et al. Robotic liver resection: a case-matched comparison. World J Surg. 2016;40(6):1422–8.
33. Morel P, Jung M, Cornateanu S, Buehler L, Majno P, Toso C, et al. Robotic versus open liver resections: a case-matched comparison. Int J Med Robot. 2017;13(3):e1800.
34. Yu YD, Kim KH, Jung DH, Namkoong JM, Yoon SY, Jung SW, et al. Robotic versus laparoscopic liver resection: a comparative study from a single center. Langenbecks Arch Surg. 2014;399(8):1039–45.
35. Tranchart H, Ceribelli C, Ferretti S, Dagher I, Patriti A. Traditional versus robot-assisted full laparoscopic liver resection: a matched-pair comparative study. World J Surg. 2014;38(11):2904–9.
36. Montalti R, Scuderi V, Patriti A, Vivarelli M, Troisi RI. Robotic versus laparoscopic resections of posterosuperior segments of the liver: a propensity score-matched comparison. Surg Endosc. 2016;30(3):1004–13.
37. Chen PD, Wu CY, Hu RH, Chen CN, Yuan RH, Liang JT, et al. Robotic major hepatectomy: is there a learning curve? Surgery. 2017;161(3):642–9.
38. Efanov M, Alikhanov R, Tsvirkun V, Kazakov I, Melekhina O, Kim P, et al. Comparative analysis of learning curve in complex robot-assisted and laparoscopic liver resection. HPB (Oxford). 2017;19(9):818–24.
39. Ji WB, Wang HG, Zhao ZM, Duan WD, Lu F, Dong JH. Robotic-assisted laparoscopic anatomic hepatectomy in China: initial experience. Ann Surg. 2011;253(2):342–8.
40. Sham JG, Richards MK, Seo YD, Pillarisetty VG, Yeung RS, Park JO. Efficacy and cost of robotic hepatectomy: is the robot cost-prohibitive? J Robot Surg. 2016;10(4):307–13.
41. Daskalaki D, Gonzalez-Heredia R, Brown M, Bianco FM, Tzvetanov I, Davis M, et al. Financial impact of the robotic approach in liver surgery: a comparative study of clinical outcomes and costs between the robotic and open technique in a single institution. J Laparoendosc Adv Surg Tech A. 2017;27(4):375–82.

Cardiac Surgery Risks in Liver Dysfunction

73

Grigore Tinica, Cristina Furnica, and Raluca Ozana Chistol

Key Concepts

- The incidence of chronic liver diseases and cirrhosis is steadily increasing and is therefore common that patients with advanced liver dysfunction are addressed for cardiac surgery interventions;
- Patients in Child Pugh class A can be assimilated to the general population and are candidates to elective cardiac surgery; Patients in Child Pugh class B can undergo elective cardiac surgery with adequate preoperative preparation and adapted intraoperative strategy;
- Elective cardiac surgery is contraindicated in Child Pugh class C patients, acute hepatitis, alcoholic hepatitis, acute liver failure and in case of severe extrahepatic complications;
- Endovascular procedures (Transcatheter Aortic Valve Implantation) are associated with acceptable mortality and morbidity rates in patients with advanced liver dysfunction and are preferred to open surgery when available and technically possible.

73.1 Introduction

The incidence of chronic liver diseases and cirrhosis is steadily increasing. The age-adjusted prevalence for 2016 in 35 countries for males and females ranged from 447 (Iceland) to 1100 (Romania) cases per 100,000 inhabitants, with a median of 833 [1]. It is therefore common that patients with advanced liver dysfunction are addressed for cardiac surgery interventions. Liver disease has been long time considered an important risk factor for both major morbidity and mortality following cardiac surgery as a result of cardiovascular disorders, haemostatic and coagulation disorders, renal impairment and bacterial infection. Several risk score models have been specifically developed for cardiac surgery to assess a patient's surgical candidacy based on the potential unfavourable outcome (major complications and mortality), the most used being the Society of Thoracic Surgeons (STS) system and the European System for Cardiac Operative Risk Evaluation (EuroSCORE) model. Both scores are of limited use as they fail to include all major factors that may render patients at higher risk for surgery. It is problematic to distinguish patients who may benefit from cardiac surgery from those whose perioperative risk exceeds benefit. Consequently, for patients with advanced liver dysfunction, the operative benefit needs to be carefully weighted after a specific assessment and the therapeutic management adapted to the particular clinical picture of the individual patient.

The aims of this chapter are to reveal the impact of the pathophysiological changes induced by advanced liver dysfunction on the surgical and anaesthetic outcomes in cardiac surgery and to outline the particular aspects of the pre, intra and postoperative management used to optimize the outcome in this group of patients.

73.2 Advanced Liver Dysfunction Physiopathological Changes Relevant for Cardiac Surgery

73.2.1 Haemostasis and Coagulation Disorders

Advanced liver dysfunction is associated with various anomalies, particularly protein synthesis impairment, that affect

G. Tinica (✉) · R. O. Chistol
Cardiovascular Institute, Iasi, Romania

Grigore T. Popa University of Medicine and Pharmacy, Iasi, Romania

C. Furnica
Grigore T. Popa University of Medicine and Pharmacy, Iasi, Romania

Institute of Forensic Medicine, Iasi, Romania

F. Radu-Ionita et al. (eds.), *Liver Diseases*, https://doi.org/10.1007/978-3-030-24432-3_73

Table 73.1 Haemostasis abnormalities in cirrhotic patients

Coagulation factor defects	Thrombocytopenia and platelet dysfunction	Increased fibrinolysis	Prothrombotic changes
– Decreased liver synthesis of fibrinogen (factor I), thrombin (factor II), factors V, VII, IX, X, XI – Vitamin K deficiency in alcohol induced liver disease	– Decreased liver synthesis of thrombopoietin – Bone marrow suppression (hepatitis virus C, infection, alcohol, antiviral therapy) – Increased platelet sequestration in the spleen – Platelets dysfunction secondary to uremia, infection, endothelial cells abnormalities (platelets inhibition by NO and prostacyclin)	– Increased levels of tissue plasminogen activator (tPA) – Decreased liver synthesis of alpha 2 antiplasmin, coagulation factor XIII, thrombin-activatable fibrinolysis inhibitor (TAFI) – Fibrinolytic activity of ascitic fluid	– Decreased liver synthesis of protein S, protein C, fibrinolytic factors – Inflammatory changes in endothelial cells – Decreased liver clearance of von Willebrand factor (vWF)

almost all aspects of haemostasis and coagulation. According to Shah et al., impaired haemostasis in cirrhotic patients is due to four types of abnormalities that may coexist in the same patient: coagulation factor defects, thrombocytopenia and platelet dysfunction, increased fibrinolysis, prothrombotic changes [2] (Table 73.1).

The above-mentioned abnormalities lead to pro-haemorrhagic and procoagulant impairment of both primary and secondary haemostasis and fibrinolysis. If haemostasis abnormalities in advanced liver dysfunction are a certitude, debates still exist concerning the threshold values of laboratory tests that indicate an increased haemorrhagic risk and impose corrective measures prior to surgery. Conventionally proposed correction thresholds are PT < 50%, fibrinogen level <1 g/L or platelet count less than 50,000/mm^3, but international normalized ratio (INR) values should not be used to guide therapy.

Corrective measures may include comorbidities control (infection treatment, optimization of renal status, avoid accentuating portal hypertension), vitamin K and cryoprecipitate administration, platelets and red blood cells transfusion, administration of antifibrinolytic agents (tranexamic acid, epsilon aminocaproic acid). Recent advancements in surgical and anaesthetic approaches have led to significant reduction in blood transfusion requirements.

73.2.2 Renal Function Impairment

Renal function impairment in cirrhotic patients has a multifactorial aetiology related to hemodynamic changes (splanchnic vasodilatation, decline in renal perfusion despite activation of the renin-angiotensin system and intense renal vasoconstriction, balance alteration between vasoconstrictor and vasodilator mediators) that alter renal vascular reactivity. Other causes of renal dysfunction (prerenal, renal or postrenal) must be systematically excluded. Prerenal causes related to true or relative hypovolemia frequently occur in cirrhotic patients due to diuretic treatment, diarrhoea, ascites drainage. Nephrotoxic drugs and those inducing a decrease in renal blood flow (eq. anti-inflammatory drugs) should be avoided in cirrhotic patients. Patients with alcoholic cirrhosis may develop mesangial nephropathy with IgA deposits, while a patient with post-hepatitis C cirrhosis may develop cryoglobulinemia related nephropathy. An important aspect to be signalled is the overestimation of the renal function in cirrhotic patients, urea and creatinine synthesis are usually diminished (decrease in lean body mass and hypoproteinemia) and do not reflect glomerular filtration ratio (GFR).

The most severe form of renal dysfunction is represented by the hepatorenal syndrome (HRS).

Definition
Hepatorenal syndrome combines functional renal failure (anuria secondary to diminished blood pressure), a decrease in sodium levels and irreducible ascites.

The hepatorenal syndrome occurs in advanced stage of cirrhosis, spontaneously or caused by complications (haemorrhages, infections, ascites puncture). Hepatorenal syndrome may be acute and short-term lethal or with a slower progression, the latter responding to vasoactive drugs or transjugular intrahepatic portosystemic shunt (TIPS) placement.

Therapeutic management generally relies on prevention (avoidance of nephrotoxic agents, drugs that induce arterial hypotension, diuretics, infection screening) and early recognition. If severe acute kidney injury/hepatorenal syndrome installs, patients should be treated with vasoconstrictors in combination with intravenous albumin according to the revised consensus recommendations of the International Club of Ascites [3].

73.2.3 Cardiovascular Alterations

Advanced liver dysfunction is associated with cardiovascular changes secondary to neurohumoral and vascular dysregulations, portal hypertension and portosystemic shunts. These changes include hyperdynamic circulation (increased cardiac output), decreased blood pressure, decreased vascular resistance and cirrhotic cardiomyopathy. The importance of cardiovascular abnormalities is associated with the degree of liver failure.

Arteriolar vasodilation is the hallmark of cardiovascular alterations and finally leads to decreased circulating blood volume. A vicious cycle (compensatory vasoconstrictor mechanisms that promote water and salt retention) is initiated as baroreceptors are stimulated.

An authentic cirrhotic cardiomyopathy has also been identified, different from other cardiomyopathies that may occur in patients with advanced liver dysfunction such as alcoholic cardiomyopathy.

Definition
Cirrhotic cardiomyopathy is defined as the presence of structural and functional cardiac abnormalities in patients with cirrhosis, without other associated heart disease.

Cirrhotic cardiomyopathy is characterized by systolic and diastolic dysfunction, as well as by conduction disorders that may become clinically evident following physiological or surgical stress, and cause heart failure. Pathogenic mechanisms include alteration of the β-adrenergic signalling pathway and exposure to cardiodepressant factors.

Decreased cardiac contractility as a response to stressors and the degree of impairment is similar regardless of the etiology of liver disease.

The exact prevalence of cirrhotic cardiomyopathy remains unknown, however one of the typical anomalies, QT interval prolongation, appears to be present in the majority of patients with Child B or C cirrhosis. No specific treatment was suggested for these changes and the recommendations for the treatment of liver disease and heart failure should be followed [4].

73.2.4 Disorders of the Immune System

The incidence of bacterial infections during hospitalization of cirrhotic patients is 4 times higher than the one registered in the general population (40% versus 10%) [5]. This phenomenon is due to reticuloendothelial system abnormalities, humoral and cellular immunity as well as neutrophil dysfunction. In cirrhotic patients, the reduced phagocytosis capacity of the Kupffer cells together with intrahepatic vascular shunts that bypass the Kupfferian system contribute to bacteraemia secondary to bacterial translocation. The toxic action of alcohol further contributes to accentuating immune disorders. An appropriate empirical antimicrobial treatment should be promptly initiated when bacteraemia is proved.

73.2.5 Pulmonary Disorders

Pulmonary and pleural disorders occurring in patients with advanced liver dysfunction are generally represented by hydrothorax, hepatopulmonary syndrome and portopulmonary hypertension.

Definition
Hepatic hydrothorax defines the pleural effusion occurring in cirrhotic patients in the absence of any lung, pleural or cardiac disease.

The hepatic hydrothorax occurs in 5–10% of patients with ascites and results from the passage of ascitic fluid from the peritoneal cavity into the pleural cavity through diaphragmatic gaps due to the pressure gradient between the two cavities [6]. Pleural effusion is mostly right-sided and its volume can cause dyspnoea. A low-salt diet is mandatory for controlling this condition associated or not with a combination of furosemide and spironolactone.

Definition
The hepatopulmonary syndrome is a rare complication associating severe hypoxemia ($PaO_2 < 70$ mHg), pulmonary vasodilatation and an increased in the alveo-capillary oxygen gradient (>20 mmHg) [7].

Pulmonary vasodilation (precapillary and capillary vasodilatation, arteriovenous shunt bypassing the alveoli) is the man cause of this hypoxemia. Vascular abnormalities predominate in the middle and lower lung fields, leading to a worsening of hypoxemia in orthostatism. This condition is generally managed with drugs inhibiting NO synthesis and endothelin-1 inactivation.

Definition
Portopulmonary hypertension (PPHTN) is reported in 2–16% of cirrhotic patients with portal hypertension depending on the study and is a complication of portal hypertension involving pulmonary arterial vasoconstriction [8].

The mean pulmonary arterial pressure (mPAP) increases (>25 mmHg), pulmonary capillary wedge pressure decreases (<15 mmHg) and these changes result in an increase in transpulmonary gradient (the difference between the pulmonary artery pressure and the pulmonary capillary wedge pressure) and pulmonary vascular resistance (>120 dynes per s/cm^{-5}). The cause of PPHTN is unknown, most authors pleading for a vasoactive humoral substance reaching the pulmonary circulation through portosystemic collaterals. Portopulmonary hypertension causes dyspnea only when the mPAP exceeds 40–50 mmHg.

Blood gases are normal or show moderate hypoxemia. The prognosis for this condition is particularly severe and usually represents a contraindication to liver transplantation. Patients are generally treated with anticoagulants and diuretics part of the general measures to prevent pulmonary thromboembolism and volume overload. Patients that do not respond to general measures are treated with agents used for severe pulmonary hypertension (epoprostenol, iloprost, bosentan, sildenafil).

73.2.6 Liver Function Deterioration

Cirrhosis is associated with an increase in resistance to venous flow, especially at a post-sinusoidal level, which decreases the total hepatic flow at the expense of portal flow. The arterial self-regulation system is also significantly altered with little or no compensation of low-flow situations. Because of these changes, the oxygenation of centrilobular hepatocytes can be severely compromised in the circumstances of a cardiac surgery intervention with cardiac arrest and major hemodynamic stress.

The vulnerability of centrilobular hepatocytes to hypoperfusion and associated metabolic changes are explained by the particular architecture of the liver. The hepatic lobule is the *anatomical unit* of the hepatic parenchyma, centered by the centrilobular vein and limited at the periphery by portal spaces containing the portal triad (portal venule, hepatic arteriole, bile ductule). The functional organization of the liver parenchyma is not modeled on the anatomical structure represented by the hepatic lobule. The concept of hepatic acinus, the *functional unit* of the liver, is based on the vascular architecture, the central axis being represented by the line connecting two portal triads and the periphery by two adjacent centrilobular veins. The hepatic acinus can be divided in three metabolic zones from central axis to the center of the lobule. The periportal zone [1] is well oxygenated and less susceptible to ischemia, the centrilobular zone [3] is poorly oxygenated and very susceptible to ischemia, and the transition zone [2] has an intermediate susceptibility. The central zone of the acinus is specialized in oxidative metabolism and gluconeogenesis; the peripheral zone preferentially ensures glycolysis, biotransformation of xenobiotics (cytochrome P450) and alcohol metabolisation. This particular architecture explains the increase of centrilobular necrosis and deterioration of liver function in the early postoperative period.

All these cirrhosis associated disorders can alter the intraoperative and postoperative course in cardiac surgery worsening the outcome, but advanced liver dysfunction is not an absolute contraindication to cardiac surgery. With adequate patient selection, perioperative and anaesthetic management the outcome can be significantly improved.

73.3 Cardiac Surgery Risks and Outcome in Patients with Advanced Liver Dysfunction

It is estimated that approximately 10% of cirrhotic patients undergo surgery within the last 2 years of their life [9]. An increased surgical risk in this group of patients is indisputable due to difficult abdominal surgical conditions, anaesthesiologic issues, haemostatic and coagulation disorders, and increased risk of infection.

Cirrhotic patients can generally undergo two types of surgery: interventions related to their liver disease (resection of hepatocellular carcinoma, treatment of umbilical hernias) and extrahepatic interventions. In the first case, the perioperative management of these patients assumes a good knowledge of the specific complications such as refractory ascites, renal impairment or postoperative worsening of hepatic function with a major risk of decompensation.

The second type of surgery to which the cirrhotic patient is confronted is extrahepatic surgery for various cancers, orthopaedic issues, valvular or coronary heart diseases, or other thoracic diseases.

In practice, the postoperative morbidity in cirrhotic patients is not only related to the complications of the surgical site like infection or haemorrhage but also to long-term complications, more frequent than the first ones. Generally, there is an increase in the risk of infection in these patients. Surgical stress combined with a potential postoperative infection create the circumstances for hepatic decompensation, under the form of refractory ascites, renal impairment, digestive haemorrhage or hepatocellular function alteration.

The occurrence of postoperative hepatocellular insufficiency is associated with a mortality rate superior to 70% in the absence of transplantation.

Between 2.5% and 27% of patients with advanced liver disease present coronary heart disease [10]. A higher incidence of adverse events related to catheterization has been observed in cirrhotic, especially related to vascular access (severe bleeding, pseudoaneurysms, hematoma).

Cardiac surgery in cirrhotic patients is associated with an increased mortality, reaching 19.3% on the short term and 42% within 1 year [11].

Preoperative assessment of the individual surgical risk for each patient suffering from advanced liver disease allows separating patients who may benefit from cardiac surgery from those whose perioperative risk exceeds surgical benefits. Several risk evaluation systems have been developed and, in this section, we will analyse their ability to predict operative mortality in cirrhotic patients that need a cardiac surgery intervention.

In cardiac surgery, several specific scoring models have been developed to assess the risk of operative mortality, the most used being EuroSCORE II and STS.

EuroSCORE II has been developed in 2011 to update the original EuroSCORE model. The scoring system includes a limited number of patient related factors like age, gender, renal impairment, extracardiac arteriopathy, poor mobility, previous cardiac surgery, chronic lung disease, active endocarditis, critical preoperative state, diabetes on insulin, and omits all parameters relevant for liver function.

STS includes liver disease among the evaluated parameters as a binary selection (Yes or No) irrespective to the type and severity of the disease ("Indicate whether the patient has a history of hepatitis B, hepatitis C, cirrhosis, portal hypertension, oesophageal varices, chronic alcohol abuse or congestive hepatopathy").

Considering all severity stages, early postoperative morbidity and mortality after cardiac surgery in cirrhotic patients ranges from 31% to 66% and 10–25%, respectively. There appears to be an almost linear relationship between severity of liver damage, morbidity and mortality.

The surgical risk in cirrhotic patients is evaluated according to three main factors: liver function assessment, type and urgency of the procedure. Cirrhotic patients are at high surgical risk not only because of the cirrhosis itself but by the presence of coagulopathy, malnutrition, immune disorders, cardiomyopathy, pulmonary and renal impairment. Elective surgery is generally contraindicated in patients with acute hepatitis (especially if INR > 1.5), alcoholic hepatitis and acute liver failure (10–50% mortality rate).

In order to estimate the surgical risk in cirrhotic patients different scoring systems have been proposed. Developed in 1964 by Child and Turcotte and modified by Pugh in 1973 (prothrombin time assessment), the Child Turcotte Pugh (CTP) score is mostly used to assess the liver functional reserve prior to derivative surgery (porto-systemic and spleno-renal shunts). Formulated more than 50 years ago, without evidence base, CTP score lacks discriminatory capacity and is not adequate for non-derivative surgery where morbidity and mortality have a more significant relationship with other factors than those included in the CTP score (total bilirubin, albumin, prothrombin time/INR, ascites, encephalopathy).

Due to the subjectivity of the CTP score, a new prognostic index in advanced liver disease called MELD (Model for End-Stage Liver Disease) has been developed by the Mayo clinic by using mathematical modelling. MELD is generalized, verifiable and can be computed with easily obtained variables (dialysis, creatinine, bilirubin, INR, sodium). MELD-XI is an adapted version of the original MELD score excluding INR and is of particular use in patients with cardiovascular diseases.

To date, the prognostic value of MELD score has been validated in different groups of patients with advanced liver disease, initially in candidates for liver transplantation and afterwards for another types of surgery.

Cardiac surgery is not contraindicated in cirrhotic patients but the risk-benefit ratio should be carefully evaluated. The performance of cardiac surgical interventions in patients with advanced liver diseases increased with 22% from 1998 to 2006 according to the New York State Department of Health Cardiac Surgery Registry review [12]. A better understanding of both diseases and prophylaxis (beta-blockers for portal hypertension, endoscopic treatment of oesophageal varices, transjugular intrahepatic portosystemic shunts, spontaneous bacterial peritonitis prophylaxis, suppression of viral replication) led to this decrease.

Compared to other types of extra-hepatic surgery, cardiac surgery is associated with major hemodynamic and circulatory changes due to significant bleeding requiring blood transfusion, hypoperfusion and hypotension, changes that impair hepatic function. Moreover, CPB circuit activates factor XII, stimulates inflammation and platelet aggregation (further detailed in subchapter Cardiopulmonary bypass and liver dysfunction).

The first study to analyse the predictive value of CTP class, CTP score and MELD score after cardiac surgery with cardiopulmonary bypass (CPB) as performed by Suman et al. in 2004. The reference outcomes were considered death within 3 months from surgery and hepatic decompensation. A CTP score >7 emerged as the strongest predictor of postoperative mortality but the authors did not manage to establish a threshold value for the MELD score. The results were confirmed in 2007 by Filsoufi et al. who added preoperative thrombocytopenia as a poor prognostic factor for hospital mortality. MELD score regained interest in 2009 when Ailawadi et al. determined that a MELD score >15 is a predictor of mortality in cirrhotic patients undergoing tricuspid valve surgery. In 2010, Thielmann et al. retrospectively evaluated 57 cirrhotic patients who underwent cardiac surgery with CPB and compared the predictive value of CTP class, MELD score and EuroSCORE and showed that MELD was superior to both CTP and EuroSCORE [13]. Several research groups proposed threshold values for MELD score ranging between 13 and 15 and corresponding to the transition from CTP B to C class.

Until 2012, most studies were unicentric and on limited number of patients.

In 2015, there was published a meta-analysis performed on 22 reports including 939 patients from eight countries in order to assess the value of advanced liver dysfunction graded according to CTP score as a risk factor for mortality and morbidity in cardiac surgery. We only considered studies that analysed cirrhotic patients that underwent valve surgery (repair or replacement of a single or multiple valves), CABG (coronary artery bypass grafting), pericardiectomy, ascending aorta surgery, patch repair of a septal defect or of the free ventricular wall. The mean in hospital mortality rates were 8.92%, 31.38%, and 47.62% for patients in CTP class A, B and C compared to mean late mortality rates of 20.58%, 43.58%, and 56.48% respectively. Patients in class A had significantly lower in hospital (OR 0.30) and late (OR 0.34) mortality rate compared to patients in class B. When compared to class C, mortality rate was even lower (OR 0.16 for early mortality and 0.07 for late mortality). When comparing class B versus class C, the difference was not statistically significant. Morbidity rates were also analysed with quantification of a 4.37% mean reexploration rate, 3.83% mean neurological complication rate, 2.67% mean cardiovascular complication rate, 16.51% mean pulmonary complication rate, 22.15% mean renal complication rate, 5.75% mean hepatic complication rate, 8.09% mean gastrointestinal complication rate, 5.64% mean sepsis and multiple organ failure syndrome rate, 5.54% mean haemorrhage and cardiac tamponade rate, 9.16% mean infection rate [13]. Morbidity risk related to CTP class could not be assessed as not all studies reported results accordingly. These findings indicate that both in hospital and late mortality rates increase in accordance with CTP classification the lower rates being registered in class A patients. With adequate preparation, perioperative and anaesthetic management, cardiac surgery can be safely performed in CTP class A patients. Other studies confirmed our findings that patients in CTP class C register significantly higher mortality rates. The need for a surgical treatment should be carefully analysed in these patients and if it considered mandatory with no medical or interventional alternatives, liver function should be optimized prior to surgery as much as possible. For patients in CTP class B, further studies are necessary to determine if it is safe to conduct cardiac surgery in this group. The most frequent complications reported in cirrhotic patients are renal (21.15%), pulmonary (16.51%) and cardiovascular (12.67%). Hepatic failure accounts for less than 6% of complications but is associated with a more than 70% mortality rate. Compared to cirrhotic patients, a large recent study performed in 2017 on 40,652 patients with isolated CABG irrespective to comorbidities (general population) reported a 1.6–2.8% mortality rate depending on study year and a major complication rate between 3.8% and 7.8% [14].

Jacob et al. performed a similar meta-analysis on 19 studies published up to February 2014 and reached similar results—9% early mortality rate in CTP class A patients, 37.7% in class B and 52% in class C. They also quantified a within 1-year mortality rate of 27.2% in class A patients, 66.2% in class B and 78.9% in class C but did not evaluate postoperative morbidity [11].

The predictive value of the MELD score was evaluated by fewer studies compared to CTP class. In 2010, Thielman proposes 13.5 as a cut-off value for postoperative in-hospital morbidity and considers MELD score as having a superior predictive value compared to CTP classification and EuroSCORE [13]. In 2017, Sabry et al. proposed a MELD score of 12 as a threshold value for postoperative morbidity after analysing 90 adult patients with chronic hepatitis C virus undergoing cardiac surgery with CPB [15]. As one can notice, MELD threshold value varies largely among studies given the heterogeneity of the evaluated population (from general population to patients awaiting liver transplantation). MELD score predicts short term mortality in cirrhotic patients undergoing cardiac surgery but further studies on homogeneous populations are needed to reach a consensus regarding the threshold value for considering the patient at high risk.

Risk stratification, preoperative evaluation and preparation, adequate operative and postoperative care are mandatory in cirrhotic patients to maintain an optimal risk-benefit ratio.

73.4 Preoperative Preparation of Cirrhotic Patients Prior to Major Cardiac Surgery

In cirrhotic patients, surgery should ideally be elective as these patients are at risk especially in case of urgent surgery. However, if the latter case cannot be avoided, the choice of the surgical technique is important.

Cirrhosis generally recognizes three etiologies: metabolic, cholestatic and non-cholestatic. Patients with metabolic liver disease maintain normal hepatic reserve for a long period of time and generally do not develop portal hypertension compared to cholestatic liver disease associated with portal hypertension and liver failure due to cholangitis in advanced stages, and non-cholestatic liver disease that involves portal hypertension and diminished hepatic reserve.

Patients with metabolic and cholestatic liver disease (except advanced stages) can be assimilated to the general population as they present a slightly increased risk.

Non-cholestatic liver disease (alcoholic liver disease, viral hepatitis, non-alcoholic steatohepatitis) is the major cause of cirrhosis worldwide and cardiac surgery risk should be particularly evaluated in this group of patients.

The preoperative evaluation begins with a clinical history and full physical examination. A history of jaundice, poorly controlled ascites, physical exhaustion, gastrointestinal haemorrhage generally indicates advanced liver dysfunction and high operative risk. One should pay attention to changes suggestive of portal encephalopathy like sleep disorders, concentration difficulties, confabulation, altered handwriting. Portal hypertension is suggested by thrombocytopenia (<150,000), increased prothrombin time/INR, and normochromic normocytic anemia. Transaminases can register normal values and are not to be considered an indicator of liver dysfunction severity.

Additional to laboratory tests, preoperative abdominal ultrasound examination is mandatory to evaluate ascites and exclude a hepatocellular carcinoma. In patients with viral hepatitis B, viral replication should be excluded prior to surgery as it could lead to postoperative acute hepatitis. An endoscopic examination should be performed prior to transesophageal echocardiography to exclude major varices at risk of bleeding.

The general status of these patients can be improved preoperatively. Nutritional assessment followed by renutrition strategy (high carbohydrate/lipid content and low sodium diet), vitamin K and protein administration are able to ameliorate prothrombin time/INR. Prophylactic administration of coagulation factors to correct hemostasis abnormalities is unjustified and potentially dangerous.

Portal hypertension can be managed with non-selective beta-blockers if the cardiac status allows it. The use of TIPS in candidates to cardiac surgery is a controverted measure. Although it decreases the portosystemic gradient, ascites and bleeding risk, TIPS could lead to heart failure, hepatic decompensation and exacerbate encephalopathy.

Hemodynamic optimization, adequate volemic management, and avoidance of nephrotic drugs are also fundamental points in the perioperative management of these patients. The impact of hypotension on morbidity and mortality (independently of other risk factors) suggests a particular susceptibility of the cirrhotic liver to ischemia, but excessive volume expansion is likely to aggravate ascites and lower limbs edema without an effective benefit on the circulating blood volume. Thus, hemodynamic optimization while monitoring the cardiac output or stroke volume is necessary.

Ascites, both peritoneal and pleural, leads to atelectasis and restrictive ventilatory defects in cirrhotic patients. Perioperative protective ventilation associating a tidal volume of 6 ml/kg of ideal weight and a PEEP (Positive end-expiratory pressure) of 6–8 cm H_2O appears particularly useful and reduces the incidence of postoperative pulmonary complications.

Finally, early recognition, timely and appropriate treatment of any perioperative infection can reduce postoperative morbidity and mortality.

Preoperative conversion of a CTP class C patient to CTP class B could improve postoperative survival.

73.5 Anaesthetic Management of Patients with Advanced Liver Dysfunction Undergoing Cardiac Surgery

The liver plays a major role in the metabolization, distribution and elimination of many drugs through two main mechanisms:

- Biotransformation through the cytochrome P450 pathway (oxygen-dependent—oxidation, reduction or hydrolysis) allowing the transformation of many hydrophobic compounds into hydrophilic compounds;
- Glucuronidation, glutathione or sulphate conjugation often succeeding first pathway (except for water-soluble molecules such as morphine), forming a more hydrophilic and acidic compound easily excreted in bile.

First pathway is altered in the early phases of liver dysfunction and the second phase, in the later phases. Generally, liver dysfunction interferes the metabolization of anaesthetic drugs secondary to alteration of the cytochrome P450 pathway, hypoproteinaemia (decreased binding) and decreased biliary excretion.

Many anaesthetic drugs are bound to plasma albumin and usually inactive in this phase. In case of hypo-albuminemia, the free fraction of these agents is therefore greater with a potentially increased pharmacological effect or toxicity. On the other hand, in case of portal hypertension, the first pass effect is reduced because of portosystemic shunts with, consequently, an increase in the bioavailability of drugs.

In well-compensated patients with close to normal liver function (CTP class A), the pharmacokinetics of anaesthetic drugs is almost unchanged. The more serious the cirrhosis is (portal hypertension, hepatocellular insufficiency), the more important and difficult to predict are the pharmacological changes.

Benzodiazepines, such as midazolam, should be avoided in cirrhotic patients as they could trigger hepatic encephalopathy. If such drugs are administered and the neurological state of the patient alters, flumazenil remains an effective antidote.

Propofol is not metabolised by the liver and does not suffer any major pharmacodynamic variation in cirrhotic patients. Similarly, inhaled anaesthetic agents, especially isoflurane, are poorly metabolized by the liver (0.2%) and are safe to be used in such cases [16]. Morphine on the other hand is metabolized by hepatic glucuronidation to an intermediate metabolite with renal elimination. Its half-life is prolonged in patients with CTP class B and C cirrhosis. If opioid administration is necessary, remifentanil could be safely used as it is not metabolized by the liver.

For curarisation, atracurium and doxacurium (for long interventions) are preferred as they do not undergo hepatic metabolization. Succinylcholine may have a prolonged effect due to a decrease in plasma cholinesterase activity.

73.6 Operative Management of Cirrhotic Patients Undergoing Major Cardiac Surgery. Cardiopulmonary Bypass and Liver Dysfunction

The key elements of operative management in cirrhotic patients are adequate visceral perfusion, correct hydroelectrolytic balance, thermoregulation, preventing hepatic decompensation, avoiding bleeding diathesis. Although not all centres are able to perform it, thromboelastography is a rapid method that evaluates the degree of coagulopathy and indicates potential optimization measures.

Cirrhotic patients poorly tolerate large volume oscillations and haemodilution is generally not recommended in this group of patients as its effects are unknown even if it was demonstrated to improve hepatic flow, both arterial and portal venous, in general population.

Compared to other major surgeries, most cardiac surgery interventions are performed on pump. The impact of cardiopulmonary bypass (CPB) upon liver function is incompletely elucidated. The materials used are not perfectly biocompatible and the established circulation is not physiological. CPB triggers a consumption of coagulation factors, an increase in the oxidative stress and a generalized inflammatory reaction resulting in the release of stress hormones and hepatotoxic cytokines. Finally, at the end of the intervention, when the aortic-cross clamp is removed, there is a sudden reperfusion with fully anticoagulated blood, immunologically primed and highly oxygenated.

The consequences of CPB could be summarized as follows:

- Immunological consequences
  - Activation of complement system (classical and alternative pathways) and liberation of active fractions C3a and C5a in the early phases (starting with aortic cannulation) as blood comes in contact with a foreign surface (cannulae, membrane oxygenator, circuits);
  - Neutrophils activation especially in lungs secondary to complement activation;
  - Prostaglandins augmentation—prostacyclin, thromboxane A2 secondary to free radicals liberation, complement activation, formation of heparin—protamine complexes;
  - Increase of pro-inflammatory cytokines (TNF-α, IL-6 and IL-8) 2–6 h after removal of aortic clamp;
  - Alteration of both humoral and cell-mediated immunity, quantitatively (decreased T, B and NK lymphocytes), qualitatively (decrease of CD4/CD8 ratio) and functionally. In cirrhotic patients, given the preoperative anergy, the risk of postoperative complications is particularly increased;
- Hematologic consequences:
  - Initial neutropenia secondary to hemodilution and lung accumulation of neutrophils followed by hyperleukocytosis (neutrophilia) correlated with an inflammatory response;
  - Activated neutrophils release proteases, free radicals, cytokines and lipid mediators. In the postoperative phase, neutrophils are desensitized and lose their abilities—chemotactic, phagocytosis and elastase production or free radicals—which would lead to septic risk;
  - Early thrombocytopenia secondary to hemodilution, CPB circuit and sequestration in the liver, spleen and lungs. Thrombocytopenia is aggravated by protamine administration;
  - Hemolysis particularly in case of abundant blood aspiration.
- Metabolic consequences:
  - Liberation of stress hormones (catecholamines, antidiuretic hormone, cortisol, glucagon) especially with normothermic CPB. Insulinemia is reduced with hypothermic CPB but not with normothermic CPB;
  - Increase in peripheral vascular resistance;
  - Desensitization of myocardial adrenergic receptors;
  - Hypocalcaemia;
- Visceral consequences:
  - Myocardial sideration of ischemic cause secondary to aortic clamping. Myocardial protection and cardioplegia are of particular importance in reducing ischemia-reperfusion myocardial injuries;
  - Extravascular lung water (EVLW) accumulation which may cause respiratory distress syndrome;
  - Pulmonary restrictive syndrome secondary to inflammatory reactions, sternotomy, prolonged decubitus and potential phrenic nerve lesions. Additional pulmonary injuries may be determined by complement activation, neutrophils sequestration and free radicals that damage the endothelium. Nowadays, membrane oxygenators reduce the incidence of pulmonary complications compared to ancient bubble oxygenators. The partial pressures of arterial oxygen (PaO2) and postoperative pulmonary vascular resistance are improved with normothermic CPB;
  - Neurological consequences are difficult to assess but cognitive disorders have been signalled in 22.5% of patients after CABG due to microembolism, hemodynamic or rheologic changes;
  - Renal impairment in CPB occurs secondary to hypotension with hypoperfusion, hemolysis and microembolism;
  - Hepatic dysfunction.

According to Di Tomasso et al., hepatic dysfunction secondary to CPB is due to microembolism, free radicals generation, inadequate tissue perfusion, dilutional anaemia and haemodynamic changes and we would add activation of multiple humoral (coagulation, complement, kinin-kallikrein, cytokines, fibrinolysis) and cellular (platelets, neutrophils, endothelial cells) systems [17]. Many factors contribute to these changes: blood contact with foreign surfaces, air-blood interface, hypothermia and reheating, blood cells trauma, intraoperative hypotension. Of particular interest in cirrhotic patients is the potential liberation of endotoxins secondary to intestinal ischemia.

In general population, transient elevation of bilirubin and hepatic enzymes is noticed in the early postoperative period, but in cirrhotic patients decompensation can occur. "Shocked liver" (hepatic ischemia), the extreme form of CPB related hepatic dysfunction determined by marked hypotension and haemodynamic instability (perfusion quantitative and qualitative variations, rheologic changes), could become fatal in cirrhotic patients. The centrilobular zone is particularly sensitive to ischemia compared to bile ducts affected by lobular congestion (in case of right heart failure). CPB is considered one of the major determinants of postoperative hepatic morbidity in cardiac surgery. Di Tomasso et al. signalled a higher rate of refractory coagulopathy, infections, right ventricular failure, portal hypertension and hepatorenal syndrome in patients with preoperative liver dysfunction [17].

Patients in CTP class A tolerate CPB same as the general population but in class B, CPB should be avoided if possible. If on pump surgery is unavoidable, normothermic CPB should be used and its duration reduced to the minimum under a strict hemodynamic and coagulation monitoring. Mean arterial blood pressure should be maintained above 60 mmHg in the context of a dry approach with avoidance of fluid overload. Anaesthetic considerations previously mentioned are to be considered during the intervention.

Patients in CTP class C or with a history of complications related to portal hypertension are associated with a high mortality risk in case of open cardiac surgery. Endovascular procedures and optimal medical treatment should be considered in these cases.

73.7 Postoperative Care of Cirrhotic Patients After Major Cardiac Surgery

The cirrhotic patient carries a higher risk of prolonged hospitalization in the intensive care unit. The common cause of perioperative mortality is sepsis. Bacteraemia is frequent, mostly secondary to bacterial translocation correlated with deficient immune response. At the slightest suspicion, an empiric antibiotherapy should be quickly initiated. Postoperative leucocytosis and hyperbilirubinemia further increase the mortality risk.

Postoperative hepatic dysfunction in cirrhotic patients ranges from temporary hyperbilirubinemia related to intraoperative haemolysis, to decompensation and liver failure depending on the preoperative hepatic reserve and aetiology of liver dysfunction. Hyperbilirubinemia can be marked and prolonged if the evolution is complicated with cardiogenic shock and prolonged mechanical ventilation. Cholestasis may also occur due to hepatic ischemia and congestion. Its consequences are variable, from digestion impairment to cholangitis. Prolonged cholestasis and hyperbilirubinemia correlate with postoperative morbidity and mortality.

Major supportive measures in the postoperative period include hemodynamic support to avoid hepatic ischemia, early reinitiation of adequate enteral nutrition, haemorrhage and sepsis prevention.

Fresh frozen plasma (FFP) can be used to correct identified coagulopathies while monitoring the central venous pressure to avoid fluid overload. If FFP is not sufficient or not indicated (fluid overload), cryoprecipitate or desmopressin represent alternative methods.

Fluid administration (oral or intravenous) and sodium intake restriction are recommended to prevent postoperative ascites. If the patient received a diuretic treatment with furosemide prior to surgery, the treatment should be continued postoperatively while monitoring hydroelectrolytic balance and renal function.

Postoperative pain relief is another issue to be considered. Patients in CTP class A tolerate morphine and fentanyl administration but the dose should be reduced in class B patients. Nonsteroidal anti-inflammatory drugs are to be avoided as they are nephrotoxic and increase the risk of gastrointestinal haemorrhage. Acetaminophen administration is not contraindicated, but doses should be reduced (<2 g/day). Special care should be paid not to provoke somnolence as it could mask incipient signs of hepatic encephalopathy.

Prophylaxis of gastrointestinal haemorrhage with intravenous ranitidine, somatostatin and metoclopramide is recommended especially in patients with portal hypertension.

Correct partial arterial pressure of oxygen and a haemoglobin level superior to 9 mg/dL assure a good hepatic oxygenation in the absence of hypotension.

73.8 Endovascular Procedures in Cirrhotic Patients

The emergence of endovascular cardiac interventions and especially transcatheter aortic valve implantation (TAVI) completely changed the management of aortic stenosis and expanded the range of potential candidates to aortic valve replacement. Patients previously considered at high risk for surgical aortic valve replacement (SAVR) are now potential candidates to TAVI.

In 2017, Alqahtani et al. published an extensive study comparing the outcomes of TAVI and SAR in cirrhotic patients. They analysed 1766 cirrhotic patients treated over a 12 years period, and propensity matched 268 patients (134 with TAVI and 134 with SAVR). The reported postoperative mortality was significantly lower with TAVI (8.2%) compared to SAVR (20.2%) same as blood transfusion rate and hospital length of stay [18].

Yassin et al. on the other hand, compared the outcomes of TAVI in cirrhotic and non-cirrhotic patients and found that cirrhotic patients registered no increase in the risk of in-hospital mortality or postprocedural complications [19].

All studies analysing the outcomes of TAVI in cirrhotic patients up to date are performed on small matched groups with low incidence of specific complications. Authors report decreased renal, pulmonary, infectious and neurological complication rates with TAVI compared to SAVR but with no statistical significance given the reduced number of cases. They are unanimous in stating that TAVI is a safe procedure in patients with advanced liver dysfunction being associated with lower mortality rates and length of stay.

The major advances of TAVI in cirrhotic patients are represented by the absence of CPB, shorter anaesthesia, lesser requirement of blood and blood products transfusions.

73.9 Early Ischemic Liver Injury After Cardiac Surgery

Ischemic hepatitis occurs in the presence of a combination of hepatic hypoxia and hepatic venous congestion and is a rare complication of cardiac surgery with CPB. Also called "shocked liver", it characterized by massive elevation of aspartate aminotransferases (AST) up to 20 times normal values [20]. At the cellular level, ischemic hepatitis occurs in two phases that correspond to an ischemia/reperfusion mechanism.

The reperfusion phase is crucial because it is the main cause of the majority of cellular damage. The ischemic phase is accompanied by an initially reversible edema of centrilobular hepatocytes and sinusoidal cells. If ischemia continues, cellular dysfunction occurs with activation of enzymes such as proteases and phospholipases and intracellular oxidative stress reactions.

The reperfusion phase occurs during the restoration of hemodynamics when hepatic blood flow increases and oxygen again reaches the hepatocytes.

In the case of prolonged ischemic phase, ischemia/reperfusion injury with cell necrosis will occur due to intracellular oxidative stress at the beginning of re-oxygenation, activation of Kupffer cells, and abnormalities of the sinusoidal microcirculation. Lactic dehydrogenase (LDH) is a marker of hepatic cytolysis. The xanthine/xanthine oxidase enzymatic system also plays a major role in cellular oxidative stress. Metabolites will contribute to free radicals formation (superoxide) that further activate the neutrophils which will secrete proteases. Free radicals and proteases are responsible for hepatic cytolysis mainly in the intermediate region.

Hepatic congestion secondary to increased central venous pressure also contributes to ischemic hepatitis.

"Shocked liver" syndrome generally installs in the first 48 h after the surgical intervention. The patient may present with nausea, vomiting, jaundice, turgescent jugular veins and hepatojugular reflux, hemorrhagic syndrome or even hepatic encephalopathy in patients with preexistent liver dysfunction. Laboratory testes reveal a marked increase of AST and alanine aminotransferase (ALT) up to 20 times normal values and also of LDH. Bilirubin level also increases but at a lesser extent. Coagulopathy is aggravated by hepatic ischemia with potential hemorrhagic diathesis. In non-cirrhotic patients, clinical symptoms and laboratory test results improve in a few days of normal hemodynamics is restored. In patients with prior liver dysfunction, it can evolve towards potentially fatal complications like hepatic encephalopathy, liver failure or multiple organ dysfunction syndrome (MODS).

The treatment of this condition relies mainly on prevention (maintenance of adequate blood perfusion and avoidance of major volume shifts during the intervention) and, if it occurs, the only option is represented by supportive measures (sepsis, hemorrhage and further ischemia risk minimization).

73.10 Conclusion

Pathophysiological changes associated with advanced liver dysfunction predispose to potentially fatal complications in cardiac surgery especially if the intervention is performed with CPB. Patients in CTP class A can undergo elective cardiac surgery same as the general population with almost similar outcome. In CTP class B patients, elective interventions are possible, preferably off pump after adequate preoperative preparation. In CTP class C patients, open cardiac surgery is contraindicated and endovascular treatment should be considered instead if technically possible. Anaesthetic and perioperative management have be adapted to specific metabolic, humoral, haematological and hemodynamic alterations to prevent postoperative morbidity and mortality.

Self Study

Questions

1. Which statement is true?
   (a) Cardiac surgery risk scores (STS, EuroSCORE II) correctly estimate mortality risk in cirrhotic patients.
   (b) Cardiopulmonary bypass has no impact on liver function.
   (c) In CTP class A patients the pharmacokinetics of anaesthetic drugs is almost unchanged.
   (d) Advanced liver dysfunction is an absolute contraindication to cardiac surgery.
2. Which statement is true?
   (a) Non cirrhotic patients register no changes of liver function tests in the postoperative period.

(b) Haemorrhagic complications are most common cause of postoperative mortality in cirrhotic patients undergoing cardiac surgery.
(c) TAVI is not indicated in CTP class C patients.
(d) Fresh frozen plasma (FFP) can be used to correct coagulopathies in the postoperative period.

Answers

1. Which statement is true?
   (a) EuroSCORE II system includes a limited number of patient related factors like age, gender, renal impairment, extracardiac arteriopathy, poor mobility, previous cardiac surgery, chronic lung disease, active endocarditis, critical preoperative state, diabetes on insulin, and omits all parameters relevant for liver function. STS on the other hand, includes liver disease among the evaluated parameters as a binary selection (Yes or No) irrespective to the type and severity of the disease
   (b) Hepatic dysfunction secondary to CPB is due to microembolism, free radicals generation, inadequate tissue perfusion, dilutional anaemia and haemodynamic changes and activation of multiple humoral (coagulation, complement, kinin-kallikrein, cytokines, fibrinolysis) and cellular (platelets, neutrophils, endothelial cells) systems.
   (c) CORRECT ANSWER. In well-compensated patients with close to normal liver function (CTP class A), the pharmacokinetics of anaesthetic drugs is almost unchanged. The more serious the cirrhosis is (portal hypertension, hepatocellular insufficiency), the more important and difficult to predict are the pharmacological changes.
   (d) CTP class A patients can safely undergo cardiac surgery. In class B, open cardiac surgery is possible, preferably off pump and after adequate preoperative preparation.
2. Which statement is true?
   (a) In general population, transient elevation of bilirubin and hepatic enzymes is noticed in the early postoperative period, but in cirrhotic patients decompensation can occur.
   (b) The cirrhotic patient carries a higher risk of prolonged hospitalization in the intensive care unit and the most common cause of perioperative mortality is sepsis. Bacteraemia is frequent, mostly secondary to bacterial translocation correlated with deficient immune response. At the slightest suspicion, an empiric antibiotherapy should be quickly initiated.
   (c) In CTP class C patients, open cardiac surgery is contraindicated and endovascular treatment (TAVI) should be considered instead if technically possible.
   (d) CORRECT ANSWER. Fresh frozen plasma (FFP) can be used to correct identified coagulopathies while monitoring the central venous pressure to avoid fluid overload. If FFP is not sufficient or not indicated (fluid overload), cryoprecipitate or desmopressin represent alternative methods.

References

1. Pimpin L, Cortez-Pinto H, Negro F, Corbould E, Lazarus JV, Webber L, Sheron N, EASL HEPAHEALTH Steering Committee. Burden of liver disease in Europe: epidemiology and analysis of risk factors to identify prevention policies. J Hepatol. 2018;69(3):718–35.
2. Shah NL, Intagliata N. Hemostatic abnormalities in patients with liver disease. 2018. Topic updated Aug 06, 2018. https://www.uptodate.com/contents/hemostatic-abnormalities-in-patients-with-liver-disease.
3. Angeli P, Ginès P, Wong F, Bernardi M, Boyer TD, Gerbes A, Moreau R, Jalan R, Sarin SK, Piano S, et al. Diagnosis and management of acute kidney injury in patients with cirrhosis: revised consensus recommendations of the International Club of Ascites. J Hepatol. 2015;62:968–74.
4. Ruiz-del-Árbol L, Serradilla R. Cirrhotic cardiomyopathy. World J Gastroenterol. 2015;21(41):11502–21.
5. Bunchorntavakul C, Chamroonkul N, Chavalitdhamrong D. Bacterial infections in cirrhosis: a critical review and practical guidance. World J Hepatol. 2016;8(6):307–21.
6. Light RW. New treatment for hepatic hydrothorax? Ann Am Thorac Soc. 2016;13(6):773–4.
7. Grilo-Bensusan I, Pascasio-Acevedo JM. Hepatopulmonary syndrome: what we know and what we would like to know. World J Gastroenterol. 2016;22(25):5728–41.
8. Rubin LJ. Portopulmonary hypertension. 2019. Topic updated Jan 22, 2019 https://www.uptodate.com/contents/portopulmonary-hypertension.
9. Peck-Radosavljevic M, Angeli P, Cordoba J, Farges O, Valla D. Managing complications in cirrhotic patients. U Eur Gastroenterol J. 2015;3(1):80–94.
10. An J, Shim JH, Kim SO, Lee D, Kim KM, Lim YS, Lee HC, Chung YH, Lee YS. Prevalence and prediction of coronary artery disease in patients with liver cirrhosis: a registry-based matched case-control study. Circulation. 2014;130(16):1353–62.
11. Jacob KA, Hjortnaes J, Kranenburg G, de Heer F, Kluin J. Mortality after cardiac surgery in patients with liver cirrhosis classified by the Child-Pugh score. Interact Cardiovasc Thorac Surg. 2015;20(4):520–30.
12. Diaz GC, Renz JF. Cardiac surgery in patients with end-stage liver disease. J Cardiothorac Vasc Anesth. 2014;28(1):155–62.
13. Hsieh WC, Chen PC, Corciova FC, Tinica G. Liver dysfunction as an important predicting risk factor in patients undergoing cardiac surgery: a systematic review and meta-analysis. Int J Clin Exp Med. 2015;8(11):20712–21.
14. Yuan X, Zhang H, Zheng Z, Rao C, Zhao Y, Wang Y, Krumholz HM, Hu S. Trends in mortality and major complications for patients undergoing coronary artery bypass grafting among Urban Teaching

Hospitals in China: 2004 to 2013. Eur Heart J Qual Care Clin Outcomes. 2017;3(4):312–8.
15. Sabry AM, Fouad HA, Hashem A, Khalifa AF. Risk factors in adult patients with chronic hepatitis C virus undergoing cardiac surgery with cardiopulmonary bypass: a prospective study. Res Opin Anesth Intens Care. 2017;4(4):213–25.
16. Safari S, Motavaf M, Seyed Siamdoust SA, Alavian SM. Hepatotoxicity of halogenated inhalational anesthetics. Iran Red Crescent Med J. 2014;16(9):e20153.
17. Di Tomasso N, Monaco F, Landoni G. Hepatic and renal effects of cardiopulmonary bypass. Best Pract Res Clin Anaesthesiol. 2015;29(2):151–61.
18. Alqahtani F, Aljohani S, Ghabra A, Alahdab F, Kawsara A, Holmes DR, Alkhouli M. Outcomes of transcatheter versus surgical aortic valve implantation for aortic stenosis in patients with hepatic cirrhosis. Am J Cardiol. 2017;120(7):1193–7.
19. Yassin AS, Subahi A, Abubakar H, Akintoye E, Alhusain R, Adegbala O, Ahmed A, Elmoughrabi A, Subahi E, Pahuja M, Sahlieh A, Elder M, Kaki A, Schreiber T, Mohamad T. Outcomes and effects of hepatic cirrhosis in patients who underwent transcatheter aortic valve implantation. Am J Cardiol. 2018;122(3):455–60.
20. Chacon MM, Schulte TE. Liver dysfunction in cardiac surgery - what causes it and is there anything we can do? J Cardiothorac Vasc Anesth. 2018;32(4):1719–21.

Future Approaches in Liver Disorders: Regenerative Medicine

74

Mariana Jinga, Vasile Daniel Balaban, Ecaterina Bontas, and Ion C. Tintoiu

Abbreviations

ATF5	Activating Transcription Factor 5
BAL	bioartificial liver
BMPs	bone morphogenetic protein
CEBPA	CCAAT/enhancer binding protein (C/EBP) alpha
CYP	cytochrome P450
DNMTi	DNA methylation inhibitor
EGF	epidermal growth factor
ESCs	embryonic stem cells
FGF	fibroblast growth factor
FGF	fibroblast growth factor
FOXA1	Forkhead Box A1
FOXA2	Forkhead Box A2
FOXA3	Forkhead Box A3
G-CSF	Granulocyte-colony stimulating factor
HDACi	histone deacetylase inhibitor
HGF	hepatocyte growth factor
HLCs	Hepatocyte like-cells
HNF1A	hepatocyte nuclear factor 1 alpha or hepatocyte nuclear factor 1 homeobox alpha
HNF4A	hepatocyte nuclear factor 4 alpha
HSCs	hematopoietic stem cells
IL-6	interleukin-6
iPSCs	induced pluripotent stem cells
LSPCs	liver stem/progenitor cells
MELD	Model For End-Stage Liver Disease
MIR122	MicroRNA 122
MSCs	mesenchymal stem cells
NASH	Nonalcoholic steatohepatitis
OSM	oncostatin M
PPARα	peroxisome proliferator-activated receptor α
PSCs	pluripotent stem cells
TGFα	transforming growth factor
TNFα	tumor necrosis factor alpha
β-PDGRR	platelet-derived growth factors

M. Jinga · V. D. Balaban
Central Military Emergency University Hospital "Dr. Carol Davila", Carol Davila University of Medicine and Pharmacy, Bucharest, Romania

E. Bontas (✉)
"Prof. C.C. Iliescu" Emergency Institute for Cardiovascular Diseases, Bucharest, Romania

I. C. Tintoiu
Faculty of Medicine, "Carol Davila" Central Military Emergency University Hospital, "Titu Maiorescu" University, Bucharest, Romania

Key Concepts

- The best option in severe damaged liver is liver transplantation
- Cell therapy with hepatocytes aim to restore liver parenchyma after liver injury
- The Bioartificial Liver is used for acute liver disease as a temporary bridge to liver transplant
- Stem cell transplantation together with gene therapy can correct the metabolic deficits of inherited liver disease on long time

74.1 Introduction

Orthotopic liver transplantation (OLT) is the only therapeutic choice in end-stage liver disorders such as cirrhosis, chronic hepatitis, acute liver failure, chronic hepatic failure or metabolic diseases [1]. Moreover, about 26% from inherited metabolic disease have OLT indication [2]. Liver transplantation have significant limitations such as high costs, donor shortage, allogeneic rejection, and long-term immunosuppression with side effects [3, 4].

To overcome these problems, the emerging field of regenerative medicine offers novel approaches to liver disease

F. Radu-Ionita et al. (eds.), *Liver Diseases*, https://doi.org/10.1007/978-3-030-24432-3_74

treatment based on a remarkable progress in basic biomedical research during the last 20–30 years. Nowadays, the major methods of regenerative medicine are *cell therapy*, *tissue/organ engineering* and *bioartificial liver* (BAL) devices with promising results [3].

74.2 Liver Architecture and Its Regeneration

Liver cells consist of hepatocytes, cholangiocytes and sinusoidal cells (Fig. 74.1) [5]. Further, *sinusoidal cells* are represented by endothelial cells, Kupffer cells (resident liver macrophages), hepatic stellate cells (Ito cells, fat-storing cells, lipocytes, perisinusoidal cells, or vitamin A-rich cells), pit cells (lymphoid cells, natural killer cells, granular lymphocytes), and liver stem/progenitor cells (LSPCs) [5–7]. Hepatocytes represent 80% from the liver volume with a normal turnover over several months [8]. Hepatocytes and cholangiocytes form parenchymal cells. Sinusoidal cells or non-parenchymal cells secrete the growths factors and cytokines which determine the hepatocytes replication [9].

Liver stem/progenitor cells (LSPCs) represent 0.3–0.7% of liver mass [10, 11] and they are also named oval cells in vitro studies [12]. LSPCs are inactive and located in the terminal ductules (i.e. canals of Hering) (Fig. 74.2) [5, 10, 13]. To date, Hering canals represent liver stem/progenitor cells niches in adult liver (Fig. 74.2) [9].

Presently, it is still debatable the role of resident stem cells in the regeneration of normal adult liver [8]. Furthermore, the proliferation of cells within periportal area (or around portal vein) from liver injury with regeneration is better mentioned as progenitor cells [8]. As a consequence, Miyajima et al. [8] suggest that the usage of *liver progenitor cells (LPCs)* is more suitable to delineate different populations of stem/progenitor cells activated in liver irrespective of liver injury.

LSPCs are characterized by 1) clonogenicity; and 2) bilineage differentiation or bipotential plasticity defined as the differentiation into hepatocytes and biliary duct cells [8]. In fact, an important liver injury (acute or chronic liver disorders) will activate bipotential LSPCs niches with their development and proliferation from periportal to the pericentral zones, process named ***ductular reaction*** or ***reactive ductules***

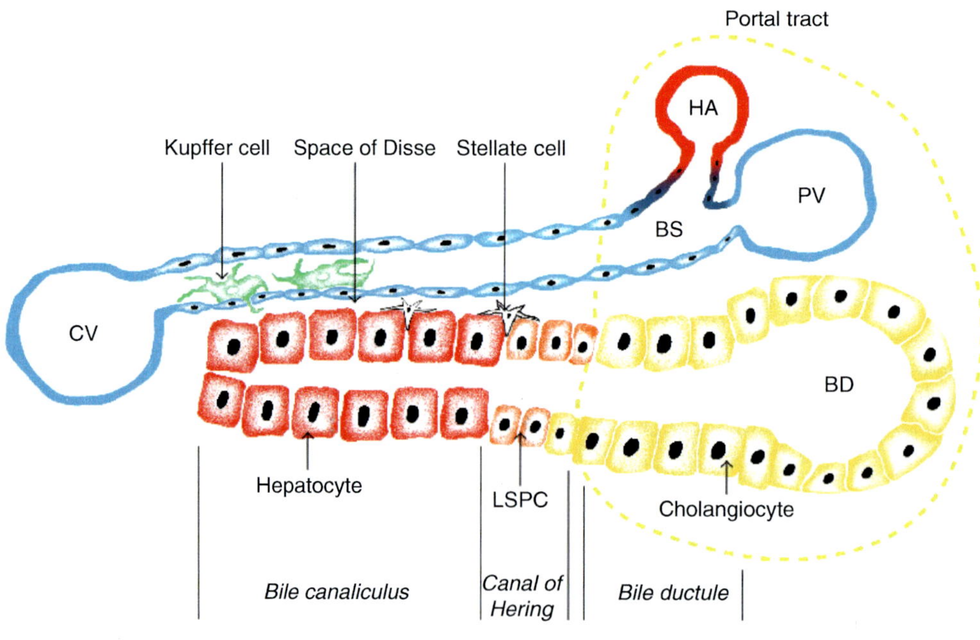

Fig. 74.1 Schematic histological structure of liver tissue. Functional units of liver tissue are formed by trabeculae and accompanying blood sinusoids. Liver tissue gets its afferent blood supply from two sources: hepatic artery and portal vein. Hepatic arterioles (HAs) and the terminal branches of portal vein (PV) merge to form blood sinusoids (BSs) lined with endotheliocytes and drained into the central veins (CVs). In the sinusoids, close to endothelium reside liver macrophages named Kupffer cells. Bile produced by hepatocytes flows in the opposite direction and is discharged into the bile ducts (BDs). Hepatic arterioles, terminal branches of portal vein, and the smallest bile ducts are drawn together forming compact structures called portal tracts shown at the right side of the figure. Liver trabeculae are built of hepatocytes. The inner cavities of trabeculae form canaliculi which are closed at the central ends of the lobules (left side of figure) and while on their way to BD they convert into bile ductules (BDLs) via a transitory zone called the canals of Hering (CH). Bile ductules drained into the bile ducts are lined with cholangiocytes, and the canals of Hering contain LSPCs. Tiny spaces between trabeculae and the endothelium of blood sinusoids are called the spaces of Disse (SD). They participate in the bidirectional traffic of different substances between blood and hepatocytes and contain stellate (Ito) cells. From [5]. [*This is an open access article distributed under the Creative Commons Attribution License, which permits unrestricted use, distribution, and reproduction in any medium, provided the original work is properly cited.*]

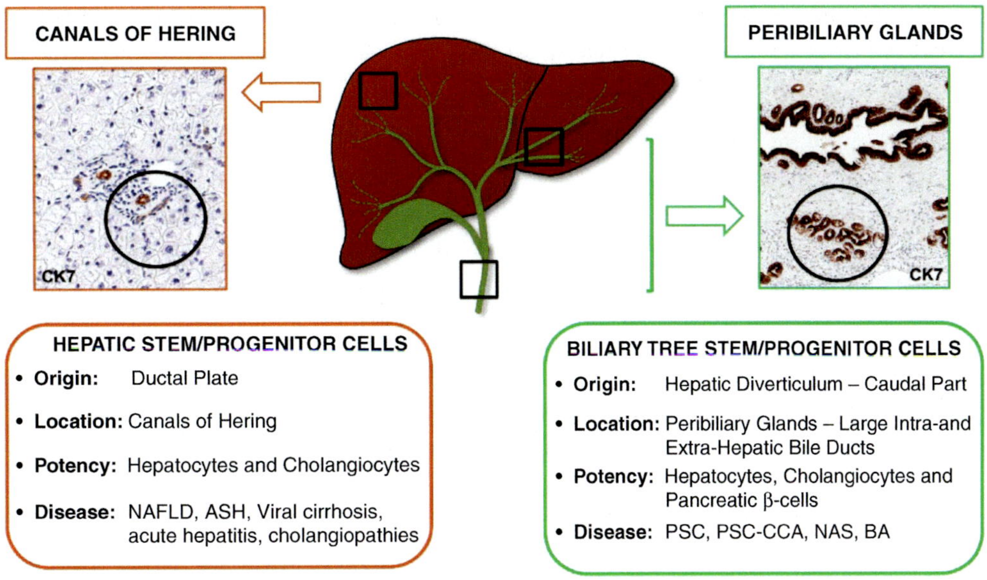

Fig. 74.2 Stem/progenitor cell niches in the human biliary tree. Canals of Hering harbor Hepatic Stem/progenitor Cells (HpSCs), while peribiliary glands (PBGs) constitute the niche for Biliary Tree Stem/progenitor Cells (BTSCs). Embryological origin, location, potency, and diseases in which cells are involved are summarized in the boxes. CK7: cytokeratin 7; NAFLD: Non-alcoholic fatty liver disease; ASH: Alcoholic steatohepatitis; PSC: Primary sclerosing cholangitis, CCA: cholangiocarcinoma; NAS: non-anastomotic strictures; BA: biliary atresia. Original Magnification: 10× (left) and 5× (right). From [13]. [*This is an open access article distributed under the Creative Commons Attribution License which permits unrestricted use, distribution, and reproduction in any medium, provided the original work is properly cited (CC BY 4.0).*]

[10, 11]. Also, LSPCs have markers CK19, EpCAM, CD133 and they can be separated with their culturing in vitro [8]. The differentiation of ***LSPCs*** into either hepatocytes or cholangiocytes needs Notch and Wnt signaling pathways [10, 11]. By "dedifferentiation, rapid proliferation, and redifferentiation", a tiny part from hepatocytes or LSPCs can induce new hepatocytes [5].

As previously discussed, some vitro populations of LSPCs from periportal areas are activated with proliferation into ***oval cells*** [14]. Hepatectomy triggers oval cells development [9]. At this stage, oval cells express intermediary phenotype with markers from hepatocytes and cholangiocytes. Oval cells can transform into hepatocytes or cholangiocytes in the presence of a right microenvironment and signaling pathways [14].

Liver Regeneration Mechanisms. Liver development may include stages of pre-hepatogenesis, liver specification (hepatoblast), proliferation (hepatoblast), and differentiation and maturation (hepatocyte, cholangiocyte) [8]. Hepatoblasts (immature hepatocytes) are liver progenitor cells which define foetal livers and neonatal livers, and their number decrease with maturity being untraceable in adult livers [15]. In vitro, hepatoblast has specific cell surface markers: $EpCAM^+$, $CD133^+$, E-$cadherin^+$, DLK^+, $Nope^+$, $CD13^+$, and $Liv2^+$ [8].

Of major interested, published evidence supports the concept that activated LSPCs regenerate hepatocytes and biliary epithelia. Current studies showed that only hepatocytes assure regeneration of parenchyma, wherein biliary epithelia do not promote regeneration and may be the result of hepatocytes de-differentiation in chronic liver disease [16]. Also, in chronic liver diseases or chronic injury, LSPCs regenerate only hepatocytes but not cholangiocytes [10, 11].

Hepatocytes have the capacity to proliferate [17]. Any liver injury triggers hepatocytes replication [9]. Of particular interest, liver regeneration is accomplished by a counterbalanced cellular mechanism such as hypertrophy and hyperplasia of all liver cell types [5]. Mature hepatocytes have great proliferation with multiple replication cycles, but when they become polyploid with reduced telomeres and chromosomal damages, their replication stops [18]. To sum up, human liver regenerative ability is influenced by 1) interconnection of hepatocytes with other cells; 2) elements of extracellular matrix liver; 3) cytokines; 4) soluble growth factors; 5) portal vein pressure; 6) injury dimension; 7) other liver diseases; and 8) age [5, 14].

Partial Hepatectomy. Sources for marginal grafts are represented mainly by living donors when right lobe is removed from young or old donors, split livers or steatotic livers [10]. After an injury including partial hepatectomy, liver can regenerate its mass. As such, both transplanted liver and donor liver develop up to normal dimension and normal mass [9]. In case of ***two-thirds of hepatectomy***, the rest of liver triggers hyperplasia with proliferation, and regenerated liver will attain 10% from initial liver mass. As a result, liver mass is reestablished but does not recuperate anatomical shape [9]. In fact, human hepatectomy is followed by immediate hepatocyte replication and delayed non-parenchymal cells replication (endothelial cells, Kupffer cells, biliary cells) [9]. Significantly, periportal cells replicate earliest [9].

At a simplistic level, it seems that hepatectomy triggers stress signaling by enhanced energy stress per unit liver volume; and liver regeneration is activated also by changed hemodynamic factors [9]. Partial hepatectomy triggers Kupffer cells to exhibit TNFα and IL-6. Serum IL-6 and HGF raise after hepatectomy [9]. Later, it is followed by the downstream signaling of HGF and TGFα [9]. It is well demonstrated that hepatectomy is associated with raised portal pressure, portal vein flow and shear stress which further trigger regeneration [9]. This leads to the liver cells proliferation hepatocytes, Kupffer cells, stellate cells, bile duct epithelium, and fenestrated endothelium of vascular sinusoids [5].

In about 8–10 days, the normal liver histology and functions are reestablished when hepatic stellate cells release β-PDGRR with blocking of hepatocyte proliferation [5].

74.2.1 Cell Therapy

The ***aim of cell transplantation*** is to provide new healthy hepatocytes which trigger liver regeneration with its restitution [5].

Cell therapy or cell-based therapy can be a choice instead of OLT [19]. Moreover, cell therapy is a life-saving choice in patients with end-stage cirrhosis, chronic hepatic failure and acute liver failure [20]. Until now, hepatocyte transplantation proved a successful bridge to OLT in case reports or uncontrolled trials either adults or children with acute liver disease [16]. Liver resection together with cell-based therapy in hepatocellular carcinoma postpone disease progression [10]. In addition, adult hepatocytes or cell-based therapy are an important tool to evaluate liver regeneration, hepatotoxicity or metabolism of xenobiotics by CYP enzymes, drug interactions [21].

Generally, conditions treated by cell transplantation in people are 1) ***congenital disorders*** (i.e. α1 antitrypsin deficiency, urea cycle defects, Crigler-Najjar syndrome type 1, familial hypercholesterolemia, congenital coagulation factor VII deficiency, glycogen storage disease type I); and 2) ***acquired disorders*** (acute liver failure—multiple etiologies, fatty liver of pregnancy, acute-on-chronic liver failure—multiple etiologies) (Table 74.1) [15, 16]. Furthermore, inherited liver disorders can be classified into two categories: 1) genetic disorders affecting a specific hepatic function with extrahepatic symptoms (Crigler-Najjar syndrome, familial hypercholesterolemia, clotting factor deficiencies) where hepatocytes are normal and can proliferate; 2) diseases in which hepatocytes are injured due to accumulation of a toxic product (α1 antitrypsin (A1AT), or copper in Wilson's disease), and hepatocytes do not proliferate) [2].

Table 74.1 Potential clinical indications for liver cell therapy[a]

A. Congenital disorders
• Alpha 1 antitrypsin deficiency[a]
• Crigler Najjar syndrome type 1[a]
• Familial hypercholesterolemia[a]
• Congenital coagulation factor VII deficiency[a]
• Hemophilia A
• Glycogen storage disease type I[a]
• Infantile Refsum disease
• Maple syrup urine disease
• Neonatal hemochromatosis
• Progressive familial intrahepatic cholestasis type 2 (PFIC2)
• Urea cycle defects—ornithine transcarbamylase carbamoylphosphate (OTC) deficiency, argininosuccinate lyase deficiency, carbamoylphosphate synthase type 1 deficiency; citrullinemia[a]
• Wilson's disease B.
Acquired disorders
• Acute liver failure (multiple etiologies)[a]
• Fatty liver of pregnancy[a]
• Acute on chronic liver failure (multiple etiologies)[a]

From [16] with **permission**

[a]Indicates conditions treated by cell transplantation in people

Hepatocyte transplantation can be frequently applied, it is not invasive as liver transplantation, and by reprogramming or gene therapy assure autologous hepatocytes [3].

General ***limitations*** of liver cell therapy include donor livers shortage, susceptible to cryopreservation, lower engraftment, allograft rejection, and immunosuppression that is a need after hepatocyte transplant [14, 16].

Importantly, ***sources of hepatocytes*** are mature primary hepatocytes, hepatocyte-like cells (HLCs), or tissue/organ engineering. Hepatocyte like-cells (HLCs) are generated in vitro, from human pluripotent stem cells (PSCs), from human ESCs, iPSCs, gestational stem cells, and mesenchymal stem cells (MSCs) [14, 22]. Hepatocytes and PSCs are the most accessible as cell therapies in liver restitution or tissue engineering [5].

Mechanisms. Simply, transplantation of hepatocytes into hepatic or extrahepatic sites is followed by engraftment and proliferation of hepatocytes [16]. Autologous transplanted liver cells have the ability to repopulate liver injury by transdifferentiation. Only 10–20% from transplanted cells get to home or engraft inside liver. Transplanted cells are homing in liver parenchyma or liver niches based on cells size and cell-cell adhesions [16]. During first 20 h, about >70% from transplanted hepatocytes are blocked in the portal spaces and sinusoids, where are finally removed by the immune system within 24–48 h. Initial engraftment of transplanted cells in vessels structure release local harmful vasoactive factors (i.e. NO, prostacyclin, complement, platelet-related thrombogenic substances, endothelin, cyclooxygenases, chemokines, cytokines) [16]. Further, these local harmful vasoactive factors increase vascular permeability facilitating surviving hepatocytes to get into the perisinusoidal space (or space of Disse) with further engraftment and proliferation [15]. Moreover, transplanted liver cells activate liver regeneration in liver resident progenitors or extrahepatic stem cells, by secretion of growth factors, noncoding RNAs, chemokines and cytokines [5]. A pre-existent liver inflammation and injury might intensify subsequently to transplanted cells in liver which trigger ischemia [16].

Cell therapy is done mainly by ***intravenous route*** to transplant suspensions of autologous hepatocytes. Basically, hepatocyte transplantation can be ensured via spleen (or intrasplenic), portal vein, extrahepatic lymph nodes or intraperitoneal administration [16]. Of note, cell therapy in a cirrhotic liver by portal vein might cause severe portal hypertension with portal thrombosis. Moreover, portal vein injection is a problematic task in patients with portal hypertension or/with coagulopathy [16]. This can be avoided by cell therapy in extrahepatic sites [20]. Transplanted hepatocytes via intrasplenic injection seed the liver in cirrhosis or after acute injury of liver [16].

The capacity of hepatocytes to engraft in extrahepatic sites is already demonstrated. Pietrosi et al. showed in an ongoing phase I–II matched case-control study in patients with end-stage chronic liver disease that administration of human foetal liver cells by intrasplenic infusion is safer with positive outcomes on MELD score and encephalopathy [23].

Finally, successful hepatocyte engraftment in metabolic liver diseases means the achievement of a therapeutic level of 5–10% from liver mass defined as the generation of absent proteins or enzymes [3].

74.2.2 Human Primary Hepatocytes

Published data demonstrate the efficacy of primary (noncultivated) hepatocytes transplantation in human liver metabolic and genetic disorders such as severe dyslipidemia, tyrosinemia, Crigler-Najjar syndrome, hepatolenticular degeneration (Wilson-Konovalov disease) and urea cycle disorders [5].

Harvested hepatocytes can be used immediately or cryopreserved. In this context, hepatocyte transplantation uses fresh or cryopreserved hepatocytes with cell viability over 60%; with ABO blood group compatibility; with immunosuppression—tacrolimus and steroids; with almost 10^9 cells per autologous infusion; with portal pressure monitoring; and it can be repeated up to 5–10% liver mass [16]. That said, donor age, ABO system compatibility, infectious risk, other liver diseases are factors taken in account when harvesting and isolate hepatocytes from donated livers [14]. Cryopreservation alters the viability and engraftment of harvested hepatocytes from livers [3].

After hepatocyte transplant, immunosuppression is a need with the mention that the hepatocyte transplant has a greater rejection risk in comparison with the whole liver [14]. Harvesting human hepatocytes from partial hepatectomy or deceased livers donors do not provide enough amounts of hepatocytes [3].

Primary or fresh hepatocytes has transplantation ***limitations*** such as lower proliferation, lesser accessibility or donor liver shortage, lower viability, and low immune tolerance with allogeneic rejection [3, 11].

Human hepatocytes are usually isolated by collagenases perfusion techniques respecting clinical Good Manufacturing Practice (GMP) terms [16]. Alternatively, human hepatocytes can be cryopreserved as cell banks being a timely option for temporary cell transplantation [15]. Presently, human hepatocytes such as allogeneic hepatocytes can be generated to be used in liver transplantation free of immunosuppression [5].

74.2.3 Hepatocyte Like-Cells (HLCs)

Hepatocytes come from endodermal lineage [5]. Hepatocyte like-cells (HLCs) are generated in vitro, from human pluripotent stem cells (PSCs), from human embryonic stem cells (ESCs), iPSCs, gestational stem cells, and mesenchymal stem cells (MSCs) (Fig. 74.3) [21, 22].

Basically, steps to maturation into HLCs are represented by 1) hepatic specification—FGFs, BMPs; 2) hepatoblast development; and 3) hepatic maturation—HGF, EGF, OSM and DEX (dexamethasone) [22]. Hepatic fate is determined by the combination of conversion factors (HNF1A, HNF4A, HNF6) with maturation factors (PROX1, ATF5, CEBPA) [24].

Importantly, HLCs have CYP5 activity being characteristic enzymes of drug and xenobiotics metabolisms. Therefore, they might represent a *gold standard* for the tests focused on drug metabolism and drug toxicity. It represents the "personalized drug administration future medicine" [22].

74.2.4 Cellular Reprogramming

Simply, a chronic liver injury displays unbalanced transcription. Also, dedifferentiated cells or diseased cells might be reset to normal function if they re-expose or re-express all important transcription factors [25].

Transcription factors. Liver development requires transcription factors with gradual activation. Therefore, transcription factors mediate the maturation of hepatocytes [21]. Examples of transcription factors are HNF4A, constitutive androstane receptor, eosinophil-associated, ribonuclease A, PPARα, Retinoid X receptor α (RXR-α, NR2B1-nuclear receptor subfamily 2, group B member 1), farnesoid X receptor; PXR, small heterodimer partner, and liver receptor homolog 1 [21]. All transcription factors interrelate. MIR122,

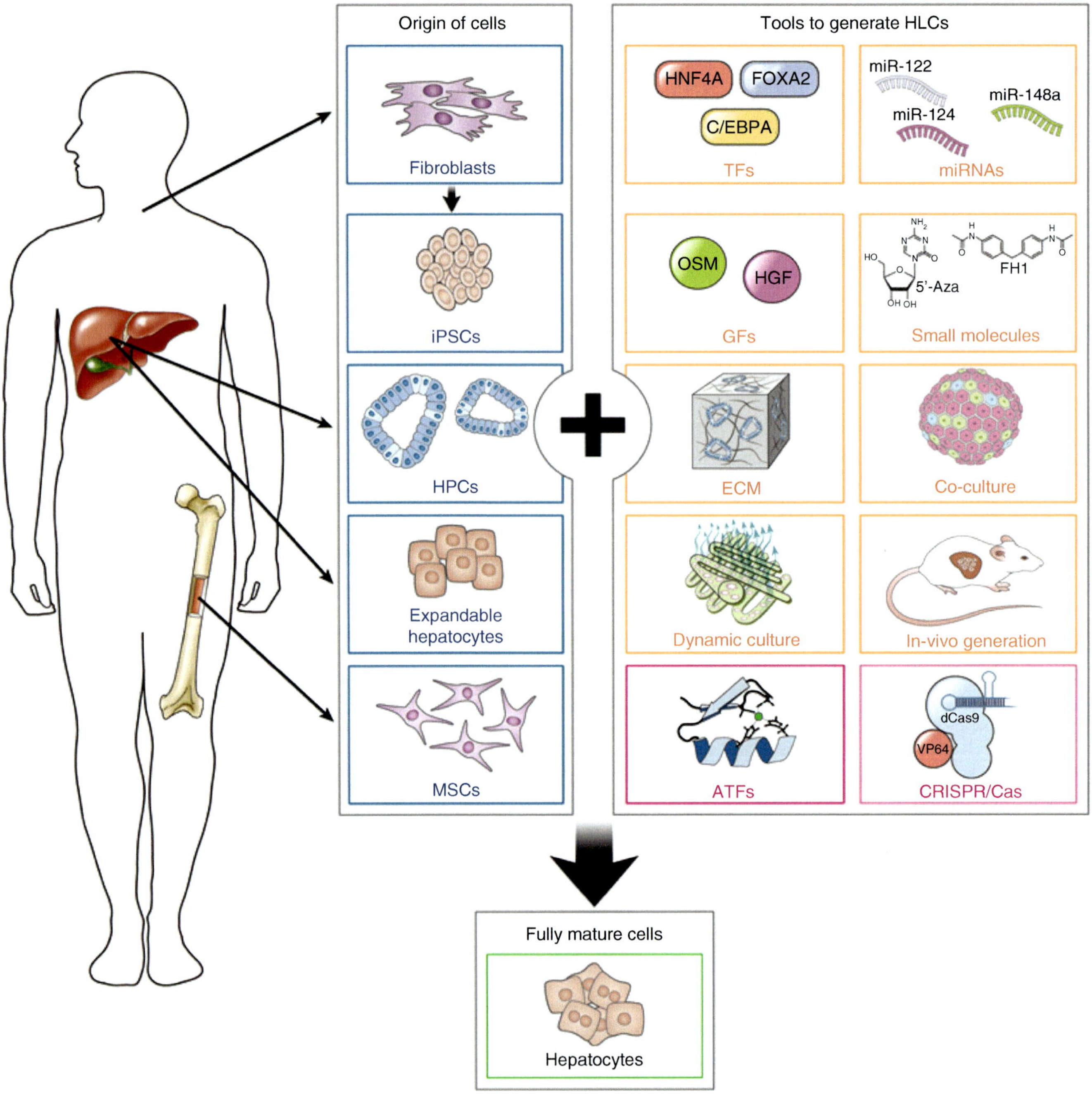

Fig. 74.3 Cells and methods to generate HLCs. Blue boxes show cells, and yellow and pink boxes show methods, used to generate HLCs. From Chen et al. [21] with permission

FOXA1 and HNF4A interrelate by upregulation in a positive feedback loop [21].

In fact, Nishigawa et al. have been shown that transcription factors such as HNF4A, forkhead box A2, CCAAT (enhancer binding protein alpha) and HNF1A, mediate the phenotype of mature hepatocyte with protein synthesis essential to lipid, biliary metabolism and coagulation [25].

In vivo, reprogramming of hepatocytes in animals, with end-stage degenerative liver diseases cause a fast recovery of liver function [25]. Therefore, transcription program assures amelioration of hepatic failure.

Small molecules (natural, synthetic) may substitute growth factors or transcription factors induced by differentiation [21]. Several small molecules can promote differentiation of PSCs and MSCs into HLCs [21]. DNMTis triggers differentiation of MSCs into HLCs [21]. HDACis act during or after differentiation into HLCs. DAPT and A8301 block differentiation of HPCs into cholangiocytes [21].

74.2.5 Pluripotent Stem Cells (PSCs)

Pluripotent stem cells (PSCs) can generate any cell as well as liver cells or hepatocytes and in this case are named induced pluripotent stem cells (iPSCs) [5]. *PSCs* comprise embryonic stem cells (ESCs) and iPSCs-derived somatic cells which can generate all cell body types having genomic stability [21].

To start with, human iPSCs can differentiate into any cell type from three primary germ layers (endoderm, mesoderm, ectoderm) [26]. Human PSCs have low immunogenicity with no immunosuppression prior engraftment, pluripotency, significant autologous activity and self-renewal [10, 27]. ***Pluripotency*** is the capacity of iPSCs to generate by differentiation any human cell body in presence of correct signaling pathways. ***Self-renewal*** means their clonogenic development with no genomic instability. In other words, human PSCs can produce infinitely "identical copies" with no chromosomal anomalies [27]. iPSCs can generate easily human HLCs using a retroviral vector and transcription factors [16]. Basically, using growth factors or by directed differentiation (transduction of FOXA2, HFNα1), iPSCs generate HLCs with main characteristics of primary hepatocytes [10]. Therefore, alternative techniques to generate iPSCs are excisable viral vectors, miRNA, mRNA transfections, or episomal plasmids transfections [22].

Importantly, human iPSCs are *promising cell source* for regenerative medicine especially in the modeling of liver infections, hepatic disease and drug toxicity testing, pharmacological screening and bio-artificial liver (Fig. 74.4) [2, 11, 21].

Genomic instability of iPSCs still represents a limitation in their use in cell therapies. Both cultured iPSCs and reprogramming of iPSCs into HLCs might assimilate genomic anomalies (i.e. variations in gene copy numbers, chromosomal abnormalities, somatic mutations). Or genomic anomalies or instability is a finding of tumorogenesis [4].

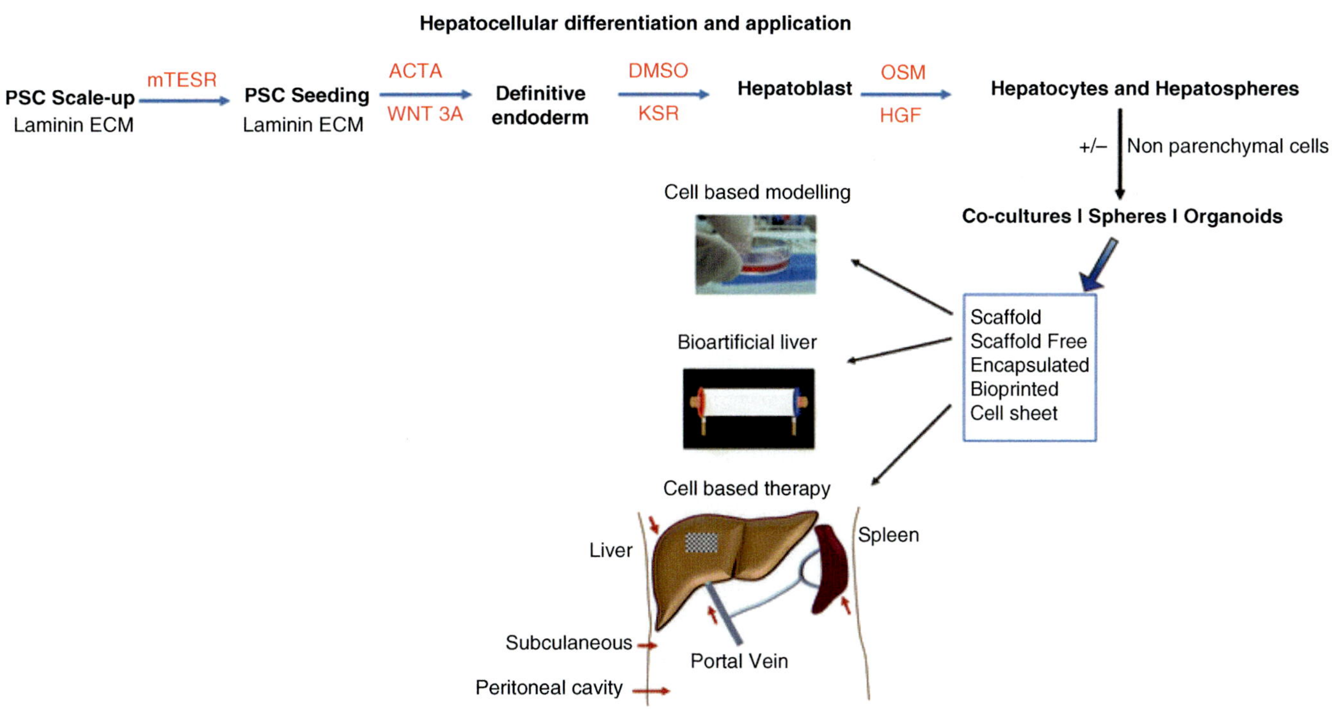

Fig. 74.4 Directed differentiation of pluripotent stem cells (PSCs) and their potential applications. PSCs were maintained on laminin extracellular matrix (ECM) and differentiated toward hepatic tissue using a four-stage process employing Activin A (ACTA), Wnt3a, and using differentiation medium (80% knockout DMEM (KO-DMEM), 20% knockout serum replacement (KSR), GlutaMAX, non-essential amino acids, β-mercaptoethanol, 1% Dimethyl sulfoxide (DMSO), and penicillin/streptomycin), and HepatoZYME maturation medium supplemented with Oncostatin M (OSM) and human hepatocyte growth factor (HGF). Following differentiation and tissue engineering, monolayer, co-culture, sphere and organoids could be applied in the future to model human biology, generate artificial liver devices, and used as cell-based therapies in vivo. The liver is shown in brown, the spleen in reddish-brown, and the liver bandage as a patch on the liver. Arrows (red) point to the site of cell delivery. From Alwahsh et al. [11]. [*Open Access This article is distributed under the terms of the Creative Commons Attribution 4.0 International License (http://creativecommons.org/licenses/by/4.0/), which permits unrestricted use, distribution, and reproduction in any medium, provided you give appropriate credit to the original author(s) and the source, provide a link to the Creative Commons license, and indicate if changes were made*]

74.2.6 Mesenchymal Stem Cells (MSCs)

MSCs are cells with mesodermal origin [5]. MSCs are isolated from adult somatic tissues such as bone marrow, lungs, liver, umbilical cord blood, placenta, adipose tissue and dental pulp [4, 21]. The best source for MSCs manufacture is human iPSCs [4].

As well, MSCs via paracrine secretion accelerate liver regeneration [5]. MSCs release growth factors, cytokines and chemokines [19]. They have stem cell-like characteristics 1) self-renewal; and 2) pluripotency (multipotent differentiation capacity) including into HLCs. MSCs differentiate into HLCs through two-steps 1) firstly, induction stage triggered by HGF and FGF; and 2) second stage is maturation induced by OSM and dexamethasone [21]. Adding growth factors (i.e. HGF, insulin-like growth factor I) to the MSCs culture generates their fate into HLCs [22].

As cell therapy, MSCs have numerous advantageous positive properties in liver disorders 1) low immunogenicity with no rejection risk and no immunosuppressive therapy; 2) increased engraftment or homing in injury locations; 3) regulate immune responses; 4) no malignant conversion; and 5) their manufacture is low-cost [5, 19].

The most used MSCs populations in studies are 1) MAPC (multipotent adult progenitor cells); 2) Muse cells (multilineage-differentiating stress-enduring); and 3) VSEL cells (very small embryonic-like stem cells) [5]. For instance, Muse cells have an important role in the repopulation of liver injury. Going into details, in liver injury, Muse cells trigger the restoration of liver injury with hepatocytes, cholangiocytes, Kupffer cells, and sinusoidal endothelial cells [5].

As stated above, MSCs represent the main part of preclinical and clinical research from human cell therapy [5]. For instance, adipose tissue-derived stem cells might be a future treatment in steatosis because improves liver function with diminishing lipid metabolism [3]. Similarly, MSCs such as human umbilical cord-derived MSC and bone marrow-derived MSC enhance liver function in cirrhosis and chronic liver failure [3].

It is already known that transplantation of autologous MSCs derived from bone marrow via intrasplenic or intrahepatic ways in patients with end-stage liver disease proved important alleviations of edema, ascites, fatigability, serum albumin with short-term efficiency [10].

Trials of MSCs transplantation has been published showing their benefits. In one published study, patients with acute-on-chronic liver failure and HBV were divided in two groups: 1) first group received immunosuppression therapy, plasma exchange and a single transplantation of MSCs derived from umbilical cord (100×10^6 cells) in suspension via hepatic artery; 2) second group were subject to immunosuppression therapy plus plasma exchange [28]. Importantly, first group with MSCs transplantation showed at 24 months: better liver function tests and superior cumulative survival rate [28].

74.2.7 Embryonic Stem Cells (ESCs)

HLCs from human ESCs are obtained from inner part of blastocyst with its destruction; and ethics of use has been questioned [16, 22]. However, even if long-term stability is unclear, it has been developed protocols for ESCs differentiation into HLCs. ESCs can be cultivated infinitely in vitro having pluripotency [2].

ESCs and iPSCs derived HLCs have a more foetal phenotype. Until now, human ESCs have been generated at GMP levels for clinical use [16]. Human ESCs or iPSCs by transduction with transcription factors are induced by differentiation into HLCs in vitro [10]. ESCs have potential indication in metabolic liver disease and liver failure but they do not have clinical use presently.

74.2.8 Hematopoietic Stem Cells (HSCs)

Hematopoietic stem cells (HSCs) can be generated from bone marrow and umbilical cord blood [29]. In case of liver transplantation, HSCs derived HLCs develop into hepatocytes by transdifferentiation [5]. Human liver disorders can be relieved by transplantation of hematopoietic cells or macrophages. Infusion with HSCs can induce liver regeneration but with the risk of teratoma development, and severe immunological reactions. These can be avoided by the usage of iPSCs derived from umbilical cord blood cells [5].

There have been published ~10 clinical trials using autologous bone marrow-derived cells in patients with liver disease, and six clinical trials have used G-CSF-mobilized mPB or direct G-CSF injections to mobilize endogenous HSC into circulation [29]. These trials comprised liver disorders patients such as hepatitis-associated cirrhosis, alcoholic liver disease, decompensated cirrhosis, cryptogenic cirrhosis, drug-induced acute liver failure, and primarily sclerosing cholangitis [29]. The endpoints of all clinical trials were serum aminotransferase levels, MELD score, Child-Pugh score and survival. Almost all studies except one showed long-term benefits over several months [29].

Other published trials support that the use of G-CSF or G-CSF mPB seems to be safe and well tolerated [29]. Moreover, G-CSF administration is associated with important therapeutic effect, with better MELD and Child-Pugh scores, better survival rates, and better SOFA (sequential organ failure assessment) score, even after 1 year treatment [29].

74.2.9 Human Fibroblasts

Adult human skin (fibroblasts, adult somatic cells) generate iPSCs with pluripotency [30]. Foetal and human fibroblast can be reprogrammed to obtain HLCs. Reprogramming is achieved with vector transfer (lentiviruses) that express transcription factors such as HNF1A, HNF4A and FOXA3 [10]. Limitations are their usage in only one infusion in a single patient. Fibroblast-derived HLCs by reprogramming may keep the epigenetic memory of source [10].

The manufacture of fibroblast-derived HLCs involves only one stage. By transdifferentiation, it can be obtained HLCs from fibroblasts [31]. Direct conversion refers to transdifferentiation of human fibroblasts to other cell lineages HLCs. This method avoids the stage of iPSCs [22].

74.3 Liver Tissue/Organ Engineering

Tissue/organ engineering (bioartificial grafts, bioartificial livers) can remove the problematic lack of donor liver and allows disease modeling. Disease modeling of liver refers to the study of infectious disease, cancer, liver fibrosis, NASH, cirrhosis [20]. In case of chronic liver disease and liver malignant tumors, ***bioartificial liver*** is a better choice in comparison with hepatocyte transplantation [14].

Newly, present scientific advances, developed and extended the tissue/organ manufacturing process by utilizing allogeneic cells or autologous cells with neutral immunological properties [5]. Consequently, liver tissues for transplantation may be produced by rather inexpensive industrial technologies [5].

To begin with, tissue/organ engineering or liver bioengineering comprises scaffold-based systems, scaffold-free systems (scaffold-free platform, scaffold-free microtissues), encapsulated techniques, liver-on-a-chip platforms, organoid technology, and bioprinted liver tissues [10, 11].

74.3.1 Scaffold-Based Systems

In ***scaffold-based systems***, the tissue/organ engineering technique is based on the generation of an extracellular matrix scaffold that reproduces the liver stromal 3D backbone. Basically, these 3D scaffolds are engineered structures which imitate the extracellular matrix of liver with porosity for recellularization, biodegradability and injectability (Fig. 74.5) [3, 20].

Sources of scaffolds are represented by biodegradable polymer matrices, 2D hepatic tissue sheets, and decellularized xenogeneic liver matrices [3]. Currently, there are many challenges to obtain manufactured implantable tissue/organ engineered organs by decellularization than reseeding or recellularization with specific cell types along with the neo-organ maturation in a bioreactor [20]. Xenogeneic (porcine or murine) liver scaffolds have highest success [3]. Xenogeneic scaffold is the decellularized native organ that undergone gamma irradiation to decrease immunogenic

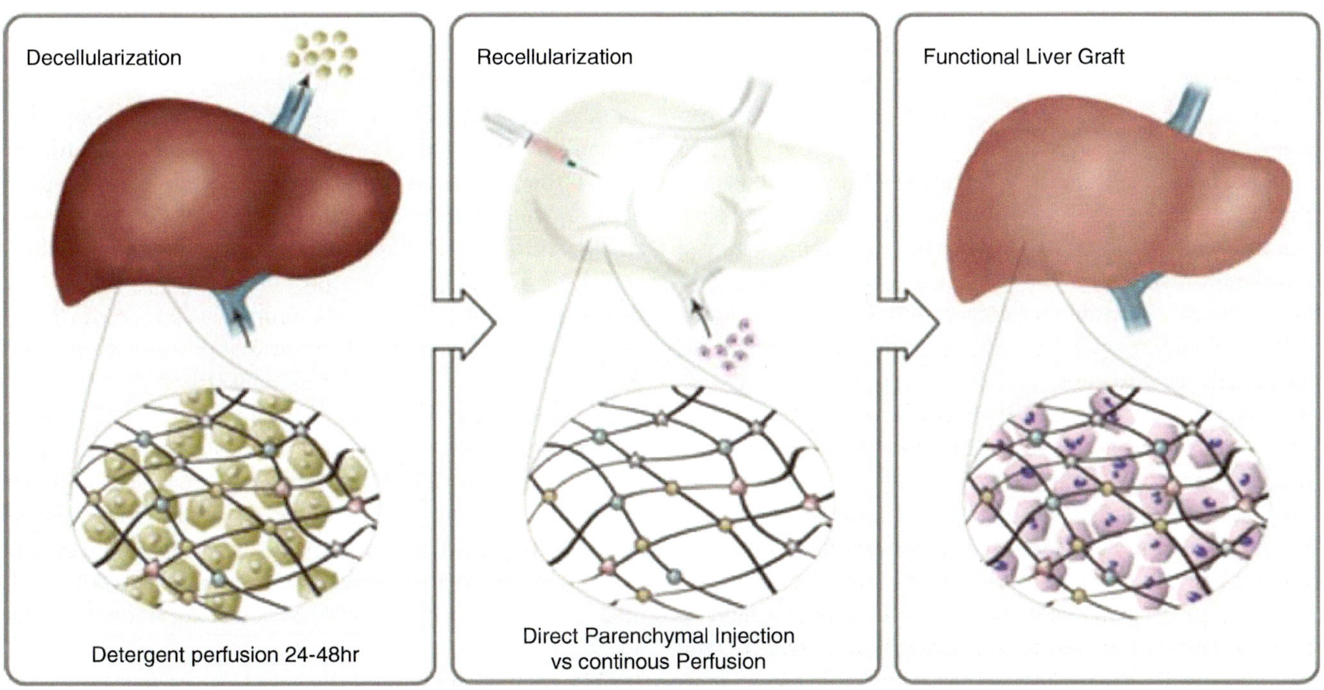

Fig. 74.5 Decellularization and recellularization process for the creation of bioengineered livers. The liver is decellularized through detergent perfusion at physiologic pressures via the native vasculature for 24-48 h. The resulting scaffold is then recellularized and reendothelialized with functional hepatocytes and endothelial cells either through direct parenchymal injections or through single or multistep continuous perfusion at physiologic pressures to produce a functional liver graft. From [3] with permission

properties; and with <50 ng double stranded DNA per scaffold in case of recellularization [20].

Further, the scaffold is recellularized or seeded with cells, and implanted with blood vessels and biliary ducts [5]. About 10–30% or 200–600 g of residual hepatic parenchyma can assure human survival. Therefore, around 2.5–7.5 billion of hepatocytes per infusion are required to guarantee survival [3]. The stage of liver scaffold recellularization still implies challenges approaches regarding the preservation of vascular network; adequate blood circulation flow; and to regenerate elements of the intrahepatic biliary tree [20]. In case of recellularization, the proliferation is checked by ki67 antibody staining; and metabolic function is verified by albumin serum level and CYP1A1/2 activity [3].

74.3.2 Organoid Technology

Organoid cell culture is defined as the 3D human microtissues or buds generated in vitro and vivo [10, 11]. Precisely, in 3D cultures, the aggregation process generates buds or organoid structures [3].

Further, ***organoids*** are 3D clusters of self-assembled cells generated in long-term 3D culture with genomic stability created on Matrigel supplemented with laminin and collagen IV. Activation of FGF signaling and inhibition of Notch and Wnt signaling pathways differentiate hepatic progenitor/stem cells into hepatocytes [21].

Sources of organoids are human adult stem cells [32]. Organoid technology supports the manufacturing of organotypic culture that is genetically stable and long-term [32]. It is a cost-effective and time-effective alternative to liver transplantation [4].

Co-culture of diverse cell types can be used to generate transplantable liver buds or organoids. It is well established that cells can self-organize in 3D spheroid structures termed liver buds or liver organoids, a feature demonstrated by vitro studies using co-cultures of human MSCs, HUVEC-human umbilical vein endothelial cells, and human iPSCs-derived human endodermal cells [10, 20]. All above mentioned cells undergo self-assembly into 3D liver buds or organoids with own vascularization. After transplantation, the organoid vessels are partly joining to host vessels and are working with liver function [11, 21]. Presently, it seems that transplanted organoids might furnish almost 1 month of functional assistance [10].

For instance, cultures of human iPSCs promote hepatocyte differentiation with expression of albumin and α1-antitrypsin. Implantation of these organoids in various liver sites or extrahepatic sites developed avascular network (HUVEC-derived blood circulation) interconnected with host circulation [14]. Human iPSCs (autologous stem cells) can generate liver buds or liver organoids with same drug metabolism of hepatocytes [3].

Isolated **Lgr5+** (leucine-rich repeat containing G-protein-coupled receptor 5) stem cells are a source for organoid cultures [31]. **Lgr5+** cells can generate organoids or liver buds in vitro and vivo [10]. These cells have chromosomal stability during lengthy culture [16].

74.3.3 Microencapsulation Technique

It defines the fixation of hepatocytes into a semipermeable polymer. As a result, it removes the side effects of immunosuppression, bleeding risk, and increases the viability and function of cryopreserved hepatocytes [16, 33].

As a side note, there are published vitro and vivo studies on acute liver failure with peritoneal transplantation of alginate microencapsulated hepatocytes technique (Fig. 74.6) [33]. Theoretically, these encapsulated hepatocytes in alginate microbeds are obtained from purified alginate, and assure metabolic function and detoxification, and defend against immunosuppression side effects [33]. Their removing after recovery is with no complications. In this context, microencapsulation technique represents a future approach in clinical transplantation [10, 33].

74.3.4 Bioprinting in the Fabrication of 3D Liver Tissues (Bioprinted Liver Tissues)

Bioprinted livers are defined as the mini-livers which present the hepatocyte functions regardless the vascular network. Hepatic 3D bioprinting is a novel technique [21]. Bioprinters produce hepatic tissues with specific cell types having an hepatic tissue design with cell allotment [21].

Inkjet printers and 3D printers are used in the maneuvering of mammalian cells [20]. Inkjet bioprinting might be used to create 2D and 3D human liver tissue [20]. Its mechanism is based on the pouring of bio-ink droplets from biomaterials by layered method (layer-by-layer) into hydrogel medium or culture medium or culture plate [20]. 3D printers produce sophisticated cell structures by using a layering process [20]. Only that, hepatocytes or cells are greatly susceptible to shear force [20]. Or bioprinting apply biochemical forces on cells. Therefore, one disadvantage is that shear-damaged cells might be locked inside bioprinted tissues with necrosis and bad shaping of the architecture [20].

One example is Novo-Gen MMX Bioprinter (Invetech, San Diego, CA) [20]. From 2014, Organovo, San Diego has commercialized bioprinted liver tissues with the aim to study liver biology, diseases modeling, and drug toxicity [20].

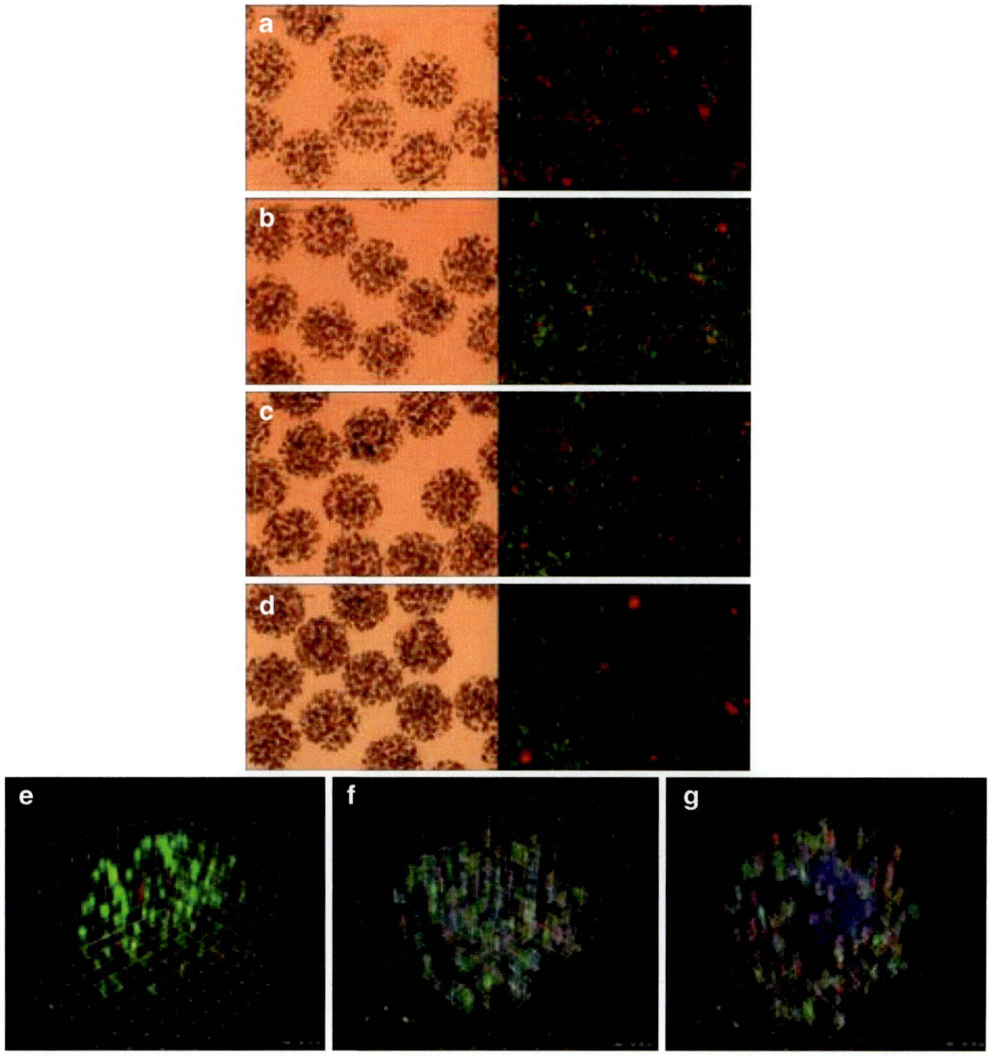

Fig. 74.6 Distribution of human hepatocytes in alginate-hepatocyte microbeads. Representative image of HMBs produced with different cell densities; 2.0, 2.5, 3.0 and 3.5 × 10^6 cells/ml alginate (**a–d** respectively) under light microscopy (left) and fluorescence microscopy (right). Representative confocal microscopy images used in 3D reconstruction to demonstrate (**e**, **f**) cell distribution and viability across the microbead, and (**g**) viability of cells within outer half vs. inner half of same microbead. Green; viable and red; dead cells. From [33]. [*This is an open-access article distributed under the terms of the Creative Commons Attribution License, which permits unrestricted use, distribution, and reproduction in any medium, provided the original author and source are properly credited.*]

74.4 Bioartificial Liver (BAL)

Cell-based extracorporeal support devices are used only as a temporary bridge for patients with acute liver failure and are represented by 1) bioartificial liver (BAL) support systems, 2) machine perfusions, and 3) hepatocyte microdevices (Fig. 74.7) [34].

BAL systems are a temporary option in therapy of acute liver failure or the treatment of acute-on-chronic liver failure [3, 4]. They also can assure for short term the endogenous regeneration of the native liver [3].

By definition, BAL system is a bioreactor with liver cells which temporarily replace the hepatic functions. Ideal BAL systems contain hepatocytes located in a mechanical artificial liver support device that assures albumin dialysis, synthetic function (albumin, coagulation factors), detoxification function (removes ammonia), diminish inflammation and enhance hepatocyte regeneration [3].

BAL support system uses as liver cells primary human hepatocytes, stem cells-derived HLCs and xenogeneic hepatocytes [3]. It has to be mentioned that there is no contact between porcine hepatocytes and patient [3]. Constant developments in hepatocyte differentiation such as iPSCs, ESCs and human fibroblasts might supply ideal HLCs for BAL systems [3]. Besides, tumorigenicity risk is diminished in a BAL system [35].

Currently, there are 11 BAL systems [4]. ***ELAD*** (the extracorporeal liver assist device) uses human hepatoblastoma cells known as HepG2/C3A cell line and is safe in acute liver failure patients [3]. The viability of HepG2/C3A is between 3 and 10 days, with synthetic function of albumin and cytochrome P-450 activity [3]. Also, ***HepatAssist*** contains porcine hepatocytes in a bioreactor [3]. Additionally, ***SRBAL*** (Spheroid Reservoir Bioartificial Liver) is based on 3D spheroids aggregates cultured cells (Fig. 74.8) [3].

Other BAL systems mentioned by published evidence are ***MELS*** (Modular Extracorporeal Liver Support), ***AMC-BAL*** (the Amsterdam Medical Center Bioartificial Liver), and ***BLSS*** (the Bioartificial Liver Support System).

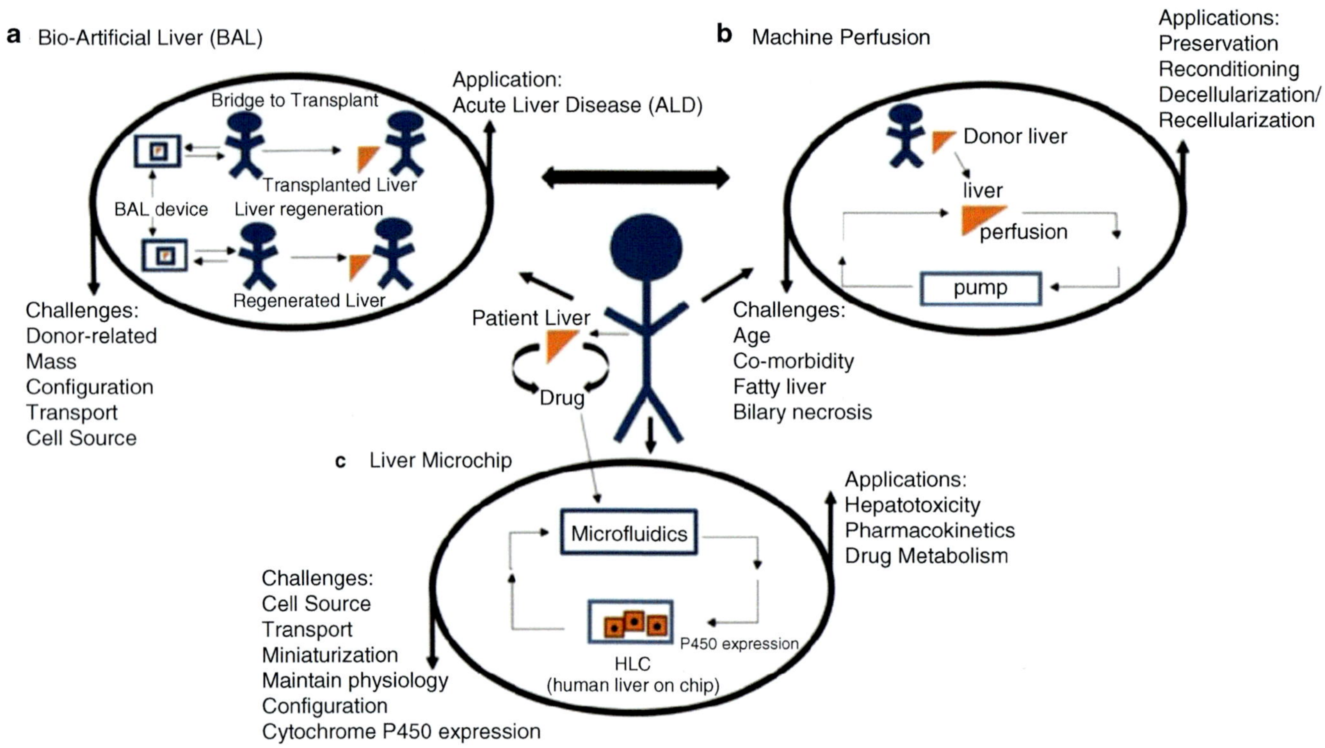

Fig. 74.7 Engineered liver devices. (**a**) **Bioartificial liver**. Engineered liver devices are at different scales and have a wide range of applications. The Bioartificial Liver (BAL) is a bioreactor system which bears hepatocytes in a variety of formats (hollow fiber vs. spheroid vs. monolayer culture). A large number of hepatocytes, approximately 10% of the adult liver, are needed to provide appropriate level of functions. Typically, the BAL is used for acute liver disease. In this case, it can be used a bridge to transplant, or as a way to regenerate acutely injured liver. The main challenges and applications are as shown. (**b**) **Machine Perfusion**. This is a technique used for several applications in animal models. The whole liver is connected to the perfusion device and perfusate is oxygenated and pumped to perfuse the whole liver under hypothermic or normothermic conditions. The technique is used to preserve organs after harvest, as opposed to storage of organs without flow in organ preservation solution. Machine perfusion is also used to condition marginal livers, for example by adding medium components to reverse fatty liver disease in a donor liver. Finally, machine perfusion can be used to understand complex, whole liver metabolic functions by measuring metabolites at inlet and outlet of the device under various experimental conditions. The main challenges and applications are as shown. (**c**) **Hepatocyte Microdevices**. This is a technique in which the hepatocytes are placed within miniature microfabricated devices so that they display physiological functions. Both animal and human liver on a chip applications are possible, and are valuable for assessing hepatotoxicity, drug metabolism, and pharmacokinetics, in the setting of drug discovery. These devices can potentially replace animals in the drug discovery pipeline. Patient-specific hepatocytes can be used to understand how genetic variations effect drug metabolism. Multiple cell types can be used in a circuit to better model the human body. The main challenges and applications are as shown [34]. [*Open Access This article is distributed under the terms of the Creative Commons Attribution 4.0 International License (http://creativecommons.org/licenses/by/4.0/), which permits unrestricted use, distribution, and reproduction in any medium, provided you give appropriate credit to the original author(s) and the source, provide a link to the Creative Commons license, and indicate if changes were made. The Creative Commons Public Domain Dedication waiver (http://creativecommons.org/publicdomain/zero/1.0/) applies to the data made available in this article, unless otherwise stated.*]

74.5 Gene Therapy

Stem cell transplantation together with gene therapy can correct the metabolic deficits of inherited liver disease on long time [3].

Advancements in liver genome editing might treat either hereditary monogenic liver disorders or viral hepatitis (hepatitis B infection) [36]. Until now, about 20 human liver transplants focused on genotyping which demonstrated the existence of chimeric genotypes or recipient genotypes in liver cell types such as sinusoidal cells, cholangiocytes, periportal liver cells, and hepatocytes [5].

Gene therapy is defined as the correction of damaged genes or "site-specific modifications" with beneficial therapeutic effects [37]. Presently, germline and somatic cells are used in gene therapy [37]. Gene therapy of somatic cells is based on the incorporation of therapeutic genes into somatic cells of patient with the final scope to remove abnormal gene [37].

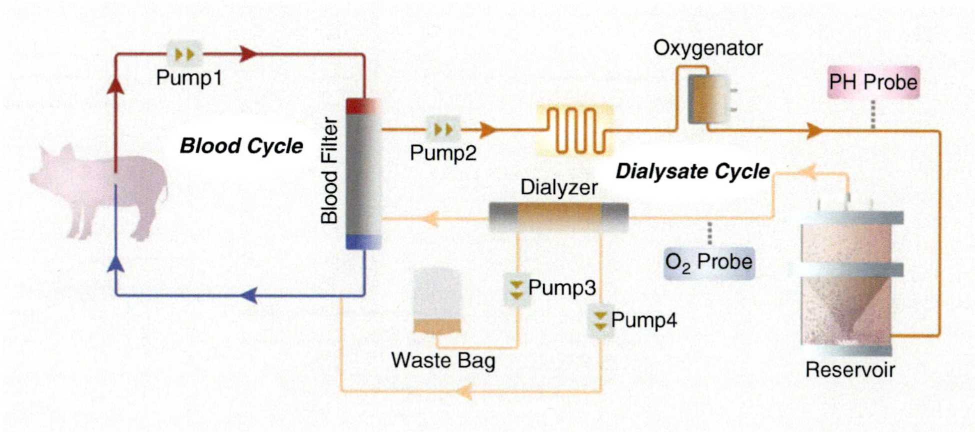

Fig. 74.8 Schematic representation of the spheroid reservoir bioartificial liver device. The red and blue lines indicate the blood compartment, while the orange line indicates the acellular albumin dialysate compartment. The blood filter consists of a hollow fiber cartridge, and the spheroid reservoir, containing over 100 g of hepatocyte spheroids, functions as a suspension bioreactor with fluid entering below and exiting above. From [3] with permission

Theoretically, gene therapy is based on the transfer of DNA into cells. It can be accomplished by gene correction, gene adding, and gene knockdown [38]. Every ***gene editing platform*** use a transfer vector that deliver genes to hepatocytes with the help of a carrier. The main transfer vectors used in gene therapy are non-viral DNA plasmids (DNA sequences) and viral vectors [38].

Gene editing platforms or *gene editing tools* have the aim to correct cells from diseases such as hereditary diseases (Crigler-Najjar syndrome, glycogen storage disease, hypercholesterolemia, Wilson's disease, and advanced cirrhosis) [10]. Presently, gene editing platforms allow accurate modifications in the genome of eukaryotic cells [36].

On the whole, gene editing platforms might be a solution for renewal with expression of absent genes; to eliminate the damaging genes; to eliminate viral genomes; or to correct mutations responsible for disease [36]. The genome-editing tools (e.g. engineered programmable endonucleases) enable corrections of gene or modifications at endogenous loci [26]. Currently, there are *four genome-editing tools* meganucleases, ZFN (zinc finger nucleases); TALENs (transcription activation-like effector nucleases); and CRISPRs (clustered regularly interspaced short palindromic repeats) which are useful to alleviate or to treat numerous diseases especially genetic disease with no effective treatment (Fig. 74.9) [26, 36].

Inside cellular genome, metabolism products can alter DNA bases with further possible replication blocking. Only that, genome has checkpoint mechanisms which repair by BER (base excision repair), NER (nucleotide excision repair), and DSBR (double-strand break repair) [26]. Repairing of DSBR can be obtained through 1) HDR pathway (high fidelity homology-directed repair); and 2) NHEJ pathway (error-prone nonhomologous end joining) [26]. Shortly, gene editing platforms insert a site-specific DSBs with different mechanisms of DNA identification [36].

A short overview of the liver diseases targeted by gene editing treatments are given in Table 74.2 [36]. The principal limitations of gene therapy are tumorigenicity and the therapeutic threshold [36].

74.6 Conclusions

The worldwide donor livers shortage stimulated and developed the regenerative medicine. Notably, there are remarkable progresses in liver regenerative medicine and ongoing experimental liver regeneration studies offer support for proper development methods of regenerative therapy such as cell therapy, tissue/organ engineering and gene therapy [5].

Unrestricted source of hepatocytes is the key need for regenerative therapy based on cell therapy [4]. Compared to organ transplantation or organ/tissue engineering, cell therapy is much less invasive and expensive [5]. Engraftment and liver repopulation are changeling for liver cell transplantation [20]. Differentiation of human ESCs and iPSCs into HLCs proved already useful as personalized medicine in drug testing or liver disease modelling. Only that, genomic instability issues have to be resolved [4].

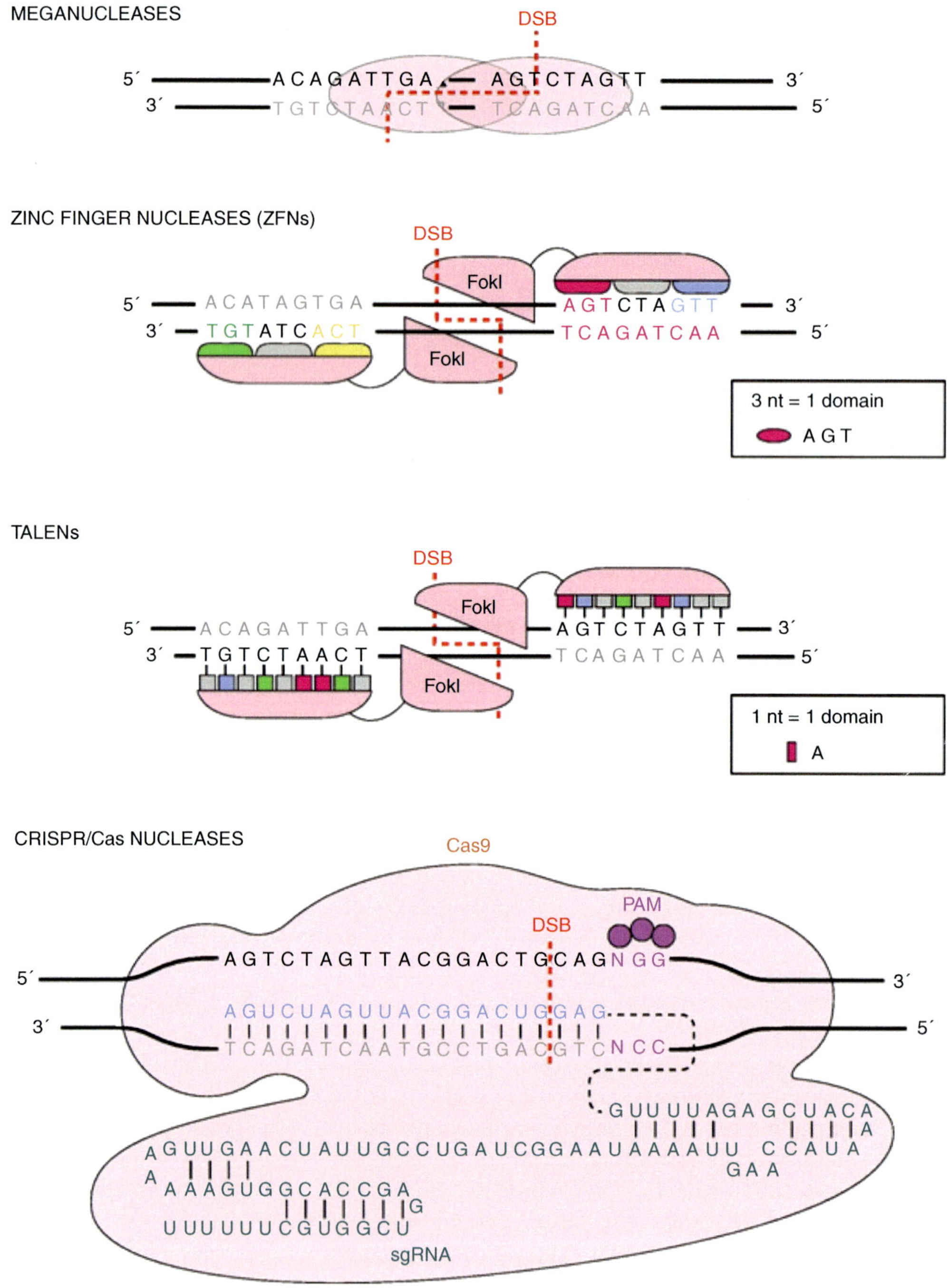

Fig. 74.9 The four main gene editing platforms. The different nucleases (pale red) bind to DNA through protein-DNA interactions (meganucleases, ZFNs, TALENs) or protein-RNA-DNA interactions (CRISPR-Cas nucleases). ZFNs and TALENs contain protein domains that can bind 3 or 1 nucleotide(s), respectively, in a sequence specific manner. The nucleases induce different types of DSBs, represented by the red lines. DSB, double-strand break; nt, nucleotide; PAM, protospacer-adjacent motif; sgRNA, single guide RNA. The vertical black bars indicate homology. From [36] with permission

Table 74.2 An overview of the liver diseases targeted by gene editing treatments [36] with permission

Disease	Type of genetic alteration	Gene editing treatment	Gene editing platform employed (preclinical)	Delivery method (preclinical)	Efficiency (preclinical)	Therapeutic threshold (preclinical)	Refs.
Haemophilia	Loss of function mutations in *Factor IX*	Correction or integration of *Factor IX* through HDR	ZFNs	AAVs	7%	Yes (>1%)	[39, 40]
Tyrosinemia	Loss of function mutations in *FAH*	Correction or integration of through HDR	CRISPR/Cas9	Hydrodynamic injections; or viral and lipid particles	0.4–6%	Yes	[41, 42]
Alpha 1 antitrypsin deficiency	Loss of function mutations in *SERPINA1*	Correction or integration of *SERPINA1* through HDR					
Hemochromatosis	Loss of function mutations in *HFE*	Correction or integration of *HFE* through HDR					
Wilson disease	Loss of function mutations in *ATP7B*	Correction or integration of *ATP7B* through HDR					
Hypercholesterolemia	Gain of function mutations in *PCSK9*	Correction or deletion of *ATP7B* through HDR and NHEJ, respectively.	CRISPR/Cas9	AAVs	50%	Yes	[43]
Hepatitis B infection	Exogenous DNA	Deletion or mutation of viral DNA through NHEJ	CRISPR/Cas9, TALENs, ZFNs	Hydrodynamic injections; AAVs	27–70%	Yes	

Self Study

Questions

1. **Which statement is true?**
   (a) An important tool to evaluate liver regeneration is cell therapy.
   (b) Hepatocyte like-cells are manufactured only from human ESCs.
   (c) Hepatocyte like-cells from human ESCs are obtained from whole blastocyst.
   (d) Co-culturing uses only human umbilical vein endothelial cells.
2. **Which statement/statements is/are true?**
   (a) Microencapsulation technique defines the fixation of hepatocytes into a semipermeable polymer.
   (b) BAL systems are a temporary option in therapy of acute liver failure.
   (c) BAL systems contain hepatocytes located in a mechanical artificial liver support device.
   (d) Stem cell transplantation together with gene therapy can correct the metabolic deficits of inherited liver disease on long time.

Answers

1. Which statement is true?
   (a) **Correct**. Cell-based therapy is an important tool to evaluate liver regeneration, hepatotoxicity or metabolism of xenobiotics by CYP enzymes, drug interactions.

(b) Hepatocyte like-cells are generated in vitro, from human pluripotent stem cells (PSCs), from human ESCs, iPSCs, gestational stem cells, and mesenchymal stem cells (MSCs).
(c) Hepatocyte like-cells from human ESCs are obtained from inner part of blastocyst.
(d) Co-culturing uses human MSCs, HUVEC-human umbilical vein endothelial cells, and human iPSCs-derived human endodermal cells.

2. Which statement/statements is/are true?
   (a) **Correct**.
   (b) **Correct**.
   (c) **Correct**.
   (d) **Correct**.

References

1. Hansel MC, Davila JC, Vosough M, Gramignoli R, Skvorak KJ, Dorko K, Marongiu F, Blake W, Strom SC. The use of induced pluripotent stem cells for the study and treatment of liver diseases. Curr Protoc Toxicol. 2016;67:14.13.1–14.13.27. https://doi.org/10.1002/0471140856.tx1413s67.
2. Dianat N, Steichen C, Vallier L, Weber A, Dubart-Kupperschmitt A. Human pluripotent stem cells for modelling human liver diseases and cell therapy. Curr Gene Ther. 2013;13(2):120–32.
3. Nicolas CT, Hickey RD, Chen HS, Mao SA, Lopera Higuita M, Wang Y, Nyberg SL. Concise review: liver regenerative medicine: from hepatocyte transplantation to bioartificial livers and bioengineered grafts. Stem Cells. 2017;35(1):42–50. https://doi.org/10.1002/stem.2500.
4. Lee CW, Chen YF, Wu HH, Lee OK. Historical perspectives and advances in mesenchymal stem cell research for the treatment of liver diseases. Gastroenterology. 2018;154(1):46–56. https://doi.org/10.1053/j.gastro.2017.09.049.
5. Kholodenko IV, Yarygin KN. Cellular mechanisms of liver regeneration and cell-based therapies of liver diseases. Biomed Res Int. 2017;2017:8910821. https://doi.org/10.1155/2017/8910821.
6. Kmiec Z. Cooperation of liver cells in health and disease. Adv Anat Embryol Cell Biol. 2001;161:III–XIII, 1–151.
7. Jacobs F, Gordts SC, Muthuramu I, De Geest B. The liver as a target organ for gene therapy: state of the art, challenges, and future perspectives. Pharmaceuticals (Basel). 2012;5(12):1372–92. https://doi.org/10.3390/ph5121372.
8. Miyajima A, Tanaka M, Itoh T. Stem/progenitor cells in liver development, homeostasis, regeneration, and reprogramming. Cell Stem Cell. 2014;14(5):561–74. https://doi.org/10.1016/j.stem.2014.04.010.
9. Kwon YJ, Lee KG, Choi D. Clinical implications of advances in liver regeneration. Clin Mol Hepatol. 2015;21(1):7–13. https://doi.org/10.3350/cmh.2015.21.1.7.
10. Lee CA, Sinha S, Fitzpatrick E, Dhawan A. Hepatocyte transplantation and advancements in alternative cell sources for liver-based regenerative medicine. J Mol Med (Berl). 2018;96(6):469–81. https://doi.org/10.1007/s00109-018-1638-5.
11. Alwahsh SM, Rashidi H, Hay DC. Liver cell therapy: is this the end of the beginning? Cell Mol Life Sci. 2018;75(8):1307–24. https://doi.org/10.1007/s00018-017-2713-8.
12. Huebert RC, Rakela J. Cellular therapy for liver disease. Mayo Clin Proc. 2014;89(3):414–24. https://doi.org/10.1016/j.mayocp.2013.10.023.
13. Overi D, Carpino G, Cardinale V, Franchitto A, Safarikia S, Onori P, Alvaro D, Gaudio E. Contribution of resident stem cells to liver and biliary tree regeneration in human diseases. Int J Mol Sci. 2018;19(10):E2917. https://doi.org/10.3390/ijms19102917.
14. Huppert SS, Campbell KM. Emerging advancements in liver regeneration and organogenesis as tools for liver replacement. Curr Opin Organ Transplant. 2016;21(6):581–7. https://doi.org/10.1097/MOT.0000000000000365.
15. Puppi J, et al. Improving the techniques for human hepatocyte transplantation: report from a consensus meeting in London. Cell Transplant. 2012;21(1):1–10. https://doi.org/10.3727/096368911X566208.
16. Forbes SJ, Gupta S, Dhawan A. Cell therapy for liver disease: from liver transplantation to cell factory. J Hepatol. 2015;62(1 Suppl):S157–69. https://doi.org/10.1016/j.jhep.2015.02.040.
17. Rezvani M, Grimm AA, Willenbring H. Assessing the therapeutic potential of lab-made hepatocytes. Hepatology. 2016;64(1):287–94. https://doi.org/10.1002/hep.28569.
18. Reid LM. Stem/progenitor cells and reprogramming (plasticity) mechanisms in liver, biliary tree, and pancreas. Hepatology. 2016;64(1):4–7. https://doi.org/10.1002/hep.28606.
19. Wang Y, Yu X, Chen E, Li L. Liver-derived human mesenchymal stem cells: a novel therapeutic source for liver diseases. Stem Cell Res Ther. 2016;7(1):71. https://doi.org/10.1186/s13287-016-0330-3.
20. Collin de l'Hortet A, Takeishi K, Guzman-Lepe J, Handa K, Matsubara K, Fukumitsu K, Dorko K, Presnell SC, Yagi H, Soto-Gutierrez A. Liver-regenerative transplantation: regrow and reset. Am J Transplant. 2016;16(6):1688–96. https://doi.org/10.1111/ajt.13678.
21. Chen C, Soto-Gutierrez A, Baptista PM, Spee B. Biotechnology challenges to in vitro maturation of hepatic stem cells. Gastroenterology. 2018;154(5):1258–72. https://doi.org/10.1053/j.gastro.2018.01.066.
22. Zakikhan K, Pournasr B, Vosough M, Nassiri-Asl M. In vitro generated hepatocyte-like cells: a novel tool in regenerative medicine and drug discovery. Cell J. 2017;19(2):204–17. https://doi.org/10.22074/cellj.2016.4362.
23. Pietrosi G, Vizzini G, Gerlach J, Chinnici C, Luca A, Amico G, et al. Phases I-II matched case-control study of human fetal liver cell transplantation for treatment of chronic liver disease. Cell Transplant. 2015;24(8):1627–38.
24. Du Y, Wang J, Jia J, Song N, Xiang C, Xu J, et al. Human hepatocytes with drug metabolic function induced from fibroblasts by lineage reprogramming. Cell Stem Cell. 2014;14(3):394–403.
25. Nishikawa T, Bell A, Brooks JM, et al. Resetting the transcription factor network reverses terminal chronic hepatic failure. J Clin Investig. 2015;125(4):1533–44.
26. Jang YY, Ye Z. Gene correction in patient-specific iPSCs for therapy development and disease modeling. Hum Genet. 2016;135(9):1041–58. https://doi.org/10.1007/s00439-016-1691-5.
27. Gieseck RL III, Colquhoun J, Hannan NR. Disease modeling using human induced pluripotent stem cells: lessons from the liver. Biochim Biophys Acta. 2015;1851(1):76–89. https://doi.org/10.1016/j.bbalip.2014.05.010.
28. Li YH, Xu Y, Wu HM, et al. Umbilical cord-derived mesenchymal stem cell transplantation in hepatitis b virus related acute-on-chronic liver failure treated with plasma exchange and entecavir: a 24-month prospective study. Stem Cell Rev. 2016;12(6):645–53. https://doi.org/10.1007/s12015-016-9683-3
29. Porada CD, Atala AJ, Almeida-Porada G. The hematopoietic system in the context of regenerative medicine. Methods. 2016;99:44–61. https://doi.org/10.1016/j.ymeth.2015.08.015.
30. Davidson MD, Ware BR, Khetani SR. Stem cell-derived liver cells for drug testing and disease modeling. Discov Med. 2015;19(106):349–58.

31. Sanal MG. Cell therapy from bench to bedside: hepatocytes from fibroblasts - the truth and myth of transdifferentiation. World J Gastroenterol. 2015;21(21):6427–33. https://doi.org/10.3748/wjg.v21.i21.6427.
32. Kretzschmar K, Clevers H. Organoids: modeling development and the stem cell niche in a dish. Dev Cell. 2016;38(6):590–600. https://doi.org/10.1016/j.devcel.2016.08.014.
33. Jitraruch S, Dhawan A, Hughes RD, Filippi C, Soong D, Philippeos C, Lehec SC, Heaton ND, Longhi MS, Mitry RR. Alginate microencapsulated hepatocytes optimised for transplantation in acute liver failure. PLoS One. 2014;9(12):e113609. https://doi.org/10.1371/journal.pone.0113609.
34. Ogoke O, Oluwole J, Parashurama N. Bioengineering considerations in liver regenerative medicine. J Biol Eng. 2017;11:46. https://doi.org/10.1186/s13036-017-0081-4.
35. Sakiyama R, Blau BJ, Miki T. Clinical translation of bioartificial liver support systems with human pluripotent stem cell-derived hepatic cells. World J Gastroenterol. 2017;23(11):1974–9. https://doi.org/10.3748/wjg.v23.i11.1974.
36. Ruiz de Galarreta M, Lujambio A. Therapeutic editing of hepatocyte genome in vivo. J Hepatol. 2017;67(4):818–28. https://doi.org/10.1016/j.jhep.2017.05.012.
37. Gonçalves GAR, Paiva RMA. Gene therapy: advances, challenges and perspectives. Einstein (Sao Paulo). 2017;15(3):369–75. https://doi.org/10.1590/S1679-45082017RB4024.
38. Kay MA. State-of-the-art gene-based therapies: the road ahead. Nat Rev Genet. 2011;12(5):316–28.
39. Li H, Haurigot V, Doyon Y, Li T, Wong SY, Bhagwat AS, et al. In vivo genome editing restores haemostasis in a mouse model of haemophilia. Nature. 2011;475:217–21.
40. Anguela XM, Sharma R, Doyon Y, Miller JC, Li H, Haurigot V, et al. Robust ZFN-mediated genome editing in adult hemophilic mice. Blood. 2013;122:3283–7.
41. Yin H, Xue W, Chen S, Bogorad RL, Benedetti E, Grompe M, et al. Genome editing with Cas9 in adult mice corrects a disease mutation and phenotype. Nat Biotechnol. 2014;32:551–3.
42. Yin H, Song CQ, Dorkin JR, Zhu LJ, Li Y, Wu Q, et al. Therapeutic genome editing by combined viral and non-viral delivery of CRISPR system components in vivo. Nat Biotechnol. 2016;34:328–33.
43. Ding Q, Strong A, Patel KM, Ng SL, Gosis BS, Regan SN, et al. Permanent alteration of PCSK9 with in vivo CRISPR-Cas9 genome editing. Circ Res. 2014;115:488–92.